CLINICAL PRACTICE
of the
DENTAL HYGIENIST

ESTHER M. WILKINS, B.S., R.D.H., D.M.D.

Department of Periodontology,
Tufts University, School of Dental Medicine,
Boston, Massachusetts
and
Forsyth School for Dental Hygienists
Boston, Massachusetts

CLINICAL PRACTICE
of the
DENTAL HYGIENIST

SEVENTH EDITION

A Lea & Febiger Book

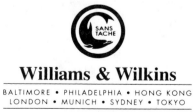

Williams & Wilkins

BALTIMORE • PHILADELPHIA • HONG KONG
LONDON • MUNICH • SYDNEY • TOKYO

A WAVERLY COMPANY

Executive Editor: Darlene Barela Cooke
Development Editor: Sharon R. Zinner
Project Editor: Denise L. Wilson
Production Coordinator: Peter Carley

Copyright © 1994
Williams & Wilkins
Rose Tree Corporate Center, Building II
1400 North Providence Road, Suite 5025
Media, PA 19063-2043 USA

Accurate indications, adverse reactions, and dosage schedules for drugs are provided in this book, but it is possible they may change. The reader is urged to review the package information data of the manufacturers of the medications mentioned.

Printed in the United States of America

First Edition, 1959
    Reprinted 1962
Second Edition, 1964
    Reprinted 1966, 1968
Third Edition, 1971
    Reprinted 1972, 1973, 1975
Fourth Edition, 1976
    Reprinted 1977, 1979, 1980, 1981
Fifth Edition, 1982
    Reprinted 1983, 1984, 1986, 1988
Sixth Edition, 1989
    Reprinted 1991, 1993
Seventh Edition, 1994
Translations:
    Fourth Edition—
        Japanese Edition by Ishiyaku Publishers, Inc., Tokyo, Japan, 1986
    Sixth Edition
        French Edition by Gaëtan Morin éditeur Itee, Boucherville, Quebec, 1991.

Library of Congress Cataloging-in-Publication Data

ISBN 0-683-09078-X

Preface

As a primary care preventive professional, the dental hygienist is a change agent with opportunities to influence the attitudes toward, and habits of, the personal oral health of many individuals. For the clinical phases of practice, responsibilities are to assess the patient's needs, to determine a dental hygiene diagnosis and treatment plan, to implement procedures to obtain predictable outcomes of treatment, and to evaluate the results for long-term continuing supervision and supplementary care. The literature of the dental hygiene profession, including *Clinical Practice of the Dental Hygienist*, has focused on these responsibilities of dental hygiene practitioners.

With increased emphasis on prevention in all areas of oral health, and special emphasis on the early recognition and treatment of periodontal infections, the demand for the dental hygienist's services has increased. Professional education, both for the new student preparing for practice and for the practitioner seeking renewal and continued proficiency, is strongly influenced by trends in the health-care delivery system and the vast increase in knowledge through research.

Additions and revisions made during preparation of the current edition of *Clinical Practice of the Dental Hygienist* have been influenced by the changes in the health-care industry, and especially by the new research. The need for individualized care has been a strong factor in delineating the content for the new edition. For examples, increased numbers of patients will present with infectious diseases; there will be more patients in the older age brackets with functionally effective natural dentitions; and patients with disabilities will have access and will survive longer with the advances in medical care available. Patients with oral, systemic, physical, or other problems that complicate treatment require specialized knowledge and frequently more skillful adaptations of basic dental hygiene procedures. Each dental hygienist must use professional clinical judgment in the selection and application of procedures appropriate for each patient's individual problem.

In younger age groups, statistics may show an improvement in the percent of children with no dental caries. However, there is still a tremendous need for preventive oral care and education for the other children not privileged by routine use of fluorides, noncariogenic diets, and early sealant placement.

The basic objective of the seventh edition of *Clinical Practice of the Dental Hygienist* has not changed from other editions, namely, to make available, in a concise manner, comprehensive information essential to the professional practice of dental hygiene. Supplementary references in the literature are included to enhance the text content. The need for specialization in the care of patients with particular physical, mental, or systemic problems has become evident.

All chapters have been revised and updated. Many new illustrations and tables have been included. A new feature is a table of KEY WORDS at the beginning of each major chapter. Development of professional vocabulary is an important objective of all education. The general Glossary near the end of the book contains words not included in the KEY WORDS, and all definitions can be located through the Index. The list of SUFFIXES AND PREFIXES still accompanies the general glossary and has been expanded.

Certain chapters have been modified, sections have been completely rewritten, and the sequence of chapters has been altered to permit groups of related topics to be together. The one entirely new chapter (Chapter 56) deals with mental disorders, an area with limited coverage in many dental hygiene curricula in the past. The completely rewritten infection control material (Chapters 2, 3, and 4) includes universal precautions and updating of information about HIV infection. In Chapter 19, *Periodontal Screening and Recording (PSR)* has been added to assist dentists and dental hygienists in the initial assessment of the severity of periodontal involvement.

Basic dental hygiene instrumentation (Chapter 31) contains information about cumulative trauma. In the attempt to prevent carpal tunnel syndrome and related problems of the working arm, shoulder, and back, exercises and preventive procedures are advised for the beginning dental hygiene student. Another new section (in Chapter 43) describes Anticipatory Guidance for parents and their infants/toddlers.

Wider use of this book by dental students and their teachers, dental assistant students, teachers, and practitioners continues. Health professionals other than members of the dental team also use the book for reference. Hospital personnel find a particular use for the sections on patient oral care, denture care, effect of chemotherapy and other drugs on the oral tissues, and xerostomia. The opportunity to assist all the health-care workers to promote the oral health of their patients is greatly appreciated.

This seventh edition has been revised and refined in response to comments and suggestions from students, teachers, and practitioners around the world. All readers are invited to send questions and ideas so that each successive edition will contain current material in an easy-to-read form.

Personal integrity and competence in patient care are the foremost factors in assuring quality control within the dental hygiene profession. It is hoped that this book will facilitate learning and, by preparing knowledgeable dental hygiene practitioners/clinicians, will continue to *elevate the image of dental hygiene*, as well as to *improve dental hygiene care and education for each patient.*

Boston, Massachusetts   Esther M. Wilkins

Acknowledgments

Many dental hygiene experts have contributed their knowledge, recommendations, time, support, and encouragement to this new edition. From students, faculty members, and practitioners, individual contributions range from a single word change or comment to the review of a whole chapter. Each is acknowledged with humble gratitude and sincere thanks.

Certain individuals contributed in a variety of ways without concentration on a particular chapter. Their participation may have consisted of reviewing specific sections, checking definitions for the Key Word tables, or expressing opinions for clarification. These people are:

Patricia Cohen, Canton, Massachusetts;
Barbara Brown, University of Rhode Island, Kingston, Rhode Island;
Tena McQueen, Columbus College, Columbus, Georgia;
Barbara Wilson, University of Rhode Island, Kingston, Rhode Island.

Special recognition goes to those who edited specific chapters. They appear here in the order of the chapters of the text:

Infection Control: **Kathy Bassett,** Pierce College, Tacoma, Washington, and **Kathy Eklund,** Forsyth School for Dental Hygienists, Boston, Massachusetts.
Cancer and Oral Cytology: **Dr. Arther Miller,** Temple University, Department of Pathology, Philadelphia, Pennsylvania.
Dental Radiographs: **Dorathea Foote,** Springfield Technical Community College, Springfield, Massachusetts.
Bacterial Plaque and Other Soft Deposits: **Linda Hanlon,** Forsyth School for Dental Hygienists, Boston, Massachusetts.
Toothbrushes and Toothbrushing: **Barbara Marquam,** Oregon Health Sciences University, Portland, Oregon, and **Marianne Clancy,** Dallas, Texas.
Irrigation: **Deborah Lyle,** Morris Plains, New Jersey, and **Shawn O'Neill-Hoffman,** West Linn, Oregon.
Dental Implants: **Salme Lavigne,** Wichita State University, Wichita, Kansas, and **Dale Scanlan,** Nepean, Ontario.
Fluorides: **Marianne Clancy,** Dallas, Texas.
Sealants: **Susan Brockmann-Bell,** Forsyth School for Dental Hygienists, Boston, Massachusetts.
Basic Instrumentation: **Robin Sylvis, Jean Ziegler,** and **Rosalie DiFerdinand,** Harcum Junior College, Bryn Mawr, Pennsylvania.
Cumulative Trauma and Exercises: **Claudia Michalak-Turcotte,** Tunxis Community College, Farmington, Connecticut and **Martha Atwood-Sanders,** Occupational and Sports Medicine Center, Meriden, Connecticut.
Maintenance: **Marilyn Hicks,** The Ohio State University, Columbus, Ohio.
Infant/Toddler, Anticipatory Guidance: **Patricia Griffiths,** Department of Dentistry, Columbus Children's Hospital, Columbus, Ohio.
Gerodontics: **Maryanne Lux,** Department of Veterans Affairs Medical Center, Dental Service, Lebanon, Pennsylvania.
Homebound and Helpless: **Jessie Brown,** Medical College of Georgia, Augusta, Georgia.

Hearing Impairment: **Lorraine DePietro,** National Information Center on Deafness, Gallaudet University, Washington, District of Columbia.

Mental Illness: **Marge Reveal,** Camosun College, Victoria, British Columbia, and **Janet Towle,** Forsyth School for Dental Hygienists, Boston, Massachusetts.

Emergency Care: **Claudia Michalak-Turcotte,** Tunxis Community College, Farmington, Connecticut, and **Cynthia Biron,** Tallahassee Community College, Tallahassee, Florida.

The illustrations for this edition reflect the work of a talented artist, **Marcia Williams** of Newton Highlands, Massachusetts. Much appreciation is expressed for her personal interest and patience in preparing the new educational drawings and updating many from the previous edition.

EMW

Contents

1. **THE PROFESSIONAL DENTAL HYGIENIST** 3
   Factors Influencing Clinical Practice 6
   Objectives for Practice 6
   Factors to Teach the Patient 7

PART II
Preparation for Dental Hygiene Appointments

2. **INFECTION CONTROL: TRANSMISSIBLE DISEASES** 11
   Microorganisms of the Oral Cavity 11
   The Infectious Process 11
   Airborne Infection 14
   Autogenous Infection 15
   Pathogens Transmissible by the Oral Cavity 16
   Tuberculosis 16
   Viral Hepatitis 17
   Hepatitis A 20
   Hepatitis B 21
   Prevention of Hepatitis B 23
   Hepatitis C 24
   Hepatitis D 25
   Hepatitis E 25
   Herpesvirus Diseases 25
   Viral Latency 26
   Varicella-Zoster Virus (VZV) 26
   Epstein-Barr Virus (EBV) 27
   Cytomegalovirus (HCMV) 27
   Herpes Simplex Virus Infections 27
   Clinical Management 28
   HIV Infection 29
   Life Cycle of the HIV 30
   HIV Classification System for Adolescents and Adults 31
   Clinical Course of HIV Infection 32

Oral Manifestations of HIV Infection 33
HIV Infection in Children 35
Prevention of HIV Infection 36
Factors to Teach the Patient 36

3. **EXPOSURE CONTROL: BARRIERS FOR PATIENT AND CLINICIAN** 41
   Personal Protection of the Dental Team 41
   Immunizations and Periodic Tests 41
   Clinical Attire 42
   Use of Face Mask 43
   Use of Protective Eyewear 44
   Hand Care 45
   Handwashing Principles 46
   Methods of Handwashing 47
   Gloves and Gloving 48
   Technical Hints 50
   Factors to Teach the Patient 50

4. **INFECTION CONTROL: CLINICAL PROCEDURES** 52
   Treatment Room Features 52
   Instrument Management 54
   Presoaking/Precleaning 54
   Cleaning 55
   Packaging 55
   Sterilization 56
   Moist Heat: Steam Under Pressure 57
   Dry Heat 58
   Chemical Vapor Sterilizer 58
   Ethylene Oxide 59
   Chemical Disinfectants 59
   Recommended Chemical Disinfectants 61
   Chemical Sterilants (Immersion) 62
   Unit Water Lines 62
   Preparation for Appointment 62
   Care of Sterile Instruments 64
   Patient Preparation 64
   Universal Procedures for the Prevention of Disease Transmission 65
   Disposal of Waste 67
   Technical Hints 67
   Factors to Teach the Patient 67

5. PATIENT RECEPTION AND
POSITIONING IN THE DENTAL
CHAIR 70
Position of the Clinician 71
Position of the Patient 73
Functional Factors 76
Technical Hints 77
Factors to Teach the Patient 77

PART III
Patient Assessment

Diagnostic Workup 80
Examination Procedures 80
Tooth Numbering Systems 81

6. PERSONAL, MEDICAL AND
DENTAL HISTORIES 85
History Preparation 85
The Questionnaire 87
The Interview 87
Items Included in the History 92
Review of History 95
Immediate Applications of Patient
Histories 95
Prophylactic Premedication 102
Technical Hints 103
Factors to Teach the Patient 103

7. VITAL SIGNS 106
Body Temperature 106
Pulse 109
Respiration 111
Blood Pressure 111
Technical Hints 114
Factors to Teach the Patient 115

8. EXTRAORAL AND INTRAORAL
EXAMINATION 116
Objectives 116
Components of Examination 116
Sequence of Examination 118
Records 119
Description of Observations 121
Oral Cancer 124
Exfoliative Cytology 125
Special Applications for the
Extraoral and Intraoral
Examination 127
Child Abuse and Neglect 127
Substance Abuse 128
Factors to Teach the Patient 130

9. DENTAL RADIOGRAPHS 133
Origin and Characteristics of X Ray 133
How X Rays Are Produced 135
Characteristics of an Acceptable
Radiograph 136

Factors that Influence the Finished
Radiograph 137
Exposure to Radiation 140
Rules for Radiation Protection 142
Protection of Clinician 142
Protection of Patient 143
Clinical Applications 144
Procedures for Film Placement and
Angulation of Ray 145
Film Selection for Intraoral Surveys 146
Definitions and Principles 147
Periapical Survey: Paralleling
Technique 147
Bitewing Survey 151
Periapical Survey: Angle-Bisection
Technique 151
Occlusal Survey 152
Panoramic Radiographs 152
Child Patient Survey 153
Edentulous Survey 154
Paraclinical Procedures 154
Conventional Processing 155
Essentials of an Adequate
Darkroom 155
Processing 156
How the Image Is Produced 157
Automated Processing 157
Analysis of Completed
Radiographs 158
Technical Hints 159
Factors to Teach the Patient 161

10. STUDY CASTS 164
Clinical Preparation 165
The Interocclusal Record (Wax
Bite) 166
Preparation of Impression Trays 166
The Impression Material 169
The Mandibular Impression 169
The Maxillary Impression 170
Disinfection of Impressions 171
Paraclinical Procedures 171
Trimming the Casts 173
Technical Hints 177
Factors to Teach the Patient 178

11. THE GINGIVA 180
Objectives 180
The Treatment Area 180
The Gingiva and Related
Structures 183
The Recognition of Gingival and
Periodontal Diseases 186
The Gingival Examination 187
Factors to Teach the Patient 193

12. DISEASE DEVELOPMENT AND
    CONTRIBUTING FACTORS 195
    Development of Gingival and
       Periodontal Infections 195
    Gingival and Periodontal Pockets 197
    Tooth Surface Pocket Wall 198
    Complications of Pocket Formation 200
    Contributing Factors in Disease
       Development 201
    Xerostomia 204
    Factors to Teach the Patient 205

13. EXAMINATION PROCEDURES 207
    The Mouth Mirror 207
    Instruments for Application of Air 208
    Probe 209
       Guide to Probing 210
       Probing Procedures 213
    Clinical Attachment Level 215
    Furcations Examination 216
    Mucogingival Examination 217
    Periodontal Charting 217
    Explorers 219
       Basic Procedures for Use of
          Explorers 221
       Supragingival Procedures 222
       Subgingival Procedures 222
       Record Findings 223
    Mobility Examination 223
    Fremitus 224
    Radiographic Examination 225
    Radiographic Changes in
       Periodontal Infections 225
    Early Periodontal Disease 227
    Other Radiographic Findings 227
    Technical Hints 228
    Factors to Teach the Patient 228

14. THE TEETH 231
    The Dentitions 231
    Dental Caries 231
       Enamel Caries 232
       Nursing Caries 234
       Root Surface Caries 236
    Enamel Hypoplasia 236
    Attrition 237
    Erosion 238
    Abrasion 238
    Fractures of Teeth 238
    Clinical Examination of the Teeth 239
    Recognition of Carious Lesions 242
    Testing for Pulpal Vitality 243
    Factors to Teach the Patient 245

15. THE OCCLUSION 248
    Static Occlusion 248

    Determination of the Classification
       of Malocclusion 250
    Occlusion of the Primary Teeth 253
    Functional Occlusion 254
    Trauma from Occlusion 255
    Technical Hints 256
    Factors to Teach the Patient 256

16. BACTERIAL PLAQUE AND OTHER
    SOFT DEPOSITS 258
    Acquired Pellicle 258
    Bacterial Plaque 260
    Clinical Aspects 266
    Significance of Bacterial Plaque 267
       Dental Caries 267
       Periodontal Infections 268
    Effect of Diet on Plaque 269
    Materia Alba 269
    Food Debris 269
    Technical Hints 269
    Factors to Teach the Patient 270

17. DENTAL CALCULUS 272
    Classification and Distribution 272
    Clinical Characteristics 273
    Calculus Formation 275
    Significance of Dental Calculus 277
    Prevention of Calculus 278
    Factors to Teach the Patient 278

18. DENTAL STAINS AND
    DISCOLORATIONS 280
    Extrinsic Stains 281
    Endogenous Intrinsic Stains 283
    Exogenous Intrinsic Stains 285
    Technical Hints 285
    Factors to Teach the Patient 285

19. INDICES AND SCORING METHODS 287
    Periodontal Screening and
       Recording (PSR) 289
    Plaque Index (Pl I) 291
    Plaque Control Record 292
    Plaque-Free Score 293
    Patient Hygiene Performance
       (PHP) 295
    Oral Hygiene Index (OHI) 296
    Simplified Oral Hygiene Index
       (OHI-S) 298
    Bleeding Indices 299
       Sulcus Bleeding Index (SBI) 300
       Gingival Bleeding Index (GBI) 300
    Papillary-Marginal-Attached
       Gingival Index (P-M-A) 301
    Gingival Index (GI) 302
    The Periodontal Index (PI) 303
    The Periodontal Disease Index
       (PDI) 304

Calculus Score   306
Dental Plaque Score   306
Community Periodontal Index of
  Treatment Needs (CPITN)   307
Dental Caries Indices   308
  Decayed, Missing, and Filled
    Permanent Teeth (DMFT)   309
  Decayed, Missing, and Filled
    Permanent Tooth Surfaces
    (DMFS)   310
  Decayed, Indicated for Extraction,
    and Filled Teeth or Surfaces (dft
    and dfs) (deft and defs)   310
  Decayed, Missing, and Filled (dmft
    or dmfs)   311
Technical Hints   311
Factors to Teach the Patient   312

20. RECORDS AND CHARTING   314
Periodontal Records and Charting   315
Dental Records and Charting   317
Technical Hints   319
Factors to Teach the Patient   319

**21. THE DENTAL HYGIENE
TREATMENT PLAN**   320
Preparation of the Treatment Plan   320
Planning the Dental Hygiene
  Treatment Plan   322
  Steps in Planning   322
  Individual Appointment Sequence   323
  Sample Dental Hygiene Treatment
    Plan   325
Informed Consent   326
Technical Hints   326
Factors to Teach the Patient   327

**PART IV
Prevention**

Introduction   330
Self-Cleansing Mechanisms   330
Steps in a Preventive Program   330
Patient Counseling   331
Factors to Teach the Patient   331

**22. ORAL INFECTION CONTROL:
TOOTHBRUSHES AND
TOOTHBRUSHING**   333
Development of Toothbrushes   333
Manual Toothbrushes   334
Toothbrush Selection for the
  Patient   336
Guidelines for Toothbrushing   337
Methods for Toothbrushing   338
  The Bass Method: Sulcular
    Brushing   338

The Roll or Rolling Stroke Method   339
The Modified Stillman Method   341
The Charters Method   341
Other Toothbrushing Methods   342
Power-assisted Toothbrushes   344
Supplemental Brushing   345
Toothbrushing for Special
  Conditions   347
Toothbrush Trauma: The Gingiva   347
Toothbrush Trauma: Dental
  Abrasion   348
Care of Toothbrushes   349

**23. INTERDENTAL CARE AND
CHEMOTHERAPY**   352
The Interdental Area   352
Dental Floss and Tape   353
Tufted Dental Floss   356
Knitting Yarn   357
Gauze Strip   357
Interdental Brushes   358
Single-Tuft Brush (End-Tuft,
  Unituft)   359
Interdental Tip   359
Pipe Cleaner   360
Toothpick in Holder   360
Wood Interdental Cleaner   360
Chemotherapy   361
Oral Irrigation   361
  Description of Irrigators   362
  Delivery Methods   362
  Beneficial Effects from Irrigation   363
  Applications for Practice   364
Mouthrinses   364
  Self-prepared Mouthrinses   365
  Commercial Mouthrinse Ingredients   366
  Chlorhexidine   367
Dentifrices   367
  Basic Components   367
  Prophylactic or Therapeutic
    Dentifrices   369
American Dental Association
  Evaluation Programs   370
Technical Hints   370
Factors to Teach the Patient   370

24. CARE OF DENTAL PROSTHESES   376
Orthodontic Appliances   376
Space Maintainers   379
Fixed Partial Dentures   381
  Care Procedures   381
Removable Partial Dentures   382
  Cleaning a Removable Prosthesis   383
  The Natural Teeth   384
Complete Dentures   384
  Cleaning the Complete Denture   385
  General Cleaning Procedures   386

The Underlying Mucosa 389
Complete Overdenture 389
Dental Hygiene Care and
Instruction 390
Technical Hints 390

25. **THE PATIENT WITH ORAL
    REHABILITATION AND IMPLANTS** 393
**Characteristics of the Rehabilitated
Mouth** 394
**Self-care for the Rehabilitated
Mouth** 396
Dental Implants 399
Types of Dental Implants 399
Preparation and Placement 400
Implant Interfaces 401
Peri-implant Hygiene 401
Maintenance 402
Factors to Teach the Patient 403

26. **DISCLOSING AGENTS** 407
Technical Hints 409
Factors to Teach the Patient 410

27. **DISEASE CONTROL: HELPING
    PATIENTS LEARN** 411
Planned Patient Learning 411
The Learning Process 412
Individual Patient Planning 413
**Presentation, Demonstration,
Practice** 414
The Preschool Child 417
The Teaching System 419
Evaluation of Teaching Aids 419

28. **DIET AND DIETARY ANALYSIS** 422
Oral Relationships 422
Daily Food Requirements 424
**Counseling for Dental Caries
Control** 425
The Dietary Analysis 425
**Preparation for Counseling of
Patient** 429
Counseling Procedures 429
Evaluation of Progress 431
Factors to Teach the Patient 431

29. **FLUORIDES** 434
Fluoride Metabolism 434
Fluoride and Tooth Development 435
Tooth Surface Fluoride 436
Fluoride Action 437
Fluoridation 438
Effects and Benefits 439
Partial Defluoridation 441
School Fluoridation 441
Discontinued Fluoridation 441
Economic Benefits 441

Fluorides in Foods 442
Dietary Fluoride Supplements 442
**Professional Topical Fluoride
Applications** 443
Sodium Fluoride 444
Acidulated Phosphate-fluoride (APF) 444
Stannous Fluoride 445
Clinical Procedures for Topical
Fluoride Applications 445
Paint-on Technique: Solution or Gel 445
Tray Technique: Gel 448
Self-applied Fluorides 449
Tray Technique: Home Application 450
Fluoride Mouthrinses 450
Fluoride Dentifrices 451
Brush-on Gel 452
Combined Fluoride Program 453
Fluoride Safety 453
Technical Hints 455
Factors to Teach the Patient 456

30. **SEALANTS** 462
**Selection of Teeth for Sealant
Application** 462
Clinical Procedures 463
Penetration of Sealant 466
Retention and Replacement 467
Fluoride and Sealant 467
Technical Hints 468
Factors to Teach the Patient 468

**PART V
Treatment**

Introduction 472

31. **PRINCIPLES FOR
    INSTRUMENTATION** 473
Instrument Identification 473
Instrument Parts 474
Instrument Grasp 475
**Wrist, Arm, Elbow, Shoulder:
Neutral Positions** 477
Fulcrum: Finger Rest 477
Adaptation 479
Angulation 479
Lateral Pressure 480
Activation: Stroke 480
Visibility and Accessibility 481
Dexterity Development 481
Prevention of Cumulative Trauma 483
Technical Hints 486

32. **INSTRUMENTS AND SHARPENING** 488
Curets 488
Scalers 490

Specifications for Instruments for
Scaling and Root Planing   493
Instrument Sharpening   494
  Some Basic Sharpening Principles   495
Sharpening Curets and Sickles   496
Moving Flat Stone: Stationary
Instrument   496
Stationary Flat Stone: Moving
Instrument   498
Sharpening Cone   499
The Neivert Whittler   500
Mandrel Mounted Stones   501
Sharpening the Hoe Scaler   502
Sharpening the Chisel Scaler   503
Sharpening Explorers   503
Care of Sharpening Stones   503
Technical Hints   504

33. SCALING AND ROOT PLANING   506
Rationale   506
Preparation for Instrumentation   507
Procedure for Scaling   509
Supragingival Scaling   511
Subgingival Instrumentation   513
  Subgingival Procedures   514
Ultrasonic and Sonic Scaling   516
  Mode of Action   517
  Purposes and Uses   517
  Clinical Procedures   518
  Advantages and Limitations   519
Use of a Topical Anesthetic   519
Technical Hints   521
Factors to Teach the Patient   522

34. NONSURGICAL PERIODONTAL
THERAPY: POSTCARE AND
ADJUNCTIVE TREATMENT   525
Immediate Evaluation   525
Patient Instructions after Scaling
and Root Planing   526
Effects of Scaling and Root
Planing   527
Gingival Curettage   528
  Healing Following Curettage   530
Professional Subgingival Irrigation   531
Factors to Teach the Patient   532

35. ACUTE GINGIVAL CONDITIONS   536
Necrotizing Ulcerative Gingivitis/
Periodontitis   536
  Clinical Recognition   536
  Treatment (NUG/NUP)   539
  Dental Hygiene Care   540
Periodontal Abscess   541
Technical Hints   543
Factors to Teach the Patient   544

36. DRESSINGS AND SUTURES   545
Types of Dressings   545
Clinical Application   547
Dressing Removal and
Replacement   547
Suture Removal   549
Technical Hints   552
Factors to Teach the Patient   552

37. HYPERSENSITIVE TEETH   554
Desensitization   556
Dental Hygiene Care   557
Technical Hints   558
Factors to Teach the Patient   558

38. EXTRINSIC STAIN REMOVAL   561
Effects of Polishing   561
Indications for Stain Removal   563
Clinical Application of Selective
Stain Removal   564
Cleaning and Polishing Agents   565
Clinical Applications   566
Procedures for Stain Removal
(Coronal Polishing)   567
The Instruments   567
Use of the Prophylaxis Angle   568
Polishing Proximal Surfaces   569
Airbrasive for Polishing   571
Cleaning the Removable Denture   571
Factors to Teach the Patient   573

39. THE PORTE POLISHER   576
Technical Hints   578
Factors to Teach the Patient   579

40. AMALGAM RESTORATIONS   580
Rationale for Finishing and
Polishing   580
The Amalgam Restoration   580
  Marginal Irregularities   582
  Overhanging Restorations   583
Clinical Management: Mercury
Hygiene   584
Finishing Procedures   584
Appointment Planning   585
Margination   587
Polishing   588
Fluoride Application   589
Factors to Teach the Patient   589

41. DEBONDING   591
Clinical Procedures for Debonding   593
Postdebonding Evaluation   594
Postdebonding Preventive Care   595
Technical Hints   595
Factors to Teach the Patient   595

42. EVALUATION AND PREVENTIVE
    MAINTENANCE 597
    Periodontal Evaluation 597
    Follow-up Evaluation 597
    The Maintenance Phase 599
    Technical Hints 600
    Factors to Teach the Patient 601

PART VI
Applied Techniques for Patients with
Special Needs

    Introduction to Patients with
      Special Needs 604
    Special Oral Problems 604
    Systemic Diseases 604
    Integration of Applications to
      Special Needs 604

43. THE PREGNANT PATIENT AND
    THE INFANT/TODDLER 605
    Fetal Development 605
    Oral Findings During Pregnancy 608
    Aspects of Patient Care 608
    Dental Hygiene Care 609
    Patient Instruction 610
    Infant and Toddler Oral Health 612

44. THE PATIENT WITH A CLEFT LIP
    AND/OR PALATE 617
    Classification of Clefts 617
    Etiology 617
    Oral Characteristics 618
    General Physical Characteristics 619
    Personal Factors 620
    Treatment 620
    Dental Hygiene Care 621

45. PREADOLESCENT TO
    POSTMENOPAUSAL PATIENTS 624
    Puberty and Adolescence 624
      Oral Conditions 626
      Dental Hygiene Care 626
    Menstruation 628
    Hormonal Contraceptives 629
    Menopause and Climacteric 630

46. THE GERODONTIC PATIENT 634
    Aging 634
    Characteristics of Aging 635
    Oral Findings in Aging 637
    Personal Factors 639
    Dental Hygiene Care 639
    Technical Hints 644

47. THE EDENTULOUS PATIENT 646
    The Edentulous Mouth 646
    Denture-Related Oral Changes 649

    Denture-Induced Oral Lesions 649
    Prevention and Maintenance 650
    Denture Marking for Identification 651
    Factors to Teach the Patient 653

48. THE ORAL AND MAXILLOFACIAL
    SURGERY PATIENT 655
    Patient Preparation 655
    Dental Hygiene Care 657
    Patient with Intermaxillary
      Fixation 659
    Treatment of Fractures 660
    Dental Hygiene Care 664
    Dental Hygiene Care Prior to
      General Surgery 666
    Technical Hints 667

49. THE PATIENT WITH ORAL CANCER 669
    Description 669
    Preparation for Treatment 670
    Surgical Treatment 671
    Radiation Therapy 672
    Chemotherapy 674
    Personal Factors 674
    Dental Hygiene Care 675
    Technical Hints 677
    Factors to Teach the Patient 677

50. CARE OF PATIENTS WITH
    DISABILITIES 679
    Dental and Dental Hygiene Care 679
      Appointment Scheduling 682
    Barrier-free Environment 682
    Patient Reception: The Initial
      Appointment 684
    Wheelchair Transfers 685
    Patient Position and Stabilization 687
    Clinic Procedures for Assessment
      of Patient 688
    Oral Manifestations 689
    Dental Hygiene Treatment Plan 690
    Disease Prevention and Control 690
    Bacterial Plaque Removal 691
    Self-care Aids 692
    Instruction for Caregiver 696
    Fluorides 698
    Pit and Fissure Sealants 698
    Diet Instruction 698
    Group In-service Education 699
    Instrumentation 701

51. THE PATIENT WHO IS
    HOMEBOUND, BEDRIDDEN, OR
    HELPLESS 705
    Homebound Patients 705
    The Helpless or Unconscious
      Patient 707
    Technical Hints 709

52. THE PATIENT WITH A PHYSICAL
IMPAIRMENT   711
Spinal Cord Dysfunctions   711
Spinal Cord Injury   711
Myelomeningocele   715
Cerebrovascular Accident (Stroke)   717
Muscular Dystrophies   719
Myasthenia Gravis   720
Multiple Sclerosis   721
Cerebral Palsy   722
Bell's Palsy   725
Parkinson's Disease   725
Arthritis   726
Scleroderma (Progressive Systemic
Sclerosis)   728

53. THE PATIENT WITH A SENSORY
DISABILITY   731
Visual Impairment   731
Hearing Impairment   734
Technical Hints   740

54. THE PATIENT WITH EPILEPSY   741
Description   741
Clinical Manifestations   742
Oral Findings   743
Phenytoin-induced Gingival
Enlargement (Overgrowth)   744
Dental Hygiene Care   745
Emergency Care   746
Technical Hints   747

55. THE PATIENT WITH MENTAL
RETARDATION   749
Mental Retardation   749
Etiology of Mental Retardation   751
General Characteristics   752
Dental and Dental Hygiene Care
and Instruction   752
Down's Syndrome   752
Autistic Disorder   754
Technical Hints   756

56. THE PATIENT WITH A MENTAL
DISORDER   759
Schizophrenia   759
Mood Disorders   763
Major Depressive Disorder   763
Bipolar Disorder   764
Postpartum Mood Disturbances   766
Anxiety Disorders   766
Eating Disorders   768
Anorexia Nervosa   769
Bulimia Nervosa   770
Psychiatric Emergencies   772

57. THE PATIENT WITH ALCOHOLISM   775
Description   775
Systemic Effects   776
Withdrawal Syndrome   779
Treatment   779
Dental Hygiene Care   780
Patient Instruction   782
Factors to Teach the Patient   782

58. THE PATIENT WITH A
CARDIOVASCULAR DISEASE   784
Congenital Heart Diseases   784
Rheumatic Heart Disease   787
Infective Endocarditis   788
Hypertension   789
Hypertensive Heart Disease   791
Ischemic Heart Disease   791
Angina Pectoris   793
Myocardial Infarction   794
Congestive Heart Failure   795
Sudden Death   796
Cardiac Pacemaker   796
Anticoagulant Therapy   798
Cardiovascular Surgery   799
Technical Hints   800
Factors to Teach the Patient   800

59. THE PATIENT WITH A BLOOD
DISORDER   802
Oral Findings Suggestive of Blood
Disorders   802
Normal Blood   802
Anemias   806
Iron Deficiency Anemia   807
Megaloblastic Anemias   807
Sickle Cell Anemia   808
Polycythemias   809
White Blood Cells   810
Leukemias   811
Hemorrhagic Disorders   813
Hemophilias   814

60. THE PATIENT WITH DIABETES
MELLITUS   818
The Diabetic Syndrome:
Classification   818
Description   818
Action of Insulin   819
Effects of Diabetes   820
Treatment for Diabetes Control   822
Oral Relationships   823
Dental Hygiene Care   824
Prevention of Diabetes   825

61. EMERGENCY CARE   828
Prevention of Emergencies   828

Emergency Materials and
   Preparation 830
Basic Life Support 835
Rescue Breathing 837
External Chest Compression 837
Airway Obstruction 839
Oxygen Administration 841

Specific Emergencies 841
Technical Hints 841

PREFIXES, SUFFIXES, AND COMBINING
   FORMS 851
GLOSSARY 855
APPENDIX 865
INDEX 867

PART 1

Orientation to Clinical Dental Hygiene Practice

The Professional Dental Hygienist

The dental hygienist is a licensed primary health-care professional, oral health educator, and clinician who, as cotherapist with the dentist, provides preventive, educational, and therapeutic services supporting total health for the control of oral diseases and the promotion of oral health. Dental hygiene services are available for general and specialty dental practices, programs for research, professional education, community health, and hospital and institutional care of disabled persons, as well as federal programs, the armed services, and dental product promotion. Key words relating to dental hygienists and their practice are defined in Table 1–1.

I. TYPES OF SERVICES

The services of the dental hygienist are divided into three basic categories, namely, preventive, educational, and therapeutic. The three are inseparable and overlap as patient care is planned and accomplished.

A. Preventive

Preventive services are the methods employed by the clinician and/or patient to promote and maintain oral health.

Preventive services fall into two groups, primary and secondary. *Primary prevention* refers to measures carried out so that disease does not occur and is truly prevented. *Secondary prevention* involves the treatment of early disease to prevent further progress of potentially irreversible conditions which, if not arrested, may lead eventually to extensive rehabilitative treatment or loss of teeth.

An example of a primary preventive measure is the application of a topical fluoride preparation for dental caries prevention. Removal of subgingival calculus and debriding the root surface in a relatively shallow pocket is an example of a secondary prevention procedure in that the treatment contributes to the prevention of a deep pocket.

B. Educational

Educational services are the strategies developed for an individual or for groups to elicit behaviors directed toward health.

Educational aspects of dental hygiene service permeate the entire patient care system. The preparation for specific treatment, the success of treatment, and the long-term success of both preventive and therapeutic services depend on the patient's understanding of each procedure and daily care of the oral cavity.

C. Therapeutic

Therapeutic services are clinical treatments designed to arrest or control disease and maintain oral tissues in health.

Dental hygiene treatment services are an integral part of the total treatment procedures. All scaling and root planing, along with the steps in postoperative care, are parts of the therapeutic phases in the treatment of periodontal infection. Restorative procedures are involved in the treatment of dental caries.

II. DENTAL HYGIENE CARE

The term *dental hygiene care* is used to denote all integrated preventive and treatment services administered to a patient by a dental hygienist. This term is parallel to the commonly used term *dental care*, which refers to the services performed by the dentist.

Clinical services, both dental and dental hygiene, have limited long-range probability of success if the

TABLE 1–1
KEY WORDS AND ABBREVIATIONS: PROFESSIONAL DENTAL HYGIENIST

CEU: continuing education unit; 1 unit commonly refers to 1 clock hour of instruction.

Continuing education: postlicensure short-term educational experiences for refresher, updating, and renewal; continuing education units may be required for relicensure.

Cotherapist: term used to describe the relationships between patient, dentist, and dental hygienist when coordinating the efforts to attain and maintain the oral health of the patient.

Dental hygiene: the science and practice of the prevention of oral diseases; the profession of the dental hygienist.

Dental hygiene diagnosis: the actual or potential oral health problems that are amenable to resolution by a dental hygienist's clinical and educational performance; a dental hygiene diagnosis identifies an existing or potential oral health problem that the dental hygienist is qualified and licensed to treat.

Dental hygiene treatment plan: after assessment, the pertinent interventions are selected and a treatment plan outlined; the plan consists of those services to be performed by the dental hygienist within the total treatment plan for dental care.

Dental hygienist (hī-je'nist): dental health specialist whose primary concern is the maintenance of oral health and the prevention of oral disease (see also opening paragraph, page 3).

Ethics (eth'iks): the science of right conduct; a system of rules or principles governing the conduct of a professional group, planned by them for the common good of man; principles of morality.

Health: state of physical, mental, and social well-being, not only the absence of disease.

Health promotion: the process of enabling people to increase control and improve their health through self-care, mutual aid, and the creation of healthy environments.

Hygiene (hī'jēn): the science of health and its preservation; a condition or practice, such as cleanliness, that is conducive to the preservation of health.

　Oral hygiene: procedures for preservation of health of the oral cavity; personal maintenance of cleanliness and other measures recommended by the dental professionals.

License by credential: acceptance for licensure by a regulatory body (state, province) on the evidence from a license obtained in another state where equivalent standards and requirements are required; also called reciprocity, a mutual or cooperative exchange.

Profession: occupation or calling that requires specialized knowledge, methods, and skills, as well as preparation, from an institution of higher learning, in the scholarly, scientific, and historic principles underlying such methods and skills; a profession continuously enlarges its body of knowledge, functions autonomously in formulation of policy, and maintains high standards of achievement and conduct; members of a profession are committed to continuing study, place service above personal gain, and are committed to providing practical services vital to human and social welfare.

Supervision: term applied to the legal relationship between dentist and dental hygienist in practice. Each practice act defines the type of supervision required.

　General supervision: means that the dentist has authorized the procedure for a patient of record, but need not be present when the authorized procedure is carried out. The procedure is carried out in accordance with the dentist's diagnosis and treatment plan.

　Direct supervision: means that the dentist has diagnosed and authorized the condition to be treated, remains on the premises while the procedure is performed, and approves the work performed before dismissal of the patient.

　Indirect supervision: means that the dentist has diagnosed and authorized the procedure for a patient of record, and is on the premises while the procedure is performed.

　Personal supervision: means that while the dentist is personally treating a patient, the dental hygienist is authorized to aid in the treatment by concurrently performing a supportive procedure.

patient does not understand the need for cooperation in daily procedures of personal care and diet, and for regular appointments for professional care. Educational and clinical services, therefore, are mutually dependent and inseparable in the total dental hygiene care of the patient.

Dr. Alfred C. Fones, the "father of dental hygiene," emphasized the important role of education. In the first textbook for dental hygienists, he wrote:

　It is primarily to this important work of public education that the dental hygienist is called. She must regard herself as the channel through which dentistry's knowledge of mouth hygiene is to be disseminated. The greatest service she can perform is the persistent education of the public in mouth hygiene and the allied branches of general hygiene.[1]

Dental hygiene has been studied and the scope of practice has developed from Dr. Fones' original concept. Scientific information about the prevention of oral diseases has been advancing steadily. The public has become increasingly aware of the need for dental hygiene care and the importance of oral health instruction. The clinical practice of the dental hygienist integrates specific care with instructional services required by the individual patient.

A. Purposes in Planning Care

Planning dental hygiene care for a patient means preparing a schedule to guide the preventive, educational, and therapeutic activities. Initially, the dental hygienist plays a major role in the collection of data to be used by the dentist in formulating the diagnosis on which the total treatment plan is based.

The dental hygienist must have a clear understanding of the patient's needs, the nature of the oral illness, and the principles relating to the treatment of the illness. The dental hygienist should be aware of the patient's emotional needs and psychologic reactions to the oral conditions. It is important to create an atmosphere in which the patient can respond to instruction, carry out the necessary procedures to supplement professional treatment, and cooperate during dental and dental hygiene appointments for the specific services.

B. Role in Patient Care

The role of the dental hygienist is to implement and coordinate the treatment and preventive program prescribed for each patient. Specific clinical services are required, and the dental hygienist teaches, motivates, and guides the patient in the performance of measures for disease control. The success of each phase of treatment, whether periodontic, orthodontic, restorative, or prosthodontic, depends on the patient's cooperative daily performance of the recommended measures. Dental hygiene care as provided by the dental hygienist becomes an integral part of the total patient care.

In general, the sections of this book are arranged in an order to correspond with a sequence in which dental hygiene services may logically be performed.

Because much of the text is concerned with details of how to perform clinical services for the patient, it is important to keep services and techniques in their proper perspective. A broad range of skills, in addition to the performance of technical procedures, is used in dental hygiene practice. Communication skills and problem-solving skills, as well as a professional demeanor, are important for successful patient care.

C. The Challenge of Planning Patient Care

Advancement in dental science has forced the professional dental hygienist to adapt dental hygiene care to changing concepts with understanding and flexibility. Dental hygiene care needs to be modified intelligently according to the patient, the oral condition and disease, and the personal problems.

Each patient is an individual with specific problems of oral care that need consideration. Good dental hygiene care is patient-centered.

The professional dental hygienist must be a self-directed person who can apply scientific knowledge to problem solving. The questions are the following: What is the status of this patient's oral health? What is the *dental hygiene diagnosis*? What is the *dental hygiene treatment plan*? What can the patient learn as a result of teaching and guidance? What will be the outcome?

In the effort to deliver the most effective and comprehensive health service, a set pattern of dental hygiene care, one that was memorized or learned by rote, cannot always be used. Knowledge must be applied to meet the individual needs of each patient.

III. SPECIAL PRACTICE AREAS

A wide range of settings is available for the practice of a dental hygienist. Likewise, a wide range of patient problems brings out the need for specialized knowledge and skills.

There are eight areas of dentistry in which a dentist may conduct an ethical limited practice. They are the following: dental public health, endodontics, oral pathology, oral and maxillofacial surgery, orthodontics, pediatric dentistry (dentistry for children), periodontics, and prosthodontics.[2] Education and training for certification in the dental specialties require a minimum of 2 years of graduate or postdoctoral study and the successful completion of written and practical examinations. Masters and postdoctoral specialty degrees require 3 or more years beyond basic dental education.

Although dental hygienists have not been required to complete examinations for practice within a specialty, educational curricula exist for certain areas. For example, advanced degree programs to prepare for dental hygiene education and public health have been available for many years.

In other special areas, short-term courses have been developed, such as for instruction in the care of patients with disabilities. In-service training may be available in long-term care institutions, hospitals, and skilled nursing facilities. Some dental hygienists have learned how to practice in a specialty through private study, special conferences, and personal experience.

Dental hygienists are needed to practice with dentists in specialty areas, particularly orthodontics, pediatric dentistry, and periodontics. Others are involved in special clinics with a variety of health specialists, where patients with dental deformities, such as cleft lip and/or palate, or patients with oral cancer are under care. In other facilities, dental hygienists serve with a combined medical and dental team in the treatment of patients with severe systemic diseases, patients with physical, mental, or emotional handicapping conditions, or patients with combinations of any of the problems mentioned.

FACTORS INFLUENCING CLINICAL PRACTICE

I. LEGAL

The law must be studied and respected by each dental hygienist practicing within the state, province, or country. Although the various practice acts have certain basic similarities, differences in scope and definition exist. Terminology varies, but each practice act regulates the patient services that may be practiced by the licensed dental hygienist. Changes may be made from time to time. Frequent review of the practice acts and/or regulations is recommended to keep dental health professionals up to date.

II. ETHICAL

Professional people in the health services are set apart from others by virtue of the dignity and responsibility of their work. Service is the primary objective of the dental hygienist and is the reason for the existence of the profession. Others look to the professional person for leadership and expect more than ordinary demonstration of good human relations. Being professional requires interpersonal, professional, interprofessional, and community relationships of a high standard.

Dental hygienists are ethically and morally responsible for providing dental hygiene care to all patients, including those who have been or may have been exposed to infectious diseases.

Dental hygienists' associations have defined principles of ethics for the professional dental hygienist. Figure 1–1 shows the Principles of Ethics of the American Dental Hygienists' Association.[3] Understanding of and loyalty to these principles are essential to successful practice.

III. PERSONAL

Each dental hygienist represents the entire profession to the patient being served. The dental hygienist's expressed or demonstrated attitudes toward dentistry, dental hygiene, and other health professions, as well as toward health services and preventive measures, are apt to be reflected in the subsequent attitude of the patient toward other dental hygienists and dental hygiene care in general.

Members of health professions must exemplify the traits they hold as objectives for others if response and cooperation are to be expected. Many personal factors of general physical health, oral health, cleanliness, appearance, and mental health are to be considered. A few of these are mentioned as follows:

1. *General Physical Health*. Optimum physical health depends primarily on a well-planned diet, a sufficient amount of sleep, and an adequate amount of exercise.

   Because of the occupational hazards of dental personnel, routine examinations at least annually should include tests for hearing, sight, uri-

---

PRINCIPLES OF ETHICS OF THE AMERICAN DENTAL HYGIENISTS' ASSOCIATION

Each member of the American Dental Hygienists' Association has the ethical obligation to subscribe to the following principles:

To provide oral health care utilizing highest professional knowledge, judgment, and ability.

To serve all patients without discrimination.

To hold professional patient relationships in confidence.

To utilize every opportunity to increase public understanding of oral health practices.

To generate public confidence in members of the dental health profession.

To cooperate with all health professions in meeting the health needs of the public.

To recognize and uphold the laws and regulations governing this profession.

To participate responsibly in this professional Association and uphold its purposes.

To maintain professional competence through continuing education.

To exchange professional knowledge with other health professions.

To represent dental hygiene with high standards of personal conduct.

FIG. 1–1. Professional Principles of Ethics (under revision 1994–95)

nary mercury, and certain communicable diseases.[4,5] Immunizations are described on pages 41–42.

2. *Oral Health*. The maintenance of a clean, healthy mouth demonstrates by example that the dental hygienist follows the teachings of the dental and dental hygiene professions relative to prevention and control of disease.

3. *Mental Health*. The mental health of the dental hygienist is reflected in interpersonal relationships and the ability to inspire confidence through a display of professional and emotional maturity. Adequate physical health, recreation, and participation in professional and community activities contribute to optimum mental health.

OBJECTIVES FOR PRACTICE

The hygienist's self-assessment is essential in attaining goals of perfection in service to the patient and in collaboration with the dentist in the total dental and dental hygiene care program. Personal objectives should be outlined and reviewed frequently in a plan for continued self-improvement.

The goal with respect to patient care is *to aid individu-*

als and groups in attaining and maintaining optimum oral health. Other objectives are related to this primary one.

The professional dental hygienist will

A. Strive toward the highest degree of professional ethics and conduct.

B. Plan and carry out effectively the dental hygiene services essential to the total care program for each individual patient.

C. Apply knowledge and understanding of the basic and clinical sciences in the recognition of oral conditions and prevention of oral diseases.

D. Apply scientific knowledge and skill to all clinical techniques and instructional procedures.

E. Recognize each patient as an individual and adapt techniques and procedures accordingly.

F. Identify and care for the needs of patients who have unusual general health problems that affect dental hygiene procedures.

G. Demonstrate interpersonal relationships that permit attending the patient with assurance and presenting dental health information effectively.

H. Provide a complete and personalized instructional service to help each patient to become motivated toward changes in oral health behavioral practices.

I. Practice safe and efficient clinical routines for the application of universal precautions for infection control.

J. Apply a continuing process of self-development and self-evaluation in clinical practice throughout professional life.

 1. Be objective and critical of procedures used in order to perform the best possible service.

 2. Appreciate the need for acquiring new knowledge and skills by regular enrollment in continuing education courses.

FACTORS TO TEACH THE PATIENT

A. The role of the dental hygienist as a cotherapist in the dental profession.

B. The scope of service of the dental hygienist as defined by various practice acts.

C. The interrelationship of instructional and clinical services in dental hygiene care.

D. The individual's potential state of oral health and how it can be developed and maintained.

REFERENCES

1. **Fones,** A.C., ed.: *Mouth Hygiene,* 4th ed. Philadelphia, Lea & Febiger, 1934, p. 248.

2. **American Dental Association:** *ADA Principles of Ethics and Code of Professional Conduct,* With Official Advisory Opinions. Revised May, 1992, *J. Am. Dent. Assoc., 123,* 98, September, 1992.

3. **American Dental Hygienists' Association,** House of Delegates: *Professional Code of Ethics for the Dental Hygienist,* Revised November, 1974.

4. **Gravois,** S.L. and Stringer, R.B.: Survey of Occupational Health Hazards in Dental Hygiene, *Dent. Hyg., 54,* 518, November, 1980.

5. **Goldman,** H.S.: Hazards in the Dental Workplace. Prevention for the Dentist, *Clin. Prev. Dent., 2,* 18, September–October, 1980.

SUGGESTED READINGS

Boyer, E.M. and Gupta, G.C.: Clinical Dental Hygienists' Perceptions of Quality Dental Hygiene Care, *J. Dent. Hyg., 66,* 216, June, 1992.

Douglass, C.W.: The Effect of Recent Trends on Dental Hygiene, *J. Dent. Educ., 55,* 225, March, 1991.

Frankel, M.S.: Taking Ethics Seriously. Building a Professional Community, *J. Dent. Hyg., 66,* 386, November–December, 1992.

McFall, D.B.: The Future of Allied Health Education, *Educ. Update, 12,* 1, December, 1992.

McIntyre, L.: The Evolution of Health Promotion, *Can. Dent. Hyg./ Probe, 26,* 15, Spring, 1992.

Mickelson, L.M.: Back to the Future: Appropriating Our Traditions, *Can. Dent. Hyg./Probe, 27,* 55, March/April, 1993.

Pimlott, J.F.L.: The Changing Role for Dental Hygiene, *Can. Dent. Hyg./Probe, 23,* 89, Summer, 1989.

Uldricks, J.M., Hicks, M.J., Whitacre, H.L., Anderson, J., and Moeschberger, M.L.: Dental Hygienists' Utilization of Periodontal Assessment Skills and Perceived Collaboration with Dentist-Employer, *J. Dent. Hyg., 67,* 22, January, 1993.

Walker, B., Juchli, J., and Pimlott, J.: Self-regulation in Alberta, Canada: The Achievement of a Goal, *Can. Dent. Hyg./Probe, 27,* 59, March/April, 1993.

Professionalism and Ethics

Fleming, W.C.: The Attributes of a Profession and Its Members, *J. Am. Dent. Assoc., 69,* 390, September, 1964.

Hine, M.K.: The Professional Concept—Its History and Meaning to Health Service, *J. Am. Coll. Dent., 37,* 19, January, 1970.

Jackson, E.: An Investigation of the Determinants of Professional Image, *Ann. Dent., 40,* 7, Summer, 1981.

MacQuarrie, E.E.: Factors in the Development of Professional Attitude. *J. Am. Dent. Hyg. Assoc., 45,* 86, March–April, 1971.

Motley, W.E.: *Ethics, Jurisprudence and History for the Dental Hygienist,* 3rd ed. Philadelphia, Lea & Febiger, 1983, 217 pp.

PART II

Preparation for Dental Hygiene Appointments

Infection Control: Transmissible Diseases

The transmission of disease is an insidious process. Infection and communicable disease can lead to illness, disability, and loss of work time. In addition, patients, family members, and community contacts can become exposed and may become ill and lose productive time or suffer permanent after-effects.

In oral health-care practice, the objective is to protect patients, dental personnel, and others that may become exposed by acquiring infection in the environment of the office or clinic. Health services facilities, including dental facilities, must be places for cure and prevention, not for dissemination of disease due to inadequate precautionary measures and habits of the professional personnel.

The first responsibility of the entire dental team is to organize and maintain a system for the sterilization, disinfection, and care of instruments and equipment. The second step is to develop and maintain work practices for all appointments that will prevent direct or indirect cross-infections between dental personnel and patients, and from one patient to another.

Table 2–1 lists and defines terms that apply to the transmission of infectious agents.

The intact mucous membrane of the oral cavity protects against infection to a degree. However, when the gingival tissues are inflamed and are manipulated during instrumentation, microorganisms can be introduced into the underlying tissues by way of the gingival sulcus or periodontal pocket.

Pathogenic (disease producing), potentially pathogenic, or nonpathogenic microorganisms may be present in the oral cavity of each patient. Pathogenic organisms may be transient. Patients may be carriers of certain diseases. Inadvertent transmission to subsequent susceptible patients or to dental personnel may occur as a result of inappropriate work practices, such as careless handwashing, unhygienic personal habits, or inadequate sterilization and handling of sterile instruments and materials.

Cross-contamination refers to the spread of microorganisms from one source to another: person to person, or person to an inanimate object and then to another person. Recognition of the many possibilities for the transfer of infection in a dental office or clinic provides a basis for planning the system of sterilization, disinfection, and handling of instruments and equipment.

MICROORGANISMS OF THE ORAL CAVITY

In utero the oral cavity is sterile, but within a few hours to 1 day a simple oral flora develops.[1] The natural oral microflora of the saliva in a mature mouth can include more than 40 species.[2] Most of the salivary bacteria come from the dorsum of the tongue, but some are from other mucous membranes. Much higher counts of total microorganisms are found in bacterial plaque and in periodontal pockets than in saliva.

THE INFECTIOUS PROCESS

A chain of events is required for the spread of an infectious agent. The six essential links are shown in Figure 2–1.

I. ESSENTIAL FEATURES FOR DISEASE TRANSMISSION
   A. An *infectious agent*, the *invading organism* (bacterium, virus, fungus, rickettsia, or protozoa).

11

TABLE 2–1
KEY WORDS AND ABBREVIATIONS: DISEASE TRANSMISSION

Aerosol (ă'er-o-sol'): an artificially generated collection of particles suspended in air.
  Microbial aerosol: suspension of particles in the air that consists partially or wholly of microorganisms; it may be capable of causing an airborne infection.
Antibody (an'tĭ-bod'ē): a soluble protein molecule produced and secreted by body cells in response to an antigen; it is capable of binding to that specific antigen.
Antigen (an'tĭ jen): a substance that is capable, under appropriate conditions, of inducing a specific immune response and of reacting with the products of that response, that is, with the specific antibody.
Carrier: a person who harbors a specific infectious agent in the absence of discernible clinical disease and serves as a potential source of infection. The carrier state may be temporary, transient, or chronic.
  Asymptomatic carrier: an individual who harbors pathogenic organisms without clinically recognizable symptoms; as a carrier and distributor, contacts may become infected.
CDCP: United States Centers for Disease Control and Prevention, Department of Health and Human Services, Public Health Service, Atlanta, GA 30333.
Communicable period of a disease: the time during which an infectious agent may be transferred directly or indirectly from an infected person to another person; the communicable period may include or overlap the incubation period.
Droplet (drop'let): diminutive drop, such as the particles of moisture expelled while coughing, sneezing, or speaking that may carry infectious agents.
ELISA or EIA: an enzyme-linked immunoabsorbent assay; a laboratory test to detect antibody in the blood serum.
  Western blot (WB): a laboratory test for antibody that is more specific than EIA and is used to validate seropositive reactions to the EIA.
Endemic (en-dĕm'ik): the constant presence of a disease or infectious agent within a geographic area.
Epidemic (ep'ĭ-dem'ik): widespread occurrence of cases of an illness in a community or region; greater than the expected number of cases for the particular population.
Fomite (fo'mīt) or **fomes** (fo'mēz): an inanimate object or material on which disease-producing agents (microorganisms) may be conveyed.
HCW: health-care worker; **DHCW:** dental health-care worker.
Immunity (ĭ-mū'nĭ-tē): the resistance that a person has against disease; it may be natural or acquired.
  Passive immunity: short-duration immunity either naturally attained by transplacental transfer from the mother or artificially acquired by inoculation of specific protective antibodies.
  Active immunity: immunity either naturally attained by infection with or without clinical manifestations, or artificially acquired by inoculation of the agent in a killed, modified, or variant form of the agent; in response, the body produces its own antibodies; usually lasts for years.
Incubation period (in'kŭ-ba'shun): the time interval between the initial contact with an infectious agent and the appearance of the first clinical sign or symptom of the disease.
Infection: a state caused by the invasion, development, or multiplication of an infectious agent into the body.
  Primary infection: first time; no pre-existing antibodies.
  Latent infection: persistent infection following a primary infection in which the causative agent remains inactive within certain cells.
  Recurrent infection: symptomatic reactivation of a latent infection.
Infectious agent: organism capable of producing an infection.
Pandemic (pan-dem'ik): widespread epidemic usually affecting the population of an extensive region, several countries, or sometimes the entire globe.
Parenteral (pah-ren'ter-al): injection by a route other than the alimentary tract, such as subcutaneous, intramuscular, or intravenous.
Pathogen (path'ō-jen): a virus, microorganism, or other substance that causes disease.
  Opportunistic pathogen: capable of causing disease only when the host's resistance is lowered.
Percutaneous (per'kŭ-ta'nē-us): by way of, or through, the skin.
Permucosal (per mu cō'sal): by way of, or through, a mucous membrane.
Prodrome (prō'drōm): early or premonitory symptom (adj: prodromal).
Replication: process by which viruses reproduce and multiply.
Retrovirus (ret'rō-vi'rus): virus with RNA core genetic material; requires the enzyme reverse transcriptase to convert its RNA into proviral DNA.
Serologic diagnosis: the identification of a disease by serum markers of that specific condition.
Seroconversion (sĕ'rō-kon-ver'shun): after exposure to the etiologic agent of a disease, the blood changes from negative ("seronegative") to positive ("seropositive") serum marker for that disease; the time interval for conversion is specific for each disease.
Serum marker: a specific finding (such as an antibody or antigen) by laboratory blood analysis that identifies an existing disease state.
Shedding (viral): presence of virus in body secretions, in excretions, or in body surface lesions with potential for transmission.

TABLE 2–1   (continued)
KEY WORDS AND ABBREVIATIONS: DISEASE TRANSMISSION

STI: sexually transmitted infection.

Surveillance (sŭr-vāl′ans) (of disease): continuing scrutiny of all aspects of occurrence and spread of a disease that are pertinent to effective control.

Susceptible host: host not possessing resistance against an infectious agent.

Transmission (horizontal): passage of an infectious agent from one individual to another.

Vertical transmission: passage of an infectious agent from one generation to another by breast milk or across the placenta.

Universal precautions: an approach to infection control in which all human blood and certain human body fluids are treated as if known to be infectious for HIV, HBV, and other blood-borne pathogens.

Vector (vek′tor): a carrier that transfers an infectious microorganism from one host to another.

Biologic vector: an arthropod vector in whose body the infecting organism multiplies before

becoming infective to the recipient.

Vehicle (vē′ĭ-k′l): a substance or object that serves as an intermediate means by which an infectious agent is transported and introduced into a susceptible host through a suitable portal of entry.

Virion (vī′rē-on): complete virus particle made up of the **nucleoid** (the genetic material) and **capsid** (the shell of protein that protects the nucleoid).

Virulence (vĭr′ū-lens): the degree of pathogenicity or disease-evoking power of an infectious agent.

Virus (vī′rus): a subcellular genetic entity capable of gaining entrance into a limited range of living cells and capable of replication only within such cells; a virus contains either DNA or RNA but not both. (DNA and RNA are defined in Table 2–5.)

Window period: the time between exposure resulting in infection and the presence of detectable serum antibody; antibody test is negative but infectious agent is transmissible during the window period.

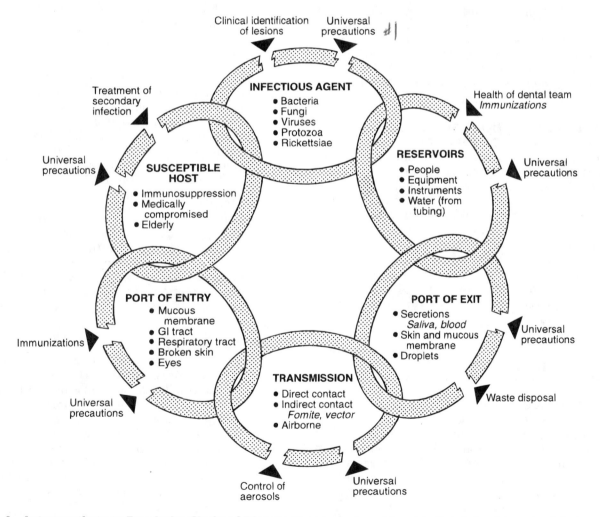

FIG. 2–1. Interventions to Break the Chain of Disease Transmission. A break in the chain of six major links is required for the spread of an infectious agent. Universal precautions are applied to interrupt the chain.

Each organism has its own specific reaction in an infected host.

B. A *reservoir* where the invading organisms live and multiply. The infectious agent has its own essential environment, which may be inanimate matter, an insect, or human cells or blood. For example, soil is the reservoir for tetanus and humans are a reservoir for herpetic infections.

C. A *mode of escape,* the port of exit from the reservoir. Organisms exit through various body systems, such as the respiratory tract, or through skin lesions. Escape from the blood stream may be through skin abrasions, hypodermic needles, or dental instruments.

D. A *mode of transmission,* which may be direct, person to person, or indirect by way of an intermediate vehicle, such as contaminated hands or hypodermic needle. Transmission by a droplet may be direct from the respiratory tract of one person to the oral cavity of the receiving host. Droplets also may pass indirectly to hands or inanimate objects to be transferred indirectly to the susceptible host.

E. A *mode of entry,* the port of entry of the infectious agent into the new host. Modes of entry may be similar to modes of escape, such as the respiratory tract, mucous membranes, or a break in the skin.

F. A *susceptible host* that does not have immunity to the invading infectious agent.

II. FACTORS THAT INFLUENCE THE DEVELOPMENT OF INFECTION

The presence of an infectious agent does not lead to infection or disease inevitably. Factors involved include, but are not limited to, the following:

A. Number of organisms and duration of exposure.
B. Virulence of the organisms: their ability to survive interim exposure.
C. Immune status of the host; antibody response; defense cell reaction.
D. General physical health and nutritional status of the host. In health, disease is resisted, whereas in a deprived state, the body can be susceptible to infection.

AIRBORNE INFECTION

I. DUST-BORNE ORGANISMS

Clostridium tetani (tetanus bacillus), *Staphylococcus aureus,* and enteric bacteria are among the organisms that may travel in the dust brought in from outside and that moves in and about dental treatment areas. When doors are opened and closed and people pass in and out, dust is set into motion that can settle on instruments, other objects, or people.

Infectious microorganisms also reach dust from the oral cavities of patients by way of large airborne particles, which are described as spatter further on. Dust-borne organisms can be sources of contamination for dental instruments and the hands of dental personnel.

Surface disinfection of all equipment contacted during an appointment contributes to control of dust-borne pathogens. Procedures for surface disinfection are described on pages 62–64.

II. AEROSOL PRODUCTION[3]

Airborne particles are usually classified by size as either *aerosols* or *splatter.* They are constantly being produced.

A. Aerosols

A particle of a true aerosol is less than 50 μ in diameter and nearly all are less than 5 μ. Aerosols are biologic contaminants that occur in solid or liquid form, are invisible, and remain suspended in air for long periods.

Aerosol particles that are 5 μ or smaller may be breathed deep into the lungs. Larger particles get trapped higher in the respiratory tree. The tiny particles may contain respiratory disease-producing organisms or traces of mercury or amalgam that collect in the lung because they are not biodegradable.

B. Spatter

Heavier, larger particles may remain airborne a relatively short time because of their own size and weight. They drop or spatter on objects, people, and the floor. The spatter is composed of particles greater than 50 μ in diameter.

In contrast to aerosols, spatter may be visible, particularly after it has landed on skin, hair, clothing, or environmental surfaces where gross contamination can result.

C. Origin

Aerosols and spatter are created during breathing, speaking, coughing, or sneezing. They are produced during all intraoral procedures, including examination and manual scaling. When produced by air-spray, air-water-spray, handpiece activity, or ultrasonic scaling, the number of aerosols increases to tremendous proportions.[3,4,5,6]

D. Contents

1. *Microorganisms.* An aerosol may contain a single organism or a clump of microorganisms adhered to a dust or debris particle. The organisms may be contained within a liquid droplet.
2. *Particles from Cavity Preparation.* Tooth fragments; microorganisms from saliva, plaque, and/or oropharynx/nasopharynx; oil from a handpiece; and water from the cooling equipment may be in aerosols following cavity preparation.
3. *Ultrasonic Scaling.* The many microorganisms found in the aerosols from ultrasonic scalers

include *Staphylococcus aureus, albus,* and *pyogenes, Streptococcus viridans,* lactobacilli, Actinomyces, pneumococci, and diphtheroids.[5,6] Viruses also may be spread by ultrasonic instruments.

E. Concentration
Bacteria-laden aerosols and spatter are in greater concentration close to the scene of instrumentation; the quantity decreases with distance. The aerosols travel with air currents and, therefore, move from room to room.

III. PREVENTION OF TRANSMISSION[3]
The control of airborne infection depends on elimination or limitation of the organisms at their source, interruption of transmission, and protection of the potentially susceptible recipient.

Carefully monitored procedures are necessary for all patients with or without a known serious communicable disease. A list of universal procedures appears on pages 65–67.

A. Limitation of Organisms
Organisms can be limited by postponement of elective treatment for a patient known to have specific communicable organisms in the oral cavity. Patients may be asked to change their appointments when they are suffering from respiratory or other communicable disease.

B. Preoperative Oral Hygiene Measures
Toothbrushing and using an antiseptic mouthrinse reduce the numbers of bacteria contained in aerosols. Preparation of the patient is described on page 64.

C. Interruption of Transmission
1. Use rubber dam, high-volume evacuation, and manual instrumentation as much as possible.
2. Install air-control methods to supply adequate ventilation, filtration, and relative humidity.
3. Employ vacuum cleaning to remove dirt and microorganisms rather than dust-arousing housekeeping methods. The cleaner must have a filter to prevent the escape of organisms after they are suctioned.[7]

D. Clean Water
Run water through all tubings to handpieces, ultrasonic scalers, and air/water spray for at least 2 minutes at the start of the day and at least 30 seconds after each appointment during the day. Contamination by spatter and aerosols is reduced by this method.[8]

E. Protection of the Clinician
The use of masks and protective eyewear can prevent direct contact of spatter and aerosols with the faces of the dental team.

AUTOGENOUS INFECTION
[handwritten: SELF PRODUCING ORIGIONATING WITHIN THE BODY]

An autogenous infection originates within a person when the normal defense mechanisms are modified. The microflora of the oral cavity may become pathogenic when, for example, the organisms are forced into the tissues during instrumentation.

I. SOURCES OF AUTOGENOUS INFECTION
A. Bacteremia
Bacteremia is a condition in which bacteria or other microorganisms are in the blood stream. In the oral cavity, bacteria can enter the blood by way of a break in the mucosa, or through a gingival or periodontal pocket. When scaling or other instrumentation is performed, the microbial flora is disturbed and may be forced into the underlying tissues.

B. Injection Site
An abscess can occur at the site of injection when microorganisms are picked up by the needle as it is carried to the injection site. Organisms from bacterial plaque or those residing on the mucosal surface can be carried into the underlying tissues as the needle is inserted.

II. FACTORS THAT ALTER NORMAL DEFENSES
The patient's complete medical and dental history must be reviewed to identify specific problems and take necessary precautions. Examples of situations that alter the normal defenses are included under the following topics.

A. Abnormal Physical Conditions
A heart valve may be defective as a result of a congenital or acquired condition. Such a valve may be susceptible to infective endocarditis resulting from a bacteremia created during dental or dental hygiene instrumentation. Prevention of infective endocarditis is described on page 102, and tables 6–5 and 6–6.

B. Systemic Diseases
Examples of systemic conditions in which susceptibility to infection is increased are diabetes mellitus, alcoholism, leukemia, glomerulonephritis, acquired immunodeficiency syndrome, and all causes of immunosuppression.

C. Drug Therapy
Certain drugs used in the treatment of systemic disease alter the body's defenses. Examples are steroids and chemotherapeutic agents that are immunosuppressive. Special precautions, such as prophylactic antibiotics, may be indicated to prevent infection.

D. Prostheses and Transplants
A patient with, for example, a joint replacement, cardiac prosthesis, ventriculoatrial shunt for hydrocephalus, or an organ transplant may require antibiotic premedication.

III. PREVENTION OF AUTOGENOUS INFECTION
A. Give Antibiotic Premedication
For the patient who is at risk for infection that may result from bacteremia, antibiotic premedication may be indicated. A list of patients who are medically compromised and potentially endangered during treatment appears on pages 102 and 103. For the American Heart Association recommendations for antibiotic premedication, see page 102 and tables 6–5 and 6–6.

B. Lower the Surface Microbial Count
Suggested procedures for lowering the numbers of microorganisms at the treatment site just prior to treatment are described on page 64. They include bacterial plaque removal procedures, particularly toothbrushing and flossing, rinsing with an antibacterial rinse, and the application of a topical antiseptic.

C. Prepare an Injection Site[9,10]
After drying the tissue surface with a sterile sponge, a topical antiseptic is swabbed over the surface (page 64). Retraction should be maintained to prevent contact of other tissues or saliva.

Disposable needles are required for disease control. Particular care must be taken to avoid contacting the needle with anything prior to injection. Contact with a tooth or tissue can contaminate the needle with microorganisms, which can then be injected as the needle is inserted.

PATHOGENS TRANSMISSIBLE BY THE ORAL CAVITY

Selected pathogens that may be transmitted by way of the oral cavity, and their disease manifestations, mode of transfer, incubation, and communicability periods, are listed in Table 2–2. Several of the so-called "children's diseases" are included.

Tuberculosis, viral hepatitis, acquired immunodeficiency syndrome, and herpetic infections are described in detail in this chapter because of the special problems they create in personal and patient care. The general preventive measures described for these diseases should be applied during all appointments.

The etiologic agents of many communicable diseases enter the body by way of the oral cavity. Many infectious diseases have specific oral manifestations from which the disease can be identified. Pathogens are often present within the oral cavity without producing oral signs or symptoms, a fact of particular importance to the total consideration of prevention of disease transmission.

TUBERCULOSIS[11]

Mycobacterium tuberculosis, the etiologic agent in tuberculosis, is a resistant organism that requires special consideration when sterilization and disinfection methods are selected and administered. Tuberculosis is a serious disease that can involve many months and years of lost time during the active stages of illness and the convalescence following. Clinical procedures must be planned to prevent exposure and infection from this debilitating disease.

Tuberculosis is a common communicable disease throughout the world. In the United States, it is no longer a leading cause of death, as it was before preventive public health and medical measures were developed. Among reportable bacterial infections, however, it has increased in recent years.

I. TRANSMISSION
A. Inhalation
Tuberculosis is contracted by the inhalation of fresh droplets containing tubercle bacilli. The organisms are disseminated from sputum and saliva of the infected individual by coughing, breathing heavily, or sneezing (figure 2–2). During the use of ultrasonic and other handpieces, and of water and air spray, aerosols are created that can carry the bacilli. Aerosol production was described on page 14.

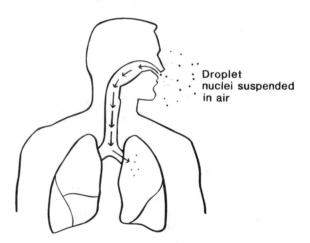

FIG. 2–2. Droplet Nuclei. Many potentially pathogenic microorganisms are disseminated by aerosols and spatter. The primary mode of transmission of tubercle bacilli is by droplet nuclei breathed directly into the lung. (Adapted from McInnes, M.E.: *Essentials of Communicable Disease,* 2nd ed. St. Louis, The C.V. Mosby Co., 1975.)

When the organisms are in tiny aerosols, they can pass readily into the lungs and the respiratory bronchioles. There, they can invade the tissue and establish an infection.

B. Factors Affecting Transmission

Transmission of tuberculosis is dependent on the following: (1) the degree to which the infected person produces infectious droplets, (2) the amount and duration of exposure, and (3) the susceptibility of the recipient. Some patients are more contagious than are others. Maximum communicability is usually just before the disease is diagnosed, when the person may have a severe cough and other respiratory symptoms.

C. Other Modes of Transmission

The tubercle bacillus may enter the body by ingestion or direct inoculation, as well as by inhalation. Infection of the lungs is most common, but the tubercle bacillus also infects lymph nodes, meninges (tuberculous meningitis), kidneys, bone, skin, and the oral cavity.

Extrapulmonary tuberculosis rates are high in patients with HIV infection. Tuberculosis is considered an AIDS-defining illness.[12]

II. DISEASE PROCESS

A. Predisposing Factors

Any debilitating or immunosuppressive condition can predispose to invasion by the tubercle bacillus. Systemic conditions that may be related to lowered resistance to infection include diabetes, congenital heart disease, chronic lung disease, alcoholism, and the acquired immunodeficiency syndrome (page 32 and table 2–7).[12]

B. Incubation Period

As shown in table 2–2, the incubation period may be as long as 12 weeks. After such an extended period, the origin of the disease is difficult or impossible to trace.

C. Early Symptoms

In the early stages before marked symptoms appear, the patient may have a low-grade fever, loss of appetite, weight loss, and may tire easily. There may be a slight cough, and eventually sputum, indicating the possible presence of tubercle bacilli in the throat and saliva.

D. Later Symptoms

Definite temperature elevation, particularly in the afternoon, night sweats, weakness, and a persistent cough become apparent. Diagnosis is by chest radiograph and tuberculin testing.

E. Reactivation Tuberculosis

A focus of an infection may remain inactive and later produce a recurrence. Treatment of a primary infection may have been incomplete. Reactivity may be related to a debilitating condition or immunosuppression.

Reactivation of latent tuberculous infection may occur after many years. Usually a patient with a healthy immune system is asymptomatic and cannot spread the disease to others. The infection can be eliminated with antituberculosis drugs.

F. Multidrug-Resistant Tuberculosis

Multiple antituberculosis drugs are taken daily or several times a week for 6 months to treat active tuberculosis (TB). Two of the principal drugs used are isoniazid and rifampin.

If medications are not prescribed properly or are not taken by the patient regularly, the tubercle bacilli can become resistant. The drug-resistant organisms can be transmitted and can cause disease in the recipient. Multidrug-resistant TB is difficult and expensive to treat.

The first line of prevention for multidrug-resistant TB is supervision of treatment so the medication is used properly. The second approach is to locate and treat persons with latent TB, particularly those at a high risk for reactivation. Direct supervision to assure completion of the full course of treatment is required.

III. CLINICAL MANAGEMENT

A. Patient History

In early disease, there may not be a suspicion of tuberculosis. Careful history-taking and review of previous histories for comparison may show the need to refer the patient to a physician.

B. Extraoral and Intraoral Examination

Tuberculosis is primarily a lesion of the lungs, but any organ or tissue may be involved.
1. *Lymphadenopathy.* Regional lymph nodes may be enlarged.
2. *Oral Lesions.*[13,14] Oral lesions are relatively rare, but when they occur, they are usually ulcers. They may be located on the soft or hard palate and, occasionally, on the tongue.

C. Patient Under Treatment

Chemotherapy can control the patient's contagious condition. Isoniazid is used for long periods, sometimes in combination with rifampin. After a few weeks from the beginning of therapy, bacilli in the sputum, the cough, and the infectivity are decreased.

VIRAL HEPATITIS

Hepatitis means inflammation of the liver. Viruses cause a variety of types of hepatitis. Some of the viruses have been specifically identified, and hepatitis A, hepa-

**TABLE 2–2
INFECTIOUS DISEASES**

Infectious Agent	Disease or Condition	Route or Mode of Transmission	Incubation Period	Communicable Period	Vaccine
Human immunodeficiency virus (HIV)	Acquired immuno-deficiency syndrome (AIDS) HIV-infection	Blood and blood products (infected IV needles) Sexual contact Transplacental and perinatal	3 months to 12 years or more	From asymptomatic through life	*
Hepatitis A virus (HAV)	Type A hepatitis "Infectious" hepatitis	Fecal-oral Food, water, shellfish	15 to 50 days (average 28 to 30 days)	2 to 3 weeks before onset (jaundice) through 8 days after	Yes
Hepatitis B virus (HBV)	Type B hepatitis "Serum" hepatitis	Blood Saliva and all body fluids Sexual contact Perinatal	2 to 6 months (average 60 to 90 days)	Before, during, and after clinical signs Carrier state: indefinite	Yes
Hepatitis C virus (HCV) PT-NANB	Type C hepatitis Parenterally transmitted nonA, nonB	Percutaneous Blood Needles	2 weeks to 6 months (6 to 9 weeks)	1 week before onset of symptoms Carrier state: indefinite	No
Delta hepatitis virus (HDV) Delta agent	Delta hepatitis	Coinfection with HBV Blood Sexual contacts Perinatal	2 to 10 weeks	All phases	HBV vaccine
Hepatitis E virus (HEV) ET-NANB	Type E hepatitis Enterically transmitted nonA, nonB	Fecal-oral Contaminated water	15 to 64 days	Similar to HAV	No
Herpes simplex virus Type 1 (HSV-1) Type 2 (HSV-2)	Acute herpetic gingivostomatitis Herpes labialis Ocular herpetic infections Herpetic whitlow	Saliva Direct contact (lip, hand) Indirect contact (on objects, limited survival) Sexual contact	2 to 12 days	Labialis: 1 day before onset until lesions are crusted Acute stomatitis: 7 weeks after recovery Asymptomatic infection: with viral shedding Reactivation period: with viral shedding	No
Varicella-zoster virus (VZV)	Chickenpox Herpes zoster (shingles)	Direct contact Indirect contact Airborne droplet	2 to 3 weeks	5 days prior to onset of rash until crusting of vesicles	*
Epstein-Barr virus (EBV)	Infectious mononucleosis	Direct contact Saliva	4 to 6 weeks	Prolonged Pharyngeal excretion 1 year after infection	No
Cytomegalovirus (CMV)	Neonatal cytomegalo-virus infection Cytomegaloviral disease	Perinatal Direct contact (most body secretions) Blood transfusion Saliva	3 to 12 weeks after delivery 3 to 8 weeks after transfusion	Months to years	No

* Vaccine progress.

TABLE 2-2 (Continued)
INFECTIOUS DISEASES

Infectious Agent	Disease or Condition	Route or Mode of Transmission	Incubation Period	Communicable Period	Vaccine
Mycobacterium tuberculosis	Tuberculosis	Droplet nuclei Sputum Saliva	4 to 12 weeks	As long as viable bacilli are discharged in sputum	B.C.G.
Treponema pallidum	Syphilis Congenital syphilis	Direct contact Transplacental	10 days to 3 months	Variable and indefinite May be 2 to 4 years	No
Neisseria gonorrhoeae	Gonorrhea Gonococcal pharyngitis	Direct contact Indirect (short survival of organisms)	2 to 7 days	During incubation Continued for months and years if untreated	No
Bordetella pertussis	Whooping cough Pertussis	Direct contact with discharges	7 to 10 days	Not treated: from early catarrhal stage to 3 weeks after paroxysmal cough	Yes
Mumps virus (Paramyxovirus)	Infectious parotitis (mumps)	Direct contact (saliva) Airborne droplet	12 to 25 days (average 18 days)	12 to 25 days after exposure From 6 to 7 days before symptoms until 9 days after swelling	Yes
Poliovirus types 1, 2, 3	Poliomyelitis	Direct contact (saliva) Droplet Fecal-oral	7 to 14 days	Probably most infectious 7 to 10 days before and after onset of symptoms	Yes
Influenza viruses (A, B, C)	Influenza	Nasal discharge Respiratory droplets	1 to 5 days	3 days from clinical onset	Yes
Measles virus (*Morbillivirus*)	Rubeola (measles)	Direct contact Saliva Airborne droplet	7 to 18 days to fever, 14 days to rash	Few days before fever to 4 days after rash appears	Yes
Rubella virus (Togavirus)	Rubella (German measles)	Nasopharyngeal secretions Direct contact Airborne droplets	16 to 23 days	From 1 weeks to at least 4 days after rash appears Highly communicable	Yes
	Congenital rubella syndrome	Maternal infection first trimester		Infants shed virus for months after birth	
Group A streptococci (Beta-hemolytic) *Streptococcus pyogenes*	Streptococcal sore throat Scarlet fever Impetigo Erysipelas	Respiratory droplets Direct contact	1 to 3 days	10 to 21 days, untreated Many nasal oropharyngeal carriers	No
Staphylococcus aureus *Staphylococcus epidermidis*	Abscesses Boils (furuncle) Impetigo Bacterial pneumonia	Saliva Exudates Nasal discharge	4 to 10 days Variable and indefinite	While lesions drain and carrier state persists	No
Candida albicans	Candidiasis	Secretions Excretions (oral, skin, vagina)	Variable 2 to 5 days for "thrush" in children	While lesions are present	No
Streptococcus pneumoniae	Pneumonia Pneumococcal pneumonia	Droplet Direct contact Indirect	1 to 3 days Not well determined	While virulent organisms are discharged	Yes

titis B, hepatitis C, hepatitis D (delta), and hepatitis E are described in this section.

The incidence of hepatitis B has increased significantly over the past 20 years. It has been a serious occupational hazard for health-care workers. Among professional personnel, both medical and dental, the use of strict sterilization of equipment and materials, aseptic techniques, and self-protection measures is mandatory. With the advent of the hepatitis B vaccine, immunization for health workers and other frequently exposed individuals is available.[15]

Table 2–3 lists the hepatitis terminology with abbreviations and significance.

HEPATITIS A[16]

Hepatitis A occurs much more frequently in children and young adults than in older adults. It is more severe in adults. Early immunization is indicated.

I. TRANSMISSION
A. Fecal-Oral Route
The most common transmission is through close contact in unsanitary conditions. Unwashed hands of an infected person can contaminate anything touched.

TABLE 2–3
VIRAL HEPATITIS: ABBREVIATIONS

Abbreviation	Term	Significance
Hepatitis A		
HAV	Hepatitis A virus	Etiologic agent Hepatitis A
anti-HAV	Antibody to hepatitis A virus	Immunity to infection
IgM anti-HAV	IgM antibody to hepatitis A virus	Recent HAV infection
Hepatitis B		
HBV	Hepatitis B virus (Dane particle)	Etiologic agent hepatitis B
HBsAg	Hepatitis B surface antigen (Australian antigen)	Current HBV infection. Surface marker in acute disease and carrier state
anti-HBs	Antibody to hepatitis B surface antigen	Indicates (1) Active immunity to HBV (past infection) (2) Passive immunity from HBIG (3) Immune response from HB vaccine
HBeAg	Hepatitis B e antigen	High titer HBV in serum indicates high infectivity. Persists into carrier state
anti-HBe	Antibody to hepatitis B e antigen	Low titer HBV. Low degree infectivity
HBcAg	Hepatitis B core antigen	No test available
anti-HBc	Antibody to hepatitis B core antigen	Indicates prior HBV infection
IgM anti-HBc	IgM class antibody to hepatitis B core antigen	Indicates recent HBC infection
Hepatitis C		
HCV	Hepatitis C virus (formerly parentally transmitted non-A, non-B)	Etiologic agent for hepatitis C
anti-HCV	Antibody to hepatitis C virus	Indicates acute disease and chronic state. Resembles hepatitis B
Hepatitis D		
HDV	Hepatitis D virus	Etiologic agent hepatitis D with HBsAg
anti-HDV	Antibody to hepatitis D virus	Indicates past or present infection
Hepatitis E		
HEV	Hepatitis E virus (formerly enterically transmitted non-A, non-B)	Etiologic agent hepatitis E
anti-HEV	Antibody to hepatitis E virus	Resembles hepatitis A
Immune Globulins		
IG	Immune globulin	Contains antibodies to HAV and low titer HBV antibodies
HBIG	Hepatitis B immune globulin	Contains high titer antibodies to HBV

B. Waterborne and Food-borne

Epidemics may occur when sanitation is inadequate. Contaminated water may carry hepatitis A virus directly to those using the water, or it may contaminate shellfish grown in the water.

Infected food handlers can contaminate uncooked food or food handled after cooking.

C. Blood

In the earliest days of active disease, the blood contains transient hepatitis A viruses; however, transmission by blood transfusion is rare.

II. DISEASE PROCESS

A. Incubation and Communicability

The incubation period is from 15 to 50 days, with an average of 28 to 30 days. During the 2- to 3-week period before the onset of jaundice, the infection is communicable. Shortly after jaundice appears, the communicability begins to diminish. A carrier state has not been demonstrated.

B. Signs and Symptoms

The stages are defined by the incidence of jaundice as preicteric (before jaundice appears) and icteric (while jaundice is present). Hepatitis A without jaundice (anicteric) is two to three times more prevalent than icteric. A diagnosis of hepatitis is not always made, because without jaundice, symptoms may resemble influenza or other diseases.

1. *Preicteric Phase.* Typically, there is an abrupt onset of an influenza-like illness, with fever, headache, fatigue, nausea, vomiting, and abdominal pain. The liver may be enlarged and tender to palpation.
2. *Icteric Phase.* Jaundice may appear in adults, but rarely in children. Other symptoms become prolonged, and the patient may be ill for a few days to a month. Occasionally, chronic hepatitis follows, but 85 to 90% of patients recover completely.

III. IMMUNITY

Anti-HAV is usually detectable in the serum within 2 weeks of onset. Immunity to reinfection follows with recovery.

In addition to those who are known to have had the disease, many more people acquire immunity from undetected disease.

Vaccine for active immunization is available.[17,18]

IV. PREVENTION

A. Sanitation and Personal Hygiene

Because the principal means of transmission is by way of the feces, prevention on that level is indicated.

1. Public health control of food handlers and of water contamination.

2. Personal hygiene control through scrupulous handwashing by a patient and all contacts, as well as by all health-care workers involved in patient care.

B. Application in Dental Setting

Instrument sterilization, use of disposable materials, and all related precautions for persons and objects contacted by the patient. Such procedures must be the same for all patients, because the presence of hepatitis A viruses is not usually known. Clinic procedures are described in Chapter 4.

V. PASSIVE IMMUNIZATION[19]

A. IG

Standard immune globulin (IG) is used for the prevention or modification of hepatitis A in a person known to be susceptible, who is accidentally exposed. Because the incubation period may be as short as 15 days, IG must be given within the first few days following exposure.

B. Indications

1. *Individual Exposure.* Exposure sufficient for the person to need IG requires close personal, physical contact, such as by the members of the patient's household and other intimate contacts.
2. *Institution for Custodial Care* (Examples: prisons, facilities for developmentally disabled). Hepatitis A may be endemic in certain institutions. IG may be used during outbreaks, for new admissions, and for all employees who have direct contact.
3. *Day-Care Centers.* When there is evidence of HAV transmission in a day-care center, particularly where children are in diapers, IG should be administered to staff, children, and family members with whom the children reside. Thorough handwashing after diaper changing is emphasized.
4. *Traveler to Endemic Area.* If a stay is to be longer than 3 months, and especially outside ordinary tourist routes, in a tropical area, or in an area known to have endemic hepatitis A, IG may be indicated. A second dose may be recommended for a stay longer than 5 months. A subclinical infection may be acquired that would confer immunity.

HEPATITIS B[16,19,20]

Hepatitis B differs in many respects from hepatitis A, particularly in mode of transmission, the length of the incubation period, the onset, and the existence of a chronic carrier state. Hepatitis B occurs at any age. Figure 2–3 shows a diagram of the hepatitis B virus.

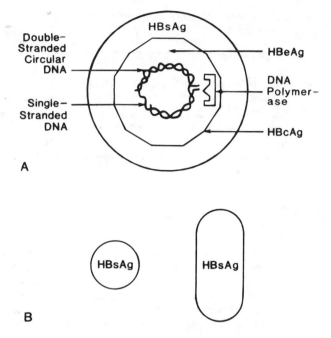

FIG. 2–3. Diagram of the Hepatitis B Virus. A. The virus is composed of an outer component of HBsAg and an inner component of HBcAg. Inside the core particle is a single molecule of circular, partially double-stranded DNA, an endogenous DNA polymerase, and HBeAg. **B.** Spherical and tubular particles of HBsAg circulate in infected blood in great numbers. (Redrawn from Hoofnagle, J.H. and Schafer, D.F.: Serologic Markers of Hepatitis B Virus Infection, *Semin. Liver Dis., 6,* 1, No. 1, 1986.)

I. TRANSMISSION
A. Blood and Other Body Fluids
Nearly all body fluids carry the virus, but only blood, saliva, semen, and vaginal fluids have been shown infectious. Hepatitis viruses also have been found in gingival sulcus fluid, menstrual blood, tears, urine, perspiration, and nasopharyngeal secretions.

B. Modes of Transmission
Hepatitis B is transmitted by percutaneous and permucosal exposure.
1. Percutaneous (intravenous, intramuscular, subcutaneous).
2. Accidents with needle stick or other sharp instruments.
3. Perinatal exposure.
4. Exchanging of contaminated needles, syringes, and other paraphernalia by users of intravenous drugs.
5. Sexual exposure.
6. Infection from blood transfusion and blood products (extremely rare because all donors are screened and all blood has been tested since 1985).

C. Perinatal Transmission
During pregnancy, transmission of the hepatitis virus to the fetus can occur, and the newborn may be exposed during birth. An infant infected perinatally is at a high risk for chronic infection, which can lead to chronic liver disease or cancer of the liver later in life. Preventive measures are possible when pregnant women are tested for HBsAg and HBeAg.

II. INDIVIDUALS AT RISK OR WITH RISK BEHAVIORS FOR HEPATITIS B[20]
Risk populations are those that have an increased prevalence of infection, increased chances or likelihood of infection, and increased prevalence of disease carriers. High risk in HBV infection can be related to a variety of factors, including occupation, place of residence, life style, confinement to an institution, other diseases and their treatments, and parenteral drug abuse. A person may belong to more than one of the risk groups listed here.

Health-care workers are included in the list; however, when they adhere to universal precautions with the use of protective barriers (gloves, masks, eyewear) and follow essential precautions for blood and other body fluid infection control, as well as have immunity following vaccination or acquired antibody to hepatitis B, they are really at a low risk.

A. Infants born to HIV-infected mothers.
B. Users of parenteral drugs (swapping contaminated needles).
C. Homosexually active men not using safe sex practices.*
D. Heterosexually active persons with multiple partners, including prostitutes, not using safe sex practices.*
E. Persons who have repeatedly contracted sexually transmitted diseases.
F. Clients and staff in institutions for the mentally retarded and current or former residents, particularly individuals with Down's syndrome.
G. Patients and staff in hemodialysis units.
H. Recipients of blood products used for treating clotting disorders, particularly before all blood was screened (prior to 1985).
I. Patients with active or chronic liver diseases.
J. Health-care workers with frequent blood contact are at a higher risk than are other health-care workers who have no or infrequent blood contact. Included are emergency room staff, hospital surgical staff, dental hygienists, dentists, and blood bank and plasma fractionation workers.
K. Household contacts of HBV carriers.
L. Male prisoners.

* "Safe sex practices" is meant to include barrier protection and no exchange of body fluids (saliva, semen, vaginal secretions), in accord with recommended guidelines.

M. Military populations stationed in countries with high endemic HBV.

N. Returned travelers from areas of endemic HBV who stayed longer than 3 months or who were treated medically by transfusion while there.

O. Morticians and embalmers.

P. Immigrants/refugees from areas of high endemic HBV.

III. DISEASE PROCESS

A. Incubation and Communicability

The incubation period is longer than that for hepatitis A and ranges from 2 to 6 months, with an average of 60 to 90 days. The period of communicability varies, but HBsAg may be detected in the blood as early as 30 days after exposure to the disease.

The presence of serum HBsAg indicates communicability. HBsAg may no longer be detected in the blood from a few days to 3 months after the icteric or jaundice stage of illness.

B. Transient Subclinical Infection

The majority of patients do not have an icteric stage, but have subclinical disease. Many remain undiagnosed for hepatitis, but develop antibodies and permanent immunity.

The infection is transient because the individual has a rapid, strong immune response to the hepatitis virus, and the HBV is cleared before it can become established.

C. Acute Type B Hepatitis

Hepatitis B cannot be distinguished from other viral hepatitis infections on the basis of the clinical signs and symptoms. The onset or preicteric stage with fever, malaise, and influenza-like symptoms is typical of all types of acute viral hepatitis. The onset may be slower and more insidious for hepatitis B, and may include skin rash, itching, and joint pains.

The period of illness extends from 4 to 6 weeks for hepatitis A and usually longer for hepatitis B.

Convalescence begins with the disappearance of jaundice. During this period, serum antibody (anti-HBs) rises except in those who become permanent carriers.

D. Carrier State

A chronic carrier of HBV is defined as an individual with the HBsAg marker in the blood serum for more than 6 months. From 5 to 10% of infected persons develop a chronic carrier state.

A carrier state may also result following a subclinical undiagnosed exposure and, therefore, may be unknown to the individual. Many carriers eventually develop cirrhosis or cancer of the liver.

E. Immunity

The presence of anti-HBs in the serum shows that the person had a previous exposure to hepatitis B and is, therefore, immune to reinfection. The anti-HBs may be present, although unknown, because immunity may have been acquired following a subclinical, anicteric, or otherwise unrecognized case of hepatitis B. Pretesting for antiHBs prior to vaccination for hepatitis may be indicated.

PREVENTION OF HEPATITIS B

Hepatitis B viruses cause serious illness, including acute and chronic hepatitis, cirrhosis, and liver cancer, that sometimes leads to disability and death. Hepatitis is a critical occupational hazard for dental personnel because of their close association with the potentially infected body fluids of patients. Every health-care individual should be immunized so that the possibilities of disease acquisition and transmission can be minimized.

I. COMPREHENSIVE PREVENTIVE PROGRAM[16,21]

A. Eliminate Transmission During Infancy and Childhood

1. Prenatal testing of all pregnant women for HBsAg.
   a. To locate newborns who require immunoprophylaxis to prevent perinatal infection.
   b. To identify household contacts who should be vaccinated.
2. Universal immunization of infants and children to be accomplished during routine health-care visits when vaccinations are usually administered. Hepatitis vaccine can be combined with diphtheria-tetanus-pertussis (DTP) or with influenza vaccine to reduce the number of injections.[21]
3. Immunization of uninfected children in special education classes.
4. Immunization of adolescents and adults, particularly those at high risk.[19] Eventually, if the universal vaccination of children continued, adult requirements would become limited.

B. Enforce Blood Bank Control Measures[16]

1. Screening of donors; rejection of individuals who have a history of viral hepatitis, who show evidence of drug addiction, or who have received a blood transfusion or tattoo within the preceding 6 months.
2. Strict testing for all donated blood.

C. Enforce Sterilization or Use of Disposable Syringes and Needles

1. For acupuncture, skin testing, parenteral inoculations, and all types of clinic treatments available to the public.
2. Education of public to expect certain standards.

II. ACTIVE IMMUNIZATION: THE VACCINES[16,19,21]

Two hepatitis B vaccines are available for pre- and postexposure prophylaxis. Both are administered intramuscularly in 3 doses, the first at the outset, then at 1 and 6 months.

The vaccine should be given only in the deltoid muscle for adults and children and in the anterolateral thigh muscle for infants and neonates.

A. Plasma-derived HB Vaccine*

The original vaccine was prepared using purified and formalin-treated HBsAg from the plasma of chronic HBsAg carriers. In its preparation, the treatment steps inactivate all classes of viruses so that transmission of any other disease becomes impossible.

B. Recombinant DNA HB Vaccine†

Recombinant DNA technology has been used to synthesize HBsAg in a culture of *Saccharomyces cerevisiae*, a yeast. The HBsAg is purified and sterilized.

C. Effectiveness

1. Both vaccines act in a comparable manner to stimulate antibody, and both convey the same degree of immunity.
2. In healthy 20- to 39-year-old adults, immunity is conferred in more than 95%. In children, protective antibodies are shown in 99%.
3. Postvaccination testing for anti-HBs within 1 to 6 months is recommended for a hemodialysis patient or other risk person having frequent exposure, including dental personnel.
4. Lower responses have been noted in older people, in hemodialysis patients, and in people receiving the injection in the buttock rather than in the deltoid muscle.[22]
5. The vaccines have no effect on a person who is already a carrier,[23] and no effect on a person who already has antibodies.
6. Immunization is not contraindicated during pregnancy. An HBV infection during pregnancy can be severe, and the newborn can become a permanent carrier.[19]

D. Booster[19,21]

1. The higher initial peak of response usually means longer persistence of antibody. Even when the antibody level drops there can still be protection.
2. A 7-year booster is suggested; however, the antibody level can be tested to determine individual needs.
3. For certain risk patients, particularly hemodialysis patients, annual antibody testing has been recommended.[19]

III. POSTEXPOSURE PROPHYLAXIS[19]

A. Indications for Prophylaxis

1. Newborn of HBsAg-positive mother.
2. Significant hepatitis B exposure to HBsAg-positive blood (page 65).

B. Hepatitis B Immune Globulin (HBIG)

High-titer anti-HBs immune globulin (HBIG) is available. Its primary use is for postexposure prophylaxis.

IG, described for passive immunization for hepatitis A (page 21), contains low-titer anti-HBs of varying amounts. It is effective against HBV to a lesser degree than is HBIG, but should be used when HBIG is not available. IG is recommended when protection for exposure to hepatitis C and E is needed.

C. Procedure for Newborn of HBsAg-Positive Mother[19]

1. *Immediate Treatment.* HBIG and HBV vaccine intramuscularly within 12 hours of birth and subsequently as recommended for a specific vaccine.
2. *Effect.* The combined treatment prevents up to 94% of infants from developing a carrier state.[24]
3. *Risk.* Breast-feeding poses no risk of infection when prophylaxis has been started.

D. Procedure for Needlestick or Wound from a Contaminated Instrument

(see pages 65–66 and table 4–7)

HEPATITIS C[16,20]

Hepatitis that developed as a result of transfusion but could not be classified with hepatitis A or B was originally called hepatitis non-A, non-B. When studied over time, two patterns of non-A, non-B were recognized. The first, associated with blood transfusion and the use of contaminated needles, became hepatitis C. The second type was associated with water-borne epidemics and is now called hepatitis E.

Hepatitis C, caused by the hepatitis C virus (HCV), has been recognized as the former chief cause of transfusion-associated non-A, non-B hepatitis. HCV also has a role in many cases of chronic liver disease. Now, a serologic test for antibody to HCV has been developed and is an established test for blood donors. This ad-

---

* Heptavax, Merck Sharp & Dohme.
†Recombivax HB, Merck Sharp & Dohme; (Engerix B, Smith Kline Biologicals).

vance in making blood transfusion safe is highly significant.[25]

I. TRANSMISSION
Hepatitis C can be acquired by percutaneous exposure to contaminated blood and plasma derivatives, contaminated needles and syringes, transfusion, or accidental needlestick. HCV has been demonstrated in saliva. Nonpercutaneous routes include sexual transmission and perinatal exposure.

II. DISEASE PROCESS
The onset of viral hepatitis C can be insidious, with no clinical symptoms, whereas in other exposures, the patient can have abdominal discomfort, nausea, and vomiting, and can progress to jaundice. Chronic infection is more common than with hepatitis B.

III. PREVENTION AND CONTROL
Measures recommended for hepatitis B can be applied to hepatitis C. Testing of all donated blood is basic to control.[20]

HEPATITIS D[16]

The delta hepatitis virus, also called the delta agent, cannot cause infection except in the presence of HBV infection. The diagram in figure 2–4 shows the delta antigen surrounded by HBsAg.

I. TRANSMISSION
Most frequently, the delta infection is superimposed on HBsAg carriers. It occurs primarily in persons who have multiple exposures to HBV, particularly patients with hemophilia and intravenous drug abusers.

Transmission is similar to that of HBV, that is, by direct exposure to contaminated blood and serous body fluids, contaminated needles and syringes, sexual contacts, and perinatal transfer.

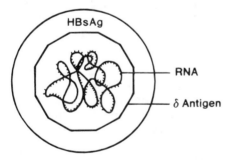

FIG. 2–4. Diagram of the Hepatitis Delta Virus. The delta agent antigen is surrounded by the hepatitis B surface antigen. (Redrawn from Hoofnagle, J.H.: Type D Hepatitis and the Hepatitis Delta Virus, in Thomas, H.C. and Jones, E.A.: *Recent Advances in Hepatology.* Edinburgh, Churchilll Livingstone, 1986.)

II. DISEASE PROCESS
Delta hepatitis is more severe and the mortality rate is greater than with hepatitis B. The onset is abrupt and signs and symptoms resemble hepatitis B. Infection can occur in the following ways.

A. Coinfection
Acute delta hepatitis occurring with acute HBV infection may lead to resolution of both types. Clearance of HBV may lead to clearance of delta virus.

B. Superinfection
Acute delta hepatitis is superimposed on an existing carrier HBV state. The HBV carrier state remains unchanged, and a delta carrier state may develop in addition.

C. Superimposition
Chronic delta hepatitis superimposes on the chronic HBsAg carrier.

III. PREVENTION
All measures used to prevent hepatitis B prevent delta hepatitis because HDV is dependent on the presence of HBV. Immunization with hepatitis B vaccine also protects the recipient from delta hepatitis infection.

HEPATITIS E[16]

Hepatitis E (HEV) was formerly known as enterically transmitted non-A, non-B hepatitis. The clinical course and distribution are like those of hepatitis A.

I. TRANSMISSION
Hepatitis E is transmitted by contaminated water, as well as person-to-person by the fecal-oral route. Reported large outbreaks have been associated with fecally contaminated water sources after heavy rains where sewage disposal was inadequate. Adults have been affected more than have children. The mortality rate in pregnant women has been high.

II. PREVENTION AND CONTROL
   A. Sanitary disposal of wastes.
   B. Handwashing, especially before handling food.

HERPESVIRUS DISEASES[26]

The herpesvirus infections represent a wide variety of disease entities that are highly infectious. Each virus is antigenically distinct. Herpesviruses produce diseases with latent, recurrent, and sometimes malignant tendencies. For example, herpes simplex type 2 has been implicated in cervical cancer and herpes simplex type 1 in oral cancer.

TABLE 2–4
HERPESVIRUS

Abbreviation	Name of Virus	Infections
VZV	Varicella-zoster	Varicella (chickenpox) Herpes zoster (shingles)
EBV	Epstein-Barr	EBV mononucleosis
HCMV	Human cytomegalovirus	Cytomegalovirus disease Fetal infection
HSV-1 HSV-2	Herpes simplex virus	Herpes labialis Herpetic gingivostomatitis Herpetic kerato-conjunctivitis Herpetic whitlow Encephalitis Neonatal herpes
HHV-6	Human herpesvirus 6	Mononucleosis-like rash

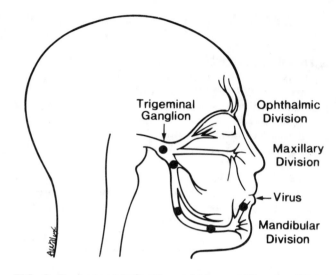

FIG. 2–5. Latent Infection of Herpes Simplex Virus. Path of the virus traced from point of viral penetration on lip to establishment of latent infection in the trigeminal ganglion.

Immunosuppressed patients have more frequent and severe herpes infections. Herpesviruses are among the opportunistic organisms in acquired immunodeficiency syndrome (AIDS) (pages 31, 32, 34 and table 2–7).

Table 2–4 lists herpesviruses, their abbreviations, and some of the infections they cause.

VIRAL LATENCY

I. GANGLIA
The herpesviruses have the ability to travel along sensory nerve pathways to specific ganglia. The specific ganglia are usually the following:
A. Herpes simplex 1 (HSV-1) travels to the trigeminal nerve ganglion (figure 2–5).
B. Herpes simplex 2 (HSV-2) goes to the thoracic, lumbar, and sacral dorsal root ganglia.
C. Varicella-zoster (VZV) goes to the sensory ganglia of the vagal, spinal, or cranial nerves.

II. PRIMARY INFECTION: SEQUENCE OF EVENTS[27]
A. Exposure of person to the virus at the mucosal surface or abraded skin.
B. Replication begins in the cells of the dermis and epidermis.
C. Infection of sensory or autonomic nerve endings.
D. Virus travels along the nerve to the ganglion.
E. After primary disease resolves, the virus becomes latent in the ganglion.
F. Reactivation at a later date is precipitated by a stimulus, such as sunlight, immunosuppression, infection, or stress (physical or emotional).
G. Virus transports along the nerve to the body surface where replication takes place and a lesion forms, usually in the same spot as the previous activation.

VARICELLA-ZOSTER VIRUS (VZV)[28]

Chickenpox (varicella) and shingles (herpes zoster) are caused by the same virus, the varicella-zoster.

I. CHICKENPOX
A. Transmission
Chickenpox is a highly contagious disease transmitted by direct contact, droplet (possibly airborne), or by indirect contact with articles soiled by discharges from the vesicles and the respiratory tract.

B. Disease Process
Primarily a disease of children, chickenpox is occasionally found in adults not previously exposed. Chickenpox can be life threatening in children who are immunocompromised, such as children with HIV infection.

When primary maternal VZV occurs during pregnancy or during the peripartum period, fetal infection may result in congenital malformations.

The disease is characterized by a maculopapular rash that becomes vesicular in a few days and then scabs. The lesions appear anywhere on the body, more abundantly on the covered than on the exposed parts. When oral lesions occur, they may spread into the upper respiratory tract.

If the itchy, crusted lesions of the skin are scratched, a secondary bacterial infection can result. Other complications are rare, but neurologic and ocular disorders are possible.

II. SHINGLES
A. Recurrent Infection
Chickenpox leaves a lasting immunity, but the VZV remains latent in the dorsal root ganglia. Reactivation in adulthood may result from immunosuppression, such as from drug therapy or from HIV infection, and in people with advanced neoplastic disease.

B. Disease Process
Shingles consists of localized unilateral eruptions associated with the nerve endings of the area innervated by the infected sensory nerves. When the second division of the trigeminal nerve is involved, intraoral lesions may occur. Pain, burning, and itching are characteristic. Eye infections and complications of the lungs, central nervous system, liver, and pancreas have been secondary developments.

EPSTEIN-BARR VIRUS (EBV)[29]

One type of infectious mononucleosis is caused by infection with the EBV. It has also been shown that the EBV replicates within the epithelial cells in hairy leukoplakia, the lesion associated with subsequent development of the acquired immunodeficiency syndrome (page 34).[30] EBV is also a factor in the development of certain lymphomas.

Infectious mononucleosis is generally a disease of adolescents and young adults. It is characterized by fever, lymphadenopathy, and sore throat, and is identified by specific atypical lymphocytes called mononucleosis cells.

The disease is transmitted orally by direct contact and by droplet. Viruses are excreted through the saliva even when the patient has no symptoms of disease, so there may be a long period of communicability or a lasting carrier state. EBV can remain latent and become reactivated, particularly when the immune system is compromised by disease or drug therapy.

CYTOMEGALOVIRUS (HCMV)[31]

Cytomegalovirus infections appear in various forms. The most affected age groups are from 1 to 2 years and from 16 to 50 years. The infections are sometimes latent or subclinical in adults. HCMV has been found in the tumor cells of Kaposi's sarcoma.

I. TRANSMISSION
A. Congenital and Neonatal
The virus from the mother's primary or recurrent infection may infect the infant *in utero,* in the birth canal, or through breast milk.

B. Direct Infections
The virus is excreted in urine, saliva, cervical secretions, and semen. Infection can result from the following:
1. Blood transfusion.
2. Graft transplant from a donor with latent infection.
3. Sexual transmission through semen, vaginal fluid, or saliva.
4. Respiratory droplet, especially among children. Children attending day-care centers have a high prevalence of HCMV infection.[32]

II. DISEASE PROCESS
A. Infants
Cytomegalic inclusion disease in a fetus is the most severe form of the infection. Survivors may be premature, anemic, and have mental retardation, microcephaly, motor disabilities, deafness, and chronic liver disease.

B. Adult Infection
Symptomatic infection is relatively rare, but infectious mononucleosis, pneumonitis, and other infections may be caused by HCMV.

C. Immunosuppression and Debilitation
HCMV, an opportunistic agent, is a common cause of both primary and reactivated infections in immunodeficient or immunosuppressed patients. Infection with HCMV is a serious complication of the acquired immunodeficiency syndrome.

III. PREVENTION
A. Personal hygiene: handwashing.
B. Universal precautions by health-care workers.
C. Seropositivity of donor checked before organ transplant.

HERPES SIMPLEX VIRUS INFECTIONS[26,33]

Primary infection usually occurs in children but may occur at any age.[34] Antibodies (anti-HSV) are produced but do not guarantee immunity to recurrent herpes or to other herpesvirus infections.

Sulcular epithelium serves as a reservoir for the viruses.[35,36] Anti-HSV is present in the gingival sulcus fluid.[37] The possibility exists that trauma to the oral area during a dental or dental hygiene appointment may bring about herpetic recurrence.[38,39]

Acyclovir, an antiviral drug, has been used in topical, oral, and intravenous forms. Acyclovir is a selective inhibitor of replication of HSV and VZV. It is established as the drug of choice for treatment of a wide range of infections caused by HSV and VZV.[40]

I. PRIMARY HERPETIC GINGIVOSTOMATITIS

The primary infection may be asymptomatic. When clinical disease is evident, gingivostomatitis and pharyngitis are the most frequent manifestations, with fever, malaise, inability to eat, and lymphadenopathy for 2 to 7 days. Painful oral vesicular lesions may occur on the gingiva, mucosa, tongue, and lips. Both first-episode HSV-1 and HSV-2 can cause pharyngitis.

A patient may be a subclinical carrier, and reactivation from the trigeminal ganglia (figure 2–5) may be followed by asymptomatic excretion of the viruses in the saliva. On the other hand, reactivation may lead to herpetic ulcerations of the lip, the typical "cold sore."

II. HERPES LABIALIS (COLD SORE, FEVER BLISTER)

Both HSV-1 and HSV-2 cause genital and oral-facial infections that cannot be distinguished clinically. Reactivations of oral-facial HSV-1 infections are more frequent than of oral-facial HSV-2 infections. Reactivations of genital HSV-2 are more frequent than of genital HSV-1 infections.[41]

Recurrent (HSV) lesions occur at or near the primary lesion at indefinite intervals. They are usually triggered by stress, sunlight, illness, or trauma. Not infrequently, they relate to the patient's dental appointment, when emotional stress and oral trauma may be involved.

A. Prodrome

Before the local lesion appears, there may be burning or slight stinging sensations with slight swelling as a forewarning or prodrome. Most frequently, the recurrent lesion is at the vermillion border of the lower lip, although less commonly, the lesions may occur intraorally on the gingiva or the hard palate.

B. Clinical Characteristics

A group of vesicles forms and eventually ruptures and coalesces. Crusting follows, and healing may take up to 10 days. The lesions are infectious, with viral shedding. Care must be taken by the patient because autoinfection (to the eye, nose, or genitals, for example) is possible, as is infection of others.

III. HERPETIC WHITLOW[26]

Herpetic whitlow is the herpes simplex infection of the fingers that results from the virus entering through minor skin abrasions. The most frequent location is around a fingernail, where cracks in the skin often occur.

A. Transmission

A whitlow may be a primary or recurrent infection of HSV-1 or HSV-2. Transmission results from direct contact with a vesicular lesion on a patient's lip or with saliva that contains the viruses.

Members of the dental team who do not wear protective gloves will have whitlow on the index fingers and thumbs that are in close contact with the patient's saliva where instrumentation and retraction are performed.[42]

Autoinfection from a lip or intraoral herpetic lesion is possible while nailbiting.

B. Disease Process

The whitlow usually starts suddenly as an area of irritation that becomes tender and painful. Groups of vesicles coalesce and the whole healing process may last up to 2 weeks. The lesions are infectious and transmissible even before the whitlow appears and is diagnosed. Recurrences are not unusual.

IV. OCULAR HERPES[26]

Herpes simplex lesions in the eye can be a primary or recurrent infection of HSV-1 or HSV-2.

A. Transmission

1. Splashing saliva or fluid from a vesicular lesion directly into an unprotected eye.
2. Extension of infection from a facial lesion.
3. Infection of an infant's eye *in utero* or during birth.

B. Disease Process

Symptoms include fever, pain, blurring of vision, swelling, excess tears, and secondary bacterial infection. Herpes keratoconjunctivitis can cause deep inflammation and, when left untreated, is a leading cause of loss of sight.

CLINICAL MANAGEMENT[43,44]

I. PATIENT HISTORY

All patient histories need questions to determine experiences with herpesviruses. Terminology may be a problem, so such terms as "fever blisters" or "cold sores" need to be used to assure patient understanding.

II. POSTPONE APPOINTMENT WITH PATIENT WITH ACTIVE LESION

A. Problems of Transmission

Explain the following to patient:
1. Contagiousness, with possible transmission to other patients.
2. Autoinoculation possible from instrumentation that can splash viruses to the patient's eye or extend lesion to nose.

B. Irritation to Lesions

Irritation to the lesions can prolong the course and increase the severity of the infection.

C. Prodromal State May Be the Most Contagious

The patient should be requested to call ahead to change an appointment when it is known that a lesion is developing.

III. UNIVERSAL PRECAUTIONS

All high-level techniques must be consistently applied for all patients because not all patients infected with a contagious disease have clinically recognizable lesions. For certain lesions, the prodromal stage is the most infectious. Disposable and sterilizable materials should be used exclusively, not only when active lesions are present.

HIV INFECTION

The *acquired immunodeficiency syndrome* (AIDS) is a severe condition caused by infection with the *human immunodeficiency virus* (HIV). HIV-infected patients may present with manifestations that range from mild abnormalities in immune response without apparent

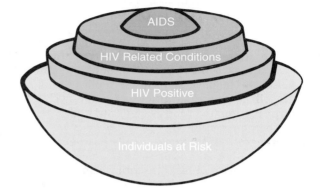

FIG. 2-6. Stages and Progression of HIV Infection. The large group at the base represents the population "at risk" but not infected; the next group, seropositive for HIV, may remain asymptomatic for 12 or more years; and the two upper groups represent populations with disease evidence with those in the uppermost group displaying AIDS-indicator conditions (C1, C2, C3, table 2–6). (Adapted from Wilson, H.S. and Kneisl, C.R.: *Psychiatric Nursing, 4th ed.* Redwood City, Addison-Wesley, 1992, p. 586.)

TABLE 2-5
HIV AND AIDS: ABBREVIATIONS/DEFINITIONS

AIDS: acquired immunodeficiency syndrome.

AZT (ZDV): zidovudine, retrovir; drug used for the treatment of HIV infection and AIDS; first antiviral drug approved by the United States Food and Drug Administration (FDA).

CD4+: T-helper lymphocyte; primary target cell for HIV infection; CD4+ count decreases with the severity of HIV-related illness.

DNA: deoxyribonucleic acid; a nucleic acid found in a cell nucleus; is a carrier of genetic information.

HIV: human immunodeficiency virus; causes AIDS.

HIV-1 antibody: antibody to human immunodeficiency virus type 1; antibody can be detected in the blood 6 to 8 weeks after infection.

HL: hairy leukoplakia.

IDU: injecting drug user.

KS: Kaposi's sarcoma; a malignant vascular tumor; an opportunistic neoplasm that may occur in people with HIV infection.

LAV: lymphadenopathy-associated virus; one of the former names for HIV.

MMWR: *Morbidity and Mortality Weekly Report;* publication of the United States Centers for Disease Control and Prevention **(CDCP),** Atlanta, GA.

PCP: pneumocystis pneumonia; caused by *Pneumocystis carinii;* an opportunistic infection that occurs in people with HIV infection.

PGL: persistent generalized lymphadenopathy.

PWA: person with AIDS.

RNA: ribonucleic acid; a nucleic acid found in cytoplasm and in the nuclei of certain cells; RNA directs the synthesis of proteins, and replaces DNA as a carrier of genetic codes in some viruses.

---

signs and symptoms to profound immunosuppression associated with a variety of life-threatening infections and rare malignant conditions. Table 2–5 provides abbreviations and terminology relating to HIV infections and AIDS.

The potential progression of HIV infection can be described by the diagrammatic representation shown in figure 2–6. Starting at the base are the individuals at risk, those who are most likely to contract HIV infection. In the next group are those who are seropositive, but are without signs or symptoms. This stage may extend an unpredictable number of years, for some individuals 12 years or more.

In the third phase, HIV-related conditions may become apparent with physical and neurologic effects of immune system deterioration. For persons in the top, or fourth, category, AIDS, as determined by the formal definition provided by the United States Centers for Disease Control and Prevention,[45] causes many complications.

People from each of these categories, as well as their families, friends, significant others, and personal caregivers, will be patients in oral health-care settings. All these individuals have personal concerns that in turn add a special dimension to the need for the entire dental team to show kindness, understanding, and support.

A person with advanced HIV disease may have experienced loss of work and career, many hospitalizations, lack of support from family and friends because of fear of disease and social stigma, and loss of physical appearance and strength. The professional person's attitude and conduct should reflect support, acceptance, and empathy.

LIFE CYCLE OF THE HIV[46,47]

Viruses are parasites and replicate by using the mechanisms of a host cell to synthesize and assemble new components. The basic steps in the replication of a retrovirus will be described briefly. The life cycle of the HIV virus is complex. Many details are not known and are still being researched.

HIV is a retrovirus. Regular cells have DNA, but in a retrovirus, RNA is the core genetic material, and enzymes, including reverse transcriptase, are essential for replication. A diagram of the HIV virus is shown in Figure 2–7.

The ability to control the epidemic/pandemic of HIV infection by means of a vaccine to immunize susceptible individuals depends on the ability to interrupt the life cycle of the HIV. Likewise, research to find antiviral drugs for relief or cure after infection must be directed toward prevention or arrest of viral replication. Each link in the life cycle of the virus may provide the area in which the life cycle can be altered or stopped.

The life cycle of the HIV can be divided into two phases: the establishment of infection, and the production of new virus particles.

I. ESTABLISHMENT OF INFECTION
A. Attachment to a Target/Host Cell
1. HIV enters the body and passes by way of the blood to a target cell surface, where it binds to a specific cellular receptor, CD4+.

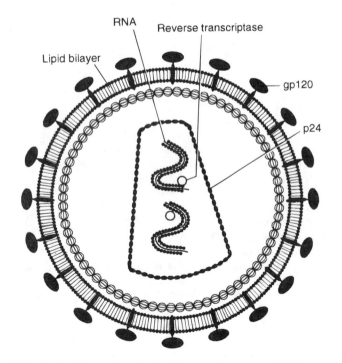

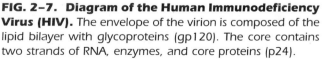

FIG. 2–7. Diagram of the Human Immunodeficiency Virus (HIV). The envelope of the virion is composed of the lipid bilayer with glycoproteins (gp120). The core contains two strands of RNA, enzymes, and core proteins (p24).

2. Target cells that have CD4+ receptors include T-helper lymphocytes, monocytes, macrophages, and certain neurons and glial cells of the brain tissue.

B. Penetration into Wall of the Target/Host Cell
Fusion occurs between the virion and the target cell membrane, and the virus becomes uncoated. Only the viral RNA and the enzymes enter the cell.

C. Transcription
1. Viral RNA is changed into single-stranded DNA by the enzyme *reverse transcriptase.* Another enzyme, *ribonuclease,* destroys the RNA, which is no longer needed. Single-stranded DNA is then translated to a double-stranded DNA, which is called the *provirus.*
2. The provirus migrates to the nucleus of the host cell, enters the nucleus, and becomes permanently integrated with host DNA.

D. Infection Is Established
Once the viral DNA enters the host nucleus, infection is established. Succeeding progeny of the host cell are HIV infected.

E. Latent Period
The integrated proviral DNA stays latent indefinitely.

II. PRODUCTION OF NEW VIRUS
A. Stimulation of the Host Cell
The mechanisms of stimulation that cause activation are not clear, but the DNA of the infected host cell can form new viral RNA and protein.

B. Assembly of Viral Proteins
1. Viral proteins are broken down to form "building blocks" for progeny viral particles.
2. DNA is transcribed into RNA for the new virus.

C. Budding from Host Cell: Release
1. Host cell membrane is used to make a new viral envelope.
2. Free new virion is released into the blood stream; it proceeds to find another CD4+ for attachment.

D. Host Cell Outcome
1. Loss of normal function.
2. Destruction; reduced numbers of host CD4+ cells lead to immune suppression.
3. The CD4+, or T-helper lymphocyte, is the primary target cell for HIV infection. A decrease in the number of these cells correlates with the risk and severity of HIV-related illnesses.

HIV CLASSIFICATION SYSTEM FOR ADOLESCENTS AND ADULTS

The CDC classification system emphasizes the importance of the CD4+ lymphocyte count in the clinical management of HIV-infected individuals. The AIDS surveillance case definition includes all HIV-infected persons with less than 200 CD4+ lymphocytes/mm^3.[45]

Measures of CD4+ counts are used to guide clinical and/or therapeutic treatment using antimicrobial prophylaxis and antiretroviral therapies. Antiretroviral therapy is recommended for all patients with a CD4+ lymphocyte count of less than 500/mm^3, and prophylaxis against *Pneumocystis carinii* pneumonia, the most common opportunistic infection diagnosed in HIV-infected patients, is recommended for all persons with CD4+ lymphocyte counts of less than 200/mm^3.

The system, charted in table 2–6, is based on **3 laboratory** categories numbered 1, 2, and 3, and **3 clinical** categories, lettered A, B, and C.

I. LABORATORY CATEGORIES
Category 1: ≥ 500 CD4+ lymphocytes/mm^3
Category 2: 200 to 499 CD4+ lymphocytes/mm^3
Category 3: < 200 CD4+ lymphocytes/mm^3

II. CLINICAL CATEGORIES
Category A: Asymptomatic (acute primary) HIV or PGL
One or more of the following conditions. (Conditions in categories B and C must not have occurred.)

- Asymptomatic HIV infection
- Persistent generalized lymphadenopathy (PGL)
- Acute (primary) HIV infection or history of acute HIV infection

Category B: Symptomatic (not A or C)
Examples of conditions in category B follow. They must be attributed to HIV infection, indicative of a defect in cell-mediated immunity, and not listed under category C.

- Bacillary angiomatosis
- Candidiasis, oropharyngeal (thrush)
- Candidiasis, vulvovaginal: persistent, frequent, or poorly responsive to therapy
- Cervical dysplasia (moderate or severe)/cervical carcinoma in situ
- Constitutional symptoms, such as fever (38.5° C) or diarrhea lasting > 1 month
- Hairy leukoplakia, oral
- Herpes zoster (shingles), involving at least two distinct episodes or more than one dermatome
- Idiopathic thrombocytopenic purpura
- Listeriosis
- Pelvic inflammatory disease, particularly if complicated by tubo-ovarian abscess
- Peripheral neuropathy

Category C: AIDS-Indicator Conditions
Conditions that follow in category C are strongly associated with severe immunodeficiency, occur frequently in HIV-infected individuals, and cause serious morbidity or mortality.

- Candidiasis of bronchi, trachea, or lungs
- Candidiasis, esophageal
- Cervical cancer, invasive*
- Coccidioidomycosis, disseminated or extrapulmonary
- Cryptococcosis, extrapulmonary
- Cryptosporidiosis, chronic intestinal (>1 month's duration)
- Cytomegalovirus disease (other than liver, spleen, or nodes)
- Cytomegalovirus retinitis (with loss of vision)

* Added in the 1993 expansion of the AIDS surveillance case definition.

TABLE 2–6
1992 REVISED CLASSIFICATION SYSTEM FOR HIV INFECTION AND EXPANDED AIDS SURVEILLANCE CASE DEFINITION FOR ADOLESCENTS AND ADULTS*

CD4+ Cell Categories	Clinical Categories		
	[A] Asymptomatic, or PGL†	[B] Symptomatic, not (A) or (C) conditions	[C] AIDS-indicator conditions‡
(1) ≥500/mm^3	A1	B1	C1
(2) 200–499/mm^3	A2	B2	C2
(3) <200/mm^3 AIDS-indicator cell count	A3	B3	C3

* The shaded boxes illustrate the expansion of the AIDS surveillance case definition. Persons with AIDS-indicator conditions (category C) are currently reportable to the health department in every state and U.S. territory. In addition to persons with clinical category C conditions (categories C1, C2, and C3), persons with CD4+ lymphocyte counts of less than 200/mm^3 (categories A3 or B3) also have been reportable as AIDS cases in the United States and its territories since April 1, 1992.
† PGL = persistent generalized lymphadenopathy. Clinical category A includes acute (primary) HIV infection.
‡ See text.

- Encephalopathy, HIV-related
- Herpes simplex: chronic ulcer(s) (>1 month's duration); or bronchitis, pneumonitis, or esophagitis
- Histoplasmosis, disseminated or extrapulmonary
- Isosporiasis, chronic intestinal (>1 month's duration)
- Kaposi's sarcoma
- Lymphoma, Burkitt's (or equivalent term)
- Lymphoma, immunoblastic (or equivalent term)
- Lymphoma, primary, of brain
- *Mycobacterium avium* complex or *M. kansasii*, disseminated or extrapulmonary
- *Mycobacterium tuberculosis*, any site (pulmonary* or extrapulmonary)
- *Mycobacterium*, other species or unidentified species, disseminated or extrapulmonary
- *Pneumocystis carinii* pneumonia
- Pneumonia, recurrent*
- Progressive multifocal leukoencephalopathy
- *Salmonella* septicemia, recurrent
- Toxoplasmosis of brain
- Wasting syndrome caused by HIV

CLINICAL COURSE OF HIV INFECTION

I. TRANSMISSION

The AIDS virus (HIV) has been found in most body fluids. Transmission has been demonstrated primarily by way of blood, semen, vaginal secretions, and breast milk.

A. Routes of Transmission

Sexual, blood, and perinatal contacts are the principal routes. The virus reaches the blood stream by the following:

1. *Intimate Unprotected Sexual Contact* (both homosexual and heterosexual). The virus from an infected person's blood, semen, or vaginal secretions enters the blood through tiny breaks in the rectum, vagina, or penis.
2. *Exposure to Infected Blood or Blood Products.*
   a. Inoculation during intravenous use of drugs: sharing of needles, syringes, or other invasive implements by drug users.
   b. Transfusion and use of blood products by patients with blood disorders; serologic testing of all donor blood has nearly eliminated the threat of infection from transfusion.
3. *Maternal Fetal or Perinatal Contact.* Viruses can be transmitted across the placenta. Exposure to infection can occur *in utero*, during delivery, and after birth through breast milk or other close contact.

B. High-Risk Individuals

1. Sexually active homosexual and bisexual men having multiple sex partners without using safe sex practices.*
2. Users or former users of intravenous drugs, when contaminated needles are shared.
3. Recipients of blood transfusions or blood products prior to mandatory testing for HIV antibodies in 1985. This includes people with hemophilia or other coagulation disorders.
4. Male and female prostitutes who do not use safe sex practices.*
5. Health-care workers who do not adhere to strict barrier procedures and do not follow essential blood and other body fluid precautions for infection control.
6. Females artificially inseminated with HIV-infected semen.
7. Recipients of HIV-infected organ transplants.
8. Steady sexual partners of all those previously listed who do not use safe sex practices.*
9. Steady sexual partners of those infected with AIDS or at high risk for AIDS who do not use safe sex practices.*
10. Infants born to HIV-infected mothers.
11. Infants fed breast milk from HIV-infected mothers.

C. Serologic Tests for Antibodies

Persons exposed to the HIV develop detectable antibody levels within 3 to 12 weeks. Antibody presence indicates infection, but there may be no clinical symptoms.

Blood banks are required to test all blood received for hepatitis B and C, syphilis, and the HIV antibody. Frequently used tests for HIV antibody have been the EIA (ELISA) and the WB (Western Blot). When the test result is positive, the blood is rejected and the person is notified and counseled.

II. INCUBATION PERIOD

The incubation period ranges from 3 months to 12 years or more.[48]

III. CLINICAL PROGRESSION OF HIV INFECTION

The course of HIV infection is shown by the flow chart in figure 2–8. The HIV affects the immune system so that the infected person is vulnerable to a wide range of clinical disorders.

A. Primary HIV Infection

An acute retroviral infection may be experienced within 12 to 18 weeks after exposure. At

---

* Added in the 1993 expansion of the AIDS surveillance case definition.

* "Safe sex practices" is meant to include barrier protection and no exchange of body fluids (saliva, semen, vaginal secretions) in accord with recommended guidelines.

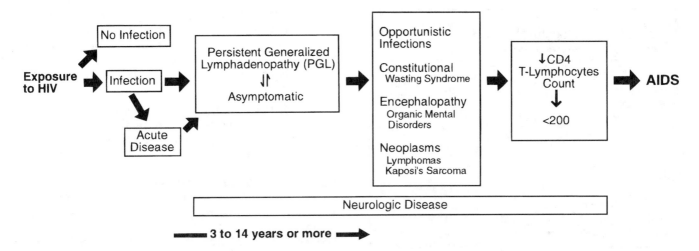

FIG. 2-8. Flow Chart Showing the Course of Infection with Human Immunodeficiency Virus. The steps are described in the text.

the time, symptoms are not identified as specific for HIV infection. The acute infection is followed or accompanied by the development of HIV antibodies that circulate in the blood stream, and transmission is possible at this stage. The symptoms of primary infection may include the following:

1. Mononucleosis-like syndrome.
2. Fever, rash, fatigue, diarrhea.
3. Muscle and joint pains.

B. Asymptomatic Latent Period

For months to years after exposure, many HIV-infected people have no apparent symptoms. Antibodies have developed, and the virus can be transmitted to others.

C. Persistent Generalized Lymphadenopathy (PGL)

Some infected patients develop PGL. The enlarged lymph nodes may be noticed during routine extraoral clinical examination.

D. Symptomatic Period

AIDS is the advanced stage of HIV infection. Severe indicator diseases or opportunistic infections may not be evident for many years after becoming infected. In both the B and C clinical categories (table 2–6), symptoms from each of the four general categories described here may be evident.

1. *Opportunistic Infections.* An opportunistic infection is caused by a microorganism that is capable of taking advantage of a compromised immune system as an opportunity to develop in a person in whom the disease would not otherwise develop. When the immune reactions of the person with HIV infection decrease, as monitored by the lowered CD4+ lymphocyte count, opportunistic infections can become more frequent, extensive, and severe.

2. *Constitutional Disease: HIV Wasting Syndrome.* Long-term fever, severe weight loss, anemia, chronic diarrhea, and chronic weakness are all effects of loss of immune response and repeated opportunistic diseases. The wasting syndrome symptoms, along with organic mental disorders (HIV dementia), contribute to the severe degeneration during the terminal AIDS illness.

3. *Encephalopathy: Organic Mental Disorders.* Disabling cognitive and/or motor dysfunction may develop with symptoms of apathy, inability to concentrate, poor memory, and depression.

4. *Neoplasms.* Several neoplasms, related to the underlying immunodeficiency, are common indicators of HIV infection and AIDS. These include Kaposi's sarcoma, primary B-cell lymphoma of the brain, and nonHodgkin's lymphoma.

ORAL MANIFESTATIONS OF HIV INFECTION

Many HIV-infected patients have head and/or neck manifestations. Certain oral findings have been identified as possible indicators of HIV infection.

Oral symptoms can be integrated with information from the patient's medical history. From the complete assessment, an early recognition, or at least a suspicion, of HIV infection may result. Referral for medical evaluation and testing can be recommended.

Early recognition of a HIV seropositive condition is important because drugs available for treatment can slow down the process of the disease. With early intervention, severe complications may be prevented and the long-term quality of life can be improved.

Table 2–7 lists oral lesions according to whether the condition is strongly associated, less commonly associated, or possibly associated with HIV infection.

TABLE 2-7
ORAL LESIONS ASSOCIATED WITH HIV INFECTION CLASSIFICATION

Group I. Lesions Strongly Associated with HIV Infection	Group III. Lesions seen with HIV Infection
Candidiasis 　Erythematous 　Pseudomembranous Hairy Leukoplakia Kaposi's sarcoma Non-Hodgkin's lymphoma Periodontal disease 　Linear gingival erythema 　Necrotizing (ulcerative) 　　gingivitis 　Necrotizing (ulcerative) 　　periodontitis	Bacterial Infections 　*Actinomyces israelii* 　*Escherichia coli* 　*Klebsiella pneumoniae* 　Cat-scratch disease Drug reactions (ulcerative, 　erythema multiforme, 　lichenoid, toxic 　epidermolysis) Epithelioid (bacillary) 　angiomatosis Fungal infection other than 　candidiasis 　*Cryptococcus 　　neoformans* 　*Geotrichum candidum* 　*Histoplasma capsulatum* 　*Mucoraceae 　　(mucormycosis/ 　　zygomycosis)* 　*Aspergillus flavus* Neurologic disturbances 　Facial palsy 　Trigeminal neuralgia Recurrent aphthous 　stomatitis Viral infections 　Cytomegalovirus 　Molluscum contagiosum
Group II. Lesions Less Commonly Associated with HIV Infection	
Bacterial infections 　*Mycobacterium avium- 　　intracellulare* 　*Mycobacterium 　　tuberculosis* Melanotic 　hyperpigmentation Necrotizing (ulcerative) 　stomatitis Salivary gland disease 　Dry mouth due to 　　decreased salivary flow 　　rate 　Unilateral or bilateral 　　swelling of major 　　salivary glands Thrombocytopenic purpura Ulceration NOS (not 　otherwise specified) Viral Infections 　Herpes simplex virus 　Human papillomavirus 　　(warty-like lesions) 　Condyloma 　　acuminatum 　Focal epithelial 　　hyperplasia 　Verruca vulgaris 　Varicella-zoster virus 　Herpes zoster 　Varicella	

(From European Commission Clearinghouse on Oral Problems Related to HIV Infection and World Health Organization Collaborating Centre on Oral Manifestations of the Human Immunodeficiency Virus, 1990, with revisions, 1992.)

I. EXTRAORAL EXAMINATION

A careful extraoral assessment is important and must be conducted for each patient as part of the maintenance program.

A. Lymphadenopathy

Palpation for enlarged lymph nodes is a routine part of every extraoral examination. In Chapter 8 (pages 118–119), procedures for palpation are described; the location of nodes is shown in figure 8–4.

B. Skin Lesions

Several conditions listed in table 2–7 develop in the skin. Examples are Kaposi's sarcoma, purpura, and herpetic lesions.

II. INTRAORAL EXAMINATION

Of the intraoral lesions listed as strongly associated with HIV infection (group I in table 2–7), candidiasis,[49] Kaposi's sarcoma,[50,51] and hairy leukoplakia[52] have been highly correlated with the subsequent development of advanced HIV infection. All three lesions are readily observable during an oral examination.

A. Fungal Infections[53]

Oral candidiasis, the most frequently occurring oral infection, appears in various forms. They are listed in table 2–7.

Although usually recognized by clinical examination, the dentist may request the use of exfoliative cytology for differential distinction (Chapter 8, pages 125–127).

B. Viral Infections[53]

Herpes simplex, hairy leukoplakia, oral lesions of chickenpox, verruca vulgaris, condyloma acuminatum, and cytomegalovirus ulcer are all examples of lesions that may be seen.

C. Bacterial Infections: Gingival and Periodontal Infections

As with other oral manifestations, gingival changes may be an initial indicator of undiagnosed HIV infection. On the other hand, there may not be any unusual gingival or periodontal changes that can be associated with HIV infection, especially when the patient maintains a high level of personal and professional oral care.[54,55]

The general clinical sequelae are that periodontal infections associated with HIV infection tend to show more severe symptoms and to progress more rapidly than do periodontal conditions in people who are not immunosuppressed.

1. *Gingivitis: Linear Gingival Erythema.* Unusual degrees of severity of gingivitis may be observed. A 2- to 3-mm red band may appear along the gingival margin with petechia-like and/or diffuse red lesions of the attached gingiva. Spontaneous bleeding and bleeding on gentle probing occur. Scaling, root planing, and an increased bacterial plaque control effort on a frequent maintenance plan are especially important, but may not reach the degree of health usually expected.

2. *Necrotizing Ulcerative Gingivitis (NUG).* An in-

creased incidence of NUG has been observed in HIV-positive patients. Ulceration and destruction of interdental papillae with spontaneous bleeding and pain may develop rapidly.

3. *Periodontal Infection.*[56] A range of severity of periodontal involvement may be observed in HIV-infected patients. Severe soft tissue necrosis and rapid destruction of periodontal attachment characteristic of a rapidly progressive periodontitis can occur in a few months. In extreme cases, loss of crestal alveolar bone has led to bone exposure and sequestration.

Severe pain and difficulty in mastication contribute to patient discomfort and malnutrition.

D. Dental Examination
Dental caries and dental erosion can be problems for patients medicated with zidovudine (AZT) or retrovir. Common side effects of AZT are nausea and vomiting. The patient who uses the medication several times each day and vomits each time could have dissolution of the enamel in the form of dental erosion. Personal daily and periodic professional fluoride must be included in the preventive oral hygiene program.

E. Xerostomia
Xerostomia, as a result of salivary gland diseases (table 2–7, Group II) or as a side effect of medications, can contribute to dental caries and discomfort from dry mucosa. In addition to fluoride therapy for dental caries control, the patient's diet should be reviewed and instruction should be given in the selection of noncariogenic food and snack items. Other information on xerostomia can be reviewed on page 204.

HIV INFECTION IN CHILDREN

An increasing number of patients with HIV infection are children younger than 13 years of age. Children aged 13 years and older are diagnosed and treated as adults.[57]

I. CHILDREN AT RISK
A. Infants born to mothers infected with HIV (perinatal transmission). Approximately 25 to 40% of infants born to HIV-seropositive mothers become infected. The risk of transmission can be related to the severity of the mother's illness and to the CD4+ cell count level.
1. *Intrauterine (Vertical Transmission).* HIV infection can cross over the placenta.
2. *Intrapartum.* Infection acquired while passing through the birth canal.
3. *Postpartum.* Exposure to breast milk.[58]
   HIV has been demonstrated in human milk,

and postpartum transmission does occur. Most breastfed infants born to HIV-positive women remain uninfected, however. Human milk contains components, such as immunoglobulins and leukocytes, that could reduce the infectivity of the HIV. Many questions remain unanswered.
B. Infants or children who received transfusions with infected blood or blood products. This mode of transfer is under control in countries where blood donors are screened and all donated blood is tested.
C. Children who have been sexually abused by an infected perpetrator.[59]

II. CLINICAL MANIFESTATIONS
The classification system for HIV infection in children younger than 13 years of age has been developed by the United States Centers for Disease Control and Prevention. In the revised 1994 system infected children are classified by three parameters: the infection status, the clinical status, and the immunologic status.[60]

Many of the organ systems are severely affected. The AIDS-indicator diseases of adult HIV infection are also found in the infected children.

A. Incubation or Latent Period
The incubation period may be shorter than that in adults. The time before clinical symptoms appear is variable and may range from months after birth to several years.

B. Diagnosis
Initial diagnosis is based on blood screening for the presence of virus or HIV antibody. Diagnosis of HIV infection in the neonate during the first year is complicated by the persistence of maternal antibody, which has been passively transferred across the placenta to the fetus. Several tests have been used in the attempt to make as early a diagnosis of HIV infection as possible. Because the core protein p24 (shown in figure 2–7) induces antibody response that can be detected early in infection, testing for p24 has been one of the tests that has been developed.

With the seropositivity of the child determined, antiretroviral therapy can be started. When the mother is without symptoms and has never been tested for HIV, the child's diagnosis may be the index case in the family. Testing of family members and parental counseling may reveal a parent in a risk category.

C. Clinical Findings[61,62]
The wide range of symptoms includes disorders of nearly every body organ system. Oral lesions are common clinical signs of HIV infection in children. Bacterial infections tend to be more frequent and more severe than those in adults. Following is a partial list of frequently found conditions:
1. Failure to thrive; developmental delay.
2. Hepatomegaly; splenomegaly.

3. Generalized lymphadenopathy.
4. Opportunistic infections
   a. Persistent oral candidiasis; *Candida* esophageal.
   b. Localized infections (such as sinusitis, otitis media, impetigo).
   c. Parotiditis; swelling of the parotid glands.
   d. Herpetic gingivostomatitis; sore mouth and poor oral intake lead to malnutrition and dehydration.
   e. *Pneumocystis carinii* pneumonia and lymphocytic interstitial pneumonia.

III. TREATMENT/MANAGEMENT[63,64]
A. Counseling

Family counseling can be an important part of the patient's care. Family and caregivers of the child need to watch for symptoms that are significant to disease progression. They also need to understand the reasons for frequent follow-up for testing and to attend faithfully to the medications program.

Counseling for oral health becomes an important part of the child's care. The healthy mouth, free from pain, can allow comfort during eating and thereby contribute to the nutritional status and the overall welfare and quality of life.

B. Medications: Threat to Dental Caries[65,66]

Children with HIV infection and AIDS take many types of medications. Many children's medications have a base with a high percentage of sucrose. Retrovir, the antiretroviral medication, may be taken by the child several times each day. It is prepared for the children as an elixir, in a sweet, sticky form to disguise its unpleasant flavor.[65]

Other children's preparations with high sucrose are the nutritional supplements. Multivitamins, given as drops for infants and toddlers, contain high quantities of sucrose. Mycostatin (for oral candidiasis) may be recommended for several applications a day, and may have a sucrose content as great as 50%.[66]

All these preparations can contribute to the initiation of dental caries. Infants and toddlers with HIV infection can be at great risk for nursing caries (page 234). When a parent is counseled concerning oral care, recommendations must be given relative to the nursing bottle and pacifiers, as well as to cleaning the mouth immediately after giving the various medications (pages 613 and 614).

PREVENTION OF HIV INFECTION

Until a vaccine is available, prevention depends to a large degree on community education for attitudinal and behavioral changes. People need to understand the modes of transmission of the HIV and the preventive measures necessary to halt its transmission. Dental personnel must keep well informed with accurate, current information that can be applied in practice and give support to community health programs.

The goal of *primary prevention* (for those not infected) is to lower the rate at which new cases of HIV infection appear. Programs for women, particularly of childbearing age, intravenous drug users who share needles, and teenagers are focused to reach the most vulnerable groups. HIV testing should be offered for all pregnant women, and all newborns should be tested in the attempt to control the increasing numbers of children with HIV infection.

The goals of *secondary prevention* (for seropositive individuals) are to reduce the rate of transmission and to introduce treatment early. Early intervention may postpone severe clinical manifestations of advanced illness. A leading part of the program is to counsel the HIV-infected individuals to use safe sex practices* and to cooperate with the program to screen and counsel their sexual contacts and families.

Ongoing programs include strict testing for blood donors and all tissue organ donors, as well as identification and counseling of recipients of blood transfusions before 1985 and their sexual partners. The incubation period has been shown to be much longer than was originally thought. With early diagnosis and medical intervention, people with HIV infection can be symptom free, healthy, and live longer than was possible earlier in the epidemic.

FACTORS TO TEACH THE PATIENT

I. Reasons for postponing an appointment when a herpes lesion ("fever blister" or "cold sore") is present on the lip or in the oral cavity.
   A. Importance of not touching or scratching the lesion because of self-infection to fingers or eyes, for example.
   B. How the viruses can survive on objects and transfer infection to other people.
II. How to help by keeping the medical history up-to-date by informing of additional exposures and immunizations to communicable diseases for self and family members.
III. Preparation for a dental or dental hygiene appointment by thorough mouth cleaning with toothbrush and dental floss to lower the bacterial count and thus lessen aerosol contamination in the treatment room.

---

* "Safe sex practices" is meant to include barrier protection and no exchange of body fluids (saliva, semen, vaginal secretions) in accord with recommended guidelines.

REFERENCES

1. **Miller,** C.H.: Microbial Ecology of the Oral Cavity, in Schuster, G.S., ed.: *Oral Microbiology and Infectious Disease,* 3rd ed. Philadelphia, B.C. Decker, 1990, pp. 465–467.

2. **Hardie,** J.: Microbial Flora of the Oral Cavity, in Schuster, G.S., ed.: *Oral Microbiology and Infectious Disease,* 2nd student ed. Baltimore, Williams & Wilkins, 1983, p. 168.

3. **Miller,** R.L. and Micik, R.E.: Air Pollution and Its Control in the Dental Office, *Dent. Clin. North Am., 22,* 453, July, 1978.

4. **Miller,** R.L.: Generation of Airborne Infection—by High Speed Dental Equipment, *J. Am. Soc. Prev. Dent., 6,* 14, May/June, 1976.

5. **Larato,** D.C., Ruskin, P.F., and Martin, A.: Effect of an Ultrasonic Scaler on Bacterial Counts in Air, *J. Periodontol., 38,* 550, November–December, 1967.

6. **Holbrook,** W.P., Muir, K.F., MacPhee, I.T., and Ross, P.W.: Bacteriological Investigation of the Aerosol from Ultrasonic Scalers, *Br. Dent. J., 144,* 245, April 18, 1978.

7. **Pokowitz,** W. and Hoffman, H.: Dental Aerobiology, *N.Y. State Dent. J., 37,* 337, June–July, 1971.

8. **Gross,** A., Devine, M.J., and Cutright, D.E.: Microbial Contamination of Dental Units and Ultrasonic Scalers, *J. Periodontol., 47,* 670, November, 1976.

9. **Crawford,** J.J.: Sterilization, Disinfection and Asepsis in Dentistry, in Block, S.S., ed.: *Disinfection, Sterilization and Preservation,* 3rd ed. Philadelphia, Lea & Febiger, 1983, pp. 517–518.

10. **Malamed,** S.F.: *Handbook of Local Anesthesia,* 3rd ed. St. Louis, The C.V. Mosby Co., 1990, p. 131.

11. **Benenson,** A.S., ed.: *Control of Communicable Diseases in Man,* 15th ed. Washington, D.C., American Public Health Association, 1990, pp. 457–465.

12. **Barnes,** P.F., Bloch, A.B., Davidson, P.T., and Snider, D.E.: Tuberculosis in Patients With Human Immunodeficiency Virus Infection, *N. Engl. J. Med., 324,* 1644, June 6, 1991.

13. **Robinson,** H.B.G. and Miller, A.S.: *Colby, Kerr, and Robinson's Color Atlas of Oral Pathology,* 5th ed. Philadelphia, J.B. Lippincott Co., 1990, p. 91.

14. **Fehrenbach,** M.J., Lemborn, U.E., and Phelan, J.A.: Immunity, in Ibsen, O.A.C. and Phelan, J.A.: *Oral Pathology for the Dental Hygienist.* Philadelphia, W.B. Saunders Co., 1992, pp. 185–186.

15. **Szmuness,** W., Stevens, C.E., Harley, E.J., Zang, E.A., Oleszko, W.R., William, D.C., Sadovsky, R., Morrison, J.M., and Kellner, A.: Hepatitis B Vaccine. Demonstration of Efficacy in a Controlled Clinical Trial in a High-risk Population in the United States, *N. Engl. J. Med., 303,* 833, October 9, 1980.

16. **Benenson:** op. cit., pp. 197–212.

17. **Werzberger,** A., Mensch, B., Kuter, B., Brown, L., Lewis, J., Sitrin, R., Miller, W., Shouval, D., Wiens, B., Calandra, G., Ryan, J., Provost, P., and Nalin, D.: A Controlled Trial of a Formalininactivated Hepatitis A Vaccine in Healthy Children, *N. Engl. J. Med., 327,* 453, August 13, 1992.

18. **Bancroft,** W.H.: Hepatitis A Vaccine (Editorial), *N. Engl. J. Med., 327,* 488, August 13, 1992.

19. **United States Centers for Disease Control:** Protection Against Viral Hepatitis. Recommendations of the Immunization Practices Advisory Committee, (ACIP), *MMWR, 39,* 1–26, No. RR-2, February 9, 1990.

20. **United States Centers for Disease Control:** Public Service Inter-agency Guidelines for Screening Donors of Blood, Plasma, Organs, Tissues, and Semen for Evidence of Hepatitis B and Hepatitis C, *MMWR, 40,* 1–17, No. RR-4, April 19, 1991.

21. **United States Centers for Disease Control:** Hepatitis B Virus: A Comprehensive Strategy for Eliminating Transmission in the United States Through Universal Childhood Vaccination, *MMWR, 40,* 1–25, No. RR-13, November 22, 1991.

22. **United States Centers for Disease Control:** Suboptimal Response to Hepatitis B Vaccine Given by Injection into the Buttock, *MMWR, 34,* 105, March 1, 1985.

23. **Dienstag,** J.L., Stevens, C.E., Bhan, A.K., and Szmuness, W.: Hepatitis B Vaccine Administered to Chronic Carriers of Hepatitis B Surface Antigen, *Ann. Intern. Med., 96,* 575, May, 1982.

24. **Stevens,** C.E., Taylor, P.E., and Tong, M.J.: Yeast-recombinant Hepatitis B Vaccine: Efficacy With Hepatitis B Immune Globulin in Prevention of Perinatal Hepatitis B Virus Transmission, *JAMA, 257,* 2612, May 15, 1987.

25. **Donahue,** J.G., Muñoz, A., Ness, P.M., Brown, D.E., Yawn, D.H., McAllister, H.A., Reitz, B.A., and Nelson, K.E.: The Declining Risk of Post-transfusion Hepatitis C Virus Infection, *N. Engl. J. Med., 327,* 369, August 6, 1992.

26. **Merchant,** V.A.: Herpesviruses and Other Microorganisms of Concern in Dentistry, *Dent. Clin. North Am., 35,* 283, April, 1991.

27. **Corey,** L. and Spear, P.G.: Infections with Herpes Simplex Viruses, *N. Engl. J. Med., 314,* 686, March 13, 1986 (first part); *314,* 749, March 20, 1986 (second part).

28. **Benenson:** op. cit., pp. 83–86.

29. **Benenson:** op. cit., pp. 291–293.

30. **Greenspan,** J.S., Greenspan, D., Lennette, E.T., Abrams, D.I., Conant, M.A., Petersen, V., and Freese, U.K.: Replication of Epstein-Barr Virus Within the Epithelial Cells of Oral "Hairy" Leukoplakia, An AIDS-associated Lesion, *N. Engl. J. Med., 313,* 1564, December 19, 1985.

31. **Chesseman,** S.H.: Cytomegalovirus, in Gorbach, S.L., Bartlett, J.G., and Blacklow, N.R.: *Infectious Diseases.* Philadelphia, W.B. Saunders Co., 1992, pp. 1715–1720.

32. **Adler,** S.P.: Molecular Epidemiology of Cytomegalovirus: Evidence for Viral Transmission to Parents from Children Infected at a Day Care Center, *Pediatr. Infect. Dis., 5,* 315, May–June, 1986.

33. **Benenson:** op. cit., pp. 212–215.

34. **Rees,** T.D. and Matheson, B.R.: Primary Herpetic Gingivostomatitis in a 56-year-old Male, *Gerodontics, 2,* 28, February, 1986.

35. **Zakay-Rones,** Z., Ehrlich, J., Hochman, N., and Levy, R.: The Sulcular Epithelium as a Reservoir for Herpes Simplex Virus in Man, *J. Periodontol., 44,* 779, December, 1973.

36. **Amit,** R., Morag, A., Ravid, Z., Hochman, N., Ehrlich, J., and Zakay-Rones, Z.: Detection of Herpes Simplex Virus in Gingival Tissue, *J. Periodontol., 63,* 502, June, 1992.

37. **Zakay-Rones,** Z., Hochman, N., and Rones, Y.: Immunological Response to Herpes Simplex Virus in Human Gingival Fluid, *J. Periodontol., 53,* 42, January, 1982.

38. **Rones,** Y., Hochman, N., Ehrlich, J., and Zakay-Rones, Z.: Sensitivity of Oral Tissues to Herpes Simplex Virus—*in vitro, J. Periodontol., 54,* 91, February, 1983.

39. **Ehrlich,** J., Cohen, G.H., and Hochman, N.: Specific Herpes Simplex Virus Antigen in Human Gingiva, *J. Periodontol., 54,* 357, June, 1983.

40. **Whitley,** R.J. and Gnann, J.W.: Acyclovir: A Decade Later, *N. Engl. J. Med., 327,* 782, September, 1992.

41. **Lafferty,** W.E., Coombs, R.W., Benedetti, J., Critchlow, C., and Corey, L.: Recurrences After Oral and Genital Herpes Simplex Virus Infection. Influence of Site of Injection and Viral Type, *N. Engl. J. Med., 316,* 1444, June 4, 1987.

42. **Manzella,** J.P., McConville, J.H., Valenti, W., Menegus, M.A., Swirkosz, E.M., and Arens, M.: An Outbreak of Herpes Simplex Virus Type 1 Gingivostomatitis in a Dental Hygiene Practice, *JAMA, 252,* 2019, October 19, 1984.

43. **Tolle,** S.L.: Herpes, *RDH, 5,* 17, April, 1985.

44. **McMechen,** D.L. and Wright, J.M.: A Protocol for the Management of Patients with Herpetic Infections, *Dent. Hyg., 59,* 546, December, 1985.

45. **United States Centers for Disease Control:** Revised Classification System for HIV Infection and Expanded Surveillance Case Definition for AIDS Among Adolescents and Adults, *MMWR, 41,* 1–19, No. RR-17, December 18, 1992.

46. **Glick,** M. and Garfunkel, A.A.: HIV Disease: Pathogenesis and Disease Progression—An Update, *Compendium, 13,* 80, February, 1992.

47. **Hazeltine,** W.A.: The Molecular Biology of HIV-1, in DeVita, V.T., Helman, S., and Rosenberg, S.A., eds.: *AIDS. Etiology, Diagnosis, Treatment, and Prevention,* 3rd ed. Philadelphia, J.B. Lippincott Co., 1992, pp. 39–44.

48. **Benenson:** op. cit., p. 4.

49. **Klein,** R.S., Harris, C.A., Small, C.B., Moll, B., Lesser, M., and Friedland, G.H.: Oral Candidiasis in High-risk Patients as the Initial Manifestation of the Acquired Immunodeficiency Syndrome, *N. Engl. J. Med., 311,* 354, August 9, 1984.

50. **Silverman,** S., Migliorati, C.A., Lozada-Nur, F., Greenspan, D., and Conant, M.A.: Oral Findings in People With or at High Risk for AIDS: A Study of 375 Homosexual Males, *J. Am. Dent. Assoc., 112,* 187, February, 1986.

51. **Keeney,** K., Abaza, N.A., Tidwel, O., and Quinn, P.: Oral Kaposi's Sarcoma in Acquired Immune Deficiency Syndrome, *J. Oral Maxillofac. Surg., 45,* 815, September, 1987.

52. **Greenspan,** D., Greenspan, J.S., Hearst, N.G., Pan, L.-Z., Conant, M.A., Abrams, D.I., Hollander, H., and Levy, J.A.: Relation of Oral Hairy Leukoplakia to Infection With the Human Immunodeficiency Virus and the Risk of Developing AIDS, *J. Infect. Dis., 155,* 475, March, 1987.

53. **Greenspan,** D., Greenspan, J.S., Schiødt, M., and Pindborg, J.J.: *AIDS and the Mouth. Diagnosis and Management of Oral Lesions.* Copenhagen, Munksgaard, 1990, pp. 91–102, 113–134.

54. **Drinkard,** C.R., Decher, L., Little, J.W., Rhame, F.S., Balfour, H.H., Rhodus, N.L., Merry, J.W., Walker, P.O., Miller, C.E., Volberding, P.A., and Melnick, S.L.: Periodontal Status of Individuals in Early Stages of Human Immunodeficiency Virus Infection, *Community Dent. Oral Epidemiol., 19,* 281, October, 1991.

55. **Riley,** C., London, J.P., and Burmeister, J.A.: Periodontal Health in 200 HIV-positive Patients, *J. Oral Pathol. Med., 21,* 124, March, 1992.

56. **Winkler,** J.R. and Robertson, P.B.: Periodontal Disease Associated with HIV Infection, *Oral Surg. Oral Med. Oral Pathol., 73,* 145, February, 1992.

57. **MacDonald,** M.G., Ginzberg, H.M., and Bolan, J.C.: HIV Infection in Pregnancy: Epidemiology and Clinical Management, *J. Acquired Immune Deficiency Syndrome, 4,* 100, February, 1991.

58. **Ruff,** A.J., Halsey, N.A., Coberly, J., and Boulos, R.: Breastfeeding and Maternal-infant Transmission of Human Immunodeficiency Virus Type I; *J. Pediatr., 121,* 325, August, 1992.

59. **Gutman,** L.T., St. Claire, K.K., Weedy, C., Herman-Giddens, M.E., Lane, B.A., Niemeyer, J.C., and McKinney, R.E.: Human Immunodeficiency Virus Transmission by Sexual Abuse, *Am. J. Dis. Child., 145,* 137, February, 1991.

60. **United States Centers for Disease Control and Prevention:** 1994 Revised Classification System for Human Immunodeficiency Virus Infection in Children Less Than 13 Years of Age, *MMWR, 43,* 1–19, No. RR-12, September 30, 1994.

61. **Hoyt,** L.G. and Oleske, J.M.: The Clinical Spectrum of HIV Infection in Infants and Children: An Overview, in Yogev, R. and Connor, E.: *Management of HIV Infection in Infants and Children.* St. Louis, The C.V. Mosby Co., 1992, pp. 227–245.

62. **Butler,** K.M., and Pizzo, P.A.: HIV Infection in Children, in DeVita, V.T., Helman, S., and Rosenberg, S.A., eds.: *AIDS Etiology, Diagnosis, Treatment, and Prevention,* 3rd ed. Philadelphia, J.B. Lippincott Co., 1992, pp. 285–312.

63. **Scott,** G.B.: HIV Infection in Children: Clinical Features and Management, *J. Acquired Immune Deficiency Syndrome, 4,* 109, February, 1991.

64. **Connor,** E., McSherry, G., and Yogev, R.: Antiviral Treatment of Pediatric HIV Infection, in Yogev, R. and Connor, E.: *Management of HIV Infection in Infants and Children.* St. Louis, The C.V. Mosby Co., 1992, pp. 505–531.

65. **Gehrke,** F.S. and Johnsen, D.S.: Bottle Caries Associated with Anti-HIV Therapy (Letter), *Pediatr. Dent., 13,* 73, January/February, 1991.

66. **Howell,** R.B. and Houpt, M.: More Than One Factor Can Influence Caries Development in HIV-positive Children (Letter), *Pediatr. Dent., 13,* 247, July/August, 1991.

SUGGESTED READINGS

Tuberculosis

Brick, P.: Tuberculosis: A New Look at an Old Foe, *Access, 6,* 10, December, 1992.

Faecher, R.S., Thomas, J.E., and Bender, B.S.: Tuberculosis: A Growing Concern for Dentistry?, *J. Am. Dent. Assoc., 124,* 94, January, 1993.

Schieffelbein, C.W. and Snider, D.E.: Tuberculosis Control Among Homeless Populations, *Arch. Intern. Med., 148,* 1843, August, 1988.

Small, P.M., Schecter, G.F., Goodman, P.C., Sande, M.A., Chaisson, R.E., and Hopewell, P.C.: Treatment of Tuberculosis in Patients with Advanced Human Immunodeficiency Virus Infection, *N. Engl. J. Med., 324,* 289, January 31, 1991.

Stead, W.W., Senner, J.W., Reddick, W.T., and Lofgren, J.P.: Racial Differences in Susceptibility to Infection by *Mycobacterium tuberculosis, N. Engl. J. Med., 322,* 422, February 15, 1990.

United States Centers for Disease Control: Tuberculosis Among Foreign-Born Persons Entering the United States, *MMWR, 39,* 1, No. RR-18, December 28, 1990.

United States Centers for Disease Control: Tuberculosis Transmission Along the U.S.-Mexican Border, *MMWR, 40,* 373, June 7, 1991.

United States Centers for Disease Control: National Action Plan to Combat Multidrug-Resistant Tuberculosis, *MMWR, 41,* 1–70, No. RR-11, June 19, 1992.

Hepatitis B

Cottone, J.A.: The Global Challenge of Hepatitis B: Implications for Dentistry, *Int. Dent. J., 41,* 131, June, 1991.

Eddleston, A.: Modern Vaccines. Hepatitis, *Lancet, 335,* 1142, May 12, 1990.

Hardie, J.: Recent Recommendations for Hepatitis B Vaccination, *Can. Dent. Hyg./Probe, 26,* 70, Summer, 1992.

Iwarson, S.: The Main Five Types of Viral Hepatitis. An Alphabetical Update, *Scand. J. Infect. Dis., 24,* 129, No. 2, 1992.

Maseman, D.C.: Hepatitis: Types, Protection and Legal Ramifications, *Semin. Dent. Hyg., 1,* 1, May, 1989.

Hepatitis C

Alter, M.J., Margolis, H.S., Krawczynski, K., Judson, F.N., Mares, A., Alexander, W.J., Hu, P.Y., Miller, J.K., Gerber, M.A., Sampliner, R.E., Meeks, E.L., and Beach, M.J.: The Natural History of Community-acquired Hepatitis C in the United States, *N. Engl. J. Med., 327,* 1899, December 31, 1992.

Kelen, G.D., Green, G.B., Purcell, R.H., Chan, D.W., Qaquish, B.F., Sivertson, K.T., and Quinn, T.C.: Hepatitis B and Hepatitis C in Emergency Department Patients, *N. Engl. J. Med., 326,* 1399, May 21, 1992.

Lynch-Salamon, D.I. and Combs, C.A.: Hepatitis C in Obstetrics and Gynecology, *Obstet. Gynecol., 79,* 621, April, 1992.

Pereira, B.J.G., Milford, E.L., Kirkman, R.L., Quan, S., Sayre, K.R., Johnson, P.J., Wilber, J.C., and Levey, A.S.: Prevalence of Hepatitis C Virus RNA in Organ Donors Positive for Hepatitis C Antibody and in the Recipients of Their Organs, *N. Engl. J. Med., 327,* 910, September 24, 1992.

Pereira, B.J.G., Milford, E.L., Kirkman, R.L., and Levey, A.S.: Transmission of Hepatitis C Virus by Organ Transplantation, *N. Engl. J. Med., 325,* 454, August 15, 1991.

Porter, S.R. and Scully, C.: Non-A, Non-B Hepatitis and Dentistry, *Br. Dent. J., 168,* 257, March 24, 1990.

Weintrub, P.S., Veereman-Wauters, G., Cowan, M.J., and Thaler, M.M.: Hepatitis C Virus Infection in Infants Whose Mothers Took Street Drugs Intravenously, *J. Pediatr., 119,* 869, December, 1991.

HIV: General

Cohen, P.A. and Wilkins, E.M.: A Hospital-based Dental Clinic for Patients With HIV Infection in the United States, *Can. Dent. Hyg./Probe, 26,* 65, Summer, 1992.

Friedland, G., Kahl, P., Saltzman, B., Rogers, M., Feiner, C., Mayers, M., Schable, C., and Klein, R.S.: Additional Evidence for Lack of Transmission of HIV Infection by Close Interpersonal (Casual) Contact, *AIDS, 4,* 639, July, 1990.

Gershon, R.R.M., Vlahov, D., and Nelson, K.E.: The Risk of Transmission of HIV-1 Through Non-percutaneous Non-sexual Modes—A Review, *AIDS, 4,* 645, July, 1990.

Glick, M.: Evaluation of Prognosis and Survival of the HIV-infected Patient, *Oral Surg. Oral Med. Oral Pathol., 74,* 386, September, 1992.

Glick, M., Muzyka, B.C., and Garfunkel, A.A.: Viability, Transmissibility, and Risk Assessment of HIV, *Compendium, 13,* 374, May, 1992.

Graham, N.M.H., Zeger, S.L., Park, L.P., Vermund, S.H., Detels, R., Rinaldo, C.R., and Phair, J.P.: The Effects on Survival of Early Treatment of Human Immunodeficiency Virus Infection, *N. Engl. J. Med., 326,* 1037, April 16, 1992.

Grinspoon, S.K. and Bilezikian, J.P.: HIV Disease and the Endocrine System, *N. Engl. J. Med., 327,* 1360, November 5, 1992.

Gruninger, S.E., Siew, C., Chang, S.-B., Clayton, R., Leete, J.K., Hojvat, S.A., Verrusio, A.C., and Neidle, E.A.: Human Immunodeficiency Virus Type 1 Infection Among Dentists, *J. Am. Dent. Assoc., 123,* 57, March, 1992.

Higgins, D.L., Galavotti, C., O'Reilly, K.R., Schnell, D.J., Moore, M., Rugg, D.L., and Johnson, R.: Evidence for the Effects of HIV Antibody Counseling and Testing on Risk Behaviors, *JAMA, 266,* 2419, November 6, 1991.

Homan, C., Krogsgaard, K., Pedersen, C., Andersson, P., and Nielsen, J.O.: High Incidence of Hepatitis B Infection and Evolution of Chronic Hepatitis B Infection in Patients With Advanced HIV Infection, *J. Acquired Immune Deficiency Syndrome, 4,* 416, April, 1991.

Letvin, N.L.: Vaccines Against Human Immunodeficiency Virus—Progress and Prospects, *N. Engl. J. Med., 329,* 1400, November 4, 1993.

Perry, S.: Organic Mental Disorders Caused by HIV: Update on Early Diagnosis and Treatment, *Am. J. Psychiatry, 147,* 696, June, 1990.

Salmaso, S., Conti, S., and Sasse, H.: Drug Use and HIV-1 Infection. Report from the Second Italian Multicenter Study, *J. Acquired Immune Deficiency Syndrome, 4,* 607, June, 1991.

Scully, C. and Porter, S.: The Level of Risk of Transmission of Human Immunodeficiency Virus Between Patients and Dental Staff, *Br. Dent. J., 170,* 97, February 9, 1991.

Selwyn, P.A., Alcabes, P., Hartel, D., Buono, D., Schoenbaum, E.E., Klein, R.S., Davenny, K., and Friedland, G.H.: Clinical Manifestations and Predictors of Disease Progression in Drug Users With Human Immunodeficiency Virus Infection, *N. Engl. J. Med., 327,* 1697, December 10, 1992.

Sobieralski, M.F., Miller, C.S., and Jones, S.E.: Subtle Manifestations of AIDS, *J. Dent. Hyg., 64,* 63, February, 1990.

Wooley, C.: Canada's First Hospital Dental Clinic for Patients With HIV Infection, *Can. Dent. Hyg./Probe, 26,* 59, Summer, 1992.

HIV: Older Patients

Blaxhult, A., Granath, F., Lidman, K., and Giesecke, J.: The Influence of Age on the Latency Period to AIDS in People Infected by HIV Through Blood Transfusion, *AIDS, 4,* 125, February, 1990.

Fillitt, H., Fruchtman, S., Sell, L., and Rosen, N.: AIDS in the Elderly: A Case and Its Implications, *Geriatrics, 44,* 65, July, 1989.

Phillips, A.N., Lee, C.A., Elford, J., Webster, A., Janossy, G., Timms, A., Bofill, M., and Kernoff, P.B.A.: More Rapid Progression to AIDS in Older HIV-Infected People: The Role of CD4+ T-Cell Counts, *J. Acquired Immune Deficiency Syndrome, 4,* 970, October, 1991.

HIV: Saliva

Barr, C.E., Miller, L.K., Lopez, M.R., Croxson, T.S., and Schwartz, S.A.: Recovery of Infectious HIV-1 From Whole Saliva. Blood Proves More Likely Virus Transmitter, *J. Am. Dent. Assoc., 123,* 37, February, 1992.

Fox, P.C.: Saliva and Salivary Gland Alterations in HIV Infection, *J. Am. Dent. Assoc., 122,* 46, November, 1991.

Fox, P.C., Wolff, A., Yeh, C.-K., Atkinson, J.C., and Baum, B.J.: Salivary inhibition of HIV-1 Infectivity: Functional Properties and Distribution in Men, Women, and Children, *J. Am. Dent. Assoc., 118,* 709, June, 1989.

HIV: Periodontal Disease

Felix, D.H., Wray, D., Jones, G.A., and Smith, G.L.F.: Oro-antral Fistula: An Unusual Complication of HIV-associated Periodontal Disease, *Br. Dent. J., 171,* 61, July 20, 1991.

Friedman, R.B., Gunsolley, J., Gentry, A., Dinius, A., Kaplowitz, L., and Settle, J.: Periodontal Status of HIV-seropositive and AIDS Patients, *J. Periodontol., 62,* 623, October, 1991.

Glick, M., Pliskin, M.E., and Weiss, R.C.: The Clinical and Histologic Appearance of HIV-associated Gingivitis, *Oral Surg. Oral Med. Oral Pathol., 69,* 395, March, 1990.

Greenspan, D. and Greenspan, J.S.: Oral Manifestations of Human Immunodeficiency Virus Infection, *Dent. Clin. North Am., 37,* 21, January, 1993.

Klein, R.S., Quart, A.M., and Small, C.B.: Periodontal Disease in Heterosexuals with Acquired Immunodeficiency Syndrome, *J. Periodontol., 62,* 535, August, 1991.

Levine, R.A. and Glick, M.: Rapidly Progressive Periodontitis as an Important Clinical Marker for HIV Disease, *Compendium, 12,* 478, July, 1991.

Robinson, P.: Periodontal Diseases and HIV Infection. A Review of the Literature, *J. Clin. Periodontol., 19,* 609, October, 1992.

Scully, C., Epstein, J.B., and Porter, S.: Recognition of Oral Lesions of HIV Infection. 3. Gingival and Periodontal Disease and Less Common Lesions, *Br. Dent. J., 169,* 370, December 8/22, 1990.

Winkler, J.R., Murray, P.A., Grassi, M., and Hammerle, C.: Diagnosis and Management of HIV-associated Periodontal Lesions, *J. Am. Dent. Assoc., 119,* 25–S, Supplement, November, 1989.

HIV: Oral Treatment

Aldous, J.A.: Dental Management of HIV-infected Individuals, *Compendium, 11,* 640, November, 1990.

Aldous, J.A. and Aldous, S.G.: Management of Oral Health for the HIV-infected Patient, *J. Dent. Hyg., 65,* 143, March–April, 1991.

Barone, R., Ficarra, G., Gaglioti, D., Orsi, A., and Mazzotta, F.: Prevalence of Oral Lesions Among HIV-infected Intravenous Drug Abusers and Other Risk Groups, *Oral Surg. Oral Med. Oral Pathol., 69,* 169, February, 1990.

Engelbert, A., Schulten, J.M., ten Kate, R.W., and van der Waal, I.: The Impact of Oral Examination on the Centers for Disease Control Classification of Subjects With Human Immunodeficiency Virus Infection, *Arch. Intern. Med., 150,* 1259, June, 1990.

Epstein, J.B. and Silverman, S.: Head and Neck Malignancies Associated With HIV Infection, *Oral Surg. Oral Med. Oral Pathol., 73,* 193, February, 1992.

Eversole, L.R.: Viral Infections of the Head and Neck Among HIV-seropositive Patients, *Oral Surg. Oral Med. Oral Pathol., 73,* 155, February, 1992.

Garfunkel, A.A. and Glick, M.: HIV Disease: Therapy, Related Systemic and Oral Conditions—An Update, *Compendium, 13,* 284, April, 1992.

Glick, M.: Clinical Protocol for Treating Patients With HIV Disease, *Gen. Dent., 38,* 418, December, 1990.

Glick, M., Trope, M., Bagasra, O., and Pliskin, M.E.: Human Immunodeficiency Virus Infection of Fibroblasts of Dental Pulp in Seropositive Patients, *Oral Surg. Oral Med. Oral Pathol., 71,* 733, June, 1991.

Greenspan, J.S. and Greenspan, D.: Oral Hairy Leukoplakia: Diagnosis and Management, *Oral Surg. Oral Med. Oral Pathol., 67,* 396, April, 1989.

Greenspan, J.S., Barr, C.E., Sciubba, J.J., and Winkler, J.R.: Oral Manifestations of HIV Infection, Definitions, Diagnostic Criteria, and Principles of Therapy, *Oral Surg. Oral Med. Oral Pathol., 73,* 142, February, 1992.

Phelan, J.A., Freedman, P.D., Newsome, N., and Klein, R.S.: Major Aphthous-like Ulcers in Patients with AIDS, *Oral Surg. Oral Med. Oral Pathol., 71,* 68, January, 1991.

Reichl, R.B.: Oral Candidiasis: An Old Disease of Growing Concern, *Gen. Dent., 38,* 114, March–April, 1990.

Scully, C. and McCarthy, G.: Management of Oral Health in Persons with HIV Infection, *Oral Surg. Oral Med. Oral Pathol., 73,* 215, February, 1992.

Scully, C., Porter, S.R., and Luker, J.: An ABC of Oral Health Care in Patients with HIV Infection, *Br. Dent. J., 170,* 149, February 23, 1991.

Shuman, D.: AIDS: Implications for Dental Hygienists, *Semin. Dent. Hyg., 1,* 1, December, 1989.

Tilliss, T.S.I. and Stach, D.J.: Recognition of HIV/AIDS-associated Oral Lesions by the Dental Team, *Clin. Prev. Dent., 13,* 5, November/December, 1991.

van der Waal, I., Schulten, E.A.J.M., and Pindborg, J.J.: Oral Manifestations of AIDS: An Overview, *Int. Dent. J., 41,* 3, February, 1991.

AIDS: Prenatal and Children

Barbacci, M., Repke, J.T., and Chaisson, R.E.: Routine Prenatal Screening for HIV Infection, *Lancet, 337,* 709, March 23, 1991.

European Collaborative Study: Children Born to Women With HIV-1 Infection: Natural History and Risk of Transmission, *Lancet, 337,* 253, February 2, 1991.

Ketchem, L., Berkowitz, R.J., McIlveen, L., Forrester, D., and Rakusan, T.: Oral Findings in HIV-seropositive Children, *Pediatr. Dent., 12,* 143, May/June, 1990.

Leggott, P.J.: Oral Manifestations of HIV Infection in Children, *Oral Surg. Oral Med. Oral Pathol., 73,* 187, February, 1992.

Palumbo, P., Jandinski, J., Connor, E., Fenesy, K., and Oleske, J.: Medical Management of Children With HIV Infection, *Pediatr. Dent., 12,* 139, May/June, 1990.

Persuad, D., Chandwani, S., Rigaud M., Leibovitz, E., Kaul, A., Lawrence, R., Pollack, H., DiJohn, D., Krasinski, K., and Borkowsky, W.: Delayed Recognition of Human Immunodeficiency Virus Infection in Preadolescent Children, *Pediatrics, 90,* 688, November, 1992.

Rotheram-Borus, M.J., Koopman, C., Haignere, C., and Davies, M.: Reducing HIV Sexual Risk Behaviors Among Runaway Adolescents, *JAMA, 266,* 1237, September 4, 1991.

Tovo, P-A., Palomba, E., Gabiano, C., Galli, L., and DeMartmo, M.: Human Immunodeficiency Virus Type 1 (HIV-1) Seroconversion During Pregnancy Does Not Increase the Risk of Perinatal Transmission, *Br. J. Obstet. Gynaecol., 98,* 940, September, 1991.

Herpesvirus

Friedman, H.M.: Herpes Simplex Virus Infections: Diagnosis and Clinical Features, *Compendium, 9,* S300, Supplement No. 9, 1988.

Gibbs, R.S. and Mead, P.B.: Preventing Neonatal Herpes—Current Strategies (Editorial), *N. Engl. J. Med., 326,* 946, April 2, 1992.

Greenberg, M.S.: Oral Herpes Simplex Infections in Immunosuppressed Patients, *Compendium, 9,* S289, Supplement No. 9, 1988.

Katz, J., Marmary, I., Ben-Yehuda, A., Barak, S., and Danon, Y.: Primary Herpetic Gingivostomatitis: No Longer a Disease of Childhood?, *Community Dent. Oral Epidemiol., 19,* 309, October, 1991.

Katz, J.A., Phero, J.C., McDonald, J.S., and Green, D.B.: Herpes Zoster Management, *Anesth. Prog., 36,* 35, March/April, 1989.

Kulhanjian, J.A., Soroush, V., Au, D.S., Bronzan, R.N., Yaswkawa, L.L., Weylman, L.E., Arvin, A.M., and Prober, C.G.: Identification of Women at Unsuspected Risk of Primary Infection With Herpes Simplex Virus Type 2 During Pregnancy, *N. Engl. J. Med., 326,* 916, April 2, 1992.

Pruksananonda, P., Hall, C.B., Insel, R.A., McIntyre, K., Pellett, P.E., Long, C.E., Schnabel, K.C., Pincus, P.H., Stamey, B.A., Dambaugh, T.R., and Stewart, J.A.: Primary Human Herpesvirus 6 Infection in Young Children, *N. Engl. J. Med., 326,* 1446, May 28, 1992.

Shipman, C.: Strategies for the Chemotherapy of Oral Herpes, *Compendium, 9,* S305, Supplement No. 9, 1988.

Exposure Control: Barriers for Patient and Clinician

Exposure control refers to all procedures during clinical care necessary to provide top-level protection from exposure to infectious agents for members of the dental team and their patients. Dental health-care workers (DHCW) have a professional obligation to serve *all* patients with comprehensive oral care, including patients with known or unknown communicable diseases. The practice of *universal precautions* means that the body fluids of all patients are treated as if they were infectious.

An organized system for exposure control is needed. First, a written exposure control plan is prepared to serve as a guide for the entire team.[1] Consistency between DHCWs is necessary to maintain standards of asepsis and to prevent cross-contamination. The written plan can be the basis for training new personnel. As new research and commercial products become available, the written protocol must be revised.

Using the protocol and transferring the objectives and overall aims to the clinical setting are the responsibilities of each member of the dental team. It should be realized that physical barriers and other requirements of the protocol provide safety for both the DHCW and the patient. Selected terms from the application of exposure control and immunizations are defined in table 3–1.

PERSONAL PROTECTION OF THE DENTAL TEAM

The continuing health and productivity of dental health personnel depend to a large degree on the control of cross-contamination. Loss of work time, personal suffering, long-term systemic effects, and even

exclusion from continued practice are possible results from communicable diseases. The only safe procedure is to practice defensively at all times, with specific precautions for personal protection.

In this section, topics include immunizations and periodic tests, clothing, barriers to infectious microorganisms, such as face mask and protective eyewear, personal hygiene, handwashing, gloves, and habits.

IMMUNIZATIONS AND PERIODIC TESTS

Dental personnel in a hospital setting are subject to the rules and regulations for all hospital employees. Policies usually require certain immunizations for new employees if written proof of immunizations is not available and tests for antibodies prove to be negative.

In private dental practices, individual initiative is required to maintain standards of safety for all dental team members. All staff members should be well aware of the signs and symptoms of diseases that are occupational hazards. All must be encouraged to seek early diagnosis and treatment of a seemingly minor condition that could be the initial symptom of a more serious communicable disease.

At the time of employment, it is reasonable for a dentist-employer to request of employees a record of current immunizations and their most recent updating, as well as specific tests, such as for tuberculosis. Immunization for rubella is particularly important for female employees of childbearing age.

Following are listed the infectious diseases for which immunization is usually provided during infancy and childhood. Booster or reimmunization requirements are specific for each disease and apply throughout life.

TABLE 3-1
KEY WORDS AND ABBREVIATIONS:
EXPOSURE CONTROL

Antimicrobial soap: a soap containing an active ingredient against skin microorganisms.

Barrier protection: refers to placing a physical barrier between the patient's body fluids (such as blood and saliva) and the health-care worker (HCW) to prevent disease transmission.

 Barriers for HCW: include gloves, mask, protective eyewear, and uniform.

 Barriers for patient: include protective eyewear, headcover during surgeries, and rubber dam during restorative and sealant procedures.

Booster dose: amount of immunogen (vaccine, toxoid, or other antigen preparation), usually smaller than the original amount, injected at an appropriate interval after the primary immunization to sustain the immune response to that immunogen.

Exposure incident: a specific eye, mouth, mucous membrane, nonintact skin, or parenteral contact with blood or other potentially infectious material that results from the performance of one's usual professional duties.

Immunization (im'u-nĭ-zā'shun): the process of rendering a subject immune to a particular disease by stimulation with a specific antigen to promote antibody formation in the body.

Inoculation (ĭ-nok'u-lā'shun): introduction of antigenic material or vaccine; more frequently used to refer to introduction of material into a culture medium.

Occupational exposure: reasonably anticipated skin, eye, mucous membrane, or parenteral contact with blood or other potentially infectious materials that may result from the performance of one's usual duties.

PPD: purified protein derivative for tuberculin intracutaneous skin test for tuberculosis; positive reaction means previous infection with *Mycobacterium tuberculosis* (mī'kō-bak-te'rē-um too-ber'kū-lo'sis).

Toxoid (tok'soid): toxin treated by heat or chemical agent to destroy its deleterious properties without destroying its ability to combine with, or stimulate the formation of, antitoxin; examples of toxoids used for active immunization are tetanus and diphtheria.

Tuberculin test (Mantoux) (too-ber'kū-lin test [Man-too']): a test for the presence of active or inactive tuberculosis; a positive test is denoted by redness and induration at the injection site by 48 to 72 hours after injection.

Vaccination (vak'si-nā'shun): process of introducing a vaccine into the body to produce immunity to a specific disease.

Vaccine (vak'sēn): a suspension of attenuated or killed microorganisms administered for the prevention or treatment of an infectious disease.

I. IMMUNIZATIONS
A. Basic Schedule[2,3]
The immunization schedule for infants and children may include protection against poliomyelitis, diphtheria, tetanus, pertussis (whooping cough), measles, mumps, rubella (German measles), influenza, and hepatitis B.[4]

Reimmunization of children against measles either at school entry or at entry into middle or junior high school (at 5 to 6 years or 11 to 12 years of age) has been found necessary to cope with outbreaks.[5]

B. Booster and Reimmunization
Each agent requires booster or reimmunization on a specific plan, which may range from 1 to 10 years, or reimmunization only upon intimate contact or exposure. The needs differ in different climates, countries, and locations. Persons moving or traveling need to become aware of specific precautions.

For tetanus boosters, intervals of 10 years are indicated. If an injury occurs, however, a booster should be given on the day of the injury.[6]

C. Adult Immunizations
Table 3–2 summarizes the vaccines and toxoids recommended for most adults by age groups.[7] Hepatitis B vaccine is also recommended, especially for members of risk groups (page 22) and all DHCWs.

II. MANAGEMENT PROGRAM
A. Recommended Tests
1. Annual tuberculin test (Mantoux); chest radiograph as indicated.
2. Periodic throat culture for possible hemolytic streptococcus carrier.

B. Obtaining Tests
Obtain tests promptly when exposed to certain infectious diseases and seek prophylactic immunization as indicated and available.

C. Written Records
Keep written records of immunizations, boosters, and reimmunizations; plan for regular follow-up. When the status of current immunizations is known, time is saved by not needing a susceptibility test prior to initiating passive immunizations when accidental exposure occurs.

CLINICAL ATTIRE

The wearing apparel of clinicians and their assistants is vulnerable to contamination from splash, spatter, aerosols, and patient contact. The gown or uniform should be designed and cared for in a manner that minimizes cross-contamination.

I. GOWN, UNIFORM, OR SCRUBSUIT
Gowns, uniforms, or scrubsuits are expected to be clean and maintained as free as possible from contamination. Wearing clinic coats over street clothes cannot

TABLE 3-2
VACCINES AND TOXOIDS RECOMMENDED FOR ADULTS, BY AGE GROUPS, UNITED STATES

Age group (years)	Vaccine/toxoid					
	Td*	Measles	Mumps	Rubella	Influenza	Pneumococcal Polysaccharide
18–24	X	X	X	X		
25–64	X	X†	X†	X		
≥65	X				X	X

* Td = Tetanus and diphtheria toxoids, adsorbed (for adult use), which is a combined preparation containing < 2 flocculation units of diphtheria toxoid.
† Indicated for persons born after 1956.
(From United States Centers for Disease Control: Update on Adult Immunization Recommendations of the Immunization Practices Advisory Committee (ACIP), *MMWR, 40,* 56, No. RR-12, November 15, 1991.)

be recommended because of the exposure of the street clothes to infectious material.

A. Solid, Closed Front

The garment should be closed at the neck and tie in back, preferably. The fabric should be disposable or able to be washed commercially and withstand washing with bleach.

B. No Pockets

Pockets are too readily available for placing contaminated objects, such as writing implements or keys. Gloved hands, prepared for patient treatment, must be kept from touching objects or being placed in pockets.

C. Long Sleeves

Long sleeves with fitted cuffs permit protective gloves to extend over the cuffs.

II. HAIR AND HEAD COVERING

A. Hair must be worn off the shoulders and fastened back away from the face. When longer, it should be held within a head cover. Because the hair is exposed to much contamination, an appropriate head cover is advised when using handpieces and ultrasonic or airbrasive instruments.

B. Facial hair should be covered with a face mask and/or face shield.

III. PROTECTION OF UNIFORM

A plastic washable or a disposable apron may be used when clinical services are performed that usually involve blood, spatter, or aerosols.

IV. OUTSIDE WEAR

Clinic uniforms and shoes should not be worn outside the clinic practice setting.[8] When clinic clothing is worn outside, contamination can be carried from, and contamination brought into, the treatment area.

Another problem is that contamination is taken into the home when uniforms are worn to and from the work area. When laundered at home, the items from a dental office or clinic should be kept separate and treated with household bleach for disinfection.

USE OF FACE MASK

Basic personal barrier protection is composed of face mask, protective eyewear, and gloves. The use of the face mask is described first because it should be positioned first when preparing for clinical care procedures. The protective eyewear is placed second. After that, the hands can be properly washed prior to gloving.

Dispersion of particles of debris, polishing agents, calculus, and water, all of which are contaminated by the patient's oral flora, occurs regularly during all instrumentation. The greatest aerosols are created following the use of a handpiece, prophylaxis angle, or ultrasonic scaler. Evidence of the spread of particles appears on the splashed face, protective eyewear, and uniform, and on the coverall placed over the patient for protection from the spray. Aerosol production was described on page 14.

I. MASK EFFICIENCY
A. Criteria: Essential Characteristics

1. *Filtration* (measured in BFE = bacterial filtration effectiveness). Standard masks block filtration of particles as small as 3 μ. Particles of 3 μ and smaller can penetrate to the alveoli of the lower respiratory tract, where their infectivity is increased. Droplet nuclei (*Mycobacterium tuberculosis*) range from 1 to 5 μ and are a risk in health-care settings.[9]

2. *Fit.* Proper fit over face is vital to protect against inhaling droplet nuclei in aerosols.

3. *Moisture Absorption.* Soak through is an important factor. Lining should be impervious. Mask must be changed for each patient and not worn longer than 1 hour.

4. *Comfort.* Degree of comfort should encourage compliance in wearing.

5. *Cost.* Cost should be economical.

B. Materials

Various materials have been used for masks, including gauze and other cloth, plastic foam, fiberglass, synthetic fiber mat, and paper. In one research study, foam, paper, and cloth were found to be the least adequate filters of aerosols, whereas glass fiber and synthetic fiber mat were shown to be the most effective.[10,11]

II. USE OF A MASK

A. Tie on the mask and position eyewear before a scrub or handwash.

B. Use a fresh mask for each patient.
1. Change mask each hour or when it becomes wet.
2. Chin-cover face shield needs to be supplemented with fitted mask if it does not provide peripheral protection for sides of face under chin.

C. Keep the mask on after completing a procedure, while still in the presence of aerosols. Particles smaller than 5 μm remain suspended longer (up to 24 hours) than do larger particles and can be inhaled directly into terminal lung alveoli. Removal of a mask in the treatment room immediately following the use of aerosol-producing procedures permits direct exposure to airborne organisms.

USE OF PROTECTIVE EYEWEAR

Eye protection for the dental team members and patients is necessary to prevent physical injuries and infections of the eyes. A list of measures for eye accident prevention is included on page 829 in conjunction with emergency treatment.

Severe and disabling eye accidents and infections have been reported.[12,13,14,15] Eye involvement may lead to pain, discomfort, loss of work time, and, in certain instances, permanent injury. Accidents can occur at any time, and as with most accidents, they occur when least prepared for or expected.

Eye infections can follow the accidental dropping of an instrument on the face or the splashing of various materials from a patient's oral cavity into the eye. Contamination can be introduced from saliva, plaque, carious material, pieces of old restorative materials during cavity preparation, bacteria-laden calculus during scaling, and any other microorganisms contained in aerosols or spatter as described on page 14. An aerosol created by an ultrasonic scaler can be heavily contaminated with oral microorganisms.

Careful, deliberate techniques and instrument management, with evacuation and other procedures for the control of oral fluids, contribute to the prevention of accidents and infections of the eyes. All measures described for prevention of airborne disease transmission by aerosols and spatter apply to eye protection. The most effective defense is the use of protective eyewear by all concerned, dental team and patients.

I. INDICATIONS FOR USE OF PROTECTIVE EYEWEAR

A. Dental Team Members

Protective eyewear should be worn at all times. For dental personnel who do not require a corrective lens for vision, protective eyewear with a clear lens should become a routine part of clinical dress.

Protective eyewear worn only when a handpiece, ultrasonic instrument, or other aerosol-producing instrument is used can easily be forgotten or misplaced. Even without power-driven instruments, pieces of calculus and spatter from air and water spray can reach the eyes.

B. Patients

Protective eyewear is recommended for each patient at each appointment. The patient's medical history should reflect types of eye surgery, implants, or other special concerns. Contact lenses should be removed.

Patients with their own prescription lenses may prefer to wear them, but for the safety of the patient's glasses, the use of the protective eyewear provided in the office or clinic is advisable.

II. PROTECTIVE EYEWEAR

A. General Features of Acceptable Eyewear

1. Wide coverage, with side shields, to protect around the eye.
2. Shatterproof; made of strong, sturdy plastic.
3. Light weight.
4. Flexible and with rounded smooth edges to prevent discomfort if pressed against the nose or ears.
5. Easily disinfected
   a. Surface areas should be smooth to prevent accumulation of infectious material.
   b. Frames and lens should not be damaged or distorted by the disinfectant used.
6. A clear or lightly tinted lens, rather than a very dark lens, on a patient permits the dental team members to watch the patient's reactions and maintain contact and response.
7. Protection against glare. Certain patients may request tinted lenses or prefer to wear their own sunglasses when their eyes are especially sensitive to the dental light.

B. Types of Eyewear

Many styles, including regular eyeglass shapes and those described as follows, have been used.
1. *Goggles* (figure 3–1A). Shielding on all sides of the glasses may give the best protection, provided they fit closely around the edges. Goggle-style coverage is especially necessary for protection during laboratory work.
2. *Eyewear with Side Shields* (figure 3–1B and C). A side shield can provide added protection. For the member of the dental team who de-

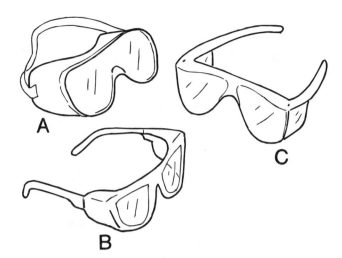

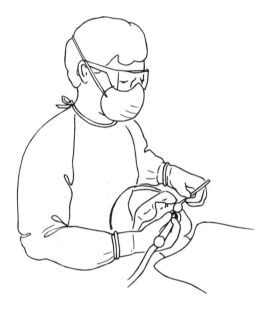

FIG. 3–1. Protective Eyewear. Protective cover for both patient and clinician may be **A.** goggles-style, or **B.** and **C.** glasses with side shields.

pends on a prescription lens, separate side shields are available that can be connected to the bow on each side.

3. *Eyewear with Curved Frames.* When the sides of the eyewear are curved back, they may provide a protection somewhat similar to that offered by those with the side shield.

4. *Postmydriatic Spectacles Used by Ophthalmologist.* Disposable glasses are available that are made of flexible plastic.

5. *Child-Sized.* Child-sized sunglasses and children's play spectacles have been used.

C. Availability

Several pairs of goggles or protective eyewear are maintained to facilitate cleaning and disinfection after each use.

III. SUGGESTIONS FOR CLINICAL APPLICATION

A. Patient Instruction

A patient who has not been asked to wear protective eyewear before needs a simple explanation of the reasons for doing so.

B. Contact Lens

1. Dental team members who wear contact lenses should always wear protective eyewear over them.

2. Patients with contact lenses should be asked to remove them and then use the protective eyewear that is provided.

C. Care of Protective Eyewear

1. Run eyewear under water stream to remove abrasive particles. Rubbing an abrasive agent over the plastic lens creates scratches.

2. Immerse in 2% alkaline glutaraldehyde for disinfection (pages 59–62).[16]

3. Rinse thoroughly after immersion because glutaraldehyde is irritating to eyes and skin.

4. Check periodically for scratches on the lens, and replace appropriately.

HAND CARE

In the infectious process of disease transmission (figure 2–1, page 13), the hands may serve as a *means of transmission* of the blood, saliva, and bacterial plaque from a patient, and the hands, especially under the fingernails, may serve as a *reservoir* for microorganisms. Skin breaks in the hands may serve as a *port of entry* for potentially pathogenic microorganisms.

By caring properly for the hands, using effective washing procedures, and following the basic rules for gloving, primary cross-contamination can be controlled. A conscious effort must be made to keep the gloved hands from touching objects other than the instruments and disinfected parts of the equipment prepared for the immediate patient.

I. BACTERIOLOGY OF THE SKIN[17]

A. Resident Bacteria

Many relatively stable bacteria inhabit the surface epithelium or deeper areas in the ducts of skin glands or depths of hair follicles; they are ultimately shed with the exfoliated surface cells, or with excretions of the skin glands. The flora may be altered by newly introduced pathogens, or reduced by washing. Resident bacteria tend to be less susceptible to destruction by disinfection procedures.

B. Transient Bacteria

Transient bacteria reflect continuous contamination by routine contacts; some bacteria are pathogens and may act temporarily as residents.

They may be washed away or, in the event that a skin break exists, may cause an autogenous infection. Most transients can be removed with soap and water by washing thoroughly and vigorously.

II. HAND CARE
A. Fingernails
1. Maintain clean, smoothly trimmed, short fingernails with well-cared-for cuticles to prevent breaks where microorganisms can enter.
2. Effects of short nails[18]
   a. Make handwashing more effective because of fewer microorganisms harbored under the nails.[19]
   b. Prevent cuts from nail in disposable gloves.
   c. Permit selection of a closer fit of glove; longer glove fingers may be required to protect nails.
   d. Allow greater dexterity during instrumentation.
   e. Decrease chance of patient discomfort.

B. Wristwatch and Jewelry
Remove hand and wrist jewelry at the beginning of the day. Microorganisms can become lodged in crevices of rings, watchbands, and watches, where scrubbing is impossible.

C. Gloves
1. After handwashing, don gloves. Never expose open skin lesions or abrasions to a patient's oral tissues and fluids. The use of gloves is described on pages 48–50.
2. After glove removal, wash hands to remove microorganisms.

HANDWASHING PRINCIPLES

I. RATIONALE
Effective and frequent handwashing can reduce the overall bacterial flora of the skin and prevent the organisms acquired from a patient from becoming skin residents. It is impossible to sterilize the skin, but every attempt must be made to reduce the bacterial flora to a minimum.

II. PURPOSES
The objective of all scrub procedures is to reduce the bacterial flora of the hands to an absolute minimum. An effective scrub procedure can be expected to accomplish the following:
A. Remove surface dirt and transient bacteria.
B. Dissolve the normal greasy film on the skin.
C. Rinse and remove all loosened debris and microorganisms.
D. Provide disinfection with a long-acting antiseptic.

III. FACILITIES
A. Sink
1. Use a sink with a foot pedal or electronic control for water-flow control to avoid contamination to/from faucet handles.
2. For regular sink, turn on water at the beginning and leave on through the entire scrub procedure. Turn faucets off with the towel after drying hands.
3. Scrub around brim of sink with disinfectant. The sink must be of sufficient size so that contact with the inside of the wash basin can be avoided easily. A sink cannot be sterilized and can be highly contaminated.
4. Prevent contamination of uniform by not leaning against the sink.
5. Use a separate area and sink reserved for instrument washing. Contaminated instruments should be removed from the treatment room prior to preparation for the next patient.

B. Soap
1. Use a liquid surgical scrub containing an antimicrobial agent. Povidone-iodine (iodophore) has a broad spectrum of action. Chlorhexidine preparations are used extensively to provide rapid disinfection and a cumulative, persistent (residual) action.
2. Apply from a foot- or knee-activated or electronically controlled dispenser to avoid contamination to and from a hand-operated dispenser or cake soap.
3. Do not use foam hand preparations, alcohol wipes, or other substitutes for handwashing, because many pathogenic microorganisms cannot be destroyed by disinfecting preparations. Rinsing is a very important part of the handwashing procedure.

C. Scrub Brushes
1. Clean brushes with a detergent, and sterilize after each use.
2. Avoid over-vigorous use of a brush to minimize skin abrasion. Skin irritation and abrasion can leave openings for additional cross-contamination.
3. Disposable sponges are available commercially and may be preferred when a scrub brush is traumatic to the skin.
4. Identify brushes by label or color-code for handwashing to prevent mixing with instrument scrub brushes; however, both types are sterilized. Handwashing and instrument cleaning should be accomplished at separate sinks.

D. Towels
1. Obtain towel from a dispenser that requires no contact except with the towel itself,

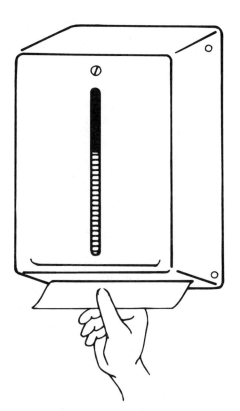

FIG. 3–2. Towel Dispenser. Correct type of dispenser that requires no contact except with the towel itself, which hangs down from the container.

which hangs down from the container (figure 3–2).

2. When a cloth towel is used, it must be used for only one patient.

METHODS OF HANDWASHING

The three methods described here are called the *short scrub, short standard handwash,* and *surgical scrub.* Handwashing methods more often are defined by numbers of latherings and rinsings. Scrub techniques, on the other hand, are best learned in time periods or specific numbers of scrub strokes applied to each area of each hand and arm. The aim of either method is to provide complete coverage and to develop a sequence of performance that can be completed efficiently.

I. SHORT SCRUB

The short scrub handwashing is recommended for the beginning of the day prior to the first gloving, and just prior to the first gloving of any series of appointments. The word "scrub" is used more from a traditional viewpoint, and does not imply that a scrub brush must be used. A sterile soft brush or nail brush may be used, but hard brushing should be avoided if breaks in the skin could result.

The objectives are to remove surface transient bacteria, dirt, and oils from the hands and wrists and to clean under the fingernails.

The procedure outlined here may be expected to take 3 to 5 minutes. Hands are held higher than forearms to allow water to run away from the clean hands.

A. Preliminary Steps
1. Don protective eyewear and mask, and fix hair securely back. Remove watch and all jewelry.
2. Wash hands and wrists briefly, using liquid surgical scrub soap. Leave water running at a moderate speed that does not allow splashing from base and sides of sink. Use cool water.
3. Clean under fingernails with orangewood stick from sterile package. Orangewood stick and soft scrub brush may be packaged together for sterilization when the use of a brush is preferred by the clinician.
4. Rinse from fingertips toward wrists. Keep hands higher than elbows through the entire procedure.

B. First Hand
1. Lather hands.
2. First hand
   a. Brush back and forth across nails and fingertips five times.
   b. Begin with the thumb, use small circular strokes (five strokes each area) on each side of thumb and each finger, then palm, and back of hand. Extend fingers to gain access to each crevice and line.
   c. Scrub wrist on all sides and move to forearm.
   d. When completed, rinse well, from fingertips on up the arm; let water run off at the elbow.

C. Second Hand
1. Rinse the brush and transfer to other hand.
2. Repeat entire procedure.
3. Rinse the hand and arm generously and thoroughly to wash away all transient microorganisms.
4. Dry hands thoroughly.
   a. Take care not to recontaminate hands while drying them.
   b. Use a separate paper towel for each hand.

D. Don Gloves

II. SHORT STANDARD HANDWASH
Handwashing is used after the first glove removal and before and after each succeeding glove application. It is the general procedure for all times except those indicated under the short scrub technique.

Handwashing is considered the most important single procedure for the prevention of cross-contamination and is a basic requirement before and after gloving.

A. Don protective eyewear and mask, and fix hair securely back. Remove watch and all jewelry.
B. Use cool water and liquid surgical scrub soap.
C. Lather hands, wrists, and forearms quickly, rubbing all surfaces vigorously. Interlace fingers and rub back and forth with pressure.
D. Rinse thoroughly, running the water from fingertips down the hands. Keep water running.
E. Repeat 2 more times. One lathering for 3 minutes is less effective than are 3 short latherings and 3 rinses in 30 seconds. The lathering serves to loosen the debris and microorganisms and the rinsings wash them away.
F. Use paper towels for drying, taking care not to recontaminate.

III. SURGICAL SCRUB

Each hospital or oral surgery clinic has rules and regulations for scrub procedures. These should be posted over the scrub sinks.

A surgical scrub performed as the initial scrub of a day should be 10 minutes and subsequent scrubs may be 3 to 5 minutes. Following treatment of a contagious or isolated patient, the scrub should be at least 5 minutes.

A. Preliminary Steps
1. Don protective eyewear, mask, and hair and beard coverings. Make sure hair is completely covered. Remove watch and jewelry.
2. Open sterile brush package to have ready.
3. Wash hands and arms, using surgical liquid soap to remove gross surface dirt before using the scrub brush. Lather vigorously with strong rubbing motions, 10 on each side of hands, wrists, and arms. Interlace the fingers and thumbs to clean the proximal surfaces.
4. Rinse thoroughly from fingertips across hands and wrists. Hold hands higher than elbows throughout the procedure. Leave water running.
5. Use orangewood stick from the sterile package to clean nails. Rinse.

B. First Hand
1. Lather the hands and arms and leave the lather on during the scrub to increase the exposure time to the antimicrobial ingredient.
2. Apply surgical liquid soap, and begin the brush procedure. Scrub in an orderly sequence without returning to areas previously scrubbed.
3. First hand and arm
   a. Brush back and forth across nails and fingertips, passing the brush under the nails.
   b. Fingers and hand. Use small circular strokes on all sides of the thumb and each finger, overlapping strokes for complete coverage.

c. Continue to wrist. Apply more soap to maintain a good lather.
d. When arm is completed, leave lather on.

C. Second Hand
1. Repeat on other arm. Some systems require the use of a second sterile brush for the second hand. When this is so, discard the first brush into the proper container and obtain second brush.
2. At one half of scrub time, rinse hands and arms thoroughly, first one and then the other, starting at the fingertips and letting water pass down over the arm.
3. Lather and repeat.
4. At end of time (or counts), rinse thoroughly, each arm separately, from fingertips. Apply towel from fingertips to elbow without reapplying to hand area.
5. Hold hands up and clasped together. Proceed to dressing area for gowning and gloving.

GLOVES AND GLOVING

Wearing gloves has become standard practice to protect both the patient and the clinician from cross-contamination.

I. CRITERIA FOR SELECTION OF TREATMENT/EXAMINATION GLOVES
A. Safety Factors
1. Effective barrier; minimal manufacturer's defects.
2. Impermeable to patient's saliva, blood, and bacteria.
3. Strength and durability to resist tears and punctures.
4. Impervious to materials routinely used during clinical procedures.
5. Nonirritating or harmful to skin; may need to use nonpowdered or nonlatex gloves when patient or clinician is allergic.

B. Comfort Factors
1. Fit hand well; no interference with motion; glove cuff extends to provide coverage over cuff of long sleeve.
2. Tactile sense minimally decreased.
3. Taste and odor not unpleasant for patient.
4. Optimum powdering with minimal stickiness after wetting.

II. TYPES OF GLOVES
A. Non-sterile examination/treatment: latex, vinyl.
B. Presterilized surgical: latex, vinyl.
C. Utility/housekeeping gloves
   1. Nitrile rubber (heavy duty, puncture resistant, autoclavable): for clinic cleanup, handling instruments during preparation for sterilization.

2. Plastic (food handler's): to wear as overgloves.
3. Copolymer: to wear as overglove.

D. Dermal underglove: to reduce irritation from latex or vinyl.

III. PROCEDURES FOR USE OF GLOVES

A. Mask and Eyewear Placement

Place mask and protective eyewear prior to handwashing and gloving to prevent the need for manipulating the mask around the face and hair after washing the hands.

B. Pregloving Handwash

1. First wash of the day is performed with the short scrub; all other times require the short standard procedure.
2. Hands must be dried thoroughly to control moisture inside glove and thus discourage growth of bacteria.

C. Glove Placement

Place gloves over the cuff of long-sleeved clinic wear to provide complete protection of arms from exposure to contamination.

D. Indications for Double Gloving

1. Clinician who is HBV or HIV positive (or has other communicable problem).

2. Clinician with dermatologic condition that could be secondarily infected by exposure to patient's saliva or blood.
3. Patient who is severely compromised and needs added protection.
4. Patient with known active infectious disease (for example, tuberculosis).

E. Avoiding Contamination

Keep gloved hands away from face, hair, clothing (pockets), telephone, patient records, operating stool, and all parts of the dental equipment that have not been predisinfected and covered with a barrier material.

F. Torn, Cut, or Punctured Glove

Remove immediately, wash hands thoroughly, and don new gloves.

G. Removal of Gloves

1. Develop a procedure whereby gloves can be removed without contaminating the hands from the exposed external surfaces of the gloves. Figure 3–3 illustrates one system for glove removal.
2. Wash hands promptly after glove removal. Organisms on the hands multiply rapidly in-

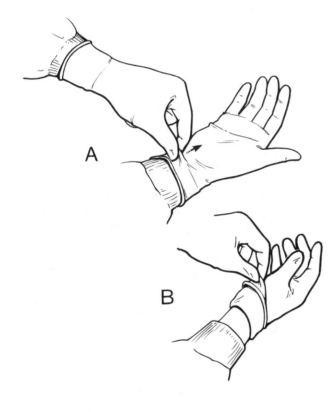
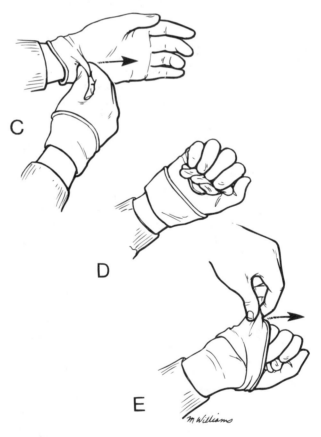

FIG. 3–3. Removal of Gloves. A. Use left fingers to pinch right glove near edge to fold back. **B.** Fold edge back without contact with clean inside surface. **C.** Use right fingers to contact outside of left glove at the wrist to invert and remove. **D.** Bunch glove into the palm. **E.** With ungloved left hand, grasp inner noncontaminated portion of the right glove to peel it off, enclosing other glove as it is inverted.

side the warm, moist environment of the glove, even when no external contamination has occurred.

H. Reuse of Gloves
Disposable, single-use gloves must not be washed or decontaminated for reuse.

TECHNICAL HINTS

I. PATIENT HISTORY
Questions to patient concerning allergies may reveal information about allergy to latex.

II. SKIN INTEGRITY
Small abrasions or cracks of the fingers should be covered with a clear liquid bandage for safety under gloves.

III. FACTORS AFFECTING GLOVE INTEGRITY
A. Length of Time Worn
New pair for each patient is the basic requirement; total time worn should be no longer than 1 hour; when gloves develop a sticky surface, remove, wash hands, and reglove with a fresh pair.

B. Complexity of the Procedure
Certain procedures are more likely to promote perforations, especially when sharp instruments must be changed frequently.

C. Packaging of the Gloves
Top gloves of a new package are tightly packed and can be torn when removed; must be handled carefully until pressure is relieved.

D. Size of Glove
When too long, the extra material at the fingertips can get caught, torn, or in the way; picking up small objects is difficult, especially sharp instruments.

E. Pressure of Time
Stress; working too fast.

F. Storage of Gloves
Keep in cool, dark place; exposure to heat, sun, or fluorescent light increases potential for deterioration and perforations.

G. Agents Used
Certain chemicals react with the glove material, for example, alcohol and products made with alcohol tend to break down the glove integrity.

H. Hazards from the Hands
Long fingernails, rings worn inside gloves.

FACTORS TO TEACH THE PATIENT

I. Importance of the patient's complete history in the protection of both the patient and the professional person.
II. Necessity for use of barriers (face mask, protective eyewear, and gloves) by the clinician for the benefit of the patient.
III. Importance of eye protection for the patient.

REFERENCES

1. **United States Department of Labor,** Occupational Safety and Health Administration: Occupational Exposure to Bloodborne Pathogens; Final Rule, *Federal Register, 56,* No. 235, December 6, 1991.
2. **United States Centers for Disease Control:** Recommendations of the Immunization Practices Advisory Committee (ACIP). General Recommendations on Immunization, *MMWR, 38,* 205, April 7, 1989.
3. **Peter,** G.: Childhood Immunizations, *N. Engl. J. Med., 327,* 1794, December 17, 1992.
4. **United States Centers for Disease Control:** Hepatitis B Virus: A Comprehensive Strategy for Eliminating Transmission in the United States Through Universal Childhood Vaccination, *MMWR, 40,* 1–25, No. RR-13, November 22, 1991.
5. **Benenson,** A.S., ed.: *Control of Communicable Disease in Man,* 15th ed. Washington, D.C., American Public Health Association, 1990, p. 272.
6. **Benenson:** op. cit., pp. 431–432.
7. **United States Centers for Disease Control:** Update on Adult Immunization. Recommendations of the Immunization Practices Advisory Committee (ACIP), *MMWR, 40,* 1–94, No. RR-12, November 15, 1991.
8. **Federation Dentaire Internationale,** Commission on Dental Practice: Technical Report: Recommendations for Hygiene in Dental Practice, *Int. Dent. J., 29,* 72, March, 1979.
9. **United States Centers for Disease Control:** Guidelines for Preventing the Transmission of Tuberculosis in Health-care Settings, With Special Focus on HIV-related Issues, *MMWR, 39,* 1–27, No. RR-17, December 7, 1990.
10. **Micik,** R.E., Miller, R.L., and Leong, A.C.: Studies on Dental Aerobiology: III. Efficacy of Surgical Masks in Protecting Dental Personnel from Airborne Bacterial Particles, *J. Dent. Res., 50,* 626, May–June, 1971.
11. **Miller,** R.L. and Micik, R.E.: Air Pollution and Its Control in the Dental Office, *Dent. Clin. North Am., 22,* 453, July, 1978.
12. **Hartley,** J.L.: Eye and Facial Injuries Resulting from Dental Procedures, *Dent. Clin. North Am., 22,* 505, July, 1978.
13. **Colvin,** J.: Eye Injuries and the Dentist, *Aust. Dent. J., 23,* 453, December, 1978.
14. **Cooley,** R.L., Cottingham, A.J., Abrams, H., and Barkmeier, W.W.: Ocular Injuries Sustained in the Dental Office: Methods of Detection, Treatment, and Prevention, *J. Am. Dent. Assoc., 97,* 985, December, 1978.
15. **Wesson,** M.D. and Thornton, J.B.: Eye Protection and Ocular Complications in the Dental Office, *Gen. Dent., 37,* 19, January–February, 1989.
16. **Gleason,** M.J. and Molinari, J.A.: Stability of Safety Glasses Dur-

ing Sterilization and Disinfection, *J. Am. Dent. Assoc., 115,* 60, July, 1987.

17. **Gröschel,** D.H.M. and Pruett, T.L.: Surgical Antisepsis, in Block, S.S.: *Disinfection, Sterilization, and Preservation,* 4th ed. Philadelphia, Lea & Febiger, 1991, pp. 642–648.

18. **Harfst,** S.A.: Personal Barrier Protection, *Dent. Clin. North Am., 35,* 357, April, 1991.

19. **Allen,** A.L. and Organ, R.J.: Occult Blood Accumulation Under the Fingernails: A Mechanism for the Spread of Bloodborne Infection, *J. Am. Dent. Assoc., 105,* 455, September, 1982.

SUGGESTED READINGS

Christensen, R.P., Robison, R.A., Robinson, D.F., Ploeger, B.J., and Leavitt, R.W.: Efficiency of 42 Brands of Face Masks and Two Face Shields in Preventing Inhalation of Airborne Debris, *Gen. Dent., 39,* 414, November/December, 1991.

Cottone, J.A., Terezhalmy, G.T., and Molinari, J.A.: *Practical Infection Control in Dentistry.* Philadelphia, Lea & Febiger, 1991, pp. 98–104.

Craig, D.C. and Quale, A.A.: The Efficacy of Face-masks, *Br. Dent. J., 158,* 87, February 9, 1985.

Edwards, K.M., Decker, M.D., Graham, B.S., Mezzatesta, J., Scott, J., and Hackell, J.: Adult Immunization With Acellular Pertussis Vaccine, *JAMA, 269,* 53, January 6, 1993.

Gardner, P. and Schaffner, W.: Immunization of Adults, *N. Engl. J. Med., 328,* 1252, April 29, 1993.

Genz, D.: Hand Care, *Dent. Teamwork, 2,* 176, September–October, 1989.

McGinley, K.J., Larson, E.L., and Leyden, J.J.: Composition and Density of Micro-flora in the Subungual Space of the Hand, *J. Clin. Microbiol., 26,* 950, May, 1988.

Miller, C.: Protection Goes Both Ways, *RDH, 11,* 34, September, 1991.

Miller, C.: Handwashing Fights Disease, *RDH, 9,* 30, December, 1989.

Miller, C.H. and Cottone, J.A.: The Basic Principles of Infectious Diseases as Related to Dental Practice, *Dent. Clin. North. Am., 37,* 1, January, 1993.

Nash, K.D.: How Infection Control Procedures Are Affecting Dental Practice Today, *J. Am. Dent. Assoc., 123,* 67, March, 1992.

Pacak-Carroll, D.: Remember Eye Protection is Necessary for Patients Too, *RDH, 12,* 14, June, 1992.

Shingleton, B.J.: Eye Injuries, *N. Engl. J. Med., 325,* 408, August 8, 1991.

Stokes, A.N., Burton, J.F., and Beale, R.P.: Eye Protection in Dental Practice, *N.Z. Dent. J., 86,* 14, January, 1990.

Wood, P.R.: *Cross Infection Control in Dentistry: A Practical Illustrated Guide.* St. Louis, The C.V. Mosby Co., 1992, pp. 37–74.

Zimmerman, R.K. and Giebink, G.S.: Childhood Immunizations: A Practical Approach for Clinicians, *Am. Fam. Physicians, 45,* 1759, April, 1992.

Gloves

Baumann, M.A.: Protective Gloves, *Int. Dent. J., 42,* 170, June, 1992.

Brownson, K.M. and Gobetti, J.P.: Fluorescein Dye Evaluation of Double-gloving, *Gen. Dent., 38,* 362, September–October, 1990.

Brunick, A.L., Burns, S., Gross, K., Tishk, M., and Feil, P.: A Comparative Study: The Effects of Latex and Vinyl Gloves on the Tactile Discrimination of First Year Dental Hygiene Students, *Clin. Prev. Dent., 12,* 21, June–July, 1990.

Burke, F.J.T. and Wilson, N.H.F.: The Incidence of Undiagnosed Punctures in Non-sterile Gloves, *Br. Dent. J., 168,* 67, January 20, 1990.

Dietz, E.R.: The Use of Gloves in Dentistry, *Dent. Assist., 58,* 6, January–February, 1989.

Field, E.A. and Jedynakiewicz, N.M.: A Practical Gloving and Handwashing Regimen for Dental Practice, *Br. Dent. J., 172,* 111, February 8, 1992.

Glang-Yetter, C., Torabinejad, M., and Torabinejad, A.: An Investigation on the Safety of Rewashed Gloves, *J. Dent. Hyg., 63,* 358, October, 1989.

Katz, J.N., Gobetti, J.P., and Shipman, C.: Fluorescein Dye Evaluation of Glove Integrity, *J. Am. Dent. Assoc., 118,* 327, March, 1989.

Klein, R.C., Party, E., and Gershey, E.L.: Virus Penetration of Examination Gloves, *Biotechniques, 9,* 197, No. 2, 1990.

Korniewiez, D., Laughon, B.E., Butz, A., and Larson, E.: Integrity of Vinyl and Latex Procedure Gloves, *Nurs. Res., 38,* 144, May–June, 1989.

Moore, R.L. and Brantley, S.W.: Frequency of Glove Perforations, *J. Clin. Orthod., 24,* 294, May, 1990.

Munksgaard, E.C.: Permeability of Protective Gloves to (di)Methacrylates in Resinous Dental Materials, *Scand. J. Dent. Res., 100,* 189, June, 1992.

Otis, L.L. and Cottone, J.A.: Prevalence of Perforations in Disposable Latex Gloves During Routine Dental Treatment, *J. Am. Dent. Assoc., 118,* 321, March, 1989.

Smart, E.R., Macleod, R.I., and Lawrence, C.M.: Allergic Reactions to Rubber Gloves in Dental Patients: Report of Three Cases, *Br. Dent. J., 172,* 445, June 20, 1992.

Tolle, L.: Gloving: Practical Guidelines for Dental Hygienists, *Dentalhygienistnews, 2,* 1, Summer, 1989.

Wright, J.G., McGeer, A.J., Chyatte, D., and Ransohoff, D.F.: Mechanisms of Glove Tears and Sharp Injuries Among Surgical Personnel, *JAMA, 266,* 1668, September 25, 1991.

Infection Control: Clinical Procedures

The success of a planned system for control of disease transmission depends on the cooperative effort of each member of the dental health team. The aim is to provide the highest level of infection control possible and practical that will ensure a safe environment for both patient and professionals.

The presence of disease-producing organisms is not always known; therefore, application of protective, preventive procedures is needed prior to, during, and following *all* patient appointments. Definitions and abbreviations related to infection control are provided in table 4–1.

I. OBJECTIVES OF INFECTION CONTROL[1]

The following are necessary to prevent the transmission of infectious agents and eliminate cross-contamination:

A. Reduction of available pathogenic microorganisms to a level at which the normal resistance mechanisms of the body may prevent infection.

B. Elimination of cross-contamination by breaking the chain of infection (see figure 2–1, page 13).

C. Application of universal precautions by treating each patient as if all human blood and certain human body fluids are known to be infectious for HIV, HBV, and other blood-borne pathogens.

II. BASIC CONSIDERATIONS FOR SAFE PRACTICE

Basic factors involved in the conduct of safe practice include the material in Chapter 3 and the following, to be described in this chapter:

A. Treatment room features.

B. Instrument management.
  1. Precleaning.
  2. Sterilization and disinfection.

C. Preparation for appointment.

D. Unit water lines.

E. Environmental surfaces.

F. Care of sterile instruments.

G. Patient preparation.

H. Summary of procedures for the prevention of disease transmission.

I. Disposal of waste.

TREATMENT ROOM FEATURES

The current design of many treatment rooms may not be conducive to ideal planning for infection control. Changes can be made in routines so that updated, preferred systems can be adapted. When renovations or a new dental office or clinic are anticipated, plans must reflect the most advanced knowledge available relative to safety and disease control.

A partial list of notable features is included here. The objective is to have materials, shapes, and surface textures that facilitate the use of infection control measures.

  1. UNIT
    —Designed for easy cleaning and disinfection, with smooth, uncluttered surfaces.
    —Removable hoses that can be cleaned and disinfected.
    —Hoses that are not mechanically retractable, but are straight, not coiled, with round smooth outer surfaces.
    —Syringes with removable autoclavable tips or fitted for disposable tips.
    —Handpieces with anti-retraction valves.
    —Handpieces that can be autoclaved.

TABLE 4-1
KEY WORDS AND ABBREVIATIONS: INFECTION CONTROL

ADA: American Dental Association, 211 E. Chicago Ave., Chicago, IL 60611.

Antimicrobial agent (an′tĭ-mĭ-kro′bē-al): any agent that kills or suppresses the growth of microorganisms.

Antiseptic (an′tĭ-sep′tik): a substance that prevents or arrests the growth or action of microorganisms either by inhibiting their activity or by destroying them; term used especially for preparations applied topically to living tissue.

Asepsis (ă-sep′sĭs): free from contamination with microorganisms; includes sterile conditions in tissues and on materials, as obtained by exclusion, removing, or killing organisms.

   Chain of asepsis: a procedure that avoids transfer of infection. The "chain" implies that each step, related to the previous one, continues to be carried out without contamination.

Aseptic technique: procedures carried out in the absence of pathogenic microorganisms.

Bioburden: a microbiologic load, that is, the number of contaminating organisms present on a surface prior to sterilization or on a surface prior to disinfection.

Biofilm: the surface film that contains microorganisms and other biologic substances.

Biohazard: a substance that poses a biologic risk because it is contaminated with biomaterial with a potential for transmitting infection.

Biologic indicator: a preparation of nonpathogenic microorganisms, usually bacterial spores, carried by an ampule or a specially impregnated paper enclosed within a package during sterilization and subsequently incubated to verify that sterilization has occurred.

Broad spectrum: indicates a range of activity of a drug or chemical substance against a wide variety of microorganisms.

Chemical indicator: a color change stripe or other mark, often on autoclave tape or bag, used to monitor the process of sterilization; color change indicates that the package has been brought to a specific temperature, but is not an indicator of sterilization.

Contamination (kon-tam ĭ-nă′shun): introduction of microorganisms, blood, or other potentially infectious material or agent onto a surface or into tissue.

Decontamination (dē kon-tam-ĭ-na′shun): disinfection; use of physical or chemical means to remove, inactivate, or destroy pathogenic microorganisms on a surface or item to the extent that they are no longer capable of transmitting infectious disease; the surface or item is rendered safe for handling, use, or disposal.

Disinfectant (dis ĭn-fek′tant): an agent, usually a chemical, but may be a physical agent, such as X rays or ultraviolet light, that destroys microorganisms but may not kill bacterial spores; refers to substances applied to inanimate objects.

EPA: United States Environmental Protection Agency, Washington, DC.

   EPA registered: number on a label indicates that the product has the acceptance of EPA.

FDA: United States Food and Drug Administration, 5600 Fishers Lane, Rockville, MD 20857; regulates food, drugs, biologic products, medical devices, radiologic products.

Infection control: the selection and use of procedures and products to prevent the spread of infectious disease.

Infectious waste: contaminated with blood, saliva, or other substances; potentially or actually infected with pathogenic material; officially called "regulated" waste.

Nosocomial (nos ō-kō′mē-al) **infection:** an infection occurring in a patient while in a health-care facility that was not present at the time of admission; includes infections acquired in the health-care facility but appearing after dismissal.

OSAP: Office Sterilization and Asepsis Procedures Research Foundation, 2150 West 29th Ave., Suite 500,

OSHA: United States Occupational Safety and Health Administration, Department of Labor, Washington, DC 20210.

Sanitation: the process by which the number of organisms on inanimate objects is reduced to a safe level. It does not imply freedom from microorganisms, and generally refers to a cleaning process.

Shelf life: stability of an item after it has been prepared; length of time a substance or preparation can be kept without changes occurring in its chemical structure or other properties.

Sporicide (spō′rĭ-sīd): substance that kills spores.

Sterilization: process by which all forms of life, including bacterial spores, are destroyed by physical or chemical means.

Synergism (sin′er-jizm): the joint action of agents so that their combined effect is greater than the sum of their individual parts.

Waste:

   Infectious waste: capable of causing an infectious disease.

   Contaminated waste: items that have contacted blood or other body secretions.

   Hazardous waste: poses a risk to humans or the environment.

   Toxic waste: capable of having a poisonous effect.

   Regulated waste: contaminated, hazardous, and otherwise useless waste that requires special disposal methods outlined by the OSHA.

2. DENTAL CHAIR
   —Controls all foot-operated. If manually operated, overlay to cover buttons (switches) that can be removed for disinfection is needed.
   —Surface and seamless finish of easily cleaned plastic material that withstands chemical disinfection without discoloring; cloth upholstery to be avoided.
3. LIGHT
   —Foot-activated switches.
   —Removable handle for sterilization.
4. CLINICIAN'S STOOL
   —Smooth, plastic material that is easily disinfected and has a minimum of seams and creases.
   —Foot-operated controls. If manually operated, must have a barrier cover for the control.
5. FLOOR
   —Carpeting should be avoided.
   —Floor covering should be smooth, easily cleaned, nonabsorbent.
6. SINK
   —Wide and deep enough for effective handwashing to the elbows.
   —Water and soap with electronic, "knee," or foot-operated controls.
   —Separate room or area for contaminated instrument care.
7. SUPPLIES
   —All sterilizable or disposable.
8. WASTE
   —Receptacle with opening large enough to prevent contact with sides when material is dropped in.
   —Heavy-duty plastic bag liner to be sealed tightly for disposal.
   —Small receptacle bag near treatment area to receive contaminated sponges and other waste. Small bag to be tied tightly for disposal in large waste receiver.

INSTRUMENT MANAGEMENT

The successful practice of universal precautions to prevent cross-contamination depends on the development of, and strict adherence to, a planned program for instrument management. A good rule is to learn the most effective, safe system, and then to follow that method without exception. A specific routine is easier for the dental team group to follow, and peer review is built-in.

The basic steps in the recirculation of instruments from the time an appointment procedure is completed until the instruments are sterilized and ready for use in the next clinical appointment are shown in the flowchart in figure 4–1. Each of the steps is described in the following sections.

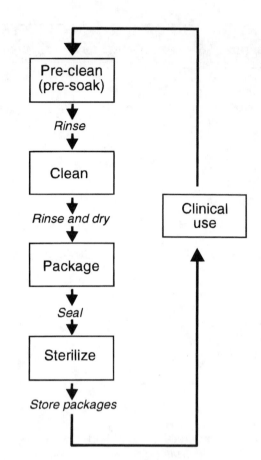

FIG. 4–1. Recirculation of Instruments. Flowchart shows step-by-step process. At the completion of treatment, instruments are cleaned, packaged, sterilized, and stored. They are kept sealed until patient appointment begins.

PRESOAKING/PRECLEANING[2]

Cleaning is more difficult when saliva and blood are left on instruments for a period of time after use in the treatment appointment. If the cleaning process cannot be accomplished immediately, a container with a holding solution of a mild disinfectant/detergent should be available in which to place the used instruments.

When a cassette is not used, the instruments can be placed directly into the basket for later submergence into the ultrasonic cleaner. The basket can be placed in the soaking solution. By doing so, one less handling of the instruments is required. When a cassette is used, the instruments are arranged in the cassette, which then carries the instruments through the entire preclean and sterilization procedure.

The presoaking/precleaning step is intended for a short period of time. Nonstainless instruments can corrode and discolor unless removed for cleaning.

Contaminated instruments and equipment must be moved to a separate area set aside for the specific purpose of infection control. Cleaning and preparation for sterilization are accomplished apart from treatment rooms.[3]

CLEANING

Ideally the instruments are contained within a cassette so that little or no handling is required. When instruments are not in a cassette, sterilized transfer forceps kept for the purpose of handling contaminated instruments can provide another means for accident prevention.

For all cleaning processes, heavy-duty, puncture-resistant gloves must be used, and a face mask and protective eyewear must be worn. The two methods for cleaning instruments are ultrasonic processing and manual cleaning.

I. ULTRASONIC PROCESSING

Ultrasonic cleaning prior to sterilization is safer than manual cleaning. Manual cleaning of instruments is a difficult and time-consuming procedure with numerous disadvantages.

When ultrasonic equipment is adjusted for optimum performance and those using it are properly informed and adhere to the manufacturer's instructions, the *quality* of cleaning is much better than that obtained by the handscrub technique. *Ultrasonic processing is not a substitute for sterilization; it is only a cleaning process.*

A. Advantages

Benefits from the use of ultrasonic cleaning include the following:
1. Increased efficiency in obtaining a high degree of cleanliness.
2. Reduced danger to clinician from direct contact with potentially pathogenic microorganisms.
3. Improved effectiveness for disinfection.
4. Elimination of possible dissemination of microorganisms through release of aerosols and droplets, which can occur during the scrubbing process.
5. Penetration into areas of the instruments where the bristles of a brush may be unable to contact.
6. Removal of tarnish.

B. Procedure
1. Guard against overloading; the solution must contact all surfaces.
2. Dismantle instruments with detachable parts, such as the mirror from the handle. Open jointed instruments.
3. Time accurately by manufacturer's guide.
4. Drain; rinse, and air dry to avoid handling; if towels are used, pat dry carefully.
5. Indications for thorough drying
   a. When sterilizing by dry heat, chemical vapor, or ethylene oxide.

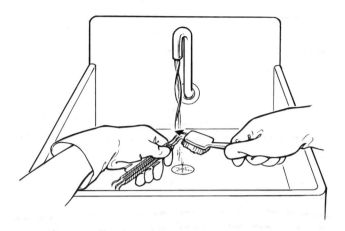

FIG. 4–2. Manual Preparation of Instruments for Sterilization. Heavy-duty gloves are worn and a long-handled brush is used to aid in the prevention of cross-contamination. Note arrow showing direction of scrub strokes away from the clinician and in a deep sink to avoid splashing.

   b. Nonstainless steel instruments require predip in rust inhibitor before steam autoclaving; water on instruments dilutes the solution.
   c. Instruments to be packaged in paper wrap.

II. MANUAL CLEANING

Ultrasonic processing is the method of choice, but when manual cleaning is the only alternative, the possibility for accidents is greater because more direct handling of the instruments is required.

A. Procedure
1. Dismantle instruments with detachable parts. Open jointed instruments.
2. Use detergent and scrub with a long-handled brush under running water; hold the instruments low in the sink (figure 4–2).
3. Brush with strokes away from the body; use care not to splash and contaminate the surrounding area.
4. Rinse thoroughly.
5. Dry on paper towels (same reasons as those listed for ultrasonic processing).

B. Care of Brushes
Soak and wash contaminated brushes in detergent; rinse thoroughly and sterilize.

PACKAGING

There are several ways of arranging instruments and equipment for sterilization after manual and/or ultrasonic cleaning. Preset cassettes, trays, or packages can be preplanned to contain all the items usually needed for a particular appointment.

Each tray or package should be dated and marked for identification of contents: for example, *Adult Scaling and Root Planing; Examination.*

I. WRAP SELECTION

Each method of sterilization has specific requirements, and the manufacturer's recommendations can be reviewed. Sturdy wrapping is necessary to prevent punctures or tears that break the chain of asepsis and require a repeat of the process.

II. PRESET ARRANGEMENTS OF INSTRUMENTS

Selected instruments for a given procedure can be arranged in a cassette, on an open tray that fits into a large see-through sterilizing bag, or in smaller bags that can be poured out, untouched, on predisinfected trays with paper covers.

Gauze sponges, cotton swabs, and other accessories can be included in the tray arrangements, or can be made up in small packages for opening as needed.

III. CHEMICAL INDICATOR FOR CYCLE MONITORING

Chemical indicator tape is used to seal all packages, except when the wrap has built-in indicators. The chemical, usually in the form of a series of stripes, changes color during the sterilization process. The change of color means that the temperature reached a designated height required for penetration and that the contact time was adequate (figure 4–3). Distinct black stripes should appear. A lighter color change may be a warning signal that the autoclave function should be checked.

Indicator tape does not serve to test for true sterilization. A biologic indicator in the form of microbial spores must be used to test each sterilizer routinely.

The striped indicator tape is left on the sealed package and thereby serves to identify those packages ready for use. Packages are kept completely sealed until unwrapped in front of the patient.

STERILIZATION

I. APPROVED METHODS

Each of the methods listed here is described in detail in the sections following. Table 4–2 summarizes the operating requirements of each.

    A. Moist heat: steam under pressure.
    B. Dry heat.
    C. Chemical vapor.
    D. Ethylene oxide.

II. SELECTION OF METHOD

All materials and items cannot be treated by the same system of sterilization. Supplement with disposable one-use products when sterilization is not possible.

The method for sterilization that is selected must provide complete destruction of all microorganisms, viruses, and spores, and yet must not damage the instruments and other materials treated. In addition, the procedures must not be complex, with many chances for errors in the processing.

Careful, specific use of sterilizing equipment in accord with the manufacturer's specifications is necessary. Incomplete sterilization most frequently results from inadequate preparation of the materials to be sterilized (cleaning, packaging), misuse of the equipment (overloading, timing, temperature selection), or inadequate maintenance.

III. TESTS FOR STERILIZATION

Sterilization is the process by which all forms of life are destroyed. That definition provides the rationale for

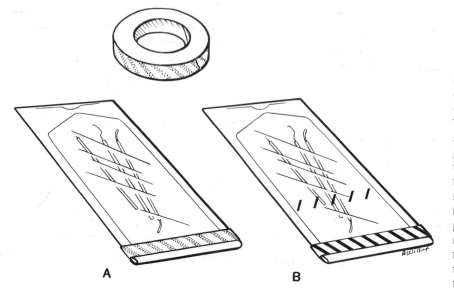

FIG. 4–3. Process Indicator Tape. A. Before autoclaving. **B.** After autoclaving. The change of color in the stripes indicates that the package has been subjected to the proper temperature for sterilization, but does not show sterilization. A biologic indicator is also needed for periodic monitoring to determine that the autoclave is functioning properly and that sterilization is actually taking place.

TABLE 4–2
METHODS OF STERILIZATION

Method	Sterilizing Requirement		
	Time	Temperature	Pressure
Moist Heat Steam under Pressure (Steam Autoclave)	15 minutes	250°F 121°C	15 psi
Dry Heat Oven	120 minutes	320°F 160°C	
Unsaturated Chemical Vapor	20 minutes	270°F 132°C	20–40 psi
Ethylene Oxide Gas	10–16 hours	75°F 25°C	

TABLE 4–3
SPORE TESTING

When	Why
Once per week	To verify proper use and functioning
Whenever a new type of packaging material or tray is used	To ensure that the sterilizing agent is getting inside to the surface of the instruments
After training of new sterilization personnel	To verify proper use of the sterilizer
During initial uses of a new sterilizer	To make sure unfamiliar operating instructions are being followed
First run after repair of a sterilizer	To make sure that the sterilizer is functioning properly
With every implantable device and hold device until results of test are known	Extra precaution for sterilization of item to be implanted into tissues
After any other change in the sterilizing procedure	To make sure change does not prevent sterilization

Adapted from Miller, C.H. and Palenik, C.J.: Sterilization, Disinfection, and Asepsis in Dentistry, in Block, S.S.: *Disinfection, Sterilization, and Preservation,* 4th ed. Philadelphia, Lea & Febiger, 1991, p. 680.

testing whether a sterilizer is working properly. The testing system requires the use of selected test microorganisms that are put through a regular cycle of sterilization and then are cultured. When no growth occurs, the sterilizer has performed adequately.

A. Microorganisms Used
1. *Steam Autoclave. Bacillus stearothermophilus* in vials, ampules, or on strips.
2. *Dry Heat Oven. Bacillus subtilis* strips.
3. *Chemical Vapor. Bacillus stearothermophilus* on strips.
4. *Ethylene Oxide. Bacillus subtilis* strips.

B. Procedures
The ampule, vial, or strip is placed in the center of a package, which in turn is placed in the middle of the load of packages to be sterilized. After the cycle has been completed at the customary time and temperature, the ampule or strip is incubated. Ampules and vials show the color change associated with no living microorganisms, whereas the strip organisms are cultured, and show no growth if the sterilizer has performed properly.

Table 4–3 shows indications for performing spore tests in dental settings. Records that are kept should show dates and outcomes.

IV. THE CHEMICAL INDICATOR
In contrast to spore testing, the chemical indicator is related only to the temperature to which the autoclave was heated. As described on page 56, a chemical indicator is used routinely when packaging instruments (figure 4–3).

MOIST HEAT: STEAM UNDER PRESSURE

Destruction of microorganisms by heat takes place as a result of inactivation of essential cellular proteins or enzymes. Moist heat causes coagulation of protein.

I. USE
Moist heat may be used for all materials except oils, waxes, and powders that are impervious to steam, or materials that cannot be subjected to high temperatures.

II. PRINCIPLES OF ACTION
A. Sterilization is achieved by action of heat and moisture; pressure serves only to attain high temperature.
B. Sterilization depends on the penetrating ability of steam.
   1. Air must be excluded, otherwise steam penetration and heat transfer are prevented.
   2. Space between objects is essential to assure access for the steam.
   3. Materials must be thoroughly cleaned; adherent material can provide a barrier to the steam.
   4. Air discharge occurs in a downward direction; load must be arranged for free passage of steam toward bottom of autoclave.

III. OPERATION
A. Packing Autoclave
Pack loosely to permit steam to reach all instruments in all packages; place jars or tall vessels on their sides to permit air to leave as steam enters.

B. Standard Procedure
121°C (250°F) at 15 pounds pressure for 15 minutes after the meters show that proper pressure and temperature have been reached. Use 30 minutes for heavy loads to assure penetration.

C. Cooling
1. *Dry Materials.* Release steam pressure, turn operating valve, and open the door; required time for drying, about 15 minutes.
2. *Liquids.* Reduce chamber pressure slowly at an even rate over 10 to 12 minutes to prevent boiling or escape of fluids into the chamber; preferable to turn off the autoclave and let the pressure fall before opening the door. Check heat sensitivity of each solution and avoid prolonged exposure, as indicated.

IV. CARE OF AUTOCLAVE
A. Daily
Maintain proper level of distilled water; wash trays and interior surfaces of chamber with water and a mild detergent; clean removable plug, screen, or strainer.

B. Weekly
Flush chamber discharge system with an appropriate cleaning solution, such as hot trisodium phosphate or a commercial cleaner.

V. EVALUATION OF STEAM UNDER PRESSURE
A. Advantages
1. All microorganisms, spores, and viruses destroyed quickly and efficiently.
2. Wide variety of materials may be treated; most economical method of sterilization.

B. Disadvantages
1. May corrode carbon steel instruments if precautions are not taken.
2. Unsuitable for oils or powders that are impervious to heat.

DRY HEAT

The action of dry heat is oxidation.

I. USE
A. Primarily for materials that cannot safely be sterilized with steam under pressure.
B. Oils and powders when they are thermostabile at the required temperatures.

C. For small metal instruments enclosed in special containers or that might be corroded or rusted by moisture, such as endodontic instruments.

II. PRINCIPLES OF ACTION
A. Sterilization is achieved by heat that is conducted from the exterior surface to the interior of the object; the time required to penetrate varies among materials.
B. Sterilization can result when the whole material is treated for a sufficient length of time at the specified temperature; therefore, timing for sterilization must start when the entire contents of the sterilizer have reached the peak temperature needed for that load.
C. Oil, grease, or organic debris on instruments insulates and protects microorganisms from the sterilizing effect.

III. OPERATION
A. Temperature
160°C (320°F) held for 2 hours; 170°C (340°F) for 1 hour. Timing must start after the desired temperature has been reached.

B. Penetration Time
Heat penetration varies with different materials, and the nature and properties of various materials must be considered.

C. Care
Care must be taken not to overheat because certain materials can be affected. Temperatures over 160°C (320°F) may destroy the sharp edges of cutting instruments; over 170°C, paper and cotton materials begin to scorch.

IV. EVALUATION OF DRY HEAT
A. Advantages
1. Useful for materials that cannot be subjected to steam under pressure.
2. When maintained at correct temperature, it is well suited for sharp instruments.
3. No corrosion as found with steam under pressure.

B. Disadvantages
1. Long exposure required; penetration slow and uneven.
2. High temperature critical to certain materials.

CHEMICAL VAPOR STERILIZER[4]

A combination of alcohols, formaldehyde, ketone, water, and acetone heated under pressure produces a gas that is effective as a sterilizing agent.

I. USE

Chemical vapor sterilization cannot be used for materials or objects that can be altered by the chemicals that make the vapor or that cannot withstand the high temperature. Examples are low-melting plastics, liquids, or heat-sensitive handpieces.

II. PRINCIPLES OF ACTION

Microbial and viral destruction results from the permeation of the heated formaldehyde and alcohol. Heavy, tightly wrapped or sealed packages would not permit the penetration of the vapors.

III. OPERATION

A. Temperature

127° to 132°C (260° to 270°F) with 20 to 40 pounds pressure in accord with the manufacturer's directions.

B. Time

Minimum of 20 minutes after the correct temperature has been attained. Time should be extended for a large load or a heavy wrap.

C. Cooling at the Completion of the Cycle

Instruments are dry. Larger instruments may need a short period for cooling.

IV. CARE OF STERILIZER

Depending on the amount of use, refilling is needed by at least every 30 cycles. In accord with manufacturer's instructions, the condensate tray is removed, the exhausted solution emptied, and the tray cleaned.

V. EVALUATION OF CHEMICAL VAPOR STERILIZER

A. Advantages

1. Corrosion- and rust-free operation for carbon steel instruments.
2. Ability to sterilize in a relatively short total cycle.
3. Ease of operation and care of the equipment.

B. Disadvantages

1. Adequate ventilation is needed; cannot use in a small room.
2. Slight odor, which is rarely objectionable.

ETHYLENE OXIDE[5]

Gaseous sterilization using ethylene oxide is not commonly found in a private dental office or clinic, but rather in hospitals and larger clinics. As compact units are developed, ethylene oxide will be more widely used in dentistry.

I. USE

Nearly all materials, whether metal, plastic, rubber, or cloth, can be sterilized in ethylene oxide with little or no damage to the material.

II. PRINCIPLES OF ACTION

Ethylene oxide vapor is effective against all types and forms of microorganisms provided sufficient time is allowed.

III. OPERATION

Specific operation is related to the type of equipment. Operation in a well-ventilated room is necessary. Overnight processing is usually the most practical.

A. Time and Temperature

The time may vary from 2 to 12 hours, depending on both the temperature and the concentration of ethylene oxide used.

B. Aeration After Completion of the Cycle

Plastic and rubber products need to be aerated at least 24 hours. Metal instruments can be used immediately.

IV. EVALUATION OF ETHYLENE OXIDE

A. Advantages

1. Many types of materials can be sterilized with minimum or no damage to the material itself. There is no damage to the finest instruments.
2. Low temperature for operation.

B. Disadvantages

1. High cost of the equipment.
2. Problems of dispersement of gaseous exhaust. Need for planned and tested ventilation.
3. Increased time of operation.
4. Gas absorption requires airing of plastic, rubber, and cloth goods for several hours.

CHEMICAL DISINFECTANTS

Disinfection does not accomplish complete destruction of all forms of microorganisms; therefore, it is not a substitute for sterilization. The object is to reduce the level of microbial contamination to a safe level. The term decontamination may also be applied.

Chemical disinfectants are used in several forms, including the surface disinfectants, immersion disinfectants, immersion sterilants, and hand antimicrobials. Each variety has specific chemicals, dilutions, and directions for application. The use of surface disinfectants is described on page 61, immersion sterilants on page 62, and hand antimicrobials on page 46.

I. CATEGORIES

Disinfectants are categorized by their biocidal activity as high level, intermediate level, or low level. Biocidal activity refers to the ability of the chemical disinfectant to destroy or inactivate living organisms.

A. High Level

High-level disinfectants inactivate spores and all forms of bacteria, fungi, and viruses. Applied at different time schedules, the high-level chemical is either a disinfectant or a sterilant.

B. Intermediate Level

Intermediate-level disinfectants inactivate all forms of microorganisms, but do not destroy spores.

C. Low Level

Low-level disinfectants inactivate vegetative bacteria and certain lipid-type viruses, but do not destroy spores, tubercle bacilli, or nonlipid viruses.

II. USES

A. Environmental Surfaces Disinfection

Following each appointment, the treatment area is cleaned and disinfected (pages 63–64).

B. Precleaning: Holding Solution

After use, instruments are placed in a disinfecting solution until cleaning and preparation for sterilization can be accomplished (page 54).

C. Dental Laboratory Impressions and Prostheses

Impressions can be carriers of infectious material to a dental laboratory, and completed prostheses must be disinfected before delivery to a patient. References may be found with the Suggested Readings at the end of Chapter 10 (page 179).

III. PRINCIPLES OF ACTION

A. Disinfection is achieved by coagulation, precipitation, or oxidation of protein of microbial cells or denaturation of the enzymes of the cells.

B. Disinfection depends on the contact of the solution at the known effective concentration for the optimum period of time.

C. Items must be thoroughly cleaned and dried, because action of the agent is altered by foreign matter and dilution.

D. A solution has a specific shelf life, use life, and reuse life. Some may be altered by changes in pH, or the active ingredient may decrease in potency. Check manufacturer's directions.

IV. CRITERIA FOR SELECTION OF A CHEMICAL AGENT

The objective is to select a product that is effective in the control of microorganisms and practical to use. Properties of an ideal disinfectant are shown in table 4–4.

The manufacturer's informational literature and container labels must provide facts about the product that assure its effectiveness. After the product has been

---

TABLE 4–4
PROPERTIES OF AN IDEAL DISINFECTANT

1. Broad spectrum:
   Should always have the widest possible antimicrobial spectrum.
2. Fast acting:
   Should always have a rapidly lethal action on all vegetative forms and spores of bacteria and fungi, protozoa, and viruses.
3. Not affected by physical factors:
   Active in the presence of organic matter, such as blood, sputum, and feces.
   Should be compatible with soaps, detergents, and other chemicals encountered in use.
4. Nontoxic
5. Surface compatibility:
   Should not corrode instruments and other metallic surfaces.
   Should not cause the disintegration of cloth, rubber, plastics, or other materials.
6. Residual effect on treated surfaces
7. Easy to use
8. Odorless:
   An inoffensive odor would facilitate its routine use.
9. Economical:
   Cost should not be prohibitively high.

From Molinari, J.A., Gleason, M.J., Cottone, J.A., and Barrett, E.D.: Comparison of Dental Surface Disinfectants, *Gen. Dent., 35,* 171, May–June, 1987.

---

selected, it is the responsibility of the dental personnel to use it as directed to obtain the best possible infection control. When the label has insufficient information, the manufacturer should be contacted and instructions obtained.

The criteria should include at least the following:

A. EPA approval.

B. Chemicals must be tuberculocidal, bacteriocidal, virucidal, and fungicidal.

C. Label must state
   1. Effectiveness and stability expressed by
      a. Shelf life: the expiration date indicating the termination of effectiveness of the unopened container.
      b. Use life: the life expectancy for the solution once it has been activated but not actually put to use with contaminated items.
      c. Reuse life: the amount of time a solution can be used and reused while being challenged with instruments that are wet or coated with bioburden.
   2. Directions for activation (mixing proportions).
   3. Type of container for storage and place (conditions such as heat and light).
   4. Directions for use
      a. Precleaning and drying of items to be submerged.
      b. Time/temperature ratio.

5. Instructions for disposal of used solution.
6. Warnings; cautions
   a. Toxic effects (that is, on eyes, skin).
   b. Specific directions for emergency care in the event of an accident (for example, splash in eye).

RECOMMENDED CHEMICAL DISINFECTANTS

The agents that have been shown adequate for use in dentistry are glutaraldehydes, chlorine compounds, iodophores, and complex phenolics. These are listed in table 4–5 and are described in sections that follow.

Alcohols and quaternary ammonium compounds are not approved for instrument or environmental surface disinfection. The alcohols, ethanol and isopropanol, have been widely accepted and used for the preparation of the skin prior to injections or blood-taking procedures. The use of alcohol for this purpose is as a cleansing agent; the length of time involved is not enough for antibacterial effect.

I. GLUTARALDEHYDES

As shown in table 4–5, the three types of glutaraldehydes are the alkaline, acidic, and neutral preparations.

A. Action

They are high-level disinfectants and act to kill microorganisms by damaging their proteins and nucleic acids.

TABLE 4–5 CHEMICAL DISINFECTING AGENTS
Chemical Classification
Glutaraldehydes Glutaraldehyde 2% neutral
Glutaraldehyde 2% alkaline
Glutaraldehyde 2% alkaline with phenolic buffer
Glutaraldehyde 2% acidic
Chlorines Chlorine dioxide
Sodium hypochlorite 5.25% household bleach
Iodophors Iodophor (1% available iodine)
Phenolics o-phenylphenyl 9% with o-benzyl-p-chlorophenol 1%

B. Preparation

The solutions become activated when the components of the two containers are mixed. The manufacturers' labels must show shelf, use, and reuse life, because the various preparations differ.

C. Limitations

1. Caustic to skin; use forceps and wear gloves.
2. Irritating to eyes; need protective eyewear.
3. Corrosive to some metal instruments.
4. Items must be rinsed in sterile water after removal from immersion bath.
5. Not used as a surface disinfectant because of toxic effects of fumes; surfaces wiped with glutaraldehyde should have residual film wiped off with sterile water.

II. CHLORINE COMPOUNDS
A. Action

Chlorine compounds have been used in a variety of ways for disinfection. Their use in water purification is well known. Solutions of sodium hypochlorite are used in cleaning dentures (page 386). Microorganisms are destroyed primarily by oxidation of microbial enzymes and cell wall components.

B. Chlorine Dioxide

The use life of chlorine dioxide is only 1 day, so new preparations must be made. The preparation is economical and generally nontoxic, but is corrosive to nonstainless steel instruments.

C. Sodium Hypochlorite

Daily fresh solutions are needed because sodium hypochlorite tends to be unstable. Use distilled water for mixing to improve the stability. The solutions can harm the eyes, skin, and clothing, and corrode certain instruments; the strong odor may be offensive. In spite of certain disadvantages, it is widely used and economical.

III. IODOPHORS
A. Action

Iodine is released slowly from the iodophor compound, and creates a disinfecting action as a broad-spectrum antimicrobial.

Povidone-iodine preparations are widely used in the forms of surgical scrubs, liquid soaps, mouthrinses, and surface antiseptics prior to hypodermic injection.

B. Environmental Surface Disinfectant

Concentrated solutions of iodophor contain less free iodine; therefore, the correct dilution for hard-surface disinfection is 1 part iodophor concentrate to 213 parts soft or distilled water. Hard water inactivates iodophors. The solution changes from amber to clear as it loses its activity.

IV. COMBINATION PHENOLICS (SYNTHETIC)

A. Action

High-concentration phenols act as protoplasmic proteins that destroy the cell wall and precipitate the protein. The lower concentrations used as surface disinfectants inactivate enzyme systems.

B. Use

Although a 10-minute disinfecting time is designated, the regulation for approval of the products containing the phenolics requests an immersion time of 20 minutes when the presence of tuberculosis is a risk.

CHEMICAL STERILANTS (IMMERSION)

Immersion in a chemical sterilant is used only for items that cannot be sterilized by heat. Because the immersion chemicals cannot be verified by spore testing, their use is limited. When ethylene oxide sterilizers are available, many of the items may be treated by that method.

A chemical that may require only 10 to 30 minutes for disinfection requires as many as 10 hours for sterilization at the same or different concentrations. Temperature may also be a factor. Manufacturer's instructions must be followed explicitly.

Instruments cannot be packaged, so maintenance of strict asepsis is not possible after chemical sterilization. Also, because of toxic effects to skin and mucosa, the chemical must be rinsed away with sterile water and dried before use on a patient.

UNIT WATER LINES

High counts of microorganisms have been found in the water line tubings after overnight standing. Tests have been made on tubings to handpieces, water syringes, and ultrasonic scalers. When the lines were flushed for 2 minutes, the microbial counts were reduced.[6]

Contaminated water should not be used for surgical purposes or during the irrigation of pocket areas, because infective microorganisms can be introduced. If contaminated water were directed forcefully into a pocket, microorganisms could enter the tissue and bacteremia result.

I. PROCEDURES FOR CLINICAL USE

A. Flush all water lines at least 5 to 6 minutes at the beginning of each day.

B. Operate handpieces and waterspray over a sink or cuspidor for 30 seconds before and 30 seconds after each patient appointment.

II. WATER RETRACTION SYSTEM

To correct saliva and debris suck-back in the water line of a handpiece, the water retraction valve should be removed and a check valve or antiretractor valve installed.[7] Originally, handpieces were made with a retraction valve to prevent dripping when the instrument was turned off. Material sucked into the line, possibly filled with microorganisms including hepatitis viruses, tubercle bacilli, and other pathogens, then is discharged when the handpiece is used for the succeeding patient.

PREPARATION FOR APPOINTMENT

The cleanliness and neatness of the treatment room reflect the character and conscientiousness of the dental personnel. The patient, with limited knowledge of dental science, may judge the ability of the dental personnel by the appearance of the office or clinic. Other patients inquire about sterilization and infection control.

The patient's attitude is important, but more important is the relationship of cleanliness to the presence of microorganisms and the need for performing techniques in a situation that minimizes cross-contamination.

The orderliness and immaculate cleanliness of the treatment rooms result from continuing care. An excellent test for the effects of care and any minor oversights is for each dental team member to sit in the dental chair occasionally and look around at what the patient sees from that vantage point.

I. OBJECTIVES

Effective care of instruments and equipment contributes to the following:

A. Control of disease transmitted by way of environmental surfaces.

B. An increase in the working efficiency of the office personnel.

C. An atmosphere of cleanliness and orderliness that will contribute to the patient's well-being.

D. An increase in the patient's confidence in the ability of the dental personnel.

E. The maintenance of the working efficiency of office equipment and instruments
   1. To prolong their span of usefulness.
   2. To contribute to patient safety.

F. A decrease in the occurrence of unpleasant odors in the office.

II. PRELIMINARY PLANNING

Preparation of the treatment room when time between appointments is limited requires an efficient procedural system. Spaulding's classification of inanimate objects (table 4–6) provides a guide for analysis.[8]

First, all surfaces and items that will be used or con-

TABLE 4–6
CLASSIFICATION OF INANIMATE OBJECTS (SPAULDING)

Surface Category	Definition	Sterilization/Disinfection	Examples
Critical Surfaces of instruments or devices	Penetrate/touch mucous membranes, oral fluids Contact normally sterile body areas	Sterilize or disposable	Needles Curets Explorers Probes
Semicritical Surfaces of instruments or devices	Touch intact mucous membrane, oral fluids (No entrance to sterile body areas) Does not penetrate	Sterilize or high-level disinfection	Radiographic biteblock Ultrasonic handpiece Amalgam condenser
Noncritical Surfaces of instruments or devices	Do not touch mucous membranes (only contact unbroken epithelium)	Cleaning and tuberculocidal intermediate-level disinfection	Light handles Certain x-ray machine parts Safety eyewear
Environmental Surfaces	No contact with patient (or only intact skin)	Cleaning and intermediate to low disinfection	Counter tops Equipment surfaces Housekeeping surface

tacted during the appointment can be categorized and listed as critical, semicritical, or noncritical. The most logical and scientific sequence for preparation for the appointment can then be outlined.

A. Hand Contacts
Only contacts essential to the service to be performed should be made. Planning ahead to have materials ready so that cabinet knobs or drawer handles do not have to be contacted is an example.

B. Sterilizable Items
Removable tips for air and water that can be cleaned and sterilized are examples. Handpieces and prophylaxis angles that can be sterilized are important additions to the list. Several handpieces are needed for rotation.

C. Disposable Items
Disposable items should be used wherever possible.

D. Items That May Be Covered
Coverings, particularly plastic-backed patient napkins, and clear plastic wrap or bags can prevent contamination from reaching surfaces. Covers for light handles, counter tops, x-ray machine parts, and water faucets are examples. Care must be taken when removing the covers not to contaminate the object beneath.

E. Items That Require Chemical Disinfection
Objects and surfaces that cannot be included in one of the preceding categories must be treated with a chemical disinfectant. If the material is not compatible with the chemical action of the disinfectant, a substitute item, which is either disposable or coverable, will be needed.

III. CLEAN AND DISINFECT ENVIRONMENTAL SURFACES
A. Agent
1. Approved effective agents are iodophors, sodium hypochlorite, or complex phenols (table 4–5).
2. The effectiveness of the disinfection procedure is the result of two actions:
   a. The physical rubbing and removal of contaminated material.
   b. The chemical inactivation of the living microorganisms.
3. Do not store gauze sponges in the solution. Use a spray bottle to dispense the disinfectant.

B. Procedure
1. Wear heavy-duty household gloves (figure 4–2).
2. Use several large gauze sponges or paper towels. The use of small sponges wastes time. A disinfectant-soaked sponge in each hand can decrease the time of cleaning certain objects, and contaminated objects, such as tubings, can be held with one sponge while scrubbing with the other sponge.

   Spraying of a disinfectant must be followed by vigorous scrubbing for cleaning. When applied only by spray without scrubbing, the agent does not penetrate or remove the film of microorganisms.
3. Scrub the disinfectant over the entire surface with attention to irregularities where contaminated material can aggregate.
4. Spray and leave the surfaces wet.

C. Surfaces to Disinfect

The list of surfaces varies from one clinic or office to another because of different equipment and availability of sterilizable and disposable items. The list must include all surfaces that are contacted if they are not sterilized, covered, or disposable.

CARE OF STERILE INSTRUMENTS

After the effort has been made to sterilize and disinfect, procedures are then conducted to prevent contamination and to control the transfer of pathogenic microorganisms. Although a strict procedure for sterile technique such as is practiced in a hospital operating room would be difficult or even impossible in a dental office, it is possible to preserve the chain of sterility through effective handling and storage procedures.

Instruments stored without sealed wrappers are only momentarily sterile because of airborne contamination.

Labeled, sterilized, and sealed packages are stored unopened in clean, dry cabinets or drawers. Paper-wrapped packages must be handled carefully to prevent tearing. All stored packages should be dated and used in rotation.

Packages wrapped and sealed in paper do not usually need resterilizing for several months to 1 year.[9] Plastic or nylon wrap with a tape or heat seal may be expected to remain sterile longer. However, the expected shelf life before resterilizing depends on the area surrounding the stored packages. A closed, protected area without exposure, such as a cabinet or drawer that can be disinfected routinely, is preferred.

PATIENT PREPARATION

The use of preoperative rinsing and toothbrushing has been shown to lower the numbers of oral bacteria and, therefore, to lower the numbers of infected aerosols created during instrumentation.

Oral procedures that require penetration of tissues, such as giving anesthesia by injection or scaling and root planing subgingival pocket surfaces, can introduce bacteria into the tissues and hence into the blood stream. Organisms injected into the tissue could multiply and create an abscess. Because of natural resistance, the body can handle and destroy invading microorganisms, provided the numbers can be kept to a minimum. Autogenous infection was described on page 15.

Practical procedures for the preparation of a patient include preoperative oral hygiene measures, rinsing with an antimicrobial mouthrinse, and the application of a surface disinfectant. These contribute to the prevention of disease transmission.

I. PREOPERATIVE ORAL HYGIENE MEASURES
A. Toothbrushing

Toothbrushing disturbs and removes microorganisms. When a patient is being trained in bacterial plaque control measures and needs supervision at each appointment, a double purpose can be accomplished. Demonstration of plaque removal from the teeth, tongue, and gingiva contributes to surface degerming prior to treatment procedures.

B. Rinsing

The numbers of bacteria on the gingival or mucosal surfaces can be reduced by the use of an antiseptic mouthrinse. In studies using a povidone-iodine mouthrinse, the bacterial counts on mucosal surfaces were reduced before and during scaling and gingivectomy.[10,11] Aerosol contamination was also reduced.[12,13] Reduction of surface and total bacteria in the oral cavity during oral procedures can contribute to surgical cleanliness and more favorable healing after treatment.

C. Chlorhexidine Rinse

The substantivity of 0.12% chlorhexidine provides a lowered bacterial count for more than 60 minutes. Preprocedural rinsing before injections is advised.[14]

II. APPLICATION OF A SURFACE ANTISEPTIC
A. Prior to Injection of Anesthetic[15,16]

As a needle is introduced into the mucosa for penetration to deeper tissues, microorganisms on the surface can be carried into the tissue (page 15). During positioning of the instrument for injection, the needle might accidentally contact a tooth surface and pick up some plaque, which could be carried to and into the injection site.

An antiseptic applied prior to the injection can decrease the risk of introducing septic material into the soft tissue.
1. Dry the surface (sponge).
2. Apply antiseptic (swab).
3. Apply topical anesthetic (swab).

B. Prior to Scaling and Other Dental Hygiene Instrumentation

1. *Instrumentation* in the sulcus or pocket and around the gingival margin can create breaks in the tissue where bacteria can enter. Subgingival instrumentation in a pocket with broken down sulcular epithelium can contribute to the entrance of bacteria into the underlying tissues. Local infection or bacteremia can be created.
2. *Procedure.* Dry the surface and swab the area prior to instrumentation. Use the antiseptic solution to irrigate the sulci and pockets carefully to prevent forcing the solution into the

tissues. Research has shown povidone-iodine to be an effective prophylactic germicide for this purpose.[10]

UNIVERSAL PROCEDURES FOR THE PREVENTION OF DISEASE TRANSMISSION

Basic procedures for clinical management are listed here. For many items, a detailed description has been provided in Chapter 3 or elsewhere in this chapter.

I. PATIENT FACTORS
A. Prepare a comprehensive patient history. Refer patients suspected of carrying infectious disease for medical evaluation.
B. Avoid elective procedures for a patient who is suffering from a communicable condition, such as a respiratory infection, or who has an open lesion on or about the lips or oral tissues for the benefit of all who would be subjected to exposure.
C. Ask the patient to rinse with germicidal mouthrinse to reduce the numbers of oral microorganisms.
D. Provide protective eyewear.

II. CLINIC PREPARATION
A. Run water through all water lines, including the air/water syringe, handpieces, and ultrasonic unit, for 5 to 6 minutes at the start of the day and for at least 30 seconds before and after each use during the day.
B. Cover or disinfect all environmental surfaces that may be touched during the appointment. Make an orderly sequence for surface disinfection.
C. Sterilize instruments and all other equipment that can be sterilized by one of the methods for complete sterilization.

III. FACTORS FOR THE DENTAL TEAM
A. Have medical examinations; keep immunizations up to date; have appropriate testing on a periodic basis.
B. Always use mask, protective eyewear, gloves, and a clean closed-front uniform.
C. Wash hands using a short scrub at the start of the day and handwashes with three latherings and thorough rinsings before and after donning gloves. Use antiseptic handwash.
D. Develop habits that minimize contacts with switches and other parts of the dental unit, dental chair, light, and operating stool, and avoid all possible environmental contacts unrelated to the procedure at hand.

IV. TREATMENT FACTORS
A. Hypodermic Needles
1. Use a safe recapping method to prevent accidental penetration or self-inoculation (figure 4–4).
2. Place used needles into a puncture-resistant container.
3. Dispose of all partially emptied carpules of anesthetics.

B. Removable Oral Appliances
Routinely, gloves should be worn to receive a septic appliance from a patient. Place appliance in a disposable cup and cover with a disinfectant. Use a fresh solution of .05% iodophor in water, or a 1:5 dilution of 5% sodium hypochlorite. Clean by ultrasonics.

When a lathe is used for cleaning the denture, wear goggles and a mask and use a sterile ragwheel and fresh pumice. Pumice is used only once and caught on a disposable paper liner in the dustbin and discarded.

V. POST-TREATMENT
A. Fold tray cover over instruments or holding solution container to transport to the sterilization area. Use heavy household gloves to handle used instruments.
B. Follow routines on pages 54–55 to disinfect, clean in ultrasonic cleaner, and prepare for sterilization.
C. Contaminated waste is secured in plastic disposal bags. See Disposal of Waste, page 67.
D. Disinfect safety eyewear for patient and dental team members.

VI. OCCUPATIONAL ACCIDENTAL EXPOSURE MANAGEMENT
Accidents happen even to the most skillful clinician. Accidental percutaneous (laceration, needlestick) or permucosal (splash to eye or mucosa) exposure to blood or other body fluids requires prompt action.

A. Significant Exposures
1. Percutaneous or permucosal stick or wound with needle or sharp instrument contaminated with blood or saliva.
2. Contamination of any obviously open wound, nonintact skin, or mucous membrane with blood, saliva, or a combination.
3. Exposure of patient's body fluids to unbroken skin is not considered a significant exposure.

B. Procedure Following Exposure[17,18]
1. Immediately wash the wound with soap and water; rinse well.
2. Obtain permission for blood testing and arrange for counseling.
3. On the same day
   a. Patient (source person) should be tested for HBsAg and anti-HIV.
   b. Exposed person should be tested for anti-HBs and anti-HIV (anti-HBs would not be needed if recent postvaccine confirmation showed positive immunization).
4. Table 4–7 outlines the necessary procedures.

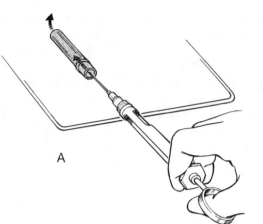

A

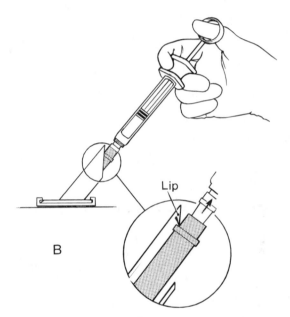

B

Lip

TABLE 4–7
HIV AND HBV POSTEXPOSURE MANAGEMENT

Patient (Source)	Exposed DHCW	Treatment
HBsAg positive or Refuses testing or Cannot be identified	Not HBV immunized	Start vaccine series Give HBIG (single dose)
	HBV vaccine received	Test for anti-HB 1. Adequate titer level: no treatment 2. Inadequate titer level: Give vaccine booster HBIG (single dose)
HBsAg Negative	Not HBV immunized	Start vaccine series
	HBV vaccine received	No treatment necessary
Has AIDS or is HIV seropositive or Refused testing or Cannot be identified	Counsel concerning the risk Test for anti-HIV	Negative for anti-HIV: Test again in 6 weeks 12 weeks 6 months 1 year Counsel: 1. Do not donate blood 2. Use appropriate protection during sexual intercourse

Key: DHCW = Dental health-care worker
HBsAg = Hepatitis B surface antigen
HBIG = Hepatitis B immune globulin
Anti-HBs = Antibody to hepatitis B surface antigen
Anti-HIV = Antibody to human immunodeficiency virus

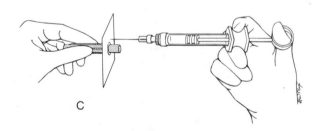

C

FIG. 4–4. Prevention of Percutaneous Injury: Needle Recapping Methods. One-handed recapping or recapping with a safety mechanical device is required. **A.** "Scoop" technique. Cap is placed on the tray and the needle is guided into it. **B.** Example of commercially available holder for cap. Device is fastened to the tray, and cap is removed and recapped by directing the needle into the cap holder. **C.** Cardboard shield retained on cap. During replacement of cap, protection is provided as shown. Needles must be discarded in a puncture-resistant container.

DISPOSAL OF WASTE

I. REGULATIONS
Investigate the regulations of each town or city sanitation division for rules concerning disposal of contaminated waste. The safety of the workers has been protected in many areas by the refusal to pick up bags of waste from hospitals and dental clinics unless the contents of the bags have been presterilized.

Figure 4–5 illustrates the universal label required by the OSHA. The labels must be attached to containers used to store or transport hazardous waste materials.

II. GUIDELINES[19]
Disposable materials, such as gloves, masks, wipes, paper drapes, or surface covers, that are contaminated with blood or body fluids should be carefully handled and discarded in sturdy, impervious plastic bags to minimize human contact. Blood, suctioned fluids, or other liquid waste may be carefully poured into a drain that is connected to a sanitary sewer system in compliance with applicable local regulations. Sharp items, such as needles and scalpel blades, should be placed intact into puncture-resistant containers.

Human tissue and contaminated solid wastes can be disposed of according to the requirements established by local or state environmental regulatory agencies and published recommendations. Infectious medical waste, including tissues and culture media, should be handled in a manner consistent with local regulations before disposal.

Liquid chemicals should be carefully poured into a drain connected to a sewer while flushing with copious amounts of water unless labeling or local regulations prohibit such a practice. Disposal methods for solid

chemicals vary with the type of chemical and local regulations governing waste management practices.

TECHNICAL HINTS

I. CLEANING THE FACE
Check and clean the exposed parts of the face not covered by mask or protective eyewear, where splatter collects, as an aid to disease control as well as for general sanitation. The face should be cleaned several times each day, and washed before eating. When washing the face, an effort should be made not to spread spatter material into the eyes or the mouth.

II. SMOKING AND EATING
Neither smoking nor eating should be permitted in treatment areas.

III. TOYS
Select toys and other reception area items that can be cleaned and disinfected.

IV. HANDPIECE MAINTENANCE
Keep records of handpiece purchase, maintenance, and other information pertinent to longevity and effectiveness. Maintain a sufficient number of handpieces to permit rotation and routine sterilization.

V. STERILIZATION MONITORING
Keep a written record of dates when processing tests and biologic monitor tests were performed for each sterilizer. Indicate advance dates for the next testing clearly on a calendar or other reference point. Tests made weekly should be performed on the same day to simplify remembering.

VI. OFFICE POLICY MANUAL
Include in the clinic or office policy manual outlines of procedures to follow for special precautions, such as for a patient who is a hepatitis carrier. Addresses for sources of various materials can be kept in a special reference section of the manual. Emergency procedures to follow when accidentally exposed should also be defined clearly (Passive Immunization, page 21).

FACTORS TO TEACH THE PATIENT

I. The meaning of "universal precautions" and what is included under the term; how these precautions protect the patient and the dental team members.
II. The contribution of the accurately completed medical and dental personal history to the provision of the best, safest treatment possible.
III. Methods for sterilization of instruments, including handpieces; how the autoclave or other sterilizer is tested daily or weekly.

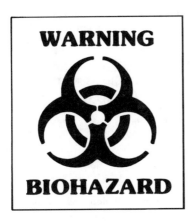

FIG. 4–5. Universal Label for Hazardous Material. A hazard-warning label should be fluorescent orange or orange-red with lettering or a symbol in a contrasting color. The label must be attached to containers used to store or transport waste. A label is not required for regulated waste that has been decontaminated (such as dental waste that has been autoclaved).

IV. Facts about the normal oral flora and the factors that influence an increased number of bacteria on the tongue, mucosa, and in the plaque.

V. Methods for personal daily control of the oral bacteria through plaque control and tongue brushing.

VI. Reasons for preprocedural rinsing.

VII. Method for thorough rinsing (page 365).

REFERENCES

1. **Bassett,** K.: *Infection Control, Hazardous Waste Management and Hazardous Materials: An Integrated Curriculum for the Dental Hygienist.* Tacoma, WA, Pierce College, Department of Dental Hygiene, 1991, p. 33.

2. **Miller,** C.H.: Sterilization and Disinfection: What Every Dentist Needs to Know, *J. Am. Dent. Assoc., 123,* 46, March, 1992.

3. **D'Autremont,** P.: Instrument Sterilization, *Dentalhygienistnews, 5,* 17, Fall, 1992.

4. **Harvey Chemiclave,** MDT Biologics Corp., 19645 Rancho Way, Rancho Dominquez, CA 90220.

5. **Parisi,** A.N. and Young, W.E.: Sterilization with Ethylene Oxide and other Gases, in Block, S.S.: *Disinfection, Sterilization, and Preservation,* 4th ed. Philadelphia, Lea & Febiger, 1991, pp. 580–595.

6. **Gross,** A., Devine, M.J., and Cutright, D.E.: Microbial Contamination of Dental Units and Ultrasonic Scalers, *J. Periodontol., 47,* 670, November, 1976.

7. **Bagga,** B.S.R., Murphy, R.A., Anderson, A.W., and Punwani, I.: Contamination of Dental Unit Cooling Water With Oral Microorganisms and Its Prevention, *J. Am. Dent. Assoc., 109,* 712, November, 1984.

8. **Favero,** M.S. and Bond, W.W.: Chemical Disinfection of Medical and Surgical Materials, in Block, S.S.: *Disinfection, Sterilization, and Preservation,* 4th ed. Philadelphia, Lea & Febiger, 1991, pp. 617–641.

9. **Butt,** W.E., Bradley, D.V., Mayhew, R.B., and Schwartz, R.S.: Evaluation of the Shelf Life of Sterile Instrument Packs, *Oral Surg. Oral Med. Oral Pathol., 72,* 650, December, 1991.

10. **Randall,** E. and Brenman, H.S.: Local Degerming with Povidone-Iodine. I. Prior to Dental Prophylaxis, *J. Periodontol., 45,* 866, December, 1974.

11. **Brenman,** H.S. and Randall, E.: Local Degerming With Povidone-Iodine. II. Prior to Gingivectomy, *J. Periodontol., 45,* 870, December, 1974.

12. **Litsky,** B.Y., Mascis, J.D., and Litsky, W.: Use of Antimicrobial Mouthwash to Minimize the Bacterial Aerosol Contamination Generated by the High-Speed Drill, *Oral Surg. Oral Med. Oral Pathol., 29,* 25, January, 1970.

13. **Wyler,** D., Miller, R.L., and Micik, R.E.: Efficacy of Self-administered Preoperative Oral Hygiene Procedures in Reducing the Concentration of Bacteria in Aerosols Generated During Dental Procedures, *J. Dent. Res., 50,* 509, March–April, 1971.

14. **Veksler,** A.E., Kayrouz, G.A., and Newman, M.G.: Reduction of Salivary Bacteria by Pre-procedural Rinses With Chlorhexidine 0.12%, *J. Periodontol., 62,* 649, November, 1991.

15. **Malamed,** S.F.: *Handbook of Local Anesthesia,* 3rd ed. St. Louis, The C.V. Mosby Co., 1990, pp. 103, 118.

16. **Connor,** J.P. and Edelson, J.G.: Needle Tract Infection, *Oral Surg. Oral Med. Oral Pathol., 65,* 401, April, 1988.

17. **United States Centers for Disease Control:** Public Health Service Statement on Management of Occupational Exposure to Human Immunodeficiency Virus, Including Considerations Regarding Zidovudine Postexposure Use, *MMWR, 39,* 1–3, No. RR-1, January 26, 1990.

18. **United States Centers for Disease Control:** Protection Against Viral Hepatitis. Recommendations of the Immunization Practices Advisory Committee (ACIP), *MMWR, 39,* 20, No. RR-2, February 9, 1990.

19. **American Dental Association,** Council on Dental Materials, Instruments, and Equipment, Council on Dental Practice, and Council on Dental Therapeutics: Infection Control Recommendations for the Dental Office and the Dental Laboratory, *J. Am. Dent. Assoc., 116,* 241, February, 1988.

SUGGESTED READINGS

Bowles, W.H. and Bowles, S.L.: A Safe and Convenient Means of Recapping Needles, *Gen. Dent., 39,* 250, July–August, 1991.

Butel, E.M. and DiFiore, P.M.: Pulp Testing While Avoiding Dangers of Infection and Cross-contamination, *Gen. Dent., 39,* 42, January–February, 1991.

Caughman, G.B., Caughman, W.F., Napier, N., and Schuster, G.S.: Disinfection of Visible-light-curing Devices, *Oper. Dent., 14,* 2, Winter, 1989.

Christensen, G.J.: Infection Control. Some Significant Loopholes, *J. Am. Dent. Assoc., 122,* 99, August, 1991.

Cochran, M.A., Miller, C.H., and Sheldrake, M.A.: The Efficacy of the Rubber Dam as a Barrier to the Spread of Microorganisms During Dental Treatment, *J. Am. Dent. Assoc., 119,* 141, July, 1989.

Cottone, J.A. and Molinari, J.A.: State-of-the-art Infection Control in Dentistry, *J. Am. Dent. Assoc., 123,* 33, August, 1991.

Dugan, W.T. and Hartleb, J.H.: Influence of a Glutaraldehyde Disinfecting Solution on Curing Light Effectiveness, *Gen. Dent., 37,* 40, January–February, 1989.

Earnest, R. and Loesche, W.: Measuring Harmful Levels of Bacteria in Dental Aerosols, *J. Am. Dent. Assoc., 122,* 55, December, 1991.

Grace, E.G., Cohen, L.A., and Ward, M.A.: Patients' Perceptions Related to the Use of Infection Control Procedures, *Clin. Prev. Dent., 13,* 30, May–June, 1991.

Johnston, M.W., Moore, W.C., and Rodu, B.: Comparison of Convection Heat Sterilization Units for the Orthodontic Office, *Am. J. Orthod. Dentofacial Orthop., 99,* 57, January, 1991.

Jones, M.L.: An Initial Assessment of the Effect of Orthodontic Pliers of Various Sterilization/Disinfection Regimes, *Br. J. Orthod., 16,* 251, November, 1989.

Lewis, D.L. and Boe, R.K.: Cross-infection Risks Associated With Current Procedures for Using High-Speed Dental Handpieces, *J. Clin. Microbiol., 30,* 401, February, 1992.

Mayo, J.A., Oertling, K.M., and Andrieu, S.C.: Bacterial Biofilm: A Source of Contamination in Dental Air-water Syringes, *Clin. Prev. Dent., 12,* 13, June–July, 1990.

Meraner, M.: The IMS Cassette: A New System for the Management of Instruments in the Dental Office, *Gen. Dent., 37,* 326, July–August, 1989.

Merchant, V.: Keeping It Clean in the Dental Office. Guidelines Help Prevent Cross-contamination, *Dent. Teamwork, 6,* 22, January–February, 1993.

Merchant, V.A. and Molinari, J.A.: Study on Adequacy of Sterilization of Air-water Syringe Tips, *Clin. Prev. Dent., 13,* 20, November–December, 1991.

Miller, C.H.: Cleaning, Sterilization and Disinfection: Basics of Microbial Killing for Infection Control, *J. Am. Dent. Assoc., 124,* 48, January, 1993.

Miller, C.H. and Hardwick, L.M.: Ultrasonic Cleaning of Dental Instruments in Cassettes, *Gen. Dent., 36,* 31, January–February, 1988.

Miller, C.H. and Palenik, C.J.: Sterilization, Disinfection, and Asepsis in Dentistry, in Block, S.S.: *Disinfection, Sterilization, and Preservation,* 4th ed. Philadelphia, Lea & Febiger, 1991, pp. 676–695.

Mills, S.E., Kuehne, J.C., and Bradley, D.V.: Bacteriological Analysis of High-speed Handpiece Turbines, *J. Am. Dent. Assoc., 124,* 59, January, 1993.

Molinari, J.A.: Controversies in Infection Control, *Dent. Clin. North Am., 34,* 55, January, 1990.

Molinari, J.A. and Molinari, G.E.: Is Mouthrinsing Before Dental Procedures Worthwhile? *J. Am. Dent. Assoc., 123,* 75, March, 1992.

Molinari, J.A. and Runnells, R.R.: Role of Disinfectants in Infection Control, *Dent. Clin. North Am., 35,* 323, April, 1991.

Overton, D., Burgess, J.O., Beck, B., and Matis, B.: Glutaraldehyde Test Kits: Evaluation for Accuracy and Range, *Gen. Dent., 37,* 126, March–April, 1989.

Palenik, C.J., Riggen, S.D., Celis, L.J., Sheldrake, M.A., and Miller, C.H.: Effectiveness of Steam Sterilization on the Contents of Sharps Containers, *Clin. Prev. Dent., 14,* 28, January–February, 1992.

Runnells, R.R.: Countering the Concerns: How to Reinforce Dental Practice Safety, *J. Am. Dent. Assoc., 124,* 65, January, 1993.

Rutala, W.A. and Weber, D.J.: Infectious Waste—Mismatch Between Science and Policy, *N. Engl. J. Med., 325,* 578, August 22, 1991.

Scully, C., Porter, S.R., and Epstein, J.: Compliance With Infection Control Procedures in a Dental Hospital Clinic, *Br. Dent. J., 173,* 20, July 11, 1992.

Siegel, L.J., Smith, K.E., Cantu, G.E., and Posnick, W.R.: The Effects of Using Infection-control Barrier Techniques on Young Children's Behavior During Dental Treatment, *ASDC J. Dent. Child., 59,* 17, January–February, 1992.

Tolle-Watts, L.: Surface Disinfectants: An Overview for Dental Hygienists, *Dentalhygienistnews, 3,* 12, Winter, 1990.

Tolle-Watts, L.: Infection Control for the Dental Hygienist of the Nineties. Part I: Personal Protection and Operatory Disinfection, *Semin. Dent. Hyg., 4,* 1, November, 1992.

Whitehouse, R.L.S., Peters, E., Lizotte, J., and Lilge, C.: Influence of Biofilms on Microbial Contamination in Dental Unit Water, *J. Dent., 19,* 290, October, 1991.

Biologic Indicators

American Dental Association, Council on Dental Materials, Instruments, and Equipment, and Council on Dental Therapeutics: Biological Indicators for Verifying Sterilization, *J. Am. Dent. Assoc., 117,* 653, October, 1988.

Hastreiter, R.J., Molinari, J.A., Falken, M.C., Roesch, M.H., Gleason, M.J., and Merchant, V.A.: Effectiveness of Dental Office Instrument Sterilization Procedures, *J. Am. Dent. Assoc., 122,* 51, October, 1991.

McErlane, B., Rosebush, W.J., and Waterfield, J.D.: Assessment of the Effectiveness of Dental Sterilizers Using Biological Monitors, *Can. Dent. Assoc. J., 58,* 481, June, 1992.

Miller, C.: Faulty Procedures Often the Culprit, *RDH, 11,* 26, November, 1991.

Miller, C.: Spore Testing of Sterilizers Ensures Patients' Protection, *RDH, 12,* 50, October, 1992.

Nickerson, A., Bhuta, P., Orton, G., and Alvin, B.: Monitoring Dental Sterilizers' Effectiveness Using Biological Indicators, *J. Dent. Hyg., 64,* 69, February, 1990.

Oxborrow, G.S. and Berube, R.: Sterility Testing—Validation of Sterilization Processes, and Sporicide Testing, in Block, S.S.: *Disinfection, Sterilization, and Preservation,* 4th ed. Philadelphia, Lea & Febiger, 1991, pp. 1047–1057.

Willette, S.J. and Fitts, K.K.: Selection and Use of Biologic Indicators, *Dentalhygienistnews, 5,* 4, Spring, 1992.

Radiographs

Brabandt, B.: Handling Radiographs With Care, *Dent. Teamwork, 4,* 25, March–April, 1991.

Brabandt, B.A.: Radiation Asepsis, *Dent. Teamwork, 3,* 16, January–February, 1990.

Ciola, B.: A Readily Adaptable, Cost-effective Method of Infection Control for Dental Radiography, *J. Am. Dent. Assoc., 117,* 349, August, 1988.

Geist, J.R., Stefanac, S.J., and Gander, D.L.: Infection Control Procedures in Intraoral Radiology: A Survey of Michigan Dental Offices, *Clin. Prev. Dent., 12,* 4, June–July, 1990.

Kelly, W.H.: Radiographic Asepsis in Endodontic Practice, *Gen. Dent., 37,* 302, July–August, 1989.

Dental Materials

Bass, R.A., Plummer, K.D., and Anderson, E.F.: The Effect of a Surface Disinfectant on a Dental Cast, *J. Prosthet. Dent., 67,* 723, May, 1992.

Bell, S.A., Brockmann, S.L., and Sackuvich, D.A.: The Effectiveness of Two Disinfectants on Denture Base Acrylic Resin with an Organic Load, *J. Prosthet. Dent., 61,* 580, May, 1989.

Dietz, E.R.: The Role of the Dental Assistant in Laboratory Asepsis, *Dent. Assist., 58,* 5, July–August, 1989.

Doundoulakis, J.H.: Surface Analysis of Titanium After Sterilization: Role in Implant-tissue Interface and Bioadhesion, *J. Prosthet. Dent., 58,* 471, October, 1987.

Ghani, F., Hobkirk, J.A., and Wilson, M.: Evaluation of a New Antiseptic-containing Alginate Impression Material, *Br. Dent. J., 169,* 83, August 11–25, 1990.

Rice, C.D., Moghadam, B., Gier, R.E., and Cobb, C.M.: Aerobic Bacterial Contamination in Dental Materials, *Oral Surg. Oral Med. Oral Pathol., 70,* 537, October, 1990.

Rosen, M. and Touyz, L.Z.G.: Influence of Mixing Disinfectant Solutions into Alginate on Working Time and Accuracy, *J. Dent., 19,* 186, June, 1991.

Witt, S. and Hart, P.: Cross-infection Hazards Associated With the Use of Pumice in Dental Laboratories, *J. Dent., 18,* 281, October, 1990.

5

Patient Reception and Positioning in the Dental Chair

The patient's well-being is the all-important consideration throughout the appointment. At the same time, the clinician must function effectively and efficiently by applying work simplification principles to reduce stress and fatigue.

The physical arrangement and interpersonal relationships provide the setting for specific services to be performed. Key words related to the positioning of patient and clinician are defined in table 5–1.

The patient's presence in the office or clinic is an expression of confidence in the dentist and the dental hygienist. This confidence is inspired by the reputation for professional knowledge and skill, the appearance of the office, and the action of the workers in it.

I. PREPARATION FOR THE PATIENT
A. Treatment Area
The procedures for the prevention of disease transmission were described in Chapters 3 and 4. The requirements are universal precautions for all patients whether or not the presence of a communicable disease is known.

1. *Environmental Surfaces.* All contact areas must be thoroughly disinfected or covered to control cross-contamination. Appointment preparation was described on pages 62–65.
2. *Instruments.* Packaged instruments remain sealed until the start of the appointment.
3. *Equipment.* Prepare and make ready other materials that will be used, such as for the determination of blood pressure and patient instruction. Anticipate specific needs for assessment procedures for a new patient.

B. Records
By leaving the record open for possible reference, the need for handling the record after handwashing and gloving for instrumentation may be avoided. Radiographs can be placed on the viewbox and the light left on.

1. Review the patient's medical and dental history for pertinent appointment information and need for updating.
2. Read previous appointment case records to focus the current treatment needs.
3. Anticipate examination procedures and new record making for a new patient.

C. Position Chair
1. Upright, in low position.
2. Chair arm adjusted for access.
3. Preadjustment of traditional chair when size of patient is known contributes to ease while making final adjustments.

D. Clear Path
Clear pathway to chair of obstacles: rheostat, clinician's stool.

II. PATIENT RECEPTION
A. Introductions
1. The dental assistant or the dentist may introduce the new patient to the dental hygienist, but more frequently, a self-introduction is in order. The patient is greeted by name and the hygienist's name is clearly stated, for example, "Good morning, Mrs. Smith; I am Miss Jones, the dental hygienist." Wearing a name-tag for the patient's convenient observation is helpful.
2. Procedure for introducing the patient to others:
   a. A lady's name always precedes a gentleman's.

70

TABLE 5-1
KEY WORDS: CHAIR POSITIONING

Body language: a set of nonverbal signals, including body movements, postures, gestures, and facial expressions, that gives expression to various physical, mental, and emotional states.

Body mechanics: the field of physiology that studies muscular actions and functions in the maintenance of the posture of the body.

Cumulative trauma: disorders of the musculoskeletal, autonomic, and peripheral nervous system caused by repeated, forceful, and awkward movements of the human body, as well as by exposure to mechanical stress, vibration, and cold temperatures.

Ergonomics (er gō-nom′iks): a branch of ecology dealing with human factors in the design and operation of machines and the physical environment; in dentistry, the science encompassing all factors that relate to quality and quantity of dental care delivered in comparison to the physical and mental fatigue generated.

Postural hypotension (pos′chu-ral hī pō-ten′shun): also called orthostatic (or thō-stat′ik) hypotension; a fall in blood pressure associated with dizziness, syncope, and blurred vision that occurs upon standing or when standing motionless in a fixed position.

Supine (soo′pīn): flat position with head and feet on the same level.

Trendelenburg (tren-del′en-berg): the modified supine position when the head is lower than the heart.

Work simplification: application to clinical procedure of time and motion studies, analysis of instruments and equipment, and body mechanics to provide the patient with a smooth, systematic, simplified approach for comprehensive dental hygiene therapy.

---

  b. An older person's name precedes the younger person's (when of the same sex and when the difference in age is obvious).
  c. In general, the patient's name precedes that of a member of the dental personnel.
 3. An older patient is not called by the first name except at the patient's request.

B. Procedures
 1. Invite patient to be seated.
  a. For the average patient, stand ready to adjust the chair.
  b. Assist the elderly, the infirm, or very small children; guide into the chair by supporting the patient's arm. Procedure for assisting a patient who is blind is described on page 733.
 2. Assist with wheelchair. Bring wheelchair adjacent to the dental chair and provide assistance when indicated. Wheelchair transfers and assistance for a patient with a walker or crutches are described on pages 685–687.
 3. Place handbag in a safe place, if possible within the patient's view.

 4. Apply drape and napkin. Stabilization aids for patients with disabilities are described on pages 702.
 5. Receive removable prosthetic appliances and cover with water in a protective container.
 6. Provide protective eyewear. For information about the types and care of protective eyewear, see pages 44–45. When a patient removes personal corrective eyeglasses to substitute those provided by the office or clinic, make sure the personal glasses are placed in their case in a safe place.

POSITION OF THE CLINICIAN

The adjustment for the position of the patient is contingent upon the position of the clinician. Attention to the patient's comfort must always be foremost, but when the working arrangement is considered, it is realistic to remember that the patient's position will be assumed for a relatively short time compared with that of the clinician, who may conduct a major portion of a full day's professional activity in close proximity to the chairside. The patient, therefore, is positioned so that a thorough, biologically oriented service may be performed conveniently and efficiently within a reasonable length of time.

I. OBJECTIVES
Objectives concern the health of the clinician, the service to be performed, and the effect on the patient. The *preferred* position attempts to accomplish the following:
  A. Contribute to rather than detract from the health of the clinician.
  B. Provide physical comfort and mental tranquility.
  C. Apply principles of body mechanics that reduce fatigue and maintain stamina for prolonged periods of peak efficiency.
  D. Contribute to ease and efficiency of performance, thereby producing complete, thorough results for effective treatment; this, in turn, has long-range benefits for the patient.
  E. Transmit to the patient a sense of well-being, security, and confidence, as well as a need for cooperation with dental personnel.
  F. Develop better patient-clinician relationships because of greater comfort, lessened physical stress, and reduced appointment time.
  G. Be flexible in relation to individual needs of patients with special health problems, where limitations of physiologic or pathologic conditions require variations in chair positions.
  H. Be flexible in relation to studying and utilizing, where applicable, new concepts of patient care and new developments in dental equipment that will contribute to all objectives of service.

II. THE SEATED CLINICIAN

In keeping with current concepts, the use of a stool is expected. Benefits can result that relate to general health, productivity, and the manner in which work is accomplished.

A. Characteristics of an Acceptable Clinician's Stool[1]

1. *Base.* Broad and heavy for stability, with no fewer than four casters. A stool with five casters has greater stability.
2. *Mobility.* Completely mobile; not connected to other dental equipment; built with free-rolling casters; without tipping hazards.
3. *Seat.* Relatively large to provide complete body support; padded firmly, yet not too hard; without a welt on the leaning edge that could dig into the upper part of the thigh.
4. *Height.* Adjustable to provide exactly the correct level for the individual so that feet can be flat on the floor and thighs parallel with the floor.
5. *Assistant's Stool.* Needs additional support at the base, with at least five casters recommended for maximum stability; should be freely adjustable for height. A footrest is needed at the base of the chair, because the assistant is positioned 4 to 6 inches higher than the clinician, and generally, the feet cannot reach the floor.

B. Use of the Clinician's Stool

Once the stool is adjusted for the individual, it does not need changing, unless other personnel also use it. Once adjusted, the height remains constant, and other dental equipment is arranged to accommodate for optimum usage. Positioning that incorporates principles of good body mechanics benefits both the clinician and the patient. Basic positioning includes the following features related to posture and the field of operation.

1. Feet are flat on the floor; thighs parallel with the floor (figure 5–1A).
2. Back is straight; head is relatively erect; shoulders are relaxed and parallel with floor.
3. Body weight is completely supported by the chair; balancing on the edge of the stool should be avoided (figure 5–1B).
4. Eyes are directed downward in a manner that prevents neck strain and eye strain; it is not necessary to bend the head.
5. Distance from the patient's mouth to the eyes of the clinician should be 14 to 16 inches (figure 5–2).
6. With elbows close to the sides, the treatment area (patient's mouth) is adjusted to elbow height.
7. Forearm and wrist are kept in a straight line.

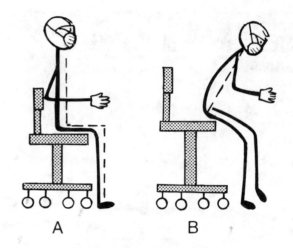

FIG. 5–1. Clinician's Use of Stool. A. Correct position, with feet flat on the floor, thighs parallel with floor, and body weight supported by the stool. **B.** Incorrect position, with seat high, body balanced on the edge of the stool, and back bent forward.

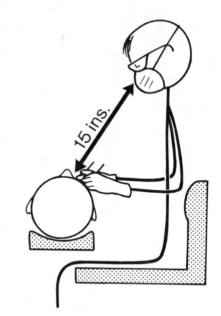

FIG. 5–2. Distance from Clinician to Patient. Acceptable positioning shows the patient at the clinician's elbow level and the oral cavity of the patient approximately 15 inches from the clinician's eyes.

III. THE STANDING CLINICIAN

As in the seated position, the standing posture also requires application of principles of good body mechanics.

A. Distribution of Balance

1. Both feet are flat on the floor with toes forward.
2. Back is straight; head relatively erect; shoulders relaxed and parallel with floor.

3. Weight is centered over the balls of the feet and distributed evenly to both feet; knees are slightly flexed.

B. Relation to Treatment Area

1. With elbows close to the sides, the treatment area (patient's mouth) is adjusted to elbow height. Forearm and wrist are in a straight line.
2. Eyes are directed downward in a manner that prevents neck strain and eye strain; it is not necessary to bend the head.
3. Distance from the patient's mouth to the eyes of the clinician should be 14 to 16 inches (figure 5–2).

POSITION OF THE PATIENT

Once the height of the treatment area is established by the height of the clinician's elbow, dental chair positioning relates directly to the type of dental chair. The sequence of procedures for effective, efficient adjustment of the traditional dental chair and of the contoured chair is outlined here.

I. GENERAL POSITIONS

Four commonly used body positions are shown in figure 5–3. Body positions are of extreme importance during emergency care; they are identified in Table 61–3, with outlines for emergency procedures.

A. Upright
This is the initial position from which chair adjustments are made.

B. Semi-upright
A patient with certain types of cardiovascular or respiratory diseases may need to be in a semi-upright position for dental and dental hygiene procedures.

C. Supine
The patient is flat, with the head and feet on the same level.

D. Trendelenburg
The patient is in the supine position and tipped back and down 35 to 45° so that the heart is higher than the head.

II. CONTOURED DENTAL CHAIR

A contoured chair provides complete body support for the patient, which increases patient relaxation. The clinician can be in a comfortable working position with good access, light, and visibility, which in turn, contribute to an efficient performance.

In a supine position, a patient is ideally situated for support of the circulation. Rarely could a patient faint while lying in a supine position.

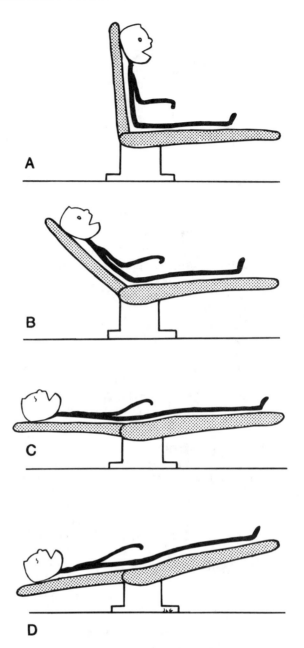

FIG. 5–3. Basic Patient Positions. A. Upright. **B.** Semi-upright. **C.** Supine or horizontal, with the brain on the same level as the heart. **D.** Trendelenburg, with the brain lower than the heart and the feet slightly elevated.

A. Characteristics of a Contoured Chair for Efficient Utilization
1. Provides complete body support.
2. Seat and leg support move as a unit; back and headrest move as a unit; both are power controlled.
3. Has a thin back without protruding adjustment devices so that the chair may be lowered close to the clinician's elbow height.
4. Has supports that hold the patient's arms as the chair is lowered into the supine position;

otherwise the hands hang down or the patient must hold them up forcibly.

5. Chair base should be shallow to permit the chair to be lowered as close to the floor as needed for correct treatment position.

6. Chair base should be power driven with pedal access from the working position on the dental clinician's stool. The controls for the back and seat should be readily available to both the assistant and clinician.

B. Prepositioning for Patient Reception
1. Chair at low level; back upright.
2. Chair arm raised on side of approach.

C. Adjustment Steps
1. Patient is seated first with back upright.
2. Chair seat and foot portion are raised first to help the patient settle back.
3. Backrest is lowered until the patient reaches the supine position for maxillary instrumentation. For mandibular teeth, chair back is adjusted to a 20° angle with the floor (figure 5–4).
4. Patient is requested to slide up until the head is at the upper edge of the backrest and on the side next to the clinician. Note patient's head position in figure 5–5, shown for a right-handed clinician.

D. Final Adjustment
1. Lower or raise the total chair until the patient's mouth is at the clinician's elbow level when the shoulder is relaxed.
2. Clinician's positions can be designated by the hours of a clock around the patient's head. Noon, or 12:00, is at the top, over the patient's forehead as shown in figure 5–5.
   a. Right-handed clinician: positioned for instrumentation between 7:30 and 12:00.
   b. Left-handed clinician: positioned between 12:00 and 4:30.

E. Conclusion of Appointment
1. Raise backrest slowly.
2. Tilt chair forward.

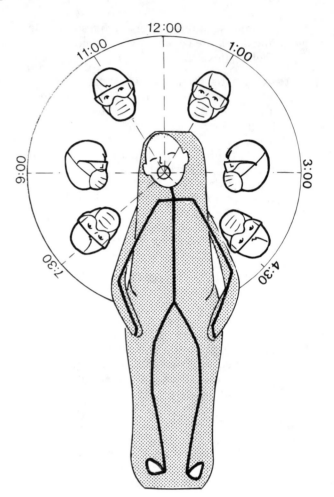

FIG. 5–5. Range of Positions for Clinician. The patient's head is placed at the upper edge of the backrest or headrest on the side next to the clinician, as shown here for the right side. The right-handed clinician is positioned between 7:30 and 12:00, whereas the left-handed clinician is positioned between 12:00 and 4:30, for side-front, side, or side-back.

3. Request that patient sit in an upright position briefly, to avoid effects of postural hypotension.

F. Contraindications for Supine Position
Most patients can be treated in the standard supine position described. Examples of conditions that may contraindicate the use of a supine position include congestive heart disease and any condition associated with breathing difficulty, such as emphysema, severe asthma, or sinusitis. During the third trimester of pregnancy, some women would be uncomfortable.

Usually when positioning is questionable, the patient volunteers a request for position varia-

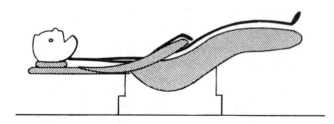

FIG. 5–4. Contoured Chair. For instrumentation in the maxillary arch, the patient is in supine position, with the back of the chair nearly parallel with the floor and the feet slightly higher than the head. For mandibular teeth, adjust the chair back to a 20° angle with the floor.

tion. Questions on the patient's history may reveal the need for adaptation.

III. TRADITIONAL DENTAL CHAIR

The back of the chair is adjusted first, then the headrest; the chair is inclined to adjust the seat; and finally, the whole chair is lowered or raised to bring the patient's mouth to the correct level and angulation. For most patients, the footrest remains in a constant position, but it should be adjusted to meet individual needs.

A. Prepositioning for Patient Reception
1. Seat parallel with floor.
2. Back slightly inclined back and away from the upright position.
3. Headrest tilted back to prevent its bumping the patient during seating.

B. Backrest
1. Raise or lower until the curvature of the chair back corresponds with the curvature in the middle of the patient's back.
2. When correctly positioned, the top border of many traditional chairs will be at a level approximating the lower third of the patient's scapulae. Other chairs have taller backs that may reach nearer the upper third of the scapulae.

C. Headrest
1. Request the patient to hold the head erect with chin slightly up.
2. Bring the headrest to a position almost touching the back of the head under the occipital protuberances before securing it.

D. Chair Seat
1. Incline the whole chair back as a unit. For the correct position, usually the chair will be tilted as far as it will go.
2. The "V" formed between the seat and the back prevents the patient from sliding forward (figure 5–6A).

E. Final Adjustment
1. *The Seated Clinician*
   a. Lower the chair to its lowest level and incline the chair back as far as it will go.
   b. To lower the patient further, it may be necessary to lower the back of the chair.
2. *The Standing Clinician.* With the chair inclined as far back as possible, raise or lower the whole chair until the patient's mouth is at elbow height of the clinician.
3. *Basic Position of the Patient.* When correctly positioned, the spinal cord of the patient should be straight from the brain to the hips. An imaginary straight line can be drawn from the top of the ear to the hips to test this.

F. Effects of Chair Maladjustment
1. *Backrest Too Low or Too High.* Curvature of the spine causes muscle tension and restlessness, and the patient attempts to slide into a more comfortable posture out of the appropriate position.
2. *Headrest Too High or Too Far Forward.* Chin moves toward chest, making accessibility and visibility difficult to maintain; clinician must lean forward and bend neck sideward (figure 5–6B).
3. *Headrest Too Low or Too Far Back.* Patient's neck muscles can be stretched and become fatigued; swallowing may be difficult; patient slides down (figure 5–6C).
4. *Chair Seat Parallel with Floor.* Patient slides forward and down (figure 5–6B).

IV. CHAIR POSITION FOR SMALL CHILD
A. Traditional Chair
1. Use a portable seat or a large, firm cushion to raise seat level.
2. Cover the seat with a cloth to protect the finish from the child's shoes, or the child's shoes can be removed.

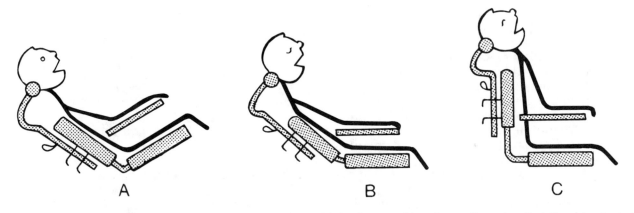

FIG. 5–6. Traditional Dental Chair. A. Correct position, with backrest and headrest adjusted so that the spine is straight from hip to top of head and the whole chair is tilted back. **B.** Incorrect position, with headrest too far forward and chair seat flat, which encourages the patient to slide forward. **C.** Incorrect position, with headrest too far back.

3. Lower back and headrest to lowest levels, with back at right angles to chair seat.
4. Incline chair back.
5. Make final adjustment so that child's head rests as near the headrest as possible; legs may be crossed to give support.

B. Contoured Chair

Adjustment the same as that for an adult. Child slides up so that the head is near the top of the backrest and on the side toward the clinician (figure 5–5).

FUNCTIONAL FACTORS

I. LIGHTING

During treatment, visibility of specific areas of the oral cavity is prerequisite to thoroughness without undue trauma to the tissues. With inadequate light, inefficiency increases and leads to prolonged treatment time, which reduces patient cooperation.

The position of the dental light or lights and the intensity of the beam affect the illumination. A study of the treatment room can be made that includes measurement of the total light at the patient's face in working position. Selection of a light that meets certain standards can assure intensity sufficient for good visibility and yet safe for the eyes.

A. Dental Light: Suggested Features

1. The light should be readily adjustable both vertically and horizontally and the beam capable of being focused.
2. The size must be small enough so that it may be brought close to the treatment area without being in the way, blocking the room light, or being a hazard for movement of people in its vicinity.
3. Intensity of room light should be sufficient to prevent a marked contrast between it and the illuminating beam of the dental light. An all luminous ceiling contributes to evenly distributed room lighting.

B. Dental Light: Location

1. *Attachment.* The most versatile arrangement is a ceiling-mounted light on a track, which permits the light to move over a range from behind a supine patient's head to a position in front of the patient's chin.
2. *Dual Lighting.* With a supine patient position in a contoured chair, advantages to the use of two operating lights have been demonstrated. One light directed from the front of the patient may be attached to the dental unit; the other light is mounted on a ceiling track as just described.

C. Dental Light: Adjustment

Direct the light first on the napkin under the patient's chin, then rotate the light up to the mouth to avoid flashing light in the patient's eyes.

II. POSITIONS DURING TREATMENT

A. Objectives

1. The area being treated should be seen clearly without having to assume body positions that are harmful if held over long periods.
2. When an assistant participates, the patient's oral cavity must be accessible and visible to both clinician and dental assistant.
3. Instruments and equipment must be within reach without stretching.

B. Solo Clinician

1. Arrange necessary items for immediate access.
2. Cervical tray may be used and positioned conveniently around the patient.
3. Height of tray for instruments should be at or slightly below the elbow, so that no effort need be expended when instruments are changed.

C. Four-Handed Dental Hygiene

1. Assistant is seated with eye level 4 to 6 inches above the clinician's eye level and facing toward the head of dental chair (figure 5–7).
2. Assistant applies principles of good body mechanics; body weight is supported by stool; feet are rested on the base of the stool.

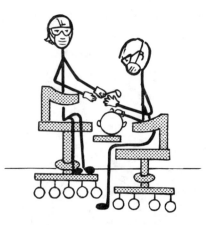

FIG. 5–7. Clinician with Assistant. The dental assistant is seated with eye level 4 to 6 inches higher than that of the clinician. The sterile tray is placed on a portable cabinet in front of the assistant within easy reach for passing instruments.

3. Instruments and other essential materials are kept within arm's length, and the portable cabinet with sterilized prepared tray is in front of the dental assistant.[2]
4. Four-handed dentistry procedures are practiced with instrument transfers and evacuation during clinical procedures.[3]

TECHNICAL HINTS

I. Prevention of cumulative trauma is based on good principles of posture, chair positions, and exercise that includes stretching hands, neck, shoulders, and back. Cumulative trauma is described on page 483 and exercises are shown in figure 31–13, page 485).

II. Keep body contact at a minimum. A good clinician does not lean on the patient, rest the forearms on the patient's shoulders, or rest the hands on the patient's face or forehead. Unnecessary contact can be unpleasant to certain patients, and more importantly, it contributes to cross-contamination.

FACTORS TO TEACH THE PATIENT

I. Orientation of patients, particularly previous patients, is important when changes in equipment and treatment procedures are introduced.

II. Give specific instruction on the parts of a dental chair or other equipment that will be of concern to the patient to prevent embarrassment or adverse reactions.

REFERENCES

1. **Sinnett,** G.M. and Wuehrmann, A.H.: The Dental Operatory of the Future, in Peterson, S., ed.: *The Dentist and His Assistant,* 3rd ed. St. Louis, The C.V. Mosby Co., 1972, pp. 392–401.
2. **Sinnett,** G.M., McDevitt, E.J., Robinson, G.E., and Wuehrmann, A.H.: Four-handed Dentistry: A New Mobile Dental Cabinet Design, *J. Am. Dent. Assoc., 78,* 305, February, 1969.
3. **Torres,** H.O.: Concepts and Practice of Four-handed, Six-handed, and Team Dentistry, in Darby, M.L. and Bushee, E.J., eds.: *Mosby's Comprehensive Review of Dental Hygiene.* St. Louis, The C.V. Mosby Co., 1986, pp. 619–636.

SUGGESTED READINGS

Armstrong, M.: Occupational Health Hazards for Dental Hygienists, *Can. Dent. Hyg./Probe, 20,* 99, September, 1986.

Barry, R.M., Woodall, W.R., and Mahan, J.M.: Postural Changes in Dental Hygienists, Four Year Longitudinal Study, *J. Dent. Hyg., 66,* 147, March–April, 1992.

Borea, G., Montebugnoli, L., and Balla, B.: The Effects of Work Posture on Muscular Electrical Activity and Circulatory Dynamics in Dentists, *Quintessence Int., 21,* 603, July, 1990.

Brodowicz, G.R. and Whiting, E.: Is Your Work a Pain in the Neck?, *Dent. Assist., 60,* 28, March/April, 1991.

Colangelo, G.A., Hobart, D.J., Belenky, M.M., and Bechtel, M.A.: Elbow Angle During a Simulated Task Requiring Fine Psychomotor Control, *J. Dent. Educ., 55,* 785, December, 1991.

Cunningham, M.A., Sharp, J.D., and Field, H.M.: Teaching Dental Students a Proper Way of Introducing Patients to Instructors, *J. Dent. Educ., 48,* 518, September, 1984.

Ettinger, R.: Office Design for Geriatric Patients, *Dentalhygienistnews, 3,* 12, Fall, 1990.

Hardage, J.L., Gildersleeve, J.R., and Rugh, J.D.: Clinical Work Posture for the Dentist: An Electromyographic Study, *J. Am. Dent. Assoc., 107,* 937, December, 1983.

Nield, J.S. and Houseman, G.A.: *Fundamentals of Dental Hygiene Instrumentation,* 2nd ed. Philadelphia, Lea & Febiger, 1988, Chapter 2.

Pruitt, C.O.: Exercises for Prevention and Alleviation of Back Pain, *Gen. Dent., 36,* 199, May–June, 1988.

Wagner, B.: Optimal Working Posture, *Quintessence Int., 15,* 77, January, 1984.

PART III

PATIENT
ASSESSMENT

DIAGNOSTIC WORK-UP

Before treatment begins, information must be obtained about the patient's general and oral health, from which a diagnosis and treatment plan can be formulated. In the dental hygiene process, assessment involves the gathering of information about the health status of the patient, the analysis and synthesis of that data, and the making of a clinical judgment. The outcome of the assessment is the formulation of a dental hygiene diagnosis.

The gathering, organizing, and assembling of all data from observations, patient questioning, and clinical and radiographic examination may be called a *diagnostic work-up*. Basically, it is a collection of all pertinent facts and materials to use during diagnosis and treatment planning and for use during all treatment as a guide. The chapters in this section, *Patient Assessment*, include descriptions for the preparation of materials that make up a diagnostic work-up.

I. PARTS OF A DIAGNOSTIC WORK-UP
A. Basic Procedures
The essential information for assessment of a patient prior to formulation of the diagnosis and treatment plan by a dentist is derived from the following:
1. Patient histories (personal, medical, and dental).
2. Determination of vital signs.
3. Extraoral and intraoral examination.
4. Radiographic survey.
5. Study casts.
6. Examination of the gingival and periodontal tissues, including clinical signs of disease involvement, probing depths and charting, and mobility evaluation.
7. Examination of the teeth to determine and record deposits, restorations, sealants, carious lesions, structural defects, pulp vitality, and occlusion factors.

B. Diagnostic Work-up for Preventive Treatment Plan
A preventive program is planned to meet individual needs. Therefore, information to be obtained depends on the particular oral problems and should include:
1. Dental or periodontal indices.
2. Bacterial plaque score.

C. Additional Procedures
In addition to the basic procedures, other parts of a diagnostic work-up are selected depending on the individual needs of a patient, as well as on the specialty area and special emphasis of the dentist. Selection of procedures to be used may be influenced by the age group to which the patient belongs.

Certain procedures may be of an emergency examination category. For example, if during the intraoral examination of the oral mucosa a suspicious lesion was found for which a biopsy was indicated, such a diagnostic procedure would take precedence over any other.

In accord with the policy or special request of the dentist, a diagnostic work-up may include some or all of the following:
1. Photographs.
2. Biopsy or cytologic smear.
3. Laboratory tests for suspected systemic conditions, such as bleeding tendencies, sickle cell anemia, or diabetes.
4. Special consultations with or referrals to medical specialists.

II. PURPOSES
The diagnostic work-up can benefit the patient, aid the dentist, and provide an overall perspective from which a patient-oriented dental hygiene care program can be formulated. Basic objectives of a diagnostic work-up are to
A. Organize information and materials for use while making the diagnosis and outlining the treatment plan for the patient.
B. Aid in
1. Planning dental hygiene preventive care and instruction for the patient.
2. Guiding instrumentation during dental hygiene appointments.
3. Correlating dental hygiene care with dental care.
C. Provide a permanent, documented, continuing record of the patient's oral and general health for
1. Evaluating the response to treatment, which may be compared with future observations at maintenance appointments.
2. Protecting the practice in case of misunderstandings or evidence in legal matters should questions arise.
D. Increase the scope of contribution of the dental hygienist to comprehensive patient care by the dental health team.

EXAMINATION PROCEDURES

A specific objective of patient examination as a part of the total diagnostic work-up is the recognition of deviations from normal that may be signs and symptoms of disease. The importance of careful, thorough examination cannot be overstressed. Concentration and attention to detail are necessary in order that each slight deviation from normal may be entered on the record for review by the dentist. Signs and symptoms of disease are the deviations from normal that must be recorded.

I. SIGNS AND SYMPTOMS
A. Sign
A *sign* is any abnormality that may be indicative of a deviation from normal or of disease that is

discovered by a professional person while examining a patient. A sign is an objective symptom.

Examples of signs are changes in color, shape, or consistency of a tissue not observable by the patient. Other signs are findings revealed by the use of a probe, explorer, radiograph, or vitality tester of the dental pulp.

B. Symptom

A *symptom* is also any departure from the normal that may be indicative of disease. Symptoms may be subjective or objective.

1. *Subjective Symptom.* Symptom observed by the patient. Examples are pain, tenderness, or itching.
2. *Objective Symptom.* Symptom observed by the professional person during an examination. As just described, objective symptoms are frequently called *signs*.

C. Pathognomonic Signs and Symptoms

Some signs and symptoms are general and may occur during various disease states. An increase in body temperature, for example, accompanies many infections.

Other signs and symptoms are *pathognomonic,* which means that the sign or symptom is unique to a particular disease and can be used to distinguish that disease or condition from other diseases or conditions.

II. TYPES OF EXAMINATION

A. Complete

A complete examination means that a thorough, comprehensive diagnostic work-up is prepared.

B. Screening

Screening implies a brief examination, using only parts of the complete diagnostic work-up. Screening is used for initial assessment and classification. In a community health program, a survey of a population made to single out people with a particular condition is called screening.

C. Limited

A limited examination is usually made for an emergency. It may be used in the management of acute conditions.

D. Follow-up

A follow-up examination is a type of limited examination. It is used to observe the effects of treatment after a period of time during which the tissue or lesion can recover and heal. Indications of the need for additional or alternate treatment are apparent at a follow-up examination.

E. Maintenance

An examination is made after a specified period of time following the completion of treatment and the restoration to health. A maintenance examination is a complete examination with a comprehensive diagnostic work-up.

III. EXAMINATION METHODS

A patient is examined by various visual, tactile, manual, and instrumental methods. General types are defined briefly here, and other specific methods are found throughout the book as they apply to a certain area under consideration.

A. Visual Examination

1. *Direct Observation.* Visual examination is made in a systematic order to note surface appearance (color, contour, size) and to observe movement and other evidence of function.
2. *Radiographic Examination.* The use of radiographs can reveal deviations from the normal not noticeable by direct observation.
3. *Transillumination.* A strong light directed through a soft tissue or a tooth to enhance examination is especially useful for detecting irregularities of the teeth and locating calculus.

B. Palpation

Palpation is examination using the sense of touch through tissue manipulation or pressure on an area with the fingers or hand. The method used depends on the area to be investigated. Types of palpation are described on page 118.

C. Instrumentation

Examination instruments, such as the explorer and probe, are used for specific examination of the teeth and periodontal tissues. They are described in detail on pages 209–217 and 219–222.

D. Percussion

Percussion is the act of tapping or striking a surface or tooth with the fingers or an instrument. Information about the status of health of the part is determined either by the response of the patient or by the sound. For example, a metal mirror handle may be used to tap each tooth successively. When a tooth is known to be painful to movement, percussion should be avoided.

E. Electrical Test

An electrical pulp vitality tester is used to detect the presence or absence of vital pulp tissue. The technique for use is described on pages 243–245.

F. Auscultation

Auscultation is the use of sound. An example is the sound of clicking or snapping of the temporomandibular joint when the jaw is moved.

TOOTH NUMBERING SYSTEMS

The three tooth designation systems in general use are the *Universal* or *Continuous Numbers 1 through 32* as adopted by the American Dental Association[1]; the *F.D.I. Two-digit,* adopted by the Fédération Dentaire Internationale[2]; and the *Palmer* or *Quadrant Numbers 1 through 8.*[3,4] Because different systems are used in dental offices and clinics, it is necessary to be familiar with all of them.

I. CONTINUOUS NUMBERS 1 THROUGH 32
This tooth numbering method is referred to as the *universal* or *ADA* system.
A. Permanent Teeth
Start with the right maxillary third molar (Number 1) and follow around the arch to the left maxillary third molar (16); descend to the left mandibular third molar (17); and follow around to the right mandibular third molar (32). Figure III–1 shows the crowns of the teeth with the corresponding numbers.

B. Primary or Deciduous Teeth
Use continuous upper case letters A through T in the same order as described for the permanent teeth: right maxillary second molar (A) around to left maxillary second molar (J); descend to left mandibular second molar (K), and around to the right mandibular second molar (T).

II. F.D.I. TWO-DIGIT
The *F.D.I.* system is also called the *International.*

A. Permanent Teeth
Each tooth is numbered by the quadrant (1 to 4) and by the tooth within the quadrant (1 to 8).
1. *Quadrant Numbers*
   1 = Maxillary right
   2 = Maxillary left
   3 = Mandibular left
   4 = Mandibular right
2. *Tooth Numbers Within Each Quadrant.* Start with number 1 at the midline (central incisor) to number 8, third molar. Figure III–2 shows each tooth number in the four quadrants.
3. *Designation.* The digits are pronounced separately. For example, "two-five" (25) is the maxillary left second premolar, and "four-two" (42) is the mandibular right lateral incisor.

B. Primary or Deciduous Teeth
Each tooth is numbered by quadrant (5 to 8) to continue with the permanent quadrant numbers. The teeth are numbered within each quadrant (1 to 5).
1. *Quadrant Numbers*
   5 = Maxillary right
   6 = Maxillary left
   7 = Mandibular left
   8 = Mandibular right
2. *Tooth Numbers Within Each Quadrant.* Number 1 is the central incisor, and number 5 is the second primary molar.
3. *Designation.* The digits are pronounced separately. For example, "eight-three" (83) is the

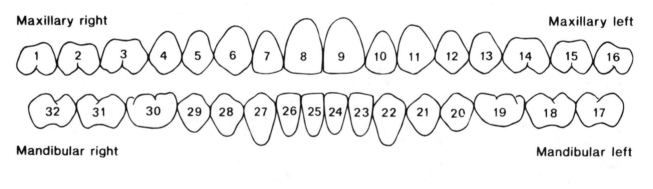

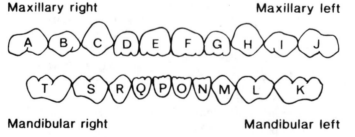

FIG. III–1. Universal Tooth Numbering (American Dental Association). *Above,* permanent dentition designated by numbers 1 through 32, starting at the maxillary right with 1 and following around to maxillary left third molar (number 16) to the left mandibular third molar (number 17) and around to the right mandibular third molar (number 32). *Below,* primary teeth are designated by letters in the same sequence.

PERMANENT TEETH

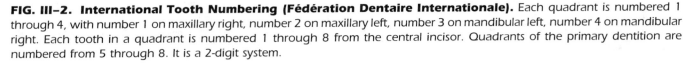

Q-1
Maxillary right

18	17	16	15	14	13	12	11	21	22	23	24	25	26	27	28
48	47	46	45	44	43	42	41	31	32	33	34	35	36	37	38

Q-2
Maxillary left

Mandibular right
Q-4

Mandibular left
Q-3

PRIMARY TEETH

Q-5
Maxillary right

55	54	53	52	51	61	62	63	64	65
85	84	83	82	81	71	72	73	74	75

Q-6
Maxillary left

Mandibular right
Q-8

Mandibular left
Q-7

FIG. III–2. International Tooth Numbering (Fédération Dentaire Internationale). Each quadrant is numbered 1 through 4, with number 1 on maxillary right, number 2 on maxillary left, number 3 on mandibular left, number 4 on mandibular right. Each tooth in a quadrant is numbered 1 through 8 from the central incisor. Quadrants of the primary dentition are numbered from 5 through 8. It is a 2-digit system.

PERMANENT TEETH

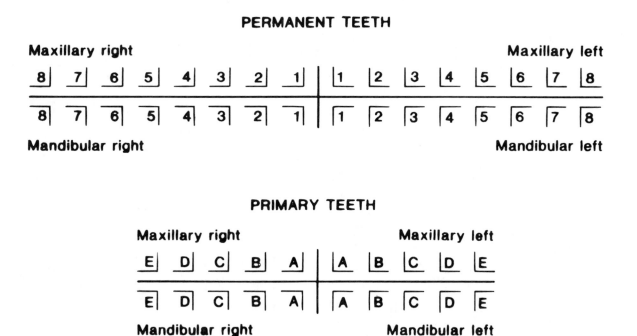

Maxillary right

Maxillary left

8	7	6	5	4	3	2	1	1	2	3	4	5	6	7	8
8	7	6	5	4	3	2	1	1	2	3	4	5	6	7	8

Mandibular right

Mandibular left

PRIMARY TEETH

Maxillary right

Maxillary left

E	D	C	B	A	A	B	C	D	E
E	D	C	B	A	A	B	C	D	E

Mandibular right

Mandibular left

FIG. III–3. Palmer System Tooth Numbering. Each permanent tooth is designated by number 1 through 8, starting at the central incisor of each quadrant. Quadrants are designated by horizontal and vertical lines. Primary teeth are identified by the letters A through E, starting at the central incisor.

mandibular right primary canine, and "six-five" (65) is the maxillary left second primary molar.

III. QUADRANT NUMBERS 1 THROUGH 8

Names to identify this method are the *Palmer system* or *Set-square.*

A. Permanent Teeth

With number 1 for each central incisor, the teeth in each quadrant are numbered to 8, the third molar (figure III–3). To identify individual teeth, horizontal and vertical lines are drawn to indicate the quadrant. For example, the left maxillary first pre-molar is ⌊4, the right mandibular first and second molars are 76̅⌋. An entire quadrant may be represented by the use of the letter Q, for example, the maxillary right quadrant is Q̲⌋.

B. Primary or Deciduous Teeth

Upper case letters A through E are used instead of the numbers. Examples are the mandibular left canine ⌈C̲ and the maxillary right first primary molar D̲⌋.

REFERENCES

1. **American Dental Association:** System of Tooth Numbering and Radiograph Mounting, Approved by the American Dental Association House of Delegates, October, 1968.

2. **Fédération Dentaire Internationale:** Two-digit System of Designating Teeth, *Int. Dent. J., 21,* 104, March, 1971.

3. **American Dental Association:** Proceedings of Dental Societies, *Dent. Cosmos, 12,* 522, October, 1870.

4. **Palmer,** C.: Palmer's Dental Notation, *Dent. Cosmos, 33,* 194, 1891.

SUGGESTED READINGS

Allen, D.L., McFall, W.T., and Jenzano, J.W.: *Periodontics for the Dental Hygienist,* 4th ed., Philadelphia, Lea & Febiger, 1987, pp. 93–136.

American Dental Association, Council on Dental Care Programs: Code on Dental Procedures and Nomenclature, *J. Am. Dent. Assoc., 122,* 91, March, 1991.

Carranza, F.A.: *Glickman's Clinical Periodontology,* 7th ed., Philadelphia, W.B. Saunders Co., 1990, pp. 476–540.

Caton, J.: Periodontal Diagnosis and Diagnostic Aids, in *Proceedings of The World Workshop in Clinical Periodontics.* Chicago, American Academy of Periodontology, 1989, pp. I-1 to I-32.

Elderton, R.J.: Keeping Up-to-date With Tooth Notation, *Br. Dent. J., 166,* 55, January 21, 1989.

Krysinski, Z.: The Three-digit System of Designating Supernumerary Teeth, *Quintessence Int., 17,* 127, February, 1986.

Peck, S. and Peck, L.: A Time for Change of Tooth Numbering Systems, *J. Dent. Educ., 57,* 643, August, 1993.

Villa Vigil, M.A., Arenal, A.A., and Gonzalez, M.A.R.: Notation of Numerical Abnormalities by an Addition to the F.D.I. System, *Quintessence Int., 20,* 299, April, 1989.

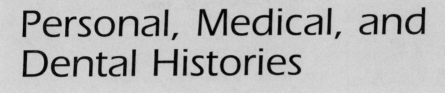

Personal, Medical, and Dental Histories

For safe, scientific dental and dental hygiene care, a meaningful, complete patient history is necessary. The history directs and guides steps to be taken in preparation for, during, and following appointments.

At least a part of the history is needed before oral examination procedures with periodontal probe and explorer are carried out. The use of instruments that would manipulate the soft tissue around the teeth may be contraindicated in certain instances until after a medical consultation to determine whether protective, precautionary measures are needed.

When a question exists about the medical history as described by the patient or when an unusual or abnormal condition is observed, consultation with the patient's physician or referral for examination of the patient who does not have a physician is mandatory. Even emergency treatment, such as for the relief of pain, should be postponed tentatively or kept to a minimum until the patient's status is determined.

I. SIGNIFICANCE

The significance of the history cannot be overestimated. Oral conditions reflect the general health of the patient. Dental procedures may complicate or be complicated by existing pathologic or physiologic conditions elsewhere in the body. General health factors influence response to treatment, such as tissue healing, and thereby affect the outcomes that may be expected from oral care.

The state of the patient's health is constantly changing. Therefore, the history represents only the period in the patient's life during which the history was made. With successive appointments, the history must be reviewed and considered along with other new findings. Key words relating to the preparation and use of the histories are defined in table 6–1.

II. PURPOSES OF THE HISTORY

Carefully prepared personal, medical and dental histories are used in comprehensive patient care to

A. Provide information pertinent to the etiology and diagnosis of oral conditions and the total treatment plan.

B. Reveal conditions that necessitate precautions, modifications, or adaptations during appointments to assure that dental and dental hygiene procedures will not harm the patient and that emergency situations will be prevented.

C. Aid in the identification of possible unrecognized conditions for which the patient should be referred for further diagnosis and treatment.

D. Permit appraisal of the general health and nutritional status, which, in turn, contributes to the prognosis of success in patient care and instruction.

E. Give insight into emotional and psychologic factors, attitudes, and prejudices that may affect present appointments as well as continuing care.

F. Document records for reference and comparison over a series of appointments for periodic follow-up.

G. Furnish evidence in legal matters should questions arise.[1]

HISTORY PREPARATION

The general methods in current use for obtaining a health history are the *interview*, the *questionnaire*, or a combination of the two. There are several systems for obtaining the history.

TABLE 6–1
KEY WORDS AND ABBREVIATIONS: PERSONAL, MEDICAL, AND DENTAL HISTORIES

Allergy (al′er-je): state of abnormal and individual hypersensitivity acquired through exposure to a particular allergen.

Antibiotic premedication (an′tĭ-bī-ot′ik): provision of an effective antibiotic before invasive clinical procedures that can create a transient bacteremia, which, in turn, can cause infective endocarditis or other serious infection.

Bacteremia (bak′tĕr-ē′mē-ah): presence of microorganisms in the blood stream.

Drug interaction: a change in the effect of one drug when a second drug is introduced concomitantly; the change may be desirable, adverse, or inconsequential.

Forensic (fo-ren′zik): pertaining to or applied in legal proceedings.

    Forensic dentistry: dentolegal science; the relation and application of dental facts to legal problems, as in using the teeth for identifying the dead.

Immunocompromised (im′ū-nō-kom′prō-mizd): when the immune response is attenuated by administration of immunosuppressive drugs, by irradiation, by malnutrition, or by certain disease processes.

Informed consent: a medicolegal document that holds providers responsible for ensuring that patients understand the risks and benefits of a procedure or medication before it is administered.

OTC: over the counter; nonprescription drug; pertains to distribution of drugs directly to the public without prescription.

PDR: *Physicians' Desk Reference;* contains current information about the actions, side effects, and interactions of drugs; a new edition is published annually.

Premedication: preliminary medication; may be for the purpose of allaying apprehension, preventing bacteremia, or otherwise facilitating the clinical procedure.

SBE: subacute bacterial endocarditis.

I. SYSTEMS

A. Preappointment Information

Basic information obtained prior to the initial assessment appointment can save time and facilitate the process. A brief telephone screening interview can help to determine potential medical problems and need for premedication, and can identify medically compromised patients for whom modifications in routine care may be needed.

B. Brief History

A brief history of vital items is obtained at the initial visit; a complete history is obtained at a succeeding appointment.

1. Purposes of brief history are to prepare for emergency care and to learn of any condition that may contraindicate instrumentation.
2. Brief history may be in the form of a ques-

tionnaire; an interview for follow-up provides opportunity for individual evaluation.

C. Self-history

Because this history is prepared at home, the history form may be mailed to the patient in advance or given at the first appointment to complete and bring in at the second appointment. Such a form might include some checking, as in a questionnaire, and some space to allow free expression by the patient.

D. Complete History

Complete history is made at the initial visit and may be a combination of interview and questionnaire.

II. RECORD FORMS

A. Types

Many varying forms are in current use. Forms are available commercially or from the American Dental Association (ADA),[2] but many dentists and dental hygienists prefer to develop their own and have a form printed to their specifications.

B. Characteristics of an Adequate Form

The number of items or questions included is not necessarily indicative of the value of the form. The extensive and involved form may be as practical or impractical as the brief checklist that permits no detailed description. Success in use depends on function and a clear common understanding of the meaning of the recorded information to all who refer to it.

Some characteristics of an adequate form are that it should

1. Provide for conventional notation of important details in a logical sequence.
2. Permit quick identification of special needs of a patient when the history is reviewed prior to each appointment.
3. Allow ample space to record the patient's own words whenever possible in the interview method, or for self-expression by the patient on a questionnaire.
4. Have space for notes concerning attitudes and knowledge as stated or displayed by the patient during the history-taking or other later appointments.
5. Be of a size consistent with the complete patient record forms for filing and ready availability.

III. INTRODUCTION TO THE PATIENT

The patient needs to realize why the information requested in the histories is essential before treatment can be undertaken. Dental personnel must convey the idea that oral health and general health are interrelated, without creating undue alarm concerning potential ill effects or harmful sequelae from required treatment.

For building rapport, children may participate in their history preparation, but most of the information will need to be supplied by a parent. The signature of the responsible adult on the record is advisable.

IV. LIMITATIONS OF A HISTORY[3,4,5]

Many patients cannot or will not provide complete or, in certain cases, correct information when answering medical or dental history questions. There may be problems related to the method of obtaining the histories, how the questions are worded, or an inadvertent lack of neutrality in the attitude of the person preparing the history. Some patients may have difficulty in comprehending a self-administered test, or there may be a language barrier.

Where the questionnaire is completed may influence answers. A crowded reception area where other patients can see the form and the checks made does not provide sufficient privacy.

Another reason for inaccuracy or incompleteness is that patients may not understand the relationship between certain diseases or conditions and dental treatment. Information may seem irrelevant, so it is withheld. Occasionally, a patient will not want to tell about a condition that may be embarrassing to discuss. The patient may fear refusal of treatment, particularly if such had been a previous experience in other dental practices.

THE QUESTIONNAIRE

Positive findings on a completed questionnaire need supplementation in a personal interview. A questionnaire by itself cannot be expected to satisfy the overall purposes of the history, but can be adapted best to phases of the personal history, some aspects of the dental history, and factual information in the medical history.

I. TYPES OF QUESTIONS

The Health Questionnaire available from the American Dental Association (figure 6–1) provides useful examples of questions essential to patient evaluation.[2]

A. System-oriented

Direct questions or topics that check whether the patient has had a disease of, for example, the digestive system, respiratory system, or urinary system may be used. The questions may contain references to body parts, for example, the stomach, lungs, kidneys. Questions can then be directed to the specific disease state and the dates and duration.

B. Disease-oriented

A typical set of questions for the patient to check may start with "Do you have, or have you had, any of the following diseases or problems?" A listing under that question contains such items as diabetes, asthma, or rheumatic fever arranged alphabetically or grouped by systems or body organs.

Follow-up questions can determine dates of illness, severity, and outcome.

C. Symptom-oriented

In the absence of previous or current disease states, questions may lead to a suspicion of a condition, which, in turn, can provide an opportunity to recommend and encourage the patient to schedule an examination by a physician. Examples of the symptom-oriented questions are "Are you thirsty much of the time?" "Does your mouth frequently become dry?" or "Do you have to urinate (pass water) more than six times a day?" Positive answers could lead to tests for diabetes detection.

II. ADVANTAGES OF A QUESTIONNAIRE

A. Broad in scope; useful during the interview to identify positive areas that need additional clarification.

B. Time-saving.

C. Consistent; all selected questions are included, and none is omitted because of time or other factors.

D. Patient has time to think over the answers; not under pressure, nor under the eyes of the interviewer.

E. Patient may write information that might not be expressed directly in an interview.

F. Legal aspects of a written record with patient's signature.

III. DISADVANTAGES OF A QUESTIONNAIRE (IF USED ALONE WITHOUT A FOLLOW-UP INTERVIEW)

A. Impersonal; no opportunity to develop rapport.

B. Inflexible; no provision for additional questioning in areas of specific importance to an individual patient.

THE INTERVIEW

In long-range planning for the patient's health, much more is involved than asking questions and receiving answers. The rapport established at the time of the interview contributes to the continued cooperation of the patient.

I. PARTICIPANTS

The interviewer is alone with the patient or parent of the child patient. The history should never be taken in a reception area when other patients are present.

Medical History Form

Date _____

Name _____ Home Phone (_____) _____
      Last   First   Middle

Address _____ Business Phone (_____) _____
      Number, Street

City _____ State _____ Zip Code _____

Occupation _____ Social Security No. _____

Date of Birth ___/___/___ Sex M F Height _____ Weight _____ Single _____ Married _____
      mo. day yr.

Name of Spouse _____ Closest Relative _____ Phone (_____) _____

If you are completing this form for another person, what is your relationship to that person? _____

Referred by _____

For the following questions, *circle yes or no*, whichever applies. Your answers are for our records only and will be considered confidential. Please note that during your initial visit you will be asked some questions about your responses to this questionnaire and there may be additional questions concerning your health.

1. Are you in good health? . . . . Yes   No
2. Has there been any change in your general health within the past year? . . . . Yes   No
3. My last physical examination was on _____
4. Are you now under the care of a physician? . . . . Yes   No
   If so, what is the condition being treated? _____
5. The name and address of my physician(s) is _____
   _____
   _____
6. Have you had any serious illness, operation, or been hospitalized in the past 5 years? . . . . Yes   No
   If so, what was the illness or problem? _____
7. Are you taking any medicine(s) including non-prescription medicine?. . . . . Yes   No
   If so, what medicine(s) are you taking? _____
8. Do you have or have you had any of the following diseases or problems?
   a. Damaged heart valves or artificial heart valves, including heart murmur or rheumatic heart disease . . . . Yes   No
   b. Cardiovascular disease (heart trouble, heart attack, angina, coronary insufficiency, coronary occlusion, high blood
      pressure, arteriosclerosis, stroke) . . . . Yes   No
        1. Do you have chest pain upon exertion? . . . . Yes   No
        2. Are you ever short of breath after mild exercise or when lying down?. . . . . Yes   No
        3. Do your ankles swell? . . . . Yes   No
        4. Do you have inborn heart defects? . . . . Yes   No
        5. Do you have a cardiac pacemaker? . . . . Yes   No
   c. Allergy . . . . Yes   No
   d. Sinus trouble . . . . Yes   No
   e. Asthma or hay fever . . . . Yes   No
   f. Fainting spells or seizures . . . . Yes   No
   g. Persistent diarrhea or recent weight loss . . . . Yes   No
   h. Diabetes . . . . Yes   No
   i. Hepatitis, jaundice or liver disease . . . . Yes   No
   j. AIDS or HIV infection . . . . Yes   No
   k. Thyroid problems . . . . Yes   No
   l. Respiratory problems, emphysema, bronchitis, etc. . . . . Yes   No
   m. Arthritis or painful swollen joints . . . . Yes   No
   n. Stomach ulcer or hyperacidity . . . . Yes   No
   o. Kidney trouble . . . . Yes   No
   p. Tuberculosis . . . . Yes   No
   q. Persistent cough or cough that produces blood . . . . Yes   No
   r. Persistent swollen glands in neck . . . . Yes   No
   s. Low blood pressure . . . . Yes   No
   t. Sexually transmitted disease . . . . Yes   No
   u. Epilepsy or other neurological disease . . . . Yes   No
   v. Problems with mental health . . . . Yes   No
   w. Cancer . . . . Yes   No
   x. Problems of the immune system . . . . Yes   No

(over)

FIG. 6–1. Medical History Form. From American Dental Association, Council on Dental Therapeutics. Reprinted with permission.

9. Have you had abnormal bleeding?. . . . .   Yes   No
    a. Have you ever required a blood transfusion? . . . .   Yes   No
10. Do you have any blood disorder such as anemia? . . . .   Yes   No
11. Have you ever had any treatment for a tumor or growth? . . . .   Yes   No
12. Are you allergic or have you had a reaction to:
    a. Local anesthetics . . . .   Yes   No
    b. Penicillin or other antibiotics . . . .   Yes   No
    c. Sulfa drugs . . . .   Yes   No
    d. Barbiturates, sedatives, or sleeping pills . . . .   Yes   No
    e. Aspirin . . . .   Yes   No
    f. Iodine . . . .   Yes   No
    g. Codeine or other narcotics . . . .   Yes   No
    h. Other _____
13. Have you had any serious trouble associated with any previous dental treatment? . . . .   Yes   No
    If so, explain _____
_____

14. Do you have any disease, condition, or problem not listed above that you think I should know about? . . . .   Yes   No
    If so, explain _____
_____

15. Are you wearing contact lenses? . . . .   Yes   No
16. Are you wearing removable dental appliances? . . . .   Yes   No

Women

17. Are you pregnant? . . . .   Yes   No
18. Do you have any problems associated with your menstrual period? . . . .   Yes   No
19. Are you nursing? . . . .   Yes   No
20. Are you taking birth control pills? . . . .   Yes   No

Chief Dental Complaint _____
_____

I certify that I have read and understand the above. I acknowledge that my questions, if any, about the inquiries set forth above have been answered to my satisfaction. I will not hold my dentist, or any other member of his/her staff, responsible for any errors or omissions that I may have made in the completion of this form.

_____
Signature of Patient

For completion by the dentist.
Comments on patient interview concerning medical history: _____
_____
_____

Significant findings from questionnaire or oral interview: _____
_____
_____

Dental management considerations: _____
_____
_____

_____   _____
(Date)   Signature of Dentist

Medical history update:

Date	Comments	Signature

FIG. 6-1. (continued)

MEDICAL HISTORY INTERVIEW

Date_____

Part I *(to be completed by patient or guardian)*

Name_____ Home Phone (_____) _____

Address_____ Business Phone (_____) _____

City_____ State_____ Zip Code_____

Occupation_____ Social Security No._____

Date of Birth_____ Sex M F Height_____ Weight_____ Single___ Married___

Name of Spouse_____ Closest Relative_____ Phone (_____) _____

If the person completing this form is other than the patient, what is his/her relationship to the patient?_____

Referred by_____

Part II *(to be completed by dentist)*

A. CHIEF COMPLAINT

_____

B. DENTAL HISTORY

Frequency of visits to dentist_____

Type of care received_____

Difficulties with past treatment_____

Adverse reactions to local anesthetics, latex gloves, rubber dam_____

Date of most recent dental radiographic exam_____

C. MEDICAL HISTORY

Are you now or have you been under the care of a physician during the past 12 months?_____

Last time at physician_____ For what purpose?_____

Physician_____ Physician's Phone No._____

Do you have any known allergies or sensitivities?_____

Do you take any medications at the present time?_____

Females only: Do you take oral contraceptives?_____ Are you pregnant?_____

Have you noted a change in your menstrual pattern?_____

D. FAMILY HISTORY

(Have any members of your family ever been treated for the conditions listed or any other medical problems?)

Diabetes_____ High blood pressure_____ Heart problem_____ Seizures_____

Other_____

E. SOCIAL HISTORY

Smoking_____ Alcohol_____ Other_____

S-502

FIG. 6-2. Medical History Interview. From American Dental Association, Council on Dental Therapeutics. Reprinted with permission.

F. REVIEW OF SYSTEMS (Have you ever had or do you now have any of the conditions listed?)

I. Skin
Itching_____
Rash_____
Ulcers_____
Pigmentations_____
Lack or loss of body hair_____

II. Extremities
Varicose veins_____
Swollen, painful joints_____
Muscle weakness, pain_____
Bone deformity, fracture_____
Prosthetic joints_____

III. Eyes
Blurring of vision_____
Double vision_____
Drooping of eyelid_____
Glaucoma_____

IV. Ear, Nose, Throat
Earache_____
Hearing loss_____
Frequent nosebleeds_____
Sinusitis)_____
Frequent sore throat_____
Hoarseness_____

V. Respiratory
Cough, blood in sputum_____
Emphysema, bronchitis_____
Wheezing, asthma_____
Tuberculosis, exposure to_____

VI. Cardiac
Shortness of breath_____
Pain, pressure in chest_____
Swelling of ankles_____
High, low blood pressure_____
Rheumatic, scarlet fever_____
Heart murmur, attack_____
Prosthetic valves/pacemakers_____

VII. Gastrointestinal
Difficulty swallowing_____
Abdominal pain, ulcers_____
Hepatitis, jaundice_____
Liver disease_____

VIII. Genitourinary
Difficulty, pain on urination_____
Blood in urine_____
Excessive urination_____
Kidney infections_____
Sexually transmitted diseases_____

IX. Endocrine
Thyroid trouble_____
Weight change_____
Diabetes_____
Excessive thirst_____

X. Hematopoietic
Easy bruising, excessive bleeding_____
Persistent lymphadenopathy_____
G6PD deficiency_____
Anemia_____
HIV infection, AIDS_____
Leukemia, problems with immune system____
Spleen problems_____

XI. Neurologic
Frequent headaches_____
Dizziness, fainting_____
Epilepsy, fits_____
Neuritis, neuralgia_____
Parasthesias, numbness_____
Paralysis_____

XII. Psychiatric
Nervousness_____
Irritability_____
Depression, excessive worry_____
Nervous breakdown_____

XIII. Growth or Tumor
Radiotherapy/chemotherapy_____

I certify that any and all questions I had about the inquiries above have been answered to my satisfaction. I was asked all of the questions on this form and I have answered these questions truthfully and completely. I will not hold my dentist, or any other member of his/her staff, responsible for any errors or omissions that I may have made.

_____   _____
date   signature of patient

_____   _____
date   signature of guardian (where applicable)

Comments on patient interview concerning medical history:_____

_____

Significant findings from questionnaire or oral interview:_____

_____

Dental management considerations:_____

_____

_____   _____
(date)   (signature of dentist)

Medical History Update:

Date   Comments   Signature

_____   _____   _____

_____   _____   _____

_____   _____   _____

FIG. 6-2. (continued)

II. SETTING

A. A consultation room or office is preferred; the patient should be away from the atmosphere of the treatment room where thoughts may be on the techniques to be performed.

B. Treatment room may be the only available place where privacy is afforded.

1. Seat patient comfortably in upright position.
2. Turn off running water and dental light, and close the door.
3. Sit on operating stool to be at eye level with the patient.

III. POINTERS FOR THE INTERVIEW

Interviewing involves communication between individuals. Communication implies the transmission or interchange of facts, attitudes, opinions, or thoughts, through words, gestures, or other means. Through tactful but direct questioning, communication can be successful and the patient will give such information as is known. Frequently, the patient is unaware of a health problem.

The attitude of the dental personnel should be one of friendly understanding, reassurance, and acceptance. Genuine interest and willingness to listen when a patient wishes to describe symptoms or complaints not only aids in establishing the rapport needed, but frequently provides insight into the patient's real attitudes and prejudices. By asking simple questions at first, and more personal questions later after rapport has developed, the patient will be more relaxed and frank in answering.

Self-confidence and gentle efficiency on the part of the interviewer help to give the patient a feeling of confidence. Skill is required, because tact, ingenuity, and judgment are taxed to the fullest in the attempt to obtain both accurate and complete information from the patient.

IV. INTERVIEW FORM

The interviewer may use a structured form with places to check and fill in, such as the ADA form S-502 shown in figure 6–2. Another method is to record on blank sheets from questions created from a guide list of essential topics. Either may involve reference to the positive or negative answers on a previously completed questionnaire.

Familiarity with the items on the history permits the interviewer to be direct and informal without reading from a fixed list of topics, a method that may lack the personal touch necessary to gain the patient's confidence. When appropriate, the patient's own words are recorded.

V. ADVANTAGES OF THE INTERVIEW

A. Personal contact contributes to development of rapport for future appointments.

B. Flexibility for individual needs; details obtained can be adapted for supplementary questioning.

VI. DISADVANTAGES OF INTERVIEW

A. Time-consuming when not prefaced with questionnaire.

B. Unless a list is consulted, items of importance may be omitted.

C. Patient may be embarrassed to talk about personal conditions and may hold back significant information.

ITEMS INCLUDED IN THE HISTORY

Information obtained by means of the history is directly related to how the goals for patient care can and will be accomplished. In tables 6–2, 6–3, and 6–4, items are listed with possible medications and other treatments the patient may have or has had, along with suggested influences on appointment procedures.

In specialized practices, objectives may require increased emphasis on certain aspects. The age group most frequently served would influence the material needed. Parental history and pre- and postnatal information may take on particular significance for the treatment of a small child; in a pedodontist's practice, a special form could be devised to include all essential items.

Insight and awareness shown while preparing the patient history depend on background knowledge of the manifestations of systemic diseases and the medications for various conditions. Objectives for the items to include in the various parts of the history are listed here.

I. PERSONAL HISTORY (table 6–2)

The basic objectives in gathering personal information about the patient are

A. Data essential for appointment planning and business aspects.

B. Approval of care of a minor and other legal aspects.

C. For consultation with the patient's physician relative to interrelations between general and oral health.

II. DENTAL HISTORY (table 6–3)

The dental history should contribute to knowledge of

A. The immediate problem, chief complaint, cause of present pain, or discomfort of any kind in the oral cavity.

B. The previous dental care as described by the patient, including extent of restorative and prosthetic replacement, as well as any adverse effects.

C. The attitude of the patient toward oral health and care of the mouth as may be indicated by previous periodic dental and dental hygiene treatments.

D. The personal daily care exercised by the patient as evidence of knowledge of the purposes of con-

TABLE 6–2
ITEMS FOR THE PERSONAL HISTORY

Items to Record in Patient History	Considerations	Influences on Appointment Procedures
1. Name Addresses: Residence and Business Telephone Numbers Sex Marital Status For Child: Name of Parent or Guardian For Parent: Ages and Sex of Children	Accurate recording necessary for business aspects of dental practice	Aids in establishing rapport Instruction applicable to entire family Advice concerning fluorides for children
2. Birthdate	Whether of age or a minor Oral conditions related to age changes; diseases, healing, and other possible characteristics	Approval of parent or guardian necessary for care of minor or person with a mental handicap; signature must be obtained Approach to patient instruction
3. Birthplace and Residence in Early Years	Presence of fluoride in drinking water Food and eating patterns Conditions endemic to certain areas	Effects of fluoride on teeth Instruction in dietary needs adapted to cultural practices
4. Occupation: Present and Former Spouse's Occupation For Children: Parent's Occupation	May be a factor in etiology of certain diseases, dental stains, occlusal wear May affect diet, oral habits, general health	Instruction applied to specific needs Dexterity in use of self-care devices related to dexterity gained from occupation Influence on oral care of entire family For child: which parent will supervise and assist child in oral care
5. Physician	Name, address, and telephone number For consultation	Consultation indicated: (1) for condition that may require premedication (2) when disease symptoms are suspected but patient does not state (3) in an emergency
6. Referred by and Address	To whom to send referral acknowledgment and appreciation	Contribution to rapport with patient Patient referred by another patient may have concept of the office procedures

tinuing care and of the value placed on the teeth and their supporting structures.

III. MEDICAL HISTORY (table 6–4)
Objectives of the medical history are to determine whether the patient has or has had any conditions in the following categories:

A. Diseases that May Complicate Certain Kinds of Dental and Dental Hygiene Treatment
Examples. Leukemia, because of lowered resistance to infection; uncontrolled hypertension, with blood pressure reading 180/105 or greater; congestive heart failure, which requires treatment before stressful procedures, particularly surgery, can be performed.

B. Diseases that Require Special Precautions or Premedication Prior to Treatment
Examples. Antibiotic coverage for patient with a history of rheumatic fever or congenital heart defect, to prevent infective endocarditis; possible need for increased sedation in patients subject to convulsions to prevent a seizure if treatment is to be stressful.

TABLE 6–3
ITEMS FOR THE DENTAL HISTORY

Items to Record in the History	Considerations	Influences on Appointment Procedures
1. Reason for Present Appointment	Chief complaint in patient's own words Pain or discomfort Onset, symptoms, duration of an acute condition	Need for immediate treatment Attitude toward dentistry and preventive care
2. Previous Dental Appointments	Date last treatment Services performed Regularity	Patient knowledge concerning regular dental care Cooperation anticipated
3. Anesthetics Used	Local, general Adverse or allergic reactions	Choice of anesthetic
4. Radiation History	Type, number, dates of dental and medical radiographs Therapeutic radiation Availability of dental radiographs from previous dentist Amount of exposure considered with exposure for medical purposes	Amount of exposure; limitations Patient's appreciation for need and use of radiographs
5. Family Dental History	Parental tooth loss or maintenance	Attitude toward saving teeth and preventive dentistry
6. Previous Treatment A. Periodontal B. Orthodontic C. Endodontic D. Prosthodontic E. Other	Type of treatment; frequency maintenance appointments Whether referred to specialist History of acute infection (necrotizing ulcerative gingivitis) Surgery; postoperative healing Age during treatment; completion Previous problem Habit correction Dates, etiology Types of prostheses Extent of restorations Tooth loss Implants	Attitude toward specialized care Previous familiarity with role of dental hygienist Attitude toward self-care and disease control For current treatment, consultation with orthodontist needed to determine instructions Periodic recheck Care of prostheses and abutment teeth Understanding of prevention
7. Injuries to Face or Teeth	Causes and extent Fractured teeth or jaws	Limitation of opening Special care during healing
8. Temporomandibular Joint	History of injury, discomfort, disease, dislocation Previous treatment	Effect on opening; accessibility during instrumentation
9. Habits	Clenching, bruxism Mouth breathing Biting objects: fingernails, pipe stem, thread, other Cheek or lip biting Patient awareness of habits	Tension of patient Instruction relative to effects of habits
10. Tobacco Use	Form of tobacco, amount used Frequency Knowledge of effects on oral tissues	Instruction concerning oral effects Need for frequent observation to detect tissue changes if patient continues at same rate (periodontal risk) Dental stains; dentifrice selection

TABLE 6–3 *(continued)*
ITEMS FOR THE DENTAL HISTORY

Items to Record in the History	Considerations	Influences on Appointment Procedures
11. Fluorides	Systemic, topical, dates Residences during tooth development years Amount of fluoride in drinking water	Current preventive procedures and need for re-evaluation

12. Plaque Control Procedures	Toothbrushing: current procedures
	    Type of brush (manual or powered)
	    Texture of filaments
	    Frequency of use
	    Age of brush; frequency of having a new brush
	Dentifrice
	    Name
	    How selected; reason
	Additional cleansing devices and frequency of use
	    Dental floss
	    Water irrigation
	    Implants care
	Mouthrinse or other agents: frequency, purpose
	Source of instruction in care of oral cavity
		Present practices and previous instruction
		New instruction needed; reception by patient
		Relation of techniques to prevention of dental caries and periodontal infections
		Supervision of child by parent: current practices
		Problems of habit change

C. Diseases Under Treatment by a Physician that Require Medicating Drugs that May Influence or Contraindicate Certain Procedures

Examples. Tranquilizers in daily use could contraindicate premedication with sedatives; anticoagulant therapy requires consultation with physician; antihypertensive drugs may alter the choice of general or local anesthetic used.

D. Allergic or Untoward Reactions to Drugs

Examples. All drugs that may possibly be used or recommended to the patient for postoperative care should be checked with the patient as to previous use and reaction.

E. Diseases and Drugs with Manifestations in the Mouth

Examples. Hematologic disorders; phenytoin-induced gingival overgrowth.

F. Communicable Diseases that Endanger the Dental Personnel

Examples. Active tuberculosis; viral hepatitis; herpes; syphilis.

G. Physiologic State of the Patient

Examples. Pregnancy; puberty; menopause.

REVIEW OF HISTORY

Updating the history at each maintenance appointment is essential. Changes in health status revealed by interim medical examinations or evidenced by reported illness or hospitalizations must be recorded and considered during continuing treatment.

Following a review of the previously recorded history, questions can be directed to the patient to compare the present condition with the previous one and to determine at least the following:

A. Interim illnesses; changes in health.
B. Visits to physician; reasons and results.
C. Laboratory tests performed and the results; blood, urine, or other analyses.
D. Current medications.
E. Changes in the oral soft tissues and the teeth observed by the patient.

IMMEDIATE APPLICATIONS OF PATIENT HISTORIES

Together with information from all other parts of the diagnostic work-up, the patient histories are essential for the preparation of the treatment plan. Treatment planning for an individual patient is described on pages 322–326.

Immediate evaluation of the histories is necessary before proceeding to succeeding steps in the preparation of materials for the complete diagnostic work-up. Any objective for the medical history could alter the procedures to be accomplished.

The list that follows is not intended to be exhaustive, but rather suggestive. From these items, the dental personnel should be alerted to precautions that may be needed.

(text continues on page 101)

**TABLE 6–4
ITEMS FOR THE MEDICAL HISTORY**

Item to Record in History	Considerations	Possible Medications and Treatment Modalities	Influences on Appointment Procedures
1. General Health and Appearance	Disabilities Overall impression of well-being Patient's appraisal of own health		Response, cooperation, and attitude to expect during appointments
2. Medical Examination	Date most recent examination Reason for the examination Tests performed; results Anticipated surgery	New prescriptions received Previous prescriptions continued	Verification with physician for added information Need for superior state of oral health in advance of surgery (1) when long recovery is expected and patient may miss maintenance appointments (2) prior to transplant, heart surgery, or prosthesis
3. Major Illnesses, Hospitalizations, Operations	Causes of illness Type and duration of treatment Anesthetics used Convalescence Course of healing: normal, not normal	Medications, treatments	Influence of illnesses on health and care of the oral cavity Anesthetic choice Expected outcome from gingival treatment
4. Age Factors	Problems of health in different age groups Geriatric: multiple disease entities. Patient may need to bring the containers for identification of their medications		Effects on dental and dental hygiene procedures and personal care
5. Height and Weight	Weight changes over past years or months Obesity Undernourishment Child growth pattern	"Diet pills" Substance abuse	Marked weight change may be a symptom of undiagnosed disease; suggest referral for medical examination Influence on dietary instructions for oral health
6. Medications Prescribed by Physician	Reasons: relation to dental care Frequency Patient's regularity of taking Sugar content of liquid medicines, threatening to dental caries (also true of over-the-counter [OTC] items)	List all drugs by name Ask patient for drugs, medicine, injections, tonics, vitamins, pills, capsules, to get a complete answer	Consultation with physician concerning adjustments in dosage for dental or dental hygiene appointments Indications for premedication Side effects of drugs
7. Self-Medication	Type, frequency OTC preparations Substance abuse	Pain relievers Sleeping tablets Cough syrup Antacids Cathartics Vitamins	Information not revealed by patient could complicate treatment Lack of interest in oral health, only pain relief

TABLE 6–4 (*continued*)
ITEMS FOR THE MEDICAL HISTORY

Item to Record in History	Considerations	Possible Medications and Treatment Modalities	Influences on Appointment Procedures
8. Family Medical History	Predisposition to certain diseases (example: diabetes) History of diseases that occur in the family	Cultural beliefs about medications	May help patient seek medical examination when symptom suggests possible disease
9. Daily Diet	Recommendations of patient's physicians, past and present Vitamin supplements Appetite Regularity of meals Food likes and dislikes	Vitamin supplements	Instructions to be given relative to oral health Prognosis for healing after treatment Need for dietary review and analysis
10. Alcohol Consumption	Frequency Amount Substance abuse	Recovering alcoholic: May be taking disulfiram, vitamins Must avoid all alcohol-containing preparations, including commercial mouthrinses.	Excessive use: effect on anesthesia; increased healing time Poor nutritional state is common; lack of oral care May result in poor patient cooperation
11. Allergies	Determine substances to which the patient is allergic: Anesthetics Penicillin Medicaments Foods Iodine	Antihistamines Inhalers Decongestants Steroids	Preparation for emergency Xerostomia Avoid use of substances to which the patient is allergic Consider allergies when planning dietary recommendations
12. Arthritis	Joint pain Immobility Temporomandibular joint involvement	Aspirin Nonsteroidal anti-inflammatory drugs Corticosteroids Total joint replacements	Antibiotic premedication Dental chair adjustment
13. Blood Disorder	Type and duration of disease Leukemia: remission, thrombocytopenia	Vitamins Minerals: Iron (iron-deficiency anemia) Folic acid supplement (sickle cell anemia) Antineoplastic drugs	Consultation with physician Need for high level of oral health Antibiotic premedication Immunosuppression Increased bleeding Oral lesions
14. Bleeding	Bleeding associated with previous dental appointments History of disorder with coagulation problem History of transfusions or other blood products Check use of aspirin (relation to bleeding tendency) Laboratory tests for bleeding time, coagulation may be needed	Anticoagulant Hemophilia factor replacement	Antibiotic premedication Emergency prevention through preappointment precautions Avoid tissue trauma May need to apply dressing after scaling to provide pressure Special measures for hemophilia

TABLE 6–4 (*continued*)
ITEMS FOR THE MEDICAL HISTORY

Item to Record in History	Considerations	Possible Medications and Treatment Modalities	Influences on Appointment Procedures
15. Cancer	Head and neck radiation effects on oral cavity, salivary glands Dental and dental hygiene therapy updated before start of surgery, radiation therapy, or immunosuppression Blood count prior to dental and dental hygiene therapy.	Radiation therapy Fluoride therapy: daily topical application Antineoplastic drugs alkylating agents, antimetabolites, antibiotics, plant alkaloids, steroids	Antibiotic premedication Bleeding; infection; poor healing response Avoid trauma to tissues Effect on oral radiographic survey: prevention of overexposure Dental caries: preventive measures Xerostomia: substitute saliva
16. Cardiovascular diseases	Consultation with physician Refer for examination when patient seems unsure of problem	Cardiac glycosides Antiarrhythmics Antianginals Antihypertensives Anticoagulants	Minimize stress Premedication for stress Ascertain that medications have been taken
Congenital Heart Disease Rheumatic Heart Disease	Susceptibility to infective endocarditis Type of problem; date of rheumatic fever	Antibiotic (prevent recurrence of rheumatic fever)	Antibiotic premedication required
Hypertension	Symptom of other disease state Monitoring blood pressure for each appointment Anesthesia: limit epinephrine or omit as recommended by physician	Diuretics Antiadrenergic agents Vasodilators Angiotensin-converting enzyme inhibitors	Postural hypotension (raise dental chair slowly) Xerostomia: saliva substitute and fluoride rinse may be needed
Angina Pectoris	Prepare for symptoms: have ready amyl nitrite vaporole or nitroglycerin tablets	Amyl nitrite, nitroglycerin, or other antianginal drugs	Allay fears and prevent stress

Heart Diseases	History of disease
	  Symptoms of fatigue, shortness of breath, or cough
	  Consult with physician
		Glycosides (digitalis)
		Anticoagulants
		Antiarrhythmic drugs
		
		Pacemaker
			Short, more frequent appointments
			Change dental chair slowly
			Patient with breathing problem (sleeps with 2 or more pillows) may need semiupright position
			Bleeding tendency associated with anticoagulant
			Avoid ultrasonic (pacemaker)
			Antibiotic premedication indicated

TABLE 6–4 (continued)
ITEMS FOR THE MEDICAL HISTORY

Item to Record in History	Considerations	Possible Medications and Treatment Modalities	Influences on Appointment Procedures
16. Cardiovascular (continued) Surgically Corrected Cardiovascular Lesions	Type, date of operation Consultation with physician Before surgical procedure, when possible: the patient needs complete oral evaluation and corrective dental work done, and needs motivation to high level of oral personal care daily	No tobacco use Anticoagulants	Antibiotic premedication vital for synthetic valves or other replacements, indefinitely Autogenous graft (bypass) needs antibiotic first 6 months Gingival bleeding can be expected
Cerebrovascular Accident (Stroke)	Date of onset; residual disabilities Speech, vision, mental function	No tobacco; low-salt diet Anticoagulants Antihypertensives Vasodilator Steroid Anticonvulsant	Gingival bleeding likely when anticoagulants are used Adapt procedures for physical disability
17. Communicable Diseases	History of diseases; immunizations Present disease; communicability Residences or extended trips in countries with high endemic incidence of certain diseases Risk group factor	Immunizations	Universal precautions
Hepatitis B	Jaundice history Clarification of type of hepatitis Laboratory clearance	Vaccine for HBV	Universal precautions
Tuberculosis	Active or passive Cough Duration of disease	Isoniazid (INH) Rifampin Pyrazinamide	Universal precautions Length of treatment: infectivity diminished after few months of treatment
Sexually Transmitted Infections (STIs)	May not obtain history of STIs Oral and pharyngeal lesions may be present	Antibiotics	Infectiousness diminishes with antibiotic therapy for gonorrhea and syphilis Refer to physician and postpone treatment when lesions or other signs suggest infection Caution for risk from previously treated diseases
Herpes	Lesions can be transmitted readily	Nondefinitive; symptomatic and palliative treatment Acyclovir	Postpone routine care when oral lesions are present
HIV Infection AIDS	Risk group identification Oral manifestations	Wide variety of opportunistic infections and complications require variety of drugs	Complete sterilization and barrier procedures as for all communicable diseases Universal precautions

TABLE 6-4 (*continued*)
ITEMS FOR THE MEDICAL HISTORY

Item to Record in History	Considerations	Possible Medications and Treatment Modalities	Influences on Appointment Procedures
18. Diabetes Mellitus	Uncontrolled: requires antibiotic premedication Undiagnosed: excess thirst, appetite, and urination Family incidence: help in finding susceptible, undiagnosed Severe advanced diabetes: complications (vision, kidney, cardiovascular, nervous system)	IDDM (Insulin-dependent): Insulin NIDDM (Noninsulin-dependent): Diet control Hypoglycemics	Prepare for emergency: insulin; sugar, frosting Appointment time related to insulin therapy and mealtime Avoid tissue trauma Need frequent maintenance appointments Periodontal disease accelerated Referral for tests for suspected undiagnosed
19. Ears	Deafness or degree of hearing impairment Infections, operations, ringing, dizziness, balance	Treatment for infection Hearing aid	Adaptations for communication and plaque control instruction
20. Endocrine	Age-group relation to certain conditions Growth, development Menstruation, menopause	Thyroid hormone supplement Antithyroid Estrogen/progestin Oral contraceptives Corticosteroids	Emphasis on high level of plaque control Any patient taking steroids may need antibiotic premedication for appointments Monitor blood pressure
21. Epilepsy	Type, frequency of seizures precipitating factors Preparation for emergency seizure	Anticonvulsant Sedative	Minimize stress Medications make patient drowsy, less alert Valproic acid requires bleeding time preoperatively
22. Eyes	Disturbance of vision Purpose for corrective eyeglasses or contact lenses Manifestations of systemic disease	Eyedrops (for example, glaucoma)	Remove contact lenses Protective eyewear during appointment Adaptations for communication with limited sight
23. Gastrointestinal	Nature and treatment of the disease Diet restrictions prescribed by physician	Antacids Antidiarrheal Laxatives Antispasmodics	Patient instruction in accord with prescribed diet and medication Xerostomia
24. Kidney	Renal disease; kidney stones Hemodialysis: hypertension, anemia, hepatitis carrier Transplant: hypertension, hepatitis	Salt restriction Many drugs are nephrotoxic Immunosuppressive drugs	Antibiotic premedication Monitor blood pressure Bleeding tendency Poor healing Susceptibility to infection Limited stress tolerance
25. Liver	History of jaundice, hepatitis Impaired drug metabolism Cirrhosis: history of alcoholism	Nutritional emphasis Abstinence from alcohol	Laboratory test for hepatitis Bleeding problems

TABLE 6-4 *(continued)*
ITEMS FOR THE MEDICAL HISTORY

Item to Record in History	Considerations	Possible Medications and Treatment Modalities	Influences on Appointment Procedures
26. Mental, Psychiatric	Emotional problems hinder oral care	Antipsychotic drugs Antianxiety drugs Tranquilizers Antidepressants Antiparkinsonism drugs	Limited stress tolerance Xerostomia (side effect)
27. Physical Activity	Overall health consciousness	Good health habits Regular exercise	Contribute to cooperative attitude in maintaining oral health
28. Physical Disabilities	Extent, cause, duration Type of treatment related to individual condition Consultation with physician or medical specialist	Pain reliever Muscle relaxant Anticonvulsant	Adjustment of physical arrangements Wheelchair accessibility and transfer Adaptations of techniques and instruction Antibiotic premedication for certain conditions: for example, prosthetic joint replacement, shunt
29. Pregnancy	Month, parturition date Possible oral manifestations History of previous pregnancies Iron deficiency anemia	Iron	Adjust physical position for comfort Frequent appointments for maintaining high level of oral hygiene
30. Respiration	Breathing problems Persistent cough Cough up blood Chest pain Precipitation of asthmatic attack	Codeine cough syrup Antihistamine Bronchial dilators Expectorants Decongestants Steroids	Dental chair position Ultrasonic and airbrasive contraindicated Anesthesia choice No aerosol agents

I. MEDICAL CONSULTATION

Dentist and physician need to consult relative to the patient's current therapy and medications or to elements of the patient's past health status that could influence present dental treatment needs.[6]

A. Telephone or Personal Contact

Immediate consultation may be needed so that urgent treatment may proceed. Follow-up in writing is essential, because without legal record of the advice or decision, a misunderstanding by the patient could result.

B. Written Request

A letter of formal request is the preferred procedure. A prepared form can be developed with spaces for filling in the specific questions and with space in the lower half for the physician or the assistant completing confidential information from the patient's medical record to provide the necessary directions.

C. Referrals

1. Patient should be referred for medical examination when signs of a possible disease condition are apparent.
2. Patient should be referred for laboratory tests when recent test results are not available or follow-up tests are needed.

II. RADIATION

When a patient is receiving radiation therapy or has had recent radiation for other purposes, a conference with the physician or oncologist involved may be necessary to discuss the quantity of radiation to be received from any necessary dental radiographs. No apparent rationale exists for precluding a properly justified dental radiographic examination because of a history of radiation therapy.[7]

III. PROPHYLACTIC PREMEDICATION

Patients susceptible to infective endocarditis must have antibiotic premedication prior to any tissue manipulation that could create a bacteremia. Other patients who may need prophylactic premedication are those with marked reduced capacity to resist infection.

Tissue manipulation, particularly the use of instruments subgingivally, must be withheld until the risk has been determined, the condition has been discussed with the patient's physician, and the prescription has been obtained. Infective endocarditis is described on pages 788–789.

PROPHYLACTIC PREMEDICATION

The American Heart Association and the American Dental Association recommend that risk patients listed below have antibiotic premedication for all dental procedures likely to induce gingival bleeding.[8] Tables 6–5 and 6–6 show the American Heart Association recommendations.

I. CARDIAC-RELATED CONDITIONS
A. Congenital heart disease; most congenital cardiac malformations.
B. Rheumatic heart disease.
C. Rheumatic fever and other febrile diseases that predispose to valvular damage. When a patient has a heart murmur, it may be necessary to determine from the patient's physician whether the murmur is considered functional or organic.

TABLE 6–5
RECOMMENDED STANDARD PROPHYLACTIC REGIMEN FOR DENTAL, ORAL, OR UPPER RESPIRATORY TRACT PROCEDURES IN PATIENTS WHO ARE AT RISK*

Drug	Dosing Regiment
Standard Regimen	
Amoxicillin	3.0 g orally 1 hour before procedure; then 1.5 g 6 hours after initial dose
Amoxicillin/Penicillin-Allergic Patients	
Erythromycin or	Erythromycin ethylsuccinate, 800 mg, or erythromycin stearate, 1.0 g, orally 2 hours before procedure; then half the dose 6 hours after initial dose
Clindamycin	300 mg orally 1 hour before procedure and 150 mg 6 hours after initial dose

* Includes those with prosthetic heart valves and other high-risk patients.
† Initial pediatric doses are as follows: amoxicillin, 50 mg/kg; erythromycin ethylsuccinate or erythromycin stearate, 20 mg/kg; and clindamycin, 10 mg/kg. Follow-up doses should be one-half the initial dose. **Total pediatric dose should not exceed total adult dose.** The following weight ranges may also be used for the initial pediatric dose of amoxicillin:<15 kg, 750 mg; 15 to 30 kg, 1500 mg; and >30 kg, 3000 mg (full adult dose)

TABLE 6–6
ALTERNATE PROPHYLACTIC REGIMENS FOR DENTAL, ORAL, OR UPPER RESPIRATORY TRACT PROCEDURES IN PATIENTS WHO ARE AT RISK

Drug	Dosing Regiment
Patients Unable to Take Oral Medications	
Ampicillin	Intravenous or intramuscular administration of ampicillin, 2.0 g, 30 minutes before procedure; then intravenous or intramuscular administration of ampicillin, 1.0 g, or oral administration of amoxicillin, 1.5 g, 6 hours after initial dose
Ampicillin/Amoxicillin/Penicillin-Allergic Patients Unable to Take Oral Medications	
Clindamycin	Intravenous administration of 300 mg 30 minutes before procedure and an intravenous or oral administration of 150 mg 6 hours after initial dose
Patients Considered High Risk and Not Candidates for Standard Regimen	
Ampicillin, gentamicin, and amoxicillin	Intravenous or intramuscular administration of ampicillin, 2.0 g, plus gentamicin, 1.5 mg/kg (not to exceed 80 mg), 30 minutes before procedure; followed by amoxicillin, 1.5 g, orally 6 hours after initial dose; alternatively, the parenteral regimen may be repeated 8 hours after initial dose
Ampicillin/Amoxicillin/Penicillin-Allergic Patients Considered High Risk	
Vancomycin	Intravenous administration of 1.0 g over 1 hour, starting 1 hour before procedure; no repeated dose necessary

* Initial pediatric doses are as follows: ampicillin, 50 mg/kg; clindamycin, 10 mg/kg; gentamicin, 2.0 mg/kg; and vancomycin, 20 mg/kg. Follow-up doses should be one half the initial dose. **Total pediatric dose should not exceed total adult dose.** No initial dose is recommended in this table for amoxicillin (25 mg/kg is the follow-

As advised by the physician, a functional murmur may not require premedication, whereas an organic murmur that is based on a defect in the structure of the heart does require antibiotic coverage.[9]
D. Prosthetic cardiac valves. Patients with vascular autografts generally do not need antibiotic premedication,[10] whereas those with prosthetic valves are susceptible to infective endocarditis.[11]
E. Previous history of infective endocarditis.
F. Indwelling transvenous cardiac pacemaker.
G. Mitral valve prolapse with insufficiency.
H. Surgically constructed systemic-pulmonary shunts.

II. OTHER INDICATIONS FOR PROPHYLACTIC PREMEDICATION

Specific recommendations are impossible to define for all patients who need antibiotic premedication. Practitioners must use clinical judgment and the advice of the patient's physician to determine the need for preventive antibiotics. The following list is not intended to be all-encompassing, but represents some of the conditions for which consideration must be given.

A. Prosthetic joint replacement.[12,13,14]

B. Reduced capacity to resist infection.
   1. Corticosteroid or other immunosuppressive therapy.
   2. Anticancer chemotherapy.
   3. Blood diseases, especially acute leukemia, agranulocytosis, and sickle cell anemia.

C. Uncontrolled, unstable diabetes mellitus. Controlled diabetes can be treated as normal (page 824).

D. Grossly contaminated traumatic facial injuries and compound fractures.

E. Renal transplant and hemodialysis; glomerulonephritis or other active renal disorder.[15]

Patients with problems of delayed healing may require additional doses of antibiotic. Bacteremia rarely persists for more than about 15 minutes after the instrumentation is terminated, and the incidence of bacteremia is less when the periodontal tissues are maintained in optimum health.

TECHNICAL HINTS

I. Date all records.

II. Keep permanent records in ink.

III. Provide a specific line on a health history form for the signature of the patient.[1] The completed history for a minor should be signed by a parent or guardian. A signature is also needed on the "Informed Consent" form (page 326).

IV. All information obtained for a patient history must be maintained in strictest confidence.

V. For patients with special health problems that require premedication, some type of coded tab can be used to alert all dental personnel to check the medical history prior to each appointment.

VI. Analyze the usefulness of items on the patient history form periodically and plan for revision as scientific research reveals new information that must be applied.

VII. A medical history update wall plaque is available for posting in an appropriate place in a dental office or clinic. It reads: *Please Advise Us of Any Change in Your Medical History Since Your Last Visit.* It is available from the American Dental Association, Department of Salable Materials, 211 East Chicago Avenue, Chicago, Illinois 60611.

FACTORS TO TEACH THE PATIENT

I. The need for obtaining the personal, medical, and dental history prior to performance of dental and dental hygiene procedures and the need for keeping the histories up to date.

II. The assurance that recorded histories are kept in strict professional confidence.

III. The relationship between oral health and general physical health.

IV. The interrelationship of medical and dental care.

V. Advantages of cooperation in furnishing information that helps dental personnel to interpret observations accurately and to assure the dentist that the correct diagnosis and treatment plan have been made.

VI. All patients who require antibiotic premedication need special attention paid to (1) the importance of preventive dentistry, (2) the imperative need for regular dental care, and (3) the necessity for taking the prescribed prescription 1 hour before the appointment starts.

REFERENCES

1. **Robbins,** K.S.: Medicolegal Considerations, in Malamed, S.F.: *Medical Emergencies in the Dental Office,* 4th ed. St. Louis, The C.V. Mosby Co., 1993, pp. 91–101.

2. **American Dental Association:** Medical History Form (S-500) and Medical History Interview (S-502), ADA Department of Salable Materials, 211 East Chicago Avenue, Chicago, IL 60611-2678.

3. **Brady,** W.F. and Martinoff, J.T.: Validity of Health History Data Collected from Dental Patients and Patient Perception of Health Status, *J. Am. Dent. Assoc., 101,* 642, October, 1980.

4. **Goebel,** W.M.: Reliability of the Medical History in Identifying Patients Likely to Place Dentists at an Increased Hepatitis Risk, *J. Am. Dent. Assoc., 98,* 907, June, 1979.

5. **Comfort,** M.B. and Wu, P.C.: The Reliability of Personal and Family Medical Histories in the Identification of Hepatitis B Carriers, *Oral Surg. Oral Med. Oral Pathol., 67,* 531, May, 1989.

6. **Chiodo,** G.T. and Rosenstein, D.I.: Consultation Between Dentists and Physicians, *Gen. Dent., 32,* 19, January–February, 1984.

7. **United States Department of Health and Human Services,** Food and Drug Administration, Center for Devices and Radiological Health: *Selection of Patients for X-Ray Examinations: Dental Radiographic Examinations.* Washington, D.C., Superintendent of Documents, HHS Publication FDA 88-8274, 1988, p. 10.

8. **Dajani,** A.S., Bisno, A.L., Chung, K.J., Durack, D.T., Freed, M., Gerber, M.A., Karchmer, A.W., Millard, H.D., Rahimtoola, S., Shulman, S.T., Watanakunakorn, C., and Taubert, K.A.: Prevention of Bacterial Endocarditis. Recommendations by the American Heart Association, *JAMA, 264,* 2919, December 12, 1990.

9. **Little,** J.W. and Falace, D.A.: *Dental Management of the Medically*

Compromised Patient, 4th ed. St. Louis, The C.V. Mosby Co., 1993, p. 134.

10. **Lindemann,** R.A. and Henson, J.L.: The Dental Management of Patients With Vascular Grafts Placed in the Treatment of Arterial Occlusive Disease, *J. Am. Dent. Assoc., 104,* 625, May, 1982.

11. **Baumgartner,** J.C. and Plack, W.F.: Dental Treatment and Management of a Patient With a Prosthetic Heart Valve, *J. Am. Dent. Assoc., 104,* 181, February, 1982.

12. **Jacobsen,** P.L. and Murray, W.: Prophylactic Coverage of Dental Patients With Artificial Joints: A Retrospective Analysis of Thirty-three Infections in Hip Prostheses, *Oral Surg. Oral Med. Oral Pathol., 50,* 130, August, 1980.

13. **Howell,** R.M. and Green, J.G.: Prophylactic Antibiotic Coverage in Dentistry: A Survey of Need for Prosthetic Joints, *Gen. Dent., 33,* 320, July–August, 1985.

14. **Mulligan,** R.: Late Infections in Patients With Prostheses for Total Replacement of Joints: Implications for the Dental Practitioner, *J. Am. Dent. Assoc., 101,* 44, July, 1980.

15. **Naylor,** G.D., Hall, E.H., and Terezhalmy, G.T.: The Patient With Chronic Renal Failure Who Is Undergoing Dialysis or Renal Transplantation: Another Consideration for Antimicrobial Prophylaxis, *Oral Surg. Oral Med. Oral Pathol., 65,* 116, January, 1988.

SUGGESTED READINGS

Carpendale, J.J.D., Dykema, R.W., Andres, C.J., and Goodacre, C.J.: Principles Governing the Prosthodontic Treatment of Patients with Cardiac Transplants, *J. Am. Dent. Assoc., 119,* 517, October, 1989.

Drinnan, A.J.: Medical Conditions of Importance in Dental Practice, *Int. Dent. J., 40,* 206, August, 1990.

Felder, R.S., Millar, S.B., and Henry, R.H.: Oral Manifestations of Drug Therapy, *Spec. Care Dentist, 8,* 119, May–June, 1988.

McCarthy, F.M., Pallasch, T.J., and Gates, R.: Documenting Safe Treatment of the Medical-risk Patient, *J. Am. Dent. Assoc., 119,* 383, September, 1989.

McClain, D.L., Bader, J.D., Daniel, S.J., and Sams, D.H.: Gingival Effects of Prescription Medications Among Adult Dental Patients, *Spec. Care Dentist, 11,* 15, January/February, 1991.

Miller, C.S., Kaplan, A.L., Guest, G.F., and Cottone, J.A.: Documenting Medication Use in Adult Dental Patients: 1987–1991, *J. Am. Dent. Assoc., 123,* 41, November, 1992.

Schein, J.: Be Wary When Taking More Than One Drug at a Time, *RDH, 13,* 46, January, 1993.

Seymour, R.A. and Heasman, P.A.: Drugs and the Periodontium, *J. Clin. Periodontol., 15,* 1, January, 1988.

Swapp, K.M.: Drugs and the Geriatric Patient. A Dental Hygiene Perspective, *J. Dent. Hyg., 64,* 326, September, 1990.

History Forms

Cooper, M.D. and Winans, G.J.: Basics of a Good Medical History Form. How to Protect the Patient and Prepare the Staff, *Dent. Teamwork, 5,* 19, January–February, 1992.

deJong, K.J.M., Abraham-Inpijn, L., Oomen, H.A.P.C., and Oosting, J.: Clinical Relevance of a Medical History in Dental Practice: Comparison Between a Questionnaire and a Dialogue, *Community Dent. Oral Epidemiol., 19,* 310, October, 1991.

deJong, K.J.M., Borgmeijer-Hoelen, A., and Abraham-Inpijn, L.: Validity of a Risk-related Patient-administered Medical Questionnaire for Dental Patients, *Oral Surg. Oral Med. Oral Pathol., 72,* 527, November, 1991.

Eubanks, S.: The Dental Assistant's Role in Risk Management. The Health History, Part 1, *Dent. Assist., 60,* 11, September/October, 1991.

Fenlon, M.R. and McCartan, B.E.: Validity of a Patient Self-completed Health Questionnaire in a Primary Care Dental Practice, *Community Dent. Oral Epidemiol., 20,* 130, June, 1992.

Frese, P.A. and Scaramucci, M.K.: Medical History Update, *Dentalhygienistnews, 4,* 9, Spring, 1991.

Levy, S.M. and Jakobsen, J.R.: A Comparison of Medical Histories Reported by Dental Patients and Their Physicians, *Spec. Care Dentist., 11,* 26, January/February, 1991.

Thibodeau, E.A. and Rossomando, K.J.: Survey of the Medical History Questionnaire, *Oral Surg. Oral Med. Oral Pathol., 74,* 400, September, 1992.

Prophylactic Antibiotic

Bahn, S.L.: Prophylactic Antibiotics Revisited, *Compendium, 12,* 492, July, 1991.

Barco, C.T.: Prevention of Infective Endocarditis: A Review of the Medical and Dental Literature, *J. Periodontol., 62,* 510, August, 1991.

Bender, I.B. and Barkan, M.J.: Dental Bacteremia and Its Relationship to Bacterial Endocarditis: Preventive Measures, *Compendium, 10,* 472, September, 1989.

Biron, C.R.: Erythromycin, *RDH, 13,* 38, January, 1993.

Browning, D.K. and Martin, M.E.: Erythromycin Preparations: Which One Should Be Prescribed for SBE Chemoprophylaxis?, *Gen. Dent., 38,* 216, May–June, 1990.

Carroll, G.C. and Sebor, R.J.: Dental Flossing and Its Relationship to Transient Bacteremia, *J. Periodontol., 51,* 691, December, 1980.

Cioffi, G.A., Terezhalmy, G.T., and Taybos, G.M.: Total Joint Replacement: A Consideration for Antimicrobial Prophylaxis, *Oral Surg. Oral Med. Oral Pathol., 66,* 124, July, 1988.

Coulter, W.A., Coffey, A., Saunders, I.D.F., and Emmerson, A.M.: Bacteremia in Children Following Dental Extraction, *J. Dent. Res., 69,* 1691, October, 1990.

DeGeest, A.F.E., Schoolmeesters, I., Willems, J.L., and DeGeest, H.: Dental Health, Prophylactic Antibiotic Measures and Infective Endocarditis: An Analysis of the Knowledge of Susceptible Patients, *Acta Cardiol., 45,* 441, No. 6, 1990.

Durack, D.T., Kaplan, E.L., and Bisno, A.L.: Apparent Failures of Endocarditis Prophylaxis. Analysis of 52 Cases Submitted to a National Registry, *JAMA, 250,* 2318, November 4, 1983.

Fédération Dentaire Internationale: Premedication in Dentistry, Technical Report No. 32, *Int. Dent. J., 39,* 55, March, 1989.

Felder, R.S., Nardone, D., and Palac, R.: Prevalence of Predisposing Factors for Endocarditis Among an Elderly Institutionalized Population, *Oral Surg. Oral Med. Oral Pathol., 73,* 30, January, 1992.

Friedlander, A.H. and Yoshikawa, T.T.: Pathogenesis, Management, and Prevention of Infective Endocarditis in the Elderly Dental Patient, *Oral Surg. Oral Med. Oral Pathol., 69,* 177, February, 1990.

Harris, R. and Kelly, M.A.: Antibiotic Prophylaxis of the Dental Patient, *Gen. Dent., 38,* 212, May–June, 1990.

Jacobson, J.J. and Mathews, L.S.: Bacteria Isolated from Late Prosthetic Joint Infections: Dental Treatment and Chemoprophylaxis, *Oral Surg. Oral Med. Oral Pathol., 63,* 122, January, 1987.

Jacobson, J.J., Millard, H.D., Plezia, R., and Blankenship, J.R.: Dental Treatment and Late Prosthetic Joint Infections, *Oral Surg. Oral Med. Oral Pathol., 61,* 413, April, 1986.

Jacobson, J.J., Schweitzer, S.O., and Kowalski, C.J.: Chemoprophylaxis of Prosthetic Joint Patients During Dental Treatment: A Decision-utility Analysis, *Oral Surg. Oral Med. Oral Pathol., 72,* 167, August, 1991.

Jacoby, G.A. and Archer, G.L.: New Mechanisms of Bacterial Resistance to Antimicrobial Agents, *N. Engl. J. Med., 324,* 601, February 28, 1991.

Kessler, D.A.: Communicating With Patients About Their Medications, *N. Engl. J. Med., 325,* 1650, December 5, 1991.

Lockhart, P.B., Crist, D., and Stone, P.H.: The Reliability of the Medical History in the Identification of Patients at Risk for Infective Endocarditis, *J. Am. Dent. Assoc., 119,* 417, September, 1989.

Lucartorto, F.M., Franker, C.F., and Maza, J.: Postscaling Bacteremia in HIV-associated Gingivitis and Periodontitis, *Oral Surg. Oral Med. Oral Pathol., 73,* 550, May, 1992.

Luce, E.B., Presti, C.F., Montemayor, I., and Crawford, M.H.: Detecting Cardiac Valvular Pathology in Patients With Systemic Lupus Erythematosus, *Spec. Care Dentist., 12,* 193, September/October, 1992.

Machen, D.E.: Legal Aspects of Orthodontic Practice: Risk Management Concepts. The Patient Requiring Antibiotic Prophylaxis, *Am. J. Orthod. Dentofacial Orthop., 100,* 190, August, 1991.

Nelson, C.L. and Van Blaricum, C.S.: Physician and Dentist Compliance With American Heart Association Guidelines for Prevention of Bacterial Endocarditis, *J. Am. Dent. Assoc., 118,* 169, February, 1989.

Nord, C.E. and Heimdahl, A.: Cardiovascular Infections: Bacterial Endocarditis of Oral Origin. Pathogenesis and Prophylaxis, *J. Clin. Periodontol., 17,* 494, August, 1990 (Part II).

Pallasch, T.J.: A Critical Appraisal of Antibiotic Prophylaxis, *Int. Dent. J., 39,* 183, September, 1989.

Sadowsky, D. and Kunzel, C.: "Usual and Customary" Practice Versus the Recommendations of Experts: Clinician Noncompliance in the Prevention of Bacterial Endocarditis, *J. Am. Dent. Assoc., 118,* 175, February, 1989.

Smith, A.J. and Adams, D.: The Dental Status and Attitudes of Patients at Risk from Infective Endocarditis, *Br. Dent. J., 174,* 59, January 23, 1993.

Thyne, G.M. and Ferguson, J.W.: Antibiotic Prophylaxis During Dental Treatment in Patients With Prosthetic Joints, *J. Bone Joint Surg.* (Br.), *73,* 191, March, 1991.

Tsevat, J., Durand-Zaleski, I., and Pauker, S.G.: Cost Effectiveness of Antibiotic Prophylaxis for Dental Procedures in Patients With Artificial Joints, *Am. J. Public Health, 79,* 739, June, 1989.

van der Bijl, P. and Maresky, L.S.: Failures of Endocarditis Prophylaxis: Selective Review of the Literature and a Case Report, *Ann. Dent., 50,* 5, Summer, 1991.

Wyatt, L., Cline, N.V., and Springstead, C.: Getting to the Heart of the Matter, *RDH, 12,* 31, April, 1992.

Wynn, R.L.: Amoxicillin Update, *Gen. Dent., 39,* 322, September–October, 1991.

7

Vital Signs

The vital signs are the body temperature, pulse and respiratory rates, and blood pressure. Table 7–1 summarizes the normal values for adults.

Recording vital signs contributes to the proper systemic evaluation of a patient in conjunction with the complete medical history. Treatment planning and appointment sequencing are directly influenced by the findings. Proficiency in determination of the vital signs is essential for monitoring during emergency treatment (see Chapter 61).

Abnormal vital signs must be regarded with suspicion, because they may indicate undetected systemic problems. For example, a patient's life may be saved because of medical treatment initiated as a result of a high blood pressure determination during a dental hygiene appointment.

When vital signs are not within normal range, they are called to the dentist's attention. The patient should be informed and the findings discussed with a physician. When the patient does not have a personal physician, a recommendation for referral or additional diagnostic procedures is indicated. Key words related to the vital signs are defined in table 7–2.

BODY TEMPERATURE

While preparing the patient history and making the extraoral and intraoral examinations, the need for taking the temperature may become apparent, or the dentist may have requested the procedure in conjunction with current oral disease. When the temperature is to be taken along with the other vital signs, the pulse and respiratory rates are determined while the thermometer is in the patient's mouth.

TABLE 7–1 ADULT VITAL SIGNS		
Vital Sign	**Values of Significance in Dental and Dental Hygiene Appointments**	
Body Temperature (oral)	Normal 37.0° C (98.6° F) Normal range 35.5° to 37.5° C (96.0° to 99.5° F)	
Pulse Rate	Normal range 60 to 100 per minute	
Respiration	Normal range 14 to 20 per minute	
Blood Pressure* Category	**Systolic mm Hg**	**Diastolic mm Hg**
Normal	<130	<85
High normal	130–139	85–89
Hypertension		
STAGE 1 (Mild)	140–159	90–99
STAGE 2 (Moderate)	160–179	100–109
STAGE 3 (Severe)	180–209	110–119
STAGE 4 (Very Severe)	≥210	≥120

* Data from *The Fifth Report of the Joint National Committee on Detection, Evaluation, and Treatment of High Blood Pressure*. National Institutes of Health, National Heart, Lung, and Blood Institute, Publication 93-1088, January, 1993.

TABLE 7–2
KEY WORDS: VITAL SIGNS

Anoxia (ah nok'se-ah): oxygen deficiency; a reduction of oxygen in the tissues can lead to deep respirations, cyanosis, increased pulse rate, and impairment of coordination.

Apnea (ap'nē-ah): temporary cessation of breathing; absence of spontaneous respirations.

Auscultation (aws'kŭl-tā'shun): listening for sounds produced within the body; may be performed directly or with a stethoscope.

Bradycardia (brād ē-kar'dē-ah): unusually slow heart beat evidenced by slowing of the pulse rate.

Core temperature: the temperature of the deep tissues of the body; remains relatively constant; contrasts with body surface temperature, which rises and falls in response to environment.

Diastole (dī as'tō-lē): the phase of the cardiac cycle in which the heart relaxes between contractions and the two ventricles are dilated by the blood flowing into them; **diastolic pressure** is the lowest blood pressure.

Diurnal (dī-er'nal): pertaining to or occurring during the daytime or period of light.

Hyperthermia (hī'per-ther'mē-ah): higher-than-normal body temperature.

Hypothermia (hī'pō-ther'mē-ah): lower-than-normal body temperature.

Korotkoff sounds (kō-rot'kof): the sounds heard during the determination of blood pressure; sounds originating within the blood passing through the vessel or produced by vibratory motion of the arterial wall.

Normotensive (nor'mō-ten'siv): normal tension or tone; of or pertaining to having normal blood pressure.

Pulse pressure (puls): the difference between systolic and diastolic blood pressure; normally 30 to 40 mm Hg.

Pyrexia (pī-rek'sē-ah): an abnormal elevation of the body temperature above 37.0° C (98.6° F).

Stethoscope (steth'ō-skōp): instrument used to hear and amplify the sounds produced by the heart, lungs, and other internal organs.

Systole (sis'tō-lē): the contraction, or period of contraction, of the heart, especially the ventricles, during which blood is forced into the aorta and the pulmonary artery; **systolic pressure** is the highest, or greatest, pressure.

Tachycardia (tăk'ē-kar'dē-ah): unusually fast heart beat; at a rate greater than 100 beats per minute.

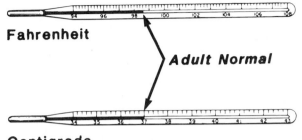

FIG. 7–1. Thermometers. Centigrade and Fahrenheit thermometers compared. Adult normal temperature is shown at 37.0° Centigrade and 98.6° Fahrenheit.

time because of illness, and for the protection of subsequent patients who may be indirectly exposed, it is important to detect the presence of a systemic, contagious condition. Screening for elevated temperature among patients may have particular significance during certain seasons or epidemics. When a definite increase in temperature is found, the patient can be dismissed by the dentist to prevent further contamination of the office or clinic. The patient can be advised to seek medical care.

I. MAINTENANCE OF BODY TEMPERATURE
A. Normal

1. *Adult.* The normal average temperature is 37.0° C (98.6° F) as illustrated in figure 7–1. The normal range is from 35.5° to 37.5° C (96.0° to 99.5° F). Over 70 years of age, the average temperature is slightly lower (36.0° C, 96.8° F).
2. *Children.*[1] There is no appreciable difference between boys and girls. Average temperatures are as follows:
   a. First year: 37.3° C (99.1° F).
   b. Fourth year: 37.5° C (99.4° F).
   c. Fifth year: 37° C (98.6° F).
   d. Twelfth year: 36.7° C (98.0° F).

B. Temperature Variations

1. *Fever (pyrexia).* Values over 37.5° C (99.5° F).
2. *Hyperthermia.* Values over 41.0° C (105.8° F).
3. *Hypothermia.* Values below 35.5° C (96.0° F).

C. Factors that Alter Body Temperature

1. *Time of Day.* Highest in late afternoon and early evening; lowest during sleep and early morning.
2. *Temporary Increase.* Exercise, hot drinks, smoking, or application of external heat.
3. *Pathologic States.* Infection, dehydration, hyperthyroidism, myocardial infarction, or tissue injury from trauma.
4. *Decrease.* Starvation, hemorrhage, or physiologic shock.

A temperature above the normal range can indicate the presence of infection. Patients can have an elevated body temperature from oral causes, such as an apical or periodontal abscess or acute pericoronitis. Determination of the temperature of a patient with an oral infection may be necessary for diagnosis and treatment planning.

For the protection of the health of the personnel in the dental office or clinic, to prevent loss of working

II. METHODS OF DETERMINING TEMPERATURE

A. Oral

Most commonly used.

1. *Indications for Use.* An oral thermometer is used for the patient who
   a. Can follow instructions.
   b. Can keep the mouth closed to hold the thermometer.
   c. Will not bite or otherwise break the thermometer (which could happen with small children or confused patients of any age).
   d. Has no mouth injuries or problems breathing through the nose.
2. *Contraindications.* The oral thermometer cannot be used for a patient who is unconscious, confused, irrational or restless; for infants or small children; or for a patient with a very dry mouth.

B. Rectal

Generally applicable when the oral thermometer is contraindicated.

C. External

Axillary and groin positions are the least accurate, but occasionally, the oral or rectal method is impossible to use.

D. Types of Thermometers

1. *Disposable.* Disposable thermometers are most frequently used. They are most effective for universal infection control procedure.
2. *Mercury-column Clinical Thermometer.* Consists of a bulb containing mercury, which, when heated by the body temperature, expands and rises in the hollow center of the glass stem. The bulb of the oral thermometer is usually tapered, whereas the bulb of the rectal thermometer is blunted and round.
3. *Electronic.* Electronic thermometers require less time for taking the temperature, are more easily cared for because of their disposable tips, and decrease the possibility of cross-contamination.

E. Comparison of Readings

Rectal readings are about 1° above oral readings, and oral readings are about 1° above axillary or groin readings.

III. PROCEDURE

A. Equipment

Clinical thermometer, tissues, clock or watch with second hand, sheath.

B. Prepare Patient

1. Tell patient what is to be done.
2. Wait 15 minutes for the patient who has just had a hot or cold beverage or has smoked within 10 minutes, because the surface temperature of the oral mucosa can alter the accuracy of the thermometer reading.

C. Prepare the Thermometer

1. Hold the thermometer only by the stem, never by the bulb.
2. Wipe with a tissue.
3. Check the reading: it must be below 35.6° C (96° F).
4. Shake down the mercury level if not already below 35.6° C (96° F). The thermometer maintains the highest temperature previously registered, and remains there until the force of shaking lowers the mercury level.
   a. Move away from furniture or other hard objects to prevent accidental forceful contact of the thermometer.
   b. Grasp stem firmly and shake with a firm, even, downward motion one or two times.
   c. Recheck the reading and reshake if indicated.
5. Place the thermometer into a thermometer sheath (a disposable cover available from a medical supply) to prevent contact with the patient's oral microflora. Figure 7–2 illustrates the procedure for preparation of a sheath.

D. Take the Temperature

1. Insert the bulb under the patient's tongue, with the stem outside the mouth.
2. Instruct patient to hold the thermometer gently with the lips, to avoid biting, and to breathe through the nose.
3. Observe watch or other timer, and remove thermometer after 3 clocked minutes.

E. Read and Record

1. Stand with back to light source and hold the thermometer by the stem at eye level to read.
2. Roll the thermometer slowly between the fingers to find the solid column of mercury.
3. Read at the point where the mercury ends. Each long line represents a degree of temperature, and short lines between are at two-tenths (0.2) of a degree.
4. Retake the temperature when the reading is unusually high or low.
   a. Reshake the mercury column down.
   b. Watch the patient to make certain that the thermometer is in position during the 3 minutes.
5. Record date, time of day, and temperature on the patient's record.
6. Inform the dentist of a temperature over 37.5° C (99.5° F).

F. Care of the Thermometer

1. *Disposable Thermometer Sheath.* Remove and dispose in waste.

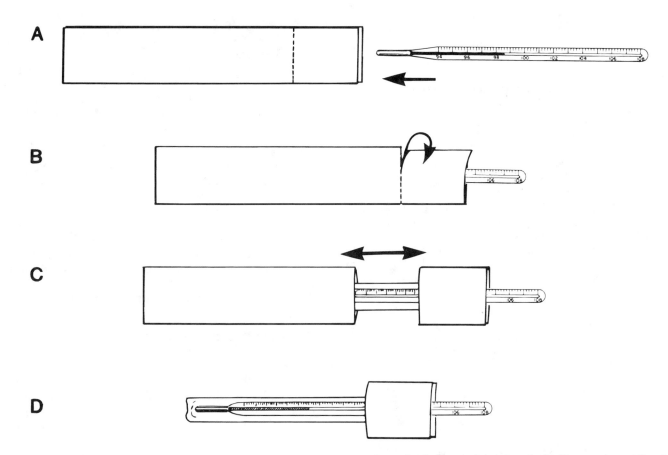

FIG. 7–2. Thermometer Sheath. A. Insert the thermometer gently to the bottom of the sheath. **B.** Tear at dotted line by twisting. **C.** Pull apart, holding by the small section of cover. **D.** Sheathed thermometer is ready for insertion under patient's tongue.

2. *Conventional*
    a. Wash with soap and slightly warm water; rinse with clear cool water; dry. Hot water can raise the temperature and force the mercury to break the thermometer.
    b. Soak in disinfectant solution, completely covered.
    c. Rinse with water and dry before placing in container or using again. Container should be sterilizable.

IV. CARE OF PATIENT WITH TEMPERATURE ELEVATION[2,3]
A. Temperature Over 41.0° C (105.8° F)
1. Treat as medical emergency.
2. Transport to a hospital for medical care.

B. Temperature 37.6° to 41.0° C (99.6° C to 105.8° F)
1. Check possible temporary or factitious cause, such as hot beverage or smoking, and observe patient while repeating the determination.
2. Review the dental and medical history.
3. Call to the attention of the dentist.

4. Provide no elective care when there are signs of respiratory infection or other possible communicable disease.

PULSE

The pulse is the intermittent throbbing sensation felt when the fingers are pressed against an artery. It is the result of the alternate expansion and contraction of an artery as a wave of blood is forced through the heart. The pulse rate or heart rate is the count of the heartbeats. Irregularities of strength, rhythm, and quality of the pulse should be noted while counting the pulse rate.

I. MAINTENANCE OF NORMAL PULSE
A. Normal Pulse Rates
1. *Adults.* There is no absolute normal. The adult range is 60 to 100 beats per minute, slightly higher for women than for men.
2. *Children.*[1] The pulse or heart rate falls steadily during childhood.
    a. *In utero*—150 beats per minute (bpm).

  b. At birth—130 bpm.
  c. Second year—105 bpm.
  d. Fourth year—90 bpm.
  e. Tenth year—70 bpm.

B. Factors That Influence Pulse Rate

An unusually fast heartbeat (over 100 beats per minute in an adult) is called *tachycardia;* an unusually slow beat (below 50) is *bradycardia.*

1. *Increased Pulse.* Caused by exercise, stimulants, eating, strong emotions, extremes of heat and cold, and some forms of heart disease.
2. *Decreased Pulse.* Caused by sleep, depressants, fasting, quieting emotions, and low vitality from prolonged illness.
3. *Emergency Situations.* Listed in table 61–3, pages 842–847.

II. PROCEDURE FOR DETERMINING PULSE RATE

A. Sequence

The pulse rate is conveniently obtained at the same time that the thermometer is in the patient's mouth to determine body temperature. Respirations are counted immediately following the pulse rate.

B. Sites

The pulse may be felt at several points over the body. The one most commonly used is on the radial artery at the wrist and is called the *radial pulse* (figure 7–3). Other sites convenient for use in a dental office or clinic are the *temporal* artery on the side of the head in front of the ear, or the *facial* artery at the border of the mandible.

The carotid pulse is used during cardiopulmonary resuscitation (page 836 and figure 61–5) for an adult, and the brachial pulse is used for an infant.

C. Prepare the Patient

1. Tell the patient what is to be done.
2. Have the patient in a comfortable position with arm and hand supported, palm down.
3. Locate the radial pulse on the thumb side of the wrist with the tips of the first three fingers (figure 7–4). Do not use the thumb because

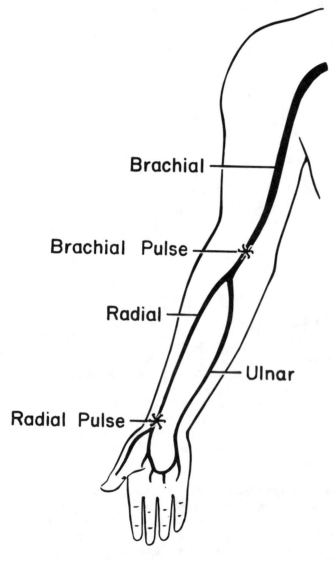

FIG. 7–3. Arteries of the Arm. Note location of radial pulse. The brachial pulse may be felt just before the brachial artery branches into the radial and ulnar arteries.

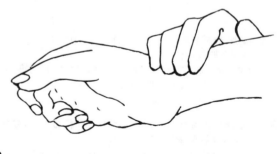

FIG. 7–4. Determination of Pulse Rate. A. Correct position of hands. **B.** The tips of the first three fingers are placed over the radial pulse located on the thumb side of the ventral surface of the wrist.

it contains a pulse that may be confused with the patient's pulse.

D. Count and Record

1. When the pulse is felt, exert light pressure and count for 1 clocked minute. Use the second hand of a watch or clock. Check with a repeat count.
2. While taking the pulse, observe the following:
   a. Rhythm: regular, regularly irregular, irregularly irregular.
   b. Volume and strength: full, strong, poor, weak, thready.
3. Record on patient's record the date, pulse rate, other characteristics.
4. Call unusual findings to the dentist's attention. A pulse rate over 90 should be considered abnormal for an adult and over 120 abnormal for a child.

RESPIRATION

The function of respiration is to supply oxygen to the tissues and to eliminate carbon dioxide. Variations in normal respirations may be shown by such characteristics as the rate, rhythm, depth, and quality and may be symptomatic of disease or emergency states.

I. MAINTENANCE OF NORMAL RESPIRATIONS

A respiration is one breath taken in and let out.

A. Normal Respiratory Rate

1. *Adults.* The adult range is from 14 to 20 per minute, slightly higher for women.
2. *Children.*[1] The respiratory rate decreases steadily during childhood. Averages are
   a. First year—30 per minute.
   b. Second year—25 per minute.
   c. Eighth year—20 per minute.
   d. Fifteenth year—18 per minute.

B. Factors That Influence Respirations

Many of the same factors that influence pulse rate also influence the number of respirations. A rate of 12 per minute or fewer is considered subnormal for an adult; over 28 is accelerated; and rates over 60 are extremely rapid and dangerous.

1. *Increased Respiration.* Caused by work and exercise, excitement, nervousness, strong emotions, pain, hemorrhage, shock.
2. *Decreased Respiration.* Caused by sleep, certain drugs, pulmonary insufficiency.
3. *Emergency Situations.* Listed in table 61–3, pages 842–847.

II. PROCEDURES FOR OBSERVING RESPIRATIONS

A. Determine Rate

1. Make the count of respirations immediately after counting the pulse.
2. Maintain the fingers over the radial pulse.
3. Respirations must be counted so that the patient is not aware, as the rate may be voluntarily altered.
4. Count the number of times the chest rises in 1 clocked minute. It is not necessary to count both inspirations and expirations.

B. Factors to Observe

1. *Depth.* Describe as shallow, normal, or deep.
2. *Rhythm.* Describe as regular (evenly spaced) or irregular (with pauses of irregular lengths between).
3. *Quality.* Describe as strong, easy, weak, or labored (noisy). Poor quality may have an effect on body color; for example, a bluish tinge of the face or nailbeds may mean an insufficiency of oxygen.
4. *Sounds.* Describe deviant sounds made during inspiration, expiration, or both.
5. *Position of Patient.* When the patient assumes an unusual position to secure comfort during breathing or prefers to remain seated upright, mark records accordingly.

C. Record

Record all findings on the patient's record.

D. Notify

Call to the attention of the dentist any unusual findings.

BLOOD PRESSURE

Information about the patient's blood pressure is essential during dental and dental hygiene appointments because special adaptations may be needed. Screening for blood pressure in dental offices has been shown to be an effective health service for all ages.

Cardiovascular diseases are described in Chapter 58, and the causes, predisposing factors, and treatment of hypertension are reviewed on pages 789–791. That information can be a helpful introduction and is recommended for reading in conjunction with this section on the techniques for obtaining blood pressure.

I. COMPONENTS OF BLOOD PRESSURE

Blood pressure is the force exerted by the blood on the blood vessel walls. When the left ventricle of the heart contracts, blood is forced out into the aorta and travels through the large arteries to the smaller arteries, arterioles, and capillaries. The pulsations extend from the heart through the arteries and disappear in the arterioles. During the course of the cardiac cycle, the blood pressure is changing constantly.

A. Systolic Pressure

Systolic pressure is the peak or the highest pressure. It is caused by ventricular contraction. The normal systolic pressure is less than 130 mm Hg.

B. Diastolic Pressure

Diastolic pressure is the lowest pressure. It is the effect of ventricular relaxation. The normal diastolic pressure is less than 85 mm Hg.

C. Pulse Pressure

The pulse pressure is the difference between the systolic and the diastolic pressures. The normal or safe difference is less than 45 mm Hg.

II. BLOOD PRESSURE CLASSIFICATION

Table 7–1 (page 106) includes the classification for blood pressure in adults. Normal average blood pressure in mm Hg at different ages is as follows:[4]

Age	Mean Systolic	Mean Diastolic
3 years	108	70
6 years	114	74
12 years	122	78
16 to 18 years	136	84

III. FACTORS THAT INFLUENCE BLOOD PRESSURE

A. Maintenance of Blood Pressure

Blood pressure depends on
1. Force of the heart beat (energy of the heart).
2. Peripheral resistance; condition of the arteries; changes in elasticity of vessels, which may occur with age.
3. Volume of blood in the circulatory system.

B. Factors That Increase Blood Pressure

1. Exercise, eating, stimulants, and emotional disturbance.
2. Use of oral contraceptives; blood pressure increases with age and length of use.

C. Factors That Decrease Blood Pressure

1. Fasting, rest, depressants, and quiet emotions.
2. Such emergencies as fainting, blood loss, shock (see table 61–3, page 843).

IV. EQUIPMENT FOR DETERMINING BLOOD PRESSURE

The mercury manometer is usually considered the most reliable recorder of blood pressure. Electronic devices are available, but additional research is needed before their reliability can be fully assured. Another type is the aneroid, which has a round gauge. It requires frequent calibration.

A. Sphygmomanometer (blood pressure machine)

Consists of an *inflatable cuff* and *two tubes,* one connected to the *pressure hand control bulb,* and the other to the *pressure gauge.*
1. *Cuff*
   a. Material. The cuff is made of a nonelastic material and is fastened by a Velcro overlap. The inflatable bladder is located within the material of the cuff.
   b. Size. The diameter of the arm, not the age of the patient, determines the size of the cuff selected. The four cuff sizes available are child size, regular adult, large adult, and thigh. The thigh size is needed for grossly obese persons.
   c. Dimension. The cuff width that is used should be 20% greater than the diameter of the arm to which it is applied (figure 7–5). It should cover approximately two thirds of the upper arm.

   When a cuff is too narrow, the blood pressure reading is too high; when the cuff is too wide, the reading is too low.[5]
2. *Mercury Manometer*
   a. Gauges are marked with long lines at each 10 mm Hg, with shorter lines at 2-mm intervals between each long line.
   b. The level of the column of mercury of the manometer should be at eye level for accurate reading and must not be tilted.

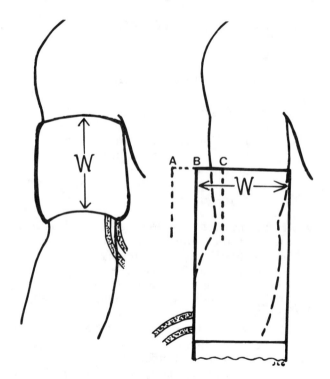

FIG. 7–5. Selection of Cuff Size. The correct width (W) is 20% greater than the diameter of the arm where applied. **A.** Too wide. **B.** Correct width. **C.** Too narrow.

B. Stethoscope (a listening aid that magnifies sound)

Consists of an *endpiece* that is connected by tubes to carry the sound to the *earpieces.*

1. *Types of Endpieces.* Bell-shaped or flat (diaphragm); the bell shape is used for medical examinations, particularly for chest examination.
2. *Care of Earpieces.* Clean by rubbing with gauze sponge moistened in disinfectant.

V. PROCEDURE FOR DETERMINING BLOOD PRESSURE

A. Prepare Patient

1. Tell patient briefly what is to be done. Detailed explanations should be avoided because they may excite the patient and change the blood pressure.
2. Seat patient comfortably, with the arm slightly flexed, with palm up, and with the whole forearm supported on a level surface at the level of the heart.
3. Use either arm unless otherwise indicated, for example, by a handicap. Repeat blood pressure determinations should be made on the same arm, because the difference between arms may be as much as 10 mm Hg.
4. Take pressure on bare arm, not over clothing. A tight sleeve should be loosened.

B. Apply Cuff

1. Apply the completely deflated cuff to the patient's arm, supported at the level of the heart. It has been shown that when the arm rests on the arm of a dental chair, higher than the heart, the diastolic pressure shows a small but significant increase.[6]
2. Place the portion of the cuff that contains the inflatable bladder directly over the brachial artery. The cuff may have an arrow to show the point that should be placed over the artery. The lower edge of the cuff is placed 1 inch above the antecubital fossa (figure 7–6). Fasten the cuff evenly and snugly.
3. Adjust the position of the gauge for convenient reading but so that the patient cannot see the mercury.
4. Palpate 1 inch below the antecubital fossa to locate the brachial artery pulse (figure 7–3). The stethoscope endpiece is placed over the spot where the brachial pulse is felt.
5. Position the stethoscope earpieces in the ears, with the tips directed forward.

C. Locate the Radial Pulse (figures 7–3 and 7–4)

Hold the fingers on the pulse.

D. Inflate the Cuff

1. Close the needle valve (air lock) attached to the hand control bulb firmly but so it may be released readily.

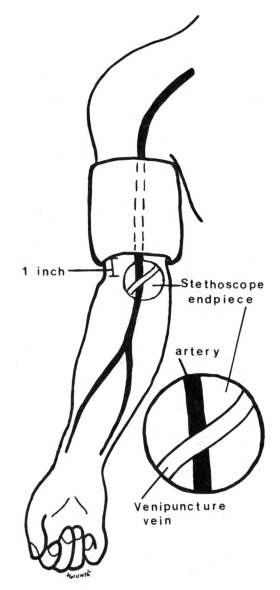

FIG. 7–6. Blood Pressure Cuff in Position. The lower edge of the cuff is placed approximately 1 inch above the antecubital fossa. The stethoscope endpiece is placed over the palpated brachial artery pulse point approximately 1 inch below the antecubital fossa and slightly toward the inner side of the arm.

2. Pump to inflate the cuff until the radial pulse stops. Note the mercury level at which the pulse disappears.
3. Look at the dial, and pump to 20 or 30 mm Hg beyond where the radial pulse was no longer felt. This is the maximum inflation level (MIL). It means that the brachial artery is collapsed by the pressure of the cuff and no blood is flowing through.

Unless the MIL is determined, the level to which the cuff is inflated will be arbitrary.

Excess pressure can be very uncomfortable for the patient.

E. Position the Stethoscope Endpiece

Place the endpiece over the palpated brachial artery, 1 inch below the antecubital fossa, and slightly toward the inner side of the arm (figure 7–6). Hold lightly in place.

F. Deflate the Cuff Gradually

1. Release the air lock slowly (2 to 3 mm per second) so that the dial drops very gradually and steadily.
2. Listen for the first sound: *systole* ("tap tap"). Note the number on the dial that is the *systolic pressure*. This is the beginning of the flow of blood past the cuff.
3. Continue to release the pressure slowly. The sound will continue, first becoming louder, then diminishing and becoming muffled, until finally disappearing. Note the number on the dial where the last distinct tap was heard. That number is the *diastolic pressure*.
4. Release further (about 10 mm) until all sounds cease. That is the second diastolic point. In some clinics and hospitals, the last sound is taken as the diastolic pressure.
5. Let the rest of the air out rapidly.

G. Repeat for Confirmation

Wait 30 seconds before inflating the cuff again. More than one reading is needed within a few minutes to determine an average and assure a correct reading.

H. Record

1. Write date and arm used.
2. Record blood pressure as a fraction, for example, 120/80. When both diastolic points are recorded, it can be written as 120/80/72.

I. Notify

Call to the prompt attention of the dentist any unusual variation from normal or from previous readings noted in the patient's permanent record.

VI. BLOOD PRESSURE FOLLOW-UP CRITERIA[4]

Table 7–3 provides a summary of recommendations at each level of blood pressure findings. Dental personnel have an obligation to advise and *refer for further evaluation*. Diagnosis of hypertension would never be made or treatment started on the basis of an isolated reading.

When the blood pressure is within normal range (130/85), it should be rechecked within 2 years. Rechecking within 1 year rather than 2 years is recommended for persons at increased risk for hypertension. The risks include family history, weight gain, obesity, black race, use of oral contraceptives, and excessive alcohol consumption.

Consultation with a patient's physician is indicated

TABLE 7–3
RECOMMENDATIONS FOR FOLLOW-UP BASED ON INITIAL SET OF BLOOD PRESSURE MEASUREMENTS FOR ADULTS AGE 18 AND OLDER[4]

Initial Screening Blood Pressure (mm Hg)*		Follow-up Recommended
Systolic	**Diastolic**	**Follow-up Recommended**
<130	<85	Recheck in 2 years
130–139	85–89	Recheck in 1 year
140–159	90–99	Confirm within 2 months
160–179	100–109	Evaluate or refer to source of care within 1 month
180–209	110–119	Evaluate or refer to source of care within 1 week
≥210	≥120	Evaluate or refer to source of care immediately

* If the systolic and diastolic categories are different, follow recommendation for the shorter time follow-up (for example, 160/85 mm Hg should be evaluated or referred to source of care within 1 month).

prior to dental or dental hygiene treatment when the blood pressure is in a moderate or higher category (table 7–1).

TECHNICAL HINTS

I. When a patient's sleeve is drawn back for blood pressure determination, observe the sleeve and the arm for small blood stains or evidence of an injection, which may reveal a mainliner drug addict. The patient may request, even insist, that a particular arm be used. When suspicion of drug abuse has been previously aroused because of physical observation or items in a medical history, determine the blood pressure on both arms to permit observation. Tell the patient that the pressure should always be measured on both sides.

II. Sources of Materials

National High Blood Pressure Education Program
High Blood Pressure Information Center
120/80 National Institutes of Health
Bethesda, MD 20205

American Heart Association
7320 Greenville Avenue
Dallas, TX 75231

FACTORS TO TEACH THE PATIENT

I. How vital signs can influence dental and dental hygiene appointments.

II. The importance of having a blood pressure determination at regular intervals.

III. For patient diagnosed as hypertensive, encourage regular continuing use of prescription drugs for control of high blood pressure.

REFERENCES

1. **Silver,** H.K.: Growth and Development, in Kempe, C.H., Silver, H.K., and O'Brien, D., eds.: *Current Pediatric Diagnosis and Treatment,* 8th ed. Los Altos, CA, Lange Medical Publications, 1984, pp. 20–24.

2. **Malamed,** S.F.: *Medical Emergencies in the Dental Office,* 4th ed. St. Louis, Mosby, 1993, pp. 27–36.

3. **McCarthy,** F.M.: Vital Signs—the Six-Minute Warnings, *J. Am. Dent. Assoc., 100,* 682, May, 1980.

4. **United States National High Blood Pressure Education Program:** *The Fifth Report of the Joint National Committee on Detection, Evaluation, and Treatment of High Blood Pressure,* Washington, D.C., National Institutes of Health, National Heart, Lung, and Blood Institute, N.I.H. Publication No. 93-1088, January, 1993, 49 pp.

5. **Geddes,** L.A. and Whistler, S.J.: The Error in Indirect Blood Pressure Measurement with the Incorrect Size of Cuff, *Am. Heart J., 96,* 4, July, 1978.

6. **Beck,** F.M., Weaver, J.M., Blozis, G.G., and Unverferth, D.V.: Effect of Arm Position and Arm Support on Indirect Blood Pressure Measurements Made in a Dental Chair, *J. Am. Dent. Assoc., 106,* 645, May, 1983.

SUGGESTED READINGS

Alexander, D. and Kelly, B.: Responses of Children, Parents, and Nurses to Tympanic Thermometry in the Pediatric Office, *Clin. Pediatr. (Phila.), 30,* 53, Supplement 4, April, 1991.

American Dental Association, Council on Community Health, Hospital, Institutional, and Medical Affairs: Hypertension Update: A Survey of the Literature of Interest to Dentists, *J. Am. Dent. Assoc., 118,* 645, May, 1989.

American Heart Association: Cardiovascular Disease in Dental Practice, (1991), American Heart Association, National Center, 7272 Greenville Ave., Dallas, TX 75231-4596.

Cline, N.V. and Springstead, M.C.: Monitoring Blood Pressure. Five Minutes Critical to Quality Patient Care, *J. Dent. Hyg., 66,* 363, October, 1992.

Cooper, K.M.: Measuring Blood Pressure The Right Way, *Nursing, 92, 22,* 75, April, 1992.

Gortzak, R.A.Th., Abraham-Inpijn, L., and Peters, G.: Non-invasive 27-hour Blood Pressure Registration Including Dental Checkups in Some Dental Practices, *Clin. Prev. Dent., 14,* 5, September/October, 1992.

Gortzak, R.A.Th. and Abraham-Inpijn, L.: Blood Pressure Measurements During Dental Checkups Representative of 26-hour Registration, *Oral Surg. Oral Med. Oral Pathol. 70,* 730, December, 1990.

Gortzak, R.A., Abraham-Inpijn, L., and Oosting, J.: Blood Pressure Response to Dental Checkup: A Continuous, Noninvasive Registration, *Gen. Dent., 39,* 339, September-October, 1991.

Little, J.W. and Halberg, F.: A New Horizon in the Prevention, Diagnosis, and Treatment of Hypertension: What Role Should Dentistry Play? *Gen. Dent., 39,* 172, May–June, 1991.

Marion, G.S., McGann, P., and Camp, D.L.: Core Body Temperature in the Elderly and Factors Which Influence Its Measurement, *Gerontology, 37,* 225, July–August, 1991.

Nordstrom, N.K., Longenecker, S., Whitacre, H.L., and Beck, F.M.: Evaluation of Two Methods of Teaching Blood Pressure Measurement, *J. Dent. Educ., 52,* 519, September, 1988.

Veerman, D.P., Van Montfrans, G.A., and Weiling, W.: Effects of Cuff Inflation on Self-recorded Blood Pressure, *Lancet, 335,* 451, February 24, 1990.

Extraoral and Intraoral Examination

A careful overall observation of each patient and a thorough examination of the oral cavity and adjacent structures are essential to total evaluation prior to treatment. A variety of lesions may be observed for which the patient may or may not report subjective symptoms. Recognition, treatment, and follow-up of specific lesions may be of definite significance to the present and future general and oral health of the patient.

Despite the occurrence of many seemingly minor lesions, the danger of oral malignancies remains a definite possibility. In the United States, approximately 3% of all male cancers and 2% of female cancers occur in the area of the oral cavity.[1] Every effort must be made to detect potentially cancerous lesions early.

Each area of the mucous membrane must be examined, and minor deviations from normal must be given prompt attention. A life may depend on an oral examination. Routine examination for each new patient and at each maintenance appointment provides a realistic approach to the control of oral disease.

The oral tissues are sensitive indicators of the general health of the individual. Changes in these structures may be the first indication of subclinical disease processes in other parts of the body.

Prerequisite to the recognition of deviations from the normal appearance of the oral cavity are knowledge and understanding of the normal morphology, anatomy, and physiology of the oral cavity and the surrounding area. Table 8–1 defines terms used for extraoral and intraoral examination.

OBJECTIVES

A thorough examination is essential to the total care of the patient as suggested by the following objectives:

I. To observe the patient overall, as well as in all areas in and about the oral cavity, and to record to call to the attention of the dentist those areas that appear to deviate from normal and that may be evidence of disease.

II. To screen each patient at each maintenance appointment assessment to detect lesions that may be pathologic, particularly cancerous.

III. To recognize a need for postponement of the current appointment because of evidence of communicable disease or in deference to the need for urgent medical consultation and/or treatment.

IV. To prevent the development of advanced, irreversible, or untreatable oral disease by early recognition of initial lesions.

V. To identify suspected conditions that require additional testing and referral for medical evaluation.

VI. To identify extraoral and intraoral deviations from normal that are related to and for which dental hygiene care and instruction may need special adaptations.

VII. To provide a means of comparison of individual oral examinations over a series of maintenance appointments, and thus to determine the effects of dental and dental hygiene care and the success of patient instruction.

VIII. To provide information for continuing records of the patient's diagnosis and treatment plan for legal purposes.

COMPONENTS OF EXAMINATION

The current concept of patient care is that the total patient is being treated, not only the oral cavity, and

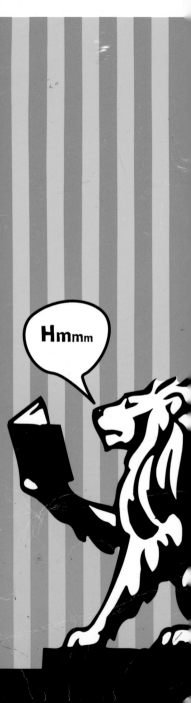

TABLE 8–1
KEY WORDS: EXTRAORAL/INTRAORAL EXAMINATION

Aphtha (af'thah): a little white or reddish ulcer.

Crust: outer scab-like layer of solid matter formed by drying of a body exudate or secretion.

Cyst (sist): a closed, epithelial-lined sac, normal or pathologic, that contains fluid or other material.

Dorsal (dor'sal): back surface; opposite of ventral.

Epidermis (ep ĭ der'mis): outermost and nonvascular layers of the skin composed of basal layer, spinous layer, granular layer, and horny layer.

    Corium (kō'rē-um): the dermis or true skin just beneath the epidermis; well supplied with nerves and blood vessels.

Erosion (e-rō'zhun): soft tissue slightly depressed lesion in which the epithelium above the basal layer is denuded.

Erythema (er'ĭ-the'mah): red area of variable size and shape; reaction to irritation, radiation, or injury.

Exophytic (ek' so-fit'ik): growing outward.

Exostosis (ek' sos-tō'sis): a benign bony growth projecting from the surface of bone.

Fissure (fish'er): a narrow slit or cleft in the epidermis; when infected ulceration, inflammation, and pain can result.

Indurated (in'du-rāt'ed): hardened; abnormally hard.

Lymphadenopathy (lim-fad'ĕ-nop'ah-the): disease of the lymph nodes; regional lymph node enlargement.

Morphology (mor fol'ō-je): science that deals with form and structure.

Palpation (pal-pa'shun): perceiving by sense of touch.

Papilla (pah-pil'ah): small, nipple-shaped projection or elevation
    (**Papillary:** adjective).

Patch: circumscribed flat lesion larger than a macule; differentiated from surrounding epidermis by color and/or texture.

Petechia (pe-te'ke-ah): minute hemorrhagic spot of pinpoint to pinhead size.

Polyp (pol'ip): any growth or mass protruding from a mucous membrane.

    Pedunculated (pē-dung'ku-lāt ed): polyp attached by a thin stalk.

    Sessile (ses'il): polyp with a broad base.

Pseudomembrane (soo' do-mem'brān): a loose membranous layer of exudate containing microorganisms, precipitated fibrin, necrotic cells, and inflammatory cells produced during an inflammatory reaction on the surface of a tissue.

Punctate (punk'tāt): marked with points or punctures differentiated from the surrounding surface by color, elevation, or texture.

Purulent (pu'roo-lent): containing, forming, or discharging pus.

Rubefacient (roo'bĕ-fa'shent): reddening of the skin.

Scar (skar): cicatrix; mark remaining after healing of a wound or healing following a surgical intervention.

Sclerosis (sklĕ-ro'sis): induration or hardening.

Temporomandibular disorder (TMD): a collective term that includes a wide range of disorders of the masticatory system characterized by one or more of the following: pain in the preauricular area, temporomandibular joint (TMJ), and muscles of mastication, with limitation or deviation in mandibular motion and TMJ sounds during mandibular function.

Torus (tō'rus): bony elevation or prominence usually located on the midline of the hard palate (torus palatinus) and the lingual surface of the mandible in the premolar area (torus mandibularis).

Trismus (triz'mus): motor disturbance of the trigeminal nerve, especially spasm of the masticatory muscles with difficulty in opening the mouth.

Ventral (ven'tral): anterior or inferior surface; opposite of dorsal.

Verruca (vĕ-roo'kah): a wart-like growth.

---

particularly not only the teeth and their immediately surrounding tissues. The examination must be, therefore, all-inclusive to detect any physical, mental, or psychologic influences of the whole patient on the oral health.

Thorough examination must become a routine part of each patient appointment if treatment for the control and prevention of oral diseases is to be effective.

I. PREPARATION FOR EXAMINATION

Emphasis must be placed on patient and clinician protection from the spread of communicable disease. Therefore, examinations are made using basic gloves, mask, and protective eyewear.

A. Patient Preparation

1. Review the patient's health histories and other parts of the records.

2. Examine radiographs on viewbox.
3. Explain the procedures to be performed.

B. Instruments and Equipment

Mouth mirror	Gloves
Probe and explorer	Mask
Cotton pliers	Protective eyewear
Sponges	Hand mirror for patient
Tongue depressor	

II. METHODS OF EXAMINATION

The various examination methods were defined on page 81. The extraoral and intraoral examination is accomplished primarily by direct observation and palpation, but other methods are also used.

A. Direct Observation

Patient position, optimum lighting, and effective retraction for accessibility contribute to the accuracy and completeness of the examination. Visual examination is made in conjunction with other methods.

B. Palpation

Gloved hands are used to move or press tissue to detect changes in consistency and size. Types of palpation include the following:

1. *Digital.* Use of a single finger. Example: index finger applied to inner border of the mandible beneath the canine-premolar area to determine the presence of a torus mandibularis.
2. *Bidigital.* Use of finger and thumb of the same hand. Example: palpation of the lips (figure 8–1).

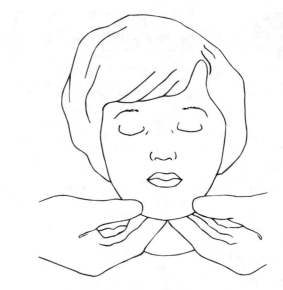

FIG. 8–3. Bilateral Palpation. Bilateral palpation is used to examine corresponding structures on opposite sides of the body.

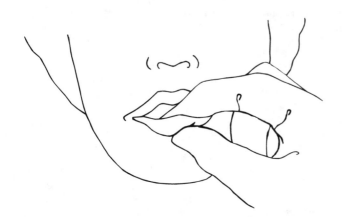

FIG. 8–1. Bidigital Palpation. Palpation of the lip to illustrate the use of a finger and thumb of the same hand.

3. *Bimanual.* Use of finger or fingers and thumb from each hand applied simultaneously in coordination. Example: index finger of one hand palpates on the floor of the mouth inside, while a finger or fingers from the other hand press on the same area from under the chin externally (figure 8–2).
4. *Bilateral.* The two hands are used at the same time to examine corresponding structures on opposite sides of the body. Comparisons may be made. Example: fingers placed beneath the chin to palpate the submandibular lymph nodes (figure 8–3).

SEQUENCE OF EXAMINATION

A recommended order for examination is outlined in table 8–2, in which factors to consider during appointments are related to the actual observations made and recorded. The sequence presented in table 8–2 is adapted from the *Oral Cancer Examination Procedure* available from the American Cancer Society.[2]

I. SYSTEMATIC SEQUENCE FOR EXAMINATION

The advantages of following a routine order for examination include the following:

A. Minimal possibility of overlooking an area and missing details of importance.
B. Increased efficiency and conservation of time.
C. Maintenance of a professional atmosphere, which inspires the patient's confidence.

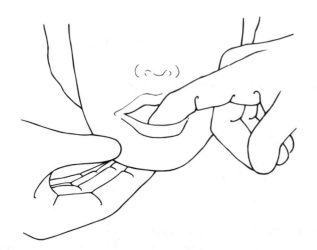

FIG. 8–2. Bimanual Palpation. Examination of the floor of the mouth by simultaneous palpation with fingers of each hand in apposition.

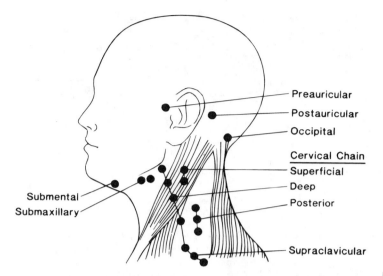

FIG. 8–4. **Lymph Nodes.** The location of the major lymph nodes into which the vessels of the facial and oral regions drain.

II. STEPS FOR THOROUGH EXAMINATION (TABLE 8–2)

A. Extraoral

1. Observe patient during reception and seating to note physical characteristics and abnormalities, and make an overall appraisal.
2. Observe head, face, eyes, and neck, and evaluate the skin of the face and neck.
3. Palpate the salivary glands and lymph nodes. Figure 8–4 shows the location of the major lymph nodes of the face, oral regions, and neck.

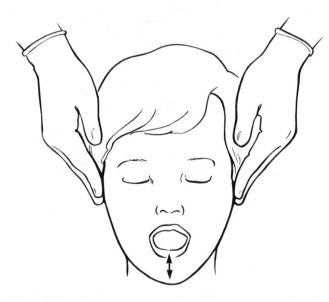

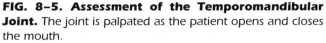

FIG. 8–5. **Assessment of the Temporomandibular Joint.** The joint is palpated as the patient opens and closes the mouth.

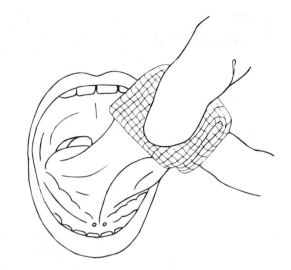

FIG. 8–6. **Examination of the Tongue.** To observe the posterior third of the tongue and the attachment to the floor of the mouth, hold the tongue with a gauze sponge, retract the cheek and move the tongue out, first to one side and then the other, as each section of the mucosa is carefully examined.

4. Observe mandibular movement and palpate the temporomandibular joint (figure 8–5). Relate to items from questions in the medical/dental history.[3,4]

B. Intraoral

1. Make a preliminary examination of the lips and intraoral mucosa, using a mouth mirror or a tongue depressor.
2. View and palpate lips, labial and buccal mucosa, and mucobuccal folds.
3. Examine and palpate the tongue, including the dorsal and ventral surfaces, lateral borders, and base. Retract to observe posterior third, first to one side then the other (figure 8–6).
4. Observe mucosa of the floor of the mouth. Palpate the floor of the mouth (figure 8–2).
5. Examine hard and soft palates, tonsillar areas, and pharynx. Use mirror to observe oropharynx, nasopharynx, and larynx.
6. Note amount and consistency of the saliva and evidences of dry mouth.

RECORDS

I. RECORD FORM

A. Contain adequate space for complete descriptions of lesions observed; not merely a check sheet.
B. Contain spaces for successive examinations at follow-up and maintenance appointments.

TABLE 8–2
EXTRAORAL AND INTRAORAL EXAMINATION

Order of Examination	To Observe	Influences on Appointments
1. Overall Appraisal of Patient	Posture, gait General health status; size Hair; scalp Breathing; state of fatigue Voice, cough, hoarseness	Response, cooperation, attitude toward treatment Length of appointment
2. Face	Expression: Evidence of fear or apprehension Shape; twitching; paralysis Jaw movements during speech Injuries; signs of abuse	Need for alleviation of fears Evidence of upper respiratory or other infections Enlarged masseter muscle (related to bruxism)
3. Skin	Color, texture, blemishes Traumatic lesions Eruptions, swellings Growths	Relation to possible systemic conditions Need for supplementary history Biopsy or other treatment Influences on instruction in diet
4. Eyes	Size of pupil (figure 8–11) Color of sclera Eyeglasses (corrective) Protruding eyeballs	Dilated pupils or pinpoint may result from drugs, emergency state (Table 61–3, pages 842–847) Eyeglasses essential during instruction Hyperthyroidism

5. Nodes (palpate) (figure 8–4)
  a. Pre- and postauricular
  b. Occipital
  c. Submental; submaxillary
  d. Cervical chain
  e. Supraclavicular
	Adenopathy; lymphadenopathy
	Induration
		Need for referral
		Medical consultation
		Coordinate with intraoral examination

6. Temporomandibular joint (Palpate) (figure 8–5)	Limitations or deviations of movement Tenderness; sensitivity Noises: clicking, popping, grating.	Disorder of joint; limitation of opening Discomfort during appointment and during personal plaque control

7. Lips
  a. Observe closed, then open
  b. Palpate (figure 8–1)
	Color, texture, size
	Cracks, angular cheilosis
	Blisters, ulcers
	Traumatic lesions
	Irritation from lip-biting
	Limitation of opening; muscle elasticity; muscle tone
	Evidences of mouthbreathing
	Induration
		Need for further examination: referral
		Immediate need for postponement of appointment when a lesion may be communicable or could interfere with procedures
		Care during retraction
		Accessibility during intraoral procedures
		Patient instruction: dietary, special plaque control for mouthbreather

8. Breath Odor	Severity Relation to oral hygiene, gingival health	Possible relation to systemic condition Alcohol use history; special needs

II. INFORMATION TO RECORD

A complete description of each finding includes the location, extent, size, color, surface texture or configurations, consistency, morphology, and history.

A. Location and Extent

When a lesion is first seen, its location is noted in relation to adjacent structures. A printed diagram of parts of the oral cavity drawn into the record form can be a valuable aid for marking the location (figure 8–7). Descriptive words to define the location and extent include the following:

1. *Localized.* Lesion limited to a small focal area.
2. *Generalized.* Involves most of an area or segment.
3. *Single Lesion.* One lesion of a particular type with a distinct margin.
4. *Multiple Lesions.* More than one lesion of a particular type. Lesions may be

TABLE 8-3
DESCRIPTION OF ELEVATED SOFT TISSUE LESIONS

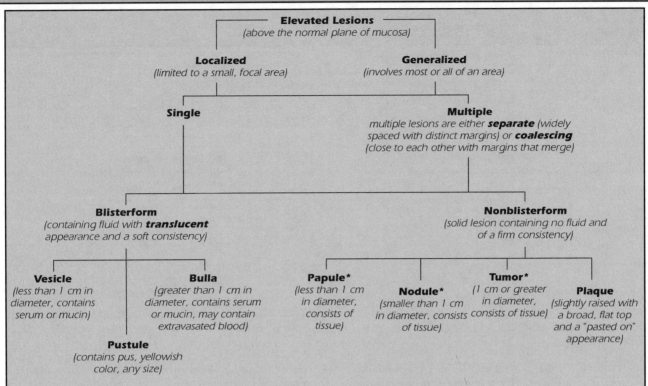

Elevated Lesions
(above the normal plane of mucosa)

Localized
(limited to a small, focal area)

Generalized
(involves most or all of an area)

Single

Multiple
*multiple lesions are either **separate** (widely spaced with distinct margins) or **coalescing** (close to each other with margins that merge)*

Blisterform
*(containing fluid with **translucent** appearance and a soft consistency)*

Nonblisterform
(solid lesion containing no fluid and of a firm consistency)

Vesicle
(less than 1 cm in diameter, contains serum or mucin)

Bulla
(greater than 1 cm in diameter, contains serum or mucin, may contain extravasated blood)

Pustule
(contains pus, yellowish color, any size)

Papule*
(less than 1 cm in diameter, consists of tissue)

Nodule*
(smaller than 1 cm in diameter, consists of tissue)

Tumor*
(1 cm or greater in diameter, consists of tissue)

Plaque
(slightly raised with a broad, flat top and a "pasted on" appearance)

* May be **pedunculated** (on a stem or stalk) or **sessile** (base or attachment is the greatest diameter of the lesion)
(From McCann, A.: Describing Soft Tissue Lesions of the Oral Cavity, *Dentalhygienistnews, 5,* 9, Spring, 1992. Used with permission.)

TABLE 8-4
DESCRIPTION OF DEPRESSED SOFT TISSUE LESIONS

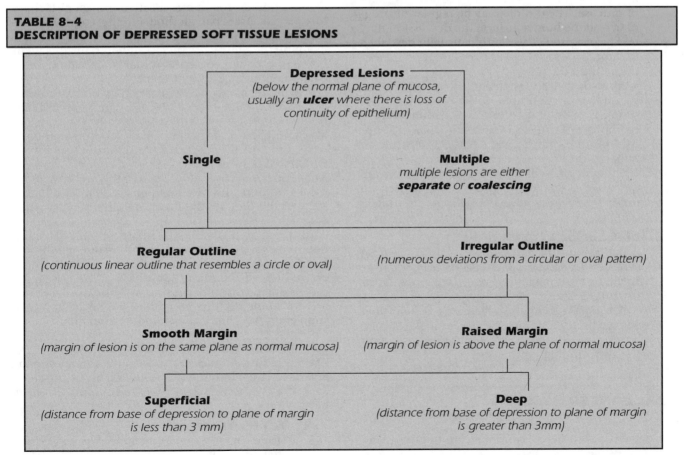

Depressed Lesions
*(below the normal plane of mucosa, usually an **ulcer** where there is loss of continuity of epithelium)*

Single

Multiple
*multiple lesions are either **separate** or **coalescing***

Regular Outline
(continuous linear outline that resembles a circle or oval)

Irregular Outline
(numerous deviations from a circular or oval pattern)

Smooth Margin
(margin of lesion is on the same plane as normal mucosa)

Raised Margin
(margin of lesion is above the plane of normal mucosa)

Superficial
(distance from base of depression to plane of margin is less than 3 mm)

Deep
(distance from base of depression to plane of margin is greater than 3mm)

(From McCann, A.: Describing Soft Tissue Lesions of the Oral Cavity, *Dentalhygienistnews, 5,* 10, Spring, 1992. Used with permission.)

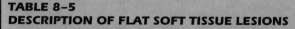

TABLE 8-5
DESCRIPTION OF FLAT SOFT TISSUE LESIONS

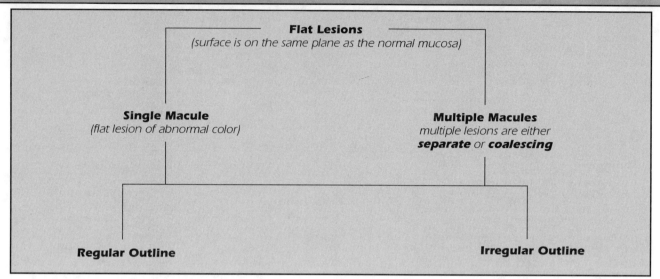

(From McCann, A.: Describing Soft Tissue Lesions of the Oral Cavity, *Dentalhygienistnews*, 5, 9, Spring, 1992. Used with permission.)

culated lesion is attached by a narrow stalk or pedicle, whereas the sessile lesion has a base as wide as the lesion itself.

B. Depressed Lesions (table 8-4)

A depressed lesion is below the level of the skin or mucosa. The outline may be regular or irregular, and the border around the depression may be flat or raised. The depth is usually described as superficial or deep. A deep lesion is greater than 3 mm deep.

Most depressed lesions are ulcers and represent a loss of continuity of the epithelium. The center is often gray to yellow, surrounded by a red border. An ulcer may result from the rupture of an elevated lesion (vesicle, pustule, or bulla).

Other depressed lesions are erosions. They are described as shallow, depressed lesions that do not extend through the epithelium into underlying tissue.

C. Flat Lesions (table 8-5)

A flat lesion is on the same level as the normal skin or oral mucosa. Flat lesions may occur as single or multiple lesions and have a regular or irregular form.

A *macule* is a circumscribed area not elevated above the surrounding skin or mucosa. It may be identified by its color, which contrasts with the surrounding normal tissues.

ORAL CANCER

The objective is to detect cancer of the mouth at the earliest possible stage. Discovered early, it is likely to have a high survival rate, whereas when a cancer extends into adjacent structures and to the lymph nodes of the neck, the prognosis is less favorable.

Because the early lesions are generally symptomless, they may go unnoticed and unreported by the patient. Observation by the dentist or dental hygienist, therefore, is the principal method for the control of oral cancer. The first step in accomplishing this task is to examine the entire face, neck, and oral mucous membrane of each patient at the initial examination and at each maintenance appointment.

The dental hygienist needs to know how to conduct the oral examination, where oral cancer occurs most frequently, what an early cancerous lesion may look like, and what to do when such a lesion is found.

I. LOCATION

Neoplasms may arise at any site in the oral cavity. The most common sites are the floor of the mouth, lateral parts of the tongue, the lower lip, and the soft palate complex.

Although patients may be instructed in self-examination to watch for changes in oral tissues, it is difficult for persons to see their own tissues, particularly the entire floor of the mouth and base of the tongue, by the usual mirror and lighting systems available in a private home. Self-examination should be routinely supplemented with professional examination.

II. APPEARANCE OF EARLY CANCER

Early oral cancer takes many forms and may resemble a variety of common oral lesions. All types should be looked at with suspicion. Five basic forms are listed here.

A. White Areas

These may vary from filmy, barely visible change in the mucosa to heavy, thick, heaped up areas of dry white keratinized tissue. Fissures, ulcers, or areas of induration in a white area are most indicative of malignancy.

Leukoplakia is a white patch or plaque that cannot be characterized as any other disease. It may be associated with physical or chemical agents and the use of tobacco.

B. Red Areas

Lesions of red, velvety consistency, sometimes with small ulcers, should be identified.

The term *erythroplakia* is used to designate lesions of the oral mucosa that appear as bright red patches or plaques that cannot be characterized as any specific disease.

C. Ulcers

These may have flat or raised margins. Palpation may reveal induration.

D. Masses

Papillary masses, sometimes with ulcerated areas, occur as elevations above the surrounding tissues. Other masses may occur below the normal mucosa and may be found only by palpation.

E. Pigmentation

Brown or black pigmented areas may be located on mucosa where pigmentation does not normally occur.

III. PROCEDURE FOR FOLLOW-UP OF A SUSPICIOUS LESION

As designated by the dentist, a lesion may be biopsied immediately, a cytologic smear may be obtained, or the patient may be referred for additional diagnosis and biopsy.

A. Biopsy

1. *Definition.* Biopsy is the removal and examination, usually by microscope, of a section of tissue or other material from the living body for the purposes of diagnosis. A biopsy is either *excisional,* when the entire lesion is removed, or *incisional,* when a representative section from the lesion is taken.
2. *Indications for Biopsy*[6,7]
   a. Any unusual oral lesion that cannot be identified with clinical certainty must be biopsied.
   b. Any lesion that has not shown evidence of healing in 2 weeks should be considered malignant until proved otherwise.
   c. A persistent, thick, white, hyperkeratotic lesion and any mass (elevated or not) that does not break through the surface epithelium should be biopsied.
   d. Any tissue surgically removed should be submitted for microscopic examination.

B. Cytologic Smear

1. *Definition.* The cytologic smear technique is a diagnostic aid in which surface cells of a suspicious lesion are removed for microscopic evaluation.
2. *Indications for Smear Technique*[6]
   a. In general, a lesion for which a biopsy is not planned may be examined by smear. An exception is a keratotic lesion that is not suitable for exfoliative cytology.
   b. A lesion that looks like potential cancer should be examined by smear if the patient refuses to have a biopsy specimen taken. A positive report from a smear should convince the patient of the need for treatment or biopsy.
   c. The smear technique is used for follow-up examination of patients with oral cancer treated by radiation. The treated tissue may heal inadequately and cause persistent ulceration.
   d. Cytology is useful for identifying *Candida albicans* organisms in patients with suspected candidiasis (moniliasis).
   e. Cytology may be useful in identifying herpesvirus by taking a smear from an intact vesicle.
   f. In mass screening programs for cancer detection, smears may be taken. However, all lesions of high suspicion should be referred for biopsy.
   g. Research studies to show changes in surface cells, for example, the effects of topical agents, may use a smear technique.
3. *Limitations of Smear Technique*
   a. When a clear-cut lesion, recognized as pathologic, is present, treatment must not be delayed by waiting for cytologic smear analysis.
   b. The smear detects only surface lesions.
   c. It is difficult or impossible to scrape deep enough to obtain representative cells from a heavily keratinized lesion.
   d. Except for candidiasis, treatment cannot be determined by smear technique results only. After a positive smear, a biopsy is needed for definitive diagnosis.
   e. Because research has shown that the smear technique is not diagnostically reliable (there can be "false negatives," which turn out to be positive biopsies), a negative report should not be considered conclusive.

EXFOLIATIVE CYTOLOGY

Stratified squamous cells are constantly growing toward the epithelial surface of the mucous membrane, where they are exfoliated. Exfoliated cells and cells beneath them are scraped off, and when prepared on a slide, changes in the cells can be detected by staining and studying them microscopically. The malignant cells stain differently from normal cells and take on unusual, abnormal forms.

I. PROCEDURE

A. Materials

Gauze sponges
Glass microscopic slides with frosted end
Plain lead pencil
Paper clips
Blade to scrape lesion (flexible metal spatula)
Fixative (70% alcohol)
Protective mailing container
History form or data sheet

B. Steps

1. *Prepare Materials.* Write the patient's name on the frosted ends of two glass slides (two for each lesion) in pencil, and place a paper clip on the end of one slide to prevent contact between the slides when packaged for mailing to the laboratory.

2. *Prepare the Lesion.* Irrigate the surface to remove debris. Wipe the surface gently with a wet gauze sponge as needed to remove debris or blood. Do not dry.

3. *Scrape the Lesion.* Use a flexible metal spatula. Scrape the entire surface of the lesion firmly several times (all strokes in the same direction) (figure 8–10A). When a wooden tongue depressor is used, it must be wet before taking the sample so the material will not be absorbed into the wood. For intact vesicles, carefully rupture the vesicle so the fluid flows onto the glass slides.

4. *Smear the Glass Slide.* Spread the collected material on the glass slide. Start at the center of the clear end of the slide and smear evenly across the surface. Cover an area approximately 20-mm wide. Handle all glass slides by their edges to prevent fingerprints or other contamination (figure 8–10B).

5. *Fix the Cells.* Immediately, to prevent drying of the cells, place the slide on a flat surface and flood with generous drops of 70% alcohol or use prepared commercial fixative spray.

6. *Obtain Second Smear.* Duplicate previous smear technique. Apply fixing agent immediately.

7. *Complete the Fixation.* Leave slides for 30 minutes. After 20 minutes, tip the slide to let remaining alcohol run off. Air dry where dust or other foreign material cannot contaminate the smear.

8. *Prepare History or Data Sheet.* Basic information includes the following:
   a. Dentist. Name and address.
   b. Patient. Name and address.

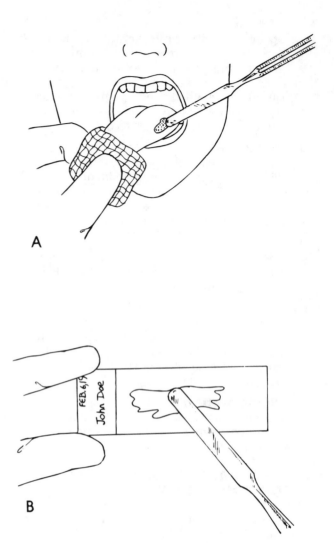

FIG. 8–10. Oral Cytology Technique. A. Tongue is held out with gauze sponge while a metal spatula is used to scrape a lesion. **B.** Collected material is spread evenly on a glass slide. See text for details.

   c. Lesion. Description (size, color, location, shape, consistency, and duration).
   d. Other. Additional related clinical findings or pertinent history.

9. *Prepare for Mailing.* Wrap slides to prevent breakage. Pack with the history or data sheet. Mailing containers, provided by most laboratories list specific instructions.

II. LABORATORY REPORT

The pathologist makes the microscopic examination and classifies the specimen in one of the following categories:

Unsatisfactory   Slide is inadequate for diagnosis. The specimen may have been too thick or thin, or the cells may have dried before fixation. Another smear should be made promptly.

Class I	Normal.
Class II	Atypical, but not suggestive of malignant cells.
Class III	Uncertain (possible for cancer).
Class IV	Probable for cancer.
Class V	Positive for cancer.

III. FOLLOW-UP

A. Report of Class IV or V
Refer for biopsy.

B. Report of Class III
Re-evaluate clinical findings; biopsy usually indicated.

C. Report of Class I or II
1. The patient must not be dismissed until the lesion has healed.
2. When lesion persists, the dentist either re-evaluates the clinical findings and requests a repeat cytologic smear or performs a biopsy.

D. Negative Report
Either biopsy or smear requires careful follow-up when a negative report is obtained for an oral lesion that appears suspicious by clinical examination. False-negative reports are possible, that is, a malignancy may be present, but the sample examined in the smear or biopsy may not have included cancerous cells.

SPECIAL APPLICATIONS FOR THE EXTRAORAL AND INTRAORAL EXAMINATION

In Part VI of this book, many types of patients with special needs for adapted techniques are described. Some of them have general physical and oral characteristics that can be identified during an extraoral and intraoral examination. Facial and oral tissue examinations for pathology apply to all patients.

With certain patients, the recognition of particular characteristics has another dimension, which may have social and legal implications. One example is the group of intraoral and extraoral signs that may reveal a child who is a victim of abuse or neglect. The physical or emotional abuse, neglect, or exploitation of the elderly has also become a problem of growing significance.[8,9,10]

Another patient who may not be identified by questions from a medical and dental history is a substance abuser. A variety of treatment problems are related to the care of a patient who misuses drugs. Identification of the patient's addiction can be essential to successful treatment. Characteristics for recognition of certain special patients are described here.

CHILD ABUSE AND NEGLECT

Recognition of a child who has been abused or neglected should be important to the entire dental team. There is a need to be aware of the problem of child abuse, to be able to identify and report suspected cases, and to document the injuries observed for future reference and comparison.

During the extraoral and intraoral examination, various findings may lead to a suspicion of child abuse. Head, facial, or oral trauma occurs in many child abuse cases. Some of the patients may be seen in dental offices or clinics, whereas others are taken to a hospital emergency clinic because other serious bodily injuries have been inflicted.

Children ranging from infants through teenagers are involved. Several thousands a year die as a result of the severe physical damage inflicted, whereas others suffer permanent brain damage or physical deformities.

I. DEFINITIONS[11]
Maltreatment of children may be categorized as abuse and neglect.

A. Abuse
Abuse refers to nonaccidental physical, sexual, or emotional acts against a child by a parent or caregiver that are beyond the acceptable norms of child care. Characteristically, the injury is more severe than might be expected from the explanation provided by the parent or caregiver.

B. Neglect
Child neglect can be defined as the failure of a parent or other person legally responsible for the child to provide for basic needs at an adequate level of care. Basic needs include food, clothing, health care, safety, and education.

C. Dental Neglect
Dental neglect is the willful failure of parent or guardian to seek and follow through with treatment necessary to ensure a level of oral health essential for adequate function and freedom from pain and infection.[12]

II. RECOGNITION[13,14,15]
Recognition of signs of suspected neglect or abuse is the first step toward protection of the child. As the child enters the reception area and then goes into the treatment room, identifiable characteristics may be displayed that are suggestive of abuse.

A. General Signs
1. *Behavioral.* An abused child may be very fearful and cry excessively, show no fear at all, or appear unhappy and withdrawn. The child

may act differently when the parent is present than when alone, which may provide clues to the type of relationship that exists. Frequently, evidence exists of developmental delays, including those of language or motor skills.

2. *Overall appearance.*
   a. Failure to thrive; malnutrition.
   b. Uncleanliness and other signs of lack of care.
   c. Clothing with long sleeves and long pants, even in warm weather, may suggest that bruises and lacerations are being covered.

3. *Wounds.* Abrasions and lacerations of varying degrees of healing inconsistent with explanations given by the parent.

4. *Signs of Trauma.* Burns; bite marks; trauma to the eyes, external ears, or neck.

B. Oral Signs

1. Bruised and swollen lips; scars on lips may show previous trauma.
2. Abrasions at the corners of the mouth, such as from a gag tied around the head.
3. Lacerations of lingual and labial frena, possibly from forced feeding or related to external traumatic blows.
4. Teeth
   a. Avulsed, fractured, darkened.
   b. Radiographic signs of fractures in different degrees of healing.
5. Jaw fracture.
6. Tongue injuries; evidence of scarring and recent healing.
7. Signs of dental neglect.
   a. Untreated disease, including rampant dental caries, pain, inflammation, bleeding gingiva.
   b. Lack or irregularity of professional care. Appointments may have been primarily for tooth removal.

C. Parental Attitude

Parents who abuse their children are frequently immature and not prepared to accept the responsibilities of parenting. On the other hand, they may have been abused by their own parents. Drug abuse and alcoholism are sometimes involved.

Child abuse is very complex. A few of the possible parental attitudes and behavior patterns are mentioned here.

1. Disinterest or denial in relationship to the child; may be critical, scolding, or belittling in front of others, including dental personnel.
2. Lack of interest in proposed dental and dental hygiene treatment plan, with a tendency to want only pain relief for the child. Such an attitude may not be shown toward other children in the family.

3. Unavailable for consultation. Does not usually accompany the child for dental appointments, but sends the child with another sibling.
4. Provides inconsistent information about the sources and causes of damaged teeth, bruises, or other signs of trauma.

III. REPORTING

Professional people have a particular responsibility to report suspected child abuse to the proper authorities. Each state in the United States has laws defining and governing child abuse and neglect. In certain states, the failure to report can lead to legal involvement. The failure to recognize and act in behalf of the child may be dangerous, even fatal, for the child involved. Telephone numbers for specific reporting should be kept current and readily available.

SUBSTANCE ABUSE

It is usually not possible to determine from a patient's medical and dental histories whether the patient uses alcohol and/or unprescribed drugs regularly, perhaps to the level of dependency. The general categories of the drugs of abuse are listed with examples in table 8–6, along with their "street" names. When a history is being prepared, more information may be obtained about drug use if the common street names of products are used.

Problems related to the use of alcohol and alcoholism are considered in Chapter 57.

Patients who use drugs recreationally may "premedicate" themselves when a stressful situation, such as a dental appointment, is anticipated. Because the day-to-day use of drugs varies, questioning at each appointment may be necessary to prevent complications. Certain precautions must be taken during patient care.

When no information is provided by the patient, awareness by dental personnel of the characteristics that suggest the possible use of drugs is important. A few of the common features that may aid in general identification are included in this section.

I. DEFINITIONS
A. Drug
A drug is a chemical substance used for diagnosis, prevention, or treatment of disease. Drugs are classified by biochemical action, physiologic effect, or the organ system involved.

B. Substance Abuse
Substance or drug abuse is the regular use of a drug other than for its accepted medical purpose or in doses greater than those considered appropriate.

C. Chemical Dependence
Dependence refers to the interaction between a drug and the individual when there is a compul-

9

Dental Radiographs

Radiographs are essential adjuncts to other means of assessment for treatment planning in the complete care program for a patient. The dentist is responsible for determining the need for radiographs. Designation of the number and types of dental exposures must be made selectively only after a review of the patient's health history and a complete clinical examination.[1]

A history of oral and body exposures to radiation is needed. Excessive dental exposure to low levels of ionizing radiation cannot be justified.[2]

The objective in radiography is to use procedures that require the least amount of radiation exposure possible to produce radiographs of the greatest interpretive value. The first consideration is to limit the number of exposures to those that have been determined necessary. Quality assurance then can be accomplished by application of known safety measures for the patient and the clinician and by following precise steps for exposure and processing. Continuing study is needed to keep informed of research developments.[3]

This chapter provides a summary of terminology, fundamentals of x-ray production, procedures for film exposure and processing, safety factors, analysis of the completed radiographs, and suggestions for patient instruction. A comprehensive bibliography for additional suggested reading is included.

Selected terms used in the study of radiography are listed and defined in table 9–1. Other terms are described throughout the chapter.*

---

* All definitions in this chapter are taken from or adapted from and in accord with the *Glossary of Maxillofacial Radiology,* 3rd ed. prepared by the American Academy of Oral and Maxillofacial Radiology, 1990.

ORIGIN AND CHARACTERISTICS OF X RAY

I. HISTORY
X ray is electromagnetic ionizing radiation of very short wavelength, resulting from the bombardment of a material (usually tungsten) by highly accelerated electrons in a high vacuum.

X rays were first discovered by Wilhelm C. Roentgen in 1895, who called them *x* rays after the mathematical symbol "*x*" for an unknown. "Roentgen rays" is a term often applied to mechanically generated x rays.

Professor Roentgen used a Crookes tube; it was not until 1913 that William D. Coolidge designed a tube in which electricity was used instead of gas. Modern x-ray tubes have the same principles of construction as those of the Coolidge tube. The historical development of the science of radiology and radiography provides a realistic monument to the early researchers and their efforts.[4]

II. PROPERTIES
  A. Short wavelength
    1. *Hard x rays.* Shorter wavelengths, high penetrating power.
    2. *Soft x rays.* Relatively longer wavelengths; relatively less penetrating; more likely to be absorbed into the tissue through which the x rays pass.
  B. Speed of travel same as that of visible light.
  C. Power to penetrate opaque substances.
  D. Invisible.
  E. Ability to affect the emulsion of a photographic film.

133

TABLE 9–1
KEY WORDS: RADIOGRAPHY

Attenuation (ah-ten′ū-a′shun): the process by which a beam of radiation is reduced in intensity when passing through some material; the combination of absorption and scattering processes leads to a decrease in flux density of the beam when projected through matter.

Cassette (kah-set′): a light tight container in which x-ray films are placed for exposure to x radiation; usually backed with lead to reduce the effect of backscattered radiation; may be made of cardboard or of metal with an exposure side of Bakelite, aluminum, or magnesium and containing an intensifying screen(s).

Intensifying screen: a card or plastic sheet coated with fluorescent material positioned singly or in pairs in a cassette to contact the film; when the cassette is exposed to x radiation, the visible light from the fluorescent image on the screen adds to the latent image produced directly by x radiation.

Impulse: the burst of radiation generated during a half cycle of alternating current; film exposure time is measured in impulses.

Irradiation (i-rā′dē-ā′shun): the exposure to radiation; one speaks of radiation therapy and of irradiation of a body part.

Latent image: the invisible change produced in an x-ray film emulsion by the action of x radiation or light from which the visible image is subsequently developed and fixed chemically.

Penumbra (pĕ num′brah): the secondary shadow that surrounds the periphery of the primary shadow; in radiography, it is the blurred margin of an image detail (geometric unsharpness).

Photoelectric effect: the ejection of bound electrons by an incident photon such that the whole energy of the photon is absorbed and transitional or characteristic x-ray emissions are produced.

Radiation: the emission and propagation of energy through space or a material medium in the form of waves or particles.

Bremsstrahlung radiation (white radiation) (brem′strah-lung): a distribution of x rays from very low energy photons to those produced by the peak kilovoltage applied across an x-ray tube; bremsstrahlung means "braking radiation" and refers to the sudden deceleration of electrons (cathode rays) as they interact with highly positively charged nuclei, such as tungsten.

Characteristic radiation: the radiation produced by electron transitions from higher energy orbitals to replace ejected electrons of inner electron orbitals; the energy of the electromagnetic radiation emitted is unique or "characteristic" of the emitting atom.

Electromagnetic radiation: Forms of energy propagated by wave motion as photons; the radiations differ widely in wavelength, frequency, and photon energy; examples are infrared waves, visible light, ultraviolet radiation, x rays, gamma rays, and cosmic radiation.

Gamma radiation: short-wavelength electromagnetic radiation of nuclear origin similar to x rays but usually of higher energy.

Leakage radiation: the radiation that escapes through the protective shielding of the x-ray unit tube head; it may be detected at the sides, top, bottom, or back of the tube head.

Primary radiation: all radiation coming directly from the target of the anode of an x-ray tube.

Scattered radiation: a form of secondary radiation that, during passage through a substance, has been deviated in direction; it may also have been modified by an increase in wavelength.

Backscatter: radiation deflected by scattering processes at angles greater than 90° to the original direction of the beam of radiation.

Compton scatter radiation: the incident radiation has sufficient energy to dislodge a bound electron, but attacks a loosely bound electron, and the remaining radiation energy proceeds in a different direction as scatter radiation.

Thompson scattering (coherent or unmodified): scattering of relatively low-energy x rays by elastic collisions without loss of photon energy.

Secondary radiation: particles or photons produced by the interaction of primary radiation with matter.

Stray radiation: radiation that serves no useful purpose; it includes leakage, secondary, and scattered radiation.

Radiograph: a visible image on a radiation-sensitive film emulsion produced by a chemical processing after exposure of the film emulsion to ionizing radiation that has passed through an area, region, or substance of interest.

Radiography: the art and science of making radiographs.

Radiologic health: the art and science of protecting human beings from injury by radiation, as well as of promoting better health through beneficial applications of radiation.

Radiology: that branch of science that deals with the use of radiant energy in the diagnosis and treatment of disease.

Rare earth: commonly used to refer to intensifying screens that contain rare earth elements; it may also refer to a screen-film system used for x-ray imaging; the systems are considered "fast" exposure systems.

Rectification: conversion of alternating current (AC) to direct current (DC); a **rectifier** changes AC to DC.

Subtraction radiography: A photographic or digital method of eliminating background anatomic structures from the final image, thus bringing out the differences between the pre- and postprocedure radiographic images.

Digital subtraction radiography: a radiographic image subtraction method in which the pre- and postprocedure radiographic images are digitized into the computer memory; these images are subtracted from each other within the computer memory, and the resultant subtracted image is displayed on the monitor.

Xeroradiography (zē′rō-rā′dē-og′rah-fē): a dry process that produces prints of x-ray images by means of a selenium plate, which records an image through the radiation-induced discharge of a positive electrostatic potential.

F. Ability to produce fluorescence on contact with certain crystals.

G. Ability to stimulate or destroy living cells.

HOW X RAYS ARE PRODUCED[5,6]

With reference to the preceding definition of x ray, essential to x-ray production are (1) a source of electrons, (2) a high voltage to accelerate the electrons, and (3) a target to stop the electrons. The parts of the tube and the circuits within the machine are designed to provide these elements.

I. THE X-RAY TUBE (Figure 9–1)
A. Protective Tube Housing
X-ray tube enclosure that reduces the primary radiation to permissible exposure levels; highly vacuated glass tube surrounded by a specially refined oil with high insulating powers.

B. Cathode (−)
1. Tungsten filament, which is heated to give off a cloud of electrons.
2. Molybdenum cup around the filament to focus the electrons toward the anode.

C. Anode (+)
1. Copper arm containing a tungsten button, the target, positioned opposite the cathode at an angle.
2. Focal spot, the part of the target on the anode bombarded by the focused electron stream when the tube is energized.

D. Aperture
Where the useful beam emerges from the tube; covered with a permanent seal of glass or aluminum.

II. CIRCUITS
A circuit is the path over which a current (flow of electricity) may flow.

A. Low-voltage filament circuit.
B. High-voltage cathode-anode circuit.

III. TRANSFORMERS
A transformer increases or decreases the incoming voltage.

A. Autotransformer
A voltage compensator that corrects minor variations in line voltage.

B. Step-down Transformer
Decreases the line voltage to approximately 3 volts to heat the filament and form the electron cloud.

C. Step-up Transformer
Increases the current (110 volts) to 65,000 to 90,000 volts to give electrons the required high speed to produce x-ray particles.

IV. MACHINE CONTROL DEVICES
Machines vary, but, in general, when operating an x-ray machine, there are four factors to control: the line switch (to electrical outlet), the kilovoltage, the milliamperage, and the time.

A. Voltage Control
Voltage is the unit of measurement used to describe the force that pushes an electric current through a circuit.
1. *Circuit Voltmeter.* Registers line voltage before voltage is stepped up by the transformer (with alternating current, this is 110 volts) or may register the kilovoltage that results after step-up.
2. *kVp (kilovoltage Peak) Selector.* Used to change the line voltage to a selected kilovoltage (65 to 90 kVp).

B. Milliamperage Control
1. *Ampere.* The unit of intensity of an electric current produced by 1 volt acting through a resistance of 1 ohm. A milliampere is 1/1000 of an ampere.

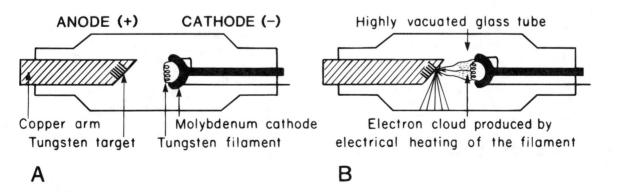

ANODE (+)   CATHODE (−)

Copper arm
Tungsten target   Molybdenum cathode
Tungsten filament

A

Highly vacuated glass tube

Electron cloud produced by electrical heating of the filament

B

FIG. 9–1. X-Ray Tube. A. Inactive. **B.** In function. *Highly accelerated electrons are propelled from the cathode to the anode. X rays are produced as the electrons strike the tungsten target.*

2. *Milliammeter.* Instrument used to select the actual current through the tube circuit during the time of exposure.

C. Time Control
1. *X-ray Timer.* A time switch mechanism used to complete the electrical circuit so that x rays are produced for a predetermined time.
2. *Mechanical Timer.* Spring-activated device; range from $\frac{1}{4}$ to 10 or 15 seconds; does not reset itself; does not accommodate new high-speed film and techniques.
3. *Electronic Timer.* Vacuum tube device; resets itself automatically to the last-used exposure time. The timer is calibrated in seconds, with 60 *impulses* in each second (in a 60-cycle AC current).

V. STEPS IN THE PRODUCTION OF X RAYS[6,7]
A. Tungsten filament is heated and a cloud of electrons is produced.
B. Difference in electrical potential is developed between the anode and the cathode.
C. Electrons are attracted to the anode from the cathode at high speed during the intervals of the alternating current, when the anode is charged positive and the cathode negative. (During the alternating half of the cycle, the electrons are attracted back into the filament in a self-rectifying tube.)
D. Curvature of the molybdenum cup controls the direction of the electrons and causes them to be projected on the focal spot.
E. Reaction of the electrons as they strike the tungsten target results in loss of energy.
   1. Approximately 1% of the energy of electrons is converted to electromagnetic energy of an x ray (larger percent at higher kilovoltages).
   2. Approximately 99% of the energy is converted to heat, which is dissipated through the copper anode and oil of the protective tube housing.
F. X rays leave the tube through the aperture to form the useful beam.
G. The beam is an emission of electromagnetic radiation.
   1. *Useful Beam.* The part of the primary radiation that is permitted to emerge from the tube head aperture and the accessory collimating devices.
   2. *Central Beam* (central ray). The center of the beam of x rays emitted from the tube.

CHARACTERISTICS OF AN ACCEPTABLE RADIOGRAPH

A *radiograph* is the visible image on a radiation-sensitive film emulsion. The image is produced by chemical processing after exposure of the film emulsion to ionizing radiation that has passed through an area, or, specifically for dentistry, through teeth or a part of the oral cavity. A *radiographic survey* refers to a series of radiographs.

Before making a radiograph, it is important to know the characteristics necessary to result in a finished radiograph that is of maximum value and truly useful for diagnosis. The basic essentials are the appearance of the image itself, the area covered, and the quality of the processed radiograph.

I. PARTS OF THE IMAGE
All parts of the image must be shown as close to their natural size and shape as possible with a minimum of distortion and superimposition.

II. AREA TO BE EXAMINED
The area being examined for assessment must be shown completely with sufficient surrounding tissue included for comparative interpretation.

III. QUALITY OF THE RADIOGRAPH
The quality depends on its density, contrast, and definition.

A. Radiolucency and Radiopacity
A radiograph has graduations from white to black that are referred to as radiopaque or radiolucent. For example, a dense material, such as a metallic restoration, prevents the passage of x rays and appears white on the processed radiograph. Soft tissue does not resist passage of x rays, and thus appears from black to gray.
1. *Radiopacity.* The appearance of light (white) images on a radiograph as a result of the lesser amount of radiation that penetrates the structures and reaches the film. A *radiopaque* structure inhibits the passage of x rays.
2. *Radiolucency.* The appearance of dark images on a radiograph as a result of the greater amount of radiation that penetrates the structures and reaches the film. A *radiolucent* structure permits the passage of radiation with relatively little attenuation by absorption.

B. Density
The density of a radiograph refers to the degree of darkening of the exposed and processed x-ray film. The term "background density" is used when referring to factors other than radiation that may have affected the appearance of the finished radiograph. Examples are exposure to white light or film used after its expiration date.

C. Contrast
Contrast means the visual differences in image density appearing between adjacent areas on a radiograph. Types of contrast are referred to as follows:

1. *Film Contrast.* A characteristic inherent in the type of film used.
2. *Long Scale Contrast.* An increased range of grays between the blacks and whites on a radiograph. Higher voltages increase the range.
3. *Short Scale Contrast.* A reduced range of grays between the blacks and whites on a radiograph. Lower kilovoltages decrease the range.
4. *Subject Contrast.* The relative difference in density and thickness of the components of the radiographed subject. Subject contrast relates to radiopacity and radiolucency.

D. Definition

Definition refers to the property of an image that pertains to the sharpness, distinctness, or clarity of outline. Inadequate definition may be related to movement of the patient, the film, or the tube head during exposure.

FACTORS THAT INFLUENCE THE FINISHED RADIOGRAPH

As the beam leaves the x-ray tube it is collimated, filtered, and allowed to travel a designated source-film (or focal spot-film) distance before reaching the film of a selected speed. The quality or diagnostic usefulness of the finished radiograph, as well as the total exposure of the patient and clinician, are influenced by the *collimation, filtration, source-film distance, film speed, kilovoltage,* and *milliampere seconds.*

Film processing (pages 156–158) also influences directly the quality of the radiograph and indirectly the total exposure, because re-exposure would be necessary should the film be rendered inadequate during processing.

I. COLLIMATION[7,8]

Collimation is the technique or mechanism for controlling the size and shape of the beam of radiation emitted through the aperture of the tube. A *collimator* is a diaphragm or system of diaphragms made of an absorbing material designed to define the dimensions and direction of a beam of radiation.

A. Purposes
1. Eliminate peripheral or more divergent radiation.
2. Minimize exposure to patient's face.
3. Minimize secondary radiation, which can fog the film and expose the bodies of patient and clinician.

B. Methods
1. *Diaphragm.* A diaphragm usually is made of lead and pierced with a central aperture of the smallest practical diameter for making radiographic exposure; it is located between the x-ray tube and the position-indicating device (PID).
   a. Recommended thickness of lead: $\frac{1}{8}$ inch.
   b. Recommended size of aperture: to permit a diameter of the beam of radiation equal to $2\frac{3}{4}$ inches at the end of the PID next to the patient's face.
2. *Rectangular Collimation.* As shown in figure 9–2, a patient receives much less unnecessary radiation with the use of a rectangular PID, because the size of the beam is greatly reduced. When a rectangular diaphragm is used, it should be approximately $1\frac{1}{2} \times 2$ inches at the skin. A rectangular diaphragm must be rotated to accommodate for films positioned horizontally or vertically.
3. *Lead-lined Cylindrical PID.**
4. *Cylindrical Scatterguard.* A steel cylinder inserted by the manufacturer into the center of the PID, where the PID attaches to the aperture of the tube head to prevent scatter rays from reaching parts of the film not being exposed by the primary x-ray beam.

C. Relation to Techniques
The dimensions of the largest periapical film are $1\frac{1}{4} \times 1\frac{5}{8}$ inches. Precise angulation techniques are required to eliminate "cone-cut" of film,** particularly when rectangular collimation is used.

II. FILTRATION[7,8]
Filtration is the insertion of absorbers or filters for the preferential attenuation of radiation of certain wavelength from a primary beam of x radiation.

A. Purpose
To minimize exposure of the patient's skin to unnecessary radiation that will not reach and expose the film.

B. Methods
1. *Inherent Filtration.* Includes the glass envelope encasing the x-ray tube and the glass window in the tube housing.
2. *Added Filtration.* Thin, commercially pure aluminum disks inserted between the lead diaphragm and the x-ray tube.
3. *Total Filtration.* The sum of inherent and added filtration.
   a. Recommended total is the equivalent of 0.5 mm (below 50 kVp); 1.5 mm (50 to 70 kVp); and 2.5 mm (over 70 kVp) of aluminum.

---

* The PID was formerly called the "cone" or "plastic cone." Research has shown that the PID must be a lead-lined, open-ended cylinder to prevent secondary radiation.

** "Cone-cut" refers to an error of technique that results when the PID is not angled for the beam of radiation to cover completely the film being exposed. The term "cone-cut" is still commonly used and is used in this chapter.

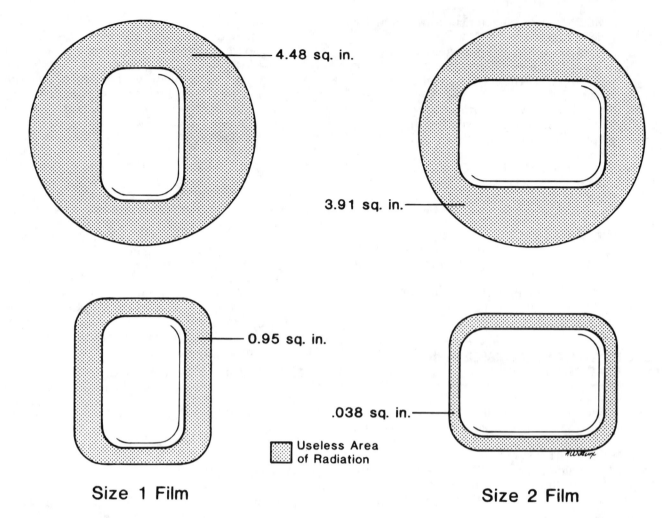

4.48 sq. in.

3.91 sq. in.

0.95 sq. in.

.038 sq. in.

▓ Useless Area
of Radiation

Size 1 Film   Size 2 Film

FIG. 9–2. Cylindrical and Rectangular Position-Indicating Devices. The useless areas of radiation are greatly lessened when rectangular collimation is used. The patient can be spared exposure to excess radiation. (Redrawn from Shannon, S.A.: Rectangular Versus Cylindrical Collimation, *Dent. Hyg., 61,* 173, April, 1987; copyright 1987 by the American Dental Hygienists' Association.)

b. Check the inherent filtration of the individual x-ray machine; then add a sufficient amount of commercially pure aluminum to bring the total to the recommended level.

C. Disadvantage of Added Filtration
Some secondary radiation is produced and scatters in all directions.

III. KILOVOLTAGE
Kilovoltage is the potential difference between the anode and cathode of an x-ray tube. The kilovoltage peak (kVp) refers to the crest value (in kilovolts) of the potential difference of a pulsating generator. When only one half of the wave is used, the value refers to the useful half of the cycle.

A. Amount of Kilovoltage
Determines the quality of the x radiation.
1. Kilovoltage creates a difference in potential

between the anode and the cathode for the production of x rays.
2. The higher the kilovoltage, the greater the acceleration of the electrons, the greater the force with which they bombard the target, and, therefore, the shorter the wavelength.
3. The shorter the wavelength, the greater the penetrating power at the skin surface.

B. Use of High Kilovoltage (90 kVp)[8]
1. Density of the finished radiograph increases with increased kilovoltage (other factors remaining constant).
2. To maintain the proper film density, the milliampere seconds must be decreased as the kVp is increased.
3. Variation in contrast
   a. Low kilovoltage. High contrast, with sharp black-white differences in densities between adjacent areas, but small range

of distinction between subject thicknesses recorded.

    b. High kilovoltage. Low contrast, with wide range of subject thicknesses recorded; greater range of densities from black to white (more gray tones), which, when examined under proper viewing conditions, provide more interpretive details.

4. Advantages
   a. Permits shorter exposure time.
   b. Reduces exposure to tissues lying in front of the film packet.

5. Disadvantages
   a. Increased radiation to tissues outside the edges of the film.
   b. More internal scattered radiation at 90 kVp than at 65 kVp once the primary beam has hit the film, but more scatter at the face with 65 kVp.

IV. MILLIAMPERE SECONDS

A. Milliamperage

The measure of the electron current passing through the x-ray tube; it regulates the heat of the filament, which determines the number of electrons available to bombard the target.

B. Quantity of Radiation

Quantity of radiation is expressed in milliampere seconds (mAs).

1. Definition: mAs are the milliamperes multiplied by the exposure time in seconds.
2. Example: At 10 milliamperes for $\frac{1}{2}$ second, the exposure of the film would be 5 mAs.

C. Radiographic Density

Radiographic density increases with increased milliamperage and/or time of exposure (other factors remaining constant).

V. DISTANCE

Several distances are involved in x-ray film exposure. The source-surface, the source-film, and the object-film distances must be considered for film placement.

A. Object-Film Distance

The object-film distance refers to the distance between the object (tooth or skin) and the film.

With the paralleling technique and the use of a film holder, the object-film distance is increased for most radiographs. A collimated beam and increased source-film distance compensate to preserve definition and film quality.

B. Source-Film Distance

The PID on the x-ray machine is designed to indicate the direction of the central axis of the x-ray beam and to serve as a guide in establishing a desired source-surface and source-film distance. Techniques using 8- and 16-inch source-film distances are common.

The source-film distance is the sum total of the distance from the source to the PID within the tube housing, the length of the PID, and the distance from the end of the PID (at the face) to the film. Directions in technique call for lightly touching the skin with the end of the PID to standardize the source-film distance.

Principles related to source-film distance are as follows:

1. The intensity of the x-ray beam varies inversely as the square of the source-film distance. For example, if 2 films of the same speed were used, one at a 16-inch source-film distance and one at an 8-inch distance, with all other factors, such as kVp and mAs, remaining constant, the film at 16 inches would require 4 times the exposure (time) to maintain the same density in the finished radiograph.
2. The exposure decreases as the distance increases; when the distance is made twice as great, the radiation exposure to the patient is reduced to one fourth.
3. To maintain film density when distance is increased, an increase in mAs, kVp, or film speed is required.

C. Advantages in the Use of an Extended Source-Film Distance

1. Definition or distinctness and clarity of detail improve (because the image is produced by the more central rays).
2. Enlargement or magnification of image decreases (because at shorter distances the outer, more divergent rays tend to enlarge or magnify the image).
3. Skin exposure of the patient is reduced.
4. Less tissue is within the primary beam of radiation, because less spreading of the x-ray beam occurs.

VI. FILMS[9]

With optimum filtration, collimation, and fast film, the skin dose to the face can be reduced significantly. Within recent years, the manufacture of very slow-speed films has been discontinued, the speed of many films has been doubled, and the use of higher speed films has gained increasing acceptance by the dental profession.

A. Film Composition

A film is a thin, transparent sheet of cellulose acetate or similar material coated on one or both sides with an emulsion sensitive to radiation and light.

1. *Emulsion.* Gelatin containing a suspension of countless tiny crystals of silver halide salts (mostly silver bromide).
2. *Film Packet.* Small, light-proof, moisture-resistant, sealed paper envelope containing an x-ray film (or two) and a thin sheet of lead foil.

a. Two-film packet: Useful for processing one film differently from the other to make diagnostic comparisons; for sending to specialist to whom patient may be referred; for legal evidence.

b. Purpose of lead foil backing: To prevent exposure of the film by scattered radiation that could enter from back of packet, and to protect the patient's tissues lying in the path of the x ray.

B. Film Speed

Film speed or film emulsion speed refers to the sensitivity of the film to radiation exposure. The speed is the amount of exposure required to produce a certain image density.

1. *Factors Determining*
   a. Grain size: The smaller the grain size, the slower the film speed.
   b. Use of double or single emulsion: Slower films have a single emulsion on one side only. Nearly all present-day films have two emulsions.
2. *Classification.* Films have been classified by the American National Standard Institute (ANSI) in cooperation with the American Dental Association (ADA). The ANSI/ADA Specification No. 22 designates 6 groups, A through F. Speed groups A, B, and C, the slowest, are associated with excess radiation exposure and are not used. Only film speeds D or faster are used for dental purposes. E film requires up to one-half the exposure time used for D film.
3. *Choice.* E film is recommended for use with rectangular collimation for marked reduction in radiation exposure.[10]

EXPOSURE TO RADIATION

Several factors influence the biologic effects of radiation, including the quality of the radiation, the chemical composition of the absorbing medium, the tissues irradiated, the dose (total and rate per unit of time), the blood supply to the tissues, and the size of the area exposed. Biologic effects of radiation are either somatic (of the general body cells) or genetic (heritable changes, chiefly mutations, produced by the absorption of ionizing radiation by reproductive cells).

I. IONIZING RADIATION

Ionizing radiation is electromagnetic radiation (for example, x rays or gamma rays) or particulate radiation (for example, electrons, neutrons, protons) capable of ionizing air directly or indirectly.

The phenomenon of separation of electrons from molecules to change their chemical activity is called ionization. The organic and inorganic compounds that make up the human body may be altered by exposure to ionizing radiation. The biologic effects following irradiation are secondary effects in that they result from physical, chemical, and biologic action set in motion by the absorption of energy from radiation.

II. EXPOSURE
A. Types of Exposure

Exposure is a measure of the x radiation to which a person or object, or a part of either, is exposed at a certain place; this measure is based on its ability to produce ionization.

1. *Threshold Exposure.* The minimum exposure that produces a detectable degree of any given effect.
2. *Entrance or Surface Exposure.* Exposure measured at the surface of an irradiated body, part, or object. It includes primary radiation and backscatter from the irradiated underlying tissue. The term skin exposure is used with reference to the exposure measured at the center of an irradiated skin surface area.
3. *Erythema Exposure.* The radiation necessary to produce a temporary redness of the skin.

B. Exposure Units[7,11]

The units of absorbed dose are expressed in *joules*/kilogram (1 rad = 0.01 j/kg). The units shown in table 9–2 are the recommendations of the International Commission on Radiation Units and Measurements.

The unit of measurement is the *gray* (Gy). An

**TABLE 9–2.
RADIATION UNITS**

Definition	Traditional Unit	S.I. Unit*	Equivalent
Unit of Radiation Exposure	Roentgen (R)	Coulomb per kilogram (C/kg)	$1 \text{ R} = 2.58 \times 10^{-4} \text{ C/kg}$
Unit of Absorbed Dose	Rad	Gray (Gy)	100 rad = 1 Gy
Unit of Dose Equivalent	Rem	Sievert (Sv)	100 rem = 1 Sv
Unit of Radioactivity	Curie (Ci)	Becquerel (Bq)	$1 \text{ Ci} = 3.7 \times 10^{10} \text{ Bq}$

* S.I. (System International) is from the French *Système International d'Unités.*

absorbed dose of 1 gray is equal to 1 j/kg; therefore, an absorbed dose of 1 Gy is equal to 100 rads.

The unit of biologic equivalence is the *sievert* (Sv). 1 Sv = 100 rem.

C. Dose

The radiation dose is the amount of energy absorbed per unit mass of tissue at a site of interest. The kinds of doses are defined in table 9–3.

D. Permissible Dose

The amount of radiation that may be received by an individual within a specified period without expectation of any significantly harmful result is called the *permissible dose*.

Assumptions on which permissible doses are calculated include the following:

1. No irradiation is beneficial.
2. There is a dose below which no somatic change can be produced.

TABLE 9–3
TYPES OF RADIATION DOSES

Absorbed dose: the amount of energy imparted by ionizing radiation to a unit mass of irradiated material at a specific exposure point; The unit of absorbed dose is the rad or gray (Gy).

Cumulative dose: the total dose resulting from repeated exposures to radiation of the same region or of the whole body

Dose: the amount of energy absorbed per unit mass of tissue at a site of interest.

Dose equivalent: the product of absorbed dose and modifying factors, such as the quality factor, distribution factor, and any other necessary factors; different types of radiation cause differing biologic effects; the traditional unit of dose equivalence is the rem (Sievert).

Erythema dose: the minimum quantity of x or gamma radiation that produces the appearance of redness (erythema).

Exit dose: the absorbed dose delivered by a beam of radiation to the surface through which the beam emerges from an object.

LLD50/30 dose: the dose of radiation that is lethal for 50% of a large population in a specified period of time, usually 30 days.

Lethal dose: the amount of radiation that is, or could be, sufficient to cause death of an organism.

Maximum permissible dose: the maximum dose equivalent that a person (or specified parts of that person) is allowed to receive in a stated period of time; the dose of radiation that would not be expected to produce any significant radiation effects in a lifetime.

Skin dose (surface absorbed dose): the absorbed dose delivered by a radiation beam and backscatter at the point where the central ray passes through the superficial layer of the object.

Threshold dose: the minimum dose that produces a detectable degree of any effect.

---

3. Children are more susceptible than older people.
4. There is a dose below which, even though it is delivered before the end of the reproductive period, the probability of genetic effects is slight.

E. Radiation Hazard

A condition under which persons might receive radiation in excess of the maximum permissible dose. Exposure would be a risk in an area where x-ray equipment is being used or where radioactive materials are stored.

F. National Council on Radiation Protection and Measurements[12]

1. *Limits for Dentists and Dental Personnel.* See table 9–4.
2. *Limits for Patients.* Exposure to x-ray radiation shall be kept to the minimum level consistent with clinical requirements. This limitation is determined by the professional judgment of the dentist.
3. *ALARA Concept.* Radiation exposures must be kept **A**s **L**ow **A**s **R**easonably **A**chievable. This concept is accepted and enforced by all regulatory agencies.

III. SENSITIVITY OF CELLS[13,14]
A. Factors Affecting

1. *Maturity of Cell.* Immature cells are most sensitive.
2. *Reproductive Capacity.* Rapidly reproducing cells are more sensitive; most sensitive when undergoing mitosis.
3. *Metabolism.* Cells are more sensitive in periods of increased metabolism.

B. Radiosensitive Tissues

Blood-forming tissues, reproductive cells, lymphatic tissues, young bone tissue, and skin are the most radiosensitive.

TABLE 9–4
MAXIMUM PERMISSIBLE DOSE EQUIVALENT VALUES (MPD)* TO WHOLE BODY, GONADS, BLOOD-FORMING ORGANS, LENS OF EYE[12]

Average Weekly Exposure†	Maximum 13-week Exposure	Maximum Yearly Exposure	Maximum Accumulated Exposure‡
0.1 R	3 R	5 R	5(N-18)R§

 * Exposure of persons for dental or medical purposes is not counted against their maximum permissible exposure limits.

 † Used only for the purpose of designating radiation barriers.

 ‡ When the previous occupational history of an individual is not definitely known, it shall be assumed that the full dose permitted by the formula 5(N-18) has already been received.

 § N = Age in years and is greater than 18. The unit for exposure is the roentgen (R).

C. Radioresistant Tissues
Most glandular tissues, muscle tissue, nerve tissue, and mature bone tissue are radioresistant.

D. Tissue Reaction
1. *Latent Period.* Lapse between the time of exposure and the time when effects are observed. (May be as long as 25 years, or relatively short, as in the case of the production of a skin erythema.)
2. *Cumulative Effect*
   a. Amount of reaction depends on dose; reaction is less when radiation is received in fractional doses than in one large dose.
   b. Partial or total repair occurs as long as destruction is not complete.
   c. Some irreparable damage may be cumulative as, little by little, more radiation is added (for example, hair loss, skin lesions, falling blood count).

RULES FOR RADIATION PROTECTION

Dental X-ray Protection, prepared by the National Council on Radiation Protection and Measurements,[12] provides specific information about radiation barriers, film speed group rating, film badge service sources, x-ray equipment data, and operating procedure regulations.

In the application of procedures for protecting the clinician and the patient from excessive radiation, particular attention should be paid to unnecessary radiation that may result from the need for an unusual number of retakes because of inadequate technical procedures. Perfecting techniques contributes to the accomplishment of minimum exposure for maximum safety.

PROTECTION OF CLINICIAN

I. PROTECTION FROM PRIMARY RADIATION
A. Stand behind a protective barrier.
B. Avoid the useful beam of radiation.
C. Never hand-hold the film during exposure.
D. Do not use fluorescent mirrors in dental examination.

II. PROTECTION FROM LEAKAGE RADIATION
A. Do not hand-hold the tube housing or the PID of the machine during exposures.
B. Test machine for leakage radiation.
C. Wear monitoring device for testing exposure.

III. PROTECTION FROM SECONDARY RADIATION
The major sources of secondary radiation are the filter and the irradiated soft tissues of the patient. Formerly when a pointed plastic cone was used for the PID, the cone was a major source of scatter radiation. Other sources may be the leakage from the tube housing, or furniture and walls contacted by the primary beam. Methods of protection are related to these sources.

A. Minimization of Total X Radiation
1. Use high-speed films. When attempting to use high-speed films with older x-ray machines, the original mechanical timers may prove inadequate. Replacement timers are available.
2. Replace older x-ray machines with modern shockproof equipment.

B. Collimation of Useful Beam
Use diaphragms or PIDs to collimate the useful beam to an area no longer than 2.75 inches in diameter at the patient's skin. Rectangular collimation has been shown to be more effective than round (figure 9–2, page 138).

C. Type of PID
Use a rectangular, long, open-ended, shielded (lead-lined) cylinder or other form of rectangular collimation.

D. Position of Clinician While Making Exposures
The clinician shall stand behind the patient's head behind the major sources of secondary radiation to prevent direct exposure.
1. *Exposure of the Region of the Central Incisors.* Stand at a 45° angle to the path of the central ray. This position is approximately behind either the left or the right ear of the patient (figure 9–3).
2. *Exposure of Other Regions.* Stand behind the patient's head and at an angle of 45° to the path of the central ray of the x-ray beam.

E. Distance
1. Safety increases with distance.
2. The correct position for the clinician is behind an appropriate radiation-resistant barrier wall, preferably with a leaded window to permit a view of the patient during exposures.
3. When protective barrier shielding is not available, the clinician shall stand as far as practical from the patient, at least 6 feet (2 meters)[15] in the zone between 90 and 135° to the primary central ray as shown in figure 9–3.

IV. MONITORING
Monitoring refers to the periodic or continuous determination of the amount of ionizing radiation or radioactivity present at a given location, usually for considerations of health protection.

The amount of x-ray radiation that reaches the dental personnel can be measured economically with a film badge. Badges can be obtained from one of several

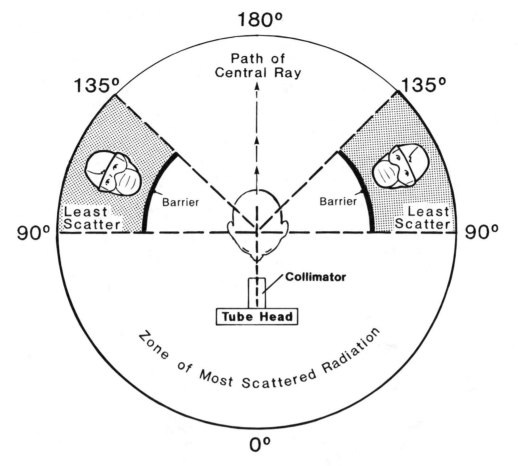

FIG. 9–3. Safe Position for Clinician. *While making an exposure, the clinician must stand behind the patient's head, at an angle of 45° to the central ray.*

laboratories. The film badge is worn on the clothing for 1, 2, or 4 weeks and is then returned by mail to the laboratory from which it was purchased. At the laboratory, the film in the badge is carefully processed and its exposure evaluated. The amount of radiation recorded by the film badge is a measure of the exposure of the wearer, who is notified by mail of the amount of exposure.

PROTECTION OF PATIENT

I. FILMS
Use high-speed films.

II. COLLIMATION
Use diaphragms and an open-ended, shielded (lead-lined), rectangular cylinder to collimate the useful beam.

III. FILTRATION
Use filtration of the useful beam to recommended levels (page 137).

IV. PROCESSING
Process films according to the manufacturer's directions. When a choice of two periods of development is offered, the exposure of the patient can be reduced if the longer development time is employed.

V. FILM SIZE
Use the largest intraoral film that can be skillfully placed in the mouth. Maximum coverage is provided in this manner with one exposure, whereas two exposures may be required if smaller films are used to examine the same area of the mouth. This factor is especially important when examining the mouths of children.

VI. TOTAL EXPOSURE
Do not expose the patient unnecessarily. There must be a good and valid reason for each exposure.

VII. PATIENT BODY-SHIELDS
The use of leaded body-shields for each patient is required by law in many states and countries. The purpose of the shield is to absorb scattered rays. Shields contain the equivalent of 0.25- or 0.3-mm lead thickness.

A. Leaded Apron

1. *Types*
   a. General body coverage with extensions over the shoulders and down over the gonadal area.
   b. Body coverage, with cervical thyroid collar attached.
   c. Body coverage, with added coverage for the patient's upper back for wear during panoramic radiography.
2. *Care.* Leaded aprons and collars should not be folded. If folded and creased, cracks eventually can develop and decrease the effective protection, as well as decrease the length of usefulness of the apron. A hanging device or hooks on the wall near the dental chair can provide a convenient arrangement for keeping the apron flat (figure 9–4). Disinfecting the apron is facilitated.

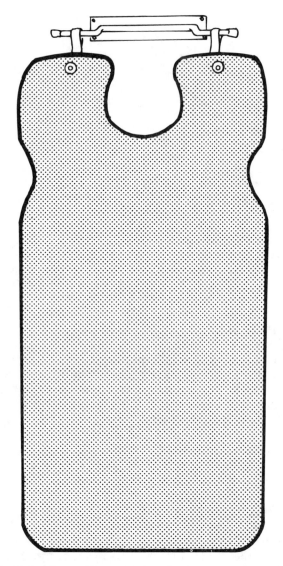

FIG. 9–4. Care of Leaded Apron. The apron can be kept on hooks or a hanging device near the x-ray machine to prevent cracks and prolong the usefulness of the apron.

B. Thyroid Cervical Collar

Thyroid cancer can result from long-term exposure of the gland to x rays.[16] The gland should be covered during dental radiographs throughout life. Figure 9–5 shows the position of a thyroid collar over the neckline of a body apron. The gland is positioned over the trachea approximately halfway between the chin and the clavicles.

CLINICAL APPLICATIONS

I. ASSESSMENT FOR NEED OF RADIOGRAPHS
A. Review health history.
B. Prepare or review radiation exposure history.
   1. Medical diagnostic or therapeutic radiation.
   2. Dates of dental surveys and availability of previous radiographs.
C. Perform clinical examination.[1]
D. Obtain dentist's prescription for number and type of radiographs.

II. PREPARATION OF CLINIC FACILITY: INFECTION CONTROL ROUTINE (pages 62–65)
A. Surface disinfection must include x-ray equipment.
B. Use barrier single-use plastic covers for all surfaces to be contacted, including x-ray machine controls.
C. Use disposable materials wherever possible.
D. Specific radiography materials
   1. Wear examination gloves or overgloves for handling.
   2. Store PID in sealed sterilizing bag or keep disposable devices in clean cup.
   3. Place films readied in clean cup kept from contamination; keep second cup available for receiving exposed films.

III. PREPARATION OF CLINICIAN
A. Use full barrier protection that includes mask, protective eyewear, gloves.
B. Maintain aseptic procedure throughout.

IV. PREPARATION OF PATIENT
A. Apply paper neck protection before positioning lead apron and thyroid collar.
B. Provide cup for holding removable dental prostheses.
C. For panoramic radiographs, ask patient to remove all jewelry and other metallic objects.
D. Provide oral antiseptic mouthrinse to lower bacterial contamination of radiographs and aerosols.

V. INTRAORAL EXAMINATION
A. Purpose
To determine necessary adaptations during film placement.

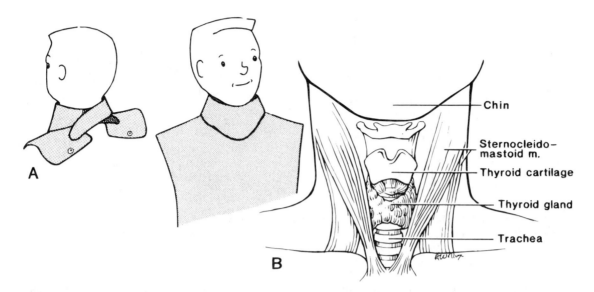

FIG. 9–5. Thyroid Cervical Collar. A. Thyroid collar in position, covering the neck and overlapping the leaded apron used for general body coverage. Velcro tabs facilitate overlap fastening at back of neck. Collars are available in child and adult sizes. **B.** The thyroid gland is located over the trachea approximately half way between the chin and the clavicles. Drawing shows anatomic relationship to the sternocleidomastoid muscle.

B. Factors of Particular Interest

1. Accessibility, determined by height and shape of palate, flexibility of muscles of orifice, floor of the mouth, possible gag reflex, size of tongue.
2. Position of teeth and edentulous areas.
3. Apparent size of teeth as compared with average size of teeth.
4. Unusual features, such as tori, sensitive areas of the mucous membranes.

VI. PATIENT COOPERATION: PREVENTION OF GAGGING

Gagging may be the result of psychologic or physiologic factors. It may present some problem in the placement of all films for molar radiographs and may be initiated in the patient who ordinarily does not gag if techniques are not carried out efficiently. Many of the factors related to the prevention of gagging may be applied for the comfort and cooperation of all patients.

A. Causes of Gagging

1. *Hypersensitive Oral Tissues.* Particularly common in posterior region of oral cavity.
2. *Anxiety and Apprehension*
   a. Fear of unknown, of the film touching a sensitive area.
   b. Previous unpleasant experiences with radiographic techniques.
   c. Failure to comprehend the clinician's instructions.
   d. Lack of confidence in the clinician.
3. *Techniques.* Film moved over the oral tissues or retained in the mouth longer than necessary.

B. Preventive Procedures

1. Inspire confidence in ability to perform the service.
2. Alleviate anxiety; explain procedures carefully. Smile and be cheerful.
3. Minimize tissue irritation.
   a. Request patient to swallow before opening for film placement.
   b. Place film firmly and positively without sliding the film over the tissue.
   c. Use a film holder on which the patient can bite to distract from the procedure.
   d. Instruct patient to breathe through the nose with quick, short breaths during film placement and to hold the breath during exposure.
4. Use a premedicating agent prescribed by the dentist.
5. Use a topical anesthetic.
   a. Cold water or ice cube: hold in the mouth for a short time before film placement to dull the sensory nerve endings.
   b. Salt: Place one-half teaspoonful on the tongue for an anesthetic effect; it may be swallowed or rinsed after radiographs are made.
   c. Prepared topical anesthetics: Apply in the form of an ointment with cotton swab or give patient a troche, or rinse to provide up to 20 minutes of surface anesthesia (pages 519–521).

PROCEDURES FOR FILM PLACEMENT AND ANGULATION OF RAY

The characteristics of the acceptable finished radiograph have been listed (page 136), and certain techni-

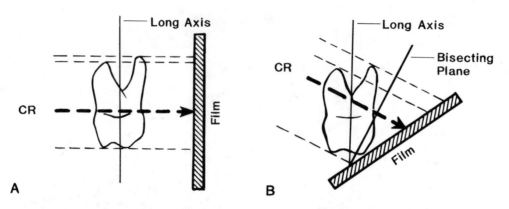

FIG. 9–6. Comparison of Paralleling and Angle Bisection Techniques. A. Paralleling technique. The film is parallel with the long axis of the tooth and the central ray (CR) is directed perpendicularly both to the film and to the long axis of the tooth. **B.** Angle bisection. The central ray (CR) is directed perpendicularly to an imaginary line that bisects the angle formed by the film and the long axis of the tooth.

cal factors, including collimation, filtration, kilovoltage, milliampere seconds, distance, and films, have been described. For consideration next in the procedure for preparation of radiographs is the placement of the film and the angulation of the useful beam.

Basic intraoral procedures for periapical, bitewing, and occlusal radiographs are included in this chapter. The principles and uses of panoramic radiographs are also described.

Two fundamental periapical procedures are used in practice: the *paralleling* or right-angle and the *angle bisection*. The principles for film placement are shown in figure 9–6.

Clinicians vary in their application of the principles of the two techniques. Basically, the primary ray should pass through the region to be examined, and the film should be placed in relation to the ray so that all parts of the image are shown as close to their natural size and shape as possible with a minimum of distortion in the finished radiograph.

As with other oral procedures, the development of a systematic procedure is essential. A comfortable, smooth operation saves time and energy for both patient and clinician, increases the confidence of the patient, and allows for consistency in technique, which produces consistent results. A basic objective during radiographic technique is to minimize the length of time the film packet remains in the patient's mouth.

FILM SELECTION FOR INTRAORAL SURVEYS

I. PERIAPICAL
A. Purpose
To obtain a view of the entire tooth and its periodontal supporting structures.

B. Films
1. *Child Size.* No. 0 (1.0) ($\frac{7}{8} \times 1\frac{3}{8}$ inches) for primary teeth and small mouths.
2. *Anterior.* No. 1 (1.1) ($\frac{15}{16} \times 1\frac{9}{16}$ inches) for anterior regions where width of arch makes positioning of standard film difficult or impossible.
3. *Standard.* No. 2 (1.2) ($1\frac{1}{4} \times 1\frac{5}{8}$ inches) may be used for all positions.

C. Number of Films Used in a Complete Survey
For the adult mouth, from 14 to 30 films may be used, depending on the clinician's preferences, objectives for showing specific areas, anatomy of the patient's mouth, and size of the films used. For children, see page 153.

II. BITEWING (INTERPROXIMAL)
A. Purposes
1. *Horizontal Film.* To show the crowns of the teeth, the alveolar crest, and the interproximal area.
2. *Vertical Film.* To show deeper periodontal information, including furcation involvement and bony defects.

B. Films
1. *Adult Posterior Survey (horizontal or vertical)*
   a. Standard No. 2 film. Tab is attached or tab with loop is slipped over the film.
   b. Four films, one for molar region and one for premolar on each side.
2. *Adult Posterior Survey Using No. 3 Film* ($1\frac{1}{16} \times 2\frac{1}{8}$ inches). Designed to include molars and premolars, one film on each side.
3. *Child Survey No. 2 Film.* With first permanent molars erupted, one film on each side.
4. *Child Survey No. 1 Film.* With primary teeth, one film on each side.

III. OCCLUSAL
A. Purpose
To show large areas of the maxilla, mandible, or floor of the mouth.

B. Film
No. 4 ($2\frac{1}{4} \times 3$ inches) for use in self packet or in intraoral cassette.

C. Standard Film

($1\frac{1}{4} \times 1\frac{5}{8}$ inches) for child or individual areas of adult.

DEFINITIONS AND PRINCIPLES

I. PLANES

A. Sagittal or Median

The plane that divides the body in the midline into right and left sides.

B. Occlusal

The mean occlusal plane represents the mean curvature from the incisal edges of the central incisors to the tips of the occluding surfaces of the third molars. The occlusal plane of the pre-molars and first molar may be considered as the mean occlusal plane.

When it is specified in techniques that the occlusal plane of the teeth being radiographed shall be parallel to the floor, at least three head positions are involved for the maxillary: for anterior teeth, the head must be tipped forward; for premolars, held at the mean occlusal plane; and for molars, tipped back.

II. ANGULATION

A. Horizontal

The angle at which the central ray of the useful beam is directed within a horizontal plane. Inadequate horizontal angulation results in *over-lapping* or *superimposition* of parts of adjacent teeth in the radiograph.

B. Vertical

The plane at which the central ray of the useful beam is directed within a vertical plane. Less vertical angulation than necessary results in *elongation,* and more angulation than necessary creates *foreshortening* of the image.

III. LONG AXIS OF A TOOTH

The long axis can be represented by an imaginary line passing longitudinally through the center of the tooth. Because of marked variations in tooth position and root curvature, estimation of the long axis of a tooth is difficult. Clinically, it can be considered that the long axis of a posterior tooth is at right angles to the occlusal surface plane.

For single-rooted teeth, the long axis would ordinarily pass from the center of the incisal edge to the tip of the apex, but it is not possible to observe such a line during clinical examination. The line from the incisal edge to the cervical third on the labial surface must not be confused with the long axis.

PERIAPICAL SURVEY: PARALLELING TECHNIQUE

The paralleling or right-angle technique is based on the principles that *the film is placed as nearly parallel to the long axis of the tooth as the anatomy of the oral cavity permits,*
and the central ray is directed at right angles to the film. In figure 9–6A, the parallel relationship of the film with the long axis of the tooth and the right-angle direction of the central ray are shown.

The distance between the crown of the tooth and the film is increased to attain parallelism.

I. PATIENT POSITION

As long as the film is parallel to the long axis of the tooth and the central ray is directed at right angles to the film, the head may be in any position convenient to the clinician and comfortable for the patient. Slight modification of positioning may be needed for making radiographs in a supine position.

The use of film holder (fig. 9–7) facilitates obtaining

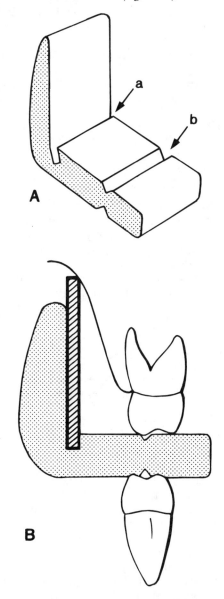

FIG. 9–7. Styrofoam Disposable Film Holder. A. Empty holder to show *a,* slot for insertion of the film, and *b,* break-off point to shorten the bite surface for use in the mandibular posterior positions. **B.** Film placement for maxillary molar radiograph for patient with a high palatal vault.

the correct angulation of the ray, because the PID for the central ray can be lined up with the part of the film holder that extends from between the teeth and that is designed to be at right angles to the film.

For the inexperienced clinician, horizontal angulation may be visualized more readily when the occlusal plane of the teeth being radiographed is parallel with the floor and the sagittal plane is perpendicular to the floor.

II. FILM PLACEMENT
A. Film Position and Angulation of the Central Ray
Instructions for film placement and angulation are included in this section. In addition to the references associated with specific parts of this section, further study may be helpful to perfect techniques.[17,18]
1. *Basic Principles.* Principles for film placement and angulation of the central ray are shown in figures 9–8 and 9–9. The image objective in the completed radiograph is also illustrated.
2. *Horizontal Angulation.* The ray is directed approximately at the center of the film and through the interproximal area.
3. *Vertical Angulation.* The ray is directed at right angles to the film.

B. Film Positioning Devices
1. *Purposes.* The use of a beam-guiding, field-size-limiting film-holding instrument provides important advantages, including dose reduction, film quality, and consistently adequate diagnostic radiographs without frequent retakes. Sanitation is improved, and lack of need for patient involvement in holding films is helpful.
2. *Characteristics.* An effective film positioning device has such characteristics as the following:
   a. Adaptable to all necessary positions for obtaining diagnostic radiographs of the entire dental arches.
   b. Weight and other properties do not hinder placement or holding, and do not require the patient to hand-hold the device.
   c. Comfortable for the patient during the necessary time interval.
   d. Simplicity of placement; minimal complexity for learning.
   e. Aid in alignment of x-ray beam for correct exposure of film.
   f. Disposable or conveniently sterilized. To this end, more than one device should be maintained to permit sterilization between patients.
3. *Types*[18,19]
   a. Hemostat. Insert the hemostat through a rubber bite block, and position and hold film in the claws of the hemostat. The film

is positioned in the mouth and held by the patient biting on the bite block.
   b. Bite blocks. Plastic or wooden (short and long for different areas of the mouth).
   c. Styrofoam disposable film holder (Stabe).[20] Simple, comfortable, lightweight device; assists in beam alignment by the end that protrudes after the teeth are closed down to hold the device in place (figure 9–7).
   d. Precision x-ray device. Has a facial shield attached to the bar, which holds the film in position parallel to the shield. A rectangular hole in the shield permits the passage of only those x rays that will reach the film. (Distributed by the Precision X-ray Company.)
   e. Snap-A-Ray. Plastic film holder with two ends for positioning anterior and posterior films. It is held between the teeth. (Rinn Corporation.)
   f. X-C-P (X-tension C-one P-aralleling). Has an adjustable circular ring that permits film alignment with the primary beam by bringing the open end of the cone in contact with the ring. (Rinn Corporation.)
   g. V.I.P. (Versatile Intraoral Positioner). Film-holding, beam-directing, with a target attachment for alignment of the open-end tube. It is called versatile because it has holders to accommodate three film sizes and it can be used for periapical and bitewing surveys. (UP-RAD Corporation.)
4. *Supplements*
   a. Removable denture may be needed in opposite jaw to stabilize a film holder.
   b. A cotton roll between the film holder or bite block and the biting surface can aid in paralleling when teeth are short and/or the palatal vault is low.

III. PARALLELING TECHNIQUE: FEATURES
A. Accuracy
The paralleling technique gives truer size and shape of dental structures with less distortion than when angle bisection is used.
1. Facial and lingual aspects can be shown in proper relation to each other.
2. Zygomatic bone can be shown in its normal position above the root apices of the molars and premolars.

B. Bitewing Radiographs May Not Be Required
In a complete survey, the right-angle view of proximal surfaces in paralleling technique radiographs is the same as that in the bitewing. Time and effort, as well as radiation to patient, may be saved.

C. Horizontal Ray Direction
No rays are directed toward the thyroid, whereas with angle bisection, several radio-

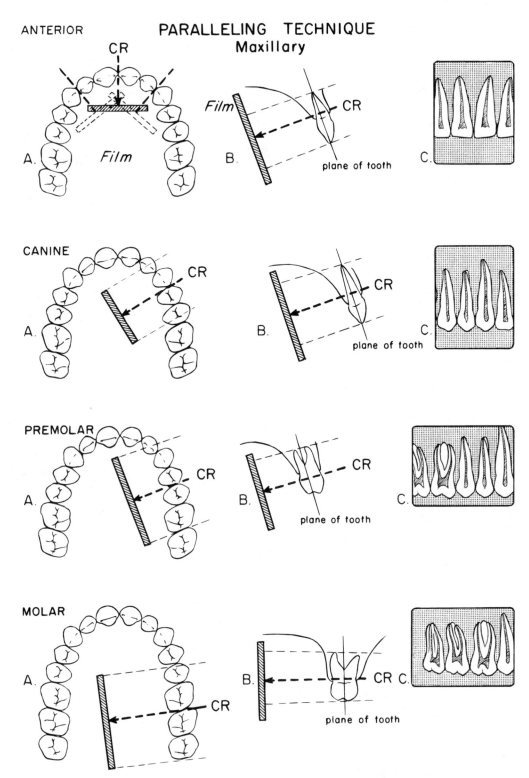

FIG. 9–8. Paralleling Technique. Film positioning for the major maxillary positions. **A.** Horizontal angulation, with film placed parallel to the long axes of the teeth; central ray (CR) directed parallel with a line through the interproximal space. **B.** Vertical angulation, with central ray (CR) directed at right angles to the film. **C.** Image objective for the completed radiograph.

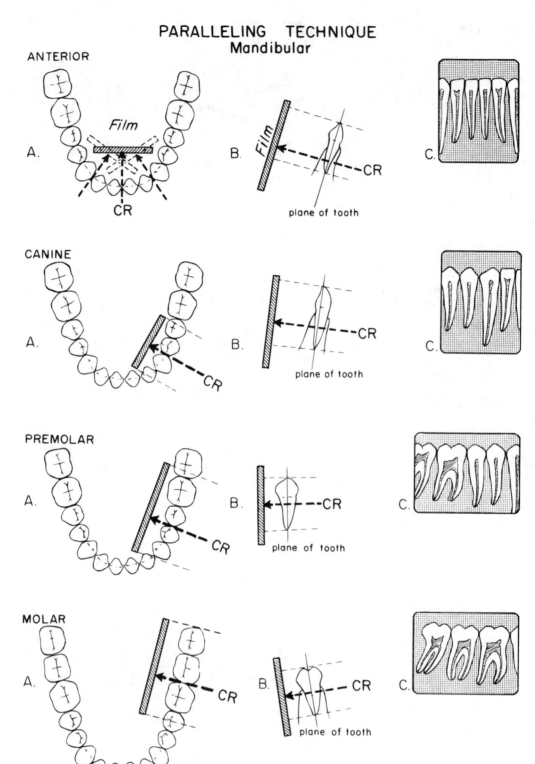

PARALLELING TECHNIQUE
Mandibular

FIG. 9–9. Paralleling Technique. Film positioning for the major mandibular positions. **A.** Horizontal angulation, with film placed parallel to the long axes of the teeth; central ray (CR) directed through the interproximal space. **B.** Vertical angulation, with central ray (CR) directed at right angles to the film. **C.** Image objective for the completed radiograph.

graphs require a relatively steep vertical angulation.

BITEWING SURVEY

The bitewing or interproximal survey is used as an adjunct to the periapical survey. It has been used at the time of the maintenance appointment to detect proximal surface caries.

As with all other radiographic surveys, a bitewing survey should be made only when a need is demonstrated for specific diagnostic purposes.

When the angle-bisection technique is used for the periapical radiographs, the bitewing survey is essential, because an accurate view of all proximal surfaces cannot otherwise be obtained. The angulation for the bitewing radiographs is based on the same principle as that for periapical surveys made with the paralleling or right-angle technique.

I. PREPARATION FOR FILM PLACEMENT
A. Patient Position
1. *Traditional.* Sagittal plane perpendicular to the floor and occlusal plane parallel with the floor.
2. *Patient in Supine Position.* The planes are reversed in their relation to the floor.

B. Vertical Angulation
Set at +8 to +10°.

C. Patient Instruction
Request patient to practice closing on posterior teeth prior to positioning film for posterior bitewings, and to practice edge-to-edge closure (figure 15–4, page 251) for anterior bitewings.

II. FILM PLACEMENT AND CENTRAL RAY ANGULATION
Figure 9–10 shows in diagram form the position of the molar bitewing film in relation to the teeth, the horizontal and vertical angulation, and the image objective for both the premolar and the molar completed radiographs when standard film is used.

A. Position of Film
1. *Molar* (standard film). Mesial border of film at mesial of maxillary second premolar or

more distal as needed to include the distal surface of the third molar when it is erupted and in position.
2. *Premolar* (standard film). Mesial border of film at center or mesial of maxillary canine.
3. *Anterior.* Center of film at mesial surface of maxillary canine for the two lateral bitewings; center of film at midline for central bitewing.

B. Position of Directing PID
With the vertical angulation at +8 to +10°, the horizontal angulation is adjusted to direct the central ray to the center of the film. The ray must pass through the interproximal space or parallel to a line through the interproximal space.

C. Maintain Film Flat During Exposure
Although slight curving of the film may be needed for certain patients, depending on the oral anatomy and tissue sensitivity, the basic rule is to keep the film as flat as possible to prevent distortion.

PERIAPICAL SURVEY: ANGLE-BISECTION TECHNIQUE

The angle-bisection technique is based on the geometric principle that *the central ray is directed perpendicularly to an imaginary line that is the bisector of the angle formed by the long axis of the tooth and the plane of the film.* Figure 9–6B illustrates in diagram form the relationship of the long axis of the tooth, the film, and the bisector of the angle formed by these two.

I. PATIENT POSITION
A. Sagittal Plane
Perpendicular to the floor.

B. Occlusal Plane
Parallel with the floor.

II. FILM PLACEMENT AND POSITION
A. Center of Film
At center of teeth being radiographed. The exception to this rule is the maxillary canine film,

FIG. 9–10. Bitewing Radiograph. A. Film position showing horizontal angulation for molar viewing, with central ray (CR) directed through the interproximal space to the center of the film. **B.** Vertical angulation set at +8 to +10°. **C.** Image objective for molar (above) and premolar (below) regions.

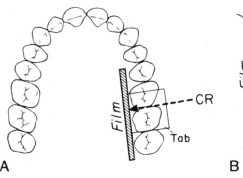
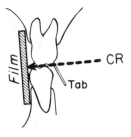
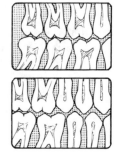

A   B   C

which is placed slightly distal to accommodate film positioning.

B. Border of Film
Located ⅛ to ¼ inch beyond the occlusal or incisal surface.

C. Film Must Be Kept as Flat as Possible
A cotton roll may be used with the anterior and maxillary molar films to aid in accomplishing this goal.

III. DIRECTION OF THE CENTRAL RAY
A. Direct the Ray Through the Apical Third of the Teeth Being Radiographed
1. *Maxillary.* To determine location of the apices of the teeth, draw an imaginary line from the ala of the nose to the tragus of the ear; the apices are approximately at that level.
2. *Mandibular.* Apices are located approximately ½ inch above the lower border of the mandible.

B. Horizontal Angulation
The ray should pass through the interproximal space or parallel to a line through the interproximal space, at approximately the center of the area being radiographed.

C. Vertical Angulation
Bisect the angle formed by the film and the long axes of the teeth, and direct the ray perpendicular to this line.

OCCLUSAL SURVEY

The use of occlusal films is particularly important for observing areas that cannot be completely or conveniently shown on other films, in cases where positioning periapical films is difficult or impossible, to supplement the angulation provided by other films for such conditions as fractures, impacted teeth, or salivary duct calculi, and as a specific part of a complete survey for edentulous or very young patients.

The central midline films for maxillary and mandibular arches are described in this section. A variety of positions for the occlusal films is possible, depending on the area to be examined. Additional references will be helpful as a guide.[21,22]

I. MAXILLARY MIDLINE PROJECTION
A. Position of Patient's Head
The line from the tragus of the ear to the ala of the nose is parallel with floor.

B. Position of Film
The emulsion side is toward the palate; posterior border of film is brought back close to third molar region; film is held between the teeth with edge-to-edge closure.

C. Angulation
The PID is directed toward the bridge of the nose at a 65° angle.

D. Exposure
Consult chart of film manufacturer's specifications for exposure related to source-film distance, kilovoltage, and milliamperage. When a cassette is used, exposure time is reduced, an advantage in prevention of movement of the film.

II. MANDIBULAR MIDLINE PROJECTION
A. Position of Patient's Head
The head is tilted directly back.

B. Position of Film
The emulsion side is toward the floor of the mouth, the posterior border of the film is in contact with the soft tissues of the retromolar area, and the film is held between the teeth in an edge-to-edge bite.

C. Angulation
For the incisal region, the PID is pointed at the tip of the chin at an angle of approximately 55°. For the floor of the mouth, the PID is directed from under the chin, perpendicular to the film.

D. Exposure
Consult chart of film manufacturer's specifications.

PANORAMIC RADIOGRAPHS

Panoramic radiography or pantomography refers to methods that produce continuous radiographs showing the maxillary and mandibular arches with adjacent structures on a single radiograph. The x-ray source may be placed intra- or extraorally.

This type of radiograph is a supplement to a periapical survey, but not a substitute because of less sharpness and detail in the panoramic radiograph. The derived benefit must be weighed against the additional exposure to a wide area of tissues outside the oral tissues.

I. TYPES OF PANORAMIC TECHNIQUES[23,24]
A. Tomography
Lamina means layer, and in this technique, a single layer of the teeth and surrounding structures appears in the radiograph. Other structures do not appear superimposed as they do in traditional extraoral techniques.

The head is stabilized with a chin support or one of several types of head holders characteristic of each machine. The film and x-ray source rotate around the patient's head.

B. Still-Picture Technique

The film in a cassette is molded to the face, using separate films for the mandible and the maxilla. Head and film positioners are used to make a series of lateral jaw radiographs.

II. USES

Because definition and detail are inferior to those attained with periapical radiographs, and because distortion occurs, panoramic radiographs provide an overall, but not a detailed, view. They do not show proximal carious lesions except for large cavities, which can be seen by direct examination. They are also inadequate for examination of periodontal supporting structures.

Routine use of panoramic radiographs for patients seeking general oral care cannot be recommended as a substitute for a periapical survey.

A. Oral Pathology

The area surveyed increases with the use of a panoramic radiograph. Radiolucent or radiopaque areas outside the border of possibility in periapical views can be seen.

B. Edentulous Patient

A panoramic survey prepared prior to making complete dentures can usually provide sufficient information for most patients.

C. Orthodontics

The overall view of growth and development at the beginning of orthodontic observation, diagnosis, and treatment, and during the treatment to assess periodic progress, can be helpful to the orthodontist.

D. Patients for Whom Conventional Radiographs Cannot Be Used

For patients with disabilities or systemic conditions that hinder cooperation, such as trismus, temporomandibular joint disorder, Parkinson's disease, facial paralysis, intermaxillary fixation, or facial trauma, and do not allow examination by intraoral techniques.

III. LIMITATIONS

A. Inferiority of Definition and Detail

Causes of poor definition are
1. Use of intensifying screens.
2. Increased object-film distance.
3. Movement of x-ray tube and film.

B. Distortion

1. Magnified images are produced because of increased film-object distance.
2. Overlapping. In periapical techniques, each film is angulated with the central ray so that when a tooth is out of line, adjustment is made to prevent overlapping. With panoramic technique, the head and teeth remain fixed, and the ray and film are positioned for the average only.

IV. PROCEDURES

Learning to use panoramic equipment is not difficult. Each machine has its own characteristics that can be learned readily from the manufacturer's instructions.

A. Patient Preparation

The use of a leaded apron with a thyroid shield is important. A special shield for panoramic radiography is available with coverage over the shoulders and part way down the back.

B. Film

Film sizes are usually either 5 × 12 or 6 × 12 inches. Speed film should be used to minimize radiation.

C. Processing

Regular processing solutions are used for panoramic film. Special film holders may be obtained.

CHILD PATIENT SURVEY

For all ages, the frequency of making radiographic surveys, as well as the selection of type, size, and number of films to be used, is based on individual patient evaluation. The objective is to minimize exposure of children to radiation. Low levels of x radiation are associated with the induction of cancer, and growing tissues are more sensitive.

The need for radiographs in a healthy child is limited when the oral cavity appears free from disease as shown by direct clinical examination. This is especially true when teeth are spaced.

A specific rule of frequency for making complete surveys is not in keeping with current knowledge of radiation hygiene and safety. The aim for a young child is to make as thorough a clinical evaluation of the teeth and the surrounding structures as possible. The real need for radiographs can then be determined.

I. INDICATIONS

With consideration for risk and benefit, six categories are suggested as indications for radiographs.
A. Detection of congenital anomalies in the mixed dentition of children undergoing complete dental care or needing orthodontic treatment.
B. Detection of proximal surface dental caries when close contacts do not permit direct examination.
C. Third molar assessment.
D. Pulpal disease; infections.
E. Trauma to the teeth or jaws.
F. Periodontal assessment is needed when probing reveals bone loss and periodontal pockets. Prepubertal periodontitis, although relatively rare, may be generalized or localized and may be evident at as early as 4 years of age. Severe bone destruction is characteristic.[25,26]

II. PRIMARY DENTITION

When radiographs are indicated, various combinations of periapical, bitewing, occlusal, panoramic, and extraoral films are possible. Film size should be consistent with the size of the mouth, the cooperation of the patient, and the ability of the clinician. Examples of number and size of films for three effective surveys are listed here.

A. Occlusal views of anterior maxillary and mandibular arches (standard film) and posterior bitewings (child or adult anterior film); total of four films.

B. Occlusal views of anterior maxillary and mandibular and maxillary posterior (standard film), posterior bitewings (child or standard film), and extraoral lateral jaw films (5 × 7 inches).

C. Periapical views for each posterior quadrant and one each for anterior (child-size film); total of six films.

III. MIXED DENTITION (6 TO 9 YEARS)

When a complete survey is determined necessary, 12 to 14 exposures using standard film are suggested. These include 2 posterior bitewings, 4 molar (to include first permanent and primary molars), 4 canine, and 2 or 4 incisor periapical views.

IV. TECHNIQUE WITH CHILDREN[27]

A. Use of Leaded Apron and Thyroid Collar

Children are more susceptible than are adults to low-level radiation.

B. Orientation to Lessen Apprehension

1. For a young child's first visit to the dental office, the radiographic survey may be a necessary first procedure. When the child is not able to cooperate, the survey may be delayed until the second or even the third visit, except in an emergency.

2. Explain procedures carefully; rehearse to show what is to be done; repeat instructions with each film placement.

C. Sequence

Make the easiest, most comfortable exposures first (extraoral, panoramic, occlusal).

D. Periapical Films

Use film holder.

EDENTULOUS SURVEY

I. INDICATIONS

Periapical, occlusal, and panoramic surveys have been used alone and together for edentulous patients. Radiographic examination of an edentulous mouth is frequently used to detect residual pathologic conditions, foreign bodies, and retained teeth or root tips prior to denture construction.

The need for radiographs for edentulous patients should be reviewed in light of the patient's health history, as well as of the history of radiation exposure and of the clinical examination. Edentulous patients who have previously worn dentures and now need new dentures do not require radiographs routinely.[28]

II. PROCEDURES FOR PERIAPICAL SURVEY[29]

The periapical series, usually of 14 films, has been considered to be the most complete and accurate for diagnosis.

A. Paralleling Technique

A film holder adjusted to provide a wider biting area is needed.

1. Turn the rubber bite block on a hemostat around so that the broader dimension is in the vertical plane.

2. Film holder can be padded with cotton rolls.

B. Angle Bisection Technique

Use cotton rolls to aid in positioning the films, and increase the angulation to accommodate flattened film.

PARACLINICAL PROCEDURES

Supplemental to the chairside clinical procedures are the processing of the films and the mounting of radiographs for diagnostic and clinical use. Standard procedures are outlined in the following sections.[30,31]

I. DEFINITION

Film processing is the chemical transformation of the latent image, produced in a film emulsion by exposure to radiation, into a stable image visible by transmitted light. The usual procedure is basically a selective reduction of affected silver halide salts to metallic silver grains (development), followed by the selective removal of unaffected silver halide (fixation), washing to remove the processing chemicals, and drying.

II. INFECTION CONTROL

A written policy for infection control during film exposure, processing, and mounting and during management of the completed radiographs during clinical treatment appointments is necessary.[32] Prevention of cross-infection during film exposure was addressed on page 144 with other clinical applications. Additional procedures must be followed to prevent cross-contamination during transport to the darkroom and during the use of the processing equipment.

Research has shown that bacteria on radiographic film can survive the processing procedures.[33] Processing procedures may reduce the bacterial counts, but the potential for cross-contamination still exists.

Personnel of each office or clinic must work out a specific protocol appropriate to their facility and the type of processing used.

The following are basic to all procedures:[34,35]

A. Films become covered with contaminated saliva and should be confined to a disposable cup after exposure.

B. Gloved hands fresh from contamination from the patient's mouth should not contact walls, doors, light switches, and other environmental surfaces when transporting a cup of contaminated exposed films to the darkroom.

C. The darkroom work area is prepared by the disinfection of all touch surfaces, and the counter is covered with clean paper. When a daylight loader is used, the interior of the daylight loader must be disinfected.

D. Under appropriate safelight, pull open packets by their tabs; allow films to drop out onto the clean barrier surface. Take care not to touch the film.

E. Dispose of wrappers and contaminated gloves with contaminated waste.

F. Gloves are not needed to mount the films on hangers for a conventional system nor to feed the films into an automatic processor.

CONVENTIONAL PROCESSING

Standardization of processing procedure goes hand in hand with standardized exposure techniques if consistently acceptable radiographs are to be prepared. Processing should be treated as an exacting chemical operation in which each step has specific objectives for the finished product. Fast and extra-fast films are even more sensitive to variations in temperature, light, and processing chemicals than were the medium and slow films formerly in general use. Hence the need for fastidious attention to detail is obvious.

ESSENTIALS OF AN ADEQUATE DARKROOM

Cleanliness and orderliness are mandatory. Because the films are handled in near darkness, materials must be available at the fingertips and each piece of equipment must be kept in its own place.

The work area must be free from chemicals, water, dust, and other substances that could contaminate the film either by splashing or by direct contact should a film touch the bench. The processing room should not be used as a storage room nor for other dental procedures in which dust or fumes might be produced.

Convenience and ease in carrying out precision procedures can be accomplished through good planning for the location and arrangement of equipment.

I. LIGHTING

A. Darkroom Completely Void of White Light

1. Find and eliminate all possible light leaks.
2. Do not use fluorescent overhead light because of afterglow.

B. Safelight

Safelight is the illumination used in the darkroom that does not affect (fog) the film emulsion. By following the manufacturer's instructions on a film package, the correct safelighting can be used.

Different films require different light filters. A 7.5-watt bulb is used in a light fixture 4 feet above the working surface, and a filter is selected for the light in accord with the type of film.

1. Filter Type GBX-2 (red filter) is designed for both intraoral and extraoral film.
2. Filter Type ML-2 (orange filter) is for intraoral films only.

C. Safelighting Test[36]

1. Unwrap a film in totally dark darkroom.
2. Place film on work tabletop and place a coin on the film.
3. Turn on safelight and leave for maximum amount of time (such as 5 minutes) typical of that required when preparing a survey to be processed.
4. Turn off safelight, remove coin, process film.
5. Observe the radiograph; if any evidence exists of a light circle where the coin was placed, the darkroom safelight is excessive.

D. Lock on Door of Darkroom

A signal light should be on the outside to show that the room is in use.

II. BASIC EQUIPMENT AND FACILITIES

A. Tanks

For developer and fixer, with water bath between.

1. Removable tanks made of stainless steel with joints welded and polished to prevent reactions with the processing chemicals.
2. Close-fitting, light-proof cover for tank.
3. Stirring paddles identified specifically for developer and fixer.
4. Water bath with connecting water flow and temperature control indicator.
5. Floating tank thermometer (kept in developer tank).

B. Workbench

Covered with linoleum or Formica for easy cleaning.

C. Drying Facilities

Rod to hold hangers over drip pan; electric fan to facilitate drying.

D. Utility Sink

E. Interval Timing Clock

F. Storage Area

Beneath workbench for materials to change solutions.

G. Waste Receiver

Conveniently located for ready disposal of film wrappers to prevent losing films in midst of paper wrappers.

III. CARE OF SOLUTION
A. Factors Affecting Life of Solution
1. Original quality (care in preparation).
2. Age.
3. Care received (temperature, whether kept covered, contamination).
4. Number of films processed.

B. Changing Solutions
At least every 3 weeks, depending on the number of radiographs processed.

C. Preparation of New Solution
1. Tanks must be thoroughly scrubbed with water and a soft brush and then thoroughly rinsed.
2. Label tanks, as well as stirrers and mixing jars, to prevent possibility of interchange.
3. Follow manufacturer's specifications and directions precisely.

IV. PROTECTION OF SOLUTION
A. Tank Cover
Use same position for tank cover so that same cover routinely is used for the same solution.

B. Purposes for Covering Tanks
1. *Prevent Evaporation.* Evaporation can change the concentration of the solutions and lower the level so the top film on hanger is not covered during processing.
2. *Prevent Oxidation.* Reduces useful life of solution.
3. *Prevent Contamination.* Dust, drippings.

C. Temperature
Keep cool when not in use; heated solutions can oxidize rapidly.

D. Replenisher
Between changing of solutions, freshness may be maintained by replenishment according to manufacturer's specifications.

PROCESSING

I. PREPARATION
A. Stir solutions and check temperature of solutions and water bath: all should be 20° C (68° F) (within 2°)

1. Lower temperatures. Chemical reactions too slow.
2. Higher temperatures. Cause fogging and may soften the emulsion.

B. Check cleanliness of workbench and film hangers; wash hands to prevent film contamination.

C. Plan number of films to be processed so that facilities will not be overcrowded; films must hang individually, out of possible contact with other films, sides of tanks, or wall in drying area.

D. Prepare labels for identification of radiographs.

E. Extinguish white lights; turn on safelight; lock door.

F. Load film hangers.
1. Hold film by edges to avoid finger marks, scratches, or bending.
2. Clip firmly; test by pulling gently on film.

II. DEVELOPING
A. Set timer. (Refer to time-temperature chart provided by the film manufacturer.*)

B. Completely immerse hanger with films in developer; turn on timer.

C. Agitate hangers (without splashing) to eliminate air bubbles and assure contact of solution with all film surfaces.

D. When timer rings, remove hangers to water or to a stop bath.

III. RINSING
A. Immerse in freely running water for at least 30 seconds; agitate to provide contact of water with film.

B. A stop bath of 10% acetic acid may be preferred in place of running water; immerse for 30 to 45 seconds.

C. Remove and drain for several seconds to prevent carrying an excess of water or acetic acid to the fixing bath.

IV. FIXING
A. Immerse completely; set and start timer.

B. Agitate hangers to remove air bubbles and assure contact of the solution with all parts of the film surfaces.

C. Clearing time is time needed for complete disappearance of white or milky opaqueness.

D. Total fixing time is minimum of twice clearing time
1. Check manufacturer's specifications.
2. Minimum of 10 minutes and maximum of 1 hour are safe; excess time produces a light radiograph.

E. Wet readings can be made after fixing 2 to 3 minutes. Rinse in water before taking to the

* The time-temperature method of processing is the only way to be assured of dependable results. Processing by the "visual inspection" method is not recommended because of the lack of standardization.

viewbox. Return to the fixer for completion of the fixing process.

V. WASHING

A. Place in running water bath for minimum of 20 minutes.
B. Temperature at 20° C (68° F)
  1. When too warm, gelatin swells, thus hindering diffusion.
  2. Drastic temperature changes cause reticulation (network of wrinkles or corrugations in the emulsion); retake necessary.

VI. DRYING

A. Drain off water and place in dryer.
B. Radiographs become brittle when left in a heated drying cabinet too long.

HOW THE IMAGE IS PRODUCED

I. THE CHEMISTRY OF PROCESSING

A. Film emulsion contains crystals of silver halides (bromide and iodide).
B. X-ray exposure changes the silver halides to silver and halide ions.
C. Developer reacts with the halide ions, leaving only the metallic silver in a specific arrangement corresponding with the radiolucency and radiopacity of the tissue being radiographed.
D. Fixer removes only those crystals of silver halide that were not affected by the action of the x rays. Fixer has no effect on the black metallic silver produced by the developer.
E. End result is a negative, showing various degrees of lightness and darkness (microscopic grains of black metallic silver).

II. DEVELOPER ACTION

A. Purpose

To remove the halides from the metallic silver.

B. Constituents

1. *Developing Agents (Reducers). Elon* brings out detail and *hydroquinone* reacts slowly and brings out contrast.
2. *Preservative. Sodium sulfite* protects the developing agents from oxidizing rapidly in air.
3. *Restrainer. Potassium bromide* inhibits the fogging tendency of the solution and slows the reaction of the reducers.
4. *Activator (Alkali). Sodium carbonate* initiates the action of the reducers with the halides.

C. Transfer to Water Bath at Completion of Developing Time

If hangers are shaken or allowed to drip over the developer, the solution falling back into the tank will be highly oxidized, thus shortening the life of the solution.

III. RINSING PURPOSES

A. To stop the developing process.
B. To remove the developing solution from the emulsion to reduce carry-over of alkaline developer to the acid fixing bath.
C. To preserve the acidity of the fixer and, hence, make a more efficient, longer-lasting fixing bath.

IV. FIXER ACTION

A. Purpose

To remove the undeveloped halide salts.

B. Constituents

1. *Fixing Agent. Sodium thiosulfate* ("hypo") dissolves the silver halides.
2. *Acidifier. Acetic acid* neutralizes the alkali from the developer.
3. *Hardener. Potassium alum* shrinks and hardens the emulsion.
4. *Preservative. Sodium sulfite* counteracts surface oxidation and stabilizes the solution.

V. WASHING PURPOSE

To remove residual chemicals from the negative.

AUTOMATED PROCESSING

Automatic film processing refers to the use of equipment designed to transport film mechanically through a series of solutions under controlled conditions.

I. OBJECTIVES AND ADVANTAGES

Although cost and maintenance factors may be greater than those of a traditional darkroom procedure, an automated and/or rapid processing machine has advantages, including the following.

A. Conservation of time by dental personnel.
B. Finished radiographs in 5 to 8 minutes, depending on the machine used. Some have dryers.
C. Consistency of results through automated control of temperature and time.
D. Radiographs available for immediate use during diagnosis, which is particularly important in emergencies, during endodontic therapy, and in certain surgical procedures.

II. PRINCIPLES OF OPERATION

Manufacturer's instructions must be followed and routine care and cleaning attended to for maintenance of equipment.

Automated or accelerated processing (or both) is accomplished by one or a combination of the following.

A. Automated Film Transport

Rollers or tracks are used to carry the film through development, washing, and fixing, then washing again, and, finally, forced drying. Certain machines produce wet films and do not have hot-air drying chambers. The various machines available are built to carry different sizes of film. Some machines may process only standard intraoral films, whereas others may also accommodate extraoral sizes.

B. High Temperature

Increased temperature decreases processing time. Special solutions are needed for the rapid processors, because with conventional solutions, the excess temperature causes deterioration and fogging of the film. Solution temperatures in the automated and rapid processors may be from 17° to 38° C (62° to 100° F), and with drying temperatures up to 65° C (150° F). The total processing and drying may take about 5 minutes.

C. Use of Special Films and Processing Solutions

1. *Concentrated Processing Solution.* Solutions with increased chemical reactivity decrease developing time. In one type of machine, a combined developer-fixer is used that eliminates the need for film to pass through two solutions. The diagnostic quality of the film is generally less with the special solutions.
2. *Films.* Films with special emulsions have been developed that process best at higher temperatures and with the special processing solutions.

D. Agitation

Mechanically controlled movement of the film and/or movement of the solution is built into some units to provide fresh solution continuously at the film surface. This decreases the processing time.

ANALYSIS OF COMPLETED RADIOGRAPHS

The completed radiographs are mounted and examined at a viewbox with an adequate light source. Interpretation of radiographs is difficult for the dentist and the determination of a pathologic condition requires keen evaluation, but to attempt to base interpretation on inadequate, insufficient radiographs is guesswork rather than true, timely diagnosis.

I. USE OF REFERENCE RADIOGRAPHS

The characteristics of acceptable finished radiographs (page 136) serve as the basis for analysis. Nothing less than the ideal should satisfy, and errors must be studied so that techniques can be improved for future surveys.

A. Available Ideal Radiographs

1. Tape a periapical or bitewing radiograph to a viewbox for continuing reference and comparison.

2. Note changes in density, contrast, or other features so that techniques can be adjusted.
3. Use information to determine the need for changes in processing solutions and timing.

B. Complete Surveys

Examples of ideal surveys for periapical, bitewing, panoramic, edentulous, or other special radiographs can be maintained for study and review. New staff members can benefit by learning what is expected.

II. MOUNTING

A. Legibly mark the mount with the name of patient, age, date, name of dentist; printing is preferred.
B. Handle radiographs only by the edges with clean, dry hands, or wear clean cotton gloves.
C. Keep films clean and free from dust, liquids, or other contaminants.
D. Place a clean, dry towel or paper in front of the illuminator where mounting is to be done; arrange radiographs on this or mount one by one directly as they are removed from the hanger.
E. The embossed dot near the edge of the negative is the guide to mounting; the depressed side of the dot is on the lingual side.
F. Identify individual negatives by the teeth and other anatomic landmarks.
G. Approved mounting system is as follows. Looking at the teeth from outside the mouth, the teeth are viewed and mounted in the same manner as the approved numbering system (figure III–1, page 82).

III. ANATOMIC LANDMARKS

A. Definition

An anatomic landmark is an anatomic structure, the image of which may serve as an aid in the localization and identification of the regions portrayed by a radiograph. The teeth are the primary landmarks.

B. Landmarks That May Be Seen in Individual Radiographs

1. *Maxillary Molar.* Maxillary sinus, zygomatic process, zygomatic (malar) bone, hamular process, coronoid process of the mandible, maxillary tuberosity.
2. *Maxillary Premolar.* Maxillary sinus.
3. *Maxillary Canine.* Maxillary sinus, junction of the maxillary sinus and nasal fossa (Y-shaped, radiopaque).
4. *Maxillary Incisors.* Incisive foramen, nasal septum and fossae, anterior nasal spine (V-shaped), median palatine suture, symphysis of the maxillae.
5. *Mandibular Molar.* Mandibular canal, internal oblique line, external oblique ridge, mylohyoid ridge.

6. *Mandibular Premolar.* Mental foramen.
7. *Mandibular Incisors.* Lingual foramen, mental ridge, genial tubercles, symphysis of the mandible. Nutrient canals are seen most frequently in this radiograph.

IV. IDENTIFICATION OF INADEQUACIES IN RADIOGRAPHS

Table 9–5 outlines the more common inadequacies, their causes, the keys to correction.

A. Causes

Inadequacies and errors may be related to any step in the entire procedure, including film placement, angulation, exposure, processing, and care and handling of the film.

B. Types

Errors appear as problems of improper density or contrast, incomplete or distorted images, fogging, artifacts, or stains.

1. *Distortion.* An inaccuracy in the size or shape of an object in the radiograph. Distortion is brought about by misalignment of the PID relative to the object. Vertical distortion produces elongation or foreshortening of the object.
2. *Fog.* A darkening of the whole or part of a radiograph by sources other than the radiation of the primary beam to which the film was exposed. Types of fog include chemical, light, and radiation.
3. *Artifact.* A blemish or an unintended radiographic image that can result from faulty manufacture, manipulation, exposure, or processing of an x-ray film.

V. INTERPRETATION

Radiographs are used in conjunction with clinical examination for a complete program of treatment. Periodic radiographs permit continuing evaluation. As part of the permanent record, radiographs help to document the oral condition for comparative, as well as legal, purposes.

The quality of the radiographs determines their usability for diagnostic interpretation. Procedures for the preparation of radiographs must be perfected in order that radiographs have maximum interpretability with minimum radiation exposure of the patient.

A. Prerequisites for Interpretation

1. *Mounting.* Mount radiographs in an opaque mount to prevent light between each radiograph from creating glare and producing a blinding effect.
2. *Viewbox.* Use an adequately lighted viewbox. Dimmed room light improves visibility for contrasting radiolucent and radiopaque areas.

 Holding the radiographs up to view by window, room, or unit light is inadequate, and only gross interpretation can be accom-

plished. When a viewbox is larger than the amount used, cover the edges to block out peripheral light.
3. *Hand Magnifying Glass.* Examine radiographs on a viewbox through a magnifying glass. A viewbox is available with a built-on magnifying glass.

B. Systematic Examination

1. Observe one radiographic feature at a time. Examine all of the radiographs in a survey for that feature, rather than taking each radiograph separately to find everything. It is important to note comparisons for each change over the entire survey.
2. When examining a particular tooth, compare the appearance of that tooth in each radiograph in which it appears, including bitewings. At different angulations, different findings may become apparent.

C. Coordination with Clinical Examination

A description of radiographic examination of the teeth may be found on pages 242 and 243 and of the periodontal tissues on pages 225–227. Correlation of radiographic findings with the clinical examination, using probe and explorer, is basic to an understanding of the true oral condition of the patient.

TECHNICAL HINTS

I. HOLDING FILM

Never hold a film in a patient's mouth during exposure.

II. QUESTION RADIATION EXPOSURE

Inquire whether the patient is receiving or has recently received radiation treatment. It may be necessary to minimize the number of exposures. The patient's physician should be consulted (page 101).

III. FILM PLACEMENT

Dot on film packet is placed toward the occlusal surface or incisal edge to prevent the embossed dot on the film from superimposing over the image on the negative.

IV. CHECK STATE RADIATION PROTECTION LAWS

Many states have regulations concerning x-ray unit registration, inspection, safety requirements, and limitations for use of x rays.

V. RECORD IN PATIENT'S PERMANENT RECORD

A. Radiation Services Exposure Record

A continuing record for each patient is kept to show the date, number of exposures, and the area.

TABLE 9–5.
ANALYSIS OF RADIOGRAPHS: CAUSES OF INADEQUACIES

	Inadequacy	Cause: Factors in Correction
Image	Elongation	Insufficient vertical angulation
	Foreshortening	Excessive vertical angulation
	Superimposition (overlapping)	Incorrect horizontal angulation (central ray not directed through interproximal space)
	Partial image	Cone-cut (incorrect direction of central ray or incorrect film placement)
		Incompletely immersed in processing tank
		Film touched other film or side of tank during processing
	Blurred or double image	Patient, tube, or packet movement during exposure
		Film exposed twice
	Stretched appearance of trabeculae or apices	Bent film
	No image	Machine malfunction from time-switch to wall-plug
		Failure to turn on the machine
		Film placed in fixer before developer
Density	Too dark	Excessive exposure
		Excessive developing
		Developer too warm
		Unsafe safelight
		Accidental exposure to white light (may be completely black)
	Too light	Insufficient exposure
		Insufficient development or excessive fixation
		Solutions too cool
		Use of old, contaminated, or poorly mixed solutions
		Film placement: leaded side toward teeth
		Film used beyond expiration date
Fog	Chemical fog	Imbalance or deterioration of processing solutions
	Light fog	Unintentional exposure to light to which the emulsion is sensitive, either before or during processing
		(1) Unsafe safelight
		(2) Darkroom leak
		(3) Holding unprocessed films too close to the safelight too long
	Radiation fog	Improper storage of unused film
		Film exposed prior to processing
Reticulation	(puckered or pebbly surface)	Sudden temperature changes during processing, particularly from warm solutions to very cold water
Artifacts	Dark lines	Bent or creased film
		Static electricity
		(1) Film removed from wrapper with excessive force
		(2) Wrapper sticking to film, when opened with wet fingers, or if there was excessive moisture from patient's mouth
		Fingernail used to grasp film during placement on hanger
	Herringbone pattern (light film)	Packet placed in mouth backwards with foil next to teeth
Discoloration	Stains and spots	Unclean film hanger
		Splatterings of developer, fixer, dust
		Finger marks
		Insufficient rinsing after developing before fixing
		Splashing dry negatives with water or solutions
		Air bubbles adhering to surface during processing (insufficient agitation)
		Overlap of film on film in tanks or while drying
		Paper wrapper stuck to film (film not dried when removed from patient's mouth)
	At later date after storage of completed radiographs	Incomplete processing or rinsing
		Storage in too warm a place
		Storage near chemicals

B. Patient Signature

When a patient refuses to have radiographs made, record such in the patient's permanent record. Obtain patient's signature to a statement indicating such refusal in the event a legal issue should arise.

VI. WHO OWNS DENTAL RADIOGRAPHS?

They are part of the dentist's record and remain as professional property, the same as do other parts of the case record. The first rule is never to give radiographs to a patient. If they are to be loaned to another dentist, they should be sent or delivered directly, preferably with a letter indicating, if known, when they will next be needed and should be returned. When possible, a duplicate set can be made by using a two-film packet. It is also possible to duplicate the mounted set so that the originals can be kept with the patient's complete record.

VII. FILM STORAGE

Film should always be stored in a clean, cool, dry place. Keep in lead-lined container. Watch expiration dates. Store oldest film in front for next use. Purchase as needed, not in excess quantity.

VIII. STUDY INFORMATIONAL SHEETS

It is important to study the informational sheets provided in the film package, particularly when a new brand of film is being used.

IX. STAIN REMOVAL FROM CLOTHES

A. Do not launder before spot removal.
B. Commercially prepared spot removers are available from dental supply companies.
C. Removal of spots in nylon materials
  1. Prepare solution containing

Sodium hypochlorite (5% solution) (household bleach)	½ oz. (15 ml)
Acetic acid (5% solution) (household vinegar)	½ oz. (15 ml)
Water at about 38° C (100° F)	1 gal (3.8 L)

  2. Soak the stained portion in the solution for 5 to 10 minutes, then soak in *fresh* fixer.
  3. Rinse thoroughly in plain water. Dry.

X. DISPOSAL OF LIQUID CHEMICALS

Governmental regulations must be checked.

FACTORS TO TEACH THE PATIENT

I. WHEN THE PATIENT ASKS ABOUT THE SAFETY OF RADIATION

Patients ask questions about safety factors, and occasionally, a patient may refuse to have any radiographs made. The patient must be reassured with confidence, be instructed as to why radiographs are necessary at this time, and be informed about how modern equipment and techniques are in accord with radiation standards.

A. Adapt the answer to the patient. Certain patients have more fear; others have more knowledge about x rays. The clinician who expresses confidence aids in allaying fears. Hesitation increases the patient's doubt.
B. Radiographs are essential to diagnosis and treatment. Without the information provided, the dentist can only guess at conditions not visible clinically.
C. The benefits resulting from the intelligent use of x rays outweigh any possible negative effects.
D. Modern x-ray machines are equipped for safety. For the patient who understands, details about filtration, collimation, film speed, and short exposure times can be explained.

II. EDUCATIONAL FEATURES IN DENTAL RADIOGRAPHS

A. Position of unerupted permanent teeth in relation to primary teeth.
B. Detection of early carious lesions not visible by clinical examination.
C. Effects of loss of teeth and the importance of having replacements.
D. Periodontal changes and other pathologic conditions appropriate to an individual patient.

REFERENCES

1. **United States Food and Drug Administration,** Center for Devices and Radiological Health: *Selection of Patients for X-ray Examinations: Dental Radiographic Examinations.* Washington, D.C., Government Printing Office, No. 017-015-00236-5.
2. **United States National Research Council:** *Health Effects of Exposure to Low Levels of Ionizing Radiation.* BEIR-V, Washington, D.C., National Academy Press, 1990.
3. **American Dental Association,** Council on Dental Materials, Instruments, and Equipment: Recommendations in Radiographic Practices: An Update, 1988, *J. Am. Dent. Assoc., 118,* 115, January, 1989.
4. **Goaz,** P.W. and White, S.C.: *Oral Radiology, Principles and Interpretation,* 2nd ed., St. Louis, Mosby, 1987, pp. 1–17.
5. **Manson-Hing,** L.R.: *Fundamentals of Dental Radiography,* 3rd ed. Philadelphia, Lea & Febiger, 1990, pp. 1–15.
6. **Wuehrmann,** A.H. and Manson-Hing, L.R.: *Dental Radiology,* 5th ed. St. Louis, Mosby, 1981, pp. 4–21.
7. **Goaz** and White: op. cit., pp. 18–43.
8. **Wuehrmann** and Manson-Hing: op. cit., pp. 35–53, 76–85.
9. **Goaz** and White: op. cit., pp. 97–101.
10. **Gratt,** B.M., White, S.C., and Halse, A.: Clinical Recommendations for the Use of D-speed Film, E-speed Film, and Xeroradiography, *J. Am. Dent. Assoc., 117,* 609, October, 1988.
11. **International Commission on Radiation Units and Measurements (ICRU):** *Radiation Quantities and Units,* ICRU Report No. 33, Washington, D.C., 1980.
12. **United States National Council on Radiation Protection**

and Measurements: *Dental X-ray Protection.* Washington, D.C., NCRP Report No. 35, March 9, 1970.

13. **Manson-Hing:** op. cit., pp. 108–130.
14. **Goaz** and White: op. cit., pp. 44–58.
15. **Féderation Dentaire Internationale,** Commission on Dental Products: *Recommendations on Radiographic Procedures,* Technical Report No. 8 (Revision), *Int. Dent. J., 39,* 147, June, 1989.
16. **Herrmann,** H.J. and Myall, R.W.T.: Observations on the Significance of the Thyroid Gland to the Dentist, *Spec. Care Dentist., 3,* 13, January-February, 1983.
17. **Manson-Hing:** op. cit., pp. 53–62.
18. **Goaz** and White: op. cit., pp. 200–227.
19. **Manson-Hing:** op. cit., pp. 82–87.
20. **Stabe Disposable Periapical X-ray Filmholder,** Rinn Corporation, 1212 Abbott Drive, Elgin, IL 60121-1819.
21. **Manson-Hing:** op. cit., pp. 140–144.
22. **Goaz** and White: op. cit., pp. 254–260.
23. **Manson-Hing:** op. cit., pp. 160–185.
24. **Goaz** and White: op. cit., pp. 314–338.
25. **Myers,** D.R., O'Dell, N.L., Clark, J.W., and Cross, R.L.: Localized Prepubertal Periodontitis: Literature Review and Report of Case, *ASDC J. Dent. Child., 56,* 107, March-April, 1989.
26. **Watanabe,** K.: Prepubertal Periodontitis: A Review of Diagnostic Criteria, Pathogenesis, and Differential Diagnosis, *J. Periodont. Res., 25,* 31, January, 1990.
27. **Manson-Hing:** op. cit., pp. 193–196.
28. **Lyman,** S. and Boucher, L.J.: Radiographic Examination of Edentulous Mouths, *J. Prosthet. Dent., 64,* 180, August, 1990.
29. **Manson-Hing:** op. cit., pp. 191–193.
30. **Frommer,** H.H.: *Radiology for Dental Auxiliaries,* 5th ed. St. Louis, Mosby, 1992, pp. 95–104.
31. **Goaz** and White: op. cit., pp. 129–137.
32. **American Academy of Oral and Maxillofacial Radiology:** Infection Control Guidelines for Dental Radiographic Procedures, *Oral Surg. Oral Med. Oral Pathol., 73,* 248, February, 1992.
33. **Bachman,** C.E., White, J.M., Goodis, H.E., and Rosenquist, J.W.: Bacterial Adherence and Contamination During Radiographic Processing, *Oral Surg. Oral Med. Oral Pathol., 70,* 669, November, 1990.
34. **American Dental Association:** Infection Control Recommendations for the Dental Office and Dental Laboratory, *J. Am. Dent. Assoc., 123,* 6, Supplement, August, 1992.
35. **Katz,** J.O., Cottone, J.A., Hardman, P.K., and Taylor, T.S.: Infection Control Protocol for Dental Radiology, *Gent. Dent., 38,* 261, July-August, 1990.
36. **Manson-Hing:** op. cit., pp. 24, 244.

SUGGESTED READINGS

Curtis, P.M., von Fraunhofer, A., and Farman, A.G.: The Radiographic Density of Composite Restorative Resins, *Oral Surg. Oral Med. Oral Pathol., 70,* 226, August, 1990.

Goren, A.D., Sciubba, J.J., Friedman, R., and Malamud, H.: Survey of Radiologic Practices Among Dental Practitioners, *Oral Surg. Oral Med. Oral Pathol., 67,* 464, April, 1989.

Haring, J.I.: X-ray Vision, *RDH, 10,* 18, July, 1990.

Jones, G.A.: Considerations for the Apprehensive X-ray Patient, *Gen. Dent., 35,* 102, March-April, 1987.

Kantor, M.L., Hunt, R.J., and Morris, A.L.: An Evaluation of Radiographic Equipment and Procedures in 300 Dental Offices in the United States, *J. Am. Dent. Assoc., 120,* 547, May, 1990.

Kantor, M.L., Zeichner, S.J., Valachovic, R.W., and Reiskin, A.B.: Efficacy of Dental Radiographic Practices: Options for Image Reception, Examination Selection, and Patient Selection, *J. Am. Dent. Assoc., 119,* 259, August, 1989.

Kidd, E.A.M. and Pitts, N.B.: A Reappraisal of the Value of the Bitewing Radiograph in the Diagnosis of Posterior Approximal Caries, *Br. Dent. J., 169,* 195, October 6, 1990.

Lyman, S. and Boucher, L.J.: Radiographic Examination of Edentulous Mouths, *J. Prosthet. Dent., 64,* 180, August, 1990.

Matteson, S.R., Philips, C., Kantor, M.L., and Leinedecker, T.: The Effect of Lesion Size, Restorative Material, and Film Speed on the Detection of Recurrent Caries, *Oral Surg. Oral Med. Oral Pathol., 68,* 232, August, 1989.

Monsour, P.A.J., Kruger, B.J., Barnes, A., and MacLeod, A.G.: A Survey of Dental Radiography, *Aust. Dent. J., 33,* 9, February, 1988.

Packota, G.V. and Kolbinson, D.A.: Patient Selection Criteria for Dental Radiography, *Can. Dent. Assoc. J., 55,* 643, August, 1989.

Waggoner, W.F. and Ashton, J.J.: Predictability of Cavitation Based Upon Radiographic Appearance: Comparison of Two Film Types, *Quintessence Int., 20,* 55, January, 1989.

White, S.C., Gratt, B.M., and Bauer, J.G.: A Clinical Comparison of Xeroradiography and Film Radiography for the Detection of Proximal Caries, *Oral Surg. Oral Med. Oral Pathol., 65,* 242, February, 1988.

White, S.C., Kaffe, I., and Gornbein, J.A.: Prediction of Efficacy of Bitewing Radiographs for Caries Detection, *Oral Surg. Oral Med. Oral Pathol., 69,* 506, April, 1990.

Infection Control

Cottone, J.A., Terezhalmy, G.T., and Molinari, J.A.: *Practical Infection Control in Dentistry.* Philadelphia, Lea & Febiger, 1991, pp. 167–175.

Hubar, J.S., Etzel, K.R., and Dietrich, C.B.: Effects of Glove Powder on Radiographic Quality, *Can. Dent. Assoc. J., 57,* 790, October, 1991.

Jefferies, D., Morris, J.W., and White, V.P.: KVP Meter Errors Induced by Plastic Wrap, *J. Dent. Hyg., 65,* 91, February, 1991.

Neaverth, E.J. and Pantera, E.A.: Chairside Disinfection of Radiographs, *Oral Surg. Oral Med. Oral Pathol., 71,* 116, January, 1991.

Parks, E.T. and Farman, A.G.: Infection Control for Dental Radiographic Procedures in U.S. Dental Hygiene Programmes, *Dentomaxillofac. Radiol., 21,* 16, February, 1992.

Tullner, J.B., Zeller, G., Hartwell, G., and Burton, J.: A Practical Barrier Technique for Infection Control in Dental Radiology, *Compendium, 13,* 1054, November, 1992.

Wolfgang, L.: Analysis of a New Barrier Infection Control System for Dental Radiographic Film, *Compendium, 13,* 68, January, 1992.

Techniques

Benn, D.K.: Frequent, Low-dose, Improved-contrast Radiographic Images With the Use of Narrow X-ray Beams, *Oral Surg. Oral Med. Oral Pathol., 74,* 221, August, 1992.

Clark, D.E., Danforth, R.A., Barnes, R.W., and Burtch, M.L.: Radiation Absorbed from Dental Implant Radiography: A Comparison of Linear Tomography, C.T. Scan, and Panoramic and Intra-oral Techniques, *J. Oral Implantol., 16,* 156, No. 3, 1990.

Domon, M. and Yoshino, N.: Factors Involved in the High Radiographic Sensitivity of E-speed Films, *Oral Surg. Oral Med. Oral Pathol., 69,* 113, January, 1990.

Espelid, I.: The Influence of Viewing Conditions on Observer Performance in Dental Radiology, *Acta Odontol. Scand., 45,* 153, June, 1987.

Hedin, M.: Developing Solutions for Dental X-ray Processors, *Swed. Dent. J., 13,* 261, No. 6, 1989.

Herzog, A.: Dental Radiography. A Review for Dental Hygiene Practitioners, *J. Dent. Hyg., 62,* 242, May, 1988.

Jarvis, W.D., Pifer, R.G., Griffin, J.A., and Skidmore, A.E.: Evaluation of Image Quality in Individual Films of Double Film Packets, *Oral Surg. Oral Med. Oral Pathol., 69,* 764, June, 1990.

Kaplan, I. and Dickens, R.L.: Lightening of Dark Radiographs With a Superproportional Reducing Agent, *Quintessence Int., 21,* 737, September, 1990.

Maddalozzo, D., Knoeppel, R.O., and Schoenfeld, C.M.: Performance of Seven Rapid Radiographic Processing Solutions, *Oral Surg. Oral Med. Oral Pathol., 69,* 382, March, 1990.

Parks, E.T.: Errors Generated With the Use of Rectangular Collimation, *Oral Surg. Oral Med. Oral Pathol., 71,* 509, April, 1991.

Sewerin, I.B. and Stoltze, K.: Blackening of Unprotected Dental X-ray Films Due to Scattered Radiation, *Scand. J. Dent. Res., 96,* 161, April, 1988.

Shrout, M.K., Hildebolt, C.F., and Vannier, M.W.: The Effect of Alignment Errors on Bitewing-based Bone Loss Measurements, *J. Clin. Periodontol., 18,* 708, October, 1991.

Svenson, B. and Petersson, A.: Influence of Different Developing Solutions and Developing Times on Radiographic Caries Diagnosis, *Dentomaxillofac. Radiol., 19,* 157, November, 1990.

Thorogood, J., Homer, K., and Smith, N.J.D.: Quality Control in the Processing of Dental Radiographs. A Practical Guide to Sensitometry, *Br. Dent. J., 164,* 282, May 7, 1988.

Thunthy, K.H.: Technique for Using Films Accidentally Exposed to Light, *Oral Surg. Oral Med. Oral Pathol., 65,* 371, March, 1988.

Wallace, J.A. and Cohen, B.D.: Accurate Radiographs With Intravenous Sedation or General Anesthesia, *Oral Surg. Oral Med. Oral Pathol., 65,* 240, February, 1988.

Wood, R.E., Bristow, R.G., Clark, G.M., Nussbaum, C., and Taylor, K.W.: Technique-dependent Decrease in Thyroid Absorbed Dose for Dental Radiography, *Health Phys., 56,* 893, June, 1989.

Zappa, U., Simona, C., Graf, H., and van Aken, J.: *In Vivo* Determination of Radiographic Projection Errors Produced by a Novel Filmholder and an X-ray Beam Manipulator, *J. Periodontol., 62,* 674, November, 1991.

Radiation Exposure Control

Borrman, H. and Holmberg, P.: Radiation Doses and Risks in Dentomaxillofacial Radiology, *Proc. Finn. Dent. Soc., 85,* 457, No. 6, 1989.

Farman, A.G.: Concepts of Radiation Safety and Protection: Beyond BEIR, *Dent. Assist., 60,* 11, January/February, 1991.

Horner, K. and Hirschmann, P.N.: Dose Reduction in Dental Radiography, *J. Dent., 18,* 171, August, 1990.

Monsour, P.A., Kruger, B.J., Barnes, A., and Sainsbury, A.: Measures Taken to Reduce X-ray Exposure of the Patient, Operator and Staff, *Aust. Dent. J., 33,* 181, June, 1988.

Preston-Martin, S. and White, S.C.: Brain and Salivary Gland Tumors Related to Prior Dental Radiography: Implications for Current Practice, *J. Am. Dent. Assoc., 120,* 151, February, 1990.

Preston-Martin, S., Thomas, D.C., White, S.C., and Cohen, D.: Prior Exposure to Medical and Dental X-rays Related to Tumors of the Parotid Gland, *J. Natl. Cancer Inst., 80,* 943, August 17, 1988.

Serman, N.J.: Exposure to Dental Radiation—a Perspective, *Quintessence Int., 21,* 331, April, 1990.

Soh, G. and Chong, Y.H.: Variability of Two Methods of Measuring Absorbed Dose in Dental Radiography, *Clin. Prev. Dent., 14,* 17, November-December, 1992.

Underhill, T.E., Chilvarquer, I., Kimura, K., Langlais, R.P., McDavid, W.D., Preece, J.W., and Barnwell, G.: Radiobiologic Risk Estimation from Dental Radiology. Part I. Absorbed Doses to Critical Organs, *Oral Surg. Oral Med. Oral Pathol., 66,* 111, July, 1988.

Underhill, T.E., Kimura, K., Chilvarquer, I., McDavid, W.D., Langlais, R.P., Preece, J.W., and Barnell, G.: Radiobiologic Risk Estimation from Dental Radiology. Part II. Cancer Incidence and Fatality, *Oral Surg. Oral Med. Oral Pathol., 66,* 261, August, 1988.

White, S.C.: 1992 Assessment of Radiation Risk from Dental Radiography, *Dentomaxillofac. Radiol., 21,* 118, August, 1992.

Gagging

Donkor, P. and Wong, J.: A Mandibular Block Technique Useful in "Gaggers," *Aust. Dent. J., 36,* 47, February, 1991.

Fleece, L., Linton, P., and Dudley, B.: Rapid Elimination of a Hyperactive Gag Reflex, *J. Prosthet. Dent., 60,* 415, October, 1988.

Ramsey, D.S., Weinstein, P., Milgrom, P., and Getz, T.: Problematic Gagging: Principles of Treatment, *J. Am. Dent. Assoc., 114,* 178, February, 1987.

Zach, G.A.: Gag Control, *Gen. Dent., 37,* 508, November-December, 1989.

Pediatric Radiography

Curbox, S.C. and Long, W.R.: Radiation Reduction Technique for Pediatric Dental Panoramic Radiographs, *Pediatr. Dent., 13,* 319, September/October, 1991.

Harrison, R. and Richardson, D.: Bitewing Radiographs of Children Taken With and Without a Film-holding Device, *Dentomaxillofac. Radiol., 18,* 97, August, 1989.

McKnight-Hanes, C., Myers, D.R., Dushku, J.C., Thompson, W.O., and Durham, L.C.: Radiographic Recommendations for the Primary Dentition: Comparison of General Dentists and Pediatric Dentists, *Pediatr. Dent., 12,* 212, July/August, 1990.

Myers, D.R., McKnight-Hanes, C., Dushku, J.C., Thompson, W.O., and Durham, L.C.: Radiographic Recommendations for the Transitional Dentition: Comparison of General Dentists and Pediatric Dentists. *Pediatr. Dent., 12,* 217, July/August, 1990.

Nowak, A.J. and Miller, J.W.: High-yield Pedodontic Radiology, *Gen. Dent., 33,* 45, January-February, 1985.

Panoramic

Hintze, H. and Wenzel, A.: Accuracy of Clinical DIagnosis for the Detection of Dentoalveolar Anomalies with Panoramic Radiography as Validating Criterion, *ASDC J. Dent. Child., 57,* 119, March-April, 1990.

Ignelzi, M.A., Fields, H.W., and Vann, W.F.: Screening Panoramic Radiographs in Children: Prevalence Data and Implications, *Pediatr. Dent., 11,* 279, December, 1989.

Kantor, M.L. and Slome, B.A.: Efficacy of Panoramic Radiography in Dental Diagnosis and Treatment Planning, *J. Dent. Res., 68,* 810, May, 1989.

Kapa, S.F. and Tyndall, D.A.: A Clinical Comparison of Image Quality and Patient Exposure Reduction in Panoramic Radiography With Heavy Metal Filtration, *Oral Surg. Oral Med. Oral Pathol., 67,* 750, June, 1989.

Lew, K.K.K.: The Prediction of Eruption-sequence from Panoramic Radiographs, *ASDC J. Dent. Child., 59,* 346, September-October, 1992.

Rohlin, M., Åkesson, L., Håkansson, J., Håkansson, H., and Nåsstrom, K.: Comparison Between Panoramic and Periapical Radiography in the Diagnosis of Periodontal Bone Loss, *Dentomaxillofac. Radiol., 18,* 72, May, 1989.

Seals, R.R., Williams, E.O., and Jones, J.D.: Panoramic Radiographs: Necessary for Edentulous Patients?, *J. Am. Dent. Assoc., 123,* 74, November, 1992.

Skoczylas, L.J., Preece, J.W., Langlais, R.P., McDavid, W.D., and Waggener, R.G.: Comparison of X-radiation Doses between Conventional and Rare Earth Panoramic Radiographic Techniques, *Oral Surg. Oral Med. Oral Pathol., 68,* 776, December, 1989.

Webb, N.B.: Panoramic Radiography, *Semin. Dent. Hyg., 2,* 1, October, 1990.

10

Study Casts

As reproductions of the teeth, gingiva, and adjacent structures, study casts can be useful and frequently indispensable adjuncts in the care of a patient. Accurate and esthetically acceptable casts have a special use as visual aids for patient instruction.

The study casts, radiographs, and clinical examination with recordings and chartings, together with the medical and dental histories, are utilized in the diagnosis, total treatment planning, treatment, and subsequent maintenance by the dentist and the dental hygienist.

I. PURPOSES AND USES OF STUDY CASTS

A. To serve as a permanent record of the patient's present condition.

B. To give sharper delineation to and corroboration of the observations made during the oral examination.

C. To observe normal conditions and the variations of and departures from the normal at the outset of treatment, and, by comparison with subsequent periodic casts, to compare and evaluate certain aspects of treatment.

D. During charting of the teeth, to note missing teeth, anomalies of size, shape, or number, partial eruption, tooth positions, such as drifting, tilting, rotation, and open or closed spacing, and other factors.

E. During examination of the occlusion, to observe the static relations (Angle's classification, malrelations of groups of teeth, and malpositions of individual teeth; pages 248–253) and other features, such as wear patterns and the effects of premature loss of teeth.

F. During periodontal charting, to record anatomic features, such as the position, size, and shape of the gingiva and interdental papillae, and the position of freni.

G. To be an effective visual aid to use when the oral conditions are explained and the dental and dental hygiene treatment plan is presented; to enable the patient to visualize and understand the need for the specific care outlined.

H. To serve as a guide to clinical treatment procedures.

I. To supplement clinical observations when the bacterial plaque control program for the patient's own treatment is explained and to serve as a visual aid in teaching aims and procedures of the recommended measures to the patient.

II. STEPS IN THE PREPARATION OF STUDY CASTS

Terms used to describe study casts and their preparation are defined in table 10–1.

The steps noted here are detailed in the sections following.

A. Clinical Procedures

1. Assemble materials and equipment.
2. Prepare the patient.
3. Select and prepare the impression trays.
4. Make the mandibular impression.
5. Make the maxillary impression.
6. Make the interocclusal record for occluding the casts.

B. Paraclinical Procedures

1. Assemble materials and equipment.
2. Prepare the impressions for pouring.
3. Pour the casts.
4. Trim and finish the casts.
5. Polish the casts.

TABLE 10-1
KEY WORDS: STUDY CASTS*

Cast (model): a positive life-size reproduction of the teeth and adjacent tissues usually formed by pouring dental plaster or stone into a matrix or impression.

Diagnostic or study cast: used in the study of a patient's oral condition in preparation for treatment planning and patient instruction.

Master cast: used to fabricate a dental restoration or prosthesis.

Centric occlusion or **habitual occlusion** (ō kloo'zhun): the usual maximum intercuspation or contact of the teeth of the opposing arches.

Dental plaster: the beta-form of calcium sulfate hemihydrate; a fibrous aggregate of fine crystals with capillary pores that are irregular in shape and porous in character; also referred to as plaster of Paris.

Dental stone: the alpha-form of calcium sulfate hemihydrate with physical properties superior to those of the beta-form (dental plaster); the alpha-form consists of cleavage fragments and crystals in the form of rods and prisms, and is therefore more dense than the beta-form.

Impression (im-presh'un): a negative imprint of an oral structure used to produce a positive replica of the structure; used as a permanent record or in the production of a dental restoration or prosthesis; usually identified by the type of material used, such as "hydrocolloid impression," "alginate impression," or "rubber base impression."

Interocclusal record: a registration of the positional relationship of the opposing teeth or dental arches made in a plastic material, such as a soft baseplate wax; also called the **maxillomandibular relationship record** or "wax bite."

Occlusal plane: the average plane established by the incisal and occlusal surfaces of the teeth; generally not actually a plane, but the planar mean of the curvature of those surfaces.

Polish: to make smooth and glossy usually by friction; the act or process of making a casting smooth and glossy.

Prosthesis (pros-thē'sĭs): an artificial replacement of an absent part of the human body; a therapeutic device to improve or alter function.

* Definitions in this chapter are taken or adapted from and in accord with *The Glossary of Prosthodontic Terms,* 6th ed. Academy of Prosthodontics Foundation, 1993.

CLINICAL PREPARATION

The need for and uses of study casts are explained to the patient when the steps in diagnosis and treatment planning are outlined. As with any procedure not familiar to the patient, an explanation is in order. The reactions of patients who have had an impression made previously may range from indifference to dread, and the conversation and approach can be directed accordingly.

When the radiographic survey has been made for the new patient prior to the study casts, the clinician will have already determined whether precautions to prevent gagging require special application. With all patients, a calm approach, an exhibition of confidence, a direct and efficient procedure, and a gentle handling of the patient's oral tissues increase rapport and contribute to a satisfactory result.

I. ASSEMBLE MATERIALS AND EQUIPMENT
A. Coverall (plastic drape), towel, and mouthrinse.
B. Impression trays
   1. Perforated type generally used; small, medium, and large sizes are available.
   2. Trays for use in the patient's mouth must be disposable or clean, shiny, and sterilized metal.
C. Mixing bowl: clean, dry, flexible rubber or plastic with smooth, unscratched surface. Reserve separate bowls for each dental material; one always for impression material, another kept only for plaster or stone.
D. Spatula: clean, dry, stiff, with a smooth, rounded end that reaches every part of the bowl without scraping or cutting its surface.
E. Saliva ejector.
F. Dental materials
   1. Soft utility wax for preparation of tray rim.
   2. Alginate: irreversible hydrocolloid with manufacturer's measuring device.
   3. Soft baseplate wax for interocclusal record.
G. Water thermometer.

II. CLINICIAN PREPARATION
Protective eyewear, mask, and gloves should be worn as for all clinic procedures. A mask should always be worn when handling powder forms of dental materials to prevent inhalation.

III. PREPARE THE PATIENT
A. Antibiotic Premedication
Impression making can be planned for an appointment when the patient who is at risk for bacteremia is protected and has received antibiotic coverage for other procedures. The medical and dental histories must be reviewed for all possible precautionary needs.

B. Explain the Procedure to be Performed
The impression material has a slight, pleasant flavor; it may feel cold when first placed.

C. Position the Patient
Position the patient upright for maximum visibility and accessibility and to minimize gagging. Stabilize the patient's head on the headrest.

D. Receive Removable Appliances
Provide a container with water in which the patient can place removable oral appliances.

E. Drape the Patient

Drape patient with a protective coverall and towel.

F. Examine the Oral Cavity

Note labially and buccally displaced teeth, height of palate, undercut areas, mandibular tori, and other factors that may influence the size or preparation of the impression tray and the procedures to be carried out during impression making.

G. Free the Mouth of Debris

1. Request patient to rinse vigorously; use dental floss.
2. When excess, tenacious debris is present, plaque control instruction should be started so that debris and plaque can be removed during brushing by the patient.

H. Request Patient to Use Mouthrinse

1. To aid in the removal of saliva and debris and lessen the numbers of surface microorganisms.
2. To lower the surface tension; aids in preventing bubbles in the impression.
3. To provide a pleasant taste and feeling for the patient.
4. To distract an anxious patient while the trays are being prepared.

I. Dry the Teeth

Use a cotton roll or compressed air stream to remove saliva from the teeth to prevent irregularities in the surface of the study cast.

J. Prevent Gagging

1. Approach with confidence to reassure the patient.
2. Work as quickly and efficiently as possible.
3. Use a topical anesthetic (pages 519–521).
   a. Cold water or an ice cube held in the mouth has some anesthetic effect.
   b. A small amount (¼ teaspoon) of salt on the tongue to swallow just before the tray is to be inserted may relieve tissue reactions.
   c. Apply topical anesthetic to posterior palatal area, or patient may rinse with a commercial topical agent. A spray topical preparation is contraindicated because of proximity to throat, where coughing may be initiated.
4. Technique considerations
   a. Avoid excessive impression material in the tray.
   b. Seat the maxillary tray from posterior to anterior as described on page 167.
   c. Instruct patient to breathe deeply through the nose before the tray is inserted and to continue after insertion; bring head forward.

THE INTEROCCLUSAL RECORD (WAX BITE)

I. PURPOSES

A. To relate the maxillary and mandibular casts correctly. Many, if not most, maxillary and mandibular casts orient to each other readily in only one position, but when such problems as openbite, crossbite, edentulous areas, and end-to-end or edge-to-edge relations interfere with direct occlusion of the casts, a wax bite is generally needed.

B. To place between the casts during trimming and storage to prevent breakage of teeth.

II. PROCEDURE

A. Request patient to practice opening and closing on the posterior teeth to assure that the habitual position can be obtained easily.

B. Ask patient to rinse with cold water.

C. Shape a double layer of soft baseplate wax in the form of the arch, warm slightly over a gas burner or soften in warm water, and place over the maxillary occlusal surfaces.

D. Guide patient to close in habitual occlusion; press the wax against the facial surfaces of the teeth to shape it accurately to the arch.

E. Remove carefully to prevent distortion; chill in cold water.

PREPARATION OF IMPRESSION TRAYS

I. SELECTION OF PROPER SIZE AND SHAPE

A. Width

1. Objective is to allow an adequate thickness of impression material on the facial and lingual surfaces of each tooth to provide strength and rigidity to the impression.
2. Tray flanges may be spread to accommodate for extra width in the molar regions, particularly lingual to the mandibular molars in the mylohyoid region.
3. When a tooth is in prominent labio-, bucco-, or linguoversion, a minimum thickness of ⅛ to ¼ inch is suggested, but even then, the fragility of the impression material in that area is increased.
4. The tray that is too wide may appear in correct relation to the facial surfaces but may impinge on the lingual or palatal cusps of molars.

B. Length

1. Objective is to allow coverage of the retromolar area of the mandible and the tuberosity of the maxilla.

2. Anteriorly there should be at least ¼ inch clearance labial to the most protruded incisor without impingement on lingual or palatal gingiva.

II. MAXILLARY TRAY TRY-IN
A. Position of Clinician
Side back of patient.

B. Retraction
1. With index finger of nondominant hand, retract the patient's lip and cheek.
2. At the same time, use the side of the tray to distend the other side of the patient's mouth to gain entry (figure 10–1).

C. Insertion
1. With a rotary motion, insert the tray.
2. Orient the tray beneath the arch and center it by using the tray handle and the midline (usually between the central incisors and in line with the middle of the nose) as guides for positioning.
3. Bring the front of the tray to a position ¼ inch labial to the most labially inclined incisor.
4. Seat the tray by bringing the posterior up before the anterior; retract the lip as the anterior is brought into place.

D. Evaluation
Evaluate the size of the tray; gently lower the front of the tray while holding the posterior border in place (figure 10–2), and examine the relationship of the posterior border to the most posterior molars and the tuberosity areas to determine whether the coverage will be ample. By moving the tray up and down, it is possible to

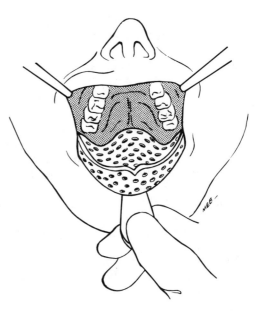

FIG. 10–2. Selection of Impression Tray. Adequate coverage is determined as the posterior border of the tray is held in position while the front of the tray is lowered to observe the relationship of the posterior border to the maxillary tuberosity areas to be covered by the impression. The mandibular tray position is examined by lifting the tray to observe coverage of the retromolar areas.

observe the relation to the facial surfaces of all teeth, malaligned teeth, protuberances, and other features to assay the space allowed for the impression material.

III. MANDIBULAR TRAY TRY-IN
A. Position of Clinician
At side front of patient.

B. Retraction
1. With index and middle fingers of nondominant hand, retract the patient's lip and cheek.
2. At the same time, use the side of the tray to distend the side of the mouth to gain entry, similar to the procedure illustrated in figure 10–1 for the maxillary tray.

C. Insertion
1. With a rotary motion, insert the tray.
2. Orient the tray over the dental arch and center it by using the tray handle and the midline (usually between the central incisors and in line with the center of the chin) as guides for positioning.
3. Bring the tray rim to about ¼ inch anterior to the most labially positioned incisor; instruct the patient to raise the tongue to permit the lingual flange of the tray to pass by the lateral borders of the tongue without interference.

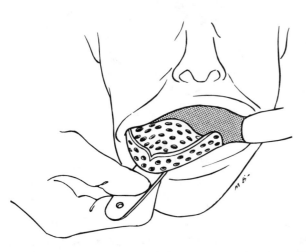

FIG. 10–1. Maxillary Tray Insertion. The patient's lip and cheek are retracted with the fingers of the nondominant hand while the side of the tray is used to distend the other lip and cheek to gain entry. The tray is inserted with a rotary motion. The procedure for the mandibular tray is similar.

4. As the tray is lowered, retract the cheeks in the posterior regions to make certain the buccal mucosa is not caught beneath the edge of the tray; hold the lip out to ascertain that there is clearance to the base of the vestibule.

D. Evaluation

1. Evaluate the size of the tray. Lift the tray handle while keeping the posterior border of the tray in position, similar to the procedure illustrated in figure 10–2 for the maxilla, to determine whether the coverage will be ample posteriorly to include the retromolar areas and laterally to allow for ¼-inch thickness of impression material on the facial and lingual aspects of the teeth.
2. Reselect larger or smaller trays as indicated and repeat try-in. When in doubt, use the larger tray rather than the smaller.

IV. APPLICATION OF WAX RIM AROUND BORDERS OF TRAYS (BEADING)

A. Purposes

1. To prevent the metal tray rims from causing discomfort to the soft tissues.
2. To seat the vestibular periphery firmly into position with reduced pressure on the displaced tissues.
3. To prevent penetration of the incisal or occlusal surfaces through the impression material and thus to prevent a defective cast.
4. To provide a slight undercut at the rim as an aid in the retention of the alginate in the tray during placement and removal
5. To create a posterior palatal seal to aid in preventing excess material from passing into the throat.

B. Procedure

1. *Application of Wax.* Attach a strip of soft utility wax firmly around the entire periphery of each tray (figure 10–3).
2. *Mandibular Tray.* Add extra layers from canine to canine labially and notch the wax to fit about the labial frenum.
3. *Maxillary Tray*
   a. Add extra layers as needed to extend the tray into the vestibule above the anterior teeth and notch the wax to fit about the labial frenum (figure 10–4).
   b. Apply extra thickness across the posterior palatal seal area.
   c. When a patient has a high palatal vault, apply extra wax to support the impression material in that area.
4. *Try-in.* Try the rimmed trays in the mouth and examine by retraction of the lips and cheeks and by use of a mouth mirror for lingual areas; hold the tray in position.
5. *Characteristics of the Completed Molding.* When the tray is held firmly, the wax contacts all

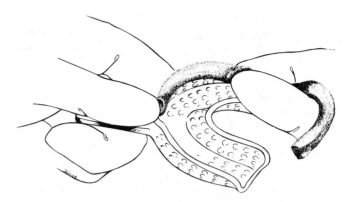

FIG. 10–3. Beading the Tray. *A strip of soft utility wax is applied around the periphery of each tray.*

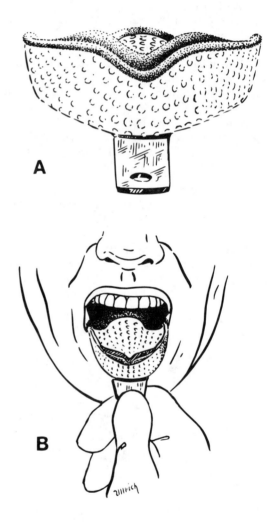

FIG. 10–4.   Check the Beading Wax. A. Tray with double layer of beading wax about the labial frenum. The extra wax extends the tray, protects the soft tissue from the metal rim, and provides a more complete impression of the area. **B.** Try-in after beading. The wax should contact all borders of the mucous membrane, displace the soft tissue outward, and prevent the teeth from contacting the tray.

borders of the mucous membrane, displaces the soft tissue outward and upward, and the teeth do not touch the tray.

THE IMPRESSION MATERIAL

I. FACTORS RELATED TO THE IMPRESSION MATERIAL THAT CONTRIBUTE TO A SATISFACTORY IMPRESSION

Texts on dental materials should be reviewed for complete information about the irreversible hydrocolloids.[1,2,3] Properties related to the clinical procedures essential to making an accurate impression are listed here. The manufacturer's directions are followed.

A. Powder

The alginate material deteriorates on standing, particularly at higher temperatures and humidity.

1. Keep metal container tightly closed; store in a cool place.
2. Use individually sealed packages to eliminate the problems of heat and moisture.
3. Individual package may be refrigerated in hot weather, provided the powder is used immediately on opening. If left exposed, water condenses on the powder. The bulk container cannot be refrigerated for that reason.

B. Water

Temperature controls gelation time.

1. At room temperature, 20° to 21° C (68° to 70° F), an ideal gelation time between 3 to 4 minutes provides adequate working time.
2. Temperature of the water should be measured with a thermometer at the time of mixing.
3. For control in hot, humid weather, use cooler water and refrigerate the bowl and spatula.

C. Strength and Quality

The strength and quality of the finished impression depend on the following factors:

1. Powder-water ratio accurately weighed and measured.
2. Spatulation (1 minute) to allow chemical reactions to proceed uniformly.
3. Holding the impression material in position for an optimum period in accord with manufacturer's specifications. The elasticity of most alginates improves with time; therefore, a superior reproduction can be obtained by waiting. Distortion can result when the impression is left in the mouth too long.

D. Surface Accuracy

The cast must be poured immediately to prevent loss of water from the impression. Permanent distortion can result.

II. MIXING THE IMPRESSION MATERIAL

Follow manufacturer's specifications precisely; total time lapse for mixing and insertion is approximately 2 minutes.

A. Place measured water 20° to 21° C (68° to 70° F, measured with a thermometer) in a clean, dry mixing bowl.
B. Sprinkle measured powder (from individually sealed package or premeasured from large container) into the water.
C. Quickly incorporate the powder and water, using a clean, dry, stiff spatula.
D. Mix for 1 minute (clocked) vigorously, incorporating powder into the water, until a smooth, creamy mix is obtained.

III. TRAY PREPARATION

The mandibular impression is made first to introduce the patient to the procedure in an area where discomfort or gagging may be the least likely.

A. Working Time

The working time is 30 seconds.

B. Filling the Tray

1. Fill the tray from one end to the other, being careful not to trap air bubbles.
2. Adapt the material to the tray thoroughly; press slightly through the perforations in the tray.
3. Do not overload; fill to a level just below the edge of the wax rim.
4. Wet index finger with cold water and pass lightly over the surface of the impression material; smooth the surface and make a slight indent where the teeth will insert.

C. Excess Material

Quickly gather the excess material from the bowl and bring the material on the spatula near to patient.

THE MANDIBULAR IMPRESSION

I. PRECOAT POTENTIAL AREAS OF AIR ENTRAPMENT

This precoat prevents air bubbles in the finished impression.

A. Take a small amount of impression material from the spatula onto the index finger.
B. Apply quickly with a positive pressure to
   1. Undercut areas, such as distal surfaces of teeth adjacent to edentulous areas, cervical areas of erosion or abrasion, or gingival surfaces of fixed partial dentures.
   2. Vestibular areas, particularly anterior areas about the freni.
   3. Occlusal surfaces.

II. STEPS FOR INSERTION OF TRAY

A. Follow mandibular tray try-in (page 167). In summary, the procedure is as follows.

1. From 8 o'clock position (4 o'clock if left-handed), retract lip and cheek with fingers of nondominant hand.
2. Use side of tray to distend the other lip and cheek.
3. Rotate the tray into position, center it over the teeth, and introduce the tray ¼ inch anterior to the facial surface of the most anterior incisor.
4. Instruct patient to raise the tongue while tray is lowered; retract cheeks and lip to clear the way for impression material to reach the base of the vestibule.

B. Seat the tray directly downward with a slight vibratory motion to aid in filling all crevices between the teeth.

C. Instruct the patient to extrude the tongue briefly to mold the lingual borders of the impression.

D. Apply equal bilateral pressure firmly, holding the middle fingers over the premolar regions and using the thumbs to support the mandible; or, if equal pressure can be maintained with one hand, place an index finger over the patient's premolar area on one side and the middle finger over the opposite side, with the thumb under the edge of the mandible for stabilization. Mold cheeks around facial buccal.

E. When the impression tray is held with one hand or when assistance is available, slip the saliva ejector in over the tray and then remove it before the tray is removed.

F. When the leftover material on the spatula has lost its surface stickiness (tackiness), hold the impression in position 2 more clocked minutes.

III. THE COMPLETED IMPRESSION

A. Removal of Impression

1. Hold tray with thumb and fingers.
2. Retract cheek and lip with fingers and release the edge of the impression by depressing the buccal mucosa.
3. Do not rock the impression back and forth to release it because these movements may cause permanent distortion of the final impression.
4. Remove the impression with a sudden jerk or snap.

B. Rinse

Rinse under cool running water to remove saliva, blood, and bacteria. Rinse carefully to prevent splashing contaminated saliva or blood over surroundings.

C. Examine and Evaluate the Impression

Observe surface detail, proper extension over retromolar area, and peripheral roll (rounded border of the impression) generally.

D. Repeat Procedure When Necessary

Correct mistakes rather than be satisfied with a substandard impression.

E. Storage

Wrap mandibular impression in a wet towel while making the maxillary impression.

THE MAXILLARY IMPRESSION

I. PREPARATION

A. Request Patient to Rinse

To clear particles left from the mandibular impression and to relax the oral muscles.

B. Examine the Maxillary Teeth

Teeth should be examined for particles of mandibular impression material; if found, remove. Request patient to use mouthrinse.

C. Prepare the Alginate

Fill the tray as described previously for the mandibular impression.

D. Precoat Undercut Areas

Precoat undercut areas, vestibular areas, and occlusal surfaces (see procedure for mandibular impression).

II. STEPS FOR INSERTION OF TRAY

A. Follow maxillary tray try-in (page 167). In summary, the procedure is as follows:

1. From 11 o'clock position (1 o'clock if left-handed), retract lip with fingers of nondominant hand.
2. Use side of tray to distend the lip and cheek.
3. Insert the tray with a rotary motion; center it over the teeth by using the small gap in the red wax border to relate to the labial frenum.
4. Introduce the material to the teeth so the wax rim is ¼ inch facial to the most anterior incisor.

B. Seat the tray from posterior to anterior to direct the impression material forward and thus prevent irritation to the soft palate area.

C. Retract the lip and bring the tray to place with a slight vibratory motion to allow the material to flow into crevices and proximal areas.

D. The middle finger of each hand is placed over the premolar region to support and guide the tray; the index fingers and thumbs hold the lip out.

E. Request the patient to form a tight "O" with the lips to mold the impression material.

F. Maintain equal pressure on each side of the tray throughout the setting of the alginate. If assistance is available or if the pressure to hold the tray can be maintained with one hand, a saliva ejector can be inserted.

G. When the leftover material on the spatula has lost its surface stickiness, hold the impression in place for 2 more clocked minutes.

III. THE COMPLETED IMPRESSION

A. Remove Impression
Hold the tray handle with the thumb and fingers of the dominant hand and retract the opposite lip and cheek with the fingers of the other hand. Elevate the cheek over the edge of the impression to break the seal, and remove the impression with a sudden jerk.

B. Rinse
Rinse under cool running water to remove saliva, blood, and bacteria. Rinse carefully to prevent dissemination of contaminated saliva and blood.

C. Examine
Examine surface detail and proper extension to include tuberosity areas and a complete reproduction of the height of the vestibule.

D. Repeat Procedure When Necessary
Repeat procedure rather than be satisfied with a substandard impression.

E. Disinfection
Proceed with disinfection for maxillary and mandibular casts.

DISINFECTION OF IMPRESSIONS[4,5,6]

To prevent cross-contamination during laboratory procedures, impressions should be disinfected in an approved disinfectant after rinsing. The dimensional stability of some impression materials may be affected by certain disinfectants, so research and manufacturer's information must be heeded.

When impressions are to be sent to a laboratory, they should be isolated in a package. A "zip-lock" bag can be used.

I. DISINFECTANTS
Iodophore (1:213) and sodium hypochlorite (1:10) have been tested and are effective with no distortion of an alginate impression when used for 10 to 15 minutes before pouring.

II. PROCEDURE
A. Apply universal precautions; wear protective gloves, eyewear, and mask to handle contaminated impressions and to protect against chemical disinfectants.

B. Immerse to assure maximum contact of the agent with all undercut areas. Impression then can be placed in the solution in a plastic zip-lock bag for 10 to 15 minutes.

C. Discard disinfectant solution and rinse the impression under running water before pouring.

PARACLINICAL PROCEDURES

Supplemental to the chairside clinical procedures is the laboratory work involved in the production of the study casts from the impressions. These duties may be the responsibility of the dental laboratory technician or other dental team member, as directed by the dentist.

The most frequent error in the use of the alginates for impressions is delay in pouring the cast. Undue dehydration or water loss from the alginate causes permanent distortion, an uneven surface, and hence an inaccurate cast. Regard for the sensitive properties of the dental materials, precision and practice in laboratory procedures, and pride in the production of neat, smooth, well-proportioned study casts determine the finished product's appearance, usefulness, and accuracy.

I. EQUIPMENT AND MATERIALS
A. Mixing bowl: clean, dry, flexible rubber or plastic, with smooth, unscratched surface. Separate bowls are reserved for each dental material.

B. Spatula: clean, dry, stiff, metal with a smooth, rounded end that can reach every part of the bowl without scraping or cutting its surface.

C. Plaster knife: sharp.

D. Vibrator with protective covering.

E. Mechanical mixer.

F. Model-base formers, glass or ceramic slab, waxed paper or other nonabsorbent-surfaced material.

G. Dental materials.
1. Baseplate wax (and wax spatula).
2. White dental stone.

H. Water at room temperature, with measuring container.

I. Model trimmer.

J. Compass or dividers.

K. Plastic ruler.

L. Waterproof sandpaper.

M. Soap solution.

II. PREPARATION OF THE IMPRESSIONS
A. Rinse impressions under cool running water to remove residual disinfection that may affect the plaster or stone surface after pouring; shake out excess water gently and apply gentle blast of compressed air.

B. Create an artificial floor of the mouth in the mandibular impression to facilitate pouring and trimming of the cast.
  1. Trim the lingual impression material all around so that the height is consistent from the occlusal and incisal surfaces to the base of the impression.
  2. Using alginate
    a. Mix a small portion of alginate.
    b. Hold the mandibular impression upright in the nondominant hand, with the middle and ring fingers extended from under the tray into the tongue area.
    c. Apply alginate over the fingers to form a flat bridge slightly above the lingual flanges of the impression.
    d. Smooth the surface with a finger moistened with cool water; hold until the alginate sets.
    e. When assisted at the chair, the floor of the mandibular impression can be made while the maxillary impression is being held for setting. There is usually sufficient alginate mixed with that for the maxillary impression to use for this purpose.
  3. Using baseplate wax
    a. Cut a piece of baseplate wax to the shape of the lingual periphery of the impression.
    b. Seal into place with a warm spatula, taking care that no heat is applied to the anatomic portions of the impression.
    c. Cool under running water.

III. MIXING THE STONE
A. Factors Related to Dental Stone That Contribute to the Successful Cast

Texts on dental materials should be reviewed for complete information about gypsum products.[7,8,9] Some pertinent properties are listed here as reference points.
  1. *Dental Stone.* Sensitive to changes in the relative humidity of the atmosphere.
    a. Store in airtight container; close soon after use; do not let water enter the container.
    b. Keep the spoon or scoop (used to remove the powder) clean and dry.
  2. *Water.* Controls the strength, rigidity, and hardness of the cast.
    a. Temperature. Generally, cooler water decreases the setting time and warmer water increases it.
    b. Quantity. Follow manufacturer's proportions exactly. Increasing the water over the specifications prolongs the setting time and reduces the strength.

  3. *Spatulation.* Prolonged or very rapid mixing can hasten the chemical reaction and shorten the setting time.

B. The Mix
  1. Measure the water and powder by the manufacturer's specifications.
    a. White stone is generally preferred for study casts. Plaster produces a cast more susceptible to breakage.
    b. Ratio of 30 to 40 ml water to 100 g stone.
  2. Place measured water (room temperature) in a clean, dry mixing bowl.
  3. Sift in the powder gradually to prevent air trapping and to allow each particle to become wet.
  4. Wait briefly until all powder is wet, then vibrate to release large bubbles.
  5. Use vacuum mixer (follow manufacturer's directions).
  6. The result is a smooth, homogeneous, creamy mix.

IV. POURING THE CAST
The finished cast has two connected parts, the anatomic portion and the base or art portion (see figure 10–6, page 175).

A. Pouring the Anatomic Portion
  1. Shake water out of the impression.
  2. Hold the impression tray by the handle and press handle against the vibrator.
  3. With a small amount of stone mix on the end of the spatula, start at one posterior corner and allow the mix to flow through the impression. Use small amounts and vibrate continually.
    a. Tip the impression so the material passes into the tooth indentations and flows slowly down the side, across the occlusal surface or the incisal edge, and up the other side of the impression of each tooth.
    b. Air is trapped when the process is hurried or when too large a quantity of mix is poured in at one time without attentive control of the flow.
  4. When all tooth indentations are covered, add larger amounts of mix to fill the impression slightly over the periphery. Vibrate.

B. One-Step Method for Forming the Base of the Cast
  1. Fill rubber model-base former with the remainder of the mix, or form a mass of stone on a glass or ceramic slab or other nonabsorbent surface (waxed paper on a smooth surface). Add excess stone at the heel areas.
  2. Invert the poured impression onto the base.
    a. Use a slight back-and-forth motion to secure the two parts together.

b. Avoid the common error of inverting the impression before the stone is firm. The mix can flow out of the impression.

3. Adjust tray to proper position

a. Occlusal plane (at premolars) should be parallel with the base of the model-base former or tabletop.

b. Midline (anterior as judged by handle of impression tray) centered at the midline of the model-base former.

c. Accommodate position so that a tooth in labio- or buccoversion does not protrude over the trimming line of the art portion (see figure 10–6).

4. Add stone on peripheral and heel areas to provide a smooth surface; remove excess so that wax periphery of the tray is visible. When excess stone above the edge of the tray rim is permitted to set, the tray is difficult to separate, and the use of a knife to carve the excess from the tray may damage the cast.

5. Final set occurs within 1 hour. Separate 1 hour after pouring to preserve the accuracy and prevent damage to the surface of the cast.

C. Other Methods for Forming the Base of the Cast

1. *Two-step or Double-pour.* Both maxillary and mandibular impressions are poured and left upright (see "Pouring the Anatomic Portion," page 172). Stone is then prepared separately for the bases, and the model-base formers are filled or the mass is placed on the smooth nonabsorbent surface.

   The impression is inverted and held on the surface of the new stone while the sides and periphery are shaped and smoothed. An advantage to this method is that there is no danger of inverting the poured impression too soon. If the cast is turned before it starts to set, the unset stone can fall away from the occlusal and incisal portions and leave bubbles in strategic places.

2. *Boxing Technique.* The object is to form a wall around the impression before pouring to provide a shape for the base as well as to prevent the need for inverting the poured impression. A strip of utility (beading) wax is attached slightly below the periphery of the impression and completely around the impression. Boxing wax or baseplate is applied around the strip of utility wax and attached to it by means of a warm spatula at a height that allows for proper thickness of the final cast, about ½ inch. Care must be taken not to displace the impression dimensionally nor to touch the anatomic portions with the warm spatula. Pouring is carried out as described previously.

Work-model formers with side walls to provide the boxing effect are available. Such a mold has a slot through the rubber where the handle of the impression tray can be inserted.

V. SEPARATION OF THE IMPRESSION AND THE CAST

A. Objective is to remove tray and impression material without breaking the teeth.

B. When model-based former is used, remove it first.

C. Cut away stone from the periphery to free the margin of the tray.

D. Remove the tray by itself.

E. Cut the impression material along the line of the occlusal surfaces and peel off the impression material (with care not to scratch the stone cast during cutting).

F. Direct removal is possible when the teeth are in reasonably normal alignment; remove the tray and the impression material with a straight pull after first releasing the anterior portion by a slight downward and forward movement. When this method is used, do not apply lateral pressures or rock the tray back and forth, because the teeth are broken easily by such forces.

G. Trimming is started promptly, or if delayed, the cast must be thoroughly soaked in water before trimming.

TRIMMING THE CASTS

The exact proportions of the study casts and the steps required to accomplish the trimming and finishing depend on several factors, including the measurements of the patient's dental arches, the positions of the teeth, and the preferences of the dentist. Development of a routine, systematic procedure for trimming can lead to the production of consistent, attractive, and useful diagnostic casts.

The method described here depends on the use of a precision-type model trimmer. No specific directions are provided for the use of angulators that are available to fit on the table of the model trimmer to give average set angles for trimming the margins of the casts; when these are available, directions are usually supplied by the manufacturer.

When a mechanical model trimmer is not available, greater skill must be developed to produce well-proportioned and smooth casts. The use of the model-base formers or a boxing method can be developed to a higher degree of precision. Trimming with a plaster knife must be started as soon as the impression is separated. Plaster files are available to aid in cutting the borders of the base.

TABLE 10-2
CRITERIA FOR AN ACCEPTABLE CAST

Cast Feature	Criteria	Figure Number
Overall base shape	See figure 10–5 with labels	10–5
Proportions	⅓ art portion ⅔ anatomic portion	10–6A
Bases	Mean occlusal plane of the related casts = parallel with both bases Bases are parallel with each other	10–6A

Posterior borders	(1) At a right angle with bases
	(2) Stand on the posterior borders: the casts rest together in natural intercuspation
	(3) Posterior borders are perpendicular
	    (a) to median line from the incisors through palate
	    (b) to middle of tongue
		10–6B
		10–6B
		
		10–7A
		10–7B

Sides	Symmetrical angulation with posterior border and heel cuts Parallel with line through the occlusal grooves of the premolars of each side	10–7 10–10A
Heels	½-inch cuts parallel with the mesiodistal plane of the opposite canine	10–10B
Anterior	Maxillary: pointed with the cuts extending from canine area Mandibular: arc shape	10–11A 10–11B
Borders	Posterior: includes retromolar area and tuberosity Sides: ¼ to 5/16 inch from protuberance over premolars and molars; anatomy of mucobuccal fold included Anterior: ¼ to 5/16 inch from the most protruded tooth or from depth of the mucobuccal fold, whichever is most facial	10–7 10–11
Surfaces of the cast	Smooth and polished with air bubbles removed or filled	

I. OBJECTIVES: CHARACTERISTICS OF THE FINISHED CASTS

Before the step-by-step description of the trimming procedure, an outline of the characteristics of the finished casts is provided as an overall guide. Table 10–2 lists the criteria for each cast feature.

II. PRELIMINARY STEPS TO TRIMMING THE CAST

  A. Casts must be wet; soak at least 5 minutes.
  B. Remove bubbles of stone on or about the teeth with a small sharp instrument; use care not to scar the cast.
  C. Level down excess stone that is distal to the retromolar area and tuberosity so casts may be occluded. Do not shorten the cast anteriorly-posteriorly at this time.
  D. Trim casts conservatively on the sides to make a smooth surface for marking.

III. TRIMMING THE BASES
  A. Objectives
    1. To make bases parallel with the mean occlusal plane and to each other.
    2. To make correct proportions for the height of

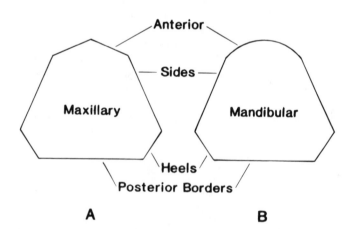

FIG. 10–5. Base Shapes for Finished Study Casts. Maxillary and mandibular casts are trimmed at the labeled areas. See text for procedures.

the casts; art portion one-third and anatomic portion two-thirds (figure 10–6A).

  B. Mandibular Cast Is Trimmed First
    1. Measure the greatest height of the anatomic portion (usually this is from the tip of the canine to the depth of the vestibule) with a plastic ruler (figure 10–8).

6. **Wood,** P.R.: *Cross Infection Control in Dentistry: A Practical Illustrated Guide.* St. Louis, Mosby, 1992, pp. 159–163.
7. **McCabe:** op. cit., pp. 28–33.
8. **Craig:** op. cit., pp. 347–373.
9. **Phillips:** op. cit., pp. 69–92.

SUGGESTED READINGS

Andrieu, S.C. and Springstead, M.C.: A Simplified Guide To Taking Accurate Alginate Impressions and Trimming Diagnostic Study Casts, *J. Practical Hygiene, 1,* 11, September, 1992.

McCance, A.M., Perera, S., and Woods, S.J.W.: Trimming Study Models for Photocopying, *J. Clin. Orthod., 25,* 445, July, 1991.

Pratten, D.H. and Novetsky, M.: Detail Reproduction of Soft Tissue: A Comparison of Impression Materials, *J. Prosthet. Dent., 65,* 188, February, 1991.

Schiele, R.J. and Aucoin, L.: Pouring Impressions, *Dental Assistant Update, 1,* 4, Second Quarter, 1992.

Torres, H.O. and Ehrlich, A.: *Modern Dental Assisting,* 3rd ed. Philadelphia, W.B. Saunders Co., 1990, pp. 478–487.

von Krammer, R.: Avoidance of Cast Breakage During Removal from the Impression, *Quintessence Int., 21,* 217, March, 1990.

Woodall, I.R., Dafoe, B.R., Young, N.S., Weed-Fonner, L., and Yankell, S.L.: *Comprehensive Dental Hygiene Care,* 3rd ed. St. Louis, Mosby, 1989, pp. 289–314.

Infection Control

Brauner, A.W.: *In Vitro* and Clinical Examination of the Effect of an Antimicrobial Impression Material on the Oral Microflora, *Dental Materials, 6,* 201, July, 1990.

Chia, W.K., Stevens, L., and Basford, K.E.: Dimensional Change of Impressions on Sterilization, *Aust. Dent. J., 35,* 23, February, 1990.

Davis, D.R., Curtis, D.A., and White, J.M.: Microwave Irradiation of Contaminated Dental Casts, *Quintessence Int., 20,* 583, August, 1989.

Gerhardt, D.E. and Williams, H.N.: Factors Affecting the Stability of Sodium Hypochlorite Solutions Used to Disinfect Dental Impressions, *Quintessence Int., 22,* 587, July, 1991.

Ishida, H., Nahara, Y., Tamamoto, M., and Hamada, T.: The Fungicidal Effect of Ultraviolet Light on Impression Materials, *J. Prosthet. Dent., 65,* 532, April, 1991.

Merchant, V.A.: Disinfection of Dental Impressions, *Dent. Teamwork, 3,* 13, January-February, 1990.

Peutzfeldt, A. and Asmussen, E.: Effect of Disinfecting Solutions on Accuracy of Alginate and Elastomeric Impressions, *Scand. J. Dent. Res., 97,* 470, October, 1989.

Peutzfeldt, A. and Asmussen, E.: Effect of Disinfecting Solutions on Surface Texture of Alginate and Elastomeric Impressions, *Scand, J. Dent. Res., 98,* 74, February, 1990.

Samaranayake, L.P., Hunjan, M., and Jennings, K.J.: Carriage of Oral Flora on Irreversible Hydrocolloid and Elastomeric Impression Materials, *J. Prosthet. Dent., 65,* 244, February, 1991.

Sicurelli, R.J. and Boylan, R.J.: Bacterial Contamination in Reversible Hydrocolloid Conditioning Units, *J. Prosthet. Dent., 65,* 16, January, 1991.

Tebrock, O.C., Engelmeier, R.L., Mayfield, T.G., and Adams, H.J.U.: Managing Dental Impressions and Casts of Patients With Communicable Diseases, *Gen. Dent., 37,* 490, November-December, 1989.

Touyz, L.Z.G. and Rosen, M.: Disinfection of Alginate Impression Material Using Disinfectants as Mixing and Soak Solutions, *J. Dent., 19,* 255, August, 1991.

The Gingiva

The true test of successful treatment, the real evaluation of the effects of scaling and related instrumentation, is the *health* of the gingival tissues. The objective of all treatment is to bring the diseased gingiva to a state of health that can be maintained by the patient. To do this, the first objective is to learn to recognize normal healthy tissue; to observe certain characteristics of color, texture, and form; to test for bleeding; and to apply this knowledge to the treatment and supervision of the patient's gingiva until health is attained.

An outline of the clinical features of the periodontal tissues in health and disease is included in this chapter. Key words are defined in table 11–1.

OBJECTIVES

The ultimate objective is to apply the dental hygienist's knowledge and skill in examination and evaluation of the periodontal tissues to patient care so that each patient attains and maintains optimum oral health. The dental hygienist must know when the treatment provided by dental hygiene services is definitive in restoring health and when additional treatment is needed. The patient can be properly informed so that complete treatment can be provided.

Specific objectives for the dental hygienist are to be able to

I. Recognize normal periodontal tissues.
II. Know the clinical features of the periodontal tissues that must be examined for a complete assessment.
III. Recognize the markers that are the basic signs of periodontal infections and classify them by type and degree of severity.
IV. Identify the dental hygiene treatment and instruction needed.
V. Outline the patient's preventive periodontal program (pages 330 and 331).

THE TREATMENT AREA

The treatment procedures of dental hygiene are applied directly to the teeth, the gingiva, and the gingival sulcus. Detailed knowledge and understanding of the anatomy and normal clinical appearance of the hard and soft oral tissues are prerequisite to meaningful examination and treatment.

I. THE TEETH

A. Clinical Crown
The part of the tooth above the attached periodontal tissues. It can be considered the part of the tooth where clinical treatment procedures are applied (figure 11–1).

B. Clinical Root
The part of the tooth below the base of the gingival sulcus or periodontal pocket. It is the part of the root to which periodontal fibers are attached.

C. Anatomic Crown
The part of the tooth covered by enamel.

D. Anatomic Root
The part of the tooth covered by cementum.

Questions ?
- Oral Hygiene

How they want presented
all we handing it in
Hand in procedure cards.

- How does self aspirating
syringe work.

Questions

Topical Local Anesth

SYRINGE *

Rubber dam

TABLE 11–2 (continued)
EXAMINATION OF THE GINGIVA. CLINICAL MARKERS.

	Appearance in Health	Changes in Disease Clinical Appearance	Causes for Changes
Surface Texture	Free gingiva: smooth Attached gingiva: stippled	Acute condition: smooth, shiny gingiva Chronic: hard, firm, with stippling, sometimes heavier than normal	Inflammatory changes in the connective tissue; edema, cellular infiltration Fibrosis
Position of Gingival Margin	Fully erupted tooth: margin is 1–2 mm above cementoenamel junction, at or slightly below the enamel contour	Enlarged gingiva: margin is higher on the tooth, above normal, pocket deepened Recession: margin is more apical; root surface is exposed	Edematous or fibrotic Junctional epithelium has migrated along the root; gingival margin follows
Position of Junctional Epithelium	During eruption: along the enamel surface Fully erupted tooth: the junctional epithelium is at the cementoenamel junction	Position, determined by use of probe, is on the root surface	Apical migration of the epithelium along the root
Mucogingival Junctions	Make clear demarcation between the pink, stippled, attached gingiva and the darker alveolar mucosa with smooth shiny surface	No attached gingiva: (1) color changes may extend full height of the gingiva; mucogingival line obliterated (2) Probing reveals that the bottom of the pocket extends into the alveolar mucosa (3) Frenal pull may displace the gingival margin from the tooth	Deepening of the pocket Apical migration of the junctional epithelium Attached gingiva decreases with pocket deepening Inflammation extends into alveolar mucosa
Bleeding	No spontaneous bleeding or upon probing	Spontaneous bleeding Bleeding on probing: Bleeding near margin in acute condition; bleeding deep in pocket in chronic condition	Degeneration of the sulcular epithelium with the formation of pocket epithelium Blood vessels engorged Tissue edematous
Exudate	No exudate on pressure	White fluid, pus, visible on digital pressure Amount not related to pocket depth	Inflammation in the connective tissue Excessive accumulation of white blood cells with serum and tissue fluid makes up the exudate (pus)

patients and among teeth for an individual, from 1 to 9 mm.[5]

b. Wider in maxilla than mandible; broadest zone related to incisors, narrowest at the canine and premolar regions.

B. Changes in Disease

1. *Free Gingiva and Papillae.* Become enlarged. May be localized or limited to specific areas or generalized throughout the gingiva. The col deepens as the papillae increase in size.

2. *Attached Gingiva.* Decreases in amount as the pocket deepens. Measurement of the amount of attached gingiva is described on page 217 and figure 13–10.

C. Enlargement from Drug Therapy

Certain drugs used for specific systemic therapy cause gingival enlargement as a side effect. Examples of such drugs are phenytoin, cyclosporin, and nifedipine. They are described on page 203 along with other contributing factors to disease development.

III. SHAPE (FORM OR CONTOUR)
A. Signs of Health
1. *Free Gingiva*
   a. Follows a curved line around each tooth; may be straighter along wide molar surfaces.
   b. The margin is knife-edged or slightly rounded on facial and lingual gingiva; closely adapted to the tooth surface.
2. *Papillae*
   a. Teeth with contact area. Facial and lingual gingiva are pointed or slightly rounded papillae with a col area under the contact (figure 11–8).
   b. Spaced teeth (with diastemas). Interdental gingiva is flat or saddle-shaped (figure 12–4D, page 203).

B. Changes in Disease
1. *Free Gingiva.* Rounded or rolled.
2. *Papillae.* Blunted, flattened, bulbous, cratered (figure 11–10).
3. *Festoon ("McCall's festoon").* An enlargement of the marginal gingiva with the formation of a lifesaver-like gingival prominence. Frequently, the total gingiva is very narrow, with associated apparent recession as shown in figure 11–10D.
4. *Clefts*
   a. "Stillman's cleft" (figure 11–11). A localized recession may be V-shaped, apostrophe-shaped, or form a slit-like indentation. It may extend several millimeters toward the mucogingival junction or even to or through the junction.
   b. Floss cleft. A cleft created by incorrect floss positioning appears as a vertical linear or V-shaped fissure in the marginal gingiva.[6] It usually occurs at one side of an interdental papilla. The injury can develop when dental floss is curved repeatedly in an incomplete "C" around the line angle so the floss is pressed across the gingiva. Correct flossing positioning is shown in figure 23–1 on page 355.

IV. CONSISTENCY
A. Signs of Health
1. Firm when palpated with the side of a blunt instrument (probe).
2. Attached gingiva is bound down firmly to the underlying bone.

B. Changes in Disease
1. *To Determine Consistency.* Gently press side of probe on free gingiva. Soft, spongy gingiva dents readily; firm, hard tissue resists.

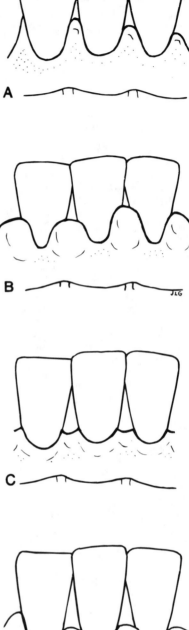

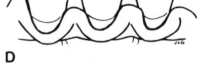

FIG. 11–10. Gingival Shape or Contour. A. Blunted papillae. **B.** Bulbous papillae. **C.** Cratered papillae. **D.** Rolled, lifesaver-shaped "McCall's festoons."

2. *Soft, Spongy Gingiva.* Related to acute stages of inflammation with increased infiltration of fluid and inflammatory elements. The tissue appears red, may be smooth and shiny with loss of stippling, has marginal enlargement, and bleeds readily on probing.

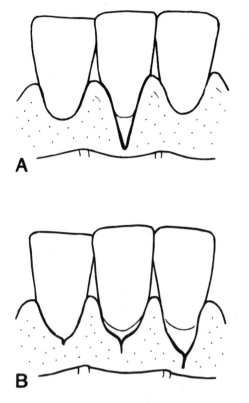

A

B

FIG. 11–11. Gingival Clefts. A. *V-shaped Stillman's cleft.* **B.** *Slit-like Stillman's clefts of varying degrees of severity in relation to the mucogingival junction.*

3. *Firm, Hard Gingiva.* Related to chronic inflammation with increased fibrosis. The tissue may appear pink and well stippled. Bleeding, when probed, usually occurs only in the deeper part of a pocket, not near the margin.
4. *Retraction of the Margin Away from the Tooth.* Normally, the free gingiva fits snugly about the tooth. When the margin tends to hang slightly away or is readily displaced with a light air blast, the gingival fibers that support the margin have been destroyed (figure 11–3).

V. SURFACE TEXTURE
A. Signs of Health
1. *Free Gingiva.* Smooth.
2. *Attached Gingiva.* Stippled (minutely "pebbled" or "orange peel" surface).
3. *Interdental Gingiva.* The free gingiva is smooth; the center portion of each papilla is stippled.

B. Changes in Disease
1. *Inflammatory Changes.* May be loss of stippling, with smooth, shiny surface.
2. *Hyperkeratosis.* May result in a leathery, hard, or nodular surface.
3. *Chronic Disease.* Tissue may be hard and fibrotic, with a normal pink color and normal or deep stippling.

VI. POSITION
The *actual* position of the gingiva is the level of the attached periodontal tissue. It is not directly visible, but can be determined by probing.

The *apparent* position of the gingiva is the level of the gingival margin or crest of the free gingiva that is seen by direct observation.

A. Signs of Health
For the fully erupted tooth in an adult, the apparent position of the gingiva margin is normally at the level of, or slightly below, the enamel contour or prominence of the cervical third of a tooth.

B. Changes in Disease
1. *Effect of Gingival Enlargement.* When the gingiva enlarges, the gingival margin may be high on the enamel, partly or nearly covering the anatomic crown.
2. *Effect of Gingival Recession*
   a. Definition. Recession is the exposure of root surface that results from the apical migration of the junctional epithelium (figure 11–12).
   b. Actual recession. The actual recession is shown by the position of the attachment level. The "receded area" is from the cementoenamel junction to the attachment.

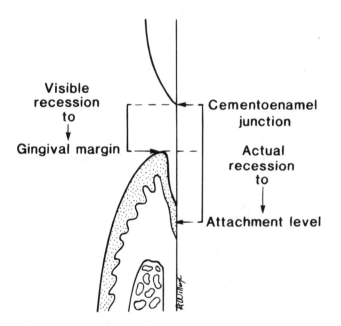

FIG. 11–12. Gingival Recession. Left, *Clinically visible recession of the gingival margin with root surface apparent to the eye.* **Right,** *The actual recession exposes the root surface as the periodontal attachment migrates along the root surface.*

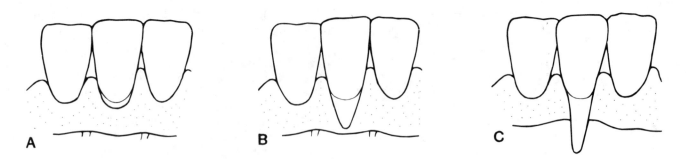

FIG. 11–13. Localized Recession. A single tooth may show narrow or wide, deep or shallow recession. **A.** Wide, shallow. **B.** Wide, deep, with narrow attached gingiva. **C.** Narrow, deep, with missing attached gingiva.

c. Apparent recession. The apparent recession is the exposed root surface that is visible on clinical examination. It is seen from the gingival margin to the cementoenamel junction.

d. Localized recession (figure 11–13). A localized recession may be narrow or wide, deep or shallow. The root surface is denuded, and the apparent recession may extend to or through the mucogingival junction.

e. Measurement. Both actual and apparent recession can be measured with a probe from the cementoenamel junction. Total recession is the actual and apparent positions added together.

VII. BLEEDING
A. Signs of Health
1. No bleeding spontaneously or on probing.
2. Healthy tissue does not bleed.

B. Changes in Disease
1. Bleeding occurs spontaneously or when probed.
2. Sulcular epithelium becomes diseased *pocket epithelium.* The ulcerated pocket wall bleeds readily on gentle probing. Development of inflammation and pocket formation is described on pages 195–197.

VIII. EXUDATE
A. Signs of Health
There is no exudate except slight gingival sulcus fluid (page 184). Gingival sulcus fluid cannot be seen by direct observation.

B. Changes in Disease
1. *Suppuration.* Formation or secretion of pus.
2. *White Fluid* (pus and subgingival bacterial plaque). May appear at the entrance to the pocket or may be squeezed out of the pocket by light finger pressure on the external wall of the pocket.

3. *Amount of Exudate.* Related to the severity of the acute inflammation, not to the depth of the pocket.

IX. THE GINGIVA OF YOUNG CHILDREN[7]
A. Signs of Health
1. *Primary Dentition*
   a. Color. Pink or slightly red.
   b. Shape. Thick, rounded, or rolled.
   c. Consistency. Firm, but not tightly adapted to the teeth; it may be easily displaced with a light air jet.
   d. Surface texture: May or may not have stippling; high percentage of patients has shiny gingiva.
   e. Width of attached gingiva in children ages 3 to 5. Between 1 and 6 mm.[5]
   f. Interdental gingiva.
      i. Anterior: diastemas are frequently present and the papillae are flat or saddle-shaped.
      ii. Posterior: col between facial and lingual papillae when teeth are in contact (figure 11–8).
2. *Mixed Dentition*
   a. Constant state of change related to exfoliation and eruption.
   b. Free gingiva may appear rolled or rounded, slightly reddened, shiny, and with a lack of firmness.
   c. The gingiva covers a varying portion of the anatomic crown, depending on the stage of eruption (figure 11–7).

B. Changes in Disease
Examination of the periodontal tissues of a child is not different from that of an adult. A complete examination is necessary, including probing around each tooth.

Gingivitis occurs frequently in children.

Although relatively rare, periodontitis can occur in primary dentition. Prepubertal periodontitis is described on page 198, in table 12–3.

Mucogingival problems occur in children.[8,9] The recognition of deficiencies of attached gingiva has particular significance for the child who will need orthodontic treatment.

X. THE GINGIVA AFTER PERIODONTAL SURGERY

The characteristics of "normal healthy gingiva" take on different dimensions for the patient who has completed treatment for pockets, bone loss, and other signs of a periodontal disease. The junctional epithelium is apical to the cementoenamel junction. After healing, the sulcus depth may be within normal range and no bleeding should occur when probed.

Depending on the exact treatment performed, examination shows changes from the initial evaluation. For example, where the initial examination showed a deficiency of attached gingiva with frenal pull, mucogingival surgery may have been designed and treatment satisfactorily completed to create new attached gingiva. With each maintenance appointment, a thorough, careful examination is necessary to control factors that may permit recurrence of disease.

FACTORS TO TEACH THE PATIENT

I. Characteristics of normal healthy gingiva.
II. The significance of bleeding; healthy tissue does not bleed.
III. Relationship of findings during a gingival examination to the personal daily care procedures for infection control.
IV. The special attention needed for an area of gingival recession to prevent abrasion, inflammation, and further involvement.
V. How the method of brushing, stiffness of toothbrush filaments, abrasiveness of a dentrifice, and pressure applied during brushing can be factors in gingival recession.
VI. Eight Warning Signs of Periodontal Disease*
  1. Gums that bleed when you brush your teeth.
  2. Gums that are red, swollen, or tender.
  3. Gums that have pulled away from the teeth.
  4. Pus between the teeth and gums when the gums are pressed.
  5. Permanent teeth that are loose or separating.
  6. Any change in the way your teeth fit together when you bite.
  7. Any changes in the fit of your partial dentures.
  8. Bad breath.

* From *Gum Disease: The Warning Signs.* American Dental Association, Department of Salable Materials, 211 E. Chicago Avenue, Chicago, IL 60611.

REFERENCES

1. **Avery,** J.K. and Steele, P.F.: *Essentials of Oral Histology and Embryology. A Clinical Approach.* St. Louis, Mosby, 1992, pp. 131–134.
2. **Ainamo,** J. and Löe, H.: Anatomical Characteristics of Gingiva. A Clinical and Microscopic Study of the Free and Attached Gingiva, *J. Periodontol.,* 37, 5, January-February, 1966.
3. **Orban,** B.: Clinical and Histologic Study of the Surface Characteristics of the Gingiva, *Oral Surg. Oral Med. Oral Pathol., 1,* 827, September, 1948.
4. **Bhaskar,** S.N., ed.: *Orban's Oral Histology and Embryology,* 11th ed. St. Louis, Mosby, 1991, pp. 323–325.
5. **Bowers,** G.M.: A Study of the Width of Attached Gingiva, *J. Periodontol.,* 34, 201, May, 1963.
6. **Hallman,** W.W., Waldrop, T.C., Houston, G.D., and Hawkins, B.F.: Flossing Clefts. Clinical and Histologic Observations, *J. Periodontol.,* 57, 501, August, 1986.
7. **Carranza,** F.A.: *Glickman's Clinical Periodontology,* 7th ed. Philadelphia, W.B. Saunders Co., 1990, pp. 286–292.
8. **Maynard,** J.G. and Ochsenbein, C.: Mucogingival Problems, Prevalence and Therapy in Children, *J. Periodontol.,* 46, 543, September, 1975.
9. **Andlin-Sobocki,** A., Marcusson, A., and Persson, M.: 3-Year Observations on Gingival Recession in Mandibular Incisors in Children, *J. Clin. Periodontol.,* 18, 155, March, 1991.

SUGGESTED READINGS

Ainamo, A., Ainamo, J., and Poikkeus, R.: Continuous Widening of the Band of Attached Gingiva From 23 to 65 Years of Age, *J. Periodont. Res.,* 16, 595, November, 1981.

Carranza, F.A.: *Glickman's Clinical Periodontology,* 7th ed. Philadelphia, W.B. Saunders Co., 1990, pp. 14–50.

Caton, J., Polson, A., Bouwsma, O., Blieden, T., Frantz, B., and Espeland, M.: Associations Between Bleeding and Visual Signs of Interdental Gingival Inflammation, *J. Periodontol.,* 59, 722, November, 1988.

Fedi, P.F., ed.: *The Periodontic Syllabus,* 2nd ed. Philadelphia, Lea & Febiger, 1989, pp. 1–13.

Gliksberg, J.H., Mintz, A., Hochberg, M.S., and Sher, M.R.: The Incidence of Mucogingival Defects: Report of Case, *J. Am. Dent. Assoc., 119,* 625, November, 1989.

Grant, D.A., Stern, I.B., and Listgarten, M.A., eds.: *Periodontics,* 6th ed. St. Louis, Mosby, 1988, pp. 3–75.

Hicks, M.J., Uldricks, J.M., Whitacre, H.L., Anderson, J., and Moeschberger, M.L.: A National Study of Periodontal Assessment by Dental Hygienists, *J. Dent. Hyg.,* 67, 82, February, 1993.

Hoag, P.M. and Pawlak, E.A.: *Essentials of Periodontics,* 4th ed. St. Louis, Mosby, 1990, pp. 1–18.

Melfi, R.C.: *Permar's Oral Embryology and Microscopic Anatomy,* 8th ed. Philadelphia, Lea & Febiger, 1988, pp. 217–231.

Gingiva of Children

Andlin-Sobocki, A.: Changes of Facial Gingival Dimensions in Children. A 2-year Longitudinal Study, *J. Clin. Periodontol.,* 20, 212, March, 1993.

Andlin-Sobocki, A. and Bodin, L.: Dimensional Alterations of the Gingiva Related to Changes of Facial/Lingual Tooth Position in Permanent Anterior Teeth of Children. A 2-year Longitudinal Study. *J. Clin. Periodontol.,* 20, 218, March, 1993.

Bimstein, E. and Eidelman, E.: Longitudinal Changes in the Width of Attached Gingiva in Children, *Pediatr. Dent., 10,* 22, March, 1988.

Bimstein, E., Machtei, E., and Eidelman, E.: Dimensional Differences in the Attached and Keratinized Gingiva and Gingival Sulcus in the Early Permanent Dentition: A Longitudinal Study, *J. Pedod., 10,* 247, Spring, 1986.

Keszthelyi, G.: The Width of Plaque-free Zones on Primary Molars With Attachment Loss, *J. Clin. Periodontol., 18,* 94, February, 1991.

Keszthelyi, G. and Szabo, I.: Attachment Loss in Primary Molars, *J. Clin. Periodontol., 14,* 48, January, 1987.

Tenenbaum, H. and Tenenbaum, M.: A Clinical Study of the Width of the Attached Gingiva in the Deciduous, Transitional and Permanent Dentitions, *J. Clin. Periodontol., 13,* 270, April, 1986.

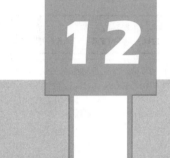

Disease Development and Contributing Factors

Early in the process of case assessment in preparation for treatment planning, the presence and severity of periodontal infection must be determined. Is the patient's disease limited to the gingival tissue without loss of periodontal attachment? Does the patient have bone loss, pocket formation, or other signs of periodontitis?

Table 12–1 shows the clinical case types. The case type designation for a patient is determined by first noting the gingival markers by direct observation (table 11–2, page 188), and then using the probe and studying the radiographs. The probe is utilized for many parts of the examination, one of which is assessment of the gingival and periodontal probing depths.

When the disease is limited to the gingiva, the possibility of reversal of the infection is considered first in the treatment planning objectives. Can the patient be guided to learn new habits of self-treatment through daily infection control supplemented by periodic professional scaling? On the other hand, if there is apical positioning of the periodontal attachment with alveolar bone loss and other indications of periodontitis, can conservative procedures of *nonsurgical periodontal therapy* provide sufficient professional treatment? Is more complex periodontal therapy required?

Individual differences and the particular clinical features of each patient must be recognized. The oral tissues need treatment that can bring them to a state of maximum health that can be maintained by the patient.

Except in cases of advanced periodontitis, the need for additional treatment after initial nonsurgical periodontal therapy is rarely possible to predict. A reassessment of the treated tissues must be built into the treatment plan. The patient must be given a clear understanding of the purpose of such a re-evaluation.

In this chapter, gingival and periodontal pockets and their development are described. Contributing factors in disease progression are outlined. Key words are defined in table 12–2.

DEVELOPMENT OF GINGIVAL AND PERIODONTAL INFECTIONS

The stages of development of gingivitis are divided into the *initial lesion,* the *early lesion,* and the *established lesion.*[1] With an accumulation of bacterial plaque on the cervical tooth surface adjacent to the gingival margin, an inflammatory reaction is set up, and the natural defense mechanisms respond. Plaque formation is described in Chapter 16.

I. THE INITIAL LESION

A. Inflammatory Response to Bacterial Plaque
Occurs within 2 to 4 days.
1. Migration and infiltration of white blood cells into the junctional epithelium and gingival sulcus.
2. Increased flow of gingival sulcus fluid.
3. Early breakdown of collagen; fluid fills the spaces in the connective tissue.

B. Clinical Appearance
No evidence of change appears in the earliest phases.

II. THE EARLY LESION

A. Inflammatory Response
Continues.
1. Bacterial plaque becomes older and thicker (7 to 14 days).

195

Case Type I—Gingival disease
Inflammation of the gingiva characterized clinically by changes in color, gingival form, position, surface appearance, and presence of bleeding and/or exudate.

Case Type II—Early periodontitis
Progression of the gingival inflammation into the deeper periodontal structures and alveolar bone crest, with slight bone loss. There is usually a slight loss of connective tissue attachment and alveolar bone.

Case Type III—Moderate periodontitis
A more advanced stage of the preceding condition, with increased destruction of the periodontal structures and noticeable loss of bone support, possibly accompanied by an increase in tooth mobility. There may be furcation involvement in multirooted teeth.

Case Type IV—Advanced periodontitis
Further progression of periodontitis with major loss of alveolar bone support usually accompanied by increased tooth mobility. Furcation involvement in multirooted teeth is likely.

Case Type V—Refractory periodontitis
Includes those patients with multiple disease sites that continue to demonstrate attachment loss after appropriate therapy. These sites presumably continue to be infected by periodontal pathogens no matter how thorough or frequent the treatment provided. Also includes those patients with recurrent disease at single or multiple sites.

(From American Academy of Periodontology: *Current Procedural Terminology for Periodontics and Insurance Reporting Manual,* 6th ed. Chicago, 1991.)

2. Infiltration of fluid, lymphocytes, and a few plasma cells into the connective tissue.
3. Breakdown of collagen fiber support to the gingival margin.
4. Epithelium proliferates and epithelial extensions and rete ridges are formed.

B. Clinical Appearance
1. Early signs of gingivitis become apparent with slight gingival enlargement; will become an established lesion if undisturbed.
2. Early gingivitis is reversible when plaque is controlled and inflammation is reduced. Healthy tissue may be restored.

III. THE ESTABLISHED LESION
A. Progression from the Early Lesion
1. Fluid increases; the predominant inflammatory cells are plasma cells (figure 59–1, page 803). Plasma cells are related to areas of chronic inflammation.

Cicatrix (sĭk'ah-triks): the fibrous tissue left after the healing of a wound; adj. cicatricial.
Collagen (kŏl'ah-jen): white fibers of the connective tissue.
Collagenase (kŏl-laj'ĕ-nās): enzyme that catalyzes the degradation (hydrolysis) of collagen.
Desquamation (des'kwah-mā'shun): shedding of the outer epithelial layer of the stratified squamous epithelium of skin or mucosa.
Diastema (dī-ahs'tē-mah): a space or abnormal opening; as a dental term, it is a space between two adjacent teeth in the same dental arch.
Edema (ĕ-dē'mah): an accumulation of excessive fluid in cells, tissues, or a serous cavity.
Enzyme (en'zīm): a protein secreted by body cells that acts as a catalyst to induce chemical changes in other substances, but remains unchanged itself.
Food impaction: forceful wedging of food into the periodontium by occlusal forces.
Gingivitis (jin'-jī-vī'tis): inflammation of the gingival tissues.
Iatrogenic (ī-at'rō-jen'ik): resulting from treatment by a professional person.
Infiltration (in'fil-trā'shun): the diffusion or accumulation in a tissue or cells of substances not normal to it or in amounts in excess of normal.
Lesion (lē'zhun): any pathologic or traumatic discontinuity of tissue or loss of function of a part; broad term including wounds, sores, ulcers, tumors, and any other tissue damage.
Nonsurgical periodontal therapy: includes bacterial plaque removal and plaque control (patient and clinician), supra- and subgingival scaling, root planing, and the adjunctive use of chemotherapeutic agents for control of bacterial infection, desensitizing hypersensitive exposed root surfaces, and dental caries prevention as related to the health of the periodontium.
Periodontitis (per'ē-ō-don-tī'tis): inflammation in the periodontium affecting gingival tissues, periodontal ligament, cementum, and supporting bone.
Permeable (per'mē-ah-b'l): permitting passage of a fluid.
Refractory (rē-frak'tō-rē): not readily responsive to treatment.
Toxin (tok'sin): a poison; protein produced by certain animals, higher plants, and pathogenic bacteria.
  Bacterial toxin: poison produced by bacteria; includes exotoxins, endotoxins, and toxic enzymes.
Xerostomia (ze'ro-stō'mē-ah): dryness of the mouth from a lack of normal secretions.

2. Formation of *pocket epithelium.*
   a. Proliferation of the junctional and sulcular epithelium continues.
   b. Areas of ulceration of the lining epithelium develop.
   c. Gingival pocket results.
3. Collagen destruction continues; connective tissue fiber support lost.

4. Progression to early periodontal lesion may occur, or some established lesions may remain stable for extended periods of time.

B. Clinical Appearance

Clear evidence of inflammation is present with marginal redness, bleeding on probing, and spongy marginal gingiva. Later, chronic fibrosis develops.

IV. PERIODONTITIS

Bacteria from supragingival plaque enter the sulcus and provide the source for subgingival plaque bacteria.

A. Extension of Inflammation

1. Plaque microorganisms produce irritants.
2. Inflammatory response continues.
3. Inflammation spreads through the loose connective tissue along (beside) the blood vessels to the alveolar bone.[2]
4. Most commonly the inflammation enters the bone through small vessel channels in the alveolar crest.
5. Inflammation spreads through the bone marrow and out into the periodontal ligament.

B. Progressive Destruction of Connective Tissue.

1. Connective tissue fibers below the junctional epithelium are destroyed; the epithelium migrates along the root surface.
2. Coronal portion of junctional epithelium becomes detached.
3. Exposed cementum where Sharpey's fibers were attached becomes altered by inflammatory products of bacteria and the sulcus fluid.
4. Diseased cementum contains a thin superficial layer of endotoxin from the bacterial breakdown.
5. Without treatment, the pocket becomes progressively deepened.

C. Characteristics of the Advanced Lesion

1. Persistence of the chronic inflammatory process.
2. Periodontal pockets develop; calculus formation progresses.
3. Periods of inactivity alternating with periods of activity can be expected.

V. CLASSIFICATION

Periodontal disease is not a single pathologic entity. It is a term used to describe a variety of inflammatory and degenerative diseases that affect the supporting structures of the teeth. A widely used system for classifying the types and severity of periodontal disease has been prepared by the American Academy of Periodontology as shown in table 12–3.[3]

GINGIVAL AND PERIODONTAL POCKETS

A pocket is a diseased sulcus. It is the presence or absence of infection that distinguishes a pocket from a sulcus and the level of attachment on the tooth that distinguishes a gingival pocket from a periodontal pocket. A pocket has an *inner wall, the tooth surface,* and an *outer wall, the sulcular or pocket epithelium* of the free gingiva. The two walls meet at the base of the pocket.

The base of the pocket is the coronal margin of the attached periodontal tissues. Histologically, the base of a healthy sulcus is the coronal border of the junctional epithelium, whereas the base of a pocket (diseased sulcus) may be at the coronal border of the connective tissue attachment (pages 212 and 213).

Pockets are divided into *gingival* and *periodontal* types to clarify the degree of anatomic involvement. They are then further categorized by their position in relation to the alveolar bone, that is, whether their pocket base is suprabony or intrabony (figure 12–1).

I. GINGIVAL POCKET

A. Definition: a pocket formed by gingival enlargement without apical migration of the junctional epithelium (figure 12–1B).
B. The margin of the gingiva has moved toward the incisal or occlusal without the deeper periodontal structures becoming involved.
C. The tooth wall is enamel.
D. During eruption, the base of the sulcus is at various levels along the enamel. The base of the sulcus of a fully erupted tooth is near the cementoenamel junction (figure 11–7, page 185).
E. All gingival pockets are suprabony; that is, the base of the pocket is coronal to the crest of the alveolar bone.

II. PERIODONTAL POCKET

A. Definition: a pocket formed as a result of disease or degeneration that caused the junctional epithelium to migrate apically along the cementum.
B. The periodontal deeper structures (attachment apparatus) are involved, that is, the cementum, periodontal ligament, and bone.
C. The tooth wall is cementum or partly cementum and partly enamel.
D. The base of the pocket is on cementum at the level of attached periodontal tissue.
E. Periodontal pockets may be suprabony or intrabony.
   1. *Suprabony.* Pocket in which the base of the pocket is coronal to the crest of the alveolar bone (figure 12–1C).
   2. *Intrabony.* Pocket in which the base of the pocket is below or apical to the crest of the alveolar bone (figure 12–1D). "Intra" means located within the bone. The term

---

TABLE 12-3
CLASSIFICATION OF GINGIVAL AND PERIODONTAL DISEASES*

Gingival Diseases

I. Plaque-associated gingivitis
   A. Chronic gingivitis
   B. Acute necrotizing ulcerative gingivitis
   C. Gingivitis associated with systemic conditions or medications. (These forms of gingivitis are plaque-associated but the clinical presentation and therapeutic approaches may be modified by the systemic factors.)
      1. Hormone-influenced gingivitis
      2. Drug-induced gingivitis
      3. HIV gingivitis

II. Gingival manifestations of systemic diseases and mucocutaneous lesions
   A. Bacterial, viral, or fungal (for example, acute herpetic gingivostomatitis)
   B. Blood dyscrasias (for example, acute monocytic leukemia)
   C. Mucocutaneous diseases (for example, lichen planus, cicatricial pemphigoid)

Periodontal Diseases

I. Periodontitis
   A. Early-onset periodontitis—age of onset is usually prior to 35 years; rapid rate of progression of tissue destruction; manifestation of defects in host defense; composition of the associated flora different from that of adult periodontitis.
      1. Prepubertal—may be generalized or localized; onset between eruption of the primary dentition and puberty; may affect the primary and the mixed dentition; characterized by severe gingival inflammation, rapid bone loss, tooth mobility, and tooth loss.
      2. Juvenile—may be generalized or localized; onset during the circumpubertal period; familial distribution; relative paucity of microbial plaque; less acute signs of inflammation than would be expected based upon the severity of destruction; presence of abnormalities in leukocyte chemotaxis and bacteriocidal activity.

   B. Rapidly progressive—most of the teeth are affected; the extent of clinical signs of inflammation may be less than expected; the age of onset is usually in the early 20s through the mid 30s.
   C. Adult periodontitis.
   D. Periodontitis associated with systemic disease (for example, diabetes, HIV infection)—several systemic diseases appear to predispose the affected individuals to periodontitis, which may be of the early-onset type, but which may differ considerably from the early-onset form previously described.
   E. Necrotizing ulcerative periodontitis—severe and rapidly progressive disease that has a distinctive erythema of the free gingiva, attached gingiva, and alveolar mucosa; extensive soft tissue necrosis; severe loss of periodontal attachment; deep pocket formation may not be evident.
   F. Refractory periodontitis—includes patients who are unresponsive to any treatment provided—whatever the thoroughness or frequency—as well as patients with recurrent disease at single or multiple sites.

II. Mucogingival conditions—the anatomy and position of the gingival tissues do not allow the control of inflammation or progressive recession.

III. Occlusal trauma—an injury to the attachment apparatus as a result of excessive occlusal forces.
   A. Primary occlusal trauma—trauma resulting from excessive occlusal forces applied to a tooth or teeth with normal supporting structures.
   B. Secondary occlusal trauma—trauma that occurs when normal occlusal forces are applied to the attachment apparatus of a tooth or teeth with inadequate support.

* Based on The American Academy of Periodontology: *Proceedings of the World Workshop in Clinical Periodontics.* Chicago, The American Academy of Periodontology, 1989, I-23-24.

"infrabony" is used in some texts. "Infra" means under or beneath.

TOOTH SURFACE POCKET WALL

I. TOOTH STRUCTURE INVOLVED

A sulcus or a pocket has a gingival side, which is the sulcular epithelium, and a tooth side. In gingival pockets, the tooth surface wall is enamel, whereas in periodontal pockets, the tooth surface wall is either cementum or a combination of cementum and enamel.

The positions of the periodontal attachment and gingival margin determine whether the tooth surface wall is cementum or enamel. Pockets may be the same depth when measured with a probe, but because of the location of the attachment on the tooth surface, the tooth surface pocket wall varies.

II. CONTENTS OF A POCKET
A. Pocket Size

A pocket is narrow, and the pocket epithelial lining is adjacent to and follows the contour of the tooth. When calculus deposits are present, the pocket wall follows the contour of the calcu-

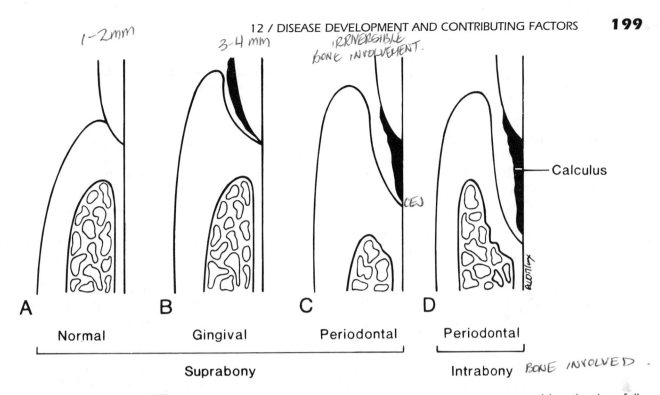

1-2mm   3-4 mm   IRREVERSIBLE BONE INVOLVEMENT.

Calculus

(CEJ)

A — Normal
B — Gingival
C — Periodontal
D — Periodontal

Suprabony   Intrabony   BONE INVOLVED.

FIG. 12–1. Types of Pockets. A. Normal relationship of the gingival tissue and the cementoenamel junction in a fully erupted tooth. **B.** Gingival pocket showing attachment at the cementoenamel junction and the pocket formed by enlarged gingival tissue. There is no bone loss. **C.** Periodontal pocket showing attachment on cementum with root surface exposed. Gingival tissue has enlarged. **D.** Periodontal intrabony pocket with the bottom of the pocket within the bone. See the text for further description of each type of pocket.

lus. The firmness of the free gingiva is influential in confining and shaping the subgingival calculus deposit.

Access of the opening of the pocket to the oral cavity provides an opportunity for bacterial plaque to collect. The deeper the pocket, the less it can be cleaned by toothbrushing or other plaque control devices.

B. Substances Found

Subgingival plaque is described in Chapter 16. Table 16–3 (page 261) lists content and features of subgingival plaque and the periodontal pocket.

The following may be inside a pocket in contact with the tooth surface on one side and with the surface of the pocket epithelium on the other side.

1. Microorganisms and their products; enzymes, endotoxins, and other metabolic products.
2. Calculus deposits and other rough areas covered with bacterial plaque.
3. Gingival sulcus fluid.
4. Desquamated epithelial cells.
5. Leukocytes, the numbers of which increase with increased inflammation in the tissues.
6. Purulent exudate made up of living and bro-

ken down leukocytes, living and dead microorganisms, and serum.

III. NATURE OF THE TOOTH SURFACE

Knowledge of the characteristics and quality of the tooth surface pocket wall is of prime importance in instrumentation. During the examination of the tooth surface with probe and explorer, the various irregularities that can occur must be differentiated. The manner in which the irregularities came into existence is important for interpretation and understanding.

A. Pocket Development Factors

1. The pocket deepens as a result of continuing action of the irritants and destructive agents from bacterial plaque.
2. The periodontal ligament fibers become detached and the junctional epithelium migrates apically.
3. The cementum becomes exposed to the open pocket and the oral fluids.
4. Physical, structural, and chemical changes alter the cementum.
5. Surface changes occur as a result of the exchange of minerals with oral fluids and exposure to plaque bacteria and their products. On different surfaces of the same teeth or different teeth in the same mouth, any of the following can occur[4]:

a. Hypermineralization of the surface cementum increases with time.
b. Demineralization.
c. Calculus formation.
d. Plaque and debris collection.

B. Tooth Surface Irregularities

Surface irregularities are detected supragingivally by drying the surface with air and observing under adequate direct or indirect light; an explorer is used as needed.

Subgingivally, examination is dependent, for the most part, on tactile and auditory sensitivity transmitted by a probe and an explorer. Causes of surface roughness include the following:

1. *Enamel Surface*
   a. Structural defects; cracks and grooves.
   b. Dental caries, demineralization.
   c. Calculus deposits and heavy stain deposits.
   d. Erosion, abrasion.
   e. Pits and irregularities from hypoplasia.
2. *Cementoenamel Junction.* Cementum overlaps enamel in 60 to 65% of teeth; cementum and enamel meet directly in 30%; and a small zone of dentin may be between the cementum and enamel in 5 to 10%.[5] The relationships of enamel and cementum at the cementoenamel junction are shown in figure 12–2.
3. *Root Surface*
   a. Diseased altered cementum.
   b. Cemental resorption.
   c. Root caries.
   d. Abrasion.
   e. Calculus.
   f. Deficient or overhanging filling.
   g. Grooves from previous incomplete instrumentation.

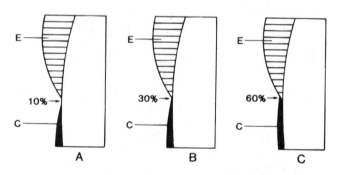

FIG. 12–2. Cementoenamel Junction. The possible relationships of the enamel and the cementum at the cementoenamel junction. **A.** The cementum and the enamel do not meet and there is a small zone of dentin exposed in 10% of teeth. **B.** The cementum meets the enamel in approximately 30% of teeth. **C.** The cementum overlaps the enamel in about 60% of teeth.

COMPLICATIONS OF POCKET FORMATION

I. FURCATION INVOLVEMENT

Furcation involvement means that the pocket and bone loss have extended into the furcation area, or furca, the area between the roots of a multirooted tooth.

A. Types of Furcation Involvement

Furcation involvement is usually classified by the amount of a furcation that has been exposed by periodontal bone destruction.

The four general classes, as shown in figure 12–3, are as follows:

1. *Class I.* Early, beginning involvement. A probe can enter the furcation area, and the anatomy of the roots on either side can be felt by moving the probe from side to side. Figure 33–2C illustrates this on page 509.
2. *Class II.* Moderate involvement. Bone has been destroyed to an extent that permits a probe to enter the furcation area but not to pass through between the roots.
3. *Class III.* Severe involvement. A probe can be passed between the roots through the entire furcation.
4. *Class IV.* Same as Class III, with exposure resulting from gingival recession.

B. Clinical Observations

1. When the gingiva over the furcation has not receded, the following may be seen:
   a. The furcation is covered by the gingival tissue pocket wall.
   b. No differences in color, size, or other tissue changes may exist to differentiate the area from adjacent gingiva, but when color changes do exist, they provide clues to supplement probe examination.
2. When the gingiva over a molar buccal furcation is receded, the root division may be seen directly.

C. Detection

A suggested procedure for probing furcations is described on page 216. Radiographic examination of furcation areas may be studied on page 226.

II. MUCOGINGIVAL INVOLVEMENT

A pocket that extends to or beyond the mucogingival junction and into the alveolar mucosa is described as *mucogingival involvement.* There is no attached gingiva in the area, and a probe can be passed through the pocket and beyond the mucogingival junction into the alveolar mucosa (figure 13–9, page 217).

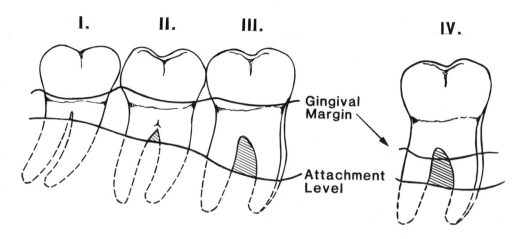

FIG. 12–3. Classification of Furcations. I. Early, beginning involvement. **II.** Moderate involvement, in which the furcation can be probed but not through and through. **III.** Severe involvement, when the bone between the roots is destroyed and a probe can be passed through. **IV.** Same as III, with clinical exposure resulting from gingival recession.

A. Significance of Attached Gingiva

1. *Functions of Attached Gingiva*
   a. Give support to the marginal gingiva.
   b. Withstand the frictional stresses of mastication and toothbrushing.
   c. Provide attachment or a solid base for the movable alveolar mucosa for the action of the cheeks, lips, and tongue.
2. *Barrier to Passage of Inflammation.* Without attachment, the inflammation from the pocket area can extend into the alveolar mucosa. The junctional epithelium (epithelial attachment) acts as a barrier to keep infection outside the body.

   With destruction of the connective tissue and periodontal ligament fibers under the junctional epithelium, the epithelium migrates along the root. A pocket is created.

   In mucogingival involvement, the bottom of the pocket extends into the alveolar mucosa. There, the unconfined inflammation can spread more rapidly in the loose connective tissue.

B. Clinical Observations

Color changes, tension test, and probe measurements are used during assessment. These are described on page 217.

1. *Width of Attached Gingiva.* A narrow zone of gingiva from gingival margin to mucogingival junction, caused by recession or occurring naturally without recession, is more susceptible to developing mucogingival involvement because there is less attached gingiva at the start.
2. *Base of Pocket at Mucogingival Junction.* When the probe measures only 1 to 2 mm and there is no bleeding on probing, but the tip of the probe is at the mucogingival junction, the area should be charted and re-evaluated at each successive maintenance review. Such an area needs specific instruction in plaque

control procedures for preventive maintenance.

When an area of minimal attached gingiva (1 to 2 mm) is placed under stress by restorative, prosthetic, or orthodontic treatment procedures, an assessment should be made of the need for periodontal treatment to increase the zone of attached gingiva.

CONTRIBUTING FACTORS IN DISEASE DEVELOPMENT

Bacterial plaque is the primary etiologic factor in the development of gingival and periodontal diseases. A variety of other factors predispose to the retention of bacterial deposits and hence to the development of disease in the soft tissues. Factors described in this section that relate to microbial plaque retention apply also to dental caries development. Dental caries is described on pages 231–236.

Although debris can be cleared away by self-cleansing, bacterial plaque adheres firmly to the tooth surface and cannot be removed completely by self-cleansing.

Retentive areas relate to rough surfaces of teeth and restorations, tooth contour and position, and gingival size, shape, and position. Iatrogenic causes, that is, factors created by professionals during patient treatment or neglect of treatment, are significant. Such factors as mastication, saliva, the tongue, cheeks, lips, and oral habits, as well as such external factors as diet, smoking, and personal plaque control techniques, contribute.

The patient's study casts can be especially useful for observing the physical factors. Irregularities, contour, position, malocclusion, and contact areas of the teeth, as well as features of the gingiva, may be partially or wholly noted. Problem areas can be explained to the patient by demonstration on the study casts. Changes in the patient's habits and daily personal care routine may be made.

I. DEFINITIONS
Complicating factors to disease development may be etiologic, predisposing, or contributing. These are delineated as follows:

1. *Etiologic Factor.* A factor that is the actual cause of a disease or condition.
2. *Predisposing Factor.* A factor that renders a person susceptible to a disease or condition.
3. *Contributing Factor.* A factor that lends assistance to, supplements, or adds to a condition or disease.

Etiologic, predisposing, and contributing factors may be local or systemic, defined as follows:

1. *Local Factor.* A factor in the immediate environment of the oral cavity or specifically in the environment of the teeth or periodontium.
2. *Systemic Factor.* A factor that results from a general physical or mental disease or condition.

II. DENTAL FACTORS
A. Tooth Surface Irregularities
Pellicle and plaque microorganisms attach to defective or rough surfaces, including the following:

1. Pits, grooves, cracks.
2. Calculus.
3. Exposed altered cementum with irregularities (page 200).
4. Dental caries and demineralization.
5. Iatrogenic
   a. Rough or grooved surfaces left after scaling.
   b. Inadequately contoured and polished dental restorations.

B. Tooth Contour
Altered shape may interfere with self-cleansing mechanisms and make personal care procedures difficult.

1. Congenital abnormalities
   a. Extra or missing cusps.
   b. Bell-shaped crown with prominent facial and lingual contours tends to provide deeper retentive area in cervical third.
2. Teeth with flattened proximal surfaces have faulty contact with adjacent teeth, thus permitting debris to wedge between.
3. Occlusal and incisal surfaces altered by attrition interrupt normal excursion of food during chewing. Marginal ridges have worn down.
4. Areas of erosion and abrasion (figure 14–7, page 239).
5. Carious lesions.
6. Heavy calculus deposits; plaque retained on rough surface.
7. Overcontoured and undercontoured restorations (figure 40–2, page 582).

C. Tooth Position
1. Malocclusion; irregular alignment of a single tooth or groups of teeth leaves areas conducive to collection of microorganisms for plaque formation.
   a. Crowded or overlapped (figure 16–5, page 266).
   b. Rotated.
   c. Deep anterior overbite
      i. Mandibular teeth force food particles against maxillary lingual surface (figure 15–10, page 251).
      ii. Lingual inclination of mandibular teeth allows maxillary teeth to force food particles against mandibular facial gingiva.
2. Tooth adjacent to edentulous area may be inclined or migrated; contact missing.
3. Opposing tooth missing; tooth may extrude beyond the line of occlusion.
4. Related to eruption
   a. Incomplete eruption; below line of occlusion.
   b. Partially erupted impacted third molar.
5. Lack of function or use of teeth eliminates or decreases effectiveness of natural cleansing.
   a. Lack of opposing teeth.
   b. Open bite.
   c. Marked maxillary anterior protrusion.
   d. Crossbite with limited lateral excursion.
   e. Unilateral chewing.
6. Food impaction
   a. Created by the combined effect of tooth contour, missing proximal contact, proximal carious lesions, irregular marginal ridge relationship.
   b. Inclination related to loss of adjacent tooth, and a plunger cusp from the opposite arch (figure 12–4A).
7. Defective contact area
   a. Restoration margin is faulty, and the contact area is missing, improperly located, or unnaturally wide (figure 12–4B).
   b. Inclined tooth; irregular marginal ridge relation (figure 12–4C).

D. Dental Prostheses
1. Orthodontic appliances provide retentive areas.
2. Fixed partial denture with deficient margin of an abutment tooth or an unusually shaped pontic (figures 25–1 and 25–2, page 395).
3. Removable partial denture; inadequately adapted clasps.

III. GINGIVA
A. Position
Deviations from normal provide retentive areas.

1. Receded; depressed area is left at cemento-enamel junction.

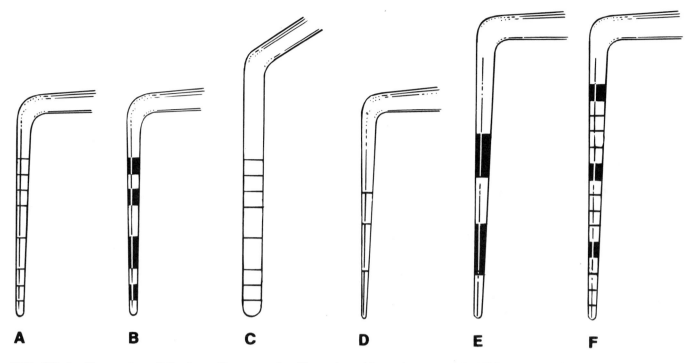

FIG. 13–1. Examples of Probes. Names and calibrated markings shown are **A.** Williams (1-1-1-2-2-1-1-1), **B.** Williams, color-coded, **C.** Goldman-Fox (1-1-1-2-2-1-1-1), **D.** Michigan O (3-3-2), **E.** Hu-Friedy or Marquis Color-coded (3-3-3-3 or 3-3-2-3) and **F.** Hu-Friedy PCPUNC 15, color coded (each millimeter to 15). See Table 13–2 for additional data on probes.

TABLE 13–2
TYPES OF PROBES

Probe Markings (mm)	Examples	Description
Marks at 1-2-3-5-7-8-9-10	Williams University of Michigan with Williams marks Glickman Merritt A and B	Round, tapered (available with color-code) Round, narrow diameter, fine Round, with longer lower shank Round, single bend to shank
Marks at 3-3-2	University of Michigan O Premier O Marquis M-1	Round, fine, tapered, narrow diameter
Marks at 3-6-9-12 3-6-8-11 (and other variations)	Hu-Friedy QULIX Marquis Nordent	Round, tapered, fine Color-coded
Marks at each mm to 15	Hu-Friedy PCPUNC 15	Round Color coded at 5-10-15
Marks at 3.5-5.5-8.5-11.5	WHO Probe (World Health Organization)	Round, tapered, fine, with ball end Color-coded (figure 19–1, page 289)
No marks	Gilmore Nabors 1N, 2N	Tapered, sharper than other probes Curved, with curved shank for furcation examination

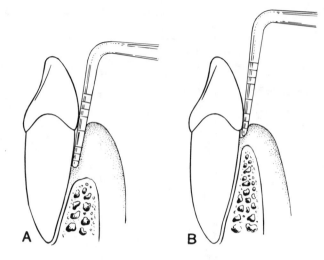

FIG. 13–2. Probing Depth. *A pocket is measured from the gingival margin to the attached periodontal tissue. Shown is the contrast of probe measurements with gingival margins at the same level.* **A.** *Deep periodontal pocket (7 mm) with apical migration of attachment.* **B.** *Shallow pocket (2 mm) with the attachment near the cementoenamel junction.*

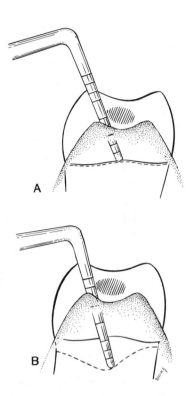

FIG. 13–3. Proximal Surface Probing. A. *Probe must be applied more than one-half way across from facial to overlap with probing from the lingual.* **B.** *Probe in area of crater formation. Probing is usually deeper on the proximal surface under the contact area than on the facial or lingual surfaces.*

B. The pocket (or sulcus) is continuous around the entire tooth, and the entire pocket or sulcus must be measured. "Spot" probing is inadequate.

C. The depth varies around an individual tooth; probing depth rarely measures the same all around a tooth or even around one side of a tooth.
   1. The level of attached tissue assumes a varying position around the tooth.
   2. The gingival margin varies in its position on the tooth.

D. Proximal surfaces must be approached by entering from both the facial and lingual aspects of the tooth.
   1. Gingival and periodontal infections begin in the col area more frequently than in other areas (figure 11–8, page 185).
   2. Probing depth may be deepest directly under the contact area because of crater formation in the alveolar bone (figure 13–3).

E. Anatomic features of the tooth-surface wall of the pocket influence the direction of probing. Examples are concave surfaces, anomalies, shape of cervical third, and position of furcations.

II. EVALUATION OF TOOTH SURFACE

During the movement of the probe, calculus and tooth surface irregularities can be felt and evaluated. The information obtained is used to plan the scaling and root planing appointments.

III. FACTORS THAT AFFECT PROBE DETERMINATIONS

The general objectives of probing are accuracy and consistency so that recordings are dependable for comparison with future probings as well as for colleagues in practice together. At the same time, patient discomfort and trauma to the tissues must be minimal. Probing is influenced by many factors, such as those that follow:

A. Severity and Extent of Periodontal Disease

With application of a light pressure, the probe passes along the tooth surface to the attached tissue level. Diseased tissue offers less resistance, so that with increased severity of disease, the probe inserts to a deeper level.[1] Average levels show that the probe is stopped as follows:
   1. *Normal Tissue.* The probe is at the base of the sulcus or crevice, at the coronal end of the junctional epithelium.
   2. *Gingivitis and Early Periodontitis.* The probe tip is within the junctional epithelium.

3. *Advanced Periodontitis.* Probe tip may penetrate through the junctional epithelium to reach attached connective tissue fibers.

B. The Probe Itself
1. *Calibration.* Must be accurately marked.
2. *Thickness.* A thinner probe slips through a narrow pocket more readily.
3. *Readability.* Aided by the markings and color-coding.

C. Technique
1. *Grasp.* Appropriate for maximum tactile sensitivity.
2. *Finger Rest.* Placed on nonmobile tooth with uniformity.

D. Placement Problems
1. *Anatomic Variations.* Tooth contours, furcations, contact areas, anomalies.
2. *Interferences.* Calculus, irregular margins of restorations, fixed dental prostheses.
3. *Accessibility, Visibility.* Obstructed by tissue bleeding, limited opening by patient, macroglossia.

E. Application of Pressure
Consistent pressure is accomplished by consistent grasp and finger rest in addition to keen tactile sensitivity.

PROBING PROCEDURES

I. PREPARATION FOR PROBE INSERTION
A. Grasp probe with modified pen grasp (page 476).
B. Establish finger rest on a neighboring tooth, preferably in the same dental arch.
C. Hold side of instrument tip flat against the tooth near the gingival margin. The cervical third of a primary tooth is more convex (figure 13–4).
D. Gently slide the tip under the gingival margin.
   1. *Healthy or Firm Fibrotic Tissue.* Insertion is more difficult because of the close adaptation of the tissue to the tooth surface; underlying gingival fibers are strong and tight.
   2. *Spongy, Soft Tissue.* Gingival margin is loose and flabby because of the destruction of underlying gingival fibers. Probe inserts readily and bleeding can be expected on gentle probing.

II. ADVANCE PROBE TO BASE OF POCKET
A. Hold side of probe tip flat against the tooth surface. Widespread roots of primary molars may make this probe position difficult unless the tissue is unduly distended by the probe (figure 13–4).

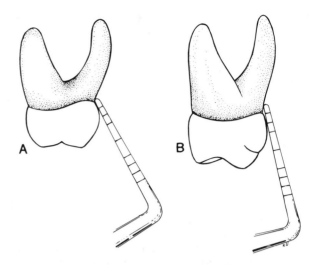

FIG. 13–4. Primary and Permanent Maxillary Molars. A. Accentuated convexity of the cervical third and widespread roots of the primary molar complicate probe placement. Probe may encounter the root. **B.** Permanent tooth with less convexity of the cervical third and roots that are less widely spread.

B. Slide the probe along the tooth surface vertically down to the base of the sulcus or pocket.
   1. Maintain contact of the side of the tip of the probe with the tooth.
      a. Gingival pocket. Side of probe is on enamel.
      b. Periodontal pocket. Side of probe is on the cemental or dentinal surface when inserted to a level below the cementoenamel junction.
   2. As the probe is passed down the side of the tooth, roughness may be felt. Evaluation of the topography and nature of the tooth surface is important to instrumentation.
   3. When obstruction by hard bulky calculus deposit is encountered, lift the probe away from tooth and follow over the edge of the calculus until the probe can move vertically into the pocket again.
   4. The base of the sulcus or pocket feels soft and elastic (compared with the hard tooth surface and calculus deposits), and with slight pressure, the tension of the attached periodontal tissue at the base of the pocket can be felt.
C. Use only the pressure needed to detect by tactile means the level of the attached tissue, whether junctional epithelium or deep connective tissue fibers. A light pressure of 10 g, or of no more than 20 g, is ample.
D. Position probe for reading.
   1. Bring the probe to position as nearly parallel

with the long axis of the tooth as possible for reading the depth.

2. Interference of the contact area does not permit placing the probe parallel for the measurement directly beneath the contact area. Hold the side of shank of the probe against the contact to minimize the angle (figure 13–3).

III. READ THE PROBE

A. Measurement for a probing depth is made from the gingival margin to the attached periodontal tissue.

B. Count the millimeters that show on the probe above the gingival margin and subtract the number from the total number of millimeters marked on the particular probe being used. A comparison of pocket measurement using probes with different calibrations is shown in figure 13–5.

C. When the gingival margin appears at a level between probe marks, use the higher mark for the final reading.

D. Dry the area being probed to improve visibility for specific reading.

IV. CIRCUMFERENTIAL PROBING
A. Probe Stroke

Maintain the probe in the sulcus or pocket of each tooth as the probe is moved in a walking stroke.

1. It is not necessary to remove the probe and reinsert it to make individual readings.

2. Repeated withdrawal and reinsertion cause unnecessary trauma to the gingival margin and hence increase postoperative discomfort.

B. Walking Stroke

1. Hold the side of the tip against the tooth at the base of the pocket.

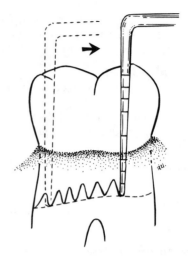

FIG. 13–6. Probe Walking Stroke. The side of the tip of the probe is held in contact with the tooth. From the base of the pocket, the probe is moved up and down in 1- to 2-mm strokes as it is advanced in 1-mm steps. The attached periodontal tissue at the base of the pocket is contacted on each down stroke to identify probing depth in each area.

2. Slide the probe up (coronally) about 1 to 2 mm and back to the attachment in a "touch . . . touch . . . touch . . ." rhythm (figure 13–6).

3. Observe probe measurement at the gingival margin at each touch.

4. Advance millimeter by millimeter along the facial and lingual surfaces into the proximal areas.

V. ADAPTATION OF PROBE FOR INDIVIDUAL TEETH
A. Molars and Premolars

1. Orient the probe at the distal line angle for both facial and lingual application.

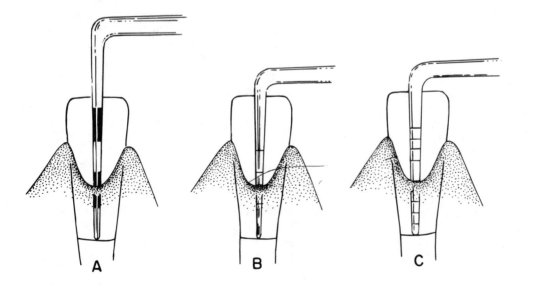

FIG. 13–5. Comparison of Probe Readings. Measurement of same 5-mm pocket with 3 different probes. **A.** Color-coded, **B.** Michigan O, **C.** Williams.

2. Insert probe at the distal line angle and probe in a distal direction; adapt the probe around the line angle; probe across the distal surface until the side of the probe contacts the contact area, then slant the probe to continue under the contact area.

3. Note the probing depth and slide the probe back to the distal line angle. Proceed in the mesial direction around the mesial line angle and across the mesial surface.

B. Anterior Teeth

1. Initial insertion may be at the distal line angle or from the midline of the facial or lingual surfaces.

2. Proceed around the distal line angle and across the distal surface; reinsert and probe the other half of the tooth.

C. Proximal Surfaces

1. Continue the walking stroke around each line angle and onto the proximal surface.

2. Roll the instrument handle between the fingers to keep the side of the probe tip adapted to the tooth surface at line angles and as the tooth contour varies.

3. Continue the strokes under the contact area. Overlap strokes from facial surface with strokes from lingual surface to assure full coverage (figure 13–3). Make sure that the col area under each contact has been thoroughly examined.

CLINICAL ATTACHMENT LEVEL

Attachment level refers to the position of the periodontal attached tissues at the base of a sulcus or pocket. It is measured from a fixed point to the attachment, whereas the probing depth is measured from a changeable point (the crest of the free gingiva) to the attachment (figure 13–7A).

I. RATIONALE

A loss of attachment occurs in disease as the junctional epithelium migrates toward the apex. Stability of attachment is characteristic in health, and treatment procedures may be aimed to obtain a gain of attachment.

Evaluation can be made of the outcome of periodontal treatment and the stability of the attachment during maintenance examinations. When periodontal disease is active, pocket formation and migration of the attachment along the cemental surface continue.

II. PROCEDURE
A. Selecting a Fixed Point

1. Cementoenamel junction is usually used.

2. Margin of a permanent restoration.

3. For animal research, a notch may be made in the tooth; in human research studies, a template or splint may be made for each patient.

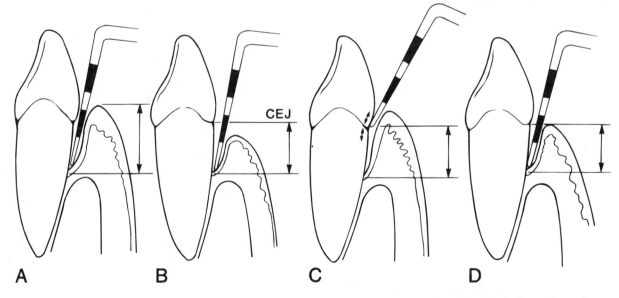

FIG. 13–7. Clinical Attachment Level. A. Probing depth: the pocket is measured from the gingival margin to the attached periodontal tissue. **B.** Clinical attachment level in the presence of gingival recession is measured directly from the cementoenamel junction (CEJ) to the attached tissue. **C.** Clinical attachment level when the gingival margin covers the cementoenamel junction: first the cementoenamel junction is located as shown, and then the distance to the cementoenamel junction is measured and subtracted from the probing depth. **D.** The clinical attachment level is equal to the probing depth when the gingival margin is at the level of the cementoenamel junction.

B. Measuring in the Presence of Visible Recession

1. Cementoenamel junction is visible directly.
2. Measure from the cementoenamel junction to the attachment (figure 13–7B).
3. The clinical attachment level is greater than the probing depth.

C. Measuring When the Cementoenamel Junction Is Covered by Gingiva

1. Slide the probe along the tooth surface, into the pocket, until the cementoenamel junction is felt (figure 13–7C).
2. Remove the calculus when it covers the cementoenamel junction.
3. Measure from the gingival crest to the cementoenamel junction.
4. Subtract the millimeters from cementoenamel junction to gingival crest from the total probing depth to the attachment.
5. Probing depth is greater than the clinical attachment level.

D. Measuring When the Free Gingival Margin Is Level with the Cementoenamel Junction

1. Apply the probe as has been described.
2. The probing depth equals the clinical attachment level (figure 13–7D).

FURCATIONS EXAMINATION

When a pocket extends into a furcation area, special adaptation of the probe must be made to determine the extent and topography of the furcation involvement. The classification of types of furcation involvement is shown on page 201 in figure 12–3.

I. ANATOMIC FEATURES

A. Bifurcation (teeth with two roots)

1. *Mandibular Molars.* The furcation area is accessible for probing from the facial and lingual surfaces (figure 13–8).
2. *Maxillary First Premolars.* The furcation area is accessible from the mesial and distal aspects, under the contact area.
3. *Primary Mandibular Molar.* Widespread roots.

B. Trifurcation (teeth with three roots)

1. *Maxillary Molars.* A palatal root and two buccal roots, the mesiobuccal and the distobuccal roots. Access for probing is from the mesial, buccal, and distal surfaces.
2. *Maxillary Primary Molars.* Widespread roots (figure 13–4, page 213).

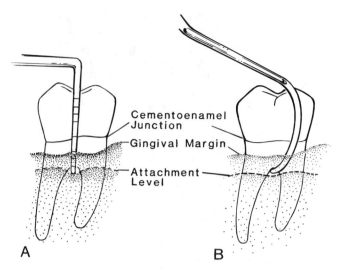

FIG. 13–8. Furcation Examination. A. Williams Probe inserted into bifurcation in area of gingival recession shows probing depth of 3 mm. **B.** Nabers Furcation Probe used to examine the topography of the furcation area.

II. EXAMINATION METHODS

A. Early Furcation

1. Measure probing depth.
2. Inspect the area by adapting the probe closely to the tooth surface and moving the end of the probe over the anatomic curvatures of the roots. An example is shown in figure 33–2C, page 509.
3. Check radiograph for early signs of furcation involvement (figure 13–18, page 225).

B. Points of Access

Measure probing depths at points of access for each bifurcation or trifurcation area. Position of gingival margin will vary. Figure 13–8A shows apparent recession and 3-mm pocket in bifurcation.

C. Probe Adaptation

Use probe in diagonal or horizontal position to examine between roots when there is gingival recession or a flexible, short, soft pocket wall that permits access.

D. Use of Furcation Probe

Use a furcation probe, such as a Nabers 1N or 2N, to examine advanced furcation (figure 13–8B).

E. Complications

Anatomic variations that complicate furcation examination are fused roots, anomalies, such as extra roots, or low or high furcations (figure 33–1, page 508).

MUCOGINGIVAL EXAMINATION

I. TENSION TEST[2]
A. Purposes
   1. To detect adequacy of the width of the attached gingiva.
   2. To locate frenal attachments and their proximity to the free gingiva.
   3. To identify promptly the mucogingival junction.

B. Procedures
   1. *Facial*
      a. Retract cheeks and lips laterally by grasping the lips with the thumbs and index fingers.
      b. Move the lips and cheeks up and down and across, creating tension at the mucogingival junction.
      c. Follow around from the molar areas on the right to molar areas on the left, both maxillary and mandibular.
   2. *Lingual (Mandible)*
      a. Hold a mouth mirror to tense the mucosa of the floor of the mouth, gently retracting the side of the tongue, so that the mucogingival junction is clearly visible.
      b. Request patient to move the tongue to the left, to the right, and up to touch the palate.

C. Observations
   1. Blanching at the mucogingival junction.
   2. Frenal attachments.
   3. Area(s) of apparent recession where there is very little keratinized gingiva and the base of the sulcus or pocket is near the mucogingival junction (figure 11–13, page 192).
   4. Area where color, size, loss of stippling, smooth shininess, or other characteristic indicates the need for careful probing to determine the amount of attached gingiva.
   5. Area where tension pulls the free gingiva away from the tooth, thereby indicating no attached gingiva.

II. GINGIVAL TISSUE EXAMINATION
When inflammation is present and a pocket extends to or through the mucogingival junction, a streak of color (red, bluish-red) that shows the inflammatory changes from the gingival margin to the mucogingival junction may be apparent. When such an area does not pull away during a tension test or does not permit passage of a probe through to the alveolar mucosa, the area should be noted in the record for examination after elimination of inflammation.

III. PROBING
When a pocket extends to or beyond the mucogingival junction, the probe may pass through the pocket di-

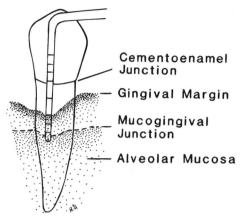

FIG. 13–9. Mucogingival Examination. Probe in position for measuring probing depth where attached gingiva is missing. Absence of attached gingiva permits the probe to pass through the mucogingival junction into the alveolar mucosa.

Labels in figure: Cementoenamel Junction; Gingival Margin; Mucogingival Junction; Alveolar Mucosa

rectly into the alveolar mucosa (figure 13–9). Mucogingival involvement is present.

IV. MEASURE THE AMOUNT OF ATTACHED GINGIVA
   A. Place the probe on the external surface of the gingiva and measure from the mucogingival junction to the gingival margin to determine the width of the total gingiva (figure 13–10A).
   B. Insert the probe and measure probing depth (figure 13–10B).
   C. Subtract the probing depth from the total gingival measurement to get the width of the attached gingiva.
   D. Record findings.

PERIODONTAL CHARTING

Charting of findings while using the probe is a part of the complete periodontal record. The summary of periodontal observations and records may be found on pages 315 and 317.

The procedure described here assumes the use of a chart form with outline drawings of teeth with both facial and lingual root drawings. The exact procedure and format are entirely the choice of an individual dentist. A composite chart that includes dental as well as periodontal findings is frequently used.

In the preparation of the charting, contrasting colors should be used. For example, when red is used to chart dental caries on a composite charting, red would not be a good color selection for drawing the gingival margin because of possible interference with a drawing of a Class V carious lesion (table 14–4, page 235). One procedure for a relatively simple charting system is described here.

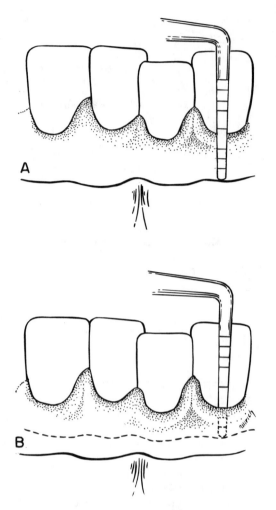

FIG. 13–10. Measuring Attached Gingiva. A. Measure the total gingiva by laying the probe over the surface of the gingiva and measuring from the free margin to the mucogingival junction. **B.** Measure the probing depth. Dotted line represents the base of the pocket. Subtract the probing depth (B) from the total gingiva (A) to obtain the width of attached gingiva. The area illustrated shows 2 mm of attached gingiva.

I. TEETH IDENTIFICATION

Mark missing, unerupted, or impacted teeth. When radiographs and study casts are available before the recording of clinical findings is scheduled, these markings can be made in advance of the patient's appointment.

II. DRAW GINGIVAL LINES

A. Gingival Margin

1. Draw the outline of the position and contour of the gingival margin on the chart form as it appears in relation to the teeth both facial and lingual.
2. Prepare in advance of the patient's appointment when new study casts are available.

B. Mucogingival Lines

1. *General Procedures*
   a. Use contrasting color to that used for drawing the gingival margin line.

b. Draw on the facial aspect for all quadrants; draw the lingual line only on mandibular chart.

2. *Three Methods.* For all, draw the gingival margin line first.
   a. Draw the lines directly, estimating distances between the gingival margin and the mucogingival junction.
   b. Measure with probe.
      i. Measure the total gingiva from gingival margin to mucogingival junction at the center of each tooth (facial and lingual). Write the millimeters on the tooth crown in light pencil to be erased later.
      ii. Place a dot on the tooth chart at the point of millimeters measured from the margin; connect the dots in a relatively straight line representing the mucogingival junction for the molars and premolars and in a scalloped line for the anterior teeth, in keeping with the actual appearance.
   c. Study casts. When parts of all of the mucogingival lines show clearly on the casts, the drawing can be made in advance of the patient's appointment.

III. RECORD PROBING DEPTHS

A. Record all diseased pockets of any depth.
B. Record deepest millimeter measurement for each of the 6 areas around a tooth as shown in figure 13–11. Areas numbered 1, 3, 4, 6 extend from the line angle to under the contact area.
C. Supplement the six recordings with additional readings to show particular areas of unusually deep pockets, furcation involvement, or mucogingival involvement.
D. Record on the charting form. Figure 13–12 shows five possible methods for recording the millimeter depth.

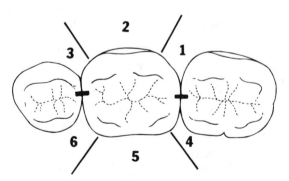

FIG. 13–11. Charting Probing Depths. The pocket/sulcus is measured completely around each tooth. Record the deepest measurement for each of the 6 areas around the tooth. Areas 1, 3, 4, and 6 extend from the line angle to under the contact area.

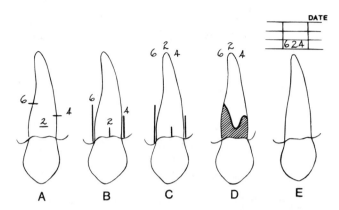

FIG. 13–12. Methods for Charting Probing Depths.
A., B. Chart forms with free-hand lines that designate relative depths. **C.** Numeric notations written at the apex of each tooth. **D.** A continuous line that defines the entire pocket and that can be shaded. **E.** Multiple spaces over the apex of each tooth, used to record the probing depths. Each row can be dated, thus allowing comparisons of measurements at successive follow-up and maintenance examinations.

IV. RECORD SPECIAL DISEASE PROBLEMS

Furcation involvement, mucogingival involvement, and frenal pull must be recorded either by a special symbol or by writing directly on the chart or in the record. See figure 20–2 (page 318) for a suggested method of charting.

EXPLORERS

I. GENERAL PURPOSES AND USES

An explorer is used to
A. Detect, by tactile sense, the texture and character of the tooth surface.
B. Examine the supragingival tooth surfaces for calculus, demineralized and carious lesions, defects or irregularities in the surfaces and margins of restorations, and other irregularities that are not apparent to direct observation. An explorer is used to confirm direct observation.
C. Examine the subgingival tooth surfaces for calculus, demineralized and carious lesions, diseased altered cementum, and other cemental changes that can result from periodontal pocket formation.
D. Define the extent of instrumentation needed and guide techniques for
1. Scaling and root planing.
2. Finishing a restoration.
3. Removing an overhanging filling.
E. Evaluate the completeness of treatment as shown by the smooth tooth surface or the smooth restoration.

II. DESCRIPTION
The basic parts of an instrument are described on page 474.

A. Working End
1. Slender, wire-like, metal *tip* that is circular in cross section and tapers to a fine sharp *point.*
2. Design
a. Single. A single instrument may be universal and adaptable to any tooth surface, or it may be designed for specific groups of surfaces. In figure 13–13, Nos. 2 through 7, 17, 18, 20, and 23 are single instruments.
b. Paired. Paired instruments are mirror images of each other, curved to provide access to contralateral tooth surfaces. In figure 13–13, Nos. 9 and 10, 11 and 12, 13 and 14, and 21 and 22 are paired.
c. Design of a balanced instrument. Middle of working end (tip of an explorer) should be centered over the long axis of the handle (figure 13–14).

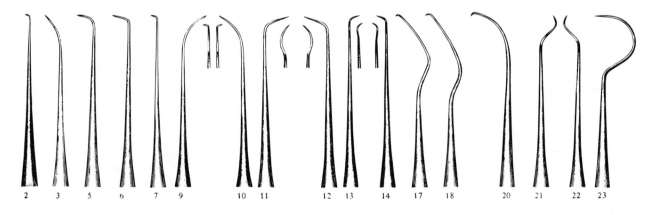

FIG. 13–13. Explorers. This series from Nos. 2 through 23 shows standard shapes of explorer tips. Nos. 2 through 7, 17, 18, 20, and 23 are single instruments. Nos. 9 and 10, 11 and 12, 13 and 14, and 21 and 22 are paired instruments. (Courtesy of the S.S. White Company, Philadelphia, PA.)

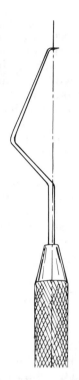

FIG. 13–14. Balanced Explorer Design. With the middle of the tip centered over the long axis of the handle (shown by broken line from tip), the explorer can be positioned in a sulcus or pocket with ease and does not cause trauma to the gingival tissue. Shown is the balanced TU-17 explorer.

B. Shank

1. *Straight, Curved, or Angulated.* Whether a shank is straight, curved, or angulated depends on the use and adaptation for which the explorer was designed. In figure 13–13, compare the straight shanks of Nos. 2, 5, 6, 7, 13, and 14 with the others in the series, which are not straight. A curved shank may facilitate application of the instrument to proximal surfaces, particularly of posterior teeth.
2. *Flexibility.* The slender, wire-like explorers have a degree of flexibility that contributes to increased sensitivity.

C. Handle

1. *Weight.* For increased acute tactile sensitivity, a lightweight handle is more effective.
2. *Diameter.* A wider diameter with serrations for friction while grasping can prevent finger cramping from too tight a grasp. With a lighter grasp, tactile sensitivity can be increased.

D. Construction

1. *Single-ended.* A single-ended instrument has one working end on a separate handle.

2. *Double-ended.* A double-ended instrument has two working ends, one on each end of a common handle. Most paired instruments are available double-ended. Other double-ended instruments combine two single instruments, for example, two unpaired explorers or an explorer with a probe.

III. PREPARATION OF EXPLORERS

Sharpen and retaper a dull explorer tip (page 503). With the explorer tip sharp and tapered, the following can be expected:

A. Increased tactile sensitivity with less pressure required.
B. Prevention of unnecessary trauma to the gingival tissue, because less pressure allows greater control.
C. Decreased instrumentation time with increased patient comfort.

IV. SPECIFIC EXPLORERS AND THEIR USES

A variety of explorers is available as shown by the examples in figure 13–13. The function of each type is related to its adaptability to specific surfaces of teeth at particular angulations. Certain explorers can be used effectively for detection of dental caries in pits and fissures, and others are designed to be adapted to examine proximal surfaces for calculus or dental caries. By other criteria, some can be used subgingivally, whereas others cannot be adapted subgingivally without inflicting damage to the sulcular epithelium. Therefore, such explorers are limited to supragingival adaptation only.

A. Subgingival Explorer

1. *Names and Numbers.* Orban No. 20, TU-17, pocket explorer.
2. *Shape.* The pocket explorer has an angulated shank with a short tip (figure 13–14). The tip should be measured to assure that it is less than 2 mm. A longer tip cannot be adapted to the line angles of narrow roots.
3. *Features for Subgingival Root Examination*
   a. Back of tip can be applied directly to the attached periodontal tissue at the base of the pocket without lacerating. When a straight or sickle explorer is directed toward the base of the pocket, the sharp tip can pass into the epithelium without resistance.
   b. The short tip can be adapted to rounded tooth surfaces and line angles. Long tips of other explorers have a tangential relationship with the tooth and cause distention and trauma to sulcular or pocket epithelium.
   c. Narrow short tip can be adapted at the base where the pocket narrows without undue displacement of the pocket soft tissue wall.

4. *Supragingival Use of No. TU-17.* It may be adapted to all surfaces and is especially useful for proximal surface examination. It is not readily adaptable to pits and fissures.

B. Sickle or Shepherd's Hook (No. 23 in figure 13-13)
1. *Use.* Examining pits and fissures and supragingival smooth surfaces; examining surfaces and margins of restorations and sealants.
2. *Adaptability*
   a. Difficult to apply to proximal surfaces because the wide hook can contact an adjacent tooth and the straight long section of the tip can pass over a small proximal carious lesion.
   b. Not adaptable for deep subgingival exploration. When the point is directed to the base of a pocket, trauma to the attachment area can result. In the attempt to prevent such damage, the clinician may not explore to the base of the pocket, thus providing incomplete service.

C. Pigtail or Cowhorn (Nos. 21 and 22 in figure 13-13).
1. *Use.* Proximal surfaces for calculus, dental caries, or margins of restorations.
2. *Adaptability.* As paired, curved tips, they are applied to opposite tooth surfaces.

D. Straight (Nos. 2, 6, 7 in figure 13-13)
1. *Use.* Supragingival, for pits and fissures, tooth irregularities of smooth surfaces, and surfaces and margins of restorations and sealants.
2. *Adaptability*
   a. For pit and fissure caries, the explorer tip is held parallel with the long axis of the tooth and applied straight into a pit.
   b. Not adaptable deep in subgingival area. Straight shanked instruments or those with long tips cannot be adapted readily in the apical portion of the pocket near the attached tissue or on line angles.

BASIC PROCEDURES FOR USE OF EXPLORERS

Development of ability to use an explorer and a probe is achieved first by learning the anatomic features of each tooth surface and the types of irregularities that may be encountered on the surfaces. The second step is repeated practice of careful and deliberate techniques for application of the instruments.

The objective is to adapt the instruments in a routine manner that relays consistent comparative information about the nature of the tooth surface. Concentration, patience, attention to detail, and alertness to each irregularity, however small it may seem, are necessary.

I. USE OF SENSORY STIMULI
Both explorers and probes can transmit tactile stimuli from tooth surfaces to the fingers. A fine explorer usually gives a more acute sense of tactile discrimination to small irregularities than does a thicker explorer. Probes vary in diameter; the narrow types may provide greater sensitivity.

II. TOOTH SURFACE IRREGULARITIES
Three basic tactile sensations must be distinguished when probing or exploring. These may be grouped as normal tooth surface, irregularities created by excess or elevations in the surface, and irregularities caused by depressions in the tooth surface. Examples of these are listed here.

A. Normal
1. *Tooth Structure.* The smooth surface of enamel and root surface that has been planed; anatomic configurations, such as cingula, furcations.
2. *Restored Surfaces.* Smooth surfaces of metal (gold, amalgam) and the softer feeling of plastic; smooth margin of a restoration.

B. Irregularities: Increases or Elevations in Tooth Surface
1. *Deposits.* Calculus.
2. *Anomalies.* Enamel pearl; unusually pronounced cementoenamel junction.
3. *Restorations.* Overcontoured, irregular margins (overhang).

C. Irregularities: Depressions, Grooves
1. *Tooth Surface.* Demineralized or carious lesion, abrasion, erosion, pits such as those caused by enamel hypoplasia, areas of cemental resorption on the root surface.
2. *Restorations.* Deficient margin, rough surface (figure 40-2, page 582).

III. TYPES OF STIMULI
During exploring and probing, distinction of irregularities can be made through auditory and tactile means.

A. Tactile
Tactile sensations pass through the instrument to the fingers and hand and to the brain for registration and action. Tactile sensations, for example, may be the result of catching on an overcontoured restoration, dropping into a carious lesion, hooking the edge of a restoration or lesion, encountering an elevated deposit, or simply passing over a rough surface.

B. Auditory
As an explorer or probe moves over the surface of enamel, cementum, a metallic restoration, a plastic restoration, or any irregularity of tooth

structure or restoration, a particular surface texture is apparent. With each contact, sound may be created. The clean smooth enamel is quiet; the rough cementum or calculus is scratchy or noisy. Sometimes a metallic restoration may "squeak" or have a metallic "ring." With experience, differentiations can be made.

SUPRAGINGIVAL PROCEDURES

I. USE OF VISION
Supragingival exploration for defects of the tooth surface differs from subgingival in that, when a surface is dried, much of the actual exploration is performed to confirm visual observation. The exceptions are the proximal areas near and around contact areas that cannot be directly observed.

Unnecessary exploration should be avoided. With adequate light and a source of air, proper retraction, and use of mouth mirror, dried supragingival calculus can generally be seen as either chalky white or brownish-yellow in contrast to tooth color. A minimum of exploration can confirm the finding.

II. FACIAL AND LINGUAL SURFACES
A. Adapt the side of tip with the point always on the tooth surface.
B. Move the instrument in short walking strokes over the surface being examined, or direct the tip gently into a suspected carious lesion.
C. Avoid deliberate exploration of cervical third areas where there is recession or where the patient has previously exhibited sensitivity. If a sensitive area must be dried, avoid an air blast, and blot with a gauze sponge or a cotton roll. Methods for desensitization are described on pages 557 and 558.

III. PROXIMAL SURFACES
A. Lead with the tip onto a proximal surface, rolling the handle between the fingers to assure adaptation around the line angle. Keep the side of the point of the explorer in contact with the tooth surface at all times.
B. Explore under the proximal contact area when there is recession of the papilla and the area is exposed. Overlap strokes from facial and lingual to assure full coverage.

SUBGINGIVAL PROCEDURES

I. ESSENTIALS FOR DETECTION OF TOOTH SURFACE IRREGULARITIES
A. Definite but light grasp.
B. Consistent finger rest with light pressure.
C. Definite contact of the instrument with the tooth.
D. Light touch as the instrument is moved over the tooth surface.

II. STEPS
A. With the tip in contact with the tooth supragingivally, hold the lower shank (the part of the shank that is next to the tip) parallel with the long axis of the tooth. Gently slide the tip under the gingival margin into the sulcus or pocket.
B. Keep the point in contact with the tooth at all times to prevent unnecessary trauma to the pocket or sulcular epithelium. Adapt the tip closely to the tooth surface by applying the side of the point.
C. Slide the explorer tip over the tooth surface to the base of the pocket until, with the back of the tip, the resistance of the soft tissue of the attached periodontal tissue is felt (figure 13–15A). Calculus deposits may obstruct direct passage of the instrument to the base of the pocket. Lift the tip slightly away from the tooth surface and follow over the deposit to proceed to the base of the pocket.
D. Use a "walking" stroke, vertical or diagonal (oblique).
  1. Lead with the tip. Move it ahead as the instrument progresses (figure 13–15B).
  2. Length of stroke depends on the depth of a pocket.
    a. Shallow pocket. The stroke may extend the entire depth, from the base of the pocket to just beneath the gingival margin.
    b. Deep pocket. Controlled strokes 2- to 3-mm long can provide more acute sensitivity to the surface and allow improved adaptation of the instrument. A deep pocket should be explored in sections. One should first explore the apical area next to the base of the pocket, then move up to a higher section, overlapping to assure full coverage.
  3. Do not remove the explorer from the pocket for each stroke on a particular surface because
    a. Trauma to the gingival margin caused by repeated withdrawal and reinsertion can cause the patient posttreatment discomfort.
    b. Concentration on the texture of the tooth surface is interrupted.
    c. More time is consumed.
E. Proximal surface
  1. Lead with tip of instrument; do not "back into" an area.
  2. Continue the strokes around the line angle. Roll the instrument handle between the fin-

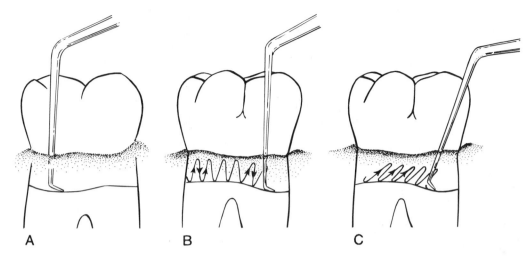

FIG. 13–15. Use of Subgingival Explorer. A. The lower shank (next to tip) is held parallel with the long axis of the tooth. The explorer is passed into the pocket and lowered until the back of the working tip meets resistance from the attached periodontal tissue at the base of the pocket. **B.** Vertical walking stroke. With the side of the tip in contact with the tooth surface at all times, the explorer is moved over the surface. **C.** Diagonal walking stroke. Complete exploration of the surface is needed; therefore, groups of strokes are overlapped.

gers to keep the tip closely adapted as the tooth contour changes.

3. Continue strokes under the contact area. Overlap strokes from facial and lingual aspects to assure full coverage.

RECORD FINDINGS

I. SUPRAGINGIVAL CALCULUS
A. Distribution
Supragingival calculus is generally localized. It is most commonly confined to the lingual surfaces of the mandibular anterior teeth and the facial surfaces of the maxillary first and second molars, opposite the openings to the salivary ducts (page 272).

B. Amount
Slight, moderate, heavy.

II. SUBGINGIVAL CALCULUS
A. Distribution
Subgingival calculus can be either localized or generalized.

B. Amount
Slight, moderate, heavy.

III. OTHER IRREGULARITIES OF TOOTH SURFACE
Note on the chart or in the record any other deviation from normal detected while using the explorer.

MOBILITY EXAMINATION

Because of the nature and function of the periodontal ligament, teeth have a slight normal mobility. Mobility can be considered abnormal or pathologic when it exceeds normal. Increased mobility can be an important clinical sign of disease.

I. CAUSES OF MOBILITY
A. Inflammation
Inflammation in the periodontal ligament leads to degeneration or destruction of the fibers.

B. Loss of Support
Loss of sufficient support by alveolar bone and periodontal ligament (destroyed by periodontal infection) can increase the mobility.

C. Trauma from Occlusion
Injury to the periodontal tissues can result from occlusal forces (page 255).

II. PROCEDURE FOR DETERMINATION OF MOBILITY
A. Position the patient for clear visibility with maximum light and ready accessibility through convenient retraction.

B. Stabilize the head. Motion of the head, lips, or cheek can interfere with a true evaluation of tooth movement.

C. Use two single-ended metal instruments with wide blunt ends, held with a modified pen grasp. Use of wooden tongue depressors or plastic mirror handles is not recommended because of their flexibility. Testing with the fingers without the metal instruments can be misleading because the soft tissue of the fingertips can move and give an illusion of tooth movement.

D. Apply specific, firm finger rests (fulcrums). A standardized finger rest pressure contributes increased consistency to the determinations. The teeth may be dried with air or sponge to prevent slipping of the instruments or the finger on the finger rest.

E. Apply the blunt ends of the instruments to opposite sides of a tooth, and rock the tooth to test horizontal mobility. Keep both instrument ends on the tooth as pressure is applied first from one side and then the other.

F. Test vertical mobility (depression of the tooth into its socket) by applying, on the occlusal or incisal surface, pressure with one of the mirror handles.

G. Test each primary abutment tooth of a fixed partial denture.

H. Move from tooth to tooth in a systematic order.

III. RECORD DEGREE OF MOVEMENT
A. Scale
N, 1, 2, 3 or I, II, III are frequently used, sometimes with a + to indicate mobility between numbers.

B. Recording
Although subjective, interpretation may be considered as follows.[3]
N = normal, physiologic
1 = slight mobility, greater than normal
2 = moderate mobility, greater than 1 mm displacement
3 = severe mobility, may move in all directions, vertical as well as horizontal.

C. The Letter N Means *Normal* Mobility
All teeth that have a periodontal ligament have normal mobility. No tooth has zero mobility except in a condition, such as ankylosis, in which there is no periodontal ligament.

D. Chart Form
A chart form should provide for a place to record mobility. Preferably more than one place should be reserved so that comparative readings may be recorded at successive maintenance appointments (figure 20–2, page 318).

FREMITUS

I. DEFINITION
Fremitus means palpable vibration or movement. In dentistry it refers to the vibratory patterns of the teeth. A tooth with fremitus has excess contact, possibly re-

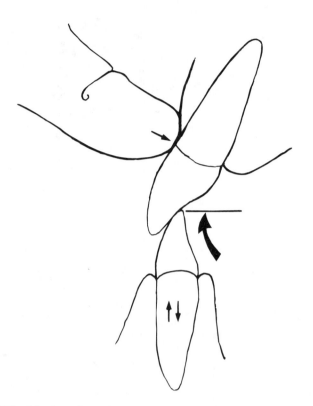

FIG. 13–16. Fremitus. With the patient seated upright and the head stabilized against the headrest, an index finger is placed firmly over the cervical third of each maxillary tooth in succession starting with the most posterior tooth on one side and moving around the arch. The patient is requested to click the posterior teeth.

lated to a premature contact. Usually, the tooth also demonstrates some degree of mobility because the excess contact forces the tooth to move. The test is used in conjunction with occlusal analysis and adjustment.

Because fremitus depends on tooth contact, determination is made only on the maxillary teeth.

II. PROCEDURE FOR DETERMINATION OF FREMITUS
A. Seat the patient upright with the head stabilized against the headrest.

B. Press an index finger on each maxillary tooth at about the cervical third (figure 13–16).

C. Request the patient to "click the back teeth" repeatedly.

D. Start with the most posterior maxillary tooth on one side and move the index finger tooth by tooth around the arch.

E. Record by tooth number the teeth where vibration is felt and the teeth where actual movement is noted. The degree recorded may be subjective, but the following range has been suggested.[4]
N = normal (without vibration or movement).
+ = One-degree fremitus; only slight vibration can be felt.

+ + = Two degree fremitus; the tooth is clearly palpable but movement is barely visible.

+ + + = Three degree fremitus; movement is clearly observed visually.

RADIOGRAPHIC EXAMINATION

Radiographs provide essential information to aid and supplement clinical findings. During other phases of the examination, and especially during probing, the mounted radiographs should be on a viewbox for viewing in conjunction with examination. When the radiographs have not been processed at the time of probing, areas of special confirmation can be marked on the record for review at the next appointment.

For observing evidence of periodontal involvement, periapical radiographs are needed. Bitewing radiographs do not show the complete periodontal tissues that extend around the roots. When bone loss is moderate to severe, the crest of the bone cannot usually be seen in a bitewing survey.

Principles for use of radiographs were described on pages 158–160. The need for mounted radiographs free from errors of technique and viewed on an adequately lighted viewbox cannot be overemphasized. A magnifying reading glass is of special assistance when studying periodontal findings.

RADIOGRAPHIC CHANGES IN PERIODONTAL INFECTIONS

I. BONE LEVEL
A. Normal Bone Level
The crest of the interdental bone appears from 1.0 to 1.5 mm from the cementoenamel junction (figure 13–17).

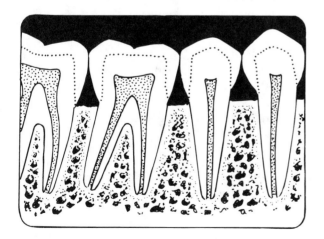

FIG. 13–17. Normal Bone Level. Drawing of a radiograph to show normal bone level, 1 to 1.5 mm from the cementoenamel junction.

B. Bone Level in Periodontal Disease
The height of the bone is lowered progressively as the inflammation is extended and bone is resorbed.

II. SHAPE OF REMAINING BONE
A. Horizontal
1. When the crest of the bone is parallel with a line between the cementoenamel junctions of two adjacent teeth, the term "horizontal bone loss" is used (figures 13–18 and 13–19).

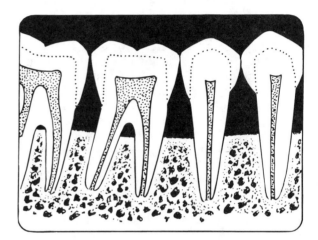

FIG. 13–18. Horizontal Bone Loss. Bone level in periodontal disease is more than 1 to 1.5 mm from the cementoenamel junction. When bone loss is horizontal, the crest of the alveolar bone is parallel with a line between the cementoenamel junctions of adjacent teeth. Note early furcation involvement in the second molar and moderate furcation involvement in the first molar.

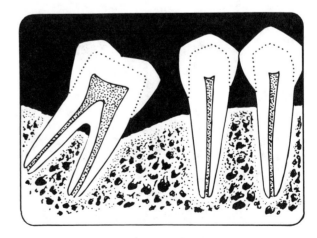

FIG. 13–19. Horizontal Bone Loss. Second molar has drifted mesially into the space created when the first molar was removed. Note that the level of the crestal bone is parallel with a line between the cementoenamel junctions of the second premolar and the tipped second molar.

2. When inflammation is the sole destructive factor, the bone loss usually appears horizontal.

3. When the amount of remaining bone is fairly evenly distributed throughout the dentition, the condition is described as *generalized* horizontal bone loss. It may be designated either by millimeters from the position of the normal bone level or by percentage. When making estimates, referral to the table of average root lengths can be helpful (Appendix, tables A–1 and A–2).

4. When bone loss is confined to specific areas, the condition is described as *localized* horizontal bone loss.

B. Angular or Vertical

1. Reduction in height of crestal bone that is irregular; the bone level is not parallel with a line joining the adjacent cementoenamel junctions (figure 13–20); bone loss is greater on the proximal surface of one tooth than on the adjacent tooth.

2. Angular bone loss is more commonly localized; rarely generalized.

3. When inflammation and trauma from occlusion are combined in causing the destruction and irregular shape of the bone, the bone may appear with "angular defects" or with "vertical bone loss."

III. CRESTAL LAMINA DURA
A. Normal

White, radiopaque; continuous with and connects the lamina dura about the roots of two adjacent teeth; covers the interdental bone (figure 13–18).

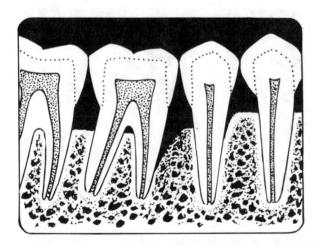

FIG. 13–20. Angular or Vertical Bone Loss; Mesial of the First Molar. The level of the crestal bone between the second premolar and the first molar is not parallel with a line between the cementoenamel junctions of the same teeth.

B. Evidence of Disease

The crestal lamina dura is indistinct, irregular, radiolucent, fuzzy.

IV. FURCATION INVOLVEMENT
A. Normal

Bone fills the area between the roots (figure 13–17).

B. Evidence of Disease

Radiolucent area in the furcation.

1. Early furcation involvement may appear as a small radiolucent black dot or as a slight thickening of the periodontal ligament space. It can be confirmed by probing. Early furcation involvement is shown in the second molar in figure 13–18.

2. Furcation involvement of maxillary molars may become advanced before radiographic evidence can be seen. Superimposition of the palatal root may mask a small area of involvement. When the proximal bone level in the radiograph appears at the level where the furcation is normally located, furcation involvement should be suspected and probed for confirmation.

3. Maxillary first premolar furcation involvement cannot be seen in a radiograph except at an unusual angulation or unusual position of the tooth. With correct vertical and horizontal angulation, the roots are superimposed.

4. Furcations may show at one angulation but not at another; variations in technique can obscure a furcation involvement. All furcations must be carefully probed.

V. PERIODONTAL LIGAMENT SPACE
A. Normal

The periodontal ligament is connective tissue and, hence, appears radiolucent in a radiograph. It appears as a fine black radiolucent line next to the root surface. On its outer side is the lamina dura, the bone that lines the tooth socket and appears radiopaque (figure 13–21).

B. Evidence of Disease

Widening or thickening.

1. *Angular Thickening or Triangulation*. The space is widened only near the coronal third, near the crest of the interdental bone.

2. *Complete Periodontal Ligament Thickened Along an Entire Side of a Root to the Apex, or Around the Root* (figure 13–21). When viewed at different angulations (in the various radiographs of a complete survey), the ligament space may reveal varying thicknesses, thus showing that the disease involvement is not

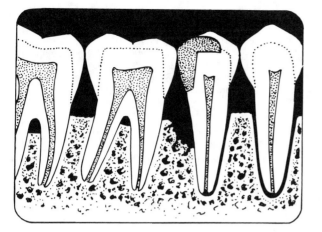

FIG. 13-21. Periodontal Ligament Space. *First and second molars have a normal periodontal ligament space, which appears as a fine black line about the roots. The first premolar shows thickening of the ligament space about the entire root, and the second premolar has thickening only about the mesial surface of the root.*

consistent around the entire root or that other structures are superimposed.

EARLY PERIODONTAL DISEASE

The real preventive service is to recognize *early signs* of periodontal involvement so that treatment can be initiated to arrest the disease and prevent more severe involvement, which could lead to tooth loss. The recognition of severe bone loss, advanced furcation involvement, and marked thickening of the periodontal ligament space is not difficult after a basic understanding has been gained. The difficult part is to watch carefully for incipient, often isolated indications of early periodontal disease. These changes can be seen in all age groups, from young children to elderly patients.

I. EARLIEST SIGNS
The earliest signs of periodontal involvement are not evident in a radiograph. Only after the inflammation has extended from the soft tissue (gingivitis) to the supporting periodontal tissues and bone resorption has become sufficient does radiographic evidence appear.

II. INITIAL BONE DESTRUCTION
A. The usual interproximal pathway of inflammation from gingivitis to periodontitis is directly from the inflamed gingival connective tissue into the crest of the interdental bone (page 197).
B. Initial bone destruction usually takes place at the crest of the interdental bone in the crestal lamina dura.

III. RADIOGRAPHIC EVIDENCE
A. Crestal lamina dura may appear slightly irregular, fuzzy, and radiolucent. At this stage it is best examined with a hand magnifying glass.
B. Angular thickening of the periodontal ligament space (triangulation) may also be apparent.

OTHER RADIOGRAPHIC FINDINGS

Any other radiographic findings that may be directly or indirectly related to periodontal involvement and its contributing factors should be noted in the record for the attention of the dentist. Certain findings have a direct relation to dental hygiene care and instruction, particularly local factors that contribute to food impaction or plaque retention.

I. CALCULUS
Gross deposits, primarily those on proximal surfaces, may be seen in radiographs. Observing these may be helpful, but the probe and explorer are needed to define the exact location and extent.

The density and contrast of the radiograph influence whether or not calculus is seen. Because all deposits are not visible, the use of radiographs has limited value for specific calculus detection.

II. OVERHANGING RESTORATIONS
Some proximal overhanging margins may be seen in radiographs. The use of an explorer is necessary to detect irregular margins and to examine all proximal margins that do not reveal irregularities in the radiographs. Superimposition can mask an overhanging margin. Types of irregularities of restoration are described on pages 582 and 583.

III. DENTAL CARIES
Clinical and radiographic identification of carious lesions is described on pages 242 and 243. Certain findings should be noted for their relationship to the periodontal tissues.
A. Large carious lesions may leave open contact areas that permit food impaction and hence damage to the periodontal tissues.
B. Carious lesions, either enamel or root caries, hold plaque and provide a rough surface for retention of food debris and materia alba.
C. Root caries and demineralization may interfere with techniques of root planing (pages 199–200).

IV. RELATIONSHIP TO POCKETS
Radiographs do not show pockets; soft tissue does not show in a radiograph. Because a pocket is measured from the gingival margin to the base of the pocket, both of which are soft tissue, pockets cannot be seen in a radiograph. Probing is necessary to identify pockets.

TECHNICAL HINTS

I. Use topical anesthetic to help to alleviate discomfort while probing.

II. Avoid the most common errors in probing:

A. Not passing the probe to the full pocket depth.

B. Not holding the probe as parallel with the long axis of a tooth as possible, and therefore obtaining a false reading.

C. Not measuring around the entire tooth and therefore missing pockets. This error most commonly applies to proximal surface probing. The probe must be passed more than halfway across from the facial aspect to overlap with the probe used on the lingual aspect which should also be passed more than halfway across.

III. Check the markings on a new probe by measuring on a standard millimeter ruler.

IV. When bleeding is readily elicited on probing or exploring and tooth surfaces are obscured so that examination is complicated, initiate toothbrushing and other appropriate disease control methods. Explain the problem to the patient, and outline a specific home care routine designed to reduce gingival inflammation. Postpone the complete examination for 1 week, after which the gingival condition should be improved.

V. Replace mirror heads frequently. Scratched mirrors obscure vision and delay procedures.

VI. Handle explorers and probes carefully. Because the tips are pliable and relatively fragile, precautions must be taken against breakage or bending (pages 54 and 55).

FACTORS TO TEACH THE PATIENT

I. The need for a careful, thorough examination if treatment is to be complete and effective.

II. Information about the instruments and how their use makes the examination complete. Examples are the complete radiographic survey, probing 360° around each tooth, and exploring each subgingival tooth surface.

III. Why bleeding can occur when probing. Healthy tissue does not bleed.

IV. Relation of probing depth measurements to normal sulci.

V. Significance of mobility.

VI. Signs of periodontal infection in radiographs.

REFERENCES

1. **Listgarten,** M.A.: Periodontal Probing: What Does it Mean?, *J. Clin. Periodontol., 7,* 165, June, 1980.

2. **Kopczyk,** R.A. and Saxe, S.R.: Clinical Signs of Gingival Inadequacy: The Tension Test, *ASDC J. Dent. Child., 41,* 352, September-October, 1974.

3. **Miller,** S.C.: *Textbook of Periodontia,* 3rd ed. Philadelphia, The Blakiston Co., 1950, p. 125.

4. **Goldman,** H.M. and Cohen, D.W.: *Periodontal Therapy,* 6th ed. St. Louis, Mosby, 1980, pp. 1092, 1107, 1110.

SUGGESTED READINGS

Caton, J.: Periodontal Diagnosis and Diagnostic Aids, in American Academy of Periodontics: *Proceedings of the Workshop in Clinical Periodontics.* Chicago, American Academy of Periodontics, 1989, pp. I-6 to I-12.

Lang, N.P. and Brägger, U.: Periodontal Diagnosis in the 1990s, *J. Clin. Periodontol., 18,* 370, July, 1991.

Machtei, E.E., Christersson, L.A., Grossi, S.G., Dunford, R., Zambon, J.J., and Genco, R.J.: Clinical Criteria for the Definition of "Established Periodontitis," *J. Periodontol., 63,* 206, March, 1992.

McKechnie, L.B.: Root Morphology in Periodontal Therapy, *Dentalhygienistnews, 6,* 3, Winter, 1993.

Nield, J.S. and Houseman, G.A.: *Fundamentals of Dental Hygiene Instrumentation,* 2nd ed. Philadelphia, Lea & Febiger, 1988, pp. 381–435.

Schulte, W., d'Hoedt, B., Lukas, D., Maunz, M., and Steppeler, M.: Periotest for Measuring Periodontal Characteristics—Correlation with Periodontal Bone Loss, *J. Periodont. Res., 27,* 184, May, 1992.

Stark, D.E. and Hoover, J.N.: Markers of Periodontal Disease Susceptibility and Activity—A Review, *Can. Dent. Assoc. J., 57,* 127, February, 1991.

Strassler, H.E.: Perio Charting Systems, *RDH, 12,* 23, January, 1992.

Waerhaug, J.: The Furcation Problem. Etiology, Pathogenesis, Diagnosis, Therapy and Prognosis, *J. Clin. Periodontol., 7,* 73, April, 1980.

Probing

Badersten, A., Nilvéus, R., and Egelberg, J.: Reproducibility of Probing Attachment Level Measurements, *J. Clin. Periodontol., 11,* 475, August, 1984.

Bergström, J. and Eliasson, S.: Prevalence of Chronic Periodontal Disease Using Probing Depth as a Diagnostic Test, *J. Clin. Periodontol., 16,* 588, October, 1989.

Chamberlain, A.D.H., Renvert, S., Garrett, S., Nilvéus, R., and Egelberg, J.: Significance of Probing Force for Evaluation of Healing Following Periodontal Therapy, *J. Clin. Periodontol., 12,* 306, April, 1985.

Claffey, N., Nylund, K., Kiger, R., Garrett, S., and Egelberg, J.: Diagnostic Predictability of Scores of Plaque, Bleeding, Suppuration and Probing Depth for Probing Attachment Loss. 3½ Years of Observation Following Initial Periodontal Therapy, *J. Clin. Periodontol., 17,* 108, February, 1990.

Heins, P.J., Fuller, W.W., and Fries, S.E.: Periodontal Probe Use in General Practice in Florida, *J. Am. Dent. Assoc., 119,* 147, July, 1989.

Moriarty, J.D., Hutchens, L.H., and Scheitler, L.E.: Histological Evaluation of Periodontal Probe Penetration in Untreated Facial Molar Furcations, *J. Clin. Periodontol., 16,* 21, January, 1989.

Neiderud, A.-M., Ericsson, I., and Lindhe, J.: Probing Pocket Depth at Mobile/Nonmobile Teeth, *J. Clin. Periodontol., 19,* 754, November, 1992.

Pattison, A.M. and Pattison, G.L.: *Periodontal Instrumentation,* 2nd ed. Norwalk, CT, Appleton & Lange, 1992, pp. 17–24.

Persson, R. and Svendsen, J.: The Role of Periodontal Probing

Depth in Clinical Decision-making, *J. Clin. Periodontol., 17,* 96, February, 1990.

Theil, E.M. and Heany, T.G.: The Validity of Periodontal Probing as a Method of Measuring Loss of Attachment, *J. Clin. Periodontol., 18,* 648, October, 1991.

Watts, T.L.P.: Probing Site Configuration in Patients with Untreated Periodontitis, A Study of Horizontal Positional Error, *J. Clin. Periodontol., 16,* 529, September, 1989.

Zappa, U., Simona, C., Schäppi, P., Graf, H., and Espeland, M.: Episodic Probing Attachment Loss in Humans: Histologic Associations, *J. Periodontol., 61,* 420, July, 1990.

Instruments

Atassi, F., Newman, H.N., and Bulman, J.S.: Probe Tine Diameter and Probing, *J. Clin. Periodontol., 19,* 301, May, 1992.

Kazmierczak, M.D., Ciancio, S.G., Mather, M., Dangler, L.V., and Troullos, E.S.: Improved Diagnostics: Clinical Evaluation of a Color-coded, Polymeric Periodontal Probe, *Clin. Prev. Dent., 14,* 24, July/August, 1992.

Keagle, J.G., Garnick, J.J., Searle, J.R., King, G.E., and Morse, P.K.: Gingival Resistance to Probing Forces. I. Determination of Optimal Probe Diameter, *J. Periodontol., 60,* 167, April, 1989.

Lukas, D., Schulte, W., König, M., and Reim, M.: High-speed Filming of the Periotest Measurement, *J. Clin. Periodontol., 19,* 388, July, 1992.

Mombelli, A., Mühle, T., and Frigg, R.: Depth-force Patterns of Periodontal Probing. Attachment-gain in Relation to Probing Force, *J. Clin. Periodontol., 19,* 295, May, 1992.

Nield, J.S.: Exploring Explorers, *Dentalhygienistnews, 3,* 16, Summer, 1990.

Van der Zee, E., Davies, E.H., and Newman, H.N.: Marking Width, Calibration from Tip and Tine Diameter of Periodontal Probes, *J. Clin. Periodontol., 18,* 516, August, 1991.

Bleeding on Probing

Abbas, F., Voss, S., Nijboer, A., Hart, A.A.M., and Van der Velden, U.: The Effect of Mechanical Oral Hygiene Procedures on Bleeding on Probing, *J. Clin. Periodontol., 17,* 199, March, 1990.

Chaves, E.S., Wood, R.C., Jones, A.A., Newbold, D.A., Manwell, M.A., and Kornman, K.S.: Relationship of "Bleeding on Probing" and "Gingival Index Bleeding" as Clinical Parameters of Gingival Inflammation, *J. Clin. Periodontol., 20,* 139, February, 1993.

Janssen, P.T.M., Faber, J.A.J., and van Palenstein Helderman, W.H.: Effect of Probing Depth and Bleeding Tendency on the Reproducibility of Probing Depth Measurements, *J. Clin. Periodontol., 15,* 565, October, 1988.

Kaldahl, W.B., Kalkwarf, K.L., Patil, K.D., and Molvar, M.P.: Relationship of Gingival Bleeding, Gingival Suppuration, and Supragingival Plaque to Attachment Loss, *J. Periodontol., 61,* 347, June, 1990.

Kalkwarf, K.L., Kaldahl, W.B., Patil, K.D., and Molvar, M.P.: Evaluation of Gingival Bleeding Following 4 Types of Periodontal Therapy, *J. Clin. Periodontol., 16,* 601, October, 1989.

Lang, N.P., Adler, R., Joss, A., and Nyman, S.: Absence of Bleeding on Probing, *J. Clin. Periodontol., 17,* 714, November, 1990.

Lang, N.P., Nyman, S., Senn, C., and Joss, A.: Bleeding on Probing as It Relates to Probing Pressure and Gingival Health, *J. Clin. Periodontol., 18,* 257, April, 1991.

Automated Probe

Agudio, G., Prato, G.P., and Bartolucci, E.G.: Computerized Charting of Probing Depths, *J. Periodontol., 56,* 766, December, 1985.

Birek, P., McCulloch, C.A.G., and Hardy, V.: Gingival Attachment Level Measurements with an Automated Periodontal Probe, *J. Clin. Periodontol., 14,* 472, September, 1987.

Borsboom, P.C.F., ten Bosch, J.J., Corba, N.H.C., and Tromp, J.A.H.: A Simple Constant-force Pocket Probe, *J. Periodontol., 52,* 390, July, 1981.

Clark, W.B., Yang, M.C.K., and Magnusson, I.: Measuring Clinical Attachment: Reproducibility of Relative Measurements with an Electronic Probe, *J. Periodontol., 63,* 831, October, 1992.

Galgut, P.N. and Waite, I.M.: A Comparison Between Measurements Made with a Conventional Periodontal Probe, an Electronic Pressure Probe and Measurements Made at Surgery, *Int. Dent. J., 40,* 333, December, 1990.

Gibbs, C.H., Hirschfeld, J.W., Lee, J.G., Low, S.B., Magnusson, I., Thousand, R.R., Yerneni, P., and Clark, W.B.: Description and Clinical Evaluation of a New Computerized Periodontal Probe—The Florida Probe, *J. Clin. Periodontol., 15,* 137, February, 1988.

Jeffcoat, M.K., Jeffcoat, R.L., Jens, S.C., and Captain, K.: A New Periodontal Probe With Automated Cemento-enamel Junction Detection, *J. Clin. Periodontol., 13,* 276, April, 1986.

Kalkwarf, K.L., Kaldahl, W.B., and Patil, K.D.: Comparison of Manual and Pressure-controlled Periodontal Probing, *J. Periodontol., 57,* 467, August, 1986.

Karim, M., Birek, P., and McCulloch, C.A.: Controlled Force Measurements of Gingival Attachment Level Made With the Toronto Automated Probe Using Electronic Guidance, *J. Clin. Periodontol., 17,* 594, September, 1990.

Magnusson, I., Fuller, W.W., Heins, P.J., Rau, C.F., Gibbs, C.H., Marks, R.G., and Clark, W.B.: Correlation Between Electronic and Visual Readings of Pocket Depths With a Newly Developed Constant Force Probe, *J. Clin. Periodontol., 15,* 180, March, 1988.

Magnusson, I., Clark, W.B., Marks, R.G., Gibbs, C.H., Manouchehr-Pour, M., and Low, S.B.: Attachment Level Measurements With a Constant Force Electronic Probe, *J. Clin. Periodontol., 15,* 185, March, 1988.

Marks, R.G., Low, S.B., Taylor, M., Baggs, R., Magnusson, I., and Clark, W.B.: Reproducibility of Attachment Level Measurements With Two Models of the Florida Probe®, *J. Clin. Periodontol., 18,* 780, November, 1991.

McCulloch, C.A.G., Birek, P., and Hardy, V.: Comparison of Gingival Attachment Level Measurements With an Automated Periodontal Probe and a Pressure-sensitive Probe, *J. Periodont. Res., 22,* 348, September, 1987.

Mombelli, A. and Graf, H.: Depth-force-patterns in Periodontal Probing, *J. Clin. Periodontol., 13,* 126, February, 1986.

Osborn, J., Stoltenberg, J., Huso, B., Aeppli, D., and Pihlstrom, B.: Comparison of Measurement Variability Using a Standard and Constant Force Periodontal Probe, *J. Periodontol., 61,* 497, August, 1990.

Osborn, J.B., Stoltenberg, J.L., Huso, B.A., Aeppli, D.M., and Pihlstrom, B.L.: Comparison of Measurement Variability in Subjects With Moderate Periodontitis Using a Conventional and Constant Force Periodontal Probe, *J. Periodontol., 63,* 283, April, 1992.

Quirynen, M., Callens, A., van Steenberghe, D., and Nys, M.: Clinical Evaluation of A Constant Force Electronic Probe, *J. Periodontol., 64,* 35, January, 1993.

Tessier, J.-F., Ellen, R.P., Birek, P., Kulkarni, G.V., and McCulloch, C.A.G.: Relationship Between Periodontal Probing Velocity and Gingival Inflammation in Human Subjects, *J. Clin. Periodontol., 20,* 41, January, 1993.

Walsh, T.F. and Saxby, M.S.: Inter- and Intra-examiner Variability Using Standard and Constant Force Periodontal Probes, *J. Clin. Periodontol., 16,* 140, March, 1989.

Watts, T.: Constant Force Probing With and Without a Stent in Untreated Periodontal Disease: The Clinical Reproducibility Problem and Possible Sources of Error, *J. Clin. Periodontol., 14,* 407, August, 1987.

Yang, M.C.K., Marks, R.G., Magnusson, I., Clouser, B., and Clark, W.B.: Reproducibility of an Electronic Probe in Relative Attachment Level Measurements, *J. Clin. Periodontol., 19,* 541, September, 1992.

Temperature Probe

Fedi, P.F. and Killoy, W.J.: Temperature Differences at Periodontal Sites in Health and Disease, *J. Periodontol., 63,* 24, January, 1992.

Haffajee, A.D., Socransky, S.S., and Goodson, J.M.: Subgingival Temperature (I). Relation to Baseline Clinical Parameters, *J. Clin. Periodontol., 19,* 401, July, 1992.

Haffajee, A.D., Socransky, S.S., and Goodson, J.M.: Subgingival Temperature (II). Relation to Future Periodontal Attachment Loss, *J. Clin. Periodontol., 19,* 409, July, 1992.

Haffajee, A.D., Socransky, S.S., Smith, C., Dibart, S., and Goodson, J.M.: Subgingival Temperature (III). Relation to Microbial Counts, *J. Clin. Periodontol., 19,* 417, July, 1992.

Kung, R.I.V., Ochs, B., and Goodson, J.M.: Temperature as a Periodontal Diagnostic, *J. Clin. Periodontol., 17,* 557, September, 1990.

Perdok, J.F., Lukacovic, M., Majeti, S., Arends, J., and Busscher, H.J.: Sulcus Temperature Distributions in the Absence and Presence of Oral Hygiene, *J. Periodont. Res., 27,* 97, March, 1992.

Radiographs

Åkesson, L., Håkansson, J., and Rohlin, M.: Comparison of Panoramic and Intraoral Radiography and Pocket Probing for the Measurement of the Marginal Bone Level, *J. Periodontol., 19,* 326, May, 1992.

Allen, D.L., McFall, W.T., and Jenzano, J.W.: *Periodontics for the Dental Hygienist,* 4th ed. Philadelphia, Lea & Febiger, 1987, pp. 118–124.

Benn, D.K.: A Review of the Reliability of Radiographic Measurements in Estimating Alveolar Bone Changes, *J. Clin. Periodontol., 17,* 14, January, 1990.

Buchanan, S.A., Jenderseck, R.S., Granet, M.A., Kircos, L.T., Chambers, D.W., and Robertson, P.B.: Radiographic Detection of Dental Calculus, *J. Periodontol., 58,* 747, November, 1987.

Carranza, F.A.: *Glickman's Clinical Periodontology,* 7th ed. Philadelphia, W.B. Saunders Co., 1990, pp. 501–516.

Deas, D.E., Pasquali, L.A., Yuan, C.H., and Kornman, K.S.: The Relationship Between Probing Attachment Loss and Computerized Radiographic Analysis in Monitoring Progression of Periodontitis, *J. Periodontol., 62,* 135, February, 1991.

Hausmann, E., Allen, K., and Clerehugh, V.: What Alveolar Crest Level on a Bite-wing Radiograph Represents Bone Loss?, *J. Periodontol., 62,* 570, September, 1991.

Jeffcoat, M.K., Page, R., Reddy, M., Wannawisute, A., Waite, P., Palcanis, K., Cogen, R., Williams, R.C., and Basch, C.: Use of Digital Radiography to Demonstrate the Potential of Naxproxen as an Adjunct in the Treatment of Rapidly Progressive Periodontitis, *J. Periodont. Res., 26,* 415, September, 1991.

Kaimenyi, J.T. and Ashley, F.P.: Assessment of Bone Loss in Periodontitis from Panoramic Radiographs, *J. Clin. Periodontol., 15,* 170, March, 1988.

Papapanou, P.N. and Wennström, J.L.: Radiographic and Clinical Assessments of Destructive Periodontal Disease, *J. Clin. Periodontol., 16,* 609, October, 1989.

The Teeth

14

Clinical examination of the teeth is essential prior to treatment to provide guidelines for treatment planning, instrumentation, instruction, and follow-up evaluation. In general, patients may tend to be more concerned about their teeth than about their gingiva. The reasons may be related to personal appearance, degree of information, which may be greater about teeth than gingiva, and sensitivity and pain associated with ailments of the teeth.

Background study of histology, dental anatomy, and oral pathology is important to this phase of clinical practice. *Suggested Readings* at the end of this chapter have been selected for additional information, reference, and review. Key words are defined in table 14–1.

With information from the patient's personal dental history (table 6–2, page 93) and a thorough clinical and radiographic examination, the dental hygienist can

A. Prepare a charting and provide a record of deviations from the normal teeth for the diagnostic work-up.
B. Identify the dental hygiene treatment and counseling needed in relation to the teeth for the particular patient.
C. Outline the patient's preventive dental program (page 330).
D. Utilize the specific data during treatment for instrument selection and adaptation.

THE DENTITIONS

Formation of the primary teeth begins *in utero*. Table 14–2 shows the weeks *in utero* when each primary tooth begins to mineralize and the average months after birth when the enamel is completely formed before the date of eruption.

Mineralization of the permanent teeth starts at birth and continues into adolescence. The chronology of development and eruption appears in table 14–3. Roots normally are completed by 3 years after eruption.

The mixed dentition, when primary teeth are being exfoliated and permanent teeth move in to take their places, occurs between the ages of 6 and 12 years. Figure 14–1 illustrates the mixed dentition of a child approximately 6 years of age.

DENTAL CARIES

The World Health Organization has defined dental caries as a "localized, post-eruptive, pathological process of external origin involving softening of the hard tooth tissue and proceeding to the formation of a cavity."[1] Dental caries is a preventable disease.

I. DEVELOPMENT OF DENTAL CARIES

Requirements for the development of a carious lesion are microorganisms, carbohydrate, primarily sucrose, and a susceptible tooth surface. Figure 28–2 (page 425) is a diagram that shows 4 overlapping circles to illustrate the essential factors in the process of dental caries initiation.

Bacterial plaque may contain numerous types of acid-forming bacteria. Mutans streptococci have been specifically implicated. The role of bacterial plaque and the factors involved in dental caries initiation are described in Chapter 16, pages 267 and 268.

231

TABLE 14-1
KEY WORDS: TEETH

Accessory root canal: a secondary canal extending from the pulp to the surface of the root; frequently found near the apex of a root but may occur higher and provide a connection to a periodontal pocket.

Amelogenesis (am′ĕ-lō-jen′ĕ-sis): production and development of enamel.

Avulsion (ah-vul′-shun): the tearing away or forcible separation of a structure or part. **Tooth avulsion** is the traumatic separation of a tooth from the alveolus.

Bruxism (bruk′sĭzm): an oral habit of grinding, clenching, or clamping the teeth; involuntary, rhythmic, or spasmodic movements outside the chewing range; may damage teeth and attachment apparatus.

Cariogenic (kăr′ē-ō-jen′ik): *adj.* conducive to dental caries.

Carious (kā′rē-us): *adj.* used to define a **carious lesion.**

Cementicle (sē-men′tĭ-kel): a calcified spherical body, composed of cementum, lying free within the periodontal ligament, attached to the cementum, or imbedded within the cementum.

Dental caries (kăr′ēz) disease of the mineralized structures of the teeth characterized by demineralization of the hard components and dissolution of the organic matrix.

  Arrested caries: carious lesion that has become stationary and does not show a tendency to progress further; frequently has a hard surface and takes on a dark brown or reddish-brown color.

  Primary caries: occurs on a surface not previously affected; also called initial caries; early lesion may be referred to as incipient caries.

  Rampant caries: widespread formation of chalky white areas and incipient lesions that may increase in size over a comparatively short time.

  Recurrent caries: occurs on a surface adjacent to a restoration; may be a continuation of the original lesion; also called secondary caries.

Dentition (den-tĭsh′un): the natural teeth in the dental arch.

  Primary (deciduous) dentition: the first teeth; normally will be shed and replaced by permanent teeth.

Permanent dentition: the natural 32 teeth that serve throughout life.

Mixed dentition: combination of primary and permanent teeth between ages 6 and 12 when primary teeth are being replaced; starts with the eruption of the first permanent tooth.

Succedaneous (suk′sē-dā′nē-us): the permanent teeth that erupt into the positions of exfoliated primary teeth.

Edentulous (ē-den′tū-lus): without teeth; referred to as partially edentulous when some, but not all, teeth are missing.

Electrolyte (ē-lek′trō-līt): a conductor; a substance that, in solution, dissociates into electrically charged particles (ions) and thus is capable of conducting an electric current.

Etiology (ē tĭ-ol′ō-jē): the science or study of the cause of a disease or disorder.

Exfoliation (eks-fō-lĭ-a′shun): loss of primary teeth following physiologic resorption of root structure.

Facet (fă-set′): a small flattened surface on a hard body, such as a tooth; a wear facet can result from attrition or repeated parafunctional contact.

Hypoplasia (hī pō-plā′zē-ah): incomplete development or underdevelopment of a tissue or organ.

  Enamel hypoplasia: incomplete or defective formation of the enamel of either primary or permanent teeth. The result may be an irregularity of tooth form, color, or surface.

Idiopathic (ĭd ē-ō-path′ik): denoting a condition of unknown cause.

Incipient (in-sip′ē-ent): beginning; coming into existence.

pH: the symbol of hydrogen ion concentration expressed in numbers corresponding to the acidity or alkalinity of an aqueous solution; the range is from 14 (pure base) to 0 (pure acid); neutral is at 7.0.

  Critical pH: the pH at which demineralization occurs; for enamel, pH 4.5 to 5.5; for cementum, pH 6.0 to 6.7.

Resorption (rē-sorp′shun): removal of bone or tooth structure; gradual dissolution of the mineralized tissue; may be internal or external; occurs during exfoliation of a primary tooth, and from the pressure of orthodontic treatment.

II. CLASSIFICATION OF CAVITIES
A. G.V. Black's Classification[2]

The standard method for classifying dental caries was developed by Dr. G.V. Black, a noted dental educator who divided the categories into classes according to surfaces of the teeth; each class is represented by a Roman numeral. These categories are customarily used for carious lesions, cavity preparations, and finished restorations. See table 14–4 for definitions and illustrations.

B. Nomenclature by Surfaces

1. *Simple Cavity.* Involves one tooth surface. *Example:* occlusal cavity.

2. *Compound Cavity.* Involves two tooth surfaces. *Example:* mesio-occlusal cavity, referred to as an "M-O" cavity.

3. *Complex Cavity.* Involves more than two tooth surfaces. *Example:* mesio-occlusal-distal, referred to as an "M-O-D" cavity.

ENAMEL CARIES

I. STEPS IN THE FORMATION OF A CAVITY
A. Phase I: Incipient Lesion

1. *Subsurface Demineralization.* Acid products from cariogenic bacterial plaque pass

TABLE 14–2
TOOTH DEVELOPMENT AND ERUPTION: PRIMARY TEETH

		Hard Tissue Formation Begins (weeks in utero)	Enamel Completed (months after birth)	Eruption (months)	Root Completed (year)
Maxillary	Central Incisor	14	1½	10 (8–12)	1½
	Lateral Incisor	16	2½	11 (9–13)	2
	Canine	17	9	19 (16–22)	3¼
	First Molar	15½	6	16 (13–19 boys) (14–18 girls)	2½
	Second Molar	19	11	29 (25–33)	3
Mandibular	Central Incisor	14	2½	8 (6–10)	1½
	Lateral Incisor	16	3	13 (10–16)	1½
	Canine	17	9	20 (17–23)	3¼
	First Molar	15½	5½	16 (14–18)	2¼
	Second Molar	18	10	27 (23–31 boys) (24–30 girls)	3

From Lunt, R.C. and Law, D.B.: A Review of the Chronology of Eruption of Deciduous Teeth, *J. Am. Dent. Assoc., 89,* 872, October, 1974.

TABLE 14–3
TOOTH DEVELOPMENT AND ERUPTION: PERMANENT TEETH

		Hard Tissue Formation Begins	Enamel Completed (years)	Eruption (years)	Root Completed (years)
Maxillary	Central Incisor	3–4 mos.	4–5	7–8	10
	Lateral Incisor	10 mos.	4–5	8–9	11
	Canine	4–5 mos.	6–7	11–12	13–15
	First Premolar	1½–1¾ yrs.	5–6	10–11	12–13
	Second Premolar	2–2¼ yrs.	6–7	10–12	12–14
	First Molar	at birth	2½–3	6–7	9–10
	Second Molar	2½–3 yrs.	7–8	12–13	14–16
	Third Molar	7–9 yrs.	12–16	17–21	18–25
Mandibular	Central Incisor	3–4 mos.	4–5	6–7	9
	Lateral Incisor	3–4 mos.	4–5	7–8	10
	Canine	4–5 mos.	6–7	9–10	12–14
	First Premolar	1¾–2 yrs.	5–6	10–12	12–13
	Second Premolar	2¼–2½ yrs.	6–7	11–12	13–14
	First Molar	at birth	2½–3	6–7	9–10
	Second Molar	2½–3 yrs.	7–8	11–13	14–15
	Third Molar	8–10 yrs.	12–16	17–21	18–25

From Ash, M.M.: *Wheeler's Dental Anatomy, Physiology, and Occlusion,* 7th ed. Philadelphia, W.B. Saunders Co., 1993, page 25.

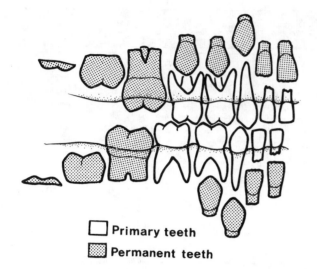

☐ Primary teeth
▨ Permanent teeth

FIG. 14–1. Mixed Dentition at Approximately Age 6 Years. The average child has 20 primary teeth in place and root resorption of the incisors has started as the developing permanent incisors move into position. The first permanent molars are partially erupted.

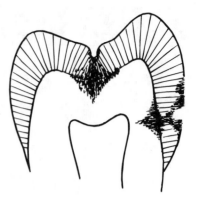

FIG. 14–2. Dental Caries. Cones of dental caries in a pit and fissure and on a smooth tooth surface. Dental caries follows the general direction of the enamel rods, spreads at the dentinoenamel junction, and then continues along the dentinal tubules.

through microchannels (pores) of the enamel.

2. *Visualization.* Area of demineralization not visible by clinical observation during initial changes; thin layer of enamel remains over the surface.

3. *First Clinical Evidence.* White spot with no breakthrough to enamel surface; with time, area may turn brown from food, beverages, or tobacco use.

4. *Remineralization.* Low concentrations of fluoride applied frequently during this phase can provide sources for uptake by the demineralized zone. The porous demineralized area readily takes up fluoride from dentifrice, mouthrinse, fluoridated drinking water, and all possible sources. Figure 29–3 (page 438) shows examples of levels of concentration of fluoride in surface enamel and in a white spot area.

B. Phase II: Untreated Incipient Lesion

1. *Breakdown of Enamel Over the Demineralized Area (White Spot).* Visible to observation and irregular to application of an explorer.

2. *Progression of Carious Lesion.* Follows general direction of enamel rods.

3. *Spread of Carious Lesion.* Spreads at dentino-enamel junction; continues along the dentinal tubules (figure 14–2).

II. TYPES OF DENTAL CARIES (described by location)

A. Pit and Fissure
Caries begins in a minute fault in the enamel.
1. Occurs where three or more lobes of the de-

veloping tooth join; closure of the enamel plates is imperfect. *Examples:* occlusal pits of molars and premolars.

2. Occurs at the endings of grooves of the teeth. *Example:* the buccal groove of a mandibular molar.

B. Smooth Surface
Caries begins in smooth surfaces where there is no pit, groove, or other fault. It occurs in areas where bacterial plaque collects, such as proximal tooth surfaces, cervical thirds of teeth, and other difficult-to-clean areas.

NURSING CARIES[3]

Nursing caries is a form of rampant caries found in very young children who routinely have been given a nursing bottle when going to sleep or who have experienced prolonged at-will breast-feeding. Other names for the same condition are nursing bottle mouth, baby bottle syndrome, baby bottle caries, and prolonged nursing habit.

I. ETIOLOGY
A. Nursing bottle that contains sweetened milk or other fluid sweetened with sucrose.
B. Pacifier dipped or filled with a sweet agent, such as honey.
C. Prolonged at-will breast-feeding.

II. EFFECTS
Maxillary anterior teeth are the most severely affected. As the baby falls asleep, pools of sweet liquid can collect about the teeth. While the sucking is active, the liquid passes beyond the teeth. The nipple covers the mandibular anterior teeth; hence, they are rarely affected.

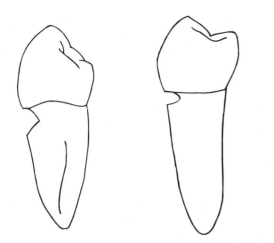

FIG. 14–7. Abrasion. Profile view of the facial surface of mandibular premolars shows shape of abrasion on the root. Note that the area of abrasion undermines the enamel.

I. CAUSES OF TOOTH FRACTURES
A. Automobile, bicycle, and diving accidents.
B. Contact sports when mouth protectors are not worn.
C. Blows incurred while fighting.
D. Iatrogenic, caused by dental treatments, such as certain endodontic or restorative procedures.

II. DESCRIPTION
A. Line of Fracture
1. Horizontal.
2. Diagonal.
3. Vertical.

B. Radiographic Signs of Recent Trauma[13]
1. Widened periodontal ligament space.
2. Radiolucent fracture line.
3. Radiopaque areas where fracture segments overlap.
4. Tooth displacement.

III. CLASSIFICATION: WORLD HEALTH ORGANIZATION[14]
Classification provided by the World Health Organization is numbered as a special section of the International Classification of Diseases. Both primary and permanent dentitions are included. Figure 14–8 illustrates fractures of a central incisor.

873.60 **Fracture of enamel of tooth only.** Includes chipping and incomplete fractures (cracks).
873.61 **Fracture of crown of tooth without pulpal involvement.**
873.62 **Fracture of crown with pulpal involvement.**
873.63 **Fracture of root of tooth.**
873.64 **Fracture of crown and root of tooth with or without pulpal involvement.**
873.65 **Fracture of tooth, unspecified.**
873.66 **Luxation (dislocation) of tooth.** This category may involve concussion, subluxation, and luxation. A tooth with concussion is sensitive to percussion but is not loosened or displaced. Loosening without displacement is subluxation, and loosening with displacement is luxation.
873.67 **Intrusion or extrusion of tooth.** Intrusion into the alveolar bone is usually accompanied by fracture of the alveolar socket. Extrusion from the socket is a partial displacement.
873.68 **Avulsion of tooth.** Avulsion is the complete displacement of the tooth out of its socket. The emergency care for a tooth forcibly displaced may be found in table 61–3.

CLINICAL EXAMINATION OF THE TEETH

Following is a list of major factors to observe when examining the teeth. Several of these are described in other chapters, for which page references are noted. Information about hypoplasia, attrition, erosion, abrasion, dental caries, and tooth vitality is included in this chapter. Table 14–5 lists factors to observe during the

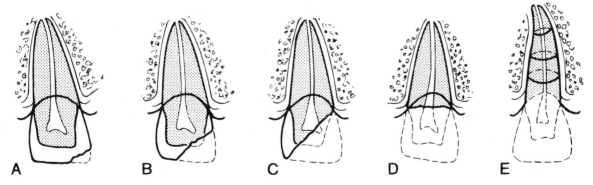

FIG. 14–8. Fractures of Teeth. A. Enamel fracture. **B.** Crown fracture without pulpal involvement. **C.** Crown fracture with pulpal involvement. **D.** Fracture of crown and root near neck of tooth. **E.** Root fractures involving cementum, dentin, and the pulp may occur in the apical, middle, or coronal third of the root.

TABLE 14–5
EXAMINATION OF THE TEETH

Feature	To Observe	Dental Hygiene Implication
Morphology	Number of teeth (missing teeth verified by radiographic examination) Size, shape Arch form Position of individual teeth Injuries; fractures of the crown (root fractures observed in radiographs)	Selection and adaptation of instruments Areas prone to dental caries initiation, particularly the difficult-to-reach areas during plaque control Pulp test for vitality may be indicated
Development	Anomalies and developmental defects Pits and white spots	Distinguish hypoplasia and dental fluorosis from demineralization Identify pits for sealants
Eruption	Sequence of eruption: normal, irregular Unerupted teeth observed in radiographs	Care in using floss in the col area where the epithelium is usually less mature in young children Orthodontic needs Procedures for preservation of primary teeth

Deposits
  Food debris
  Plaque
  Calculus
    Supragingival
    Subgingival
	Overall evaluation of self-care and plaque-control measures
	Relation of appearance of teeth to gingival health
	Extent and location of plaque, debris, and calculus
	Calculus and the tooth surface pocket wall
		Need for instruction and guidance
		
		Frequency of follow-up and maintenance appointments

Stains
  Extrinsic
  Intrinsic
	Extrinsic: colors relate to causes
	Intrinsic: dark, grayish
	
	Tobacco stain
		Need for test for pulp vitality
		Stain removal procedures; selection of polishing agent
		Dentifrice recommendation
		Plaque-control emphasis for plaque-related stains
		Provide information concerning the oral effects of tobacco use

Regressive Changes	Attrition: primary and permanent Abrasion: physical agents that may be a cause Erosion	Evaluate causes and treat or counsel for prevention Dietary analysis: for finding foods that may be related Selection of nonabrasive dentifrice Habit evaluation
Exposed Cementum	Relation to gingival recession, pocket formation Areas of narrow attached gingiva Hypersensitivity	Special care areas where only slight attached gingiva remains Nonabrasive dentifrice advised Measures to prevent root-surface caries Care during instrumentation Indication for application of desensitizing agent
Dental Caries	Areas of demineralization Carious lesions (proximal lesions observed in radiographs) Arrested caries Root caries	Charting Treatment plan Preventive program for caries control, fluoride, dietary factors Follow-up and frequency of maintenance

TABLE 14-5 (continued)
EXAMINATION OF THE TEETH

Feature	To Observe	Dental Hygiene Implication
Restorations	Contour of restorations, overhangs	
	Proximal contact (see separate heading later in this table)	Chart and correct inadequate margins
	Surface smoothness	Selection of instruments and polishing agents
	Staining	Dentifrice selection to prevent discoloration
Factors Related to Occlusion Tooth wear	Facets; worn-down cusp tips	Need for study of bruxism and other parafunctional habits
	Health of supporting structures; observation of radiographs for signs of trauma from occlusion	
Proximal contacts	Use of floss to find open contact areas Areas of food retention	Chart inadequate contacts for corrective measures Use of floss by patient
Mobility	Degree; comparison of chartings	Need for reduction of inflammatory factors that may be related
	Possible causes	Dentist will identify and treat factors related to trauma from occlusion
Classification	Position of teeth	Relationship to orthodontic treatment needs
	Angle's classification	
Habits	Nail or object biting; lip or cheek biting Observe effects on lip, cheek, teeth Tongue thrust; reverse swallow	Guidance for habit correction when indicated
Edentulous Areas	Radiographic evaluation for impacted, unerupted teeth, retained root tips, other deviations from normal	Supplemental fulcrum selection during instrumentation Applied plaque-control procedures for abutment teeth
Replacement for Missing Teeth Dentures Partial dentures	Teeth and tissue that support a prosthesis Cleanliness of a prosthesis Factors that contribute to food and debris retention	Preventive measures for harm to supporting teeth and soft tissues Instruction in personal care of fixed and removable dentures; use of floss under fixed partial denture; other appropriate care
Saliva	Amount and consistency Dryness of mouth	Relation to instruction for prevention of dental caries: more caries can be expected in a dry mouth. Use of saliva substitute; fluoride

examination of the teeth and suggests relationships to appointment procedures.

I. GENERAL CHARACTERISTICS
A. Number of teeth; eruption pattern (tables 14-2 and 14-3).
B. Anomalies of size, form, number.
C. Replacements, such as restorations for individual teeth and groups of teeth (fixed and removable).

II. DEPOSITS (table 16-2, page 260)
A. Calculus.
B. Bacterial plaque.
C. Materia alba.

III. COLOR
A. Intrinsic stains (pages 283-285).
B. Extrinsic stains (pages 281-283).

IV. DEVELOPMENTAL DEFECTS
A. Enamel hypoplasia.
B. Amelogenesis imperfecta; dentinogenesis imperfecta (page 284).

V. REGRESSIVE CHANGES
A. Attrition.
B. Erosion.
C. Abrasion.

VI. OCCLUSION (pages 248, 254)
  A. Proximal contact relation: areas of food impaction.
  B. Mobility (page 223).

VII. DENTAL CARIES AND DEMINERALIZATION

VIII. VITALITY OF PULP

IX. TOOTH FRACTURES

RECOGNITION OF CARIOUS LESIONS

Both visual and exploratory means are used to identify dental caries.

I. PREPARATION
Dry each tooth or group of teeth with compressed air and carefully inspect each surface, first visually, and then with an explorer as necessary to confirm visual findings.

II. VISUAL EXAMINATION: ENAMEL CARIES
Characteristic changes in the color and translucency of tooth structure may be observed. Such changes either are definite signs of dental caries progress or may lead the examiner to suspect dental caries, which can then be checked further with an explorer. Variations in color and translucency include the following:
  A. Chalky white areas of demineralization.
  B. Grayish-white discoloration of marginal ridges caused by dental caries of the proximal surface underneath.
  C. Grayish-white color spreading from margins of restorations caused by lesions of secondary dental caries.
  D. In relation to an amalgam restoration, dental caries appears translucent in outer portion and white and opaque adjacent to the amalgam.
  E. Open carious lesions may vary in color from yellowish-brown to dark brown.
  F. Discoloration is generally less severe when dental caries progresses rapidly than when it progresses slowly.
  G. Dull, flat white, opaque areas under direct light show loss of translucency, particularly of the enamel.
  H. Dark shadow on a proximal surface may be shown by transillumination. This type of observation is especially useful for anterior teeth and unrestored posterior teeth.

III. EXPLORATORY EXAMINATION
A. Smooth Surface Caries
  1. *Technique.* Adapt the side of the tip of the explorer closely to the tooth surface as described on page 222. Examine for hardness versus softness, roughness versus smoothness, and continuity of tooth surface versus breaks in continuity.
  2. *Restorations.* Follow the margins of all restorations around with an explorer. Overhanging margins may or may not appear in the radiographs, depending on superimposition. Types of overhangs are described on pages 582–583. Chart all irregularities of existing restorations.

B. Pit and Fissure Caries
When a pit or fissure is discolored, one cannot determine visually whether dental caries is present except when a large obvious cavity can be seen. An obvious cavity should not be explored.
  1. Direct the explorer tip so that it can pass straight into the pit or fissure. When the tip is not positioned correctly, caries in a small narrow pit can go undetected.
  2. Explorer catches when dental caries is present and softening of tooth structure is evident.

IV. RADIOGRAPHIC EXAMINATION
During the clinical examination, information revealed by radiographs is utilized for supplementation and confirmation. Neither clinical nor radiographic examination is complete without the other. A few principal items to be seen in a radiographic examination of the teeth are
  Anomalies
  Impactions
  Fractures
  Internal and root resorption
  Dental caries
  Periapical radiolucencies

A. Technique Principles
Periapical radiographs usually provide sufficient information concerning the teeth, but panoramic, extraoral, or occlusal radiographs may be needed for detecting or defining anomalies and pathologic lesions outside the scope of periapical radiographs. Bitewing radiographs or periapical radiographs made by a paralleling technique with no overlapping are most satisfactory for dental caries detection.

Principles for examination were described on pages 158–160. Mounted radiographs on an adequately lighted viewbox are a necessity during charting and treatment procedures. For the detection of early carious lesions, a hand magnifying reading glass can be of invaluable assistance.

B. Detection of Dental Caries
Radiographs are not needed for facial, lingual, or occlusal carious lesions because they are accessible and best observed by exploration and direct vision. Because of superimposition of other parts of the tooth, facial, lingual, and oc-

clusal carious lesions need to be fairly well advanced before they are definitely discernible in a radiograph.

1. *Proximal Caries.* Proximal surface lesions may be missed if radiographs are not used. Clinical skills for caries discernment need to be perfected, however, to prevent excess exposure of a patient to unnecessary radiation.
   a. Proximal lesions. Properly angulated radiographs with no overlapping are required for the detection of small lesions that involve the enamel or extend slightly into the dentin.
   b. Proximal overhanging restorations. An overhanging filling or dental caries under that filling may be present, even if none can be seen in the radiograph because of superimposition. An explorer must be passed around the complete margin to confirm the condition.
2. *Root Caries*
   a. Location. Most root carious lesions occur in the vicinity of and just beneath the cementoenamel junction.
   b. Appearance. Root caries appears as a saucer-shaped lesion in a radiograph. It may appear to undermine the enamel or it may be located beneath an overhanging filling.

TESTING FOR PULPAL VITALITY

Any tooth suspected of being nonvital must be tested for pulpal vitality or degree of vitality. Such testing is particularly significant prior to treatment involving periodontal surgery, any restorative procedures, and orthodontic appliance placement. Diagnosis of vitality is made not only on the basis of a pulp test, but also on consideration of all data from the patient history and clinical and radiographic examinations.

A tooth may become nonvital from bacterial causes, particularly invasion of the pulp from dental caries or periodontal disease. Physical causes may be mechanical or thermal injuries. Examples of mechanical injuries are trauma, such as a blow, or iatrogenic dental procedures, such as cavity preparation or too-rapid orthodontic movement.

I. OBSERVATIONS THAT SUGGEST LOSS OF VITALITY
A. Clinical
1. Discoloration of a tooth crown (intrinsic stains, pages 283 and 284).
2. Fracture (part of the crown may be missing, figure 14–8).
3. Large carious lesion or large restoration.
4. Fistula with opening into the oral cavity over the apical region of a tooth.

B. Radiographic
1. Apical radiolucency, which may indicate a granuloma, cyst, or abscess.
2. Bone loss with a widened periodontal ligament space extending to the apex.
3. Fractured root.
4. Large carious lesion or restoration that appears closely related to the pulp chamber.

II. RESPONSE TO PULP TESTING
A. Rationale
Electrical pulp testing is based on the knowledge that an electrical stimulus can create pain to which a patient can react. The pulp tester, therefore, determines the conduction of stimuli to the sensory receptors. The vitality of the pulp depends on its blood supply and not on its nerve supply. For that reason, a positive or negative pulp test may not always show the true condition of the pulp.

B. Factors That Influence a Patient's Response to a Pulp Tester
1. *Degree of Pulpal Degeneration or Inflammation.* A necrotic pulp gives no response at all, whereas an acutely or chronically inflamed pulp responds at varying degrees between no response and full normal response.
2. *Pain Perception Threshold.* The lowest perceptible intensity of pain caused by a threshold stimulus. A threshold stimulus is the minimum stimulus necessary to induce patient response.
3. *Reaction to Pain.* May vary with a patient's attitude, age, sex, emotional security, fatigue, drugs used, as well as the size of the pulp and thickness of the dentin, particularly the amount of secondary dentin.
4. *Nerve Transmission Blocks.* Injuries or lesions of nerves, and anesthetics.
5. *Adjacent Metal.* Restorations or continuous bridgework.

III. ELECTRICAL PULP TESTER (VITALOMETER)
Although thermal tests using hot or cold applications have been used, the electrical pulp testers are considered more consistent.

A. Types
1. *Battery-operated*
   a. Advantages. Hand held so a clinician can work alone; portable.
   b. Disadvantage. Battery can run down. Some types have a light to indicate current in circuit.
2. *Plug-in*
   a. Advantage. More dependable than battery-operated.
   b. Disadvantage. Not self-contained; requires house-current plug.

B. Precaution

The application of an electrical current to a patient with a cardiac pacemaker or any electronic life-support device by the use of a pulp tester, ultrasonic scaler, desensitizing equipment, or electrosurgical instrument may interfere with the function of the life-support device and may constitute a serious health hazard.[15,16] A review of the patient history and consult with the patient's cardiologist are necessary prior to application of a pulp tester.

C. Preparation and Use of Equipment

Manufacturer's instructions are provided for each pulp tester and should be followed carefully. When the tester rheostat is separate from the applicator tip, an assistant is needed.

Consistency of procedures is essential to obtain consistent readings. The same pulp tester should be used for a particular patient at continuing comparative tests. Notes in a patient's record can indicate specific directions for that patient.

D. General Procedures

1. Assemble equipment.
2. Explain briefly to the patient what is to be done, but avoid detailed description, which could create anxiety or apprehension.
3. Dry the teeth to be tested to prevent the current from passing to the gingiva; isolate with cotton rolls and insert a saliva ejector, or use rubber dam.
4. Moisten the end of the tip of the tester with a small amount of toothpaste. Another electrolyte (conductor) may be used if its consistency allows it to remain where placed and prevents it from flowing over the tooth surface.
5. Instruct the patient to signal when a sensation is felt; suggest raising a hand or making a sound.
6. Apply tester tip. For certain types of pulp testers, the patient lightly holds the handle with the gloved clinician to complete the circuit.[15]
   a. Apply first to at least one tooth other than the one in question, preferably an adjacent tooth and the same tooth on the contralateral side. Such a procedure determines a normal response for the patient.
   b. Place *without pressure* but with definite contact on sound tooth structure in a consistent location on the middle or gingival third. The middle third of the crown of a single-rooted tooth and the middle third of each cusp of a multirooted tooth are frequently used (figure 14–9).

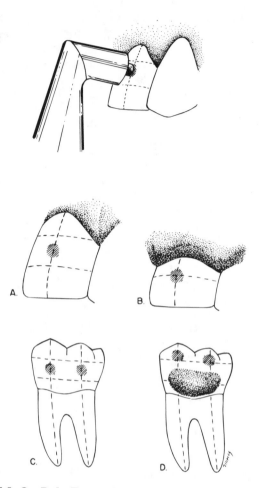

FIG. 14–9. Pulp Tester in Position. A. Correct contact point for tip of pulp tester is within the *middle third* of the crown. Avoid contact with gingiva or restorations. **B.** Adjustment of position of contact point because of gingival enlargement. **C.** Contact points on multirooted tooth. Place tip of pulp tester in the middle third over each root. **D.** Adjustment of position of contact points because of large Class V restoration.

E. Readings

1. Avoid contact with gingival or other soft tissues. A low-resistance circuit can be formed, thus allowing the circuit to by-pass the tooth.
2. Avoid contact with metallic restorations. The metal forms a more rapid conductor than does tooth structure. When approximal restorations are in contact, the circuit can be transmitted across to the adjacent tooth. The reading obtained would not pertain to the tooth in question (figure 14–10). A nonconductive clear plastic matrix strip may be inserted to separate the two metallic restorations.
3. Start with the rheostat at zero; advance slowly but steadily, stopping only momentarily after each number. Do not proceed

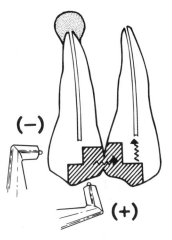

FIG. 14–10. Use of Pulp Tester. False-positive response can result when the tester is placed on a metallic restoration. The current can be transmitted across a contact area to give a reading for the adjacent tooth rather than for the tooth in question. (Redrawn from Antel, J. and Christie, W.J.: Electrical Pulp Testing, *Can. Dent. Assoc. J. 45*, 597, November, 1979.)

with such regularity that the patient can count and anticipate.

4. Test each tooth at least twice. Average the readings.
5. Record on patient's record the lowest number (average number) at which a minimal stimulus induced a response. Record for all teeth tested, not only the tooth in question.

F. Reasons for False-negative Responses[16]

1. Patient premedicated with analgesics, tranquilizers, narcotics, or alcohol.
2. Recently traumatized tooth.
3. Pulp canal narrow and calcified.
4. Newly erupted tooth with incomplete closure at the apex; immature tooth.
5. Operational factors
   a. Inadequate contact with tooth causes insufficient conduction.
   b. Wearing surgical gloves changes the conduction so that the circuit is incomplete.[15] (See General Procedures, no. 6, page 244.)
   c. Tester not turned on; batteries weak or dead.

FACTORS TO TEACH THE PATIENT

I. The cause and process of enamel or root caries formation and development for the patients at risk.
II. A description of the hardness of the enamel and of why a cavity is sometimes larger in the dentin before there is evidence from the external surface.
III. Why radiographs may be used to detect proximal incipient caries.
IV. Reasons for preservation of primary teeth.
V. Frequency of complete oral examination in relation to a continuing preventive program.
VI. Preventive measures for control and prevention of tooth abrasion, such as dentifrice selection and correction of brush selection and use.
VII. Dietary factors related to erosion.
VIII. Methods for prevention of dental caries, such as fluorides, plaque prevention and control, and control of cariogenic foods in the diet.
IX. Methods for prevention of nursing caries. Explain that nothing but plain water should be used in bedtime or naptime nursing bottles. Discourage the use of a sweetener on a pacifier. Also teach the use of a cup for milk or juice by the baby's first birthday.
X. Medicines or vitamin preparations made with heavy syrup (sucrose) have been shown to cause dental caries. Parents must learn to clean children's teeth after sugar exposures.[17]
XI. Discuss accident prevention procedures, such as always wearing a mouthguard for contact sports and wearing seat belts.

REFERENCES

1. **World Health Organization:** *The Etiology and Prevention of Dental Caries.* WHO Technical Report Series, No. 494, Geneva, World Health Organization, 1972, 19 pp.
2. **Blackwell,** R.E.: *G.V. Black's Operative Dentistry,* Volume II, 9th ed. Milwaukee, Medico-Dental Publishing Co., 1955, pp. 1–4.
3. **Ripa,** L.W.: Nursing Caries: A Comprehensive Review, *Pediatr. Dent., 10,* 268, December, 1988.
4. **American Academy of Pediatric Dentistry:** Policy Statement on Infant Dental Care, May, 1993. American Academy of Pediatric Dentistry, 211 East Chicago Avenue, Chicago, IL 60611.
5. **Bowden,** G.H.W.: Microbiology of Root Surface Caries in Humans, *J. Dent. Res., 69,* 1205, May, 1990.
6. **van Houte,** J., Jordan, H.V., Laraway, R., Kent, R., Soparkar, P.M., and DePaola, P.F.: Association of the Microbial Flora of Dental Plaque and Saliva With Human Root-surface Caries, *J. Dent. Res., 69,* 1463, August, 1990.
7. **Katz,** R.V.: The Clinical Identification of Root Caries, *Gerodontology, 5,* 21, Spring, 1986.
8. **Burt,** B.A., Ismail, A.I., and Eklund, S.A.: Root Caries in an Optimally Fluoridated and a High-fluoride Community, *J. Dent. Res., 65,* 1154, September, 1986.
9. **Stamm,** J.W., Banting, D.W., and Imrey, P.B.: Adult Root Caries Survey of Two Similar Communities With Contrasting Natural Water Fluoride Levels, *J. Am. Dent. Assoc., 120,* 143, February, 1990.
10. **Kitamura,** M., Kiyak, H.A., and Mulligan, K.: Predictors of Root Caries in the Elderly, *Community Dent. Oral Epidemiol., 14,* 34, February, 1986.

11. **Ravald,** N., Hamp, S.-E., and Birkhed, D.: Long-term Evaluation of Root Surface Caries in Periodontally Treated Patients, *J. Clin. Periodontol., 13,* 758, September, 1986.

12. **Sognnaes,** R.F., Wolcott, R.B., and Xhonga, F.A.: Dental Erosion. 1. Erosion-like Patterns Occurring in Association with Other Dental Conditions, *J. Am. Dent. Assoc., 84,* 571, March, 1972.

13. **Tyndall,** D.A.: Seminar II. The Radiology of Trauma, *Dent. Radiogr. Photogr., 57,* 17, Nos. 1–4, 1985.

14. **World Health Organization:** *Application of the International Classification of Diseases to Dentistry and Stomatology,* ICD-DA, 2nd ed. Geneva, World Health Organization, 1978, pp. 88–89.

15. **Kolbinson,** D.A. and Teplitsky, P.E.: Electric Pulp Testing With Examination Gloves, *Oral Surg. Oral Med. Oral Pathol., 65,* 122, January, 1988.

16. **Cohen,** S. and Burns, R.C., eds.: *Pathways of the Pulp,* 5th ed. St. Louis, Mosby, 1991, p. 16.

17. **Rekola,** M.: *In vivo* Acid Production From Medicines in Syrup Form, *Caries Res., 23,* 412, November-December, 1989.

SUGGESTED READINGS

Anderson, M.H., Molvar, M.P., and Powell, L.V.: Treating Dental Caries as an Infectious Disease, *Oper. Dent., 16,* 21, January-February, 1991.

Artun, J. and Thylstrup, A.: A 3-year Clinical and SEM Study of Surface Changes of Carious Enamel Lesions After Inactivation, *Am. J. Orthod. Dentofacial Orthop., 95,* 327, April, 1989.

de Vries, H.C.B., Ruiken, H.M.H.M., König, K.G., and van't Hof, M.A.: Radiographic Versus Clinical Diagnosis of Approximal Carious Lesions, *Caries Res., 24,* 364, September-October, 1990.

Hirsch, J.M., Livian, G., Edward, S., and Noren, J.G.: Tobacco Habits Among Teenagers in the City of Göteborg, Sweden and Possible Association With Dental Caries, *Swed. Dent. J., 15,* 117, No. 3, 1991.

Kidd, E.A.M., Toffenetti, F., and Mjör, I.A.: Secondary Caries, *Int. Dent. J., 42,* 127, June, 1992.

Massler, M. and Schour, I.: *Atlas of the Mouth,* 2nd ed. Chicago, American Dental Association, Plates 7–16.

McCabe, R.P., Adamkiewicz, V.W., and Pekovic, D.D.: Invasion of Bacteria in Enamel Carious Lesions, *Can. Dent. Assoc. J., 57,* 403, May, 1991.

McCormack-Brown, K.R. and McDermott, R.J.: Dental Caries: Selected Factors of Children at Risk, *Dent. Assist., 60,* 10, July/August, 1991.

Newbrun, E.: Preventing Dental Caries: Current and Prospective Strategies, *J. Am. Dent. Assoc., 123,* 68, May, 1992.

Newbrun, E.: Preventing Dental Caries: Breaking the Chain of Transmission, *J. Am. Dent. Assoc., 123,* 55, June, 1992.

Pitts, N.B. and Kidd, E.A.M.: Some of the Factors to be Considered in the Prescription and Timing of Bitewing Radiography in the Diagnosis and Management of Dental Caries, *J. Dent., 20,* 74, April, 1992.

Smith, D.J., Anderson, J.M., King, W.F., van Houte, J., and Taubman, M.A.: Oral Streptococcal Colonization of Infants, *Oral Microbiol. Immunol., 8,* 1, February, 1993.

Tappuni, A.R. and Challacombe, S.J.: Distribution and Isolation Frequency of Eight Streptococcal Species in Saliva From Predentate and Dentate Children and Adults, *J. Dent. Res., 72,* 31, January, 1993.

Wenzel, A., Fejerskov, O., Kidd, E., Joyston-Bechal, S., and Groeneveld, A.: Depth of Occlusal Caries Assessed Clinically by Conventional Film Radiographs and by Digitized, Processed Radiographs, *Caries Res., 24,* 327, September-October, 1990.

Wenzel, A., Larsen, M.J., and Fejerskov, O.: Detection of Occlusal Caries Without Cavitation by Visual Inspection, Film Radiographs, Xeroradiographs, and Digitized Radiographs, *Caries Res., 25,* 365, September-October, 1991.

Wright, J.T., Cutter, G.R., Dasanayake, A.P., Stiles, H.M., and Caufield, P.W.: Effect of Conventional Dental Restorative Treatment on Bacteria in Saliva, *Community Dent. Oral Epidemiol., 20,* 138, June, 1992.

Yusof, Z.: Proximal Tooth Surface Quality and Periodontal Status, *J. Oral Rehabil., 18,* 95, January, 1991.

Nursing Caries

Alaluusua, S.: Transmission of Mutans Streptococci, *Proc. Finn. Dent. Soc., 87,* 443, No. 4, 1991.

Barnes, G.P., Parker, W.A., Lyon, T.C., Drum, M.A., and Coleman, G.C.: Ethnicity, Location, Age, and Fluoridation Factors in Baby Bottle Tooth Decay and Caries Prevalence of Head Start Children, *Public Health Rep., 107,* 167, March-April, 1992.

Broderick, E., Mabry, J., Robertson, D., and Thompson, J.: Baby Bottle Tooth Decay in Native American Children in Head Start Centers, *Public Health Rep., 104,* 50, January-February, 1989.

Caufield, P.W., Cutter, G.R., and Dasanayake, A.P.: Initial Acquisition of Mutans Streptococci by Infants: Evidence for a Discrete Window of Infectivity, *J. Dent. Res., 72,* 37, January, 1993.

Crall, J.J., Edelstein, B., and Tinanoff, N.: Relationship of Microbiological, Social, and Environmental Variables to Caries Status in Young Children, *Pediatr. Dent., 12,* 233, July-August, 1990.

Davenport, E.S.: Caries in the Preschool Child: Aetiology, *J. Dent., 18,* 300, December, 1990.

Kamp, A.A.: Well-baby Dental Examinations: A Survey of Preschool Children's Oral Health, *Pediatr. Dent., 13,* 86, March-April, 1991.

Kaste, L.M., Marianos, D., Chang, R., and Phipps, K.R.: The Assessment of Nursing Caries and Its Relationship to High Caries in the Permanent Dentition, *J. Public Health Dent., 52,* 64, Winter, 1992.

Koranyi, K., Rasnake, L.K., and Tarnowski, K.J.: Nursing Bottle Weaning and Prevention of Dental Caries: A Survey of Pediatricians, *Pediatr. Dent., 13,* 32, January-February, 1991.

McIntosh, E.A. and Buhler, P.L.: Survey of Dentists in the Ottawa-Carleton Region Concerning Nursing Bottle Syndrome, *Can. J. Public Health, 82,* 349, September-October, 1991.

Yiu, C.K. and Wei, S.H.Y.: Management of Rampant Caries in Children, *Quintessence Int., 23,* 159, March, 1992.

Root Caries

Beck, J.: The Epidemiology of Root Surface Caries, *J. Dent. Res., 69,* 1216, May, 1990.

Beighton, D., Lynch, E., and Heath, M.R.: A Microbiological Study of Primary Root-caries Lesions With Different Treatment Needs, *J. Dent. Res., 72,* 623, March, 1993.

Faine, M.P., Allender, D., Baab, D., Persson, R., and Lamont, R.J.: Dietary and Salivary Factors Associated With Root Caries, *Spec. Care Dentist., 12,* 177, July/August, 1992.

Fure, S. and Zickert, I.: Root Surface Caries and Associated Factors, *Scand. J. Dent. Res., 98,* 391, October, 1990.

Hojo, S., Takahashi, N., and Yamada, T.: Acid Profile in Carious Dentin, *J. Dent. Res., 70,* 182, March, 1991.

Hunt, R.J., Eldredge, J.B., and Beck, J.D.: Effect of Residence in a Fluoridated Community on the Incidence of Coronal and Root Caries in an Older Adult Population, *J. Public Health Dent., 49,* 138, Summer, 1989.

Katz, R.V.: Clinical Signs of Root Caries: Measurement Issues From an Epidemiologic Perspective, *J. Dent. Res., 69,* 1211, May, 1990.

Maggio, J.J., Hausman, E.M., Allen, K., and Potts, T.V.: A Model for Dentinal Caries Progression by Digital Subtraction Radiography, *J. Prosthet. Dent., 64,* 727, December, 1990.

Mitchell, T.L. and Forgay, M.G.E.: Root Surface Caries: Implications for Dental Hygienists, *Can. Dent. Hyg./Probe, 21,* 31, March, 1987.

Newbrun, E.: *Cariology,* 3rd ed. Chicago, Quintessence, 1989, pp. 65, 67–70.

Ravald, N. and Birkhed, D.: Factors Associated with Active and Inactive Root Caries in Patients With Periodontal Disease, *Caries Res., 25,* 377, September-October, 1991.

Schaeken, M.J.M., Keltjens, H.M.A.M., and van der Hoeven, J.S.: Effects of Fluoride and Chlorhexidine on the Microflora of Dental Root Surfaces and Progression of Root-surface Caries, *J. Dent. Res., 70,* 150, February, 1991.

Scheinin, A., Pienihäkkinen, K., Tiekso, J., and Holmberg, S.: Multifactorial Modeling for Root Caries Prediction, *Community Dent. Oral Epidemiol., 20,* 35, February, 1992.

Sumney, D.L. and Jordan, H.V.: Characterization of Bacteria Isolated from Human Root Surface Carious Lesions, *J. Dent. Res., 53,* 343, March-April, 1974.

Surmont, P.A. and Martens, L.C.: Root Surface Caries: An Update, *Clin. Prev. Dent., 11,* 14, May-June, 1989.

Syed, S.A., Loesche, W.J., Pape, H.L., and Grenier, E.: Predominant Cultivable Flora Isolated From Human Root Surface Caries Plaque, *Infect. Immun., 11,* 727, April, 1975.

Thomson, W.M.: Root Surface Caries—An Overview of Aetiology, Prevalence, Prevention and Management, *N.Z. Dent. J., 86,* 4, January, 1990.

Wilkins, E.M.: Root Caries: The Problem and the Protocol. First of Two Parts, *Dentalhygienistnews, 3,* 2, Fall, 1990; Second of Two Parts, *Dentalhygienistnews, 4,* 6, Winter, 1991.

Hypoplasia/Erosion

Bevenius, J., L'Estrange, P., and Angmar-Mansson, B.: Erosion: Guidelines for the General Practitioner, *Aust. Dent. J., 33,* 407, October, 1988.

Gabai, Y., Fattal, B., Rahamin, E., and Gedalia, I.: Effect of pH Levels in Swimming Pools on Enamel of Human Teeth, *Am. J. Dent., 1,* 241, December, 1988.

Haring, J.I. and Ibsen, O.A.C.: Developmental Disorders, in Ibsen, O.A.C. and Phelan, J.A.: *Oral Pathology for the Dental Hygienist.* Philadelphia, W.B. Saunders Co., 1992, pp. 267–269.

Harrison, J.L. and Roeder, L.B.: Dental Erosion Caused by Cola Beverages, *Gen. Dent., 39,* 23, January-February, 1991.

Järvinen, V.K., Rytömaa, I.I., and Heinonen, O.P.: Risk Factors in Dental Erosion, *J. Dent. Res., 70,* 942, June, 1991.

Krutchkoff, D.J., Eisenberg, E., O'Brien, J.E., and Ponzillo, J.J.: Cocaine-induced Dental Erosions (Correspondence), *N. Engl. J. Med., 322,* 408, February 8, 1990.

Seow, W.K.: Enamel Hypoplasia in the Primary Dentition: A Review, *ASDC J. Dent. Child., 58,* 441, November-December, 1991.

Injuries/Fractures

Bakland, L.K.: Traumatic Injuries, in Ingle, J.I. and Tainter, J.F.: *Endodontics,* 3rd ed. Philadelphia, Lea & Febiger, 1985, pp. 708–769.

Camp, J.H.: Diagnosis and Management of Sports-related Injuries to the Teeth, *Dent. Clin. North Am., 35,* 733, October, 1991.

Hovland, E.J.: Horizontal Root Fractures. Treatment and Repair, *Dent. Clin. North Am., 36,* 509, April, 1992.

Pulp Testing

Bender, I.B., Landau, M.A., Fonsecca, S., and Trowbridge, H.O.: The Optimum Placement-site of the Electrode in Electric Pulp Testing of the 12 Anterior Teeth, *J. Am. Dent. Assoc., 118,* 305, March, 1989.

Butel, E.M. and DiFiore, P.M.: Pulp Testing While Avoiding Dangers of Infection and Cross-contamination, *Gen. Dent., 39,* 42, January-February, 1991.

Cailleteau, J.G. and Ludington, J.R.: Using the Electric Pulp Tester With Gloves: A Simplified Approach, *J. Endod., 15,* 80, February, 1989.

Dal Santo, F.B., Throckmorton, G.S., and Ellis, E.: Reproducibility of Data From a Hand-held Digital Pulp Tester Used on Teeth and Oral Soft Tissue, *Oral Surg. Oral Med. Oral Pathol., 73,* 103, January, 1992.

Ingle, J.I. and Tainter, J.F.: *Endodontics,* 3rd ed. Philadelphia, Lea & Febiger, 1985, pp. 456–460.

Lado, E.A., Richmond, A.F., and Marks, R.G.: Reliability and Validity of a Digital Pulp Tester as a Test Standard for Measuring Sensory Perception, *J. Endod., 14,* 352, July, 1988.

Seltzer, S. and Bender, I.B.: *The Dental Pulp. Biologic Considerations in Dental Procedures,* 3rd ed. St. Louis, Ishiyaku EuroAmerica, 1990, pp. 377–379.

Treasure, P.: Capacitance Effect of Rubber Gloves on Electric Pulp Testers, *Int. Endod. J., 22,* 236, September, 1989.

15

The Occlusion

Occlusion is the relationship of the teeth in the mandibular arch to those in the maxillary arch as they are brought together. The occlusion is examined and recorded as part of the oral examination. Knowledge of the occlusion of each patient can contribute significantly to complete care and instruction. Recognition of malocclusion assists in the referral of patients to the orthodontist, gives many valuable points of reference for patient instruction, and determines necessary adaptations in techniques. Table 15–1 defines key words relating to occlusion and occlusal factors. Recognizing a patient's occlusion and understanding the oral health problems of malocclusion can aid in accomplishing the following:

A. Providing information for the diagnostic work-up and planning dental hygiene care.
B. Planning personalized instruction in relation to such factors as oral habits, masticatory efficiency, personal oral care procedures, and predisposing factors to dental and periodontal infections.
C. Adapting techniques of instrumentation to malpositioned teeth or groups of teeth.
D. Planning the frequency of maintenance appointments for professional care on the basis of deposit retention areas, particularly those that are difficult to reach in routine personal care.
E. Providing the general features of malocclusion to consider when orthodontic referral is discussed with the patient.

STATIC OCCLUSION

Static occlusal relationships are seen when the jaws are closed in centric relation. The static occlusion can be efficiently observed in occluded study casts and seen directly in the oral cavity when the lips and cheeks are retracted. Classification of malocclusion and the variations that occur with each category are described here.

I. NORMAL (IDEAL) OCCLUSION
The ideal mechanical relationship between the teeth of the maxillary arch and the teeth of the mandibular arch.
A. All teeth in maxillary arch in maximum contact with all teeth in mandibular arch in a definite pattern.
B. Maxillary teeth slightly overlapping the mandibular teeth on the facial surfaces.

II. MALOCCLUSION
Any deviation from the physiologically acceptable relationship of the maxillary arch and/or teeth to the mandibular arch and/or teeth.

III. TYPES OF FACIAL PROFILES (FIGURE 15–1)
A. Mesognathic
Having slightly protruded jaws, which give the facial outline a relatively flat appearance (straight profile).

B. Retrognathic
Having a prominent maxilla and a mandible posterior to its normal relationship (convex profile).

C. Prognathic
Having a prominent, protruded mandible and normal (usually) maxilla (concave profile).

248

TABLE 15–1
KEY WORDS: OCCLUSION

Ankylosis (ang′kĭ-lo′sis): union or consolidation of two similar or dissimilar hard tissues previously adjacent but not attached.
  Dental ankylosis: rigid fixation of a tooth to the surrounding alveolus as a result of ossification of the periodontal ligament; prevents eruption and orthodontic movement.
Centric occlusion (ŏ-kloo′zhun): the maximum intercuspation or contact of the teeth of the opposing arches; also called habitual occlusion.
Centric relation: the most unstrained, retruded physiologic relation of the mandible to the maxilla from which lateral movements can be made.
Cephalometer (sef′ah-lom′ĕ-ter): an orienting device for positioning the head for radiographic examination and measurement.
Cephalometric analysis (sef′ah-lō-met′rik): the process of evaluating dental and skeletal relationships by way of measurements obtained directly from the head or from cephalometric radiographs and tracings made from the radiographs.
Cephalostat (sef′ah-lō-stat′): a head-holding instrument used to obtain cephalometric radiographs; head is held in a precisely defined position relative to the film and to the central ray of the x-ray source.
Diastema (dī as′tĕ mah): a space between two adjacent teeth in the same arch.
Occlusal guard: a removable dental appliance usually made of plastic that covers a dental arch and is designed to minimize the damaging effects of bruxism and other oral habits; also called bite guard, mouth guard, or night guard.

Occlusal prematurity: any contact of opposing teeth that occurs before the desirable intercuspation.
Orthodontic and dentofacial orthopedics: the specialty area of dentistry concerned with the diagnosis, supervision, guidance, and treatment of the growing and mature dentofacial structures; includes conditions that require movement of teeth and the treatment of malrelationships and malformations of the craniofacial complex.
Orthopedics (or′thō-pē′diks): correction of abnormal form or relationship of bone structures; may be accomplished surgically (orthopedic surgery) or by the application of appliances to stimulate changes in the bone structure through natural physiologic response (orthopedic therapy); orthodontic therapy is orthopedic therapy.
Parafunctional: abnormal or deviated function, as in bruxism.
Pathologic migration: the movement of a tooth out of its natural position as a result of periodontal infection; contrasts with **mesial migration,** which is the physiologic process maintained by tooth proximal contacts in the normal dental arches.
Tongue thrust: the infantile pattern of the suckle-swallow movement in which the tongue is place between the incisor teeth or alveolar ridges; may result in an anterior open bite, deformation of the jaws, and abnormal function.
Trauma from occlusion: injury to the periodontium that results from occlusal forces in excess of the reparative capacity of the attachment apparatus; also called occlusal traumatism.

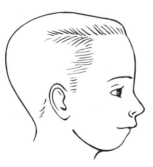 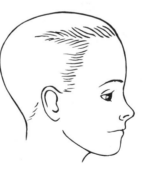

FIG. 15–1. Types of Facial Profiles.   RETROGNATHIC   MESOGNATHIC   PROGNATHIC

IV. MALRELATIONS OF GROUPS OF TEETH
A. Crossbites
  1. *Posterior.* Maxillary or mandibular posterior teeth are either facial or lingual to their normal position. This condition may occur bilaterally or unilaterally (figure 15–2).
  2. *Anterior.* Maxillary incisors are lingual to the mandibular incisors (figure 15–3).

B. Edge-To-Edge Bite
Incisal surfaces of maxillary teeth occlude with incisal surfaces of mandibular teeth instead of overlapping as in normal occlusion (figure 15–4).

C. End-to-End Bite
Molars and premolars occlude cusp-to-cusp as viewed mesiodistally (figure 15–5).

D. Openbite

Lack of occlusal or incisal contact between certain maxillary and mandibular teeth because either or both have failed to reach the line of occlusion. The teeth cannot be brought together, and a space remains as a result of the arching of the line of occlusion (figure 15–6).

E. Overjet

The horizontal distance between the labioincisal surfaces of the mandibular incisors and the linguoincisal surfaces of the maxillary incisors (figure 15–7). One way to measure the amount of overjet is to place the tip of a probe on the labial surface of the mandibular incisor and, holding it horizontally against the incisal edge of the maxillary tooth, read the distance in millimeters.

F. Underjet (maxillary teeth are lingual to mandibular teeth)

The horizontal distance between the labioincisal surfaces of the maxillary incisors and the linguoincisal surfaces of the mandibular incisors (figure 15–8).

G. Overbite (vertical overlap)

Overbite is the vertical distance by which the maxillary incisors overlap the mandibular incisors.

1. *Normal Overbite.* An overbite is considered normal when the incisal edges of the maxillary teeth are within the incisal third of the mandibular teeth, as shown in figure 15–9 in side view and in figure 15–11A in anterior view.
2. *Moderate Overbite.* An overbite is considered moderate when the incisal edges of the maxillary teeth appear within the middle third of the mandibular teeth (figure 15–11B).
3. *Deep (Severe) Overbite.* An overbite is considered deep (severe) when the incisal edges of the maxillary teeth are within the cervical third of the mandibular teeth (figure 15–11C). When in addition the incisal edges of the mandibular teeth are in contact with the maxillary lingual gingival tissue, the overbite is called very deep. A side view of very deep overbite is shown in figure 15–10.
4. *Anterior Crossbite.* The opposite situation occurs in anterior crossbite, in which the maxillary anterior teeth are lingual to the mandibular anterior teeth (figure 15–3).
5. *Clinical Examination of Overbite.* Normal, moderate, and severe anterior overbite are observed directly when the teeth are closed in occlusion. With the posterior teeth closed together, the lips can be retracted and the teeth observed as in figure 15–11. The degree of anterior overbite is judged by the position of the incisal edge of the maxillary teeth: normal (slight) within the incisal third of the mandibular incisors; moderate overbite within the middle third; and severe overbite within the cervical third. By placing a mouth mirror under the incisal edge of the maxillary teeth, one can sometimes see the mandibular teeth in contact with the maxillary lingual gingiva. When contact is not visible, an examination of the lingual gingiva may reveal teeth prints, or at least enlargement and redness from the contact.

V. MALPOSITIONS OF INDIVIDUAL TEETH

A. Labioversion

A tooth that has assumed a position labial to normal.

B. Linguoversion

Position lingual to normal.

C. Buccoversion

Position buccal to normal.

D. Supraversion

Elongated above the line of occlusion.

E. Torsiversion

Turned or rotated.

F. Infraversion

Depressed below the line of occlusion, for example, primary tooth that is submerged or ankylosed.

DETERMINATION OF THE CLASSIFICATION OF MALOCCLUSION

The determination of the classification of occlusion is based upon the principles of Edward H. Angle, presented in the early 1900s. He defined normal occlusion as "the normal relations of the occlusal inclined planes of the teeth when the jaws are closed"[1] and based his system of classification upon the relationship of the first permanent molars.

Although authorities have since agreed that the maxillary first permanent molars do not occupy a fixed position in the dental arch, Angle's system serves to provide an acceptable basis for a useful classification. A more comprehensive picture of malocclusion is made by the orthodontist, who studies the relationships of the position of the teeth to the jaws, the face, and the skull.

Three general classes of malocclusion are described in the following sections. These are designated by Roman numerals. Because the mandible is movable and the maxilla is stationary, the classes describe the relationship of the mandible to the maxilla. For example, in Distoclusion (Class II) the mandible is distal, whereas in Mesioclusion (Class III) the mandible is mesial to the maxilla, as compared to the normal position.

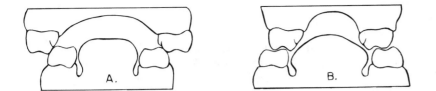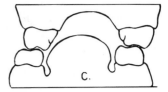

FIG. 15–2. Posterior Crossbite. A. Mandibular teeth lingual to normal position. **B.** Mandibular teeth facial to normal position. **C.** Unilateral crossbite: right side, normal; left side, mandibular teeth facial to normal position.

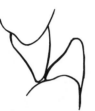

FIG. 15–3. Anterior Crossbite. Maxillary anterior teeth are lingual to the mandibular anterior teeth. Anterior crossbite occurs in Angle's Class III malocclusion.

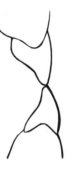

FIG. 15–4. Edge-to-Edge Bite. Incisal surfaces occlude.

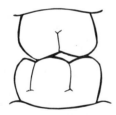

FIG. 15–5. End-to-End Bite. Molars in cusp-to-cusp occlusion as viewed from the facial.

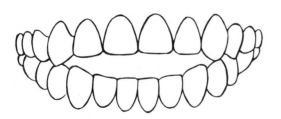

FIG. 15–6. Openbite. Lack of incisal contact. Posterior teeth in normal occlusion.

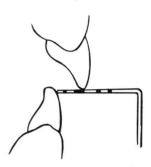

FIG. 15–7. Overjet. Maxillary incisors are labial to the mandibular incisors. Measurable horizontal distance is evident between the incisal edge of the maxillary incisors and the incisal edge of the mandibular incisors. A periodontal probe can be used to measure for recording the distance.

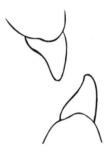

FIG. 15–8. Underjet. Maxillary incisors are lingual to the mandibular incisors. Measurable horizontal distance is evident between the incisal edges of the maxillary incisors and the incisal edges of the mandibular incisors.

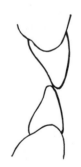

FIG. 15–9. Normal Overbite. Profile view to show position of incisal edge of maxillary tooth within the incisal third of the facial surface of the mandibular incisor.

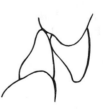

FIG. 15–10. Deep (Severe) Anterior Overbite. Incisal edge of maxillary tooth is at the level of the cervical third of the facial surface of the mandibular anterior tooth. See the facial view in figure 15–11C.

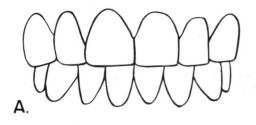

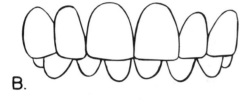

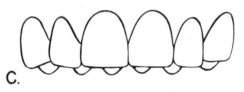

FIG. 15–11. Overbite, Anterior View. A. Normal overbite: incisal edges of the maxillary teeth are within the incisal third of the facial surfaces of the mandibular teeth. **B.** Moderate overbite: incisal edges of maxillary teeth are within the middle third of the facial surfaces of the mandibular teeth. **C.** Severe overbite: the incisal edges of the maxillary teeth are within the cervical third of the facial of the mandibular teeth. When the incisal edges of the mandibular teeth are in contact with the maxillary lingual gingival tissue, the overbite is considered very severe. See the profile view in figure 15–10.

I. NORMAL (IDEAL) OCCLUSION (FIGURE 15–12)

A. Facial Profile
Mesognathic (figure 15–1).

B. Molar Relation
The mesiobuccal cusp of the maxillary first permanent molar occludes with the buccal groove of the mandibular first permanent molar.

C. Canine Relation
The maxillary permanent canine occludes with the distal half of the mandibular canine and the mesial half of the mandibular first premolar.

II. MALOCCLUSION

A. Class I or Neutroclusion (figure 15–12)
1. *Facial Profile.* Same as normal occlusion.
2. *Molar Relation.* Same as normal occlusion.
3. *Canine Relation.* Same as normal occlusion.
4. *Malposition of Individual Teeth or Groups of Teeth.*
5. *General Types of Conditions That Frequently Occur in Class I.*
   a. Crowded maxillary or mandibular anterior teeth.
   b. Protruded or retruded maxillary incisors.
   c. Anterior crossbite.
   d. Posterior crossbite.
   e. Mesial drift of molars resulting from premature loss of teeth.

B. Class II or Distoclusion (figure 15–12)
1. *Description.* Mandibular teeth posterior to normal position in their relation to the maxillary teeth.
2. *Facial Profile.* Retrognathic; maxilla protrudes; lower lip is full and often rests between the maxillary and mandibular incisors; the mandible appears retruded or weak (figure 15–1, Retrognathic).
3. *Molar Relation*
   a. The buccal groove of the mandibular first permanent molar is distal to the mesiobuccal cusp of the maxillary first permanent molar by at least the width of a premolar.
   b. When the distance is less than the width of a premolar, the relation should be classified as "tendency toward Class II."
4. *Canine Relation*
   a. The distal surface of the mandibular canine is distal to the mesial surface of the maxillary canine by at least the width of a premolar.
   b. When the distance is less than the width of a premolar, the relation should be classified as "tendency toward Class II."
5. *Class II, Division 1*
   a. Description. The mandible is retruded and all maxillary incisors are protruded.
   b. General types of conditions that frequently occur in Class II, Division 1 malocclusion. Deep overbite, excessive overjet, abnormal muscle function (lips), short mandible, or short upper lip.
6. *Class II, Division 2*
   a. Description. The mandible is retruded, and one or more maxillary incisors are retruded.
   b. General types of conditions that frequently occur in Class II, Division 2 malocclusion. Maxillary lateral incisors protrude while both central incisors retrude,

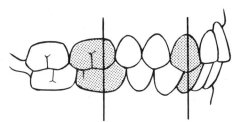

Normal (Ideal) Occlusion

Molar relationship: mesiobuccal cusp of maxillary first permanent molar occludes with the buccal groove of the mandibular first permanent molar.

Malocclusion

Class I: Neutroclusion. Molar relationship same as Normal, with malposition of individual teeth or groups of teeth.

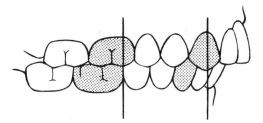

Class II: Distoclusion.

Molar relationship: buccal groove of the mandibular first permanent molar is distal to the mesiobuccal cusp of the maxillary first permanent molar by at least the width of a premolar.

Division 1: mandible is retruded and all maxillary incisors are protruded.

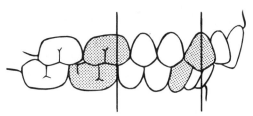

Class II: Distoclusion.

Division 2: mandible is retruded and one or more maxillary incisors are retruded.

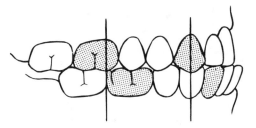

Class III: Mesioclusion.

Molar relationship: buccal groove of the mandibular first permanent molar is mesial to the mesiobuccal cusp of the maxillary first permanent molar by at least the width of a premolar.

FIG. 15–12. Normal Occlusion and Classification of Malocclusion.

crowded maxillary anterior teeth, or deep overbite.
7. *Subdivision.* One side is Class I, the other side is Class II (may be Division 1 or 2).

C. Class III or Mesioclusion (figure 15–12)

1. *Description.* Mandibular teeth are anterior to normal position in relation to maxillary teeth.
2. *Facial Profile.* Prognathic; lower lip and mandible are prominent (figure 15–1).
3. *Molar Relation*
   a. The buccal groove of the mandibular first permanent molar is mesial to the mesiobuccal cusp of the maxillary first permanent molar by at least the width of a premolar.
   b. When the distance is less than the width of a premolar, the relation should be classified as "tendency toward Class III."
4. *Canine Relation*
   a. The distal surface of the mandibular canine is mesial to the mesial surface of the maxillary canine by at least the width of a premolar.
   b. When the distance is less than the width of a premolar, the relation should be classified as "tendency toward Class III."
5. *General Types of Conditions That Frequently Occur in Class III Malocclusion*
   a. True Class III. Maxillary incisors are lingual to mandibular incisors in an anterior crossbite (figure 15–3).
   b. Maxillary and mandibular incisors are in edge-to-edge occlusion.
   c. Mandibular incisors are very crowded, but lingual to maxillary incisors.

OCCLUSION OF THE PRIMARY TEETH[2]

I. NORMAL (IDEAL)
A. Primary Canine Relation
Same as permanent dentition.
1. *With Primate Spaces**
   a. Mandibular. Between mandibular canine and first molar (figure 15–13A).
   b. Maxillary. Between maxillary lateral incisor and canine (figure 15–13B).
2. *Without Primate Spaces.* Closed arches.

* **Primate space:** a diastema or gap in the tooth row occasionally observed in the human primary dentition. It is characteristic of nearly all species of primates except man. The maxillary primate spaces accommodate the mandibular canines, and the mandibular primate spaces accommodate the maxillary canines when the teeth are in occlusion. As a reduction in the length of canines accompanied man's evolution, the canines no longer protruded beyond the occlusal level. The diastema (primate space) was no longer functional.

B. Second Primary Molar Relation

The mesiobuccal cusp of the maxillary second primary molar occludes with the buccal groove of the mandibular second primary molar.

1. *Variations in Distal Surfaces Relationships.* Terminal step.
   a. The distal surface of the mandibular primary molar is mesial to that of the maxillary, thereby forming a mesial step (figure 15–14A).
   b. Morphologic variation in molar size; maxillary and mandibular primary molars have approximately the same mesiodistal width.
2. *Variation.* Terminal plane.
   a. The distal surfaces of the maxillary and mandibular primary molars are on same vertical plane (figure 15–14B).

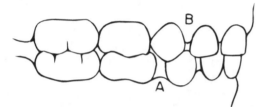

FIG. 15–13. Primary Teeth With Primate Spaces. A. Mandibular primate space between canine and first molar. **B.** Maxillary primate space between the lateral incisor and the canine.

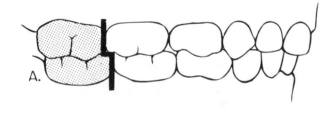

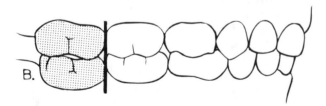

FIG. 15–14. Eruption Patterns of the First Permanent Molars. A. Terminal step. The distal surface of mandibular second primary molar is mesial to the distal surface of the maxillary primary molar. **B.** Terminal plane. The distal surfaces of the mandibular and maxillary second primary molars are on the same vertical plane; permanent molars erupt in end-to-end occlusion.

b. The maxillary molar is narrow mesiodistally than the mandibular molar (occurs in many patients).
3. *Effects on Occlusion of First Permanent Molars*
   a. Terminal step. First permanent molar erupts directly into proper occlusion (figure 15–14A).
   b. Terminal plane. First permanent molars erupt end-to-end. With mandibular primate space, early mesial shift of primary molars into the primate space occurs, and the permanent mandibular molar shifts into proper occlusion. Without primate spaces, late mesial shift of permanent mandibular molar into proper occlusion occurs, following exfoliation of second primary molar (figure 15–14B).

II. MALOCCLUSION OF THE PRIMARY TEETH
Same as permanent dentition.

FUNCTIONAL OCCLUSION

In contrast to static occlusion, which pertains to the relationship of the teeth when the jaws are closed, functional occlusion consists of all contacts during chewing, swallowing, or other normal action. Functional occlusion is associated with performance.

The pressures or forces created by the muscles of mastication are transmitted from the teeth, after contact, to the periodontium. Such forces are necessary to maintain the occlusal relationship of the teeth and guide the teeth during eruption. The forces are also necessary to provide functional stimulation for the preservation of the health of the attachment apparatus, namely the periodontal ligament, the cementum, and the alveolar bone.

I. TYPES OF OCCLUSAL CONTACTS
A. Functional Contacts
Functional contacts are the normal contacts that are made between the maxillary teeth and the mandibular teeth during chewing and swallowing. Each contact is momentary, so the total contact time is only a few minutes each day.

B. Parafunctional Contacts
Parafunctional contacts are those made outside the normal range of function.
1. They result from occlusal habits and neuroses.
2. They are potentially injurious to the periodontal supporting structures, but only in the presence of bacterial plaque and inflammatory factors.
3. They create wear facets and attrition on the teeth. A facet is a shiny, flat, worn spot on the surface of a tooth, frequently on the side of a cusp.

4. They can be divided into the following:
    a. Tooth-to-tooth contacts. Bruxism, clenching, tapping.
    b. Tooth-to-hard-object contacts. Nail biting, occupational use of such objects as tacks or pins, use of smoking equipment, such as a pipe stem or hard cigarette holder.
    c. Tooth-to-oral tissues contacts. Lip or cheek biting.

II. PROXIMAL CONTACTS

Proximal contacts serve to stabilize the position of teeth in the dental arches and to prevent food impaction between the teeth. Attrition or wear of the teeth occurs at the proximal contacts.

A. Drifting

When proximal contact is lost, teeth can drift into spaces created by unreplaced missing teeth. There is also a natural tendency for mesial migration of teeth toward the midline. In the absence of disease, the surrounding periodontal tissues adapt to repositioned teeth (figure 13–19, page 225, and figures 24–5 and 24–6, page 380).

B. Pathologic Migration

With destruction of the supporting structures of a tooth as a result of periodontal infection and with a force to move a tooth weakened by disease and bone loss, migration of the tooth can result. *Pathologic migration occurs when disease is present; in contrast, drifting is migration with a healthy periodontium.*

TRAUMA FROM OCCLUSION

Periodontal tissue injury caused by repeated occlusal forces that exceed the physiologic limits of tissue tolerance is called trauma from occlusion. Other names are periodontal traumatism, occlusal traumatism, and periodontal trauma.

I. TYPES OF TRAUMA FROM OCCLUSION
A. Primary

When the excessive occlusal force is exerted on a tooth with normal bone support, *primary trauma from occlusion* results. An example is the effect of a new restoration placed above the line of occlusion.

B. Secondary

When the excessive occlusal force is exerted on a tooth with bone loss and inadequate alveolar bone support, and the ability of the tooth to withstand occlusal forces is impaired, *secondary trauma from occlusion* results. When a tooth has lost the support of the surrounding bone, even the pressures of what are usually considered normal occlusal forces may create lesions of trauma from occlusion.

II. EFFECTS OF TRAUMA FROM OCCLUSION

The attachment apparatus (periodontal ligament, cementum, and alveolar bone) has as its main purpose the maintenance of the tooth in the socket in a functional state. In a healthy situation, occlusal pressures and forces during chewing and swallowing are readily dispersed or absorbed and no unusual effects are produced.

A. Excess Forces

When the forces of occlusion are greater than can be taken care of by the attachment apparatus, damage can result. Circulatory disturbances, tissue destruction from crushing under pressure, bone resorption, and other pathologic processes are initiated.

B. Relation to Inflammatory Factors

1. *Trauma from occlusion does not cause gingivitis, periodontitis, or pocket formation.* The steps in the development of inflammatory disease and pockets were outlined on pages 195–197.
2. In the presence of inflammatory disease, the existing periodontal destruction may be aggravated or promoted by trauma from occlusion.

III. METHODS OF APPLICATION OF EXCESS PRESSURE

To understand the nature of the occlusal forces that can cause periodontal trauma from occlusion, it is helpful to recognize types of tooth contacts that can overburden a tooth or group of teeth.[3]

A. Individual Teeth that Touch Before Full Closure

The contact is premature and may put excessive force on an individual tooth.

B. Two or Only a Few Teeth in Contact During Movement of the Jaw

The teeth involved receive a disproportionate amount of force.

C. Initial Contacts on Inclined Planes of Cusps

Following the initial contact, when the teeth are brought together in a closed position, there may be excess pressure on the teeth where initial contact was made.

D. Heavy Forces Not in a Vertical or Axial Direction

Normal occlusal relationships imply a direct cusp-to-fossa position during closure, with the force of occlusion in a vertical direction toward the tooth apex and parallel with the long axis. When pressures are exerted laterally or horizontally, excess force is placed on the periodontal attachment apparatus.

E. Increased Frequency, Intensity, and Duration of Contacts

In the presence of parafunctional habits, such as bruxism, clenching, tapping, or biting objects, many more than the usual number of tooth contacts are made each day, and the intensity and duration are altered.

IV. RECOGNITION OF SIGNS OF TRAUMA FROM OCCLUSION

No one clinical or radiographic finding clearly defines the presence of trauma from occlusion. Diagnosis of the condition is complex. The possible observations listed as follows should be looked for specifically and recorded for evaluation and correlation with the patient history and all other clinical determinations.

A. Clinical Findings That May Occur in Trauma from Occlusion

1. Tooth mobility.
2. Fremitus.
3. Sensitivity of teeth to pressure and/or percussion.
4. Pathologic migration.
5. Wear facets or atypical occlusal wear.
6. Open contacts related to food impaction.
7. Neuromuscular disturbances in the muscles of mastication. In severe cases muscle spasm can occur.
8. Temporomandibular joint symptoms.

B. Radiographic Findings

Characteristics that may occur in trauma from occlusion include:

1. Widened periodontal ligament spaces, particularly angular thickening (triangulation). This finding frequently occurs in conjunction with tooth mobility.
2. Angular (vertical) bone loss in localized areas (figure 13–20, page 226).
3. Root resorption.
4. Furcation involvement.
5. Thickened lamina dura. Although related to occlusal forces, thickened lamina dura should not be considered a detrimental or destructive effect of trauma from occlusion. It may be a defense reaction to strengthen tooth support against occlusal forces. Thickened lamina dura is frequently associated with teeth that have undergone orthodontic treatment.

TECHNICAL HINTS

I. Observe the facial profile as the patient enters and is seated in the dental chair to estimate the classification of occlusion before examination of the teeth.

II. Avoid mention of a dentofacial deformity that would make the patient feel self-conscious.

III. Avoid suggesting to the patient or a parent the possible procedures the orthodontist may use in treatment because complications become known only after the complete diagnosis.

IV. Closing to centric relation can be performed most effectively by instructing the patient to curl the tongue and to try to hold the tip of the tongue as far back as possible while closing.

V. When a small child has difficulty in occluding, the clinician may firmly but gently press the cushions of the thumbs on the mucous membrane over the pterygomandibular raphe, holding the thumbs between the cheek and buccal surfaces of the teeth as the patient is requested to close.

VI. Prepare mouth guards for patients in active sports.

VII. Study the occlusion of the patient with removable dentures with the dentures in place in the mouth.

FACTORS TO TEACH THE PATIENT

I. Interpretation of the *general* purposes of orthodontic care (function and esthetics) to patients referred by the dentist to an orthodontist.
   A. Dependence of masticatory efficiency on the occlusion of the teeth.
   B. Influence of masticatory efficiency on food selection in the diet.
   C. Influence of masticatory efficiency and diet on the nutritional status of the body and oral health.

II. Review and demonstrate suggestions for the corection of oral habits.

III. The space-maintaining function of the primary teeth in prevention of malocclusion of permanent teeth.

IV. The role of malocclusion as a predisposing factor for bacterial plaque retention in the formation of dental caries and periodontal diseases.

V. Bacterial plaque removal methods for reducing dental calculus and soft deposit retention in areas where teeth are crowded, displaced, or otherwise not in normal occlusion.

VI. The relation of the occlusion and the position of the teeth to the patient's personal oral care procedures.
   A. Selection of the proper type of toothbrush.
   B. Application of thorough toothbrushing method or methods.
   C. Use of dental floss.

VII. Specific reasons for frequency of maintenance examinations when related to malocclusion and while in the process of having orthodontic therapy.

REFERENCES

1. **Angle,** E.H.: *Malocclusion of the Teeth,* 7th ed. Philadelphia, S.S. White, 1907.
2. **Baume,** L.J.: Physiological Tooth Migration and Its Significance for the Development of the Occlusion, I. The Biogenetic Course of the Deciduous Dentition, *J. Dent. Res., 29,* 123, April, 1950; II. The Biogenesis of the Accessional Dentition, *J. Dent. Res., 29,* 331, June, 1950; III. The Biogenesis of the Successional Dentition, *J. Dent. Res., 29,* 338, June, 1950; IV. The Biogenesis of Overbite, *J. Dent. Res., 29,* 440, August, 1950.
3. **Allen,** D.L., McFall, W.T., and Jenzano, J.W.: *Periodontics for the Dental Hygienist,* 4th ed. Philadelphia, Lea & Febiger, 1987, pp. 85–86.

SUGGESTED READINGS

Baker, I.M.: Record Taking in the Orthodontic Office, *Dent. Assist., 60,* 25, March/April, 1991.

Brezniak, N. and Wasserstein, A.: Root Resorption After Orthodontic Treatment: Part 1. Literature Review, *Am. J. Orthod. Dentofacial Orthop., 103,* 62, January, 1993.

Bresniak, N. and Wasserstein, A.: Root Resorption After Orthodontic Treatment: Part 2. Literature Review, *Am. J. Orthod. Dentofacial Orthop., 103,* 138, February, 1993.

Dyer, G.S., Harris, E.F., and Vaden, J.L.: Age Effects on Orthodontic Treatment: Adolescents Contrasted with Adults, *Am. J. Orthod. Dentofacial Orthop., 100,* 523, December, 1991.

Fink, D.F. and Smith, R.J.: The Duration of Orthodontic Treatment, *Am. J. Orthod. Dentofacial Orthop., 102,* 45, July, 1992.

Khan, R.S. and Horrocks, E.N.: A Study of Adult Orthodontic Patients and Their Treatment, *Br. J. Orthod., 18,* 183, August, 1991.

Machen, D.E.: Legal Aspects of Orthodontic Practice: Risk Management Concepts. Oral Hygiene Assessment: Plaque Accumulation, Gingival Inflammation, Decalcification, and Caries, *Am. J. Orthod. Dentofacial Orthop., 100,* 93, July, 1991.

Newman, G.V.: Limited Orthodontics for the Older Population: Multidisciplinary Modalities, *Am. J. Orthod. Dentofacial Orthop., 101,* 281, March, 1992.

Robinson, H.B.G. and Miller, A.S.: *Color Atlas of Oral Pathology,* 5th ed. Philadelphia, J.B. Lippincott Co., 1990, pp. 52, 83–84, 93, 95.

Torres, H.O. and Ehrlich, A.: *Modern Dental Assisting,* 4th ed. Philadelphia, W.B. Saunders Co., 1990, pp. 596–662.

Villarosa, G.A. and Moss, R.A.: Oral Behavioral Patterns as Factors Contributing to the Development of Head and Facial Pain, *J. Prosthet. Dent., 54,* 427, September, 1985.

Wagaiyu, E.G. and Ashley, F.P.: Mouthbreathing, Lip Seal and Upper Lip Coverage and Their Relationship With Gingival Inflammation in 11–14-year-old Schoolchildren, *J. Clin. Periodontol., 18,* 698, October, 1991.

Oral Habits

Christensen, J. and Fields, H.: Oral Habits, in Pinkham, J.R., ed.: *Pediatric Dentistry. Infancy Through Adolescence.* Philadelphia, W.B. Saunders Co., 1988, pp. 301–307.

DeBiase, C.B.: *Dental Health Education Theory and Practice.* Philadelphia, Lea & Febiger, 1991, pp. 28, 66–67, 88, 133, 157.

Martinez, N.P. and Hunckler, R.J.: Managing Digital Habits in Children, *Compendium, 6,* 188, March, 1985.

Massler, M.: Oral Habits: Development and Management, *J. Pedod., 7,* 109, Winter, 1983.

Ngan, P. and Wei, S.H.Y.: Early Orthodontic Treatment in the Mixed Dentition, in Wei, S.H.Y.: *Pediatric Dentistry. Total Patient Care.* Philadelphia, Lea & Febiger, 1988, pp. 483–485.

Odenrick, L. and Brattström, V.: Nailbiting: Frequency and Association With Root Resorption During Orthodontic Treatment, *Br. J. Orthod., 12,* 78, April, 1985.

Occlusion

Ash, M.M.: *Wheeler's Dental Anatomy, Physiology and Occlusion,* 7th ed. Philadelphia, W.B. Saunders Co., 1993, pp. 414–469.

Austin, D. and Attanasio, R.: A Procedure for Making a Bruxism Device in the Office, *J. Prosthet. Dent., 66,* 266, August, 1991.

Carranza, F.A.: *Glickman's Clinical Periodontology,* 7th ed. Philadelphia, W.B. Saunders Co., 1990, pp. 264–285, 422–431.

Grant, D.A., Stern, I.B., and Listgarten, M.A., eds.: *Periodontics,* 6th ed. St. Louis, Mosby, 1988, pp. 479–509, 513–514, 977–979, 1017–1044.

Hanamura, H., Houston, F., Rylander, H., Carlsson, G.E., Haraldson, T., and Nyman, S.: Periodontal Status and Bruxism. A Comparative Study of Patients With Periodontal Disease and Occlusal Parafunctions, *J. Periodontol., 58,* 173, March, 1987.

Hoag, P.M.: Occlusal Treatment, in *Proceedings of the World Workshop in Clinical Periodontics.* Chicago, American Academy of Periodontology, 1989, pp. III-1 to III-23.

Hoag, P.M. and Pawlak, E.A.: *Essentials of Periodontics,* 4th ed. St. Louis, Mosby, 1990, pp. 95–101.

Weisgold, A.S. and Baumgarten, H.S.: Occlusal Therapy, in Genco, R.J., Goldman, H.M., and Cohen, D.W., eds.: *Contemporary Periodontics.* St. Louis, Mosby, 1990, pp. 493–504.

Bacterial Plaque and Other Soft Deposits

Dental caries and gingival and periodontal infections are caused by microorganisms in microbial/bacterial plaques. Disease-producing microorganisms attach to the tooth surfaces and colonize. They bring about carious lesions of the enamel and root surfaces, in pits and fissures, and on smooth surfaces (pages 231–236). They also bring about inflammatory changes in the periodontium that can lead to destruction of tissues and loss of attachment. The morphologic forms of bacteria are shown in figure 16–1.

During the clinical examination of the teeth and surrounding soft tissues, the soft and hard deposits that accumulate on the teeth and within the sulci or pockets must be recognized and assessed. From the findings, an initial treatment plan can be formulated based on the individual needs of the patient. Key words are defined in table 16–1.

The soft deposits are acquired pellicle or cuticle, bacterial plaque, materia alba, and food debris, each of which is an entity, and the terms should not be interchanged. The hard, calcified deposit on teeth is dental calculus, which is described in Chapter 17. A classification with definitions of the dental deposits is presented in table 16–2.[1]

ACQUIRED PELLICLE

The acquired pellicle is an amorphous, acellular, organic, tenacious membranous layer that forms over exposed tooth surfaces, as well as over restorations and dental calculus. Its thickness, which varies from 0.1 to 0.8 μm, usually is greater near the gingiva.

I. FORMATION
Within minutes after all external material has been removed from the tooth surfaces with an abrasive, the acquired pellicle begins to form. It is composed primarily of glycoproteins from the saliva that are selectively adsorbed by the hydroxyapatite of the tooth surface. The adsorbed material becomes a highly insoluble coating over the teeth, calculus deposits, restorations, and complete and partial dentures.

II. TYPES OF PELLICLES[2]
A. Surface Pellicle, Unstained
The unstained pellicle is clear, translucent, insoluble, and not readily visible until a disclosing agent has been applied. When stained with a disclosing agent, it appears thin, with a pale staining that contrasts with the thicker, darker staining of bacterial plaque.

B. Surface Pellicle, Stained
Unstained pellicle can take on extrinsic stain and become brown, grayish, or other colors as described on page 283.

C. Subsurface Pellicle
Surface pellicle is continuous with subsurface pellicle that is embedded in tooth structure, particularly where the tooth surface is partially demineralized.[3]

III. SIGNIFICANCE OF PELLICLE
A. Protective
Pellicle appears to provide a barrier against acids; thus it may aid in reducing dental caries attack.[3]

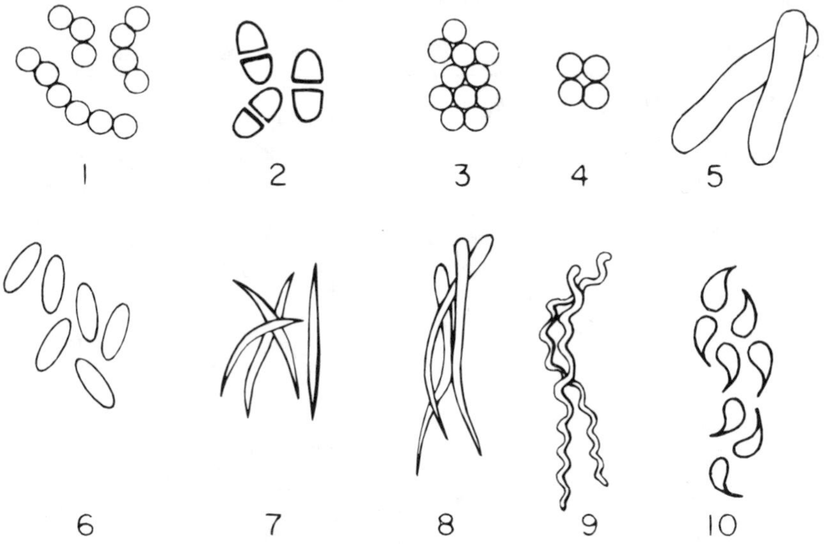

FIG. 16–1. Morphologic Forms of Bacteria. 1. Streptococci. **2.** Diplococci. **3.** Staphylococci. **4.** Sarcina. **5.** Bacilli. **6.** Coccobacilli. **7.** Fusiform bacilli. **8.** Filamentous bacilli. **9.** Spirochetes. **10.** Vibrios. (From Hammond, B.: Bacterial structure and function, in Schuster, G.S., ed.: *Oral Microbiology and Infectious Disease*, 2nd student ed. Toronto, B.C. Decker, 1988, p. 23.)

TABLE 16–1
KEY WORDS: BACTERIAL PLAQUE

Acellular (ā-sel′ū-lar): not made up of or containing cells.

Adsorption (ad-sorp′shun): attachment of one substance to the surface of another; the action of a substance in attracting and holding other materials or particles on its surface.

Aerobe (a′er-ōb): heterotrophic microorganism that can live and grow in the presence of free oxygen; some are obligate, others facultative; *adj.* aerobic.

Anaerobe (an-a′er-ōb): heterotrophic microorganism that lives and grows in complete (or almost complete) absence of oxygen; some are obligate, others facultative; *adj.* anaerobic.

Calculogenesis (kal′kū-lō-jen′ĕ-sis): formation of calculus.

Calculogenic: adjective applied to bacterial plaque that is conducive to the formation of calculus.

Cariogenesis (kār′ē-ō-jen′ĕ-sis): development of dental caries.

Cariogenic (kār′ē-ō-jen′ik): adjective to indicate a conduciveness to the initiation of dental caries, such as a cariogenic plaque or a cariogenic food.

Facultative (fak′ul-tā′tĭv): able to live under more than one specific set of environmental conditions; contrast with **obligate.**

Flora (flo′rah): the collective organisms of a given locale.

Oral flora: the various bacteria and other microscopic organisms that inhabit the oral cavity. The mouth has an indigenous flora, meaning those organisms that are native to that area. Certain organisms specifically reside in certain parts, for example, on the tongue, on the mucosa, or in the gingival sulcus.

Heterotrophic (het′er-ō-trōf′ik): not self-sustaining; feeding on others.

Leukocyte (loo′kō sīt): white blood corpuscle capable of ameboid movement; function to protect the body against infection and disease. (For a description of the various white blood cells, see pages 805–806, and figure 59–1, page 803.)

Materia alba (mah te′rē-ah al′bah): white or cream-colored cheesy mass that can collect over bacterial plaque on unclean, neglected teeth; it is composed of food debris, mucin, bacteria (see text page 269).

Maturation (mach′u-ra′shun): stage or process of attaining maximal development; become mature.

Microorganism (mī′krō-or′gan-izm): minute living organisms, usually microscopic; includes bacteria, rickettsiae, viruses, fungi, and protozoa.

Mycoplasma (mī′kō-plaz′mah): pleomorphic, gram-negative bacteria that lack cell walls; many are regular oral cavity residents; some are pathogenic.

Obligate (ob′lĭ-gāt): ability to survive only in a particular environment; opposite of **facultative.**

Parasite (par′ah-sīt): plant or animal that lives upon or within another living organism and draws its nourishment therefrom; may be obligate or facultative; *adj.* parasitic.

Pathogen (path′ō-jen): disease-producing agent or microorganism; *adj.* pathogenic.

Pleomorphism (plē′ō-mor′fism): assumption of various distinct forms by a single organism or within a species; *adj.* pleomorphic.

Saprophyte (sap′rō-fīt): any organism, such as bacteria, that lives upon dead or decaying organic matter.

TABLE 16–2
TOOTH DEPOSITS

Category	Tooth Deposit	Description	Derivation
Nonmineralized	Acquired Pellicle	Translucent, homogenous, thin, unstructured film covering and adherent to the surfaces of the teeth, restorations, calculus, and other surfaces in the oral cavity	Supragingival: saliva Subgingival: gingival sulcus fluid
	Microbial (Bacterial) Plaques	Dense, organized bacterial systems embedded in an intermicrobial matrix that adhere closely to the teeth, calculus, and other surfaces in the oral cavity Water irrigation removes only the outer layer of loose organisms	Colonization of oral microorganisms
	Materia Alba	Loosely adherent, unstructured, white or grayish-white mass of oral debris and bacteria that lies over bacterial plaque Vigorous rinsing and water irrigation can remove materia alba	Incidental accumulation
	Food Debris	Unstructured, loosely attached particulate matter Self-cleansing activity of tongue and saliva and rinsing vigorously remove debris	Food retention following eating
Mineralized	Calculus	Calcified bacterial plaque; hard, tenacious mass that forms on the clinical crowns of the natural teeth and on dentures and other appliances	Plaque mineralization
	a. Supragingival	Occurs coronal to the margin of the gingiva; is covered with bacterial plaque	Supragingival: source of minerals is saliva
	b. Subgingival	Occurs apical to the margin of the gingiva; is covered with bacterial plaque	Subgingival: source of minerals is gingival sulcus fluid

(Adapted from Schroeder, H.E.: *Formation and Inhibition of Dental Calculus*. Vienna, Hans Huber, 1969, pp. 14–15.)

B. Nidus for Bacteria
Pellicle participates in plaque formation by aiding the adherence of microorganisms.

C. Attachment of Calculus
One mode of calculus attachment is by the acquired pellicle (page 276).

BACTERIAL PLAQUE

Microbial/dental plaque, commonly referred to as bacterial plaque, is a dense, nonmineralized, complex mass of colonies in a gel-like intermicrobial matrix. It adheres firmly to the acquired pellicle and hence to the teeth, calculus, and fixed and removable restorations.
The term *microbial dental plaque* is more accurate than "bacterial plaque" because microorganisms other than

bacteria can be found. They may include mycoplasmas, yeasts, protozoa, and viruses. Characteristics of supragingival and subgingival plaques are shown in table 16–3.

I. STAGES IN THE FORMATION OF PLAQUE
Plaque is formed in three basic steps, namely, pellicle formation, bacterial colonization, and plaque maturation (figure 16–2). Plaque formation does not occur randomly but involves a series of complex interactions.

A. Formation of a Pellicle
The pellicle forms on the tooth surface by selective adsorption of protein components from the saliva.

B. Bacteria Attach to the Pellicle
Initial attachment of bacteria to the pellicle is by selective adherence of specific bacteria from the oral environment. Innate characteristics of the

TABLE 16–3
CHARACTERISTICS OF SUPRAGINGIVAL AND SUBGINGIVAL PLAQUE

Characteristic	Supragingival Plaque	Subgingival Plaque
Location	Coronal to the margin of the free gingiva	Apical to the margin of the free gingiva
Origin	Salivary glycoprotein forms pellicle Microorganisms from saliva are selectively attracted to pellicle	Downgrowth of bacteria from supragingival plaque

Distribution	Starts on proximal surfaces and other protected areas
	Heaviest collection on
	  Areas not cleaned daily by patient
	  Cervical third, especially facial
	  Lingual mandibular molars
	  Proximal surfaces
	Pit and fissure plaque
		Shallow pocket: similar to supragingival plaque
		Undisturbed; held by pocket wall
		Attached plaque covers calculus
		Unattached plaque extends to the periodontal attachment

Adhesion	Firmly attached to acquired pellicle, other bacteria, and tooth surfaces Surface bacteria (unattached): loose, washed away by saliva or swallowed	Adheres to tooth surface, subgingival pellicle, and calculus Subgingival flora: loose, floating, motile organisms in deep pocket do not adhere; they are between adherent plaque on tooth and the pocket epithelium
Retention	Rough surfaces of teeth or restorations Malpositioned teeth Carious lesions (See Chapter 12 for other factors)	Pocket holds plaque against tooth Overhanging margins of fillings that extend into pockets

Shape and Size	Friction of tongue, cheeks, lips limits shape and size
	Thickness: thicker at the cervical third and on proximal surfaces
	  Healthy gingiva: thin plaque, 15 to 20 cells thick
	  Chronic gingivitis: thick plaque, 100 to 300 cells thick
		Molded by pocket wall to shape of the tooth surface
		Follows form created by subgingival calculus
		May become thicker as the diseased pocket wall becomes less tight

Structure	Adherent, densely packed microbial layer over pellicle on tooth surface Intermicrobial matrix Onset: small isolated colonies 2 to 5 days; colonies merge to form a covering of plaque	Three layers (see figure 16–4) 1. Tooth-surface-attached plaque: many gram-positive rods and cocci 2. Unattached plaque in middle: many gram-negative, motile forms; spirochetes; leukocytes 3. Epithelium-attached plaque: gram-negative, motile forms predominate; many leukocytes migrate through epithelium
Microorganisms	Early plaque: primarily gram-positive cocci Older plaque (3 to 4 days): increased numbers of filaments and fusiforms 4 to 9 days undisturbed: more complex flora with rods, filamentous forms 7 to 14 days: vibrios, spirochetes, more gram-negative organisms	Environment conducive to growth of anaerobic population Diseased pocket: primarily gram-negative, motile, spirochetes, rods See table 16–4
Sources of Nutrients for Bacterial Proliferation	Saliva Ingested food	Tissue fluid (gingival sulcus fluid) Exudate Leukocytes

Significance	Etiology of
	  Gingivitis
	  Supragingival calculus
	  Dental caries (figure 16–6)
		Etiology of
		  Gingivitis
		  Periodontal infections
		  Subgingival calculus

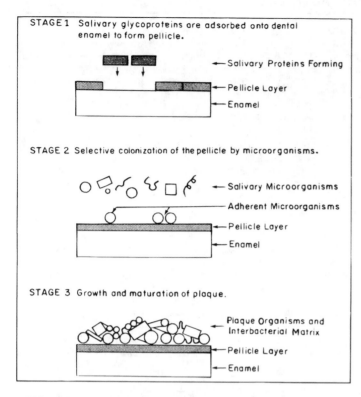

STAGE 1 Salivary glycoproteins are adsorbed onto dental enamel to form pellicle.

← Salivary Proteins Forming
← Pellicle Layer
← Enamel

STAGE 2 Selective colonization of the pellicle by microorganisms.

← Salivary Microorganisms
← Adherent Microorganisms
← Pellicle Layer
← Enamel

STAGE 3 Growth and maturation of plaque.

← Plaque Organisms and Interbacterial Matrix
← Pellicle Layer
← Enamel

FIG. 16–2. Stages of Plaque Formation. Diagrammatic representation of the three stages of bacterial plaque formation. (Redrawn from Katz, S., McDonald, J.L., and Stookey, G.K.: *Preventive Dentistry.* Upper Montclair, NJ, DCP Publishing, 1977.)

bacteria and the pellicle determine the adhesive interactions that cause a particular organism to adhere to a particular pellicle.

C. Bacterial Multiplication and Colonization

1. Microcolonies form in layers as the bacteria multiply and grow.
2. With increased size, colonies meet and coalesce to form a continuous bacterial mass.
3. Organisms of the first few hours are gram-positive cocci and rods.

D. Plaque Growth and Maturation

The increase in the mass and thickness of plaque results from
1. Continued bacterial multiplication.
2. Continuous adherence of bacteria to the plaque surface.

E. Matrix Formation

The intermicrobial substance is derived mainly from saliva for supragingival plaque and from gingival sulcus fluid and exudate for subgingival plaque. Other components of the intermicrobial substance are the polysaccharides, glucans, and fructans or levans produced by certain bacteria from dietary sucrose. The polysaccharides are sticky and contribute to the adhesion of the plaque to the teeth.

II. CHANGES IN PLAQUE MICROORGANISMS

Bacterial plaque consists of a complex mixture of microorganisms that occurs primarily as microcolonies. The population density is very high and increases as plaque ages. The probability of the development of dental caries and/or gingivitis increases as the number of microorganisms increases.

Changes in the types of organisms occur within plaque as the plaque matures. When oral hygiene practices are discontinued, the numbers of bacteria increase rapidly. The changes in oral flora follow a pattern such as that shown in figure 16–3. The changes can be described as follows:[4]

A. Days 1 to 2

Early plaque consists primarily of cocci. Streptococci, which dominate the bacterial population, include *mutans streptococcus* and *Streptococcus sanguis.*

B. Days 2 to 4

The cocci still dominate, and increasing numbers of filamentous forms and slender rods may be seen on the surface of the cocci colonies. Gradually, the filamentous forms grow into the cocci layer and replace many of the cocci. Slow plaque formers continue to form plaque comprised primarily of cocci for a longer time than do fast plaque formers.

C. Days 4 to 7

Filaments increase in numbers, and a more mixed flora begins to appear with rods, filamentous forms, and fusobacteria. Plaque near the gingival margin thickens and develops a more mature flora, with spirochetes and vibrios. As plaque spreads coronally, the new plaque has the characteristic coccal forms.

D. Days 7 to 14

Vibrios and spirochetes appear, and the number of white blood cells increases. As plaque matures and thickens, more gram-negative and anaerobic organisms appear. During this period, signs of inflammation are beginning to be observable in the gingiva.

E. Days 14 to 21

Vibrios and spirochetes are prevalent in older plaque, along with cocci and filamentous forms. The densely packed filamentous microorganisms arrange themselves perpendicular to the tooth surface in a palisade. Gingivitis is evident clinically.

III. SUBGINGIVAL MICROBIAL PLAQUE

A. Source

Subgingival plaque results from the apical proliferation of microorganisms from supragingival

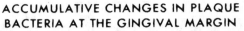

ACCUMULATIVE CHANGES IN PLAQUE
BACTERIA AT THE GINGIVAL MARGIN

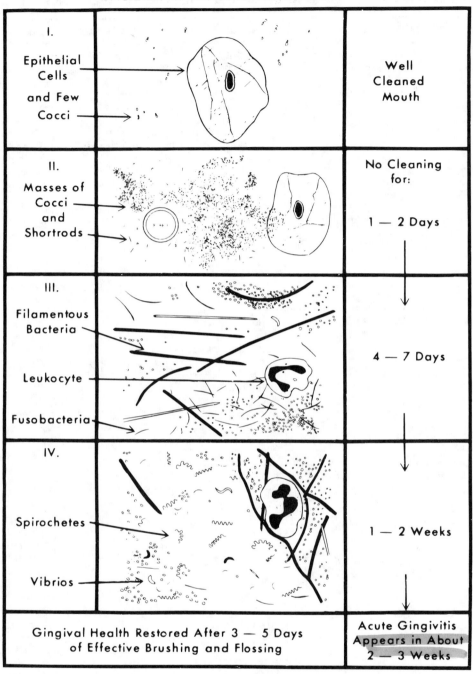

FIG. 16–3. Plaque Microorganisms. On the right are the time intervals from 1 day to 3 weeks. On the left are the changes in the plaque content that take place as plaque ages. As the numbers of microorganisms increase, the numbers of defense cells (leukocytes) also increase. (From Crawford, J.J.: Microbiology, in Barton, R.E., Matteson, S.R., and Richardson, R.E.: The Dental Assistant, 6th ed. Philadelphia, Lea & Febiger, 1988.)

plaque. In the early stages of gingivitis and periodontitis, the supragingival plaque is a strong influence on the accumulation and pathogenic features of the subgingival plaque. As the periodontal pocket deepens, the supragingival plaque only relates to the coronally situated pocket plaque.

B. Microorganisms

The flora of the subgingival plaque differs from that of the supragingival plaque. The subgingival plaque includes more anaerobic and motile organisms and they are predominantly gram negative. Table 16–4 lists significant microorganisms that occur in subgingival plaque and are

TABLE 16–4
MAJOR/DOMINANT MICROORGANISMS IN PERIODONTAL INFECTIONS*

Periodontal Condition	Bacterial and Immunologic Features	Bacterial Species
Periodontal Health	Gram-positive Coccal and rod forms Few gram-negative	Streptococcus species Actinomyces species *Rothia dentocariosa*
Gingivitis	Gram-positive and gram-negative bacteria Few motile rods and spirochetes Total numbers 10 to 20 times those in healthy tissue	Streptococcus species Actinomyces species Veillonella species Treponema species *Fusobacterium nucleatum*
Pregnancy Gingivitis	Changes may relate to hormonal changes	*Prevotella intermedia* Capnocytophaga species
Necrotizing Ulcerative Gingivitis	Spirochetes invade tissue Gram-negative bacteria primarily	Treponema species *Fusobacterium nucleatum* *Prevotella intermedia*
Prepubertal Periodontitis	Gram-negative bacteria predominate Capnophilic and anaerobic Impaired neutrophil function	*Actinobacillus actinomycetemcomitans* Capnocytophaga species *Prevotella intermedia*
Juvenile Periodontitis	Gram-negative Capnophilic and anaerobic Soft tissue invasion of bacteria Impaired neutrophil function	*Actinobacillus actinomycetemcomitans* *Eikenella corrodens* *Prevotella intermedia* Capnocytophaga species
Rapid Progressive Periodontitis	Gram-negative Anaerobic organisms Impaired neutrophil function	*Porphyromonas gingivalis* *Actinobacillus actinomycetemcomitans* *Prevotella intermedia* *Fusobacterium nucleatum* *Eikenella corrodens* *Campylobacter rectus*
Adult Periodontitis	Gram-negative Anaerobic organisms Complex flora: coccoid, spiral, and rod forms Motile	*Porphyromonas gingivalis* *Actinobacillus actinomycetemcomitans* *Prevotella intermedia* *Bacteroides forsythus* *Treponema denticola* *Treponema socranskii* *Campylobacter rectus* *Fusobacterium nucleatum* *Streptococcus intermedius* *Eikenella corrodens* Actinomyces species Eubacterium species
Refractory Periodontitis	Gram-negative Anaerobic organisms Defective host defenses Resistance to usual therapy	*Bacteroides forsythus* *Fusobacterium nucleatum* *Porphyromonas gingivalis* *Campylobacter rectus* *Prevotella intermedia* Peptostreptococcus *Actinobacillus actinomycetemcomitans* Capnocytophaga species Spirochetes Motile rods Candida

* See special listing of references for this table in Suggested Readings at end of chapter, page 270.

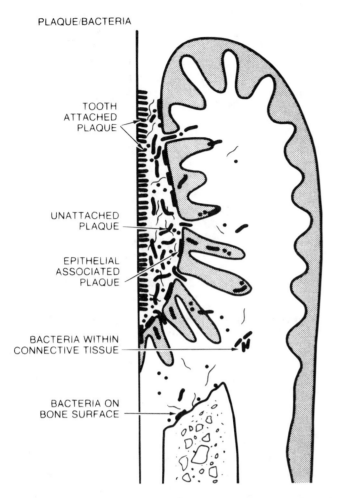

PLAQUE/BACTERIA

TOOTH ATTACHED PLAQUE

UNATTACHED PLAQUE

EPITHELIAL ASSOCIATED PLAQUE

BACTERIA WITHIN CONNECTIVE TISSUE

BACTERIA ON BONE SURFACE

FIG. 16–4. Bacterial Invasion. Diagram of a periodontal pocket shows bacteria of attached and unattached plaque bacteria within the pocket epithelium, in the connective tissue, and on the surface of the bone. (From Carranza, F.A.: *Glickman's Clinical Periodontology*, 6th ed. Philadelphia, W.B. Saunders Co., 1984, p. 368.)

associated with periodontal health and various periodontal infections.

C. Organization of Subgingival Plaque (figure 16–4)

1. *Tooth-surface Attached Plaque.* Over the pellicle, which covers the tooth surface, is a layer of densely packed microorganisms. Next to the tooth, on the innermost side of this layer, are many gram-positive rods and cocci. The plaque of this area is associated with calculus formation, root caries, and root resorption.
2. *Unattached Plaque.* Between the two layers of attached plaque are many motile, gram-negative organisms. The "fluid" plaque contains many white blood cells.
3. *Epithelium-associated Plaque.* Loosely attached to the pocket epithelium are many gram-negative microorganisms and numerous

white blood cells. Many virulent pathogenic organisms in this layer may be considered a focus for the advancement of periodontal infection. From this layer, microorganisms invade the underlying connective tissue. Figure 16–4 shows bacteria within the connective tissue and on the bone surface.

D. Invasion of Microorganisms

The invasion of spirochetes in necrotizing ulcerative gingivitis is described in Chapter 35 (page 538). Electron microscopy has made possible the detection of microorganisms within tissues.[5] Bacterial invasion provides a significant pathogenic mechanism for progress of periodontal infections.

IV. COMPOSITION OF BACTERIAL PLAQUE

Plaque is composed of microorganisms and intermicrobial matrix. Organic and inorganic solids constitute approximately 20%, and water accounts for 80%. Microorganisms make up at least 70 to 80% of the solid matter, which is higher in subgingival plaque than in supragingival.

Composition differs between individuals and between different tooth surfaces of an individual. As plaque ages, it changes.

A. Inorganic Elements[6,7]

1. *Calcium and Phosphorus.* The concentration of calcium, phosphorus, magnesium, and fluoride is higher in plaque than in saliva, thus illustrating the ability of plaque to concentrate inorganic elements.

    Plaque on the lingual surfaces of the mandibular anterior teeth contains a higher concentration of calcium and phosphate than does plaque on the other teeth, and the amount is even higher on those same surfaces in heavy calculus formers.
2. *Fluoride.* The concentration of fluoride in plaque is higher when fluoridated water is used, and is increased following professional topical applications of fluoride and the use of fluoride-containing dentifrices and mouthrinses.

B. Organic Components

The organic intermicrobial substance surrounds the microorganisms of plaque and contains primarily carbohydrates and proteins, with small amounts of lipids.

1. *Carbohydrates.* Carbohydrates, which are produced by several types of bacteria, include glucans and fructans or levans made from dietary sucrose. Dextran is a type of glucan. These carbohydrates contribute to the following:
    a. Adherence of the microorganisms to each other and the tooth. An example is *mutans streptococcus*, which may be linked to glucans.

b. Energy storage of carbohydrate for reserve use by plaque bacteria.
2. *Proteins*
   a. Supragingival plaque contains proteins
      derived from saliva.
   b. Subgingival plaque contains proteins
      from gingival exudate and sulcus fluid.
3. *Lipids.* The lipid content may include lipopolysaccharide endotoxins from gram-negative bacteria.

CLINICAL ASPECTS

I. DISTRIBUTION
A. Location
1. *Supragingival Plaque.* Plaque is coronal to the
   gingival margin.
2. *Gingival Plaque.* Plaque forms on the external
   surfaces of the oral epithelium and attached
   gingiva.
3. *Subgingival Plaque.* Plaque is located between
   the periodontal attachment and the gingival
   margin, within the sulcus or pocket.
4. *Fissure Plaque.* Plaque also develops in pits
   and fissures and is referred to as *fissure
   plaque.*

B. By Surfaces
1. *During Formation.* Supragingival plaque formation begins at the gingival margin, particularly on proximal surfaces, and increases
   rapidly when left undisturbed. It spreads
   over the gingival third and on toward the
   middle third of the crown.
2. *Tooth Surfaces Involved*
   a. Plaque occurs most frequently on proxi-
      mal surfaces and around the gingival
      third, associated with protected areas (fig-
      ure 16–5).
   b. Least amounts occur on the palatal sur-
      faces of maxillary teeth because of the ac-
      tivity of the tongue.

C. Factors Influencing Plaque Accumulation
In Chapter 12 (pages 201–205), many factors
that influence deposit accumulation and disease
development were outlined. A review of those
factors can be helpful in conjunction with the
material in this section.
1. Figure 16–5 illustrates the accumulation of
   bacterial plaque around crowded mandibular anterior teeth. Research has shown that,
   when personal plaque removal efforts are
   made conscientiously, plaque accumulation
   around crowded teeth is not greater than
   that around teeth in good alignment.[8]
2. More rapid collection occurs on rough surfaces of teeth, restorations, and calculus.

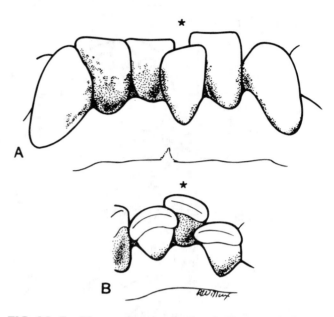

FIG. 16–5. Plaque Accumulation in Protected Areas.
Crowded mandibular anterior teeth demonstrate bacterial
plaque after use of a disclosing agent. The thickest plaque is
on the proximal surfaces and at the cervical thirds of the
teeth. Note the central incisors in facial view **(A)** and lingual
view **(B)**, with thick extensive plaque on the less accessible
protected surfaces.

3. Thick, dense deposits usually collect in difficult-to-clean areas, such as under overhanging margins of crowns or fillings, under
   ledges of calculus, and in areas associated
   with carious lesions.
4. Deposits may extend over an entire crown
   of a tooth that is unopposed, out of occlusion,
   or not used during mastication.

II. DETECTION
A. Direct Vision
1. *Thin Plaque.* May be translucent and therefore not visible.
2. *Stained Plaque.* May acquire extrinsic stains
   that make it visible, for examples, yellow,
   green, tobacco, as described on pages
   281–283.
3. *Thick Plaque.* The tooth may appear dull,
   dingy, with a matted fur-like surface. Materia alba or food debris may collect over the
   plaque.

B. Use of Explorer or Probe
1. *Tactile Examination.* When calcification has
   started, plaque may feel slightly rough;
   otherwise the surface may feel only somewhat slippery because of the coating of soft,
   slimy plaque.
2. *Removal of Plaque.* When no plaque is visible,
   an explorer can be passed over the tooth sur-

face. When present, plaque adheres to the explorer tip. This technique is used when evaluating for a Plaque Index (page 291).

C. Use of Disclosing Agent

When a disclosing agent is applied, plaque takes on the color and becomes readily visible (figure 26–1, page 408). Disclosing agent should not be applied until the evaluation of the oral mucosa and gingival color has been recorded.

D. Clinical Record

1. Record plaque by location and extent (slight, moderate, or heavy). An index or plaque score may be used (pages 291–293).
2. Plaque recordings and indices are kept for comparison in conjunction with the instructional plan for plaque control by the patient, both current and for maintenance appointments.
3. Plaque evaluation records are included with the complete charting and oral examination.

SIGNIFICANCE OF BACTERIAL PLAQUE

The role of plaque in the initiation and perpetuation of both dental caries and periodontal infections has led to a realization that all bacterial plaque is not the same, but that the content and effects vary. Two hypotheses have been used to describe plaque differences.

The "Non-specific Plaque Hypothesis" suggests that dental caries and periodontal infections result from the bacterial products of the entire plaque flora. The level or threshold of disease activity would be determined by the quantity of microorganisms and the response by host defense.

The "Specific Plaque Hypothesis," on the other hand, is based on the realization that the principal differences between plaques are brought about by specific pathogenic microorganisms. By this system, particular microorganisms must always be present in association with specific infections. Prevention or treatment procedures would then be directed at the specific plaque microorganisms.

On the basis of their pathogenic effects, the three main categories of plaques are as follows:

I. CARIOGENIC PLAQUE

Associated with the initiation of dental caries. A high-sucrose diet favors the cariogenic flora.

II. PERIODONTAL-DISEASE-PRODUCING PLAQUE

Directly involved in promoting the inflammatory responses demonstrated by gingivitis, periodontitis, and other periodontal infections.

III. CALCULUS PLAQUE OR CALCULOGENIC PLAQUE

Invites mineralization of the plaque, leading to calculus formation.

DENTAL CARIES

Dental caries is a disease of the dental calcified structures (enamel, dentin, and cementum) that is characterized by demineralization of the mineral components and dissolution of the organic matrix. Clinical characteristics and types of cavities were described in Chapter 14.

I. ESSENTIALS FOR DENTAL CARIES

The sequence of events leading to demineralization and dental caries is shown in figure 16–6.

A. Susceptible Tooth Surface

A tooth with optimum fluoride content resists the process of dental caries.

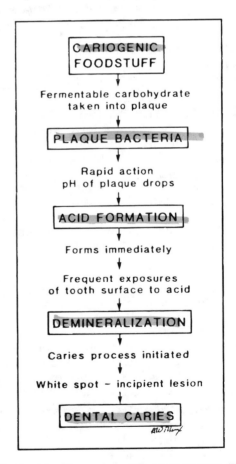

FIG. 16–6. Development of Dental Caries. Flowchart shows the step-by-step action within the microbial plaque on the tooth surface.

B. Microorganisms[9]

Mutans streptococci (*Streptococcus mutans* and *S. sobrinus*, predominantly) play a major role in caries development and progression. They appear in large numbers in carious lesions.

Historically, acidogenic lactobacilli also have been implicated. The lactobacilli may have a more important role in the progression of a carious lesion, and may be less significant in its origin.

Bacterial plaque contains many acidogenic microorganisms. In addition to mutans streptococci and lactobacilli, other predominant groups of microorganisms with acidogenic potential include nonmutans streptococci, actinomyces, and Veillonella species.

C. Cariogenic Foodstuff Source

1. Cariogenic foodstuff, particularly sucrose, enters the microbial plaque.
2. Acid-forming bacteria break down the sugar to an acid.
3. Acid on the tooth surface causes subsurface demineralization.
4. Decreased salivary flow (xerostomia) and increased dietary carbohydrate promote the growth of mutans streptococci and lactobacilli in bacterial plaque.

II. CONTRIBUTING FACTORS

A. Time

Acid formation begins *immediately* when the sucrose from food is taken into the plaque.

B. The pH of the Plaque

The pH of the plaque is lowered promptly, and 1 to 2 hours are required for the pH to return to a normal level, assuming the plaque is left undisturbed.

1. Plaque pH before eating ranges from 6.2 to 7.0; it is lower in the caries-susceptible person and higher in the caries-resistant person.
2. Immediately following sucrose intake into plaque, a rapid drop in the pH of the plaque occurs.[10,11]
3. Critical pH for enamel demineralization averages between 4.5 to 5.5, below which the enamel demineralizes. The critical pH for root surface demineralization is approximately 6.0 to 6.7.[12]
4. The amount of demineralization depends on the length of time and the frequency with which the acid with a pH below the critical pH is in contact with the tooth surface.

C. Frequency of Carbohydrate Intake

With each meal or snack that contains sucrose, the pH of the plaque is lowered (figure 28–6 page 430). Large amounts of sucrose eaten at mealtimes can be expected to be less cariogenic than small amounts eaten at frequent intervals during the day.[13] These and other related facts can be presented to the patient when the diet is discussed as a part of the basic instruction or as part of a total dental caries control program with dietary analysis (pages 425–431).

III. THE CARIOUS LESION

The incipient carious lesion begins as subsurface demineralization. Acid from bacterial action on the tooth surface passes through microchannels in the enamel, demineralization occurs, and eventually a white spot can be seen clinically. Early and continuous use of fluoride for remineralization is necessary. Dental caries formation is described on pages 231 and 232, 234 and the use of fluoride in remineralization is covered on pages 437 and 438.

PERIODONTAL INFECTIONS

Bacterial plaque is unquestionably the single most important etiologic factor in periodontal infections. The variations in clinical manifestations in different individuals can be accounted for by the differences in the bacterial activity within the plaque, as well as by the tissue response and resistance to the microorganisms and their products.

Table 16–4 lists significant microorganisms present in the bacterial plaque of the various periodontal infections. Total counts of microorganisms in diseased periodontal pockets are extremely high. Several hundred types exist. Morphologic varieties include cocci, rods, fusiforms, filaments, spirilla, and spirochetes (figure 16–1).

I. INITIATION OF GINGIVAL DISEASE

Microorganisms of the bacterial plaque at the gingival margin multiply and extend beneath the margin. A high concentration of microorganisms is in contact with the sulcular epithelium. The irritation from the bacteria and their products leads to degeneration of the sulcular epithelium. Inflammation in the adjacent connective tissue results. The steps in the development of gingivitis and pocket formation are described on pages 195–197.

II. EXPERIMENTAL GINGIVITIS[4]

Gingivitis develops in 2 to 3 weeks when plaque is left undisturbed on the tooth surfaces. The microbiologic changes were outlined on page 262. Most gingivitis is reversible, and when the gingiva are treated by plaque removal procedures, the gingiva can return to health within a few days.

An experimental gingivitis program to demonstrate the effect of plaque can be conducted as follows:

A. Observe and record characteristics of the healthy gingiva at the outset. Record a gingival index, a plaque index, and a bleeding index.
B. Withhold all plaque control procedures for a period of 3 weeks.

C. Repeat clinical observations of tissues and record indices at least weekly during the test period. Note initial evidence of gingivitis.

D. Reinstate plaque removal measures after 3 weeks. Make daily observations relative to gingival bleeding and indications that healing is taking place. In 1 week, repeat gingival and plaque indices.

III. CALCULUS FORMATION

Bacterial plaque forms a matrix for calculus formation (page 275). The significance of calculus in periodontal infections is described on page 277.

EFFECT OF DIET ON PLAQUE

I. CARIOGENIC FOODS
A. Dental Caries

The relationship of the cariogenic food content of the diet and its frequency of use to the development of dental caries is well defined in research and clinical application. Dental caries initiation is outlined in figure 16–6.

B. Effect of Sucrose on Amount and pH of Plaque

When a cariogenic diet is used, plaque forms and grows more profusely.[14] Patients fed sucrose by stomach tube had a less acidogenic plaque than did patients who were fed sucrose by mouth.[15]

II. FOOD INTAKE

Food particles are not needed in the mouth for plaque to form. In one study, neither varying the number of meals nor feeding by stomach tube affected the development of plaque.[16] In another study, less plaque developed in a group of stomach-fed patients when compared with those fed by mouth.[15]

III. TEXTURE OF DIET

The friction of mastication has been shown to affect only the occlusal and incisal thirds of the crowns of teeth. Plaque on the gingival third collected in spite of a normal diet that included coarse bread and fresh fruit,[4] or of chewing raw carrots three times daily as the only methods for personal care.[17] Chewing apples did not affect moderate amounts of plaque, but did tend to remove food debris in a group of 12-year-olds.[18]

MATERIA ALBA

Materia alba is a loosely adherent mass of bacteria and cellular debris that frequently occurs on top of bacterial plaque.

Materia alba ("white material") distinguishes itself clinically as a bulky, soft deposit that is clearly visible without application of a disclosing agent. It is white, or grayish-white, and characteristically may resemble cottage cheese.

Materia alba forms over bacterial plaque. It is a product of informal accumulation of living and dead bacteria, desquamated epithelial cells, disintegrating leukocytes, salivary proteins, and particles of food debris.

Surface bacteria in contact with the gingiva contribute to gingival inflammation. Tooth surface demineralization and dental caries are seen frequently under materia alba.

Clinical distinction between materia alba, food debris, and bacterial plaque is necessary, but patient instruction for the removal of all three involves the same basic plaque control procedures. Materia alba can be removed with a water spray or oral irrigator, whereas bacterial plaque cannot.

FOOD DEBRIS

Loose food particles collect about the cervical third and proximal embrasures of the teeth.

When there are open contact areas, mobility of teeth, or irregularities of occlusion, such as plunger cusps, food may be forced between the teeth during mastication, and vertical food impaction results. Horizontal or lateral food impaction occurs in facial and lingual embrasures, particularly when the interdental papillae are reduced or missing.

Food debris adds to a general unsanitary condition of the mouth. Cariogenic foods contribute to dental caries because liquified carbohydrate diffuses rapidly into the plaque and hence to the acid-forming bacteria.

Some self-cleansing through the action of the tongue, lips, saliva, and related factors takes place. Debris removal by toothbrushing, flossing, and other aids constitutes a total plaque control program. Cleansing of debris from about fixed prosthetic and orthodontic appliances is important to the plan for oral sanitation.

TECHNICAL HINTS

I. Check all surfaces of restorations and prosthetic appliances and remove rough areas and overhanging margins. Soft deposits accumulate on rough or irregular surfaces more rapidly and in greater quantity than on smooth surfaces.

II. Withhold the use of a disclosing agent until the intraoral mucosal and gingival examinations have been made. Coloring agents can disguise soft tissue changes and deviations from normal.

FACTORS TO TEACH THE PATIENT

I. Location, composition, and properties of bacterial plaque with emphasis on its role in dental caries and periodontal infections.

II. The cause and prevention of dental caries.

III. Effects of personal oral care procedures in the prevention of bacterial plaque and materia alba.

IV. Plaque control procedures with special adaptations for individual needs.

V. Sources of cariogenic foodstuff in the diet with suggestions for control.

VI. Relationship of frequency of eating cariogenic foods to dental caries.

REFERENCES

1. **Schroeder,** H.E.: *Formation and Inhibition of Dental Calculus,* Vienna, Hans Huber Publishers, 1969, pp. 14–15.

2. **Meckel,** A.H.: Formation and Properties of Organic Films on Teeth, *Arch. Oral Biol., 10,* 585, July-August, 1965.

3. **Meckel,** A.H.: The Nature and Importance of Organic Deposits on Dental Enamel, *Caries Res., 2,* 104, No. 2, 1968.

4. **Löe,** H., Theilade, E., and Jensen, S.B.: Experimental Gingivitis in Man, *J. Periodontol., 36,* 177, May-June, 1965.

5. **Carranza,** F.A., Saglie, R., Newman, M.G., and Valentin, P.L.: Scanning and Transmission Electron Microscopic Study of Tissue-invading Microorganisms in Localized Juvenile Periodontitis, *J. Periodontol., 54,* 598, October, 1983.

6. **Mandel,** I.D.: Relation of Saliva and Plaque to Caries, *J. Dent. Res., 53,* 246, March-April, Supplement, 1974.

7. **Grøn,** P., Yao, K., and Spinelli, M.: A Study of Inorganic Constituents in Dental Plaque, *J. Dent. Res., 48,* 799, September-October, 1969.

8. **Årtun,** J. and Osterberg, S.K.: Periodontal Status of Secondary Crowded Mandibular Incisors. Long-term Results After Orthodontic Treatment, *J. Clin. Periodontol., 14,* 261, May, 1987.

9. **Van Houte,** J., Sansone, C., Joshipura, K., and Kent, R.: Mutans Streptococci and Non-mutans Streptococci Acidogenic at Low pH, and *in vitro* Acidogenic Potential of Dental Plaque in Two Different Areas of the Human Dentition, *J. Dent. Res., 70,* 1503, December, 1991.

10. **Stephan,** R.M.: Intra-oral Hydrogen-ion Concentrations Associated with Dental Caries Activity, *J. Dent. Res., 23,* 257, August, 1944.

11. **Rosen,** S. and Weisenstein, P.R.: The Effect of Sugar Solutions on pH of Dental Plaques from Caries-susceptible and Caries-free Individuals, *J. Dent. Res., 44,* 845, September-October, 1965.

12. **Hoppenbrouwers,** P.M.M., Driessens, F.C.M., and Borggreven, J.M.P.M.: The Mineral Solubility of Human Tooth Roots, *Arch. Oral Biol., 32,* 319, No. 5, 1987.

13. **Gustafsson,** B.E., Quensel, C.E., Lanke, L.S., Lundquist, C., Grahnén, H., Bonow, B.E., and Krasse, B.: The Vipeholm Dental Caries Study. The Effect of Different Levels of Carbohydrate Intake on Caries Activity in 436 Individuals Observed for Five Years, *Acta Odontol. Scand., 11,* 232, Nos. 3–4, 1954.

14. **Carlsson,** J. and Egelberg, J.: Effect of Diet on Early Plaque Formation in Man, *Odont. Revy, 16,* 112, No. 1, 1965.

15. **Littleton,** N.W., Carter, C.H., and Kelley, R.T.: Studies of Oral Health in Persons Nourished by Stomach Tube. I. Changes in pH of Plaque Material after the Addition of Sucrose, *J. Am. Dent. Assoc., 74,* 119, January, 1967.

16. **Egelberg,** J.: Local Effect of Diet on Plaque Formation and Development of Gingivitis in Dogs. III. Effect of Frequency of Meals and Tube Feeding, *Odont. Revy, 16,* 50, No. 1, 1965.

17. **Lindhe,** J. and Wicén, P.-O.: The Effects on the Gingivae of Chewing Fibrous Foods, *J. Periodont. Res., 4,* 193, No. 3, 1969.

18. **Birkeland,** J.M. and Jorkjend, L.: The Effect of Chewing Apples on Dental Plaque and Food Debris, *Community Dent. Oral Epidemiol., 2,* 161, No. 4, 1974.

REFERENCES FOR TABLE 16–4

Choi, J.-I., Nakagawa, T., Yamada, S., Takazoe, I., and Okuda, K.: Clinical, Microbiological and Immunological Studies on Recurrent Periodontal Disease, *J. Clin. Periodontol., 17,* 426, August, Part I, 1990.

Christersson, L.A., Fransson, C.L., Dunford, R.G., and Zambon, J.J.: Subgingival Distribution of Periodontal Pathogenic Microorganisms in Adult Periodontitis, *J. Periodontol., 63,* 418, May, 1992.

Dzink, J.L., Socransky, S.S., and Haffajee, A.D.: The Predominant Cultivable Microbiota of Active and Inactive Lesions of Destructive Periodontal Diseases, *J. Clin. Periodontol., 15,* 316, May, 1988.

Falkler, W.A., Martin, S.A., Vincent, J.W., Tall, B.D., Nauman, R.K., and Suzuki, J.B.: A Clinical, Demographic and Microbiologic Study of ANUG Patients in an Urban Dental School, *J. Clin. Periodontol., 14,* 307, July, 1987.

Haffajee, A.D., Socransky, S.S., Dzink, J.L., Taubman, M.A., and Ebersole, J.L.: Clinical, Microbiological Features of Subjects with Refractory Periodontal Diseases, *J. Clin. Periodontol., 15,* 390, July, 1988.

Kornman, K.S. and Loesche, W.J.: The Subgingival Microbial Flora During Pregnancy, *J. Periodont. Res., 15,* 111, March, 1980.

Kornman, K.S. and Robertson, P.B.: Clinical and Microbiological Evaluation of Therapy for Juvenile Periodontitis, *J. Periodontol., 56,* 443, August, 1985.

Listgarten, M.A.: Electron Microscopic Observations on the Bacterial Flora of Acute Necrotizing Ulcerative Gingivitis, *J. Periodontol., 36,* 328, July-August, 1965.

Listgarten, M.A., Lai, C.-H., and Young, V.: Microbial Composition and Pattern of Antibiotic Resistance in Subgingival Microbial Samples From Patients with Refractory Periodontitis, *J. Periodontol., 64,* 155, March, 1993.

Loesche, W.J., Syed, S.A., Schmidt, E., and Morrison, E.C.: Bacterial Profiles of Subgingival Plaques in Periodontitis, *J. Periodontol., 56,* 447, August, 1985.

Loesche, W.J., Syed, S.A., Laughon, B.E., and Stoll, J.: The Bacteriology of Acute Necrotizing Ulcerative Gingivitis, *J. Periodontol., 53,* 223, April, 1982.

Mandell, R.L., Ebersole, J.L., and Socransky, S.S.: Clinical Immunologic and Microbiologic Features of Active Disease Sites in Juvenile Periodontitis, *J. Clin. Periodontol., 14,* 534, October, 1987.

Moore, W.E.C., Moore, L.H., Ranney, R.R., Smibert, R.M., Burmeister, J.A., and Schenkein, H.A.: The Microflora of Periodontal Sites Showing Active Destructive Progression, *J. Clin. Periodontol., 18,* 729, November, 1991.

Page, R.C., Altman, L.C., Ebersole, J.L., Vandesteen, G.E., Dahlberg, W.H., Williams, B.L., and Osterberg, S.K.: Rapidly Progressive Periodontitis. A Distinct Clinical Condition, *J. Periodontol., 54,* 197, April, 1983.

Preber, H., Bergström, J., and Linder, L.E.: Occurrence of Periopathogens in Smoker and Non-smoker Patients, *J. Clin. Periodontol., 19,* 667, October, 1992.

wet with saliva. With a combination of retraction, light, and drying with air, small deposits usually can be seen. An explorer may be used when visual examination is not definite (pages 221 and 222).

III. SUBGINGIVAL EXAMINATION
A. Visual Examination
Of calculus within a pocket
1. Dark edge of calculus may be seen at or just beneath the margin.
2. Diseased gingival margin does not adapt closely to a tooth surface, thus permitting a view into the pocket where calculus can be seen.
3. Gentle air blast can deflect the margin from the tooth for observation into the pocket.
4. When light shines through anterior teeth during transillumination, a dark opaque shadow-like area seen on a proximal tooth surface could be subgingival calculus. Supragingival calculus may also be found by this method. Without calculus, stain, or thick, soft deposit, the enamel is translucent.

B. Gingival Tissue Color Change
Dark calculus may reflect through a thin margin and suggest the presence of subgingival calculus.

C. Tactile Examination
1. *Probe.* While probing for sulcus/pocket characteristics, a rough subgingival tooth surface can be felt when calculus is present. Although there are other causes of roughness, subgingival calculus is the most common (page 200).
2. *Explorer.* A fine subgingival explorer is needed that can be adapted close to the root surface all the way to the bottom of a pocket. Each subgingival area must be examined carefully to the bottom of the pocket, completely around each tooth.

IV. CLINICAL RECORD
Calculus deposits are described in the examination record. The location of supra- and subgingival deposits and their extent (slight, moderate, or heavy) must be designated. A calculus index may be useful for patient evaluation and counseling at continuing maintenance appointments (page 306).

The calculus record is included with the complete charting and oral examination (page 317).

CALCULUS FORMATION[4]

Subgingival calculus does not develop by direct extension from supragingival calculus. First, subgingival bacterial plaque forms by extension of supragingival plaque. Each plaque mineralizes separately.

Calculus results from the deposition of minerals into a plaque organic matrix. Calculus formation occurs in three basic steps: *pellicle formation, plaque formation,* and *mineralization.* Mineralization of supra- and subgingival calculus is essentially the same, although the source of the elements for mineralization is not the same.

I. PELLICLE FORMATION
The formation and characteristics of pellicle were described on page 258. The pellicle, or cuticle, is composed of mucoproteins from the saliva and is an acellular material. Its thickness and contour vary on the tooth surface. It begins to form within minutes after all deposits have been removed from the tooth surface.

II. PLAQUE MATURATION
A. Microorganisms settle in the pellicle layer.
B. Colonies are formed. Originally, the colonies consist primarily of cocci and rod-shaped organisms. By the fifth day, the plaque is mostly made up of filamentous organisms.
C. The colonies grow together to form a cohesive plaque layer.

III. MINERALIZATION
A. Mineralization Foci (Centers) Form
Within 24 to 72 hours, more and more mineralization centers develop close to the underlying tooth surface. Eventually, the centers grow large enough to touch and unite.

B. Organic Matrix
Mineralization first occurs within the intermicrobial matrix. The filamentous microorganisms provide the matrix for the deposition of minerals.

A calculus-like deposit has been observed on the teeth of germ-free animals that have no bacterial plaque.[5,6,7] It may indicate that other organic substances, such as the pellicle, may mineralize.

C. Sources of Minerals
1. *Supragingival Calculus.* The source of elements for supragingival calculus is the saliva.
2. *Subgingival Calculus.* The gingival sulcus fluid and the inflammatory exudate supply the minerals for the subgingival deposits. Gingival sulcus fluid was described on page 184. Because the amount of sulcus fluid and exudate increases with increases in inflammation, more minerals are available for mineralization of subgingival plaque.

D. Crystal Formation
Mineralization consists of crystal formation, namely, hydroxyapatite, octocalcium phosphate, whitlockite, and brushite, each with a characteristic developmental pattern. The crys-

tals form in the intercellular matrix and on the surface of bacteria, and finally within the bacteria.[8,9]

E. Mechanism of Mineralization[4]

The mineralization process is considered the same for both supra- and subgingival calculus. Heavy calculus formers have higher salivary levels of calcium and phosphorus than do light calculus formers.[10] Light calculus formers have higher levels of parotid pyrophosphate.[11] Pyrophosphate is an inhibitor of calcification and is used in anticalculus dentifrices (page 278).

The process by which minerals, mainly calcium and phosphate, become incorporated from the saliva or gingival sulcus fluid into the plaque matrix is still not completely understood. Several theories may explain the complex mechanism.[4]

Current research studies point to the probability that calcification of calculus may involve the same phenomena as those of other ectopic calcifications (such as urinary or renal calculi) and may be similar to normal calcification of bone, cartilage, enamel, or dentin. For those wishing to read about this complex subject, some references are provided in the *Suggested Readings* at the end of this chapter.

IV. FORMATION TIME

Formation time means the average number of days required for the primary soft deposit to change to the mature mineralized stage. The average time is about 12 days, within a range from 10 days for rapid calculus formers to 20 days for slow calculus formers.[10] Mineralization can begin as early as 24 to 48 hours.

Formation time depends on individual tendency, but it is strongly influenced by the roughness of the tooth surface and the care and character of personal plaque control measures. Determination of the approximate formation time for an individual is important to instruction and counseling, as well as to treatment planning for professional care and frequency of maintenance appointments.

V. STRUCTURE OF CALCULUS
A. Layers

Calculus forms in layers that are more or less parallel with the tooth surface. The layers are separated by a line that appears to be a pellicle that was deposited over the previously formed calculus, and as mineralization progressed, the pellicle became imbedded.

The lines between the layers of calculus can be called incremental lines. They form around the tooth in supragingival calculus, but form irregularly from crown to apex on the root surface in subgingival calculus. The lines are evidence that calculus grows or increases by apposition of new layers.

B. Surface

The surface of a calculus mass is rough and can be detected by use of an explorer. As observed by electron microscope, the surface roughness appears as peaks, valleys, and pits.

C. Outer Layer

The outer layer of subgingival calculus is partly calcified. On the surface is a thick, mat-like soft layer of bacterial plaque. The outer surface of the plaque on the subgingival calculus is in contact with the diseased pocket epithelium. The contents of the three layers of subgingival plaque are outlined in table 16–3, page 261.

VI. ATTACHMENT OF CALCULUS

Calculus is more readily removed from some tooth surfaces than from others. The ease or difficulty of removal can be related to the manner of attachment of the calculus to the tooth surface.

Several modes of attachment have been observed by conventional histologic techniques and by electron microscopy. On any one tooth and in any one area, more than one mode of attachment may be found.

When studying the attachment types, the character of the hard, smooth enamel surface, and of the rough, porous, cemental surface should be considered. Three general modes of attachment can be identified.[12]

A. Attachment by Means of an Acquired Pellicle or Cuticle

1. The pellicle is a thin, acellular, homogeneous layer positioned between the calculus and the tooth surface.
2. Calculus attachment is superficial because no interlocking or penetration occurs.
3. Pellicle attachment occurs most frequently on enamel and newly scaled and planed root surfaces.
4. Calculus may be removed readily because of the smooth attachment.

B. Attachment to Minute Irregularities in the Tooth Surface by Mechanical Locking into Undercuts

1. Enamel irregularities include cracks, lamellae, and carious defects.
2. Cemental irregularities include tiny spaces left at previous locations of Sharpey's fibers, resorption lacunae, scaling grooves, cemental tears, or fragmentation.
3. Difficult to be certain all calculus is removed when it is attached by this method.

C. Attachment by Direct Contact Between Calcified Intercellular Matrix and the Tooth Surface

1. Interlocking of inorganic crystals of the tooth with the mineralizing bacterial plaque.

2. Distinction between calculus and cementum is difficult during root planing.

VII. COMPOSITION

Calculus is made up of inorganic and organic components and water. Although the percentage varies depending on the age and hardness of a deposit and the location from which the sample for analysis is taken, mature calculus usually contains between 75 and 85% inorganic components; the rest is organic components and water. The chemical content of supra- and subgingival calculus is similar.[13,14,15]

A. Inorganic

1. *Inorganic Components.* The components are mainly calcium (Ca), phosphorus (P), carbonate (CO_3), sodium (Na), magnesium (Mg), and potassium (K).

2. *Trace Elements.* Various trace elements have been identified, including chlorine (Cl), zinc (Zn), strontium (Sr), bromine (Br), copper (Cu), manganese (Mn), tungsten (W), gold (Au), aluminum (Al), silicon (Si), iron (Fe), and fluorine (Fl).

3. *Fluoride in Calculus*
   a. Concentration. The concentration of fluoride in calculus varies and is influenced by the amount of fluoride received from fluoride in the drinking water, topical application,[16] dentifrices,[17,18] or any form that is received by contact with the external surface of the calculus.
   b. Uptake. The surface of the cementum, which is more permeable, has a content of fluoride higher than that of the enamel surface.

4. *Crystals.* At least two thirds of the inorganic matter of calculus is crystalline, principally apatite. Predominating is hydroxyapatite, which is the same crystal present in enamel, dentin, cementum, and bone. Calculus also contains varying amounts of brushite, whitlockite, and octocalcium phosphate.[19]

5. *Calculus Compared with Teeth and Bone.* Dental enamel is the most highly calcified tissue in the body and contains 96% inorganic salts; dentin contains 65% and cementum and bone contain 45 to 50%.[20] Mature calculus has approximately 75 to 85% inorganic content. A comparison of calculus with the tooth parts provides insight into the effects of instrumentation, the difficulty of distinguishing calculus from cementum or dentin when scaling subgingivally, and the modes of attachment of calculus to the tooth surface.

B. Organic

The organic proportion of calculus consists of various types of nonvital microorganisms, desquamated epithelial cells, leukocytes, and mucin from the saliva. Substances identified in the organic matrix include cholesterol, cholesterol esters, phospholipids, and fatty acids in the lipid fraction; reducing sugars and carbohydrate-protein complexes in the carbohydrate fraction; and keratins, nucleoproteins, and amino acids in the protein portion.[21,22]

The microorganisms are predominantly filamentous. In early calculus, during the first 5 days, cocci are found with some rods.[21,23] Most of the organisms within calculus are considered nonviable. The plaque on the calculus surface contains viable organisms.

SIGNIFICANCE OF DENTAL CALCULUS

Calculus has long been considered to have an important role in the development, promotion, and recurrence of gingival and periodontal infections.

Significant to the rationale for calculus removal and the production of a smooth tooth surface are the points summarized here concerning the relationship of calculus to periodontal and gingival diseases.

I. RELATION TO BACTERIAL PLAQUE

A. Subgingival plaque develops as a result of downgrowth of supragingival plaque bacteria.

B. Subgingival plaque contains pathogenic bacteria that cause inflammation and destruction in the gingival tissue and lead to loss of attachment to the tooth surface and development and deepening of the pocket.

II. RELATION TO POCKET FORMATION

A. With increased pocket depth, greater amounts of plaque can accumulate with increased numbers of pathogenic organisms. Irritation to the pocket lining stimulates greater flow of gingival sulcus fluid, which contains minerals for subgingival calculus formation.

B. Calculus is mineralized bacterial plaque. The plaque bacteria comprise a matrix for the mineralization of the calculus.

C. Subgingival calculus is always covered by masses of active plaque bacteria. The bacterial mass is in contact with the diseased pocket epithelium and promotes gingivitis and periodontitis.

D. With its rough surface and permeable structure, calculus can act as a reservoir for toxic microbial and tissue breakdown products.

E. Calculus is a predisposing factor in pocket development in that it provides a haven for the collection of bacterial masses on the rough surface of the calculus deposit.

PREVENTION OF CALCULUS

Dental calculus can be a cosmetic problem or a periodontal health problem (or both) for many patients. Patients at risk for calculus formation need individualized counseling. Risk factors related to calculus formation are the same as those for bacterial plaque formation. The contributing factors in disease development described in Chapter 12 (pages 201–204) apply to calculus and plaque and their formation and reformation.

There are several methods for coping with the problem of calculus. The patient must understand the importance of individual daily bacterial plaque removal and how the professional maintenance appointment on a regular basis can supplement the personal care.

I. PROFESSIONAL REMOVAL OF CALCULUS
A. Removal of calculus provides a smooth tooth surface in an environment conducive to gingival healing.
B. The smooth surfaces can be easier for the patient to maintain.
C. With emphasis on good oral hygiene and routine professional removal, low levels of supra- and subgingival calculus have been demonstrated on a long-term basis.[24]

II. PERSONAL BACTERIAL PLAQUE CONTROL
Removal of bacterial plaque by appropriately selected brushing, flossing, and supplementary methods is a major factor in the control of dental calculus reformation.

III. ANTICALCULUS DENTIFRICE
Calculus-control dentifrices currently available contain either a pyrophosphate system or a zinc system. Their aim is to inhibit calculus crystal growth, which in turn should lessen the amount of calculus deposited on the teeth. The dentifrices cannot claim an effect on existing calculus deposits and are offered as a preventive measure in the formation of new calculus.

For a patient who cannot control supragingival calculus, and hence cannot achieve optimum gingival tissue health, an anticalculus dentifrice may provide motivation, as well as supplement mechanical plaque removal efforts.[25]

FACTORS TO TEACH THE PATIENT

I. What calculus is and how it forms from bacterial plaque.
II. The effect of calculus on the health of the periodontal tissues and, therefore, on the general health of the oral cavity.
III. Properties of calculus that explain the need for detailed, meticulous scaling procedures.
IV. Reasons for producing a calculus-free smooth tooth surface during scaling.
V. Plaque control measures that the patient may carry out to minimize calculus deposits.
VI. What to expect from use of an anticalculus dentifrice.
VII. Selection of only products with an ADA Seal of Acceptance (figure 23–15).

REFERENCES

1. **Suomi,** J.D., Smith, L.W., McClendon, B.J., Spolsky, V.W., and Horowitz, H.S.: Oral Calculus in Children, *J. Periodontol., 42,* 341, June, 1971.
2. **Wotman,** S., Mercadante, J., Mandel, I.D., Goldman, R.S., and Denning, C.: The Occurrence of Calculus in Normal Children, Children with Cystic Fibrosis, and Children with Asthma, *J. Periodontol., 44,* 278, May, 1973.
3. **Everett,** F.G. and Potter, G.R.: Morphology of Submarginal Calculus, *J. Periodontol., 30,* 27, January, 1959.
4. **Mandel,** I.D.: Dental Calculus (Calcified Dental Plaque), in Genco, R.J., Goldman, H.M., and Cohen, D.W., eds.: *Contemporary Periodontics.* St. Louis, Mosby, 1990, pp. 135–146.
5. **Fitzgerald,** R.J. and McDaniel, E.G.: Dental Calculus in the Germ-free Rat, *Arch. Oral Biol., 2,* 239, August, 1960.
6. **Gustafsson,** B.E. and Krasse, B.: Dental Calculus in Germfree Rats, *Acta Odontol. Scand., 20,* 135, No. 2, 1962.
7. **Theilade,** J., Fitzgerald, R.J., Scott, D.B., and Nylen, M.U.: Electron Microscopic Observations of Dental Calculus in Germfree and Conventional Rats, *Arch. Oral Biol., 9,* 97, January-February, 1964.
8. **Gonzales,** F. and Sognnaes, R.F.: Electronmicroscopy of Dental Calculus, *Science, 131,* 156, January 15, 1960.
9. **Zander,** H.A., Hazen, S.P., and Scott, D.B.: Mineralization of Dental Calculus, *Proc. Soc. Exp. Biol. Med., 103,* 257, February, 1960.
10. **Schroeder,** H.E.: *Formation and Inhibition of Dental Calculus.* Vienna, Hans Huber Publishers, 1969, pp. 73–74.
11. **Vogel,** J.J. and Amdur, B.H.: Inorganic Pyrophosphate in Parotid Saliva and Its Relation to Calculus Formation, *Arch. Oral Biol., 12,* 159, January, 1967.
12. **Canis,** M.F., Kramer, G.M., and Pameijer, C.M.: Calculus Attachment. Review of the Literature and New Findings, *J. Periodontol., 50,* 406, August, 1979.
13. **Mandel,** I.D.: Biochemical Aspects of Calculus Formation, *J. Periodont. Res., 9,* 10, No. 1, 1974.
14. **Glock,** G.E. and Murray, M.M.: Chemical Investigation of Salivary Calculus, *J. Dent. Res., 17,* 257, August, 1938.
15. **Mandel,** I.D. and Levy, B.M.: Studies on Salivary Calculus. I. Histochemical and Chemical Investigations of Supra- and Subgingival Calculus, *Oral Surg., 10,* 874, August, 1957.
16. **Schait,** A. and Mühlemann, H.R.: Fluoride Uptake by Calculus Following Topical Application of Fluorides, *Helv. Odont. Acta, 15,* 132, October, 1971.
17. **Kinoshita,** S., Schait, A., Schroeder, H.E., and Mühlemann, H.R.: Origin of Fluoride in Early Dental Calculus, *Helv. Odont. Acta, 9,* 141, October, 1965.
18. **Mühlemann,** H.R., Schait, A., and Schroeder, H.E.: Salivary Origin of Fluorine in Calcified Dental Plaques, *Helv. Odont. Acta, 8,* 128, October, 1964.

19. **Grøn,** P., van Campen, G.J., and Lindstrom, I.: Human Dental Calculus. Inorganic Chemical and Crystallographic Composition, *Arch. Oral Biol., 12,* 829, July, 1967.

20. **Melfi,** R.C.: *Permar's Oral Embryology and Microscopic Anatomy,* 8th ed. Philadelphia, Lea & Febiger, 1988, pp. 85, 111, 145.

21. **Mandel,** I.D., Levy, B.M., and Wasserman, B.H.: Histochemistry of Calculus Formation, *J. Periodontol., 28,* 132, April, 1957.

22. **Mandel,** I.D.: Histochemical and Biochemical Aspects of Calculus Formation, *Periodontics, 1,* 43, March-April, 1963.

23. **Turesky,** S., Renstrup, G., and Glickman, I.: Histologic and Histochemical Observations Regarding Early Calculus Formation in Children and Adults, *J. Periodontol., 32,* 7, January, 1961.

24. **Ånerud,** Å., Löe, H., and Boysen, H.: The Natural History and Clinical Course of Calculus Formation in Man, *J. Clin. Periodontol., 18,* 160, March, 1991.

25. **Tilliss,** T.S.I.: A Closer Look at Tartar Control Dentifrices, *J. Dent. Hyg., 63,* 364, October, 1989.

SUGGESTED READINGS

Allen, D.L., McFall, W.T., and Jenzano, J.W.: *Periodontics for the Dental Hygienist,* 4th ed. Philadelphia, Lea & Febiger, 1987, pp. 42–44.

Barnett, M.L., Charles, C.H., Gilman, R.M., and Bartels, L.L.: Correlation Between Volpe-Manhold Calculus Index Scores and Actual Calculus Area, *Clin. Prev. Dent., 11,* 3, November-December, 1989.

Brown, C.M., Hancock, E.B., O'Leary, T.J., Miller, C.H., and Sheldrake, M.A.: A Microbiological Comparison of Young Adults Based on Relative Amounts of Subgingival Calculus, *J. Periodontol., 62,* 591, October, 1991.

Carranza, F.A.: *Glickman's Clinical Periodontology,* 7th ed. Philadelphia, W.B. Saunders Co., 1990, pp. 387–399.

Christersson, L.A., Grossi, S.G., Dunford, R.G., Machtei, E.E., and Genco, R.J.: Dental Plaque and Calculus: Risk Indicators for Their Formation, *J. Dent. Res., 71,* 1425, July, 1992.

Gaare, D., Rølla, G., Aryadi, F.J., and Van der Ouderaa, F.: Improvement of Gingival Health by Toothbrushing in Individuals with Large Amounts of Calculus, *J. Clin. Periodontol., 17,* 38, January, 1990.

Giorgio, S.K.: A New Approach to Calculus Tracking, *Compendium,* Special Issue No. 1, pp. S1–26, 1991.

Grant, D.A., Stern, I.B., and Listgarten, M.A., eds.: *Periodontics,* 6th ed. St. Louis, Mosby, 1988, pp. 198–215.

Kodaka, T. and Miake, K.: Inorganic Components and the Fine Structures of Marginal and Deep Subgingival Calculus Attached to Human Teeth, *Bull. Tokyo Dent. Coll., 32,* 99, August, 1991.

Lindhe, J.: *Textbook of Clinical Periodontology,* 2nd ed. Copenhagen, Munksgaard, 1989, pp. 114–122.

Mandel, I.D.: Calculus Formation and Prevention: An Overview, *Compendium,* Special Issue No. 1, pp. S1–3, 1991.

Mandel, I.D. and Gaffar, A.: Calculus Revisited. A Review, *J. Clin. Periodontol., 13,* 249, April, 1986.

Ten Cate, J.M., ed.: *Recent Advances in the Study of Dental Calculus.* Oxford, IRL Press at Oxford University Press, 1989, pp. 7–35.

Turesky, S., Breuer, M., and Coffman, G.: The Effect of Certain Systemic Medications on Oral Calculus Formation, *J. Periodontol., 63,* 871, November, 1992.

Walsh, T.F., Figures, K.H., and Lamb, D.J.: *Clinical Dental Hygiene. A Handbook for the Dental Team.* Oxford, England, Wright, 1992, pp. 56–57, 88–89, 121–122.

Anticalculus Dentifrice

Beacham, B.E., Kurgansky, D., and Gould, W.M.: Circumoral Dermatitis and Cheilitis Caused by Tartar Control Dentifrices, *J. Am. Acad. Dermatol., 22,* 1029, June, 1990.

Chikte, U.M.E., Rudolph, M.J., and Reinach, S.G.: Anti-calculus Effects of Dentifrice Containing Pyrophosphate Compared with Control, *Clin. Prev. Dent., 14,* 29, July-August, 1992.

Disney, J.A., Graves, R.C., Cancro, L., Payonk, G., and Stewart, P.: An Evaluation of 6 Dentifrice Formulations for Supragingival Anticalculus and Antiplaque Activity, *J. Clin. Periodontol., 16,* 525, September, 1989.

Drake, D.R., Chung, J., Grigsby, W., and Wu-Yuan, C.: Synergistic Effect of Pyrophosphate and Sodium Dodecyl Sulfate on Periodontal Pathogens, *J. Periodontol., 63,* 696, August, 1992.

Edgar, W.M. and Jenkins, G.N.: Inorganic Pyrophosphate in Human Parotid Saliva and Dental Plaque, *Arch. Oral Biol., 17,* 219, January, 1972.

Gaengler, P., Kurbad, A., and Weinert, W.: Evaluation of Anticalculus Efficacy. An SEM Method of Evaluating the Effectiveness of Pyrophosphate Dentifrice on Calculus Formation, *J. Clin. Periodontol., 20,* 144, February, 1993.

Kazmierczak, M., Mather, M., Ciancio, S., Fischman, S., and Cancro, L.: A Clinical Evaluation of Anticalculus Dentifrices, *Clin. Prev. Dent., 12,* 13, April-May, 1990.

Kowitz, G., Jacobson, J., Meng, Z., and Lucatorto, F.: The Effects of Tartar-control Toothpaste on the Oral Soft Tissues, *Oral Surg. Oral Med. Oral Pathol., 70,* 529, October, 1990.

Lobene, R.R.: A Clinical Study of the Anticalculus Effect of a Dentifrice Containing Soluble Pyrophosphate and Sodium Fluoride, *Clin. Prev. Dent., 8,* 5, May-June, 1986.

Lobene, R.R., Soparkar, P.M., Newman, M.B., and Kohut, B.E.: Reduced Formation of Supragingival Calculus with Use of Fluoride-Zinc Chloride Dentifrice, *J. Am. Dent. Assoc., 114,* 350, March, 1987.

Lu, K.H., Yen, D.J.C., Zacherl, W.A., Ruhlman, C.D., Sturzenberger, O.P., and Lehnhoff, R.W.: The Effect of a Fluoride Dentifrice Containing an Anticalculus Agent on Dental Caries in Children, *ASDC J. Dent. Child., 52,* 449, November-December, 1985.

Mallatt, M.E., Beiswanger, B.B., Stookey, G.K., Swancar, J.R., and Hennon, D.K.: Influence of Soluble Pyrophosphate on Calculus Formation in Adults, *J. Dent. Res., 64,* 1159, September, 1985.

Mellberg, J.R., Petrou, I.D., Fletcher, R., and Grote, N.: Evaluation of the Effects of a Pyrophosphate-Fluoride Anticalculus Dentifrice on Remineralization and Fluoride Uptake *in situ, Caries Res., 25,* 65, January-February, 1991.

Petrone, M., Lobene, R.R., Harrison, L.B., Volpe, A., and Petrone, D.M.: Clinical Comparison of the Anticalculus Efficacy of Three Commercially Available Dentifrices, *Clin. Prev. Dent., 13,* 18, July-August, 1991.

Rugg-Gunn, A.J.: A Double-blind Clinical Trial of an Anticalculus Toothpaste Containing Pyrophosphate and Sodium Monofluorophosphate, *Br. Dent. J., 165,* 133, August 20, 1988.

Rustogi, K.N., Volpe, A.R., and Petrone, M.E.: A Clinical Comparison of Two Anticalculus Dentifrices, *Compendium, 9,* 78, January, 1988.

Scruggs, R.R., Stewart, P.W., Samuels, M.S., and Stamm, J.W.: Clinical Evaluation of Seven Anticalculus Dentifrice Formulations, *Clin. Prev. Dent., 13,* 23, January, 1991.

Segreto, V.A., Collins, E.M., D'Agostino, R., Cancro, L.P., Pfeifer, J., and Gilbert, R.J.: Anticalculus Effect of a Dentifrice Containing 0.5% Zinc Citrate Trihydrate, *Community Dent. Oral Epidemiol., 19,* 29, February, 1991.

Stephan, K.W., Saxton, C.A., Jones, C.L., Ritchie, J.A., and Morrison, T.: Control of Gingivitis and Calculus by a Dentifrice Containing a Zinc Salt and Triclosan, *J. Periodontol., 61,* 674, November, 1990.

Zacherl, W.A. and Albrecht, E.B.: Soluble Pyrophosphate as a Calculus Inhibitor, *RDH, 6,* 51, May/June, 1986.

Zacherl, W.A., Pfeiffer, H.J., and Swancar, J.R.: The Effect of Soluble Pyrophosphates on Dental Calculus in Adults, *J. Am. Dent. Assoc., 110,* 737, May, 1985.

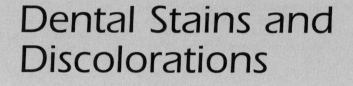

Dental Stains and Discolorations

Discolorations of the teeth and restorations occur in three general ways: (1) stain adheres directly to the surfaces, (2) stain contained within calculus and soft deposits, and (3) stain incorporated within the tooth structure or the restorative material. Instructional and clinical procedures apply to all three. The first two types may be removed by scaling or polishing. Certain stains may be prevented by the patient's routine personal care.

The significance of stains is primarily the appearance or cosmetic effect. In general, any detrimental effect on the teeth or gingival tissues is related to the bacterial plaque or calculus in which the stain occurs. Thick deposits of stain conceivably can provide a rough surface on which bacterial plaque can collect and irritate the adjacent gingiva. Certain stains provide a means of evaluating oral cleanliness and the patient's habits of personal care. Key words that relate to dental stains and discolorations are defined in table 18–1.

I. CLASSIFICATION OF STAINS
A. Classified by Location
1. *Extrinsic.* Extrinsic stains occur on the external surface of the tooth and may be removed by procedures of toothbrushing, scaling, and/or polishing.
2. *Intrinsic.* Intrinsic stains occur within the tooth substance and cannot be removed by techniques of scaling or polishing.

B. Classified by Source
1. *Exogenous.* Exogenous stains develop or originate from sources outside the tooth. Exogenous stains may be extrinsic and stay on the outer surface of the tooth or intrinsic and become incorporated within the tooth structure.

2. *Endogenous.* Endogenous stains develop or originate from within the tooth. Endogenous stains are always intrinsic and usually are discolorations of the dentin reflected through the enamel.

II. RECOGNITION AND IDENTIFICATION
More than one type of stain may occur and more than one etiologic factor may cause the stains of an individual's dentition. A differential diagnosis may be needed.

A. Medical and Dental History
Developmental complications, medications, tobacco, and fluoride histories all contribute necessary information.

Accurately prepared medical and dental histories can provide information to supplement clinical observations.

B. Food Diary
Analysis of a food diary may aid in identifying certain contributing factors.

C. Oral Hygiene Habits
The history of personal plaque removal with the type and frequency of use of toothbrush, floss, and other supplemental materials and devices may help to explain the presence of certain stains. The state of oral hygiene and oral cleanliness is significant to the occurrence of dental stains.

III. APPLICATION OF PROCEDURES FOR STAIN REMOVAL
A. Stains Occurring Directly on the Tooth Surface
1. Stains that are directly associated with the plaque or pellicle on the surface of the en-

TABLE 18–1
KEY WORDS: DENTAL STAINS AND DISCOLORATIONS

Amelogenesis imperfecta (am'ĕ-lo-jen'ĕ-sis im-per fec'tah): imperfect formation of enamel; hereditary condition in which the ameloblasts fail to lay the enamel matrix down properly or at all.

Chlorophyll (klo'rō-fĭl): green plant pigment essential to photosynthesis.

Chromogenic (krō mō-jen'ik): producing color or pigment.

Chronologic (kron ō loj'ic): arranged in order of time.

Dentinogenesis imperfecta (den'tĭ-nō-jen'ĕ-sis): hereditary disorder of dentin formation in which the odontoblasts lay down an abnormal matrix; occurs in both primary and permanent dentitions.

Endogenous (en-doj'ĕ-nus): produced within or caused by factors within.

Exogenous (eks-oj'ĕ-nus): originating outside or caused by factors outside.

Extrinsic (eks-trin'sĭk): derived from or situated on the outside; external.

Hypoplasia (hī'pō-plā'zē-ah): incomplete development or underdevelopment of an organ or a tissue.

Intrinsic (in-trin'sik): situated entirely within.

amel or exposed cementum are removed as much as possible during toothbrushing by the patient. Certain stains can be removed by scaling, whereas others require polishing.

2. When stains are tenacious, excessive polishing should be avoided. As mild an abrasive agent as possible should be used. Precautions should be taken to prevent (1) abrasion of the tooth surface or gingival margin, (2) removal of a layer of fluoride-rich tooth surface, or (3) overheating with a power-driven polisher.

B. Stains Incorporated within Tooth Deposits

When stain is included within the substance of a soft deposit or calculus, it is removed with the deposit.

EXTRINSIC STAINS

The most frequently observed stains, yellow, green, black line, and tobacco, are described first; descriptions of the less common orange, red, and metallic stains follow.

I. YELLOW STAIN
A. Clinical Appearance

Dull, yellowish discoloration of bacterial plaque appears.

B. Distribution on Tooth Surfaces

Yellow stain is associated with presence of bacterial plaque. (Note distribution of bacterial plaque, table 16–3, page 261.)

C. Occurrence

1. Common to all ages.
2. More evident when personal oral care procedures are neglected.

D. Etiology

Usually food pigments.

II. GREEN STAIN
A. Clinical Appearance

1. Light or yellowish green to very dark green.
2. Embedded in bacterial plaque.
3. Occurs in three general forms.
   a. Small curved line following contour of facial gingival crest.
   b. Smeared irregularly, may even cover entire facial surface.
   c. Streaked, following grooves or lines in enamel.
4. The stain is frequently superimposed by soft yellow or gray debris (materia alba and food debris).
5. Dark green occasionally becomes embedded in surface enamel and may be observed as an exogenous intrinsic stain when superficial layers of deposit are removed.
6. Enamel under stain is sometimes demineralized as a result of cariogenic plaque or materia alba. The rough demineralized surface encourages plaque retention, demineralization, and recurrence of green stain.

B. Distribution on Tooth Surfaces

1. Primarily facial; may extend to proximal.
2. Most frequently facial cervical third of maxillary anterior teeth.

C. Composition

1. Chromogenic bacteria and fungi.
2. Decomposed hemoglobin.
3. Inorganic elements include calcium, potassium, sodium, silicon, magnesium, phosphorus, and other elements in small amounts.[1]

D. Occurrence

1. May occur at any age; primarily found in childhood.
2. Collects on both permanent and primary teeth.

E. Recurrence

Recurrence depends on fastidiousness of personal care procedures.

F. Etiology

Green stain results from oral uncleanliness, chromogenic bacteria, and gingival hemorrhage.

1. Chromogenic bacteria or fungi are retained and nourished in bacterial plaque where the green stain is produced.
2. Blood pigments from hemoglobin are decomposed by bacteria.
3. Predisposing factors are the presence of means for retention and proliferation of chromogenic bacteria, such as bacterial plaque, materia alba, and food debris.

G. Clinical Approach

1. Do not scale the area. Often, an area of demineralized tooth structure underlies the stain and soft deposits.
2. Ask the patient to remove the soft deposits during a bacterial plaque control lesson. Initiate a daily fluoride remineralization program.
3. Polish the area gently, preferably with a porte polisher, until the area shows evidence of remineralization.

H. Other Green Stains

In addition to the clinical entity "Green Stain" just described, bacterial plaque and acquired pellicle may become stained by a variety of substances. Differential distinction may be determined by questioning the patient or from items in the medical or dental histories. Green discoloration may result from the following:
1. Chlorophyll preparations.
2. Metallic dusts of industry.
3. Certain drugs. The stain from smoking marijuana may appear grayish green.

III. BLACK LINE STAIN

Black line stain is a highly retentive black or dark brown calculus-like stain that forms along the gingival third near the gingival margin. It may occur on primary or permanent teeth.

A. Other Names

Pigmented dental plaque, brown stain, black stain.

B. Clinical Features

1. Continuous or interrupted fine line, 1-mm wide (average), no appreciable thickness.
2. May be a wider band or even occupy entire gingival third in severe cases (rare).
3. Follows contour of gingival crest about 1 mm above crest.
4. Usually demarcated from gingival crest by clear white line of unstained enamel.
5. Appears black at bases of pits and fissures.
6. Heavy deposits slightly elevated from the tooth surface may be detected with an explorer.
7. Gingiva is firm, with little or no tendency to bleed.
8. Teeth are frequently clean and shiny, with a tendency to lower incidence of dental caries.

C. Distribution on Tooth Surfaces

1. Facial and lingual surfaces: follows contour of gingival crest onto proximal surfaces.
2. Rarely on facial surface of maxillary anterior.
3. Most frequently, lingual and proximal surfaces of maxillary posterior teeth.

D. Composition and Formation[2,3]

1. Black line stain, like calculus, is composed of microorganisms embedded in an intermicrobial substance.
2. The microorganisms are primarily gram-positive rods, with other bacteria, including cocci, in smaller percentages.

   The composition of black line stain is different from the composition of supragingival calculus, in which cocci predominate. Attachment to the tooth of black line stain is by a pellicle-like structure.[4]

   Oral disease does not result from the presence of black line stain. In contrast, gingivitis is related to the formation of supragingival plaque, and in the presence of a cariogenic substrate, dental caries develops.
3. Mineralization in black line stain is similar to the formation of calculus.

E. Occurrence

1. All ages; more common in childhood.
2. More common in female patients.
3. Frequently found in clean mouths.

F. Recurrence

Black line stain tends to form again despite regular personal care, but quantity may be less when plaque control procedures are meticulous.

G. Predisposing Factors

None apparent, except a natural tendency.

IV. TOBACCO STAIN

A. Clinical Appearance

1. Light brown to dark leathery brown or black.
2. Shape
   a. Diffuse staining of bacterial plaque.
   b. Narrow band that follows contour of gingival crest, slightly above the crest.
   c. Wide, firm, tar-like band may cover cervical third and extend to central third of crown.
3. May be incorporated in calculus deposit.
4. Heavy deposits (particularly from smokeless tobacco) may penetrate the enamel and become exogenous intrinsic.

B. Distribution on Tooth Surfaces

1. Cervical third, primarily.
2. Any surface, as well as pits and fissures.
3. Most frequently on lingual surfaces.

C. Composition

1. Tar products of combustion.
2. Brown pigment from smokeless tobacco.

D. Predisposing Factors
1. Natural tendencies. The quantity of stain is not necessarily proportional to the amount of tobacco used.
2. Personal oral care procedures; increased deposits occur with neglect.
3. Extent of bacterial plaque and calculus available for adherence.

V. OTHER BROWN STAINS
A. Brown Pellicle
The acquired pellicle is smooth and structureless and recurs readily after removal.[5] The pellicle can take on stains of various colors that result from chemical alteration of the pellicle.[6]

B. Stannous Fluoride[7,8,9]
Light brown, sometimes yellowish, stain forms on the teeth in the pellicle after repeated use of a stannous fluoride gel or other product, or after having a topical fluoride application. The brown stain results from the formation of stannous sulfide or brown tin oxide from the reaction of the tin ion in the fluoride compound.

C. Foodstuffs
Tea, coffee, and soy sauce are often implicated in the formation of a brownish-stained pellicle. As with other brown pellicle stains, less stain occurs when the personal oral hygiene and plaque control are excellent.

D. Anti-plaque Agents[10,11]
Chlorhexidine and alexidine are used in mouthrinses and are effective against plaque formation (page 367). A brownish stain of the tooth surfaces results, usually more pronounced on proximal and other surfaces less accessible to routine plaque control procedures. The stain also tends to form more rapidly on exposed roots than on enamel. Tooth staining has been considered a significant side effect.

E. Betel Leaf[12]
Betel leaf chewing is common among people of all ages in eastern countries. Betel has a caries-inhibiting effect.

The discoloration imparted to the teeth is a dark mahogany brown, sometimes almost black. It may become thick and hard, with partly smooth and partly rough surfaces.

Microscopically, the black deposit consists of microorganisms and mineralized material with a laminated pattern characteristic of subgingival calculus. It should be removed by scaling.

VI. ORANGE AND RED STAINS
A. Clinical Appearance
Orange or red stains appear at the cervical third.

B. Distribution on Tooth Surfaces
1. More frequently on anterior than on posterior teeth.
2. Both facial and lingual surfaces of anterior teeth.

C. Occurrence
Rare (red more rare than orange).

D. Etiology
Chromogenic bacteria.

VII. METALLIC STAINS
A. Metals or Metallic Salts from Metal-containing Dust of Industry
1. *Clinical Appearance.* Examples of colors on teeth:
   a. Copper or brass: green or bluish-green.
   b. Iron: brown to greenish-brown.
   c. Nickel: green.
   d. Cadmium: yellow or golden brown.
2. *Distribution on Tooth Surfaces*
   a. Primarily anterior; may occur on any teeth.
   b. Cervical third more commonly.
3. *Manner of Formation*
   a. Industrial worker inhales dust through mouth, bringing metallic substance in contact with teeth.
   b. Metal imparts color to bacterial plaque.
   c. Occasionally, stain may penetrate tooth substance and become exogenous intrinsic stain.

B. Metallic Substances Contained in Drugs
1. *Clinical Appearance.* Examples of colors on teeth:
   a. Iron. Black (iron sulfide) or brown.
   b. Manganese (from potassium permanganate). Black.
2. *Distribution on Tooth Surfaces.* General, may occur on all.
3. *Manner of Formation*
   a. Drug enters plaque substance, imparts color to plaque and calculus.
   b. Pigment from drug may attach directly to tooth substance.
4. *Prevention.* Use a medication through a straw or in tablet or capsule form to prevent direct contact with the teeth.

ENDOGENOUS INTRINSIC STAINS

Stains incorporated within the tooth structure may be related to the period of tooth development or may be acquired after eruption. Occasionally, a patient, desiring an improvement in the appearance of the anterior teeth, may request removal of a discoloration. The dentist may employ one of two alternatives in the treatment of these teeth. Improvement in tooth color can be produced by bleaching in certain instances. In other cases, a cosmetic dentistry procedure is indicated to cover the discoloration.

I. PULPLESS TEETH

Not all pulpless teeth discolor. Improved endodontic procedures have contributed to the prevention of many discolorations formerly associated with that cause.

A. Clinical Appearance

A wide range of colors exists; stains may be light yellow-brown, slate gray, reddish-brown, dark brown, bluish-black, or black. Others have an orange or greenish tinge.

B. Manner of Formation

1. Blood and other pulp tissue elements may be made available for breakdown as a result of hemorrhages in the pulp chamber, root canal operations, or necrosis and decomposition of the pulp tissue.
2. Pigments from the decomposed hemoglobin and pulp tissue penetrate the dentinal tubules.

II. TETRACYCLINES

A. Tetracycline antibiotics, used widely for combatting many types of infections, have an affinity for mineralized tissues and are absorbed by the bones and teeth. They can be transferred through the placenta and enter fetal circulation.

B. Discoloration of the teeth of a child can result when the drug is administered to the mother during the third trimester of pregnancy or to the child in infancy and early childhood.

C. Color of teeth may be light green to dark yellow, or a gray-brown. The discoloration depends on the dosage, length of time the drug was used, and the type of tetracycline. After eruption, the teeth may fluoresce under ultraviolet light, but that property is lost with age and exposure.[14,15]

D. Discoloration may be generalized or limited to specific parts of individual teeth that were developing at the time of administration of the antibiotic. Reference to the Table of Tooth Development can assist in determining the patient's age at the time the drug was administered, and the patient's medical history at that age may reveal the illness for which the antibiotic was prescribed (tables 14–2 and 14–3, page 233).

III. IMPERFECT TOOTH DEVELOPMENT

Defective tooth development may result from factors of genetic abnormality or environmental influences during tooth development.

A. Hereditary: Genetic[14,15]

1. *Amelogenesis Imperfecta.* The enamel is partially or completely missing because of a generalized disturbance of the ameloblasts. Teeth are yellowish-brown or gray-brown.
2. *Dentinogenesis Imperfecta ("Opalescent Dentin").* The dentin is abnormal as a result of disturbances in the odontoblastic layer during development. The teeth appear translucent or opalescent, and vary in color from gray to bluish-brown.

B. Enamel Hypoplasia

1. *Systemic Hypoplasia* (chronologic hypoplasia resulting from ameloblastic disturbance of short duration). Teeth erupt with white spots or with pits. Over a long period of time, the white spots may become discolored from food pigments or other substances taken into the mouth. Figure 14–4 (page 237) shows an example of chronologic hypoplasia.
2. *Local Hypoplasia* (affects single tooth). White spots may become stained as in systemic hypoplasia.

C. Dental Fluorosis

Dental fluorosis was originally called "brown stain." Later, Dr. Frederick S. McKay, who studied the condition and described it in the dental literature, named it "mottled enamel" (pages 438 and 439).

1. *Manner of Formation*
   a. Enamel hypomineralization results from ingestion of excessive fluoride ion in drinking water (more than 2 parts per million) during the period of mineralization. The enamel alterations are a result of toxic damage to the ameloblasts.
   b. When the teeth erupt, they have white spots or areas that later become discolored from oral pigments and appear light or dark brown.
   c. Severe effects of excess fluoride during development may produce cracks or pitting; the discoloration concentrates in these. This condition and appearance led to the name mottled enamel.

2. *Classification*
   Dean provided the original definitions for five grades of fluorosis. They ranged from "questionable" (a few white flecks or spots) to "severe" (marked brown staining and pitting of the enamel surfaces).[16]

   More specific classifications have been developed for clinical and research purposes.[17,18] The Tooth Surface Index of Fluorosis (TSIF) is shown in table 29–2, page 440.

IV. OTHER SYSTEMIC CAUSES

Several types of tooth discolorations may result from blood-borne pigments.

Pigments circulating in the blood are transmitted to the dentin from the capillaries of the pulp. For example, prolonged jaundice early in life can impart a yellow or greenish discoloration to the teeth.

Erythroblastosis fetalis (Rh incompatibility) may leave a green, brown, or blue hue to the teeth.

EXOGENOUS INTRINSIC STAINS

When intrinsic stains come from an outside source, not from within the tooth, the stain is called exogenous intrinsic. Extrinsic stains, such as tobacco and green stains, can provide stain that becomes intrinsic.

Restorative materials cause staining of teeth, as described in the section that follows. Tooth-color restorations may become stained from the various extrinsic-staining substances mentioned in this chapter. A few references are included in the *Suggested Readings* at the end of the chapter.

I. RESTORATIVE MATERIALS
A. Silver Amalgam
1. Silver amalgam can impart a gray to black discoloration to the tooth structure around a restoration.
2. Metallic ions migrate from the amalgam restoration into the enamel and dentin.
3. Silver, tin, and mercury ions eventually contact debris at the junction of the tooth and the restoration and form sulfides, which are products of corrosion.

B. Copper Amalgam
Copper amalgam used for filling primary teeth may impart a bluish-green color.

II. ENDODONTIC THERAPY AND RESTORATIVE MATERIALS
A. Silver nitrate: bluish-black.
B. Volatile oils: yellowish-brown.
C. Strong iodine: brown.
D. Aureomycin: yellow.
E. Silver-containing root canal sealer: black.

III. DRUGS
A. Stannous Fluoride Topical Application[7]
1. Light to dark brown staining from the formation of tin sulfide.
2. Located most frequently in occlusal pits and grooves of posterior teeth and cervical third facial surfaces of anterior teeth; in carious and precarious lesions; and in margins of tooth color and amalgam restorations.
3. Staining may accompany dental caries arrestment.

B. Ammoniacal Silver Nitrate
Used in treatment of such sensitive areas as exposed cementum or for inhibition of demineralization in dental caries prevention; imparts a dark brown to black discoloration.

IV. STAIN IN DENTIN
Discoloration resulting from a carious lesion is an example.

TECHNICAL HINTS

I. Record color, type, extent, and location of stains with the patient's examination and assessment.
II. Make additions to the dental history as information is gained concerning the origin of stains such as those related to tooth development, systemic disease, occupations, or medications.
III. Avoid making patient feel self-conscious by overemphasizing the appearance of stains, particularly those that may occur in spite of conscientious bacterial plaque removal habits.
IV. Use tact when questioning patients with brown stain, because nonsmokers do not appreciate having an assumption made concerning the cause of a brown stain on the teeth.

FACTORS TO TEACH THE PATIENT

I. Predisposing factors that contribute to stain accumulation.
II. Personal care procedures that can aid in the prevention or reduction of stains.
III. Reasons for not using an abrasive dentifrice with vigorous brushing strokes to lessen or remove stain accumulation.
IV. The need to avoid tobacco, coffee, tea, and other beverages or foodstuffs that can stain, to prevent discoloration of new restorations.
V. Reasons for the difficulty of removing certain extrinsic stains during scaling and polishing.
VI. Effect of tetracyclines on developing teeth. Need to avoid use during pregnancy and by children to age 12.

REFERENCES

1. **Shay,** D.E., Haddox, J.H., and Richmond, J.L.: An Inorganic Qualitative and Quantitative Analysis of Green Stain, *J. Am. Dent. Assoc., 50,* 156, February, 1955.
2. **Theilade,** J., Slots, J., and Fejerskov, O.: The Ultrastructure of Black Stain on Human Primary Teeth, *Scand. J. Dent. Res., 81,* 528, No. 7, 1973.
3. **Slots,** J.: The Microflora of Black Stain on Human Primary Teeth, *Scand. J. Dent. Res., 82,* 484, No. 7, 1974.

4. **Theilade,** J.: Development of Bacterial Plaque in the Oral Cavity, *J. Clin. Periodontol., 4,* 1, December, 1977.

5. **Meckel,** A.H.: The Formation and Properties of Organic Films on Teeth, *Arch. Oral Biol., 10,* 585, July-August, 1965.

6. **Eriksen,** H.M. and Nordbø, H.: Extrinsic Discoloration of Teeth, *J. Clin. Periodontol., 5,* 229, November, 1978.

7. **Horowitz,** H.S. and Chamberlin, S.R.: Pigmentation of Teeth Following Topical Applications of Stannous Fluoride in a Non-fluoridated Area, *J. Public Health Dent., 31,* 32, Winter, 1971.

8. **Shannon,** I.L.: Stannous Fluoride: Does It Stain Teeth? How Does It React with Tooth Surfaces? A Review, *Gen. Dent., 26,* 64, September-October, 1978.

9. **Leverett,** D.H., McHugh, W.D., and Jensen, Ø.E.: Dental Caries and Staining After Twenty-eight Months of Rinsing with Stannous Fluoride or Sodium Fluoride, *J. Dent. Res., 65,* 424, March, 1986.

10. **Flötra,** L., Gjermo, P., Rölla, G., and Waerhaug, J.: Side Effects of Chlorhexidine Mouthwashes, *Scand. J. Dent. Res., 79,* 119, April, 1971.

11. **Formicola,** A.J., Deasy, M.J., Johnson, D.H., and Howe, E.E.: Tooth Staining Effects of an Alexidine Mouthwash, *J. Periodontol., 50,* 207, April, 1979.

12. **Reichart,** P.A., Lenz, H., König, H., Becker, J., and Mohr, U.: The Black Layer on the Teeth of Betel Chewers: A Light Microscopic, Microradiographic, and Electronmicroscopic Study, *J. Oral Pathol., 14,* 466, July, 1985.

13. **Ehrlich,** A. and Torres, H.O.: *Essentials of Dental Assisting.* Philadelphia, W.B. Saunders Co., 1992, pp. 389–393.

14. **Robinson,** H.B.G. and Miller, A.S.: *Color Atlas of Oral Pathology,* 5th ed. Philadelphia, J.B. Lippincott Co., 1990, pp. 41–47, 55.

15. **Haring,** J.I. and Ibsen, O.A.C.: Developmental Disorders, in Ibsen, O.A.C. and Phelan, J.A.: *Oral Pathology for the Dental Hygienist.* Philadelphia, W.B. Saunders Co., 1992, pp. 267–271, 395–399.

16. **Dean,** H.T.: Investigation of Physiological Effects by Epidemiological Method, in Moulton, F.R., ed.: *Fluorine and Dental Health.* Washington, D.C., American Association for the Advancement of Science, No. 19, 1942.

17. **Thylstrup,** A. and Fejerskov, O.: Clinical Appearance of Dental Fluorosis in Permanent Teeth in Relation to Histologic Changes, *Community Dent. Oral Epidemiol., 6,* 315, December, 1978.

18. **Horowitz,** H.S., Driscoll, W.S., Meyers, R.J., Heifetz, S.B., and Kingman, A.: A New Method for Assessing the Prevalence of Dental Fluorosis—the Tooth Surface Index of Fluorosis, *J. Am. Dent. Assoc., 109,* 37, July 1984.

SUGGESTED READINGS

Barta, J.E., King, D.L., and Jorgensen, R.L.: ABO Blood Group Incompatibility and Primary Tooth Discoloration, *Pediatr. Dent., 11,* 316, December, 1989.

Cohen, B.D. and Abrams, B.L.: An Unusual Case of Stained Roots of Unerupted Third Molars, *Gen. Dent., 37,* 342, July-August, 1989.

Cuff, M.J.A., McQuade, M.J., Scheidt, M.J., Sutherland, D.E., and Van Dyke, T.E.: The Presence of Nicotine on Root Surfaces of Peri-odontally Diseased Teeth in Smokers, *J. Periodontol., 60,* 564, October, 1989.

Massler, M. and Schour, I.: *Atlas of the Mouth.* Chicago, American Dental Association, Plate 12.

Tilliss, T.: Dental Stains and Chemotherapeutics: A Closer Look, *Dentalhygienistnews, 2,* 12, January/February/March, 1989.

Walsh, T.F., Figures, K.H., and Lamb, D.J.: *Clinical Dental Hygiene. A Handbook for the Dental Team.* Oxford, England, Wright, 1992, pp. 59–60.

Chlorhexidine and Antibiotics

Addy, M., Moran, J., Davies, R.M., Beak, A., and Lewis, A.: The Effect of Single Morning and Evening Rinses of Chlorhexidine on the Development of Tooth Staining and Plaque Accumulation. A Blind Cross-over Trial, *J. Clin. Periodontol., 9,* 134, March, 1982.

Addy, M., Moran, J., Griffiths, A.A., and Wills-Wood, N.J.: Extrinsic Tooth Discoloration by Metals and Chlorhexidine. I. Surface Protein Denaturation or Dietary Precipitation?, *Br. Dent. J., 159,* 281, November 9, 1985.

Addy, M. and Moran, J.: Extrinsic Tooth Discoloration by Metals and Chlorhexidine. II. Clinical Staining Produced by Chlorhexidine, Iron and Tea, *Br. Dent. J., 159,* 331, November 23, 1985.

Addy, M., Al-Arrayed, F., and Moran, J.: The Use of an Oxidising Mouthwash to Reduce Staining Associated with Chlorhexidine. Studies *in vitro* and *in vivo, J. Clin. Periodontol., 18,* 267, April, 1991.

Addy, M., Wade, W.G., Jenkins, S., and Goodfield, S.: Comparison of Two Commercially Available Chlorhexidine Mouthrinses: I. Staining and Antimicrobial Effects *in vitro, Clin. Prev. Dent., 11,* 10, September-October, 1989.

Beiswanger, B.B., Mallatt, M.E., Mau, M.S., Jackson, R.D., and Hennon, D.K.: The Clinical Effects of a Mouthrinse Containing 0.1% Octenidine, *J. Dent. Res., 69,* 454, February, 1990.

Berger, R.S., Mandel, E.B., Hayes, T.J., and Grimwood, R.R.: Minocycline Staining of the Oral Cavity, *J. Am. Acad. Dermatol., 21,* 1300, December, 1989.

Jenkins, S., Addy, M., and Newcombe, R.: Comparison of Two Commercially Available Chlorhexidine Mouthrinses: II. Effects on Plaque Reformation, Gingivitis, and Tooth Staining, *Clin. Prev. Dent., 11,* 12, November-December, 1989.

Parkins, F.M., Furnish, G., and Bernstein, M.: Minocycline Use Discolors Teeth, *J. Am. Dent. Assoc., 123,* 87, October, 1992.

Poliak, S.G., DiGiovanna, J.J., Gross, E.G., Gantt, G., and Peck, G.L.: Minocycline-associated Tooth Discoloration in Young Adults, *JAMA, 254,* 2930, November 22/29, 1985.

Discoloration of Restorations

Chan, K.C., Fuller, J.L., and Hormati, A.A.: The Ability of Foods to Stain Two Composite Resins, *J. Prosthet. Dent., 43,* 542, May, 1980.

Kidd, E.A.M.: The Caries Status of Tooth-coloured Restorations with Marginal Stain, *Br. Dent. J., 171,* 241, October 19, 1991.

Luce, M.S. and Campbell, C.E.: Stain Potential of Four Microfilled Composites, *J. Prosthet. Dent., 60,* 151, August, 1988.

Nordbö, H., Attramadal, A., and Eriksen, H.M.: Iron Discoloration of Acrylic Resin Exposed to Chlorhexidine or Tannic Acid: A Model Study, *J. Prosthet. Dent., 49,* 126, January, 1983.

Um, C.M. and Ruyter, I.E.: Staining of Resin-based Veneering Materials with Coffee and Tea, *Quintessence Int., 22,* 377, May, 1981.

Indices and Scoring Methods

Indices and scoring methods are used in clinical practice and community programs to determine and record the state of health of individuals and groups. Several indices and scoring methods are described in this chapter. Those included have been selected because they are well known and widely used in the assessment of oral health status. The *Suggested Readings* at the end of the chapter contain references to other indices. Table 19–1 defines related terminology.

Familiarity with the various types of indices may prove helpful when different evaluation criteria are needed. A distinction must be made between an individual oral health assessment score, a clinical trial, and a community health epidemiologic survey.

I. INDIVIDUAL ASSESSMENT SCORE
A. Purpose
In clinical practice, an index, plaque record, or scoring system for an individual patient can be used for education, motivation, and evaluation. The effects of personal disease control efforts, the progress of healing between professional treatments, and the maintenance of health over time can be monitored. An example is the plaque-free score described on pages 293–295 in which a patient is able to measure the effects of personal daily care efforts by the changes in the scores. This system may prove to be a valuable motivating device.

B. Uses
1. Provides individual assessment to help a patient recognize an oral problem.
2. Reveals the degree of effectiveness of present oral hygiene practices.
3. Motivates the person in preventive and professional care for the elimination and control of oral disease.
4. Evaluates the success of individual and professional treatment over a period of time by comparing index scores.

II. CLINICAL TRIAL
A. Purpose
A clinical trial is planned for the determination of the effect of an agent or procedure on the prevention, progression, or control of a disease. The trial is conducted by comparing an experimental group with a control group that is similar to the experimental group in every way except for the variable being studied.

Examples of indices used for clinical trials are the Plaque Index (Pl I) of Silness and Löe[1] and the Patient Hygiene Performance (PHP) of Podshadley and Haley.[2] These and other indices are described in this chapter.

B. Uses
1. Determines baseline data before experimental factors are introduced.
2. Measures the effectiveness of specific agents for the prevention, control, or treatment of oral conditions.
3. Measures the effectiveness of mechanical devices for personal care, such as toothbrushes, interdental cleaning devices, or irrigators.

III. EPIDEMIOLOGIC SURVEY
A. Purpose
The word epidemiology denotes the study of disease characteristics of populations. An example of an index designed for a survey of popula-

TABLE 19–1
KEY WORDS: INDICES AND SCORING METHODS

Calibration (kal'ĭ-brā'shun): determination of accuracy and consistency between examiners to standardize procedures and gain reliability of recorded findings; instrument calibration is defined in table 13–1.

Epidemiology (ep'ĭ-dē'mē-ol'ō-jē): the study of the relationships of various factors that determine the frequency and distribution of diseases in the human community; study of health and disease in populations.

Incidence (in'sĭ-dens): the rate at which a certain event occurs, as the number of new cases of a specific disease occurring during a certain period of time.

Index (in'deks): a graduated, numeric scale with upper and lower limits; scores on the scale correspond to a specific criterion for individuals or populations; *pl.* indices (in'dĭ ces) or indexes (in dek'sēs).

Pilot study: a trial run of a planned study using a small sample to pretest an instrument, survey, or questionnaire.

Placebo (plah-sē'bō): an inactive substance or preparation with no intrinsic therapeutic value given to satisfy a patient's symbolic need for drug therapy; used in controlled research studies in a form identical in appearance to the material being tested.

Prevalence (prev'ah-lens): the total number of cases of a specific disease or condition in existence in a given population at a certain time.

Reliability: ability of an index or test procedure to measure consistently at different times and under a variety of conditions; reproducibility; consistency.

Screening of a *population:* assessment of many individuals to disclose certain characteristics or a certain disease entity; *individual* screening: brief assessment for initial evaluation and classification of needs for additional examination and treatment planning.

Validity: ability of an index or test procedure to measure what it is intended to measure.

tion groups is the DMFT (Decayed, Missing, and Filled Teeth) Index.[3] It has been used with populations around the world to determine the extent of dental caries. Such a survey was not designed for evaluation of an individual patient.

B. Uses

1. Shows the prevalence and incidence of a particular condition occurring within a given population.
2. Provides baseline data to show existing dental health practices.
3. Assesses the needs of a community.
4. Compares the effects of a community program and evaluates the results.

IV. INDEX

An index is an expression of clinical observations in numeric values. It is used to describe the status of the individual or group with respect to a condition being

measured. The use of a numeric scale and a standardized method for interpreting observations of a condition results in an index score that is more consistent and less subjective than a word description of that condition.

A. Descriptive Categories of Indices

1. *General Categories*
   a. Simple index. One that measures the presence or absence of a condition. An example is an index that measures the presence of bacterial plaque without evaluating its effect on the gingiva.
   b. Cumulative index. One that measures all the evidence of a condition, past and present. An example is the DMFT Index for dental caries.
2. *Types of Simple and Cumulative Indices*
   a. Irreversible. One that measures conditions that will not change. An example is an index that measures dental caries.
   b. Reversible. One that measures conditions that can be changed. Examples are indices that measure bacterial plaque.

B. Selection Criteria

A useful and effective index

1. Is simple to use and calculate.
2. Requires minimal equipment and expense.
3. Uses a minimal amount of time to complete.
4. Does not cause patient discomfort nor is otherwise unacceptable to a patient.
5. Has clear-cut criteria that are readily understandable.
6. Is as free as possible from subjective interpretation.
7. Is reproducible by the same examiner or different examiners.
8. Is amenable to statistical analysis; has validity and reliability.

V. SYSTEMS DESCRIBED IN THIS CHAPTER

A. Screening for Periodontal Health (PSR) (page 289)

B. Bacterial Plaque

1. Plaque Index (Pl I) (page 291).
2. Plaque Control Record (page 292).
3. Plaque-free Score (page 293).

C. Plaque, Debris, Calculus

1. Patient Hygiene Performance (PHP) (page 295).
2. Oral Hygiene Index (OHI) (page 296).
3. Simplified Oral Hygiene Index (OHI-S) (page 298).

D. Gingival Bleeding

1. Sulcus Bleeding Index (SBI) (page 300).
2. Gingival Bleeding Index (GBI) (page 300).

E. Gingival Changes/Gingivitis
1. Papillary-Marginal-Attached Index (P-M-A) (page 301).
2. Gingival Index (GI) (page 302).

F. Periodontal Diseases
1. Periodontal Index (PI) (page 303).
2. Periodontal Disease Index (PDI) (page 304).
3. Community Periodontal Index of Treatment Needs (CPITN) (page 307).

G. Dental Caries
1. Decayed, Missing, and Filled Permanent Teeth (DMFT) (page 309).
2. Decayed, Missing, and Filled Permanent Tooth Surfaces (DMFS) (page 310).
3. Primary teeth indices (page 310).

PERIODONTAL SCREENING & RECORDING (PSR)
(American Academy of Periodontology and American Dental Association[4])

I. PURPOSE
To assess the state of periodontal health in a rapid and effective manner and to motivate the patient to seek necessary complete periodontal assessment and treatment.

II. SELECTION OF TEETH
The dentition is divided into sextants. Each tooth is examined. Posterior sextants begin distal to the canines.

III. PROCEDURE
A. Instrument
Specially designed probe used by World Health Organization for the CPITN (page 307).
1. *Markings.* At intervals from tip: 3.5, 2.0, 3.0, and 3.0 mm (total 11.5 mm) (figure 19–1).
2. *Working Tip.* A ball 0.5 mm in diameter. The functions of the ball are
   a. To aid in the detection of calculus, rough overhanging margins of restorations, and other tooth surface irregularities.
   b. To facilitate assessment at the probing depth and reduce risk of overmeasurement.
3. *Color Coding.* Color-coded between 3.5 and 5.5 mm.

B. Probe Application
1. Insert probe gently into a sulcus until resistance is felt.
2. Apply a circumferential walking step to probe systematically about each tooth through each sextant.
3. Observe color-coded area of the probe for prompt identification of probing depths.

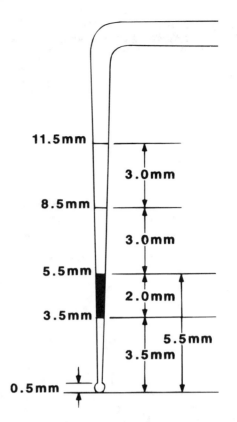

FIG. 19–1. Periodontal Probe. The probe, with markings as shown, is used to make determinations for the PSR and the Community Periodontal Index of Treatment Needs (CPITN). (From FDI: A Simplified Periodontal Examination for Dental Practices. Fédération Dentaire Internationale, 64 Wimpole Street, London W1M 8AL.)

4. Remember that each sextant receives one code number corresponding to the deepest position of the color-coded portion of the probe.

C. Criteria
1. Five codes and an asterisk are used. Table 19–2 shows the clinical findings, code significance, and patient management guidelines.
2. Each code may include conditions identified with the preceding codes; for example, Code 3 with probing depth from 3.5 to 5.5 mm also may include calculus, an overhanging restoration, and bleeding on probing.
3. One need not probe the remaining teeth in a sextant when a Code 4 is found. For Codes 0, 1, 2, and 3, the sextant is completely probed.

D. Recording
1. Use a simple six-box form to provide a space for each sextant. The form can be made into peel-off stickers or a rubber stamp to facilitate recording in the patient's permanent record.

TABLE 19–2
PERIODONTAL SCREENING AND RECORDING(PSR) *

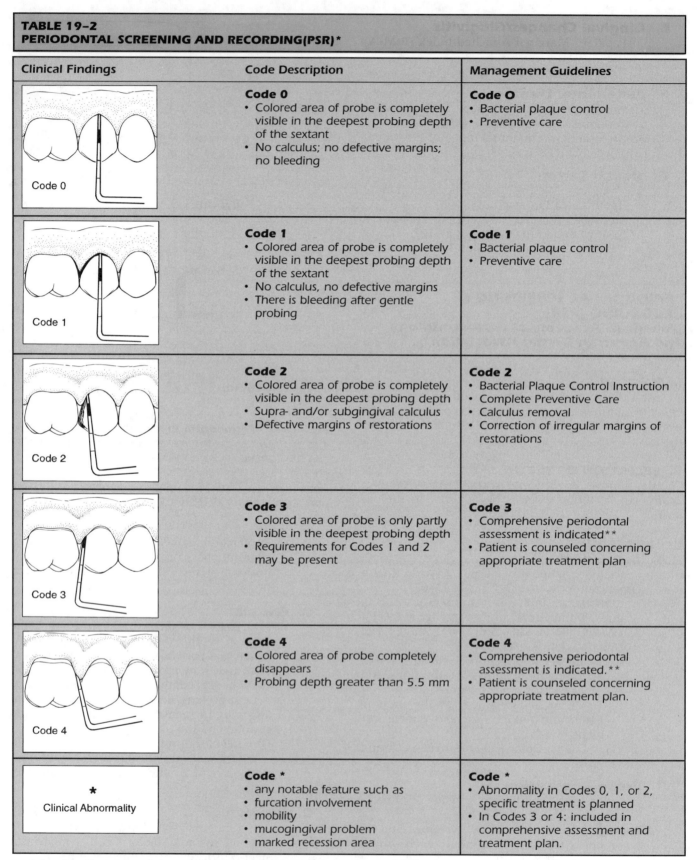

Clinical Findings	Code Description	Management Guidelines
Code 0	**Code 0** • Colored area of probe is completely visible in the deepest probing depth of the sextant • No calculus; no defective margins; no bleeding	**Code O** • Bacterial plaque control • Preventive care
Code 1	**Code 1** • Colored area of probe is completely visible in the deepest probing depth of the sextant • No calculus, no defective margins • There is bleeding after gentle probing	**Code 1** • Bacterial plaque control • Preventive care
Code 2	**Code 2** • Colored area of probe is completely visible in the deepest probing depth • Supra- and/or subgingival calculus • Defective margins of restorations	**Code 2** • Bacterial Plaque Control Instruction • Complete Preventive Care • Calculus removal • Correction of irregular margins of restorations
Code 3	**Code 3** • Colored area of probe is only partly visible in the deepest probing depth • Requirements for Codes 1 and 2 may be present	**Code 3** • Comprehensive periodontal assessment is indicated** • Patient is counseled concerning appropriate treatment plan
Code 4	**Code 4** • Colored area of probe completely disappears • Probing depth greater than 5.5 mm	**Code 4** • Comprehensive periodontal assessment is indicated.** • Patient is counseled concerning appropriate treatment plan.
* Clinical Abnormality	**Code *** • any notable feature such as • furcation involvement • mobility • mucogingival problem • marked recession area	**Code *** • Abnormality in Codes 0, 1, or 2, specific treatment is planned • In Codes 3 or 4: included in comprehensive assessment and treatment plan.

* American Dental Association and American Academy of Periodontology. 1992
** Comprehensive periodontal assessment includes but is not limited to radiographic and clinical examination (complete soft tissue record, identification of probing depths, mobility, gingival recession, mucogingival problems, and furcation involvements).

2. One score is marked for each sextant; the highest code observed is recorded. When indicated, an asterisk is added to the score in the individual space with the sextant code number.

IV. SCORING

A. Follow-up Patient Management
Patients are classified into assessment and treatment planning needs by the highest coded score of their PSR (table 19–2, right column).

B. Calculation Examples
Example 1.

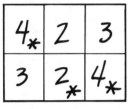

PSR Sextant Score

Interpretation: With Codes 3 and 4, a comprehensive periodontal examination is indicated. Asterisks mean furcation involvement in two quadrants, and a possible mucogingival involvement in the mandibular anterior sextant. When the patient has not been aware of the presence of periodontal involvement, counseling is important if cooperation and compliance are to be obtained.

Example 2.

PSR Sextant Score

Interpretation: An overall Code 2 can indicate calculus and overhanging restorations that must be removed. All restorations must be checked for recurrent dental caries. Appointments for instruction in bacterial plaque control are of primary concern. The asterisks in two quadrants may indicate minimal attached gingiva.

PLAQUE INDEX (Pl I)
(Silness and Löe[1,5])

I. PURPOSE
To assess the thickness of plaque at the gingival area.

II. SELECTION OF TEETH
The entire dentition or selected teeth can be evaluated.

A. Areas Examined
Examine four gingival areas (distal, facial, mesial, lingual) systematically for each tooth.

B. Modified Procedures
Examine only the facial, mesial, and lingual areas. Assign double score to the mesial reading, and divide the total by 4.

III. PROCEDURE

A. Dry the teeth and examine visually using adequate light, mouth mirror, and probe or explorer.

B. Evaluate bacterial plaque on the cervical third; pay no attention to plaque that has extended to the middle or incisal thirds.

C. Use probe to test the surface when no plaque is visible. Pass the probe or explorer across the tooth surface in the cervical third and near the entrance to the sulcus. When no plaque adheres to the probe tip, the area is scored 0. When plaque adheres, a score of 1 is assigned.

D. Use a disclosing agent, if necessary, to assist evaluation for the 0 to 1 scores. When the Pl I is used in conjunction with the Gingival Index (GI, page 302), the GI must be completed first because the disclosing agent masks the gingival characteristics.

E. Include plaque on the surface of calculus and on dental restorations in the cervical third in the evaluation.

F. Criteria

0 = No plaque.

1 = A film of plaque adhering to the free gingival margin and adjacent area of the tooth. The plaque may be recognized only after application of disclosing agent or by running the explorer across the tooth surface.

2 = Moderate accumulation of soft deposits within the gingival pocket that can be seen with the naked eye or on the tooth and gingival margin.

3 = Abundance of soft matter within the gingival pocket and/or on the tooth and gingival margin.

IV. SCORING

A. Pl I for Area
Each area (distal, facial, mesial, lingual or palatal) is assigned a score from 0 to 3.

B. Pl I for a Tooth
Scores for each area are totalled and divided by 4.

C. Pl I for Groups of Teeth
Scores for individual teeth may be grouped and totalled and divided by the number of teeth. For instance, a Pl I may be determined for specific

teeth or groups of teeth. The right side may be compared with the left.

D. Pl I for the Individual

Add the scores for each tooth and divide by the number of teeth examined. The Pl I ranges from 0 to 3.

E. Suggested Nominal Scale for Patient Reference

Rating	Scores
Excellent	0
Good	0.1–0.9
Fair	1.0–1.9
Poor	2.0–3.0

F. Pl I for a Group

Add the scores for each member of a group and divide by the number of individuals.

PLAQUE CONTROL RECORD
(O'Leary, Drake, and Naylor[6])

I. PURPOSE

To record the presence of bacterial plaque on individual tooth surfaces to permit the patient to visualize progress while learning plaque control.

II. SELECTION OF TEETH AND SURFACES

A. All teeth are included. Missing teeth are identified on the record form by a single thick horizontal line.

B. Four surfaces are recorded: facial, lingual, mesial, and distal.

C. Six areas may be recorded. The mesial and distal segments of the diagram may be divided to provide space to record proximal surfaces from the facial separately from the lingual or palatal surfaces (figure 19–2).[7]

III. PROCEDURE

A. Apply disclosing agent or give a chewable tablet. Instruct patient to swish and rub the solution over the tooth surfaces with the tongue before rinsing.

B. Examine each tooth surface for bacterial plaque at the gingival margin. No attempt is made to differentiate quantity of plaque.

C. Record by making a dash or coloring in the appropriate spaces on the diagram (figure 19–2) to indicate plaque on facial, lingual, palatal, mesial, and/or distal surfaces.

IV. SCORING

A. Total the number of teeth present; multiply by 4 (or 6 if modification is used) to obtain the

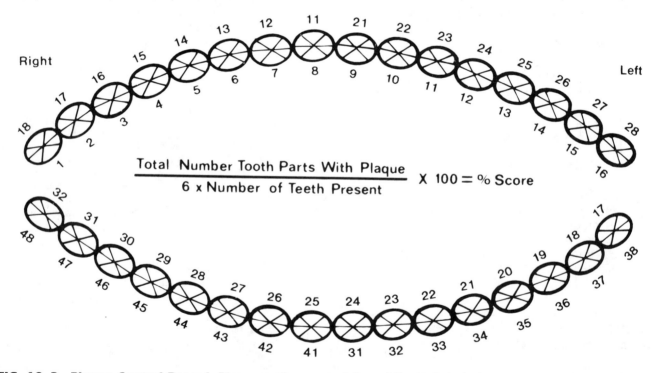

$$\frac{\text{Total Number Tooth Parts With Plaque}}{6 \times \text{Number of Teeth Present}} \times 100 = \% \text{ Score}$$

FIG. 19–2. Plaque Control Record. Diagrammatic representation of the teeth includes spaces to record plaque on six areas of each tooth. The facial surfaces are on the outer and the lingual and palatal surfaces on the inner portion of the arches. Teeth are numbered by the ADA System on the inside and by the FDI System on the outside. (Modified from Ramfjord, S.P. and Ash, M.M.: *Periodontology and Periodontics.* Philadelphia, W.B. Saunders Co., 1979, p. 273; and from O'Leary, T.J., Drake, R.B., and Naylor, J.E.: *J. Periodontol., 43,* 38, 1972.)

number of available surfaces. Count the number of surfaces with plaque.

B. Multiply the number of plaque-stained surfaces by 100 and divide by the total number of available surfaces to derive the percent of surfaces.

C. Compare over subsequent appointments as the patient learns and practices plaque control. Ten percent or fewer plaque-stained surfaces can be considered a good goal, but if the plaque is regularly left in the same areas, special instruction is indicated to prevent pocket formation.

D. Calculation example for plaque control record:

Individual findings: 26 teeth scored
8 surfaces with plaque

1. Multiply the number of teeth by 4:

$$26 \times 4 = 104 \text{ surfaces}$$

2. Percent with plaque =

$$\frac{\text{Number of surfaces with plaque} \times 100}{\text{Number of available tooth surfaces}}$$

$$= \frac{8 \times 100}{104} = \frac{800}{104} = 7.6$$

Interpretation: Although 0% is ideal, fewer than 10% plaque-stained surfaces has been suggested as a guideline in periodontal therapy. After initial therapy and when the patient has reached a 10% level of plaque control or better, necessary additional periodontal and restorative procedures may be initiated.[6] In comparison, a similar evaluation using a plaque-free score would mean that a goal of 90% or better plaque-free surfaces would have to be reached before the surgical phase of treatment could be undertaken.

PLAQUE-FREE SCORE
(Grant, Stern, Everett[8])

I. PURPOSE

To determine the location, number, and percent of plaque-free surfaces for individual motivation and instruction. Interdental bleeding can also be documented.

II. SELECTION OF TEETH AND SURFACES

A. All erupted teeth are included. Missing teeth are identified on the record form by a single thick horizontal line through the box in the chart form.

B. Four surfaces are recorded for each tooth: facial, lingual or palatal, mesial, and distal.

III. PROCEDURE
A. Plaque-free Score

1. Apply disclosing agent or give chewable tablet. Instruct patient to swish and rub the solution over the tooth surfaces with the tongue before rinsing.

2. Examine each tooth surface for evidence of plaque. Use adequate light and a mouth mirror for visualizing all surfaces. The patient needs a hand mirror to see the location of the plaque that has been missed during personal hygiene procedures.

3. Record in red the surfaces showing plaque. Use an appropriate tooth chart form or a diagrammatic form, such as that shown in figure 19–3. Red ink for recording the plaque is suggested when a red disclosing agent is used to help the patient associate the location of the plaque in the mouth with the recording.

B. Papillary Bleeding on Probing

1. The small circles between the diagrammatic tooth blocks in figure 19–3 are used to record proximal bleeding on probing.

2. Improvement in the gingival tissue health will be demonstrated over a period of time as fewer bleeding areas are noted.

IV. SCORING
A. Plaque-free Score

1. Total the number of teeth present.

2. Total the number of surfaces with plaque that appear in red on the tooth diagram.

3. Consult table 19–3:
   a. Read across the top or bottom to locate the number of teeth and total surfaces.
   b. Read down the side to locate the number of surfaces with plaque.
   c. Find the intersection of the top and side numbers; this number is the plaque-free score in percent.

4. To calculate without table 19–3 for reference
   a. Multiply the number of teeth by 4 to determine the number of available surfaces.
   b. Subtract the number of surfaces with plaque from the total available surfaces to find the number of plaque-free surfaces.
   c. Plaque-free score =

$$\frac{\text{Number of plaque-free surfaces} \times 100}{\text{Number of available surfaces}}$$

$$= \text{Percent plaque-free surfaces}$$

5. Evaluate plaque-free score. Ideally, 100% is the goal. When a patient maintains a percent under 85, check individual surfaces to determine whether plaque is usually left in the same areas. To prevent the development of

TABLE 19–3
PLAQUE-FREE SCORE

Number of Tooth Surfaces with Plaque	Number of Tooth Surfaces 32–128	31–124	30–120	29–116	28–112	27–108	26–104	25–100	24–96	23–92	22–88	21–84	
1	99.2	99.2	99.2	99.2	99.2	99.1	99.1	99.0	99.0	99.0	98.9	98.9	
4	96.9	96.8	96.7	97.6	96.5	96.3	96.2	96.0	95.9	95.7	95.5	95.3	
7	94.6	95.4	94.2	94.0	93.8	93.6	93.3	93.0	92.8	92.4	92.1	91.7	
10	92.2	92.0	91.7	91.4	91.1	90.8	90.4	90.0	89.6	89.2	88.7	88.1	
13	89.9	89.6	89.2	88.8	88.4	88.0	87.5	87.0	86.5	85.9	85.3	84.5	
16	87.5	87.1	86.7	86.3	85.8	85.2	84.7	84.0	83.4	82.7	81.9	81.0	
19	85.2	84.7	84.2	83.7	83.1	82.5	81.8	81.0	80.3	79.4	78.5	77.4	
22	83.9	82.3	81.7	81.1	80.4	79.7	78.9	78.0	77.1	76.1	75.0	73.9	
25	80.4	79.9	79.2	78.5	77.7	76.9	76.0	75.0	74.0	72.9	71.6	70.3	
28	78.2	77.5	76.7	75.9	75.0	74.1	73.1	72.0	70.9	69.6	68.2	66.4	
31	75.8	75.0	74.2	73.3	72.4	71.3	70.2	69.0	67.8	66.4	64.8	63.1	
34	73.5	72.6	71.7	70.7	69.7	68.6	67.4	66.0	64.6	63.1	61.4	59.6	
37	71.1	70.2	69.2	68.2	67.0	65.8	64.5	63.0	61.5	59.8	58.0	56.0	
40	68.8	67.8	66.7	65.6	64.3	63.0	61.6	60.0	58.4	56.6	54.6	52.4	
43	66.5	65.4	64.2	63.0	61.7	60.2	58.7	57.0	55.3	53.3	51.2	48.9	
46	64.1	63.0	61.7	60.4	59.0	57.5	55.8	54.0	52.1	50.0	47.8	45.3	
49	61.8	60.5	59.2	57.8	56.3	54.7	52.9	51.0	49.0	46.8	44.4	41.7	
52	59.4	58.1	56.7	55.2	53.6	51.9	50.0	48.0	45.9	43.5	41.0	38.1	
55	57.1	55.7	54.2	52.6	50.9	49.1	47.2	45.0	42.8	40.3	37.5	34.6	
58	54.7	53.3	51.7	50.0	48.3	46.3	44.3	42.0	39.6	37.0	34.1	31.0	
61	52.4	50.9	49.2	47.5	45.6	43.6	41.4	39.0	36.4	33.7	30.7	27.4	
64	50.0	48.4	46.7	44.9	42.9	40.8	38.5	36.0	33.4	30.5	27.3	23.9	
67	47.7	46.0	44.2	42.3	40.2	38.0	35.6	33.0	30.3	27.2	23.9	20.3	
70	45.4	43.6	41.7	39.7	37.5	35.2	32.7	30.0	27.1	24.0	20.5	16.7	
73	43.0	41.2	39.2	37.1	34.9	32.5	29.9	27.0	24.0	20.7	17.1	13.1	
76	40.7	38.8	36.7	34.5	32.2	29.7	27.0	24.0	20.9	17.4	13.7	9.6	
79	38.3	36.3	34.2	31.9	29.5	26.9	24.1	21.0	17.8	14.2	10.3	6.0	
82	36.0	33.9	31.7	29.4	26.8	24.1	21.2	18.0	14.6	10.9	6.9	2.4	
85	33.6	31.5	29.2	26.8	24.2	21.3	18.3	15.0	11.5	7.7	3.3	—	
88	31.3	29.1	26.7	24.2	21.5	18.6	15.4	12.0	8.4	4.4	0.0	—	
91	29.0	26.7	24.2	21.6	18.8	15.8	12.5	9.0	5.3	1.1	—	1.3	79
94	27.6	24.2	21.7	19.0	16.1	13.0	9.7	6.0	2.1	—	0.0	5.0	78
97	24.3	21.8	19.2	16.4	13.4	10.2	6.8	3.0	—	—	4.0	8.8	73
100	21.9	19.4	16.7	13.8	10.8	7.5	3.9	0.0	—	2.8	7.9	12.5	70
103	19.9	17.0	14.2	11.3	8.1	4.7	1.0	—	1.5	7.0	11.9	16.3	67
106	17.2	14.6	11.7	8.7	5.4	1.9	—	0.0	5.9	11.2	15.8	20.0	64
109	14.9	12.1	9.2	6.1	2.7	—	—	4.7	10.3	15.3	19.8	23.8	61
112	12.5	9.7	6.7	3.5	0.0	—	3.4	9.4	14.8	19.5	23.7	27.5	58
115	11.2	7.3	4.2	.9	—	1.8	8.4	14.1	19.2	23.7	27.7	31.3	55
118	7.9	4.9	1.7	—	0.0	7.2	13.4	18.8	23.6	27.8	31.6	35.0	52
121	5.5	2.5	—	—	5.8	12.5	18.4	23.5	28.0	32.0	35.6	38.8	49
124	3.2	0.0	—	4.2	11.6	17.9	23.4	28.2	32.4	36.2	39.5	42.5	46
128	0.0	—	2.3	10.5	17.4	23.3	28.4	32.9	36.8	40.3	43.5	46.3	43
	—	0.0	9.1	16.7	23.1	28.6	33.4	37.5	41.2	44.5	47.4	50.0	40
	—	7.5	16.0	23.0	28.9	34.0	38.4	42.2	45.6	48.7	51.4	53.8	37
	5.6	15.0	22.8	29.2	34.7	39.3	43.4	46.9	50.0	52.8	55.3	57.5	34
	13.9	22.5	29.6	35.5	40.4	44.7	48.4	51.6	54.5	57.0	59.3	61.3	31
	22.3	30.0	36.4	41.7	46.2	50.0	53.4	56.3	58.9	61.2	63.2	65.0	28
	30.6	37.5	43.2	48.0	52.0	55.4	58.4	61.0	63.3	65.3	67.2	68.8	25
	38.9	45.0	50.0	54.2	57.7	60.8	63.4	65.7	67.7	69.5	71.1	72.5	22
	47.3	52.5	56.9	60.5	63.5	66.1	68.4	70.4	72.1	73.7	75.0	76.3	19
	55.6	60.0	63.7	66.7	69.3	71.5	73.4	75.0	76.5	78.8	79.0	80.0	16
	63.9	67.5	70.5	73.0	75.0	76.8	78.4	79.7	80.9	82.0	82.9	87.5	13
	72.3	75.0	77.3	79.2	80.8	82.2	83.4	84.4	85.3	86.2	86.9	87.5	10
	80.6	82.5	84.1	85.5	86.6	87.5	88.4	89.1	89.8	90.3	90.8	91.3	7
	88.9	90.0	91.0	91.7	92.4	92.9	93.4	93.8	94.2	94.5	94.8	95.0	4
	97.3	97.5	97.8	98.0	98.1	98.3	98.4	98.5	98.6	98.7	98.7	98.8	1
	9–36	**10–40**	**11–44**	**12–48**	**13–52**	**14–56**	**15–60**	**16–64**	**17–68**	**18–72**	**19–76**	**20–80**	

(From Grant, D.A., Stern, I.B., and Everett, F.G.: *Periodontics,* 5th ed. St. Louis, Mosby, 1979.)

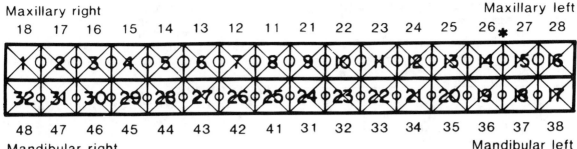

Maxillary right   Maxillary left

Mandibular right   Mandibular left

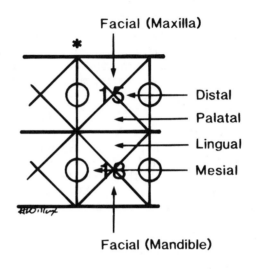

FIG. 19–3. Plaque-free Score. Diagrammatic representation of the teeth used to record plaque and papillary bleeding. Enlargement of teeth (*) shows tooth surfaces. Teeth are numbered by the ADA System inside each block and by the FDI System outside each block. (Adapted from Grant, D.A., Stern, I.B., and Listgarten, M.A.: *Periodontics*, 6th ed. St. Louis, Mosby, 1988, p. 613.)

specific areas of periodontal infection, remedial instruction in the areas usually missed is indicated.

B. Papillary Bleeding on Probing
1. Total the number of small circles marked for bleeding. A person with 32 teeth has 30 interdental areas. The mesial or distal surface of a tooth adjacent to an edentulous area is probed and counted.
2. Evaluate total interdental bleeding. In health, bleeding on probing does not occur.

C. Calculation Example for Plaque-free Score

Individual findings: 24 teeth scored
                         37 surfaces with plaque

1. With table 19–3
   a. Locate the number of teeth across the top of table 19–3 (24–96); there are 96 total surfaces.
   b. Locate the number of surfaces with plaque down the side (37); find the intersection.
   c. The percent of plaque-free surfaces is 61.5.

2. Without reference table 19–3
   a. Multiply the number of teeth by 4:

   $24 \times 4 = 96$ available surfaces

   b. Subtract the number of surfaces with plaque from total available surfaces:

   $96 - 37 = 59$ plaque-free surfaces

   c. Percent plaque-free surfaces =

   $$\frac{59 \times 100}{96} = 61.5$$

Interpretation: On the basis of the ideal 100%, 61.5% is poor. More instruction is indicated.

PATIENT HYGIENE PERFORMANCE (PHP) (Podshadley and Haley[2])

I. PURPOSE
To assess the extent of plaque and debris over a tooth surface. Debris is defined for the PHP as the soft foreign material consisting of bacterial plaque, materia alba, and food debris that is loosely attached to tooth surfaces.

II. SELECTION OF TEETH AND SURFACES
A. Teeth Examined

(FDI System tooth numbers are in parentheses.)

Maxillary	Mandibular
No. 3 (16) Right first molar	No. 19 (36) Left first molar
No. 8 (11) Right central incisor	No. 24 (31) Left central incisor
No. 14 (26) Left first molar	No. 30 (46) Right first molar

B. Substitutions
When a first molar is missing, is less than three-fourths erupted, has a full crown, or is broken down, the second molar is used. The third molar is used when the second is missing. The adjacent central incisor is used for a missing incisor.

C. Surfaces
The facial surfaces of incisors and maxillary molars and the lingual surface of mandibular molars are examined. These surfaces are the same as those used for the Simplified Oral Hygiene Index (figure 19–7, page 299).

III. PROCEDURE
A. Apply disclosing agent. Instruct the patient to swish for 30 seconds and expectorate, but not rinse.
B. Examination is made using a mouth mirror.
C. Each tooth surface to be evaluated is subdivided (mentally) into 5 sections (figure 19–4A) as follows:
   1. *Vertically.* Three divisions—mesial, middle, and distal.
   2. *Horizontally.* The middle third is subdivided into gingival, middle, and occlusal or incisal thirds.
D. Each of the 5 subdivisions is scored for the presence of stained debris as follows:

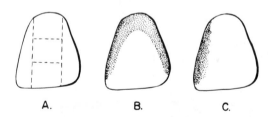

A.   B.   C.

FIG. 19–4. Patient Hygiene Performance (PHP). A. *Oral debris is assessed by dividing a tooth into 5 subdivisions, each of which is scored 1 when debris is shown to be present after use of a disclosing agent.* **B.** *Example of debris score of 3. Shaded portion represents debris stained by disclosing agent.* **C.** *Example of debris score of 1. (From Podshadley, A.G. and Haley, J.V.: A Method for Evaluating Oral Hygiene Performance,* Public Health Rep., *83, 259, 1968.)*

0 = No debris (or questionable).
1 = Debris definitely present.
Identify by *M* when all three molars or both incisors are missing.
Identity by *S* when a substitute tooth is used.

IV. SCORING
A. Debris Score for Individual Tooth
Add the scores for each of the 5 subdivisions. The scores range from 0 to 5.

B. PHP for the Individual
Total the scores for the individual teeth and divide by the number of teeth examined. The PHP ranges from 0 to 5.

C. Suggested Nominal Scale for Evaluation of Scores

Rating	Scores
Excellent	0–(no debris)
Good	0.1–1.7
Fair	1.8–3.4
Poor	3.5–5.0

D. Calculation Example for an Individual

Tooth	Debris Score
No. 3 (16)	5
No. 8 (11)	3
No. 14 (26)	4
No. 19 (36)	5
No. 24 (31)	2
No. 30 (46)	22
Total	22

$$PHP = \frac{Total\ Debris\ Score}{Number\ of\ Teeth\ Scored} = \frac{22}{6} = 3.66$$

Interpretation: According to the suggested nominal scale, this person with a PHP of 3.66 would be classified as exhibiting poor hygiene performance.

E. PHP for a Group
To obtain the average PHP score for a group or population, total the individual scores and divide by the number of people examined.

ORAL HYGIENE INDEX (OHI) (Greene and Vermillion,[9] Waggener[10])

I. PURPOSE
To measure existing debris and calculus as an indication of oral cleanliness. The OHI has two components, the *Debris Index* and the *Calculus Index.* Each is based on 12 numeric determinations that designate the amount of debris or calculus found on selected tooth surfaces. The two scores may be used singly or may be combined for an OHI.

II. SELECTION OF TEETH AND SURFACES

A. Divide the dentition into sextants. Posterior sextants begin distal to the canines.

1. Score only fully erupted permanent teeth. A tooth is considered fully erupted when it has reached the occlusal plane.

2. Exclude third molars, teeth with full crown restorations, and teeth reduced in height because of severe dental caries or trauma.

B. Select the 12 tooth surfaces, 1 facial and 1 lingual or palatal in each sextant, that are covered with the greatest amount of debris, plaque, and calculus.

1. Facial and lingual or palatal surfaces in each sextant may be taken from different teeth.

2. Include proximal surfaces to the contact area. A score represents half the circumference of the selected tooth.

III. PROCEDURE

A. Evaluation

Evaluate each sextant to record first the debris and then the calculus.

B. Sequence

Proceed in routine order from maxillary right, anterior, and left sextants to mandibular left, anterior, and right sextants.

C. Record 12 Debris Scores

1. *Definition of Oral Debris.* Oral debris is the soft foreign matter on the surfaces of the teeth that consists of bacterial plaque, materia alba, and food debris.

2. *Examination.* Run the side of the tip of a probe or explorer across the tooth surface to estimate the surface area covered by debris.

3. *Criteria* (figure 19–5)

0 = No debris or stain present.
1 = Soft debris covering not more than one third of the tooth surface being examined, or the presence of extrinsic stains without debris, regardless of surface area covered.
2 = Soft debris covering more than one third but not more than two thirds of the exposed tooth surface.
3 = Soft debris covering more than two thirds of the exposed tooth surface.

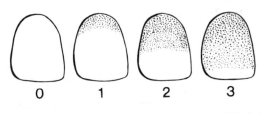

FIG. 19–5. Oral Hygiene Index. For the Debris Index, 12 surfaces are scored, 2 in each sextant. Scoring of 0 to 3 is based on tooth surfaces covered by debris as shown.

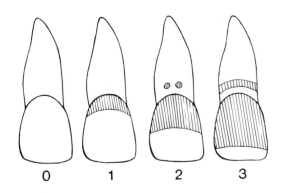

FIG. 19–6. Oral Hygiene Index. For the Calculus Index, 12 surfaces are scored, 2 in each sextant. Scoring of 0 to 3 is based on location and tooth surface area with calculus as shown. Note slight subgingival calculus recorded as 2 and more extensive subgingival calculus by 3.

D. Record 12 Calculus Scores

1. *Definition of Calculus.* Dental calculus is a hard deposit of inorganic salts composed primarily of calcium carbonate and phosphate mixed with debris, microorganisms, and desquamated epithelial cells.

2. *Examination.* Use an explorer to estimate surface area covered by supragingival calculus deposits. Identify subgingival deposits by exploring and/or probing. Record only definite deposits of hard calculus.

3. *Criteria* (figure 19–6)

0 = No calculus present.
1 = Supragingival calculus covering not more than one third of the exposed tooth surface being examined.
2 = Supragingival calculus covering more than one third but not more than two thirds of the exposed tooth surface, or the presence of individual flecks of subgingival calculus around the cervical portion of the tooth.
3 = Supragingival calculus covering more than two thirds of the exposed tooth surface or a continuous heavy band of subgingival calculus around the cervical portion of the tooth.

IV. SCORING

A. OHI for an Individual

1. Determine Debris Index (DI) and Calculus Index (CI)

a. Divide total scores by number of sextants.

i. Each selected surface has a severity score of 0 to 3 (see Criteria, previous section).

ii. The total score for debris or calculus ranges from 0 to 36 (12 scores multiplied by maximum severity of 3).

b. Debris Index (DI) or Calculus Index (CI) ranges from 0 to 6.

2. Oral Hygiene Index (OHI) = DI + CI
   a. Combine the Debris Index and the Calculus Index.
   b. The OHI ranges from 0 to 12.

B. Suggested Nominal Scale

1. DI and CI

Rating	Scores
Excellent	0
Good	0.1–1.2
Fair	1.3–3.0
Poor	3.1–6.0

2. OHI

Rating	Scores
Excellent	0
Good	0.1–2.4
Fair	2.5–6.0
Poor	6.1–12.0

C. Calculation Example for Individual OHI

Debris Scores

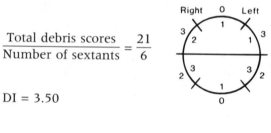

$$\frac{\text{Total debris scores}}{\text{Number of sextants}} = \frac{21}{6}$$

DI = 3.50

Calculus scores

$$\frac{\text{Total calculus scores}}{\text{Number of sextants}} = \frac{10}{6}$$

CI = 1.67

$$OHI = DI + CI = 3.50 + 1.67 = 5.17$$

Interpretation: According to the suggested nominal scale, the OHI score for this individual (5.17) indicates a fair oral hygiene status with poor plaque removal skills and a fair amount of calculus buildup.

D. OHI for a Group

1. *Group Debris Index.* Divide total DI scores by number of individuals.
2. *Group Calculus Index.* Divide total CI scores by number of individuals.
3. *Mean Oral Hygiene Index (OHI).* Divide total DI and CI scores for all individuals by the number of individuals.

SIMPLIFIED ORAL HYGIENE INDEX (OHI-S) (Greene and Vermillion[11,12])

I. PURPOSE

To assess oral cleanliness by estimating the tooth surface covered with debris and/or calculus.

A. Components

The OHI-S has two components, the Simplified Debris Index (DI-S) and the Simplified Calculus Index (CI-S). The two scores may be used separately or may be combined for the OHI-S.

B. Comparison with OHI (pages 296–298)

After experience with the Oral Hygiene Index (OHI), the need for simplification was recognized because of the length of time required to evaluate debris and calculus, as well as to make subjective decisions on tooth selection.

1. *Tooth Selection.* In the OHI, the examiner must select the tooth with the most debris or calculus in each sextant. The OHI-S assesses 6 specific teeth, 1 in each sextant.
2. *Number of Surfaces.* In the OHI, 12 surfaces are evaluated; only 6 surfaces are used in the OHI-S.
3. *Scoring.* The OHI ranges from 0 to 12; the OHI-S ranges from 0 to 6.

II. SELECTION OF TEETH AND SURFACES

A. Identify the Six Specific Teeth (figure 19–7)

1. *Posterior.* The first fully erupted tooth distal to each second premolar is examined. The facial surfaces of the maxillary molars and the lingual surfaces of the mandibular molars are used. Although usually the first molars are used, the second or third molars also may be used.
2. *Anterior.* The facial surfaces of the maxillary right and the mandibular left central incisors are used. When either is missing, the opposite central incisor is scored.

B. Extent

A score represents half the circumference of the selected tooth; includes proximal surfaces to the contact areas.

III. PROCEDURE

A. Qualification

At least two of the six possible surfaces must have been examined for an individual score to be calculated.

B. Record Six Debris Scores and Six Calculus Scores

Follow the routine and use the same criteria as those for the OHI described on page 297. Figures 19–5 (debris) and 19–6 (calculus) illustrate the extent of deposits for each score from 0 to 3.

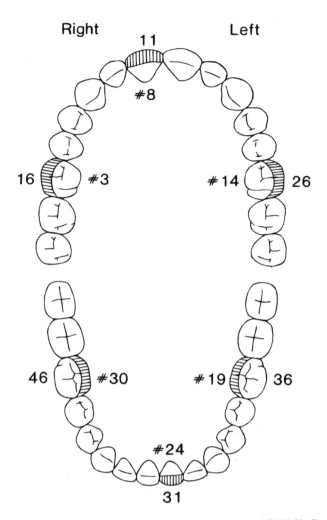

Right   Left

11

#8

16   #3   #14   26

46   #30   #19   36

#24

31

FIG. 19–7. Simplified Oral Hygiene Index (OHI-S). Six tooth surfaces are scored as follows: facial surfaces of maxillary molars and of the maxillary right and mandibular left central incisors, and the lingual surfaces of mandibular molars. Teeth are numbered by the ADA System on the lingual surface and by the FDI System on the facial surface.

IV. SCORING

A. OHI-S for an Individual

1. *Determine Simplified Debris Index (DI-S) and Simplified Calculus Index (CI-S)*
   a. Divide total scores by number of sextants.
   b. DI-S and CI-S values range from 0 to 3.
2. *Simplified Oral Hygiene Index (OHI-S)*
   a. Combine the DI-S and CI-S.
   b. OHI-S value ranges from 0 to 6.

B. Suggested Nominal Scale[12]

DI-S and CI-S

Rating	Scores
Excellent	0
Good	0.1–0.6
Fair	0.7–1.8
Poor	1.9–3.0

OHI-S

Rating	Scores
Excellent	0
Good	0.1–1.2
Fair	1.3–3.0
Poor	3.1–6.0

C. Calculation Example for an Individual

	Individual Scores	
Tooth	DI-S	CI-S
No. 3 (16)	2	2
No. 8 (11)	1	0
No. 14 (26)	3	2
No. 19 (36)	3	2
No. 24 (31)	2	1
No. 30 (46)	2	2
Total	13	9

$$DI\text{-}S = \frac{\text{Total Debris Scores}}{\text{Number of Teeth Scored}} = \frac{13}{6} = 2.17$$

$$CI\text{-}S = \frac{\text{Total Calculus Scores}}{\text{Number of Teeth Scored}} = \frac{9}{6} = 1.50$$

$$OHI\text{-}S = DI\text{-}S + CI\text{-}S = 2.17 + 1.50 = 3.67$$

Interpretation: According to the suggested nominal scale, the score for this individual (3.67) indicates a poor oral hygiene status.

D. OHI-S Group Score

Compute the average of the individual scores by totalling the scores and dividing by the number of individuals.

BLEEDING INDICES

Bleeding on gentle probing or flossing is an early sign of gingival inflammation and precedes color changes and enlargement of the gingival tissues.[13,14] Based on the principle that healthy tissue does not bleed, testing for bleeding has become a significant procedure for evaluation prior to treatment planning, after therapy to show the effects of treatment, and at maintenance appointments to determine continued control of gingival inflammation.

For patient instruction and motivation, a variety of bleeding indices and scoring methods has been developed. The Gingival Index (GI) described on page 302 includes an estimate of bleeding on probing, along with other clinical observations to score the severity of gingivitis. The GI has been used extensively in research, as well as for patient instruction and motivation.

Another example is a plaque-free score as described on page 293. The form illustrated in figure 19–3 has small circles that can be colored to illustrate interproximal bleeding. A series of diagrams made over several weeks can show the patient's progress toward health, as less and less bleeding is charted.

Two well-known bleeding indices are described here. They are the Sulcus Bleeding Index developed by Mühlemann and the Gingival Bleeding Index of Carter and Barnes.

SULCUS BLEEDING INDEX (SBI) (Mühlemann and Son[13])

I. PURPOSE

To locate areas of gingival sulcus bleeding upon gentle probing and thus recognize and record the presence of early (initial) inflammatory gingival disease.

II. AREAS EXAMINED

Four gingival units are scored systematically for each tooth: the labial and lingual marginal gingiva (M units), and the mesial and distal papillary gingiva (P units).

III. PROCEDURE

A. Use standardized lighting while probing each of the four areas.
B. Hold the probe parallel with the long axis of the tooth for M units, and direct the probe toward the col area for P units.
C. Wait 30 seconds after probing before scoring apparently healthy gingival units.
D. Dry the gingiva gently if necessary to observe color changes clearly.
E. Criteria

0 = Healthy appearance of P and M, no bleeding on sulcus probing.
1 = Apparently healthy P and M showing no change in color and no swelling, but bleeding from sulcus on probing.
2 = Bleeding on probing *and* change of color caused by inflammation. No swelling or macroscopic edema.
3 = Bleeding on probing *and* change in color and slight edematous swelling.
4 = (1) Bleeding on probing *and* change in color *and* obvious swelling.
(2) Bleeding on probing and obvious swelling.
5 = Bleeding on probing and spontaneous bleeding *and* change in color, marked swelling with or without ulceration.

IV. SCORING

A. SBI for Area

Each of the 4 gingival units (M and P) is scored 0 to 5.

B. SBI for Tooth

Scores for the 4 units are totalled and divided by 4.

C. SBI for Individual

By totalling scores for individual teeth and dividing by the number of teeth, the SBI is determined. Indices range from 0 to 5.

GINGIVAL BLEEDING INDEX (GBI) (Carter and Barnes[15])

I. PURPOSE

To record the presence or absence of gingival inflammation as determined by bleeding from interproximal gingival sulci.

II. AREAS EXAMINED

Each interproximal area has two sulci, which either are scored as one interdental unit or may be scored individually. Certain areas may be excluded from scoring because of accessibility, tooth position, diastemas, or other factors, and if exclusions are made, a consistent procedure should be followed for an individual and for a group if a study is to be made.

A full complement of teeth has 28 proximal areas. In the original studies, third molars were excluded, and 26 units were recorded.[15]

III. PROCEDURE

A. Instrument

Unwaxed dental floss is used. Floss has the advantages of being readily available, disposable, and usable by the instructed patient.

B. Steps

1. Pass the floss interproximally first on one side of the papilla and then on the other.
2. Curve the floss around the adjacent tooth (figure 23–1E and F, page 355), and bring the floss below the gingival margin.
3. Move the floss up and down for one stroke, with care not to lacerate the gingiva. Adapt finger rests to provide controlled, consistent pressure.
4. Use a new length of clean floss for each area.
5. Retract for visibility of bleeding from both facial and lingual aspects.
6. Allow 30 seconds for reinspection of an area that does not show blood immediately either in the area or on the floss.

C. Criteria

Bleeding indicates the presence of disease. No attempt is made to quantify the severity of bleeding because no bleeding represents health.

IV. SCORING

The numbers of bleeding areas and scorable units are recorded. Patient participation in observing and recording over a series of appointments can increase motivation.

PAPILLARY-MARGINAL-ATTACHED GINGIVAL INDEX (P-M-A)
(Schour and Massler[16,17])

I. PURPOSE
To assess the extent of gingival changes in large groups for epidemiologic studies.

II. SELECTION OF TEETH AND AREAS
Three gingival units are examined for each tooth (figure 19–8).

P = *Papillary* portion between the teeth
1. Number each papilla by the tooth just distal. No papilla is present when teeth are separated by a diastema or edentulous area.
2. Mild gingivitis is associated with papillary changes. Inflammation usually begins within the papilla at the col area.

M = *Marginal* collar around the tooth
1. Located between papillae, attached by junctional epithelium, and demarcated from attached gingiva by the free gingival groove (page 183).
2. Moderate gingivitis is associated with papillary and marginal gingival inflammation.

A = *Attached* gingiva overlying the alveolar bone
1. Stippled gingiva between the free gingival groove and the mucogingival junction.
2. Severe gingivitis is associated with spread of inflammation from papillary and marginal gingivitis into the attached gingiva.

III. PROCEDURE
A. Instruments and Equipment
1. Adequate lighting; headrest for stabilization.
2. Mouth mirror.
3. Probe for pressing on gingiva. In the original studies, a blunt explorer was used.

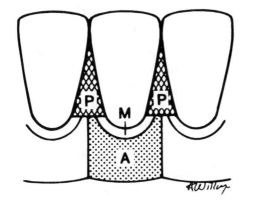

FIG. 19–8. Papillary-Marginal-Attached Gingival Index (P-M-A). Each of the 3 parts of the gingiva is scored from 0 (healthy) to 5 (marked disease characteristics). Units are scored and recorded separately to show *P* (Papillary), *M* (Marginal), and *A* (Attached) conditions.

B. Examine Facial Surfaces Only
1. Proceed in a routine order from left maxillary second molar around to right second molar; then mandibular right second molar around to left.
2. Third molars are not included.

C. Criteria

Gingival Area	Score	Criteria
Papillary	*P*	0 = Normal; no inflammation.
		1 + = Mild papillary engorgement; slight increase in size.
		2 + = Obvious increase in size of gingival papilla; bleeding on pressure.
		3 + = Excessive increase in size with spontaneous bleeding.
		4 + = Necrotic papilla.
		5 + = Atrophy and loss of papilla (through inflammation).
Marginal	*M*	0 = Normal; no inflammation visible.
		1 + = Engorgement; slight increase in size; no bleeding.
		2 + = Obvious engorgement; bleeding upon pressure.
		3 + = Swollen collar; spontaneous bleeding; beginning infiltration into attached gingiva.
		4 + = Necrotic gingivitis.
		5 + = Recession of the free marginal gingiva below the cementoenamel junction as a result of inflammatory changes.
Attached	*A*	0 = Normal; pale rose; stippled.
		1 + = Slight engorgement with loss of stippling; change in color may or may not be present.
		2 + = Obvious engorgement of attached gingiva with marked increase in redness. Pocket formation present.
		3 + = Advanced periodontitis. Deep pockets evident.

IV. SCORING
A. P-M-A for an Individual
1. Count the number of Papillary, Marginal, and Attached units scored, and record separately as follows:

$$P\text{-}M\text{-}A = 10\text{-}5\text{-}0$$

2. Keep totals separate. If added together the sum would reflect different meanings and would not represent the areas of the gingiva where the inflammation occurred.

B. Suggested Nominal Scale for the P-M-A[16]

Mild gingivitis	1 to 4 papillae
	0 to 2 margins
Moderate gingivitis	4 to 8 papillae
	2 to 4 margins
Severe gingivitis	more than 8 papillae
	more than 4 margins

C. P-M-A for a Group
Compute the average of the P, M, and A by totalling each for all individuals and then dividing each by the number of individuals examined.

GINGIVAL INDEX (GI)
(Löe and Silness[5,18])

I. PURPOSE
To assess the severity of gingivitis based on color, consistency, and bleeding on probing.

II. SELECTION OF TEETH AND GINGIVAL AREAS
A gingival index may be determined for selected teeth or for the entire dentition.

A. Areas Examined
Four gingival areas (distal, facial, mesial, lingual) are examined systematically for each tooth.

B. Modified Procedure
The distal examination for each tooth can be omitted. The score for the mesial is doubled, and the total score for each tooth is divided by 4.

III. PROCEDURE
A. Dry the teeth and gingiva; under adequate light, use a mouth mirror and probe.
B. Use the probe to press on the gingiva to determine the degree of firmness.
C. Use the probe to run along the soft tissue wall near the entrance to the gingival sulcus to evaluate bleeding (figure 19–9).
D. Criteria

    0 = Normal gingiva.
    1 = Mild inflammation—slight change in color, slight edema. *No bleeding on probing.*
    2 = Moderate inflammation—redness, edema, and glazing. *Bleeding on probing.*

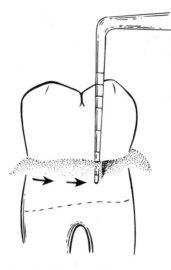

FIG. 19–9. Gingival Index (GI). Probe stroke for bleeding evaluation. The broken line represents the level of attachment of the periodontal tissues. The probe is inserted a few millimeters and moved along the soft tissue pocket wall with light pressure in a circumferential direction. The stroke shown here is in contrast with the walking stroke used for probing depth evaluation and measurement as described on page 214.

    3 = Severe inflammation—marked redness and edema. Ulceration. *Tendency to spontaneous bleeding.*

IV. SCORING
A. GI for Area
Each of the 4 gingival surfaces (distal, facial, mesial, lingual) is given a score of 0 to 3.

B. GI for a Tooth
Scores for each area are totalled and divided by 4.

C. GI for Groups of Teeth
Scores for individual teeth may be grouped and totalled, and divided by the number of teeth. A GI may be determined for specific teeth, group of teeth, quadrant, or side of mouth.

D. GI for the Individual
By totalling scores and dividing by the number of teeth examined, the GI is determined. Indices range from 0 to 3.

E. Suggested Nominal Scale for Patient Reference

Rating	Scores
Excellent (healthy tissue)	0
Good	0.1–1.0
Fair	1.1–2.0
Poor	2.1–3.0

F. Calculation Example for an Individual

(using 6 teeth for an example of screening; see figure 19–10)

Gingival Area

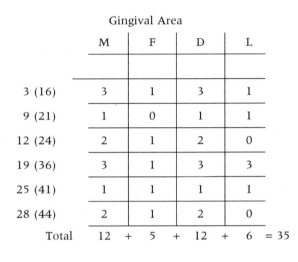

	M	F	D	L
3 (16)	3	1	3	1
9 (21)	1	0	1	1
12 (24)	2	1	2	0
19 (36)	3	1	3	3
25 (41)	1	1	1	1
28 (44)	2	1	2	0
Total	12 +	5 +	12 +	6 = 35

$$\text{Gingival Index} = \frac{\text{Total score}}{\text{Number of surfaces}} = \frac{35}{24} = 1.45 \text{ GI}$$

Interpretation: According to the suggested nominal scale, the score for this individual (1.45) indicates only fair gingival health (moderate inflammation). The ratings for each gingival area or surface can be used to help the patient compare gingival changes and improve oral hygiene procedures.

G. GI for a Group

Add the individual GI scores and divide by the number of individuals examined.

THE PERIODONTAL INDEX (PI)
(Russell[19,20])

I. PURPOSE

To assess and score the periodontal disease status of populations in epidemiologic studies.

II. SELECTION OF TEETH

Each tooth present is scored according to the condition of the surrounding tissues.

III. PROCEDURE
A. Instruments

Each tooth present is examined using a mouth mirror and explorer with adequate illumination. In the original examinations,[19] a Jacquette scaler and chip blower were used to define the presence of periodontal pockets. At present, a periodontal probe is the preferred instrument.

B. Criteria

0 = Negative	There is neither overt inflammation in the investing tissues nor loss of function caused by destruction of supporting tissue.
1 = Mild Gingivitis	There is an overt area of inflammation in the free gingiva that does not circumscribe the tooth.
2 = Gingivitis	Inflammation completely circumscribes the tooth, but there is no apparent break in the epithelial attachment.
6 = Gingivitis with Pocket Formation	The epithelial attachment has been broken and there is a pocket (not merely a deepened gingival crevice caused by swelling in the free gingiva). There is no interference with normal masticatory function; the tooth is firm in its socket and has not drifted.
8 = Advanced Destruction with Loss of Masticatory Function	The tooth may be loose; may have drifted; may sound dull on percussion with a metallic instrument; may be depressible in its socket.

IV. SCORING

A. Each tooth is assigned a score from 0 (no disease) to 8 (severe disease with loss of function).

B. Add the scores for each tooth and divide by the number of teeth examined to obtain the individual's score.

C. For PI group score, total the individuals' scores and divide by the number of individuals examined. The average ranges from 0 to 8.

D. Suggested Nominal Scale for Patient Reference follows[20]

Condition	Scores
Clinically normal supportive tissues	0–0.2
Simple gingivitis	0.3–0.9
Beginning destructive periodontal disease	0.7–1.9
Established destructive periodontal disease	1.6–5.0
Terminal disease	3.8–8.0

E. Breakdown of scores can be performed in various ways. In a population group, scores may be averaged by specific age groups, such as ages 1 to 9, 10 to 19, 20 to 29, and so forth. Scores may be calculated for each sex or for each sex within the various age groups. Data may also be used to calculate disease in relation to economic factors or educational background of the individuals.

THE PERIODONTAL DISEASE INDEX (PDI) (Ramfjord[21,22])

I. PURPOSE

To show the periodontal status of an individual or group by assessing the prevalence and severity of gingivitis and periodontitis.

The Periodontal Disease Index (PDI) combines the evaluation of gingival status with the probed attachment level (cervice depth measured from the cementoenamel junction).

Although not part of the PDI, a Calculus Index (CI) and Plaque Index (PI) usually have been included when making a survey and thus are described after the PDI.

II. SELECTION OF TEETH AND SURFACES

A. Six teeth are used to represent the six segments of the dentition (figure 19–10).

(FDI System tooth numbers are in parentheses.)

Maxillary	Mandibular
No. 3 (16) right first molar	No. 19 (36) left first molar
No. 9 (21) left central incisor	No. 25 (41) right central incisor
No. 12 (24) left first premolar	No. 28 (44) right first premolar

B. Only fully erupted teeth are used.

C. Substitutions are not made for missing teeth; scores are derived from the teeth present.

III. PROCEDURE

A. Determine Gingival Status

1. Under consistent standardized light, dry the gingiva with cotton to observe color and form.

2. Apply gentle pressure with the probe to determine consistency (density). When the color change definitely indicates the presence of inflammation, the consistency is not checked.

3. Criteria for gingival status

   0 = Absence of signs of inflammation.
   1 = Mild to moderate inflammatory gingival changes, not extending around the tooth.
   2 = Mild to moderately severe gingivitis extending all around the tooth.
   3 = Severe gingivitis characterized by marked redness, swelling, tendency to bleed, and ulceration, not necessarily extending around the tooth.

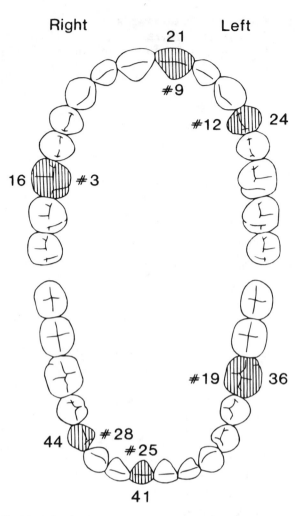

FIG. 19–10. Periodontal Disease Index (PDI). *The six shaded teeth are scored. Teeth are numbered by the ADA System on the lingual side and the FDI System on the facial side.*

4. Summary for an individual
   a. Individual teeth. Add the scores for each area and divide by the number of areas examined.
   b. Score for individual. Add the scores for all the examined teeth and divide by the total number of teeth examined. The range is from 0 to 3.

B. Determine Crevice Depth from Cementoenamel Junction (CEJ)

1. *Technique Objective.* To measure the crevice or sulcus depth from the CEJ to the bottom of the gingival crevice or pocket. This technique measures the probed attachment level and is described in detail on page 215.

2. *Instrument.* To obtain consistent readings, a probe is needed that has been calibrated for shape, thickness, angulation, and the placement and definition of reference marks.

When the index was first used, a Michigan probe No. 0 was used (figure 13–1D, page 211).

3. *Locations of Measurements*
   a. The two measurements made are at the middle of the facial surface and at the facial aspect of the mesial contact area, with the side of the probe held touching both teeth (figure 19–11).
   b. The original PDI required four measurements for each tooth, on the facial, mesial, distal, and lingual surfaces. It was later found that no significant loss in accuracy resulted from using only two measurements. Four measurements are still used for certain types of research evaluations.

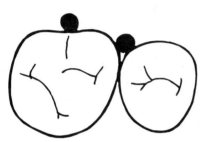

FIG. 19–11. Periodontal Disease Index (PDI). Probe positions for measuring crevice depth are shown by the black dots. One measurement is made at the middle of the facial surface and the other at the facial aspect of the mesial contact area. The side of the probe is held touching both teeth.

4. *Measurements*
   a. When the CEJ is covered by gingiva, determine the location of the CEJ by sliding the probe subgingivally (figure 19–12A), and measure the distance to the CEJ from the margin. Scale to remove calculus when deposits cover the CEJ (figure 19–12B). Measure from the gingival margin to determine the probed pocket depth (figure 19–12C) and subtract the measured distance from the gingival margin to the CEJ to determine the probed attachment level.
   b. When the CEJ is visible because of gingival recession, the crevice depth can be measured directly from the CEJ (figure 19–12D).
   c. When the gingival margin is level with the CEJ, the probed pocket depth and the probed attachment level are equal (figure 13–7D, page 215).

5. Criteria for PDI

0 to 3 (Gingivitis Index)	= When the gingival crevice or pocket in none of the measured areas extends apical to the cementoenamel junction.
4	= When the crevices (pockets) of any 2 (or 4) recorded areas extend apical to the cementoenamel junction not more than, but including, 3 mm. (The gingivitis score is then disregarded.)

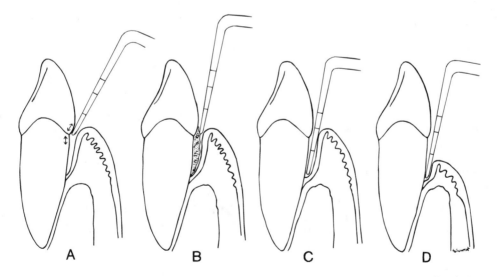

FIG. 19–12. Periodontal Disease Index (PDI). The crevice (sulcus) depth from the cementoenamel junction is determined as follows. **A.** Locate the cementoenamel junction with the probe tip and measure the distance from the gingival margin. **B.** When calculus interferes with efforts to locate the cementoenamel junction, scaling is performed. **C.** Apply probe to measure the probing depth from gingival margin to attached periodontal tissue, and subtract the distance to the cementoenamel junction. **D.** When recession is apparent, the direct reading from the cementoenamel juntion can be measured. Note use of Michigan 0 probe.

5 = When the crevices (pockets) of any of the 2 (or 4) recorded areas extend apical to the cementoenamel junction from 3 mm to 6 mm inclusive. (The gingivitis score is disregarded.)

6 = When the crevices (pockets) extend more than 6 mm apical to the cementoenamel junction in any of the 2 (or 4) measured areas. (The gingivitis score is disregarded.)

IV. SCORING

A. PDI for an Individual

Add scores for individual teeth and divide by the number of teeth examined. The PDI ranges from 0 to 6.

B. Suggested Nominal Scale for Evaluation of Scores

1. *Gingivitis.* Numbers 0 to 3 indicate gingival involvement only, with increasing severity from 0 (no disease) through 3.9 (severe gingivitis).
2. *Periodontitis.* Numbers 4 through 6 indicate periodontal involvement with migration of the junctional epithelium and bone loss of increasing degree of severity from 4 (early disease) through 6 (advanced disease).

C. Calculation Example for an Individual

Tooth	Periodontal Disease Score
No. 3 (16)	4
No. 9 (21)	0
No. 12 (24)	5
No. 19 (36)	6
No. 25 (41)	4
No. 28 (44)	2
Total	21

$$PDI = \frac{Total\ scores}{Number\ of\ teeth} = \frac{21}{6} = 3.5$$

Interpretation: For epidemiologic purposes, using the average (mean) group score of 3.5 can be acceptable for showing overall characteristics of a large population. In this example, however, the 3.5 PDI, which by the nominal score represents "severe gingivitis," would be misleading when reporting the condition of this individual. The scores for each tooth clearly show that 4 of the 6 teeth examined have measurements that show loss of attachment and loss of bone typical of periodontitis. Care must be taken when interpreting the PDI on an individual basis.

D. PDI Group Score

Total the individual PDI scores and divide by the number of individuals examined. The average ranges from 0 to 6.

CALCULUS SCORE (Used with PDI) (Ramfjord[22])

I. PURPOSE

To evaluate the presence and extent of calculus. This index is not an integral part of the PDI, but was developed and used in conjunction with the PDI.

Because calculus may have to be removed to determine the location of the cementoenamel junction for crevice and pocket measurements in the PDI, calculus should be scored first, before its removal.

II. SURFACES EXAMINED

For each of the 6 teeth (figure 19–10), 4 surfaces (facial, lingual [or palatal], mesial, and distal) are scored from 0 to 3.

III. PROCEDURE

A. Instruments

A subgingival explorer (for example, the No. TU-17, figure 13–14, page 220) may be used to locate subgingival calculus and determine its extent. The probe (such as the Michigan 0) used for crevice and pocket determinations may provide sufficient sensitivity for calculus evaluation.

B. Criteria

0 = No calculus.
1 = Supragingival calculus extending only slightly below the free gingival margin (not more than 1 mm).
2 = Moderate amount of supra- and subgingival calculus, or subgingival calculus only.
3 = Abundance of supra- and subgingival calculus.

IV. SCORING

A. Individual Teeth

Add scores for each surface and divide by the number of surfaces (4).

B. Calculus Score for an Individual

Add the scores for the individual teeth and divide by the number of teeth. The calculus score ranges from 0 to 3.

DENTAL PLAQUE SCORE (Used with PDI) (Ramfjord[22])

I. PURPOSE

To evaluate the extent of plaque on the basis of tooth surface coverage.

II. SELECTION OF TEETH AND SURFACES

For each of the 6 teeth (figure 19–10), 4 surfaces (facial, lingual, mesial, and distal) are scored from 0 to 3.

B. Criteria for Identification of Dental Caries

Same as for DMFT.

C. Criteria for def

d = number of primary teeth or surfaces with dental caries but not restored.

e = number of teeth indicated for extraction because of dental caries.

f = number of filled primary teeth on surfaces that do not have dental caries (each surface is scored once only, "d" has first score).

D. Difference Between deft/defs and dft/dfs

In the deft and defs, both "d" and "e" are used to describe teeth with dental caries. Thus, d and e are sometimes combined, and the index becomes the "dft" or "dfs."

IV. SCORING

A. Individual dft

A 2½-year old child with nursing caries (page 234) has 18 teeth. Teeth A (55) and J (65) are unerupted. There is no sign of dental caries in teeth M (73), N (72), O (71), P (81), Q (82), and R (83). All other teeth have 2 carious surfaces each, except B (54), which is broken down to the gumline.

Summary: Total teeth = 18
Caries-free = 6
"d" teeth = 12
"f" teeth = 0
dft = d + f = 12 + 0 = 12

Interpretation: 12 of 18 teeth with carious lesions indicates a serious need for dental treatment for the child.

B. Individual dfs

Using the same 2½-year-old child to calculate dfs:

Total number of carious surfaces: 11 × 2 = 22
Tooth B: 1 × 5 = 5
Total 27 dfs

Interpretation: The child has 48 anterior surfaces (12 teeth × 4 surfaces) and 30 posterior surfaces (6 teeth × 5 surfaces) to total 78 surfaces.

$$\frac{dfs}{\text{number of surfaces}} = \frac{27}{78} = \begin{array}{l} .34 \text{ or } 34\% \text{ of the} \\ \text{surfaces in need of} \\ \text{dental treatment.} \end{array}$$

C. Mixed Dentition

A DMFT or DMFS and a deft or defs are never added together. Each child is given a separate index for permanent teeth and another for primary teeth. The index for the permanent teeth is usually determined first, and then the index for the primary teeth is prepared separately.

DECAYED, MISSING, AND FILLED (dmft or dmfs)

I. PURPOSE

To determine dental caries experience past and present for children older than 7 and up to 11 or 12 years of age.

II. SELECTION OF TEETH OR SURFACES

A. dmft: 12 teeth evaluated (8 primary molars; 4 primary canines).

B. dmfs: 56 surfaces evaluated.
1. Primary molars: 8 × 5 surfaces each = 40.
2. Primary canines: 4 × 4 surfaces each = 16.

C. A primary molar or canine is presumed missing because of dental caries when it has been lost before the normal exfoliation time.

D. Each tooth is counted only once. When both dental caries and a restoration are present, the tooth or surface is listed as *d*, dental caries.

III. PROCEDURE

A. Instruments and examination are the same as for DMFT or DMFS (pages 309 and 310).

B. Criteria for dmft or dmfs

d = number of primary molars and canines or number of surfaces that are carious (*d*ecayed).

m = number of primary molars and canines *m*issing.

f = number of *f*illed primary molars and canines without caries (teeth or surfaces).

IV. SCORING

A. Individual dmf

A 10-year-old boy has all primary molars and canines present.
Examination reveals d = 2, m = 0, f = 1.

dmf = d + m + f = 2 + 0 + 1 = 3 dmf

B. Mixed Dentition

Permanent and primary teeth are evaluated separately. A DMFT or DMFS and a dmft and a dmfs are never added together.

TECHNICAL HINTS

I. Select an index or scoring method that best fits the needs of the situation or patient.

II. Calibrate criteria for each index used.

III. Implement an index at the beginning of an appointment series.

IV. Permit the patient to graph or chart the plaque or gingival index used and correlate the numeric values with the oral findings that may be seen.

V. Keep a continuing record, graph, or chart for index recording in the patient's permanent file for observation and review at each maintenance appointment.

FACTORS TO TEACH THE PATIENT

I. How an index is used and calculated and what the scores mean.

II. Correlation of index scores with current oral health practices and procedures.

III. Procedures to follow to improve index scores and bring the oral tissues to health.

REFERENCES

1. **Silness,** J. and Löe, H.: Periodontal Disease in Pregnancy. II. Correlation Between Oral Hygiene and Periodontal Condition, *Acta Odontol. Scand., 22,* 121, No. 1, 1964.

2. **Podshadley,** A.G. and Haley, J.V.: A Method for Evaluating Oral Hygiene Performance, *Public Health Rep., 83,* 259, March, 1968.

3. **Klein,** H., Palmer, C.E., and Knutson, J.W.: Studies on Dental Caries. I. Dental Status and Dental Needs of Elementary School Children, *Public Health Rep., 53,* 751, May 13, 1938.

4. **American Academy of Periodontology and American Dental Association:** *Periodontal Screening & Recording.* Sponsored by Procter & Gamble, June, 1992.

5. **Löe,** H.: The Gingival Index, the Plaque Index and the Retention Index Systems, *J. Periodontol., 38,* 610, November-December, 1967 (Part II).

6. **O'Leary,** T.J., Drake, R.B., and Naylor, J.E.: The Plaque Control Record, *J. Periodontol., 43,* 38, January, 1972.

7. **Ramfjord,** S.P. and Ash, M.M.: *Periodontology and Periodontics.* Philadelphia, W.B. Saunders Co., 1979, p. 273.

8. **Grant,** D.A., Stern, I.B., and Everett, F.G.: *Periodontics,* 5th ed. St. Louis, Mosby, 1979, pp. 529–531.

9. **Greene,** J.C. and Vermillion, J.R.: Oral Hygiene Index: A Method for Classifying Oral Hygiene Status, *J. Am. Dent. Assoc., 61,* 172, August, 1960.

10. **Waggener,** E.W.: Community Dentistry, in Steele, P.F., ed.: *Dimensions of Dental Hygiene,* 2nd ed. Philadelphia, Lea & Febiger, 1975, pp. 13–16.

11. **Greene,** J.C. and Vermillion, J.R.: The Simplified Oral Hygiene Index, *J. Am. Dent. Assoc., 68,* 7, January, 1964.

12. **Greene,** J.C.: The Oral Hygiene Index—Development and Uses, *J. Periodontol., 38,* 625, November-December, 1967 (Part II).

13. **Mühlemann,** H.R. and Son, S.: Gingival Sulcus Bleeding—A Leading Symptom in Initial Gingivitis, *Helv. Odontol. Acta, 15,* 107, October, 1971.

14. **Meitner,** S.W., Zander, H.A., Iker, H.P., and Polson, A.M.: Identification of Inflamed Gingival Surfaces, *J. Clin. Periodontol., 6,* 93, April, 1979.

15. **Carter,** H.G. and Barnes, G.P.: The Gingival Bleeding Index, *J. Periodontol., 45,* 801, November, 1974.

16. **Schour,** I. and Massler, M.: Prevalence of Gingivitis in Young Adults, *J. Dent. Res., 27,* 733, Abstract No. 33, December, 1948.

17. **Massler,** M.: The P-M-A Index for the Assessment of Gingivitis, *J. Periodontol., 38,* 592, November-December, 1967 (Part II).

18. **Löe,** H. and Silness, J.: Periodontal Disease in Pregnancy. I. Prevalence and Severity, *Acta Odontol. Scand., 21,* 533, No. 6, 1963.

19. **Russell,** A.L.: A System of Classification and Scoring for Prevalence Surveys of Periodontal Disease, *J. Dent. Res., 35,* 350, June, 1956.

20. **Russell,** A.L.: The Periodontal Index, *J. Periodontol., 38,* 585, November-December, 1967 (Part II).

21. **Ramfjord,** S.P.: Indices for Prevalence and Incidence of Periodontal Disease, *J. Periodontol., 30,* 51, January, 1959.

22. **Ramfjord,** S.P.: The Periodontal Disease Index (PDI), *J. Periodontol., 38,* 602, November-December, 1967 (Part II).

23. **Shick,** R.A. and Ash, M.M.: Evaluation of the Vertical Method of Toothbrushing, *J. Periodontol., 32,* 346, October, 1961.

24. **Fédération Dentaire Internationale:** A Simplified Periodontal Examination for Dental Practices, FDI WG6 and Joint FDI/WHO WG1, Fédération Dentaire Internationale, 64 Wimpole Street, London, WIM 8AL.

25. **Ainamo,** J., Barmes, D., Beagrie, G., Cutress, T., Martin, J., and Sardo-Infirri, J.: Development of the World Health Organization (WHO) Community Periodontal Index of Treatment Needs (CPITN), *Int. Dent. J., 32,* 281, September, 1982.

26. **Gruebbel,** A.O.: A Measurement of Dental Caries Prevalence and Treatment Service for Deciduous Teeth, *J. Dent. Res., 23,* 163, June, 1944.

SUGGESTED READINGS

Ainamo, J., Etemadzadeh, H., and Kallio, P.: Comparability and Discriminating Power of 4 Plaque Quantifications, *J. Clin. Periodontol., 20,* 244, April, 1993.

Blieden, T.M., Caton, J.G., Proskin, H.M., Stein, S.H., and Wagener, C.J.: Examiner Reliability for an Invasive Bleeding Index, *J. Clin. Periodontol., 19,* 262, April, 1992.

Blount, R.L. and Stokes, T.F.: A Comparison of the OHI-S and the PHP in an Oral Hygiene Program, *ASDC J. Dent. Child., 53,* 53, January-February, 1986.

Breur, M.M. and Cosgrove, R.S.: The Relationship Between Gingivitis and Plaque Levels, *J. Periodontol., 60,* 172, April, 1989.

Burt, B.A. and Eklund, S.A.: *Dentistry, Dental Practice, and the Community,* 4th ed. Philadelphia, W.B. Saunders Co., 1992, pp. 52–82.

Fischman, S., Cancro, L.P., Pretara-Spanedda, P., and Jacobs, D.: Distal Mesial Plaque Index. A Technique for Assessing Dental Plaque about the Gingiva, *Dent. Hygiene, 61,* 404, September, 1987.

Fischman, S.L.: Clinical Index Systems Used to Assess the Efficacy of Mouthrinses on Plaque and Gingivitis, *J. Clin. Periodontol., 15,* 506, September, 1988.

Galgut, P.N.: The Bleeding/Plaque Ratio in the Treatment of Periodontal Disease, *J. Clin. Periodontol., 15,* 606, November, 1988.

Isokangas, P., Alanen, P., and Tiekso, J.: The Clinician's Ability to Identify Caries Risk Subjects Without Saliva Tests—A Pilot Study, *Community Dent. Oral Epidemiol., 21,* 8, February, 1993.

Kallio, P., Ainamo, J., and Dusadeepan, A.: Self-assessment of Gingival Bleeding, *Int. Dent. J., 40,* 231, August, 1990.

Lobene, R.R., Mankodi, S.M., Ciancio, S.G., Lamm, R.A., Charles, C.H., and Ross, N.M.: Correlations Among Gingival Indices: A Methodology Study, *J. Periodontol., 60,* 159, March, 1989.

Marks, R.G., Magnusson, I., Taylor, M., Clouser, B., Maruniak, J., and Clark, W.B.: Evaluation of Reliability and Reproducibility of Dental Indices, *J. Clin. Periodontol., 20,* 54, January, 1993.

Palat, M., Gomez, C., Scherer, W., Hittelman, E., and LoPresti, J.: Indicators of Gingival Inflammation: The Gingival Index vs Sulcular Temperature Measurements, *J. Practical Hyg., 2,* 25, January/February, 1993.

Pendrys, D.G.: The Fluorosis Risk Index: A Method for Investigating Risk Factors, *J. Public Health Dent., 50,* 291, Fall, 1990.

Quirynen, M., Dekeyser, C., and van Steenberghe, D.: Discriminating Power of Five Plaque Indices, *J. Periodontol, 62,* 100, February, 1991.

Silness, J. and Røynstrand, T.: Partial Mouth Recording of Plaque, Gingivitis and Probing Depth in Adolescents, *J. Clin. Periodontol., 15,* 189, March, 1988.

Tal, H. and Rosenberg, M.: Estimation of Dental Plaque Levels and Gingival Inflammation Using a Simple Oral Rinse Technique, *J. Periodontol., 61,* 339, June, 1990.

Toevs, S.E. and Lukken, K.M.: Assessing Interproximal Gingival Health, *J. Dent. Hyg., 63,* 228, June, 1989.

Toevs, S.E. and Lukken, K.M.: Bleeding As An Indicator of Health or Disease. Clinical Application of this Parameter, *J. Dent. Hyg., 64,* 256, July-August, 1990.

Periodontal Disease Indices

Almas, K., Bulman, J.S., and Newman, H.N.: Assessment of Periodontal Status with CPITN and Conventional Periodontal Indices, *J. Clin. Periodontol., 18,* 654, October, 1991.

Barnes, G.P., Parker, W.A., Lyon, T.C., and Fultz, R.P.: Indices Used to Evaluate Signs, Symptoms and Etiologic Factors Associated with Diseases of the Periodontium, *J. Periodontol., 57,* 643, October, 1986.

Eaton, K.A. and Woodman, A.J.: Evaluation of Simple Periodontal Screening Technique Currently Used in the UK Armed Forces, *Community Dent. Oral Epidemiol., 17,* 190, August, 1989.

Gaengler, P., Goebel, G., Kurbad, A., and Kosa, W.: Assessment of Periodontal Disease and Dental Caries in a Population Survey Using the CPITN, GPM/T and DMF/T Indices, *Community Dent. Oral Epidemiol., 16,* 236, August, 1988.

Persson, R., Svendsen, J., and Daubert, K.: A Longitudinal Evaluation of Periodontal Therapy Using The CPITN Index, *J. Clin. Periodontol., 16,* 569, October, 1989.

Rams, T.E., Oler, J., Listgarten, M.A., and Slots, J.: Utility of Ramfjord Index Teeth to Assess Periodontal Disease Progression in Longitudinal Studies, *J. Clin. Periodontol., 20,* 147, February, 1993.

Sterrett, J.D., Hawkins, C.H., Pelletier, L., and Murphy, H.J.: The Use of Accurate Gingival Indices in Current Periodontal Literature, *Can. Dent. Hyg./Probe, 24,* 85, Summer, 1990.

Other Indices

Adams, R.A. and Nystrom, G.P.: A Periodontitis Severity Index, *J. Periodontol., 57,* 176, March, 1986.

Aherne, C.A., O'Mullane, D., and Barrett, B.E.: Indices of Root Surface Caries, *J. Dent. Res., 69,* 1222, May, 1990.

Caton, J.G. and Polson, A.M.: The Interdental Bleeding Index: A Simplified Procedure for Monitoring Gingival Health, *Compendium, 6,* 88, February, 1985.

Chosack, A.: A Dental Caries Severity Index for Primary Teeth, *Community Dent. Oral Epidemiol., 14,* 86, April, 1986.

Clarkson, J. and O'Mullane, D.: A Modified DDE Index for Use in Epidemiological Studies of Enamel Defects, *J. Dent. Res., 68,* 445, March, 1989.

Gourdon, A.M., Buyle-Bodin, Y., Woda, A., and Faraj, M.: Development of an Abrasion Index, *J. Prosthet Dent., 57,* 358, March, 1987.

Granath, L., Widenheim, J., and Birkhed, D.: Diagnosis of Mild Enamel Fluorosis in Permanent Maxillary Incisors Using Two Scoring Systems, *Community Dent. Oral Epidemiol., 13,* 273, October, 1985.

Horowitz, H.S., Driscoll, W.S., Meyers, R.J., Heifetz, S.B., and Kingman, A.: A New Method for Assessing the Prevalence of Dental Fluorosis—the Tooth Surface Index of Fluorosis, *J. Am. Dent. Assoc., 109,* 37, July, 1984.

Horowitz, H.S.: Indexes for Measuring Dental Fluorosis, *J. Public Health Dent., 46,* 179, Fall, 1986.

Katz, R.V.: Assessing Root Caries in Populations: The Evolution of the Root Caries Index, *J. Public Health Dent., 40,* 7, Winter, 1980.

Katz, R.V.: Development of an Index for the Prevalence of Root Caries, *J. Dent. Res., 63,* 814, Special Issue, May, 1984.

Koch, A.L., Gershen, J.A., and Marcus, M.: A Children's Oral Health Status Index Based on Dentists' Judgment, *J. Am. Dent. Assoc., 110,* 36, January, 1985.

Lobene, R.R., Weatherford, T., Ross, N.M., Lamn, R.A., and Menaker, L.: A Modified Gingival Index for Use in Clinical Trials, *Clin. Prev. Dent., 8,* 3, January-February, 1986.

Marcus, M., Koch, A.L., and Gershen, J.A.: A Proposed Index of Oral Health Status: A Practical Application, *J. Am. Dent. Assoc., 107,* 729, November, 1983.

Massler, M. and Schour, I.: The P-M-A Index of Gingivitis, *J. Dent. Res., 28,* 634, Abstract No. 7, December, 1949.

Nowicki, D., Vogel, R.I., Melcer, S., and Deasy, M.J.: The Gingival Bleeding Time Index, *J. Periodontol., 52,* 260, May, 1981.

Øilo, G., Dahl, B.L., Hatle, G., and Gad, A.-L.: An Index for Evaluating Wear of Teeth, *Acta Odontol. Scand., 45,* 361, No. 5, 1987.

Quigley, G.A. and Hein, J.W.: Comparative Cleansing Efficiency of Manual and Power Brushing, *J. Am. Dent. Assoc., 65,* 26, July, 1962.

Shaw, L. and Murray, J.J.: A New Index for Measuring Extrinsic Stain in Clinical Trials, *Community Dent. Oral Epidemiol., 5,* 116, May, 1977.

Silberman, S.L., Trubman, A., Duncan, W.K., and Meydrech, E.F.: A Simplified Hypoplasia Index, *J. Public Health Dent., 50,* 282, Summer, 1990.

Smith, B.G.N. and Knight, J.K.: An Index for Measuring the Wear of Teeth, *Br. Dent. J., 156,* 435, June 23, 1984.

20

Records and Charting

Patient health records provide a means of communication between the members of the health team themselves, as well as with their patients. Coordinated planning and continuity of care can be facilitated. The records serve as a basis for the evaluation of the quality of care and aid when a review is made of the effectiveness of patient care practices. Data from health records are utilized in research and education.

Comprehensive health histories, informed consent forms, and accurate documentation are essential to a safe, thorough, and caring practice. They are both business and legal documents for protection of health-care workers.

Complete and accurate examinations with proper documentation by records and chartings are basic to all patient care. All findings of the diagnostic work-up are recorded. Some systems of recording involve the completion of forms with topics and spaces to check or fill in the information, whereas others call for a prose-style summary.

Radiographs, study casts, photographs, and all other materials collected during the initial examination and during continuing patient appointments are official parts of the permanent records. Each part must be dated.

A filing system with ready accessibility to the health records by authorized personnel only is needed. The privacy of records must be maintained.

Computerized systems have many advantages for integration of the records into the total practice. Appointment schedules, medical alerts, and financial aspects all can be part of the data management by the computer.

I. PURPOSES FOR CHARTING

The purpose of each type of charting is defined by its title: the dental charting includes diagrammatic representation of existing conditions of the teeth, whereas the periodontal charting indicates clinical features of the periodontium. Separate types of chart forms may be used to record the special features of each, or the two may be combined on one chart. Neatness in the markings of symbols, drawings, and labels goes hand in hand with the accuracy of the examination itself.

An accurate, detailed, and carefully recorded charting is used as follows:

A. For Treatment Planning
The charting is a graphic representation of the existing condition of the patient's teeth and periodontium from which needed treatment procedures can be organized into a treatment plan.

B. For Counseling Treatment
During dental and dental hygiene appointments, the charting is useful for guiding specific procedures.

C. For Evaluation
The outcome and degree of lasting effects of treatment are determined by comparing the findings of the initially recorded examination with periodic follow-up examinations.

D. For Protection
In the event of misunderstanding by a patient, or if legal questions should arise, the records and chartings are realistic evidence.

E. For Identification
In the event of emergency, accident, or disaster, a patient may be identified by the teeth for which a record has been maintained.

H. Chart tooth sensitivity. The patient may report hypersensitive areas, or they may be discovered during instrumentation. Record the tooth number and surface for reference during the treatment phase.

TECHNICAL HINTS

I. Use a record form with adequate space for recording details.

II. Prepare permanent records in ink.

III. Use abbreviations and symbols only if their meaning is clear to all who read them.

IV. Check that all records are complete, accurate, clearly stated, readable, and neat.

V. Plan appointments, when possible, in order that radiographs and study casts will be available prior to and at the time of clinical charting. When the medical and dental history and the extraoral and intraoral examinations can be completed in advance, time can be saved. Necessary consultations with a patient's physician, preparation with premedication when indicated for the patient susceptible to bacteremia, or other special adaptation can be made.

FACTORS TO TEACH THE PATIENT

I. Interpretation of all recordings; meaning of all numbers used, such as for probing depths.

II. The importance of making a complete study of the patient's oral problems before beginning treatment.

III. Advantages of cooperation and patience in furnishing information that will help dental personnel to interpret observations accurately so that the correct diagnosis and appropriate treatment plan can be made.

IV. Assurance that all information received is completely confidential, and that the records are locked when the office is closed.

SUGGESTED READINGS

Allen, D.L., McFall, W.T., and Jenzano, J.W.: *Periodontics for the Dental Hygienist,* 4th ed. Philadelphia, Lea & Febiger, 1987, pp. 99–135.

Benedon, R.M.: Comprehensive Charting and Follow-up of the Periodontally Involved Patient, *Compendium, 9,* 339, April, 1988.

Carranza, F.A.: *Glickman's Clinical Periodontology,* 7th ed. Philadelphia, W.B. Saunders Co., 1990, pp. 481–500.

Ehrlich, A. and Torres, H.O.: *Essentials of Dental Assisting.* Philadelphia, W.B. Saunders Co., 1992, pp. 221–235.

Eubanks, S.: The Dental Assistant's Role in Risk Management. Patient Records, *Dent. Assist., 61,* 18, Second Quarter, 1992.

Grant, D.A., Stern, I.B., and Listgarten, M.A., eds.: *Periodontics,* 6th ed. St. Louis, Mosby, 1988, pp. 537–559.

Keselyak, N. and Maschak, L.: The Problem-oriented Dental Record: A Key to Dental Hygiene Treatment Planning and the Problem-Solving Model for Dental Hygiene Practice, *Can. Dent. Hyg./Probe, 27,* 15, January/February, 1993.

Stach, D.J.: The Complete Dental Record, in Woodall, I.R.: *Comprehensive Dental Hygiene Care,* 4th ed. St. Louis, Mosby, 1993, pp. 70–77.

Forensic Identification

Beale, D.R.: The Importance of Dental Records for Identification, *N.Z. Dent. J., 87,* 84, July, 1991.

Clark, D.H., ed.: *Practical Forensic Odontology.* Oxford, Wright, 1992, pp. 101–109 (Dental Record Interpretation).

O'Reilly, P.: An Overview of Forensic Dentistry, *Clin. Prev. Dent., 8,* 16, January-February, 1986.

Parker, L.S.: Dental Detectives, *RDH, 10,* 14, February, 1990.

The Dental Hygiene Treatment Plan

The information about the patient is organized into the dental hygiene *assessment, diagnosis, prognosis,* and *treatment plan*. Terms and key words used in conjunction with these steps are defined in table 21–1.

I. ASSESSMENT
In the dental hygiene process, assessment includes the gathering of details of the health status of the patient, the analysis and synthesis of that data, and the application of clinical judgment to arrive at a dental hygiene diagnosis. Assessment procedures have been described in Chapters 6 through 20.

II. DENTAL HYGIENE DIAGNOSIS
The dental hygiene diagnosis is based on the patient's problem. A part of the patient's problem relates to the ''chief complaint'' determined during the interview in conjunction with the patient's health histories. Another part of the patient's problem is determined by the clinician during the oral examination. Clinical findings can reveal symptoms that have not been apparent to the patient.

The fundamental parts of the dental hygiene diagnosis are the *problem,* the *cause of the problem,* and the *signs and symptoms* present. Such evidence provides direction for a plan of dental hygiene intervention consisting of patient counseling and direct clinical care.

The dental hygiene diagnosis excludes interventions that require surgery, prescription drugs, or other modes of treatment that are legally defined as dental practice.

III. DENTAL HYGIENE PROGNOSIS
The dental hygiene prognosis is a look ahead to an anticipated outcome. By using information from the assessment, an intervention can be selected with the intent to reverse the patient's problem toward health, or at least to alter the situation in a manner that, with time and continued care, can result in a state of optimum health.

Prognosis in a total treatment plan consists of an overall prognosis with reference to the entire dentition and a separate prognosis for the individual teeth.

The patient may use the prognosis to decide between proposed alternate treatment plans; the insurance company may use the prognosis as the basis on which decisions are made regarding payment for services; and the restorative dentist and periodontist use the prognosis to determine the most effective treatment plan for the existing periodontium and teeth.

IV. DENTAL HYGIENE TREATMENT PLAN
A sequential plan for treatment names those dental hygiene procedures to be carried out within the patient's total treatment plan. Except for emergency care, the dental hygiene treatment logically precedes other phases of treatment.

One primary objective of dental hygiene therapy is health of the gingival tissues. The success of restorative, prosthetic, orthodontic, and other specialty dentistry depends on obtaining and maintaining soft tissue health. The dental hygiene treatment plan has a major influence on the future oral health of the patient.

PREPARATION OF THE TREATMENT PLAN

I. OBJECTIVES
The objectives of a treatment sequence are:

A. To Eliminate and Control Etiologic and Predisposing Disease Factors
The principal etiologic agents in both dental car-

TABLE 21-1
KEY WORDS: DENTAL HYGIENE
TREATMENT PLAN

Assessment (ah-ses'ment): the critical analysis and valuation or judgment of the status or quality of a particular condition, situation, or other subject of appraisal.

Chief complaint: the patient's concern as stated during the initial health history preparation; may be the reason for seeking professional care; the complaint may require emergency dental diagnosis, such as pain or discomfort.

Consent: voluntary agreement with an action proposed by another.

   Informed consent: a patient's voluntary agreement to a treatment plan after details of the proposed treatment have been presented and comprehended by the patient.

Definitive care: complete care; end point where all treatment required at that time has been completed.

Dental hygiene diagnosis: identification of an existing or potential oral health problem that a dental hygienist is qualified and licensed to treat.

Diagnosis (di'ag-no'sis): identification of a disease or deviation from normal condition by recognition of characteristic signs and symptoms.

Differential diagnosis: determination of which one of several diseases or conditions may be producing the symptoms.

Intervention: to happen or take place between other events; to intervene, as with a specific treatment.

Prognosis (prog-no'sis): prediction of outcome; a forecast of the probable course and outcome of an attack of disease and the prospects of recovery as expected by the nature of the specific condition and the symptoms of the case.

Total treatment plan: sequential outline of the essential services and procedures that must be carried out by the dentist, the dental hygienist, and the patient to eliminate disease and restore the oral cavity to health and normal function.

   Dental hygiene treatment plan: the services within the framework of the total treatment plan to be carried out by the dental hygienist.

ies and periodontal and gingival diseases are the microorganisms of bacterial plaque. The goal should be to control the etiologic agent and, thus, to prevent future recurrences of the same conditions.

B. To Eliminate the Signs and Symptoms of Disease

Treatment planning includes measures to eliminate signs of disease, such as carious lesions, inflammation, and periodontal pockets.

C. To Restore Normal Function

This includes occlusal adjustment, restoration of teeth, replacement of missing teeth, orthodontic tooth movement, and periodontal surgical needs.

D. To Maintain Health and Prevent the Recurrence of Disease

Methods used are counseling and supervision of the patient in daily self-care and provision of regular follow-up professional supervision and care.

II. PARTS OF A TOTAL TREATMENT PLAN

A total treatment plan usually involves several interdependent areas of oral care based on an individual patient's diagnosis and disease symptoms. Divisions for a treatment plan are listed below with examples of services included in each.

A. Priority Treatment

1. Emergency care for pain or other acute condition.
2. Such procedures as biopsy of a lesion found during the extraoral and intraoral examinations, or a laboratory test for a suspected systemic condition.

B. Preventive Phase

1. Mechanisms to arrest and reverse oral diseases in the early stages.
2. Procedures for the patient's daily self-care, including microbial plaque control.
3. Introduction to self-applied fluoride.

C. Preparatory Phase

1. Initial (Phase 1) periodontal therapy includes disease control procedures performed by the patient, and professional complete scaling and root planing.
2. Dental caries may be treated initially by excavation of large carious lesions; placement of sedative temporary fillings; pulp treatment as indicated.
3. Endodontic therapy.
4. Preparation for oral surgery includes plaque control and scaling to reduce the bacterial count and inflammation.
5. Removal of hopeless teeth that cannot be successfully treated.

D. Treatment Phase

1. Gingival and periodontal treatment, including elimination of inflammation and pockets; surgical procedures; occlusal adjustment.
2. Restorative treatment.
3. Prosthetic treatment.
4. Orthodontic treatment.
5. Tissue maintenance during therapy (page 322).

E. Maintenance Phase.

1. Patient is instructed in specific daily plaque control and other preventive measures.
2. Professional appointments at designated intervals.
   a. Complete re-evaluation and updating of records, including all parts of the diagnostic work-up.

b. Maintenance treatment plan may include any service as a continuation, supplement, or addition to previous preventive, educational, or therapeutic measures. The maintenance appointment is described on pages 599 and 600.

PLANNING THE DENTAL HYGIENE TREATMENT PLAN

The dental hygienist's objective is to prepare a flexible, realistic dental hygiene plan and sequence of procedures based on the plan for total care of the patient. As described on page 3, a dental hygienist's services may be divided into preventive, educational, and therapeutic, all of which are applicable at various levels in the total treatment plan. Services to be performed depend on state or area practice acts, and any examples cited here are not intended to represent a specific location.

An objective in planning dental hygiene care is to ensure the best possible sequence of procedures that will contribute to the restoration of the patient's oral health in the shortest possible time and will pave the way to the long-range preventive program that will continue throughout the patient's lifetime. To achieve the goals of planned care, the dental hygienist must see the dental hygiene aspects within the total plan for the patient and contribute to the overall continuity of the corrective and maintenance phases.

I. CHARACTERISTICS OF A WELL-PLANNED TREATMENT PLAN
An effective plan
A. Adapts to the needs of the patient's oral condition.
B. Is orderly in sequence to allow for thoroughness in each procedure and to prevent duplication or repetition of efforts.
C. Includes purposefully selected procedures that are
1. Planned with a reasonable degree of predictability of outcome.
2. Expected to resolve the condition and reach an optimum result in a minimum of time.
3. Projected toward a state of health the patient can maintain with self-care procedures.
D. Adaptable to continuing long-term care.

II. RECORD AND EXPLAIN
The treatment plan is included in the patient's record. The patient or a parent of a young or mentally disabled patient must understand the treatment plan and be aware of the expected outcome of each appointment, as well as of the total series. The role of the patient in treatment through self-care on a daily basis must be written into the treatment plan and explained to the patient.

STEPS IN PLANNING

I. OBJECTIVES
A. Review the patient's oral problems as described in the diagnosis and total treatment plan.
B. Identify objectives that may be attained.
1. Overall objectives of the total treatment and anticipated state of oral health after treatment.
2. Dental hygiene goals, both short-term and long-term.

II. SERVICES
Preventive, educational, preparatory, and treatment procedures are selected that can be expected to meet the objectives. The services to be performed for each phase of the total treatment plan are listed in sequence for the appointment series, and time requirements for each phase are estimated and recorded.

Examples are given here for each phase of the treatment plan.

A. Preventive
A typical program includes bacterial plaque control measures, self-applied and professionally applied fluorides, diet counseling, and pit and fissure sealants.

B. Preparatory
Complete scaling and root planing may be the major services to prepare a patient for periodontal surgery. *Preparatory* treatment is in contrast to *definitive* treatment, which means the complete treatment needed by a patient to bring the oral tissues to a state of health at that time.

C. Treatment
1. *Periodontal.* Scaling and root planing that are preparatory for one patient may be the definitive and curative treatment for another patient.
2. *Periodontal Post-surgical Procedures.* Suture removal, removal and replacement of periodontal dressings, and other postoperative care and instruction are parts of the patient's treatment plan that may be performed by the dental hygienist.
3. *Restorative.* Finishing and polishing of restorations should be followed by a topical fluoride application to promote remineralization of the enamel that has been highly polished adjacent to the restoration.

D. Tissue Maintenance During Long-term Therapy
When restorative, prosthetic, orthodontic, or other treatment continues over a long period, appointments are needed for gingival reassessment, supervision of plaque control measures, calculus removal, topical fluoride applications, and other procedures specific for the patient.

III. CRITERIA FOR DETERMINATION OF SEQUENCE

Suggested treatment patterns by case type are shown in figure 21–1. Sequence planning involves first the identification of the overall treatment pattern and then an outline of a series of appointments with the specific services to be included.

The next step is to sequence the order in which the parts of an individual appointment are to be carried out. The sequence is influenced by numerous factors, including urgency of treatment, need for treating etiologic factors first, the severity and extent of the condition, and certain special patient requirements. These factors are described here with examples.

A. Urgency

When discomfort or pain is present, the area involved requires first attention. In the dental hygiene treatment plan, this could apply to an area of the gingiva that is particularly difficult to clean because of inaccessibility. Either specially adapted plaque control instruction or scaling may be needed.

B. Etiologic Factors Should Be Treated First

The factors that caused or contributed to the development of the existing condition must be arrested and controlled. In patients with gingival or periodontal infections, the continued success of treatment depends on the removal of bacterial plaque.

Infection can recur when daily control measures for the removal of the etiologic agent, plaque, are not carried out. New dental caries also can develop unless continued attention is paid to preventive measures.

Pellicle forms within minutes after a tooth surface has been completely cleaned, and disclosable plaque is present within 24 hours or less. Therefore, plaque control measures must be introduced in the treatment plan before scaling or root planing.

C. Special Patient Requirements (Items from the Patient History)

1. *Antibiotic Premedication.* A list of conditions that require antibiotic premedication appears on pages 102 and 103. For patients who need antibiotics, all instrumentation, including the examination procedures that require use of instruments (probing, exploring), as well as tooth movement for mobility determination, must be done under antibiotic coverage.

   Bacteremias have been demonstrated during brushing, flossing, and other disease control measures. Instruction and practice of the plaque-removing procedures must be carried out while the patient is premedicated.

   Appointments must be planned and conducted efficiently to prevent the need for un-necessary premedication. When a patient's physical health and strength do not contraindicate, appointments that are longer than customary may be reserved so that more can be accomplished.

2. *Systemic Diseases.* Chronic disease or physical disability may influence the content or length of appointments.

D. Severity and Extent of the Condition

Findings that indicate the severity of gingival or periodontal infection include changes in color, size, shape, consistency, and bleeding of the gingiva, probing depths, mobility of teeth, and radiographic signs. To determine the length of appointments and sequence of procedures, consideration is given necessarily to probing depths in relation to the distribution of dental calculus. The number of appointments and the length of appointments increase with severity.

A suggested division of conditions graded by the severity of infection follows.

1. *Moderate to Severe Periodontal Disease.* For the patient who requires complicated periodontal, restorative, and prosthetic treatment, the dental hygiene treatment plan includes preventive and preparatory procedures, as well as maintenance during therapy, postsurgical care, and follow-up.

2. *Moderate or Slight Periodontal Disease.* The dental hygiene treatment plan includes the preventive phase and complete scaling and planing. This treatment may be definitive, or the follow-up evaluation may show the need for surgical or other additional treatment.

3. *Gingivitis with Supra- and Subgingival Calculus.* The preventive phase and complete scaling are indicated. The treatment may be definitive.

4. *Gingivitis with Slight Supragingival Calculus or No Calculus.* Dental hygiene services usually constitute the definitive treatment. To eliminate gingival inflammation, bacterial debridement, and plaque control measures may be the total treatment, which is supplemented by scaling when calculus is present.

INDIVIDUAL APPOINTMENT SEQUENCE

I. EVALUATION

Each appointment starts with an evaluation of the gingival tissues.

A. Previously Treated Area

The area is examined for progress toward health, the signs of inflammation that may still be present, and indications for additional treatment that is needed.

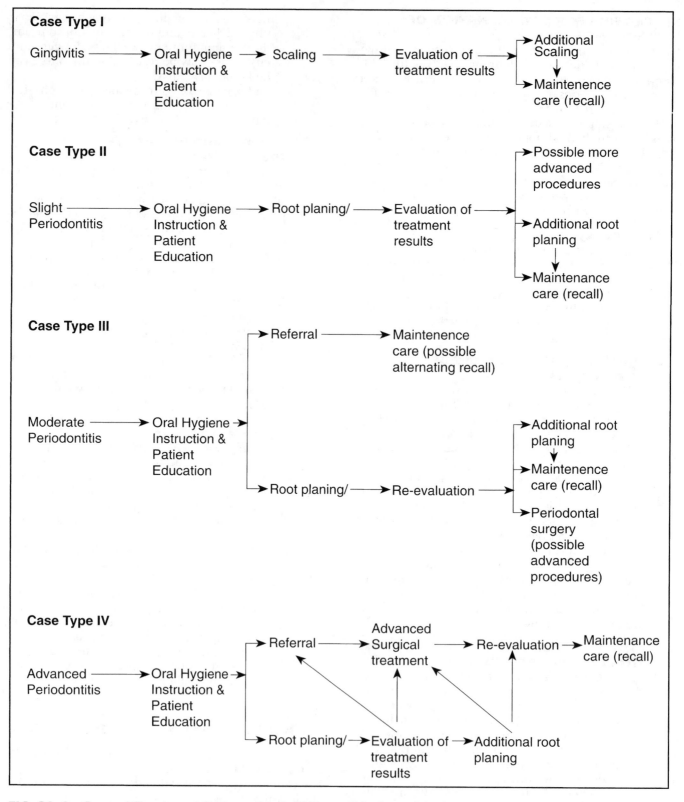

FIG. 21–1. General Treatment Patterns by Case Type. Flowcharts show suggested treatment programs for the four basic case types from gingivitis to advanced periodontitis. Note that the first step in all programs is patient instruction. (Adapted from Karch, J.D.: Diagnosing and Managing the Periodontal Patient, *Risk Management Series*, p. 19. Copyright 1986, American Dental Association. Reprinted and adapted by permission.)

B. Effects of Plaque Control Measures

The self-treatment by the patient is evaluated. After the color, size, shape, consistency, and other characteristics of the gingiva are observed, a disclosing agent is used to evaluate the degree of plaque present on the teeth. This evaluates the patient's techniques and thoroughness in plaque removal.

II. INSTRUCTION FOR DISEASE CONTROL

Instruction begins when evaluation starts, and continues throughout. Specific procedures for the use of plaque removal devices, such as toothbrush, floss, or other aid, are presented before instrumentation or other professional clinical services are performed. The reasons for this sequence are presented on page 414.

III. TISSUE CONDITIONING

Preparation or conditioning of the gingival tissue for scaling can be of particular importance when there is spongy, soft tissue that bleeds on slight provocation, and when the area is generally septic from plaque, materia alba, and debris accumulation.

Tissue conditioning is accomplished by initiating plaque control procedures and prescribing a concentrated daily program of plaque removal and hot saltwater rinsing. A quadrant that needs tissue conditioning is not selected for scaling until gingival healing and patient cooperation have been demonstrated.

Anticipated outcomes of such a program include:

A. Gingival Healing

The tissue becomes less edematous, bleeding is minimized, and scaling procedures are facilitated.

B. General Oral Cleanliness with Lowered Bacterial Accumulation

There is less likelihood that bacteremias will be produced during scaling, and there is less contamination in aerosols produced.

C. Learning by the Patient

The patient can practice and see benefits of plaque removal.

IV. CLINICAL SERVICES

The questions of which area or quadrant should be scaled first and in which order the other areas and quadrants should follow can be answered for most patients by considering the following order of choices:

A. Patient Selection

When the patient indicates an area of discomfort, that area may be treated first.

B. Apprehensive Patient

To make the first scaling less complicated and to help orient the patient to the procedures to be followed, either the quadrant with the fewest teeth or the quadrant with the least severe periodontal infection can be selected.

C. When Two Quadrants Are To Be Treated at the Same Appointment

Select a maxillary and mandibular of the same side.

SAMPLE DENTAL HYGIENE TREATMENT PLAN

A presentation of sample treatment plans is impossible for each of the wide variety of patient problems or combinations of problems encountered in practice. Each patient must be handled individually.

Examples of treatment sequences and plans are found in special areas of this book. An outline for maintenance appointments can be found on pages 599 and 600, and a treatment sequence for a patient with necrotizing ulcerative gingivitis is found on pages 540 and 541.

The diagnostic work-up for the patient whose dental hygiene treatment plan is sketched as follows was completed by the dental hygienist. The original diagnosis was generalized moderate periodontal disease. The preliminary total treatment plan included occlusal adjustment, restorative procedures, and the prosthetic replacement of two missing teeth. No emergency measures were required. None of the periodontal surgery or dental treatment was started until the dental hygiene preventive and preparatory appointments were completed and the patient's mouth was re-evaluated.

The examinations revealed slight localized supragingival calculus and generalized moderate-to-heavy subgingival calculus. Because the patient had enlarged, spongy marginal gingiva with generalized bleeding on probing and plaque on the cervical thirds of most teeth, scaling was not started on the first appointment. The importance of tissue conditioning was described in the previous section, and the rationale for introducing plaque control before scaling is described on page 414.

More detail is included in the treatment plan recorded below than probably would be written in practice. Abbreviations used must be recognized by all personnel involved in using the patient's record. For example, "Plaque I," "Plaque II," "Plaque III" might be sufficient notation for the plaque control instruction series.

APPOINTMENT I
1. Complete assessment procedures.
2. Record plaque or bleeding scores (pages 291–295, 299 and 300).
3. Give disease control instruction (*First Lesson*, page 414).
4. Introduce self-applied fluoride program.
   a. Discuss dentifrice recommendation.
   b. Explain the need for frequent brushing to gain most benefit from fluoride in dentifrice.
   c. Demonstrate use of fluoride mouthrinse.

APPOINTMENT II
1. Evaluate disease control with the patient.
   a. Assess gingival tissue (table 11–2, pages 188 and 189).
   b. Record indices.
2. Give instruction (*Second Lesson*, page 416).
3. Perform scaling
   a. First quadrant scaling and root planing with anesthesia.
   b. Postoperative instructions.

APPOINTMENT III
1. Evaluate
   a. Assess gingival tissue; record bleeding index.
   b. Examine first quadrant scaled; note healing. Explore to check for residual calculus.
   c. Evaluate plaque. Disclose for Plaque Index.
2. Instruction (*Third Lesson*, page 416).
3. Perform scaling and root planing
   a. Complete first quadrant when residual calculus is found.
   b. Second quadrant scaling with anesthesia.

APPOINTMENT IV
1. Evaluate
   a. Assess gingival tissue.
   b. Record bleeding or other indices.
   c. Examine previously scaled quadrants; explore for residual calculus.
   d. Evaluate plaque.
2. Give instruction: continue as needed.
3. Perform scaling and root planing.
   a. Complete first and second quadrants.
   b. Third quadrant scaling with anesthesia.

APPOINTMENT V
The same basic structure is followed as outlined for Appointments III and IV. Each time the previously treated quadrants must be checked and completed. Each time the instruction is continued if the patient is still not accomplishing infection control. The fourth quadrant is scaled under anesthesia.

APPOINTMENT VI
1. Evaluate four quadrants; determine probing depths compared with initial record.
2. Evaluate need for stain removal. Scaling, planing, and the patient's daily therapeutic plaque removal often remove stains so that stain removal will be highly selective.
3. Re-evaluate for periodontal referral when necessary; plan for the next phase of appointments when patient is ready as shown by the health of the gingival tissue.

APPOINTMENT VII: Maintenance During Therapy
When the restorative and prosthetic treatment extends over a period of time, periodic appointments are needed for monitoring the continued success of the patient's self-care. A gingival tissue assessment, checks with a probe to determine bleeding, plaque checks with disclosing agents, additional instruction, particularly for the care of newly fixed or removable prosthetic appliances, and motivational encouragement are essential.

APPOINTMENT VIII: Maintenance
Frequency of maintenance appointments is determined. Components of the maintenance appointment are described on pages 599 and 600.

INFORMED CONSENT

Informed consent means that the patient has been informed about the nature of the oral condition and the treatment needed, and that the patient has consented to follow the recommendations made. In other words, informed consent is the permission granted by the patient, or the patient's parent or guardian, for the professional person to proceed. Each state has its own law on this subject.

Suggested forms are available, and each dental office or clinic needs printed forms with the official name and address heading.[1,2] The forms are used with duplicate or triplicate copies so that the file, the patient, and any other required specialist can maintain a copy.

Prior to obtaining the signature on the form, the patient should receive information about the following:
   I. The health problem and its need for treatment.
   II. The diagnosis and a description of the severity, extent, and possible outcome if treatment is not done.
   III. The recommended treatment and any risks involved; optional therapy and its outcome and risks.
   IV. The responsibilities of the patient relative to supplementary personal care and follow-up.
   V. Expected outcomes.
   VI. Appointments needed and financial arrangements.

TECHNICAL HINTS

   I. Treatment plans for minors or mentally disabled patients should be discussed with the parent or guardian. Permission should be obtained by signature, particularly when anesthesia must be used or prescriptions issued.
   II. Complete records are essential. Misunderstandings can lead to legal involvements.
   III. When practice acts require that the dentist administer the anesthesia for the dental hygiene patient, record the time of the patient's appointment on the dentist's daily schedule.

FACTORS TO TEACH THE PATIENT

I. Why a treatment plan is made.

II. Explanation of unclear parts of the total treatment plan.

III. Parts of the treatment plan carried out by the patient. Interrelation of roles of patient and members of the dental team in eliminating the patient's oral infection.

IV. The long-term effects of comprehensive continuing care.

V. Why infection control measures must be learned before, and in conjunction with, scaling.

VI. Significance of the indices as guides for evaluating the health of the gingiva.

VII. What presurgical preparation means, what it consists of, and what its expected advantages are.

REFERENCES

1. **Robbins,** K.S.: Medical-legal Considerations, in Malamed, S.F.: *Handbook of Medical Emergencies in the Dental Office,* 4th ed. St. Louis, Mosby, 1993, pp. 91–101.

2. **Bailey,** B.L.: Informed Consent in Dentistry, *J. Am. Dent. Assoc., 110,* 709, May, 1985.

SUGGESTED READINGS

Coleman, G.C.: Dental Treatment Planning, in Coleman, G.C. and Nelson, J.: *Principles of Oral Diagnosis.* St. Louis, Mosby, 1993, pp. 219–248.

Fisher, E.T.: General Dentist and Periodontist Working Together, *Compendium, 11,* 454, July, 1990.

Genco, R.J., Goldman, H.M., and Cohen, D.W., eds.: *Contemporary Periodontics.* St. Louis, Mosby, 1990, pp. 348–359.

Grant, D.A., Stern, I.B., and Listgarten, M.A., eds.: *Periodontics,* 6th ed. St. Louis, Mosby, 1988, pp. 592–608.

Levine, R.A.: A Patient-centered Periodontal Program for the 1990s, Part I, *Compendium, 11,* 222, April, 1990; Part II, page 274, May, 1990.

McCullough, C.: Diagnosis and Treatment Planning, *Access, 7,* 26, April, 1993.

McGuire, M.K.: Prognosis Versus Actual Outcome: A Long-term Survey of 100 Treated Periodontal Patients Under Maintenance Care, *J. Periodontol., 62,* 51, January, 1991.

Miller, S.S.: Dental Hygiene Diagnosis, *RDH, 2,* 46, July-August, 1982.

Pattison, A.M. and Pattison, G.L.: *Periodontal Instrumentation,* 2nd ed. Norwalk, CT, Appleton & Lange, 1992, pp. 329–335.

Informed Consent

American Academy of Periodontology: *Informed Consent for Surgical Periodontics.* Chicago, American Academy of Periodontology, 1992.

Gild, W.M.: Informed Consent: A Review, *Anesth. Analg., 68,* 649, May, 1989.

Litch, C.S. and Liggett, M.L.: Consent for Dental Therapy in Severely Ill Patients, *J. Dent. Educ., 56,* 298, May, 1992.

Odom, J.G., Odom, S.S., and Jolly, D.E.: Informed Consent and the Geriatric Dental Patient, *Spec. Care Dentist., 12,* 202, September/October, 1992.

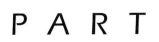

P A R T   **IV**

Prevention

INTRODUCTION

This section, *Prevention*, includes procedures for bacterial disease control, use of fluorides, application of pit and fissure sealants, diet counseling, and all related preventive measures. In planning the sequence of treatment for the patient, initiation of preventive measures precedes dental and dental hygiene clinical services except in an emergency.

Dental caries and periodontal infections are caused by microorganisms of bacterial plaque. The long-range success of professional treatment is limited unless the causes of the condition, namely the microorganisms, are eliminated or brought to a controllable level.

Preventive dentistry is the sum total of the efforts to promote, restore, and maintain the oral health of the individual. Primary prevention, which involves measures to prevent disease completely, and secondary prevention, which relates to early recognition and treatment of incipient illnesses, were described on page 3 in Chapter 1. Tertiary preventive measures go even farther and are represented in the more complex dental and periodontal therapy, even to the extent of replacement of missing teeth. Prevention is still involved as long as complete breakdown and loss of function are prevented.

SELF-CLEANSING MECHANISMS

The teeth, by their anatomy, alignment, and occlusion, function with the gingiva, tongue, cheeks, and saliva in a relationship called the self-cleansing mechanism of the oral cavity. A review of the natural self-cleansing mechanisms during and following mastication is included here as an introduction to the mechanical and other self-care preventive methods covered in the next few chapters.

The following steps are described for food particles, but the same processes apply to any substances that enter the mouth and influence oral cleanliness and the formation of deposits on the teeth.

I. FOOD ENTERS THE MOUTH
Food is carried by the tongue, assisted by the lips and cheeks, to the occlusal surfaces for grinding.
   A. Salivary flow increases as a result of sensory reflex stimulation.
   B. Saliva begins lubrication of food and oral tissues.

II. THE TEETH ARE BROUGHT TOGETHER FOR CHEWING
The food moves over the occlusal surfaces.
   A. Marginal ridges tend to force particles toward occlusal surfaces, away from the proximal region.
   B. Contact areas prevent interdental entrance.

III. FOOD IS FORCED OUT BY PRESSURE OF BITE
Food passes over the smooth facial and lingual surfaces.
   A. Embrasures provide spillways for the escape of particles.
   B. Cervical enamel ridges deflect particles away from the free gingiva onto the attached gingiva.
   C. Gingival crest prevents retention of particles by its position at a point below the height of contour of the cervical enamel ridge, by its knife-edge shape, and by its close adherence to the tooth surface.
   D. Interdental papilla fills the interproximal area and prevents particles from entering.

IV. FOOD PARTICLES ARE BROUGHT BACK BY THE TONGUE TO THE OCCLUSAL SURFACES FOR ADDITIONAL CHEWING
The process is repeated until the food is ready for swallowing.
   A. Salivary flow continues to be stimulated by repeated masticatory movements.
   B. Saliva moistens food and oral mucosa and thus reduces the adhering capacity of the food.

V. FOOD PARTICLES REMAINING ON THE TEETH ARE REMOVED
   A. Tip of tongue explores and attempts to dislodge remaining particles.
   B. Lips and cheeks in conjunction with tongue aid in natural rinsing process by forcing saliva over and between the teeth.
   C. Saliva continues to flow in increased amounts during rinsing and swallowing of particles, then gradually returns to its normal flow.

STEPS IN A PREVENTIVE PROGRAM

A *program for prevention* is composed of the cooperative steps taken by the patient and members of the dental team to preserve the natural dentition and the supporting structures by preventing the onset, progress, and recurrence of oral diseases and other destructive or disfiguring conditions.

Each patient needs a *preventive treatment plan*. Planning and carrying out the preventive program may be divided into the six basic steps reviewed in this section. Details to describe each step either were part of the diagnostic work-up described in previous chapters or will be parts of the chapters to follow.

I. ASSESS PATIENT'S NEEDS: FORMULATE THE DENTAL HYGIENE DIAGNOSIS
   A. Review all information from the history, examinations, radiographs, chartings.
   B. Identify the presence and severity of infection and predisposing factors.
   C. Utilize indices to rate the extent of the needs and provide a baseline for continuing comparisons.

II. PLAN FOR INTERVENTION

A. Apply information about the patient, such as educational level, occupation, socioeconomic background, and attitudes toward oral health.
B. Recognize the influence of physical or mental disabilities.
C. Determine the current personal oral care procedures carried out by the patient, and their frequency.
D. Outline the instruction recommended and the goals to be attained by the patient.

III. IMPLEMENTATION

A. Provide motivating demonstration and supervision for specific daily bacterial plaque removal, self-applied fluoride, and other applicable preventive measures.
B. Show methods for self-evaluation.

IV. PERFORM CLINICAL PREVENTIVE SERVICES

A. Complete scaling and bacterial debridement.
B. Apply caries-preventive agents.

V. EVALUATE CHANGES IN THE PATIENT'S ORAL HEALTH

A. Evaluate gingival tissue, bleeding, plaque, and techniques performed by the patient.
B. Use successive indices to compare progress.
C. Provide preventive counseling for corrective action when initial goals are not met.

VI. PLAN LONG-TERM MAINTENANCE

A. Re-evaluate periodically to monitor continuance of preventive practices.
B. Provide additional preventive measures when indicated, particularly following placement of new restorations or prosthetic devices.

PATIENT COUNSELING

Instruction is an essential part of the preventive program if goals for attaining a patient's oral health are to be reached. Personalized patient instruction contributes first to the knowledge, attitudes, and practices of the individual and then, through the individual, to the family and the community.

The outmoded concept that all teeth eventually must be removed has been replaced by a new concept of preservation based on current research findings. It is now known that periodontal infections and dental caries can be prevented or controlled, and therefore, teeth can be preserved throughout the lifetime of the individual.

Dental health education is the provision of oral health information to people in such a way that they can apply it in everyday living.[1] Knowledge of and belief in health facts are not enough; benefits result only when knowledge is put into action. Learning occurs when an individual changes behavior and when changes are incorporated as a part of everyday living.

I. MOTIVATION

Instruction is tailored to individual needs and motivations. An individual is motivated to practice behavior that leads to achievement of goals that are valued. Instruction can be effective if the patient considers oral health a valuable asset or goal.

Stimulation of behavior, or motivation, stems from basic physiologic and social needs. Peer group approval and the need to conform to group standards, as well as the fear of disapproval or rejection when appearance of the teeth or odor of the breath is unacceptable, are frequently much stronger motivating factors than is a health reason, such as freedom from infection or the ability to chew food for body cell maintenance.

The need for relief from pain can bring a patient to seek immediate dental care; however, additional motivation is needed to help the patient realize that future pain can be avoided through a preventive care program.

Motivation and what the patient learns and practices are proportional to the sincerity and concern of the dental team members. A motivated dental professional develops patient-centered systems of instruction that are meaningful to the patient.

II. PATIENT-CENTERED INSTRUCTION

For most patients, major emphasis must be placed on control of dental caries or periodontal infections. Attention should also be paid to prevention of oral accidents, particularly those related to mouth protectors for contact sports, safety belts for automobiles, and children's accidents that lead to fractured anterior teeth.

Whereas patient instruction of the past connoted teaching a patient how and when to use a toothbrush, usually by means of a model and in one short session, patient instruction now envelops a wide range of essential areas of learning aimed at developing a patient's knowledge, attitudes, and practices for continuing oral health. The ability to interpret and apply current dental research findings requires continuing review through reading and other educational efforts.

FACTORS TO TEACH THE PATIENT

I. The relationship between preventive measures and clinical services.
II. Why particular preventive measures were selected for the particular patient.
III. Self-assessment methods for determining health of gingiva.
IV. Objectives for bacterial plaque infection control.

REFERENCE

1. **Young,** W.O. and Striffler, D.F.: *The Dentist, His Practice, and His Community,* 2nd ed. Philadelphia, W.B. Saunders Co., 1969, p. 296.

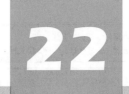

Oral Infection Control: Toothbrushes and Toothbrushing

The toothbrush is the principal instrument in general use for accomplishing bacterial plaque removal as a necessary part of disease control. Many different designs of toothbrushes and supplementary devices have been manufactured and promoted.

Patients who have not previously received professional advice concerning the best brush for their particular oral conditions probably have used brushes selected on the basis of cost, availability, advertising claims, family tradition, or habit. Because of the variety in shapes, sizes, textures, and other characteristics, dental professionals must become familiar with the many available products to advise patients appropriately.

Key words relating to toothbrushes are listed in table 22–1 with their definitions.

DEVELOPMENT OF TOOTHBRUSHES[1-4]

Crudely contrived toothpicks, presumably used for relief from food impaction, are believed to be the earliest implements devised for the care of the teeth. Excavations in Mesopotamia uncovered elaborate gold toothpicks used by the Sumerians about 3000 B.C.

The earliest record of the "chewstick," which has been considered the primitive toothbrush, dates back in the Chinese literature to about 1600 B.C. The care of the mouth was associated with religious training and ritual: the Buddhists had a "toothstick," and the Mohammedans used the "miswak" or "siwak." Chewsticks, made from various types of tasty woods by crushing an end and spreading the fibers in a brush-like manner, are still used by many Asiatic and African people.

The Ebers Papyrus, compiled about 1500 B.C. and dating probably at about 4000 B.C., contained reference to conditions similar to periodontal diseases and to preparations used as mouthwashes and dentifrices. The writings of Hippocrates (about 300 B.C.) include descriptions of diseased gums related to calculus and of complex preparations for the treatment of unhealthy mouths.

I. EARLY TOOTHBRUSHES

It is believed that the first brush made of hog's bristles was mentioned in the early Chinese literature. Pierre Fauchard in 1728 in *Le Chirurgien Dentiste* described many aspects of oral health. He condemned the toothbrush made of horse's hair because it was rough and destructive to the teeth and advised the use of sponges or herb roots. Fauchard recommended scaling of teeth and developed instruments and splints for loose teeth, as well as dentifrices and mouthwashes.

One of the earlier toothbrushes made in England was produced by William Addis about 1780. By the early nineteenth century, craftsmen in various European countries constructed handles of gold, ivory, or ebony in which replaceable brush heads could be fitted. The first patent for a toothbrush in the United States was issued to H. N. Wadsworth in the middle of the nineteenth century.

Many new varieties of toothbrushes were developed around 1900, when celluloid was available for the manufacture of toothbrush handles. In 1919, the American Academy of Periodontology defined specifications for toothbrush design and brushing methods in an attempt to standardize professional recommendations.[5]

Nylon came into use in toothbrush construction in 1938. World War II complications prevented Chinese

---

**TABLE 22–1
KEY WORDS: TOOTHBRUSHES**

Abrasion (ah-brā'zhun) **(gingiva):** lesion of the gingiva that results from the mechanical removal of the surface epithelium.

Abrasion (tooth): loss of tooth structure produced by a mechanical cause (such as a hard-bristled toothbrush used with excessive pressure and an abrasive dentifrice) abrasion contrasts with erosion, which involves a chemical process.

Bristle (bris'l): individual short stiff natural hair of an animal; historically, toothbrush bristles were taken from a hog or wild boar, but current toothbrush bristles are made of nylon and are called filaments.

End-rounded: characteristic shape of each toothbrush filament; a special manufacturing process removes all sharp edges and provides smooth, rounded ends to prevent injury to gingiva or tooth structure during use.

Filament (fil'ah-ment): individual synthetic fiber; a single element of a **tuft** fixed into a toothbrush head.

Mechanical plaque control: oral hygiene methods for removal of bacterial plaque from tooth surfaces using a toothbrush and selected devices for interdental cleaning; contrasts with chemotherapeutic plaque control in which an antimicrobial agent is used.

Power-assisted toothbrush: a brush driven by electricity or battery; also called automatic, electric, or mechanical (in contrast with manual).

Stiffness: the reaction force exerted per unit area of the brush during deflection; the term stiffness is used interchangeably with **firmness** of toothbrush bristles or filaments; the stiffness depends primarily on the length and diameter of the filaments.

Sulcular (sŭl'kŭ-lar) **brushing:** a method in which the end-rounded filament tips are activated at and just below the gingival margin for the purpose of loosening and removing bacterial plaque from the gingival sulcus.

Toothbrush head: the part of the toothbrush composed of the tufts and the **stock** (extension of the handle where the tufts are attached).

Tuft: a cluster of bristles or filaments secured together in one hole in the head of a toothbrush.

---

export of wild boar bristles, and synthetic materials were substituted for natural bristles. Since then, synthetic materials have been improved and manufacturer's specifications standardized. Many current toothbrushes are made exclusively of synthetic materials. Powered toothbrushes, although developed earlier, were not actively promoted until about 1960.

II. BRUSHING METHODS

Historically, the purpose of brushing was to provide *massage* to increase the resistance of the gingival tissue. Massage or friction from a hard-bristled brush was believed to *increase keratinization,* which, in turn, resulted in the resistance to bacterial invasion.[6]

Koecker, in 1842,[7] wrote that, after the dentist has scaled off the tartar, the patient must clean the teeth every morning and after every meal with a hard brush and an astringent powder. For the inner surfaces he recommended a conical-shaped brush of fine hog's bristles. For the outer surfaces, he believed the brush should be oblong of the "best white horse-hair." He instructed the patient to press hard against the gums so the bristles went between the teeth. . ." and between the edges of the gums and the roots of the teeth. The pressure of the brush is to be applied in the direction from the crowns of the teeth towards the roots, so the mucus, which adheres to the roots under the edges of the gums, may be completely detached, and after that, removed by the friction in a direction towards the grinding surfaces."

MANUAL TOOTHBRUSHES

I. CHARACTERISTICS OF AN EFFECTIVE TOOTHBRUSH[8]

A. Conforms to individual patient requirements in size, shape, and texture.

B. Is easily and efficiently manipulated.

C. Is readily cleaned and aerated; impervious to moisture.

D. Is durable and inexpensive.

E. Has prime functional properties of flexibility, softness, and diameter of the bristles or filaments, and of strength, rigidity, and lightness of the handle.

F. Has end-rounded filaments or bristles.

G. Is designed for utility, efficiency, and cleanliness.

II. GENERAL DESCRIPTION

A. Parts (figure 22–1)

1. *Handle.* The part grasped in the hand during toothbrushing.

2. *Head.* The working end; consists of tufts of bristles or filaments and the stock where the tufts are secured.

3. *Shank.* The section that connects the head and the handle.

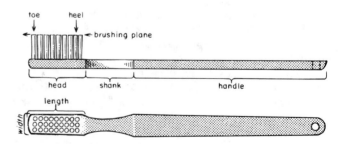

FIG. 22–1. Parts of a Toothbrush.

B. Dimensions

1. *Total Brush Length.* About 15 to 19 cm (6 to 7.5 inches); junior and child sizes may be shorter.
2. *Head.* Should be only large enough to accommodate the tufts.
   a. Length of brushing plane, 25.4 to 31.8 mm (1 to 1¼ inches); width, 7.9 to 9.5 mm (⁵⁄₁₆ to ⅜ inch).
   b. Bristle or filament height, 11 mm (⁷⁄₁₆ inch).

III. HANDLE

A. Composition

Nearly all current brush handles are plastics, which combine durability, imperviousness to moisture, pleasing appearance, low cost, sufficient rigidity, and smooth texture.

B. Shape

1. *Preferred Characteristics*
   a. Easy to grasp.
   b. Does not slip or rotate during use.
   c. No sharp corners or projections.
   d. Light weight, consistent with strength.
2. *Variations.* A twist, curve, offset, or angle in the shank with or without thumb rests may assist the patient in the adaptation of the brush to difficult-to-reach areas. Slight deviations may not complicate manipulation or affect control of the brush placement and pressure.

   Bent or thickened handles can be helpful for use by patients with certain types of disability (pages 692 and 693).

IV. HEAD

A. Design

1. *Tufted.* Is 5 to 11 tufts long and 2 to 4 rows wide, spaced for easy cleaning of the brush.
2. *Multitufted.* Is 10 or 12 tufts long and 3 or 4 rows wide, spaced closely to provide a smooth brushing plane and to allow the filaments to support each other.

B. Brushing Plane (profile)

Brushes are available with variously shaped filament profiles. The brushing plane is also referred to as the trim, which is the characteristic arrangement of the tips of the filaments at the brushing surface.

The trim may range from filaments of equal lengths (flat planes, figure 22–2) to those with variable lengths, such as dome-shaped, rippled, or bi-level. All filaments should be soft and end-rounded for safety to oral soft tissues and tooth structure. When used properly, all can reduce plaque and gingivitis. Efficiency for cleaning the hard-to-reach areas, such as extension onto proximal surfaces, malpositioned teeth, or exposed root surfaces, depends on individual patient abilities and understanding.

Flat

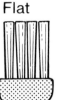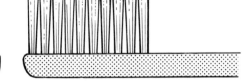

Rippled

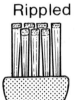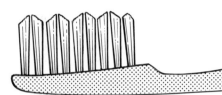

Dome

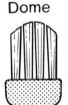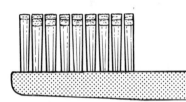

Bi-level

Bi-level-orthodontic

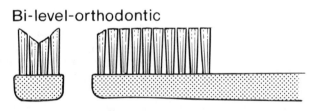

FIG. 22–2. Brush Trim Profiles. A variety of filament profiles are available. In addition to the classic flat planed brush, other trims include the rippled, dome, and bi-level. Brushes for use over orthodontic appliances are made with various bi-level shapes.

V. BRISTLES AND FILAMENTS

Most current toothbrushes have nylon filaments. Natural bristles are relatively unsanitary, and their physical qualifications cannot be standardized.

The stiffness depends on the diameter and length of the filament. Brushes designated as soft, medium, or hard are not comparatively consistent between manufacturers.

A. Factors Influencing Stiffness

1. *Diameter.* Thinner filaments are softer and more resilient.
2. *Length.* Shorter filaments are stiffer and have less flexibility.
3. *Number of Filaments in a Tuft.* Each filament gives support to the adjacent filaments; each tuft gives support to adjacent tufts.

B. Natural Bristles

1. *Source.* Historically, bristles were obtained from the hair of the hog or wild boar.
2. *Uniformity.* Bristles are not consistent in texture or wearing properties. Their inherent resiliency varies with the breed of animal, as well as with the geographic location and season when the bristles were taken.
3. *Diameter.* They vary in size from 0.087 mm (.0035 inch) to 0.475 mm (.019 inch), depending on the portion of the bristle and the age and life of the animal.
4. *Shape.* Bristles have deficient, irregular, frequently open ends.
5. *Disadvantages.*[9] Toothbrushes with natural bristles are not recommended because the bristles
   a. Cannot be standardized.
   b. Wear more rapidly and irregularly.
   c. Are hollow, thereby allowing microorganisms and debris to collect inside.
   d. Are water absorbent (water softens the bristle).

C. Filaments

1. *Composition.* Synthetic, plastic materials, primarily nylon.
2. *Uniformity.* Controlled.
3. *Diameter*
   a. Filaments may range from extra soft to hard. Diameters range from 0.15 mm (.006 inch) to 0.3 mm (.012 inch).
   b. Small interdental brushes are made with filaments of 0.075 mm (.003 inch) (page 358).
4. *Shape.* End-rounded filaments cause the least trauma to the tissues. Research has shown a direct relation between gingival damage and the absence of end-rounding.[10,11] Figure 22–3 shows examples of nonrounded and end-rounded filaments.[11]
5. *Advantages of Filaments Over Natural Bristles*
   a. Rinse clean and dry rapidly when left in open.
   b. More durable and maintain their form longer.
   c. Ends, rounded and closed, repel water and debris.
   d. More resistant to accumulation of bacteria and fungi than are natural bristles.

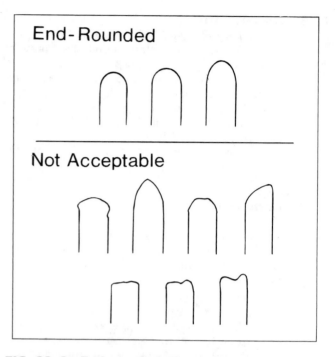

FIG. 22–3. End-rounded Filaments. Examples of the shape of acceptable end-rounding and of those that are not acceptable are shown. (From Silverstone, L.M. and Featherstone, M.J.: A Scanning Electron Microscope Study of the End Rounding of Bristles in Eight Toothbrush Types, *Quintessence Int., 19,* 3, February, 1988.)

TOOTHBRUSH SELECTION FOR THE PATIENT

I. INFLUENCING FACTORS (see also page 413)

Factors that influence the selection of the proper toothbrush for an individual patient include the following:

A. Patient

1. Ability of the patient to use the brush and remove plaque from all tooth surfaces without damage to the soft tissue or tooth structure.
2. Manual dexterity of patient.
3. Motivation, ability, and willingness to follow the prescribed procedures.

B. Gingiva

1. Status of gingival or periodontal health.
2. Anatomic configurations of the gingiva.

C. Position of Teeth

Displaced teeth require variations in brush placement.

1. Crowded teeth (figure 16–5, page 266).
2. Open contacts (figure 12–4, page 203).

D. Shape of Teeth and Exposed Roots
E. Personal Preferences
1. Professional personnel may prefer to instruct certain methods and with certain brushes.
2. Patient may have preferences and may resist change.

F. Method Selected
Method of brushing to be recommended and instructed.

II. TOOTHBRUSH SIZE AND SHAPE
The brush selected must be able to be adapted to all facial, lingual, palatal, and occlusal surfaces for bacterial plaque removal.

III. SOFT NYLON BRUSH
The following are suggested as advantages for the use of a soft end-rounded brush that is applied appropriately.
1. More effective in cleaning the cervical areas, both proximal and marginal.
2. Less traumatic to the gingival tissue; therefore, patients can brush at the cervical areas without fear of discomfort or soft tissue laceration.
3. Can be directed into the sulcus for sulcular brushing and into interproximal areas for cleaning the proximal surfaces.
4. Applicable around fixed orthodontic appliances or fixation appliances used to treat a fractured jaw.
5. Tooth abrasion and/or gingival recession can be prevented or may be less severe in an overvigorous brusher.
6. More effective use for sensitive gingiva in such conditions as necrotizing ulcerative gingivitis or severe gingivitis, or during healing stages following scaling and root planing or periodontal surgery.
7. Small size is ideal for a young child as a first brush on primary teeth.

GUIDELINES FOR TOOTHBRUSHING

Complete toothbrushing instruction for a patient involves teaching what, when, where, and how. In addition to descriptions of specific toothbrushing methods, the succeeding sections consider the grasp of the brush, the sequence and amount of brushing, the areas of limited access, and supplementary brushing for the occlusal surfaces and the tongue. The possible detrimental effects from improper toothbrushing and variations for special conditions are described. The care of toothbrushes is outlined.

I. GRASP OF BRUSH
A. Objectives
Manipulation of the brush for successful removal of bacterial plaque can be related to the manner in which the brush is held. Patients may need specific instruction in how to hold and place the brush. When they start to brush to remove the bacterial plaque that has been colored with a disclosing agent, the tenaciousness of the plaque and the need for controlled pressure can be realized. With a firm, comfortable grasp, the following can be expected:
1. Control of the brush during all movements.
2. Effective positioning at the beginning of each brushing stroke, follow-through during the complete stroke, and repositioning for the next stroke.
3. Sensitivity to the amount of pressure applied.

B. Procedure
1. Grasp toothbrush handle in the palm of the hand with thumb against the shank.
   a. Near enough to the head of the brush so that it can be controlled effectively.
   b. Not so close to the head of the brush that manipulation of the brush is hindered or that fingers can touch the anterior teeth when reaching the brush head to molar regions.
2. Direct filaments in the direction needed for placement on the teeth; direction depends on the brushing method to be used.
3. Adapt grasp for the various positions of the brush head on the teeth throughout the procedure; adjust to permit unrestricted movement of the wrist and arm.
4. Apply appropriate pressure for removal of the bacterial plaque. Too much pressure, however, bends the filaments and curves them away from the area where brushing is needed.

II. SEQUENCE
A. The procedure in brushing, for any method used, should assure complete coverage for each tooth surface.
B. Start brushing from a molar region of one arch around to the opposite side, then back around the lingual or facial. Repeat in the opposing arch.
C. Each brush placement must overlap the previous one for thorough coverage (figure 22–4).
D. Encourage the patient to begin by brushing one of the areas of greatest individual need.
   1. Areas that are most frequently missed.
   2. Areas that are most difficult for brush placement and/or manipulation, such as the right side for the right-handed brusher or the left side for the left-handed brusher.
E. Suggest that the sequence be varied at least once each day so that the same areas are not always brushed last when time may be limited and plaque removal may be less complete.

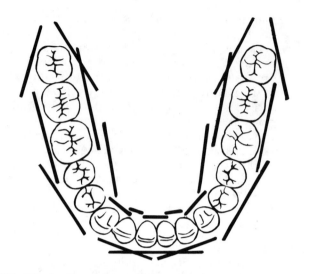

FIG. 22–4. Brushing Positions. Each brush position, as represented by a black line, should overlap the previous position. Note placement at canines, where the distal aspect of the canine is brushed with the premolars and the mesial aspect is brushed with the incisors. Short lines on the lingual anterior aspect indicate brush placed vertically (figure 22–9). The maxillary teeth require a similar number of brushing positions.

III. AMOUNT OF BRUSHING
A. The Count System
To ensure thorough coverage with an even distribution of amount of brushing and to help the patient concentrate on the performance, a system of counting is useful.
1. Count 6 strokes in each area (or 5 or 10, whichever is most appropriate for the particular patient) for modified Stillman or other method in which a stroke is used.
2. Count slowly to 10 for each brush position while brush is vibrated and filament ends are held in position for the Bass, Charters, or other vibratory method.

B. The Clock System
Some patients brush thoroughly while watching a clock or an egg timer for 3 or 4 minutes. Timed procedures cannot assure thorough coverage, because single areas that are most accessible may get more brushing time.

C. Combination
For many patients, use of the "count" system in combination with the "clock" system produces the most complete removal of bacterial plaque.

IV. FREQUENCY OF BRUSHING
Because of individual variations, one set rule for frequency cannot be applied. The emphasis in patient education should be placed on complete plaque removal daily rather than on number of brushings.

For the control of bacterial plaque, and for oral sanitation and halitosis prevention, at least two brushings, accompanied by appropriate interdental care, are recommended for each day. The longer the bacteria remain undisturbed, the greater the pathogenic potential of the plaque.

A clean mouth before going to sleep should be encouraged. Bacteria thrive in the dark, warm, moist climate of the oral environment. Patients who use a chewable fluoride tablet, mouthrinse, or gel application before going to bed should complete their plaque removal before fluoride application.

METHODS FOR TOOTHBRUSHING

Most toothbrushing methods can be classified into one of eight groups based on the motion and position of the brush. Noted beside certain categories that follow are names of methods that utilize the designated motion as part or all of their particular procedure. Some of these methods are recorded for descriptive, comparative, or historic purposes only, and are not currently recommended. A few even have been shown to be detrimental.
  A. **Sulcular:** Bass.
  B. **Roll:** Rolling stroke, modified Stillman.
  C. **Vibratory:** Stillman, Charters, Bass.
  D. **Circular:** Fones.
  E. **Vertical:** Leonard.
  F. **Horizontal.**
  G. **Physiologic:** Smith.
  H. **Scrub-brush.**

THE BASS METHOD: SULCULAR BRUSHING

The Bass method is widely accepted as an effective method for bacterial plaque removal adjacent to and directly beneath the gingival margin. This area around the tooth is the most significant in the control of gingival and periodontal infections.

I. PURPOSES AND INDICATIONS
  A. For all patients for bacterial plaque removal adjacent to and directly beneath the gingival margin.
  B. Particularly for open interproximal areas, cervical areas beneath the height of contour of the enamel, and exposed root surfaces.
  C. For the patient who has had periodontal surgery.

II. PROCEDURE[12]
A. Grasp Brush Handle
Direct the filaments apically (up for maxillary, down for mandibular teeth). Even though the

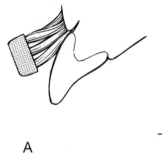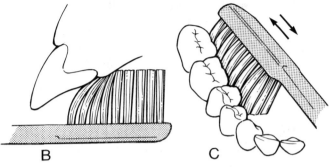

FIG. 22-5. Sulcular Brushing. A. Filament tips are directed into the gingival sulcus at approximately 45° to the long axis of the tooth. **B.** Position for palatal surface of maxillary anterior teeth. **C.** Brush in position for lingual surfaces of mandibular posterior teeth.

A B C

brush placement calls for directing the filaments at a 45° angle, it is usually easier and safer for the patient to first place the sides of the filaments parallel with the long axis of the tooth. From that position the brush can be turned slightly and brought to the gingival margin to the 45° angle (figure 22-5).

B. Angle the Filaments
Place the brush with the filament tips directed straight into the gingival sulcus. The filaments will be directed at approximately 45° to the long axis of the tooth, as shown in figure 22-5A.

C. Press Lightly Without Flexing
Press lightly so the filament tips enter the gingival sulci and embrasures and cover the gingival margin. Do not bend the filaments with excess pressure.

D. Vibrate the Brush
Vibrate the brush back and forth with very short strokes without disengaging the tips of the filaments from the sulci. Count at least 10 vibrations.

E. Reposition the Brush
Apply the brush to the next group of two or three teeth. Take care to overlap placement, as shown in figure 22-4.

F. Repeat Stroke
The entire stroke (Parts A through D) is repeated at each position around the maxillary and mandibular arches, both facially and lingually.

G. Position Brush for Lingual and Palatal Anterior Surfaces (figure 22-5B)
Hold the brush the long narrow way for the anterior components as described for the rolling stroke method. The filaments are kept straight and directed into the sulci.

III. PROBLEMS
A. An overeager brusher may convert the previously mentioned "very short strokes" into a vigorous scrub that causes injury to the gingival margin.

B. Dexterity requirement may be too high for certain patients. A 45° angle can be difficult to visualize.

C. Rolling stroke procedure may precede the sulcular brushing when a patient believes it helps to clean the teeth. The two methods should be performed separately rather than trying to combine them in what has been referred to as a "modified Bass."

The procedure of rolling the brush down over the crown after the vibratory part of the sulcular brush stroke has several disadvantages: (1) too often the brush is hastily and carelessly replaced into the sulcus position, or the opposite is true, and considerable time is consumed in the attempt to replace the brush carefully; (2) gingival margin injury by the constant replacement of the brush can result; and (3) patient may tend to roll the brush down over the crown prematurely, thereby accomplishing very little sulcular brushing.

THE ROLL OR ROLLING STROKE METHOD

I. PURPOSES AND INDICATIONS
A. Cleaning gingiva and removing plaque, materia alba, and food debris from the teeth without emphasis on gingival sulcus.
   1. For children with relatively healthy gingiva and normal tissue contour when a sulcular technique may seem difficult for the patient to master.
   2. For general cleaning in conjunction with the use of a vibratory technique (Charters, Stillman).

B. Useful for preparatory instruction (first lesson) for modified Stillman method because the initial brush placement is the same. This can be particularly helpful when there is a question as to how complicated a technique the patient can master and practice.

II. PROCEDURE[5,13]
A. Grasp Brush Handle
Direct filaments apically (up for maxillary, down for mandibular teeth).

B. Place Side of Brush on the Attached Gingiva

The filaments are directed apically. When the plastic portion of the brush head is level with the occlusal or incisal plane, generally the brush is at the proper height, as shown in figure 22–6A.

C. Press to Flex the Filaments

The sides of the filaments are pressed against the gingiva. The gingiva will blanch.

D. Roll the Brush Slowly Over the Teeth

As the brush is rolled, the wrist is turned slightly. The filaments remain flexed and follow the contours of the teeth, thereby permitting cleaning of the cervical areas. Some filaments may reach interdentally.

E. Replace and Repeat Five Times or More

The entire stroke (Parts A through D) is repeated at least five times for each tooth or group of teeth. When the brush is removed and repositioned, the wrist is rotated, the brush is moved away from the teeth, and the cheek is stretched facially with the back of the brush head. Care must be taken not to drag the filament tips over the gingival margin when the brush is returned to the initial position (figure 22–6A).

F. Overlap Strokes

When moving the brush to an adjacent position, overlap the brush position, as shown in figure 22–4.

G. Position Brush for Lingual or Palatal Surfaces

1. Use the brush the long, narrow way.
2. Hook the heel of the brush on the incisal edge (figure 22–6D).
3. Press (down for maxillary, up for mandibular) until the filaments lie flat against the teeth and gingiva.
4. Press and roll (curve up for mandibular, down for maxillary teeth).
5. Replace and repeat five times for each brush width.

III. PROBLEMS

A. Brushing too high during initial placement can lacerate the alveolar mucosa.
B. Tendency to use quick, sweeping strokes results in no brushing for the cervical third of the tooth because the brush tips pass over rather than into the area; likewise for the interproximal areas.
C. Replacing brush with filament tips directed into the gingiva can produce punctate lesions (page 348).

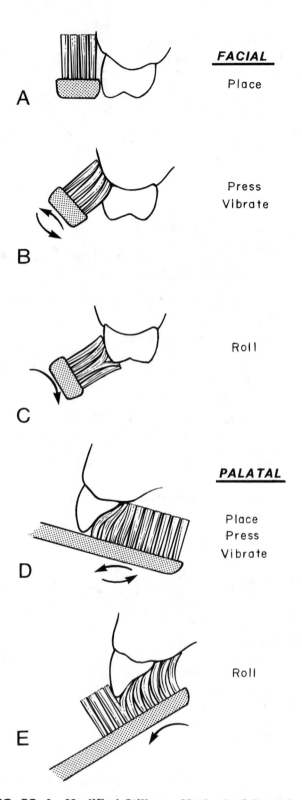

FACIAL

Place

Press
Vibrate

Roll

PALATAL

Place
Press
Vibrate

Roll

FIG. 22–6. Modified Stillman Method of Brushing.
A. Initial brush placement with sides of bristles or filaments against the attached gingiva. **B.** The brush is pressed and angled, then vibrated. **C.** Vibrating is continued as the brush is rolled slowly over the crown. **D.** Maxillary anterior lingual placement with the brush applied the long way. **E.** Vibrating continues as the brush is rolled over the crown and interdental areas. Placement is similar for the lingual surfaces of the mandibular anterior teeth. The roll or rolling stroke brushing method has the same brush positions.

THE MODIFIED STILLMAN METHOD

This method, as originally described by Stillman,[14] was designed for massage and stimulation, as well as for cleaning the cervical areas. The brush ends were placed partly on the gingiva and partly on the cervical areas of the tooth and were directed slightly apically. Pressure was applied to effect a blanching. The handle was given a slight rotary motion, and the brush ends were maintained in position on the tooth surface. After several applications, the brush was moved to the adjacent tooth.

A modified Stillman, which incorporates a rolling stroke after the vibratory (rotary) phase, frequently is used. The modifications minimize the possibility of gingival trauma and increase the plaque removal effects.[15]

I. PURPOSES AND INDICATIONS
A. Bacterial plaque removal from cervical areas below the height of contour of the crown and from exposed proximal surfaces.
B. General application for cleaning tooth surfaces and massage of the gingiva.

II. PROCEDURE (figure 22–6)
A. Grasp Brush Handle
Direct filaments apically (up for maxillary, down for mandibular teeth).

B. Place Side of Brush on the Attached Gingiva
The filaments are directed apically. When the plastic portion of the brush head is level with the occlusal or incisal plane, generally the brush is at the proper height, as shown in figure 22–6A.

C. Press to Flex the Filaments
The sides of the filaments are pressed lightly against the gingiva. The gingiva will blanch.

D. Angle the Filaments
Turn the handle by rotating the wrist so that the filaments are directed at an angle of approximately 45° with the long axis of the tooth.

E. Vibrate the Brush
Vibrate gently but firmly. Maintain light pressure on the filaments, and keep the tips of the filaments in position with constant contact. Count to 10 slowly as the brush is vibrated by a rotary motion of the handle.

F. Roll and Vibrate the Brush
Turn the wrist and work the vibrating brush slowly down over the gingiva and tooth. Make some of the filaments reach interdentally.

G. Replace Brush for Repeat Stroke
Reposition the brush by rotating the wrist. Avoid dragging the filaments back over the free gingival margin by holding the brush out, slightly away from the tooth.

H. Repeat Stroke Five Times or More
The entire stroke (Parts A through F) is repeated at least 5 times for each tooth or group of teeth. When moving the brush to an adjacent position, overlap the brush position, as shown in figure 22–4.

I. Position Brush for Lingual and Palatal Surfaces
1. Position the brush the long, narrow way for the anterior components, as described for the rolling stroke technique and shown in figure 22–6 D and E.
2. Press and vibrate, roll, and repeat.

III. PROBLEMS
A. Without careful placement using a brush with end-rounded filaments, tissue laceration can result. Light pressure is needed.
B. Patient may try to move the brush into the rolling stroke too quickly, and the vibratory aspect may be ineffective for plaque removal at the gingival margin.

THE CHARTERS METHOD

During his long productive dental career, Dr. W. J. Charters emphasized the importance of prevention. The interproximal toothbrushing method that he taught had as its objectives cleanliness through removal of the "film and mucin" from the proximal surfaces and gingival massage through mechanical stimulation.

Among his many published papers, Charters described two brush positions, one at a right angle to the long axis of the tooth[16] and another at a 45° angle with the tips of the bristles toward the occlusal plane.[17] The right-angle position might have been intended primarily for patients with interdental periodontal tissue loss, where access permitted the bristles to enter the embrasure.

For either brush position, the instructions were to force the tips into the interproximal area. "With the bristles between the teeth, as much pressure as possible is exerted, giving the brush several slight rotary or vibratory movements. This causes the sides of the bristles to come in contact with the gum margin, producing an ideal massage."[17]

The classic periodontal textbooks[18] have described the Charters method with the bristles directed toward the occlusal plane at a 45° angle with the long axis. This method is described as follows.

I. PURPOSES AND INDICATIONS
A. Loosen debris and bacterial plaque.
B. Massage and stimulate marginal and interdental gingiva.

C. Aid in plaque removal from proximal tooth surfaces when interproximal tissue is missing, for example, following periodontal surgery.

D. Adapt to cervical areas below the height of contour of the crown and to exposed root surfaces.

E. Remove bacterial plaque from abutment teeth and under the gingival border of a fixed partial denture (bridge) or from the undersurface of a sanitary bridge.

F. Cleansing orthodontic appliances (figure 24–2C, page 378).

II. PROCEDURE[17]

A. Apply Rolling Stroke Procedure
Instruct in a basic rolling stroke for general cleaning to be accomplished first.

B. Grasp Brush Handle
Hold brush (outside the oral cavity) with filaments directed toward the occlusal or incisal plane of the teeth that will be brushed. The tips are pointed down for application to the maxillary and pointed up for application to the mandibular arch. Insert the brush held in the direction it will be used.

C. Place the Brush
Place the sides of the filaments against the enamel with the brush tips toward the occlusal or incisal plane.

D. Angle the Filaments
Angle at approximately 45° to the occlusal or incisal plane. Slide the brush to a position at the junction of the free gingival margin and the tooth surface (figure 22–7B).

E. Press Lightly
Press lightly to flex the filaments and force the tips between the teeth. The sides of the filaments are pressed against the gingival margin.

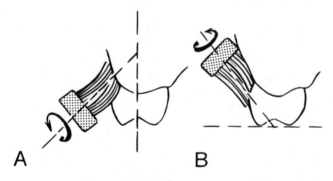

FIG. 22–7. Charters and Stillman Methods Compared. A. Stillman. The brush is angled at approximately 45° to the long axis of the tooth. **B.** Charters. The brush is angled at approximately 45° to the occlusal plane, with brush tips directed toward the occlusal or incisal surfaces.

F. Vibrate the Brush
Vibrate gently but firmly, keeping the tips of the filaments in contact. Count to 10 slowly as the brush is vibrated by a rotary motion of the handle.

G. Reposition the Brush and Repeat
Repeat Parts B through F, as described, several times in each position around the dental arches.

H. Overlap Strokes
When moving the brush to an adjacent position, overlap the brush position, as shown in figure 22–4.

I. Position Brush for Lingual and Palatal Surfaces
Because the Charters brush position is difficult to accomplish on the lingual surfaces, a modified Stillman technique is frequently advised. When the Charters method is preferred, the positions are as follows:

1. *Posterior*
   a. With brush tips pointed toward the occlusal surfaces, extend the brush handle across the incisal edge of the canine of the side opposite that to be brushed.
   b. Place the sides of the toe-end filaments against the distal surface of the most posterior tooth and subsequently at each embrasure.
   c. Press and vibrate.
2. *Anterior*
   a. With brush handle parallel with the long axis of the tooth, place the sides of the toe-end filaments over the interproximal embrasure.
   b. Press and vibrate.

J. Application of Brush for Fixed Partial Denture
When placing the brush, check that the filament tips are directed under the gingival border of the pontic.

III. PROBLEMS
A. Brush ends do not engage the gingival sulcus to remove subgingival bacterial accumulations.

B. In some areas, the correct brush placement is limited or impossible; therefore, modifications become necessary, consequently adding to the complexity of the procedure.

C. Requirements in digital dexterity are high.

OTHER TOOTHBRUSHING METHODS

The rolling stroke, modified Stillman, and Bass are probably the methods most used for patient instruction either directly or as guidelines with variations. Other methods that have been used are included here. The technique and intent of some of the methods overlap. Assessment prior to special instruction may reveal that a mixture of techniques may be in use by a patient.

I. CIRCULAR: THE FONES METHOD

Many patients, especially schoolchildren, probably received instruction in this method because it was advocated by Fones, who founded the first course for dental hygienists. He described the technique in the first dental hygiene text, which was used for many years by dental hygiene students throughout the United States.

Although now considered possibly detrimental for adults, particularly when used by a vigorous brusher, this method may be recommended as an easy-to-learn first technique for young children. A soft brush with .006- to .008-inch filament diameter is selected. In abbreviated form, the technique described by Dr. Fones includes the following[19]:

A. With the teeth closed, place the brush inside the cheek with the brush tips lightly contacting the gingiva over the last maxillary molar.

B. Use a fast, wide, circular motion that sweeps from the maxillary gingiva to the mandibular gingiva with very little pressure (figure 22–8).

C. Bring anterior teeth in end-to-end contact, and hold lip out when necessary to make the continuous circular strokes.

D. Lingual and palatal tooth surfaces require an in-and-out stroke. Brush sweeps across palate on the maxillary arch and back and forth to the molars on the mandibular arch.

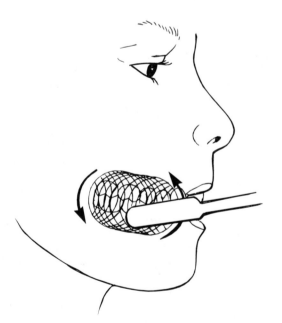

FIG. 22–8. Fones Method of Brushing. With the teeth closed, a circular motion extends from the maxillary gingiva to the mandibular gingiva using a light pressure.

II. VERTICAL: LEONARD METHOD

As described by Hirschfeld,[20] the up-and-down stroke was employed when teeth were cleaned with a primitive crude twig toothbrush. The true vertical stroke passes from the gingiva over the maxillary teeth to the gingiva over the mandibular teeth, with a vigorous sweeping motion.

Leonard described and advocated a vertical stroke in which maxillary and mandibular teeth were brushed separately. Paraphrased, he described his method as follows:[21]

A. With the teeth edge-to-edge, place the brush with the filaments against the teeth at right angles to the long axes of the teeth.

B. Brush vigorously, without great pressure, with a stroke that is mostly up and down on the tooth surfaces, with just a slight rotation or circular movement after striking the gingival margin with force.

C. Use enough pressure to force the filaments into the embrasures, but not enough to damage the brush.

D. The upper and lower teeth are not brushed in the same series of strokes. The teeth are placed edge-to-edge to keep the brush from slipping over the occlusal or incisal surfaces.

III. HORIZONTAL

Horizontal or crosswise brushing is generally recognized as detrimental. An unlimited sweep with a horizontal scrubbing motion bears pressure on teeth that are most facially inclined or prominent. With the use of an abrasive dentifrice, such brushing may produce tooth abrasion. Because the interdental areas are not touched by this method, bacterial plaque can remain undisturbed on proximal surfaces.

IV. PHYSIOLOGIC: SMITH'S METHOD

The physiologic method was described by Smith[22] and advocated later by Bell.[23] It was based on the principle that the toothbrush should follow the same physiologic pathway that food follows when it traverses over the tissues in a "natural" masticating act.

A soft brush with "small tufts of fine bristles arranged in four parallel rows and trimmed to an even length" was used in a brushing stroke directed down over the lower teeth onto the gingiva and upward over the teeth for the maxillary. Smith also suggested a few gentle horizontal strokes to clean the portion of the sulci directly over the bifurcations of the roots.

V. SCRUB-BRUSH

A scrub-brush procedure consists of vigorously combined horizontal, vertical, and circular strokes, with some vibratory motions for certain areas. Without caution, vigorous scrubbing can encourage gingival recession and, with a dentifrice of sufficient abrasiveness, can create areas of tooth abrasion.

POWER-ASSISTED TOOTHBRUSHES

Power-assisted brushes are also known as automatic, mechanical, or electric brushes. The American Dental Association Council on Dental Materials, Instruments and Equipment evaluates and classifies power-assisted brushes for the reduction of bacterial plaque and gingivitis.[24]

Comparisons have been made in research between the power-assisted and the manual brushes to determine the ability of each type to remove plaque, prevent calculus development, and reduce the incidence of gingivitis. Both types have been shown effective when used correctly.

I. DESCRIPTION
A. Motion
The action on different models may be one of the following:
1. Rotational.
2. Counter-rotational.
3. Oscillating-counter-rotational.

B. Power Source
1. *Direct.* Cord from electrical outlet connects directly to the toothbrush handle.
2. *Replaceable Batteries.* Disadvantage in the nuisance and cost of repeatedly replacing or recharging batteries; also, as the batteries lose their power, the brush is slowed. Corrosion may be a problem if water gets into the case.
3. *Rechargeable.* The instrument is placed into a stand that contains the recharger and is connected to the electrical outlet. A few models have a recharger built into the handle.
4. *Switches.* A few models require that the push button be held down during operation. This requirement may present difficulties for some patients, such as small children or persons with certain types of disabilities.

C. Speeds
Speeds vary from low to high among the different models. Some have the speed coordinated with the filament texture. The number of strokes per minute varies from, for example, as low as 1000 cycles per minute for a replaceable battery type, to about 3600 oscillations per minute for an arcuate model. The rechargeable battery types operate at approximately 2000 complete strokes per minute.

II. PURPOSES AND INDICATIONS
A. General Application
Power-assisted brushes have been developed to facilitate mechanical removal of bacterial plaque and food debris for all patients. All the general objectives that apply to the use of manual brushes can be applied to power-assisted brushes. They may be especially helpful for people who lack the manual dexterity needed to handle a manual brush successfully.

B. Special Dental Treatment
With instruction and supervision, a power-assisted brush recommended by a dental professional may be of special benefit for a patient with plaque-retentive areas or devices.
1. Those who wear orthodontic appliances (pages 376–379).
2. Those undergoing complex restorative and prosthodontic treatment (page 396).
3. Those with dental implants (pages 401 and 402).

C. Patients with Disabilities
The thick handles of power-assisted brushes have been shown to be easily handled and manipulated by patients with certain disabilities, especially when grasping is difficult to accomplish (pages 692–694).

D. Patients Unable to Brush
A power-assisted brush may be readily handled by a parent or caregiver.

III. INSTRUCTION
With a manual brush, an individual must learn to apply the brush tips in certain ways in order that each surface of each tooth can be reached, slight pressure can be applied for a thorough brushing effect, and the stroke can be repeated a number of times. With a power-assisted brush, the action is built in. The only muscle training required is turning the handle to apply the brush to each surface of each tooth and holding it on each surface for a reasonable length of time in a correct position.

IV. METHODS FOR USE
The general suggestions presented here are basic and, as with all brushing techniques, need adaptations for an individual mouth. Familiarity with the instructions provided by the manufacturers of the various power-assisted brushes is a prerequisite.
A. Select brush with soft end-rounded filaments.
B. Select dentifrice with minimum abrasivity. The extra strokes made by a power-assisted brush can increase the effects of abrasion to the tooth surface.
C. Place a small amount of dentifrice on the brush and spread the dentifrice over the teeth to prevent splashing when the power is turned on.
D. Any of the brushing methods previously described in this chapter can be applied for use with a power-assisted brush.
E. Vary the brush position for each tooth surface. Brush each tooth separately.
1. Apply the brush for sulcular brushing to the distal, facial, and mesial surfaces of each tooth as the brush is moved from the most posterior

teeth toward the anterior, quadrant by quadrant.

2. Turn the brush to reach proximal areas.
3. Angulate for access to surfaces of rotated, crowded, or otherwise displaced teeth.
4. Retract lip with fingers of other hand to give access to and visibility of anterior facial surfaces, particularly including prominent canines.
5. Modify brush positions for application to proximal surfaces when interdental papillae are missing. Brush head may be positioned parallel with the long axis and inserted vertically.

F. Make strokes slowly, with a slight steady pressure. Pressure should not be great enough at any time to bend the filaments.

G. Precautions
1. Synthetic restorations should be avoided or treated without pressure because they can wear down under repeated application of the fast-moving filaments with dentifrice.
2. Avoid pressure with abrasive dentifrice over exposed cementum or dentin.

SUPPLEMENTAL BRUSHING

I. PROBLEM AREAS

Each surface of each tooth must be brushed. Initial instruction necessarily may be limited to a basic procedure, particularly when it varies from the patient's present procedures.

At succeeding lessons, the special hard-to-get areas are shown to the patient. Suggestions are made and demonstrated for brush adaptation for areas that were missed. Methods for cleaning the interdental areas and fixed and removable appliances are described in Chapters 23 and 24.

Attention in teaching should be given to the following:

A. Facially displaced teeth, especially canines and premolars, where the zone of attached gingiva may be minimal and where toothbrush abrasion frequently occurs.
B. Inclined teeth, for example, lingual surfaces of mandibular molars that are inclined lingually.
C. Exposed root surfaces; cemental and dentinal surfaces.
D. Overlapped teeth or wide embrasures, which require use of vertical brush position (figure 22–9).
E. Surfaces of teeth next to edentulous areas (figure 23–6, page 357).
F. Exposed furcation areas (figure 23–10, page 360).
G. Right canine and lateral incisor, both maxillary and mandibular, which are commonly missed by right-handed brushers; the opposite is true for left-handed brushers.

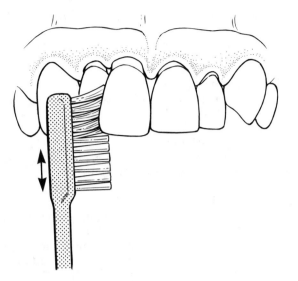

FIG. 22–9. Brush in Vertical Position. For overlapped teeth, open interproximal areas, and selected areas of recession, the bacterial plaque on proximal tooth surfaces can be conveniently removed with the brush held in a vertical position.

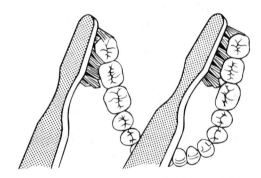

FIG. 22–10. Brushing Problems. Brush placement to remove plaque from the distal surfaces of the most posterior teeth. The distobuccal surface is approached by stretching the cheek; the distolingual surface is approached by directing the brush across from the canine of the opposite side.

H. Distal surfaces of most posterior teeth (figure 22–10). At best, the brush may reach only the distal line angles. Supplementation with dental floss, yarn, or tufted dental floss is needed for the distal surface (page 356).

II. OCCLUSAL BRUSHING
A. Objectives
1. Loosen plaque microorganisms packed in pits and fissures.
2. Remove plaque deposits from occlusal surfaces of teeth out of occlusion or not used during mastication.

3. Remove plaque from the margins of restorations.
4. Clean pits and fissures to prepare for sealants.

B. Procedure

1. Place brush on occlusal surfaces of molar teeth with filament tips pointed into the occlusal pits at a right angle. The handle should be parallel with the occlusal surface. The toe of the brush should cover the distal grooves of the most posterior tooth.
2. Two acceptable strokes are suggested.
   a. Vibrate the brush in a slight circular movement while maintaining the filament tips on the occlusal surface throughout a count of 10. Press moderately so filaments do not bend but go straight into the pits and fissures (figure 22–11).
   b. Force the filaments against the occlusal surface with sharp, quick strokes; lift the brush off each time to dislodge debris; repeat about 10 times.
3. Move brush to premolar area, overlapping previous brush position.

C. Precaution

Long scrubbing strokes from anterior to posterior on an occlusal surface may contact only the prominent parts of the cusps (figure 22–11B and C).

III. TONGUE CLEANING

Total mouth cleanliness includes tongue care.

A. Microorganisms of the Tongue

1. Main foci for oral microorganisms are
   a. Dorsum of tongue.
   b. Gingival sulci and pockets.
   c. Bacterial plaque on all teeth.
2. Microorganisms in saliva are principally from the tongue.
3. The microflora of the tongue is not constant, but changes frequently.[25]

B. Effects of Cleaning the Tongue

1. Reduction of oral debris.
2. Retardation of bacterial plaque formation and total plaque accumulation.
3. Reduction of number of microorganisms. When brushing of the tongue is discontinued, the number of organisms increases.
4. Contribution to overall cleanliness.

C. Anatomic Features of Tongue Conducive to Debris Retention

1. *Surface Papillae.* Numerous filiform papillae extend as minute projections, whereas fungiform papillae are not as high and create elevations and depressions that entrap debris and microorganisms (figure 11–2, page 182).

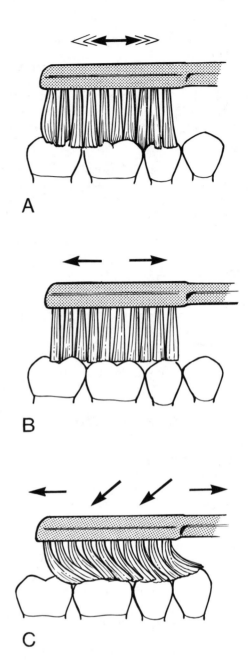

FIG. 22–11. Occlusal Brushing. A. Vibrating brush with light pressure while maintaining filament tips on the occlusal surface permits tips to work their way into pits and fissures. **B.** Long horizontal strokes contact only the cusp tips. **C.** Excess pressure curves the filaments so that tips cannot get into the pits and fissures.

2. *Fissured Tongue.* Fissures may be several millimeters deep and retain debris.

D. Brushing Procedure

1. Hold the brush handle at a right angle to the midline of the tongue and direct the brush tips toward the throat.
2. With the tongue extruded, the sides of the

filaments are placed on the posterior part of the tongue surface.

3. With light pressure, draw the brush forward and over the tip of the tongue. Repeat three or four times. Do not scrub the papillae.

E. Tongue Scraper

Tongue cleaners or scrapers may be made of plastic, stainless steel, or other flexible metal. They are curved and wide enough to fit over the tongue surface without hitting the teeth. Some are made with a single handle, whereas others have two ends to hold, as shown in figure 22–12.

1. *Purpose.* By removing debris and microorganisms, the patient can expect to contribute to overall mouth cleanliness, reduce the numbers of bacteria available for plaque formation, and lessen mouth odors. The procedure can be especially helpful for the patient who has a coated tongue or deep fissures or who smokes.

2. *Procedure.* Place the arch toward the posterior of the dorsal surface (figure 22–12). Press with a light but firm stroke, and pull forward. Repeat several times, covering the entire surface of the tongue. Wash the tongue scraper under running water.

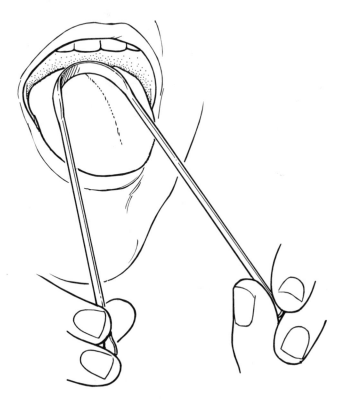

FIG. 22–12. Tongue Scraper. A variety of plastic or flexible metal scrapers are available to clean the dorsal surface of the tongue. The scraper is pressed over the tongue with a light but firm stroke.

TOOTHBRUSHING FOR SPECIAL CONDITIONS

Even when an unusual oral condition develops, a patient must be encouraged to brush whenever possible to reduce the possibility of infection and promote healing. Prolonged omission of techniques of plaque removal is never indicated. Examples of conditions that may require a temporary departure from personal care routines follow.

I. ACUTE ORAL INFLAMMATORY OR TRAUMATIC LESIONS

When an acute oral condition precludes normal brushing, the patient should be instructed to brush all areas of the mouth that are not affected and to resume regular plaque control measures on the affected area as soon as possible. When not otherwise contraindicated by instructions from the dentist, rinsing with a warm, mild saline solution can encourage healing and debris removal.

II. FOLLOWING PERIODONTAL SURGERY

Patients must receive specific instructions concerning brushing while sutures and/or a dressing are in place. Because direct, vigorous brushing of a periodontal dressing could cause its displacement, brushing of the occlusal surfaces and light strokes over the dressing may be advised. Other teeth and gingiva should be brushed as usual. Additional instructions appear in table 36–2 on pages 548 and 549.

III. ACUTE STAGE OF NECROTIZING ULCERATIVE GINGIVITIS

A major contributing factor in the development of this disease is a lack of oral cleanliness. During the acute stage, the oral tissues are sensitive to any touch, and toothbrushing therefore is neglected. Instructions for these patients are on pages 540 and 541. A soft brush is indicated along with careful brush placement to avoid trauma.

IV. FOLLOWING DENTAL EXTRACTION

Instructions may be found on page 658 and include brushing all teeth and gingiva except the surgical wound area. Teeth adjacent to the extraction site need cleaning as soon as possible to reduce bacterial collections and to promote healing.

V. FOLLOWING DENTAL RESTORATIONS

Patients tend to avoid brushing a new crown, newly placed fixed partial denture, or other prosthesis. Specific instructions should be given at the time of insertion.

TOOTHBRUSH TRAUMA: THE GINGIVA

Trauma to the gingiva occurs most frequently on the facial surfaces over teeth prominent in the dental arch.

The lesions frequently are found over canines and premolars.

Lesions are especially apt to occur after initial instruction in use of a new method of brushing. The patient may be overzealous or may have misunderstood correct brush placement. Examination of a patient's gingiva within a few days to a week after instruction can be important.

I. ACUTE ALTERATIONS
Acute lesions are usually lacerations or ulcerations. The severity of the lesion may depend on the frequency and extent of brushing, as well as on the stiffness of the filaments and the force applied.

A. Appearance
1. Scuffed epithelial surface with denuded underlying connective tissue.
2. Punctate lesions that appear as red pinpoint spots.
3. Diffuse redness and denuded attached gingiva.

B. Precipitating Factors
1. Horizontal or vertical scrub toothbrushing method.
2. Excess pressure applied using firm palm grasp of handle.[26]
3. Use of abrasive dentifrice.[27]
4. Overvigorous placement and application of the toothbrush.
5. Penetration of gingiva by filament ends.
6. Use of toothbrush with frayed, broken bristles or filaments.
7. Application of filaments beyond attached gingiva.

II. CHRONIC ALTERATIONS
A. Changes in Gingival Contour
1. *Appearance*
   a. Rolled, bulbous, hard, firm marginal gingiva, in "piled up" or festoon shape (page 190 and figure 11-10D).
   b. Gingival cleft, which is a narrow groove or slit that extends from the crest of the gingiva to the attached gingiva ("Stillman's Cleft," figure 11-11, page 191).
2. *Location*
   a. Usually appear only on the facial gingiva, because of the vigor with which toothbrush is used.
   b. Frequently inversely related to the right- or left-handedness of the patient.
   c. Areas most often involved are around canines or teeth in labioversion or buccoversion.

B. Gingival Recession
1. *Appearance.* Margin has moved apically and cementum is exposed.

2. *Predisposing Factors*
   a. Anatomic. Narrow band of attached gingiva and thin facial bone over teeth malposed in labioversion.
   b. Toothbrushing habits. Vigorous pressured brushing with abrasive dentifrice and worn brush.

C. Suggested Corrective Measures
A. Recommend use of a soft toothbrush with end-rounded filaments.
B. Correct the patient's toothbrushing method; demonstrate a toothbrushing method better suited to the oral condition.
C. Temporary cessation of brushing the traumatized area may be needed. An antiplaque rinse may assist in the healing process.

TOOTHBRUSH TRAUMA: DENTAL ABRASION

I. APPEARANCE
Wedge-shaped indentations with smooth, shiny surfaces (figure 14-7, page 239).

Abrasion is the loss of tooth substance produced by mechanical wear other than that caused by mastication. Abrasion also may be defined as the pathologic wearing away of tooth substance through some abnormal mechanical process, in contrast with erosion that generally involves a chemical process.

II. LOCATION OF ABRADED AREAS
A. Primarily on facial surfaces, especially of canines, premolars, and sometimes first molars, or, on any tooth in buccoversion or labioversion, those most available to the pressure of the toothbrush. The canines are susceptible because of their prominence on the curvature of the dental arches.
B. Most abraded areas are on the cervical areas of exposed root surfaces, but occasionally may occur on the enamel. When adjacent teeth are involved, the lesions appear in line with each other.

III. CONTRIBUTING FACTORS
A. Hard toothbrush with abrasive agent in the dentifrice.
B. Horizontal brushing with excessive pressure.
C. Form of filament ends. Abrasion is less frequent when filaments are end-rounded.
D. Prominence of the tooth surface labially or buccally.

IV. CORRECTIVE MEASURES
A. Explain the problem to the patient to assure full cooperation.

B. Advise a specific brush with end-rounded filaments.
C. Change or correct the toothbrushing procedure.
D. Recommend a less abrasive dentifrice.
E. Use a smaller amount of dentifrice.
  1. Start brushing in the area of the dentition where the most plaque and calculus are noted at a maintenance appointment.
  2. Avoid applying the dentifrice vigorously to the same tooth surfaces.

CARE OF TOOTHBRUSHES

When discussing the type and features of the brush selected for an individual patient, the number of brushes needed and the frequency of replacement should be included. Perhaps an ideal time to teach cleaning and daily care of brushes would be after a practice session when the brush has to be washed and cleaned for storage at the dental office.

The condition of a brush depends on many factors, including the amount and manner of use, the type of care, and the quality of the brush at the start.

I. SUPPLY OF BRUSHES
A. Advise at least two brushes for home use and a third in a portable container for use at work, school, or travel.
B. Purchase of brushes should be staggered so that all brushes are not new at the same time and, more important, so that they are all not old at the same time, thereby resulting in less than optimum maintenance of the gingival condition.

II. BRUSH REPLACEMENT
A. Frequent replacement recommended; at least every 2 to 3 months.
B. Brushes should be replaced before filaments become splayed, frayed, or lose resiliency. Duration of a brush is influenced by many factors, including frequency and method of use.
C. Brush contamination can occur within 1 month of use.[28,29] Contamination can cause systemic or localized infection.
D. Patients who are debilitated, immunosuppressed, have a known infection, or are about to undergo surgery for any reason can be advised to disinfect their brushes or use disposable brushes temporarily.[28]

III. CLEANING TOOTHBRUSHES
A. Clean thoroughly after each use.
B. Hold brush head under strong stream of warm water from faucet to force particles, dentifrice, and bacteria from between the filaments.
C. Tap the handle on edge of sink to remove remaining particles.
D. Use one toothbrush to clean another brush; filaments can be worked between those of the other brush to remove resistant debris.
E. Rinse completely and tap out excess water.

IV. BRUSH STORAGE
A. Brushes should be kept in open air with head in an upright position, apart from contact with other brushes, particularly those of another person.
B. Portable brush container should have sufficient holes to give air temporarily until the brush can be completely exposed for drying. A closed container encourages bacterial growth.

REFERENCES

1. **Hirschfeld,** I.: *The Toothbrush: Its Use and Abuse.* Brooklyn, NY, Dental Items of Interest, 1939, pp. 1–27.
2. **Kimery,** M.J. and Stallard, R.E.: The Evolutionary Development and Contemporary Utilization of Various Oral Hygiene Procedures. *Periodont. Abstr., 16,* 90, September, 1968.
3. **McCauley,** H.B.: Toothbrushes, Toothbrush Materials and Design, *J. Am. Dent. Assoc., 33,* 283, March 1, 1946.
4. **Weinberger,** B.W.: *An Introduction to the History of Dentistry.* St. Louis, Mosby, 1948, pp. 43, 140–144.
5. **American Academy of Periodontology,** Committee Report: The Tooth Brush and Methods of Cleaning the Teeth, *Dent. Items Interest, 42,* 193, March, 1920.
6. **Alexander,** J.F.: Toothbrushes and Toothbrushing, in Menaker, L., ed.: *The Biologic Basis of Dental Caries.* Hagerstown, MD, Harper & Row, 1980, pp. 482–496.
7. **Koecker,** L.: Principles of Dental Surgery, Exhibiting a New Method of Treating the Diseases of the Teeth and Gums. Baltimore, MD, American Society of Dental Surgeons, 1842, Chapter III, pp. 155–156.
8. **American Dental Association,** Council on Dental Therapeutics: *Accepted Dental Therapeutics,* 40th ed. Chicago, American Dental Association, 1984, pp. 386–387.
9. **Massassati,** A. and Frank, R.M.: Scanning Electron Microscopy of Unused and Used Manual Toothbrushes, *J. Clin. Periodontol., 9,* 148, March, 1982.
10. **Breitenmoser,** J., Mörmann, W., and Mühleman, H.R.: Damaging Effects of Toothbrush Bristle End Form on Gingiva, *J. Periodontol., 50,* 212, April, 1979.
11. **Silverstone,** L.M. and Featherstone, M.J.: A Scanning Electron Microscope Study of the End Rounding of Bristles in Eight Toothbrush Types, *Quintessence Int., 19,* 3, February, 1988.
12. **Bass,** C.C.: An Effective Method of Personal Oral Hygiene, *J. Louisiana State Med. Soc., 106,* 100, March, 1954.
13. **Hard,** D.: Oral Prophylaxis, in Bunting, R.W.: *Oral Hygiene,* 3rd ed. Philadelphia, Lea & Febiger, 1957, pp. 280–283.
14. **Stillman,** P.R.: A Philosophy of the Treatment of Periodontal Disease, *Dent. Digest, 38,* 315, September, 1932.
15. **Hirschfeld:** op. cit., p. 380.
16. **Charters,** W.J.: Home Care of the Mouth. I. Proper Home Care of the Mouth, *J. Periodontol., 19,* 136, October, 1948.
17. **Charters,** W.J.: Eliminating Mouth Infections with the Toothbrush and Other Stimulating Instruments, *Dent. Digest, 38,* 130, April, 1932.
18. **Miller,** S.C.: *Textbook of Periodontia,* 3rd ed. Philadelphia, The Blakiston Co., 1950, pp. 327–328.

19. **Fones,** A.C., ed.: *Mouth Hygiene,* 4th ed. Philadelphia, Lea & Febiger, 1934, pp. 299–306.
20. **Hirschfeld:** op. cit., pp. 369–371.
21. **Leonard,** H.J.: Conservative Treatment of Periodontoclasia, *J. Am. Dent. Assoc., 26,* 1308, August, 1939.
22. **Smith,** T.S.: Anatomic and Physiologic Conditions Governing the Use of the Toothbrush, *J. Am. Dent. Assoc., 27,* 874, June, 1940.
23. **Bell,** D.G.: Home Care of the Mouth. III. Teaching Home Care to the Patient, *J. Periodontol., 19,* 140, October, 1948.
24. **American Dental Association,** Council of Dental Materials, Instruments and Equipment: *Clinical Products in Dentistry. A Desktop Reference.* Chicago, American Dental Association, Revised annually.
25. **Van der Weijden,** G.A. and Van der Velden, U.: Fluctuation of the Microbiota of the Tongue in Humans, *J. Clin. Periodontol., 18,* 26, January, 1991.
26. **Niemi,** M.-L., Ainamo, J., and Etemadzadeh, H.: The Effect of Toothbrush Grip on Gingival Abrasion and Plaque Removal During Toothbrushing, *J. Clin. Periodontol., 14,* 19, January, 1987.
27. **Niemi,** M.-L., Sandholm, L., and Ainamo, J.: Frequency of Gingival Lesions After Standardized Brushing as Related to Stiffness of Toothbrush and Abrasiveness of Dentifrice, *J. Clin. Periodontol., 11,* 254, April, 1984.
28. **Glass,** R.T.: The Infected Toothbrush, the Infected Denture, and Transmission of Disease: A Review, *Compendium, 13,* 592, July, 1992.
29. **Müller,** H.P., Lange, D.E., and Müller, R.F.: Actinobacillus actinomycetecomitans Contamination of Toothbrushes from Patients Harbouring the Organism, *J. Clin. Periodontol., 16,* 388, July, 1989.

SUGGESTED READINGS

Abraham, N.J., Cirincione, U.K., and Glass, R.T.: Dentists' and Dental Hygienists' Attitudes Toward Toothbrush Replacement and Maintenance, *Clin. Prev. Dent., 12,* 28, December, 1990.

Dean, D.H., Beeson, L.D., Cannon, D.F., and Plunkett, C.B.: Condition of Toothbrushes in Use: Correlation with Behavioral and Socio-economic Factors, *Clin. Prev. Dent., 14,* 14, January/February, 1992.

Donley, T.G. and Donley, K.B.: Systemic Bacteremia Following Toothbrushing: A Protocol for the Management of Patients Susceptible to Infective Endocarditis, *Gen. Dent., 36,* 482, November–December, 1988.

Frandsen, A.: Mechanical Oral Hygiene Practices. State-of-the-Science Review, in Löe, H. and Kleinman, D.V.: *Dental Plaque Control Measures and Oral Hygiene Practices.* Washington, DC, IRL Press, 1986, pp. 93–97.

Kirk, A.D., Bowers, B.A., Moylan, J.A., and Meyers, W.C.: Toothbrush Swallowing, *Arch. Surg., 123,* 382, March, 1988.

Miyazaki, H., Kambe, M., Yamazaki, M., Yamaguchi, Y., Ansai, T., Ohtani, I., Shirahama, R., Yamashita, Y., Itoh-Andoh, M., and Takehara, T.: Learning Efficiency of a Toothbrush for Mastering Scrubbing Method, *Clin. Prev. Dent., 12,* 19, December, 1990.

Rawls, H.R., Mkwayi-Tulloch, N.J., and Krull, M.E.: A Mathematical Model for Predicting Toothbrush Stiffness, *Dent. Materials, 6,* 111, April, 1990.

Salman, R.A.: Roentgeno-oddities. Toothbrush Ingestion, *Oral Surg. Oral Med. Oral Pathol., 66,* 386, September, 1988.

Vehkalahti, M. and Paunio, I.: Remaining Teeth in Finnish Adults Related to the Frequency of Tooth-brushing, *Acta Odontol. Scand., 47,* 375, December, 1989.

Waerhaug, J: Effect of Toothbrushing on Subgingival Plaque Formation, *J. Periodontol., 52,* 30, January, 1981.

Toothbrush Trials

Agerholm, D.M.: A Clinical Trial to Evaluate Plaque Removal with a Double-head Toothbrush, *Br. Dent. J., 170,* 411, June 8, 1991.

Beatty, C.F., Fallon, P.A., and Marshall, D.D.: Comparative Analysis of the Plaque Removal Ability of .007 and .008 Toothbrush Bristles, *Clin. Prev. Dent., 12,* 22, December, 1990.

Davies, A.L., Rooney, J.C., Constable, G.M., and Lamb, D.J.: The Effect of Variations in Toothbrush Design on Dental Plaque Scores, *Clin. Prev. Dent., 10,* 3, May-June, 1988.

Dean, D.H.: Toothbrushes with Graduated Wear: Correlation With *In Vitro* Cleansing Performance, *Clin. Prev. Dent., 13,* 25, July-August, 1991.

Gibson, M.T., Joyston-Bechal, S., and Smales, F.C.: Clinical Evaluation of Plaque Removal with a Double-headed Toothbrush, *J. Clin. Periodontol., 15,* 94, February, 1988.

Mandel, I.D.: The Plaque Fighters: Choosing a Weapon, *J. Am. Dent. Assoc., 124,* 71, April, 1993.

Park, K.K., Matis, B.A., and Christen, A.G.: Choosing an Effective Toothbrush, *Clin. Prev. Dent., 7,* 5, July-August, 1985.

Stabbe, K.A., Tishk, M.N., Overman, P.R., and Love, J.W.: A Comparison of Plaque Reaccumulation and Patient Acceptance Using a Conventional Toothbrush and a Newly Designed Toothbrush, *Clin. Prev. Dent., 10,* 10, September-October, 1988.

Thevissen, E., Quirynen, M., and van Steenberghe, D.: Plaque Removing Effect of a Convex-shaped Brush Compared with a Conventional Flat Brush, *J. Periodontol., 58,* 861, December, 1987.

Volpe, A.R., Emling, R.C., and Yankell, S.L.: The Toothbrush—A New Dimension in Design, Engineering, and Clinical Evaluation, *J. Clin. Dent., 3,* C1–C33, Supplement C, 1992.

Power-assisted Brushes

Baab, D.A. and Johnson, R.H.: The Effect of a New Electric Toothbrush on Supragingival Plaque and Gingivitis, *J. Periodontol., 60,* 336, June, 1989.

Bader, H.I.: Review of Currently Available Battery-operated Toothbrushes, *Compendium, 13,* 1162, December, 1992.

Boyd, R.L., Murray, P., and Robertson, P.B.: Effect of Rotary Electric Toothbrush Versus Manual Toothbrush on Periodontal Status During Orthodontic Treatment, *Am. J. Orthod. Dentofacial Orthop., 96,* 342, October, 1989.

Boyd, R.L., Murray, P., and Robertson, P.B.: Effect on Periodontal Status of Rotary Electric Toothbrushes Versus Manual Toothbrushes During Periodontal Maintenance. I. Clinical Results, *J. Periodontol., 60,* 390, July, 1989.

Ciancio, S.G. and Mather, M.L.: A Clinical Comparison of Two Electric Toothbrushes with Different Mechanical Actions, *Clin. Prev. Dent., 12,* 5, August-September, 1990.

Efraimsen, H.E., Johansen, J.R., Haugen, E., and Holland, R.I.: Abrasive Effect of a Rotating Electrical Toothbrush on Dentin, *Clin. Prev. Dent., 12,* 13, October-November, 1990.

Hoover, J.N., Singer, D.L., Pahwa, P., and Komiyama, K.: Clinical Evaluation of a Light Energy Conversion Toothbrush, *J. Clin. Periodontol., 19,* 434, July, 1992.

Hotta, M. and Aono, M.: A Clinical Study on the Control of Dental Plaque Using an Electronic Toothbrush with Piezo-Electric Element, *Clin. Prev. Dent., 14,* 16, July-August, 1992.

Khocht, A., Spindel, L., and Person, P.: A Comparative Clinical Study of the Safety and Efficacy of Three Toothbrushes, *J. Periodontol., 63,* 603, July, 1992.

Killoy, W.J., Love, J.W., Love, J., Fedi, P.F., and Tira, D.E.: The Effectiveness of a Counter-rotary Action Powered Toothbrush and Conventional Toothbrush on Plaque Removal and Gingival Bleeding. A Short Term Study, *J. Periodontol., 60,* 473, August, 1989.

Mueller, L.J., Darby, M.L., Allen, D.S., and Tolle, S.L.: Rotary Electric Toothbrushing. Clinical Effects on the Presence of Gingivitis and Supragingival Plaque, *Dent. Hyg., 61,* 546, December, 1987.

Murray, P.A., Boyd, R.L., and Robertson, P.B.: Effect on Periodontal Status of Rotary Electric Toothbrushes vs. Manual Toothbrushes During Periodontal Maintenance. II. Microbiological Results, *J. Periodontol., 60,* 396, July, 1989.

Schifter, C.C., Emling, R.C., Seibert, J.S., and Yankell, S.L.: A Comparison of Plaque Removal Effectiveness of an Electric Versus a Manual Toothbrush, *Clin. Prev. Dent., 5,* 15, September-October, 1983.

Silverstone, L.M., Tilliss, T.S.I., Cross-Poline, G.N., Van der Linden, E., Stach, D.J., and Featherstone, M.J.: A Six-week Study Comparing Efficacy of a Rotary Electric Toothbrush with a Conventional Toothbrush, *Clin. Prev. Dent., 14,* 29, March-April, 1992.

Walsh, M., Heckman, B., Leggott, P., Armitage, G., and Robertson, P.B.: Comparison of Manual and Power Toothbrushing, With and Without Adjunctive Oral Irrigation, for Controlling Plaque and Gingivitis, *J. Clin. Periodontol., 16,* 419, August, 1989.

Chewing Sticks

Eid, M.A., Al-Shammery, A.R., and Selim, H.A.: The Relationship Between Chewing Sticks (Miswak) and Periodontal Health. II. Relationship to Plaque, Gingivitis, Pocket Depth, and Attachment Loss, *Quintessence Int., 21,* 1019, December, 1990.

Eid, M.A., Selim, H.A., Al-Shammery, A.R.: The Relationship Between Chewing Sticks (Miswak) and Periodontal Health. Part I. Review of the Literature and Profile of the Subjects, *Quintessence Int., 21,* 913, November, 1990.

Gazi, M., Saini, T., Ashri, N., and Lambourne, A.: Miswak Chewing Stick Versus Conventional Toothbrush as an Oral Hygiene Aid, *Clin. Prev. Dent., 12,* 19, October-November, 1990.

van Palenstein Helderman, W.H., Munck, L., Mushendwa, S., and Mrema, F.G.: Cleaning Effectiveness of Chewing Sticks Among Tanzanian Schoolchildren, *J. Clin. Periodontol., 19,* 460, August, 1992.

Trauma From Toothbrushing

Bergström, J. and Eliasson, S.: Cervical Abrasion in Relation to Toothbrushing and Periodontal Health, *Scand. J. Dent. Res., 96,* 405, October, 1988.

Niemi, M.-L.: Gingival Abrasion and Plaque Removal after Toothbrushing with an Electric and a Manual Toothbrush, *Acta Odontol. Scand., 45,* 367, No. 5, 1987.

Niemi, M.-L., Ainamo, J., and Etemadzadeh, H.: Gingival Abrasion and Plaque Removal with Manual Versus Electric Toothbrushing, *J. Clin. Periodontol., 13,* 709, August, 1986.

Rawls, H.R., Mkwayi-Tulloch, N.J., Casella, R., and Cosgrove, R.: The Measurement of Toothbrush Wear, *J. Dent. Res., 68,* 1781, December, 1989.

Stookey, G.K., Schemehorn, B.R., and Choi, K.L.: *In Vitro* Studies of the Hard-tissue Abrasivity of a New Home Plaque-removal Instrument, *Compendium, 6,* S152, Supplement No. 6, 1985.

Vehkalahti, M.: Occurrence of Gingival Recession in Adults, *J. Periodontol., 60,* 599, November, 1989.

Toothbrush Contamination

Denny, F.W.: Risk of Toothbrushes in the Transmission of Respiratory Infections, *Pediatr. Infect. Dis. J., 10,* 710, September, 1991.

Glass, R.T. and Lare, M.M.: Toothbrush Contamination: A Potential Health Risk?, *Quintessence Int., 17,* 39, January, 1986.

Glass, R.T. and Jensen, H.G.: More on the Contaminated Toothbrush: the Viral Story, *Quintessence Int., 19,* 713, November, 1988.

Kozai, K., Iwai, T., and Miura, K.: Residual Contamination of Toothbrushes by Microorganisms, *ASDC J. Dent. Child, 56,* 201, May-June, 1989.

23

Interdental Care and Chemotherapy

Traditionally, toothbrushing has been considered to be first in line as the method for cleaning the teeth and removing bacterial plaque for the prevention of gingival and periodontal infections. Toothbrushing cannot accomplish plaque removal for the proximal tooth surfaces and adjacent gingiva to the same degree that it does for the facial, lingual, and palatal aspects. Interdental plaque control, therefore, is essential to complete the patient's self-care program.

Objectives and procedures for devices for proximal bacterial plaque removal are included in this chapter. Key words are defined in table 23–1. Particular applications are given for care of teeth and soft tissues related to dental prostheses in Chapter 24. In Chapter 25, the necessary adaptations for a mouth with complete rehabilitation and dental implants are described.

When the preventive treatment plan is outlined for an individual, assessment is made of the oral condition, the problem areas, and the overall prognosis for health improvement or maintenance. Measures for interdental plaque control are selected to complement plaque control by toothbrushing.

At first, the simplest procedures are selected for the patient's convenience and ease of learning. The daily oral care regimen also must be kept at a realistic level with respect to the time the patient is able or willing to spend. As the values the patient places on oral health increase over time, and as the preventive maintenance program becomes a priority in the patient's lifelong self-care health goals, a more refined program can be introduced.

THE INTERDENTAL AREA

Normally, the interdental gingiva fills the gingival embrasure and the area beneath the contact area. The removal of bacterial plaque from a normal shallow sulcus and from the enamel under the proximal gingival tissue usually can be accomplished with dental floss without adding more complicated procedures.

When the interdental papilla is missing or reduced in height, the tooth surfaces are exposed, the shape of the interdental gingiva is changed, and the embrasures are open. A review of the gingival and dental anatomy of the interdental area can give meaning to and clarify the role and purpose of the various devices available for interdental care.

I. GINGIVAL ANATOMY
A. Posterior Teeth
Between adjacent posterior teeth are two papillae, one facial and one lingual or palatal. They are connected by a col, a depressed concave area that follows the shape of the apical border of the contact area (figure 11–8, page 185).

B. Anterior Teeth
Between anterior teeth in contact is a single papilla with a pyramidal shape. As shown in figure 11–8 (page 185), the tip of the papilla may form a small col under the contact area.

C. Epithelium
The epithelium covering a col is usually thin and not keratinized. It is less resistant to bacterial infection than are keratinized surfaces. When inflammation is present in the interdental tissue, the papillae become enlarged with inflammatory cells and fluids, and the col becomes deeper.

The col is in a protected area when the teeth are in alignment and the contact area is normal.

in Plaque Removal by Super Floss and Waxed Dental Floss, *J. Clin. Periodontol.*, 12, 788, October, 1985.

Irrigation

Braatz, L., Garrett, S., Claffey, N., and Egelberg, J.: Antimicrobial Irrigation of Deep Pockets to Supplement Non-Surgical Periodontal Therapy. II. Daily Irrigation, *J. Clin. Periodontol.*, 12, 630, September, 1985.

Drisko, C.L., White, C.L., Killoy, W.J., and Mayberry, W.E.: Comparison of Dark-field Microscopy and a Flagella Stain for Monitoring the Effect of a Water Pik on Bacterial Motility, *J. Periodontol.*, 58, 381, June, 1987.

Dunkin, R.T., Sumner, C.S., and Hughes, W.R.: An Effectiveness Study of a Subgingival Delivery System, *Quintessence Int.*, 20, 345, May, 1989.

Dunkin, R.T., Sumner, C.S., and Hughes, W.R.: Safety Study of a Subgingival Delivery System, *Quintessence Int.*, 20, 401, June, 1989.

Goodman, C.H. and Robinson, P.J.: Periodontal Therapy: Reviewing Subgingival Irrigations and Future Considerations, *J. Am. Dent. Assoc.*, 121, 541, October, 1990.

Greenstein, G.: Subgingival Irrigation—An Adjunct to Periodontal Therapy. Current Status and Future Directions, *J.D.H.*, 64, 389, October, 1990.

Herzog, A. and Hodges, K.O.: Subgingival Irrigation with Chloramine-T, *J.D.H.*, 62, 515, November-December, 1988.

Lang, N.P. and Räber, K.: Use of Oral Irrigators as Vehicle for the Application of Antimicrobial Agents in Chemical Plaque Control, *J. Clin. Periodontol.*, 8, 177, June, 1981.

Lang, N.P. and Ramseier-Grossman, K.: Optimal Dosage of Chlorhexidine Digluconate in Chemical Plaque Control when Applied by the Oral Irrigator, *J. Clin. Periodontol.*, 8, 189, June, 1981.

Linden, G.J. and Newman, H.N.: The Effects of Subgingival Irrigation with Low Dosage Metronidazole on Periodontal Inflammation, *J. Clin. Periodontol.*, 18, 177, March, 1991.

Macaulay, W.J.R. and Newman, H.N.: The Effect on the Composition of Subgingival Plaque of a Simplified Oral Hygiene System Including Pulsating Jet Subgingival Irrigation, *J. Periodont. Res.*, 21, 375, July, 1986.

Manhold, J.H. and Knutsen, M.: A Retrospective of Normal Oral Healthcare Procedures vs. Power Brush/Jet Lavage with a Corroborative Study, *Clin. Prev. Dent.*, 14, 10, July-August, 1992.

Stein, M.: A Literature Review. Oral Irrigation Therapy. The Adjunctive Roles for Home and Professional Use, *Can. Dent. Hyg. Assoc./Probe*, 27, 18, January/February, 1993.

Van der Ouderaa, F.J. and Cummins, D.: Delivery Systems for Agents in Supra- and Sub-gingival Plaque Control, *J. Dent. Res.*, 68 (Special Issue), 1617, November, 1989.

Vignarajah, S., Newman, H.N., and Bulman, J.: Pulsated Jet Subgingival Irrigation with 0.1% Chlorhexidine, Simplified Oral Hygiene and Chronic Periodontitis, *J. Clin. Periodontol.*, 16, 365, July, 1989.

Walsh, M., Heckman, B., Leggott, P., Armitage, G., and Robertson, P.B.: Comparison of Manual and Power Toothbrushing With and Without Adjunctive Oral Irrigation, for Controlling Plaque and Gingivitis, *J. Clin. Periodontol.*, 16, 419, August, 1989.

Wolff, L.F., Bakdash, M.B., Pihlstrom, B.L., Bandt, C.L., and Aeppli, D.M.: The Effect of Professional and Home Subgingival Irrigation with Antimicrobial Agents on Gingivitis and Early Periodontitis, *J. Dent. Hyg.*, 63, 222, June, 1989.

Zubery, Y., Machtei, E.E., and Ben-Yehouda, A.: Self-performed Subgingival Irrigation—A Case Report, *Clin. Prev. Dent.*, 12, 5, October-November, 1990.

Mouthrinses

Binney, A., Addy, M., and Newcombe, R.G.: The Effect of a Number of Commercial Mouthrinses Compared with Toothpaste on Plaque Regrowth, *J. Periodontol.*, 63, 839, October, 1992.

Brecx, M., Brownstone, E., MacDonald, L., Gelskey, S., and Cheang, M.: Efficacy of Listerine®, Meridol®, and Chlorhexidine Mouthrinses as Supplements to Regular Toothcleaning Measures, *J. Periodontol.*, 19, 202, March, 1992.

Busscher, H.J., Perdok, J.F., and Van der Mei, H.C.: Bacterial Growth Inhibition and Short-term Clinical Efficacy of a Vegetable Oil-based Mouthrinse: Preliminary Study, *Clin. Prev. Dent.*, 14, 5, May-June, 1992.

Ciancio, S.G.: Use of Mouthrinses for Professional Indications, *J. Clin. Periodontol.*, 15, 520, September, 1988.

Clark, W.B., Magnusson, I., Walker, C.B., and Marks, R.G.: Efficacy of Perimed® Antibacterial System on Established Gingivitis. I. Clinical Results, *J. Clin. Periodontol.*, 16, 630, November, 1989.

Finkelstein, P., Yost, K.G., and Grossman, E.: Mechanical Devices Versus Antimicrobial Rinses in Plaque and Gingivitis Reduction, *Clin. Prev. Dent.*, 12, 8, August-September, 1990.

Grossman, E., Meckel, A.H., Isaacs, R.L., Ferretti, G.A., Sturzenberger, O.P., Bollmer, B.W., Moore, D.J., Lijana, R.C., and Manhart, M.D.: A Clinical Comparison of Antibacterial Mouthrinses: Effects of Chlorhexidine, Phenolics, and Sanguinarine on Dental Plaque and Gingivitis, *J. Periodontol.*, 60, 435, August, 1989.

Jenkins, S., Addy, M., and Newcombe, R.: Evaluation of a Mouthrinse Containing Chlorhexidine and Fluoride as an Adjunct to Oral Hygiene, *J. Clin. Periodontol.*, 20, 20, January, 1993.

Jenkins, S., Addy, M., and Newcombe, R.: Triclosan and Sodium Lauryl Sulphate Mouthwashes. I. Effects on Salivary Bacterial Counts, *J. Clin. Periodontol.*, 18, 140, February, 1991.

Jenkins, S., Addy, M., and Newcombe, R.: Triclosan and Sodium Lauryl Sulphate Mouthrinses. II. Effects of 4-day Plaque Regrowth, *J. Clin. Periodontol.*, 18, 145, February, 1991.

Joyston-Bechal, S. and Hernaman, N.: The Effect of a Mouthrinse Containing Chlorhexidine and Fluoride on Plaque and Gingival Bleeding, *J. Clin. Periodontol.*, 20, 49, January, 1993.

Mandel, I.D.: The Mouthrinse Wars (Guest Editorial), *J. Periodontol.*, 60, 478, August, 1989.

Meiller, T.F., Kutcher, M.J., Overholser, C.D., Niehaus, C., DePaola, L.G., and Siegel, M.A.: Effect of an Antimicrobial Mouthrinse on Recurrent Aphthous Ulcerations, *Oral Surg. Oral Med. Oral Pathol.*, 72, 425, October, 1991.

Overholser, C.D., Meiller, T.F., DePaola, L.G., Minah, G.E., and Niehaus, C.: Comparative Effects of 2 Chemotherapeutic Mouthrinses on the Development of Supragingival Dental Plaque and Gingivitis, *J. Clin. Periodontol.*, 17, 575, September, 1990.

Perdok, J.F., van der Mei, H.C., and Busscher, H.J.: Physicochemical Properties of Commercially Available Mouthrinses, *J. Dent.*, 18, 147, June, 1990.

Walker, C.B.: Microbiological Effects of Mouthrinses Containing Antimicrobials, *J. Clin. Periodontol.*, 15, 499, September, 1988.

Dentifrices

Binney, A., Addy, M., and Newcombe, R.G.: The Effect of a Number of Commercial Mouthrinses Compared with Toothpaste on Plaque Regrowth, *J. Periodontol.*, 63, 839, October, 1992.

Bye, F.L., Caffesse, R.G., McLean, T.N., and Smith, B.A.: The Effect of a Microsil®-containing Dentifrice in the Prevention and Treatment of Gingivitis, *Clin. Prev. Dent.*, 11, 17, January-February, 1989.

Cutress, T., Howell, P.T., Finidori, C., and Abdullah, F.: Caries Preventive Effect of High Fluoride and Xylitol Containing Dentifrices, *ASDC J. Dent. Child.*, 59, 313, July-August, 1992.

Forward, G.C.: Role of Toothpastes in the Cleaning of Teeth, *Int. Dent. J.*, 41, 164, June, 1991.

Gillan, D.G., Newman, H.N., and Bulman, J.S.: The Effect of Strontium Chloride Hexahydrate Dentifrices on Plaque Accumulation and Gingival Inflammation, *J. Clin. Periodontol.*, 19, 737, November, 1992.

Günbay, S., Bicakci, N., Parlak, H., Güneri, T., and Kirilmaz, L.: The Effect of Zinc Chloride Dentifrices on Plaque Growth and Oral Zinc Levels, *Quintessence Int., 23,* 619, September, 1992.

Jenkins, S., Addy, M., and Newcombe, R.: The Effects of a Chlorhexidine Toothpaste on the Development of Plaque, Gingivitis and Tooth Staining, *J. Clin. Periodontol., 20,* 59, January, 1993.

Lamey, P.-J., Rees, T.D., and Forsyth, A.: Sensitivity Reaction to the Cinnamonaldehyde Component of Toothpaste, *Br. Dent. J., 168,* 115, February 10, 1990.

Marsh, P.D.: Dentifrices Containing New Agents for the Control of Plaque and Gingivitis: Microbiological Aspects, *J. Clin. Periodontol., 18,* 462, July, 1991.

Moran, J., Addy, M., and Newcombe, R.: The Antibacterial Effect of Toothpastes on the Salivary Flora, *J. Clin. Periodontol., 15,* 193, March, 1988.

Nordbö, H., Pulkkanen, U., Eriksen, H.M., and Enersen, M.: The Capacity of a New Dentifrice to Prevent and Remove Extrinsic Tooth Discoloration. A Clinical Study, *Clin. Prev. Dent., 10,* 15, September-October, 1988.

Spear, C.S. and Savisky, L.A.: A Study of Children's Taste and Visual Preferences in Dentifrices, *ASDC J. Dent. Child., 58,* 300, July-August, 1991.

Thyne, G., Young, D.W., and Ferguson, M.M.: Contact Stomatitis Caused by Toothpaste, *N.Z. Dent. J., 85,* 124, October, 1989.

Van der Ouderaa, F. and Cummins, D.: Anti-Plaque Dentifrices: Current Status and Prospects, *Int. Dent. J., 41,* 117, April, 1991.

Chlorhexidine

Addy, M., Jenkins, S., and Newcombe, R.: The Effect of Some Chlorhexidine-containing Mouthrinses on Salivary Bacterial Counts, *J. Clin. Periodontol., 18,* 90, February, 1991.

Addy, M., Jenkins, S., and Newcombe, R.: Studies on the Effect of Toothpaste Rinses on Plaque Regrowth, (1) Influence of Surfactants on Chlorhexidine Efficacy, *J. Clin. Periodontol., 16,* 380, July, 1989.

Addy, M., Wade, W., and Goodfield, S.: Staining and Antimicrobial Properties *In Vitro* of Some Chlorhexidine Formulations. *Clin. Prev. Dent., 13,* 13, January, 1991.

Addy, M., Wade, W.G., Jenkins, S., and Goodfield, S.: Comparison of Two Commercially Available Chlorhexidine Mouthrinses: 1. Staining and Antimicrobial Effects *In Vitro, Clin. Prev. Dent., 11,* 10, September-October, 1989.

Ainamo, J., Nieminen, A., and Westerlund, U.: Optimal Dosage of Chlorhexidine Acetate in Chewing Gum, *J. Clin. Periodontol., 17,* 729, November, 1990.

Bernstein, D., Schiff, G., Echler, G., Prince, A., Feller, M., and Briner, W.: *In Vitro* Virucidal Effectiveness of a 0.12% Chlorhexidine Gluconate Mouthrinse, *J. Dent. Res., 69,* 874, March, 1990.

Brecx, M.C., Liechti, T., Widmer, J., Gehr, P., and Lang, N.P.: Histological and Clinical Parameters of Human Gingiva Following 3 Weeks of Chemical (Chlorhexidine) or Mechanical Plaque Control, *J. Clin. Periodontol., 16,* 150, March, 1989.

Cline, N.V. and Layman, D.L.: The Effects of Chlorhexidine on the Attachment and Growth of Cultured Human Periodontal Cells, *J. Periodontol., 63,* 598, July, 1992.

Jenkins, S., Addy, M., and Newcombe, R.: Comparison of Two Commercially Available Chlorhexidine Mouthrinses. II. Effects on Plaque Reformation, Gingivitis, and Tooth Staining, *Clin. Prev. Dent., 11,* 12, November-December, 1989.

Jenkins, S., Addy, M., and Wade, W.: The Mechanism of Action of Chlorhexidine, *J. Clin. Periodontol., 15,* 415, August, 1988.

Kalaga, A., Addy, M., and Hunter, B.: Comparison of Chlorhexidine Delivery by Mouthwash and Spray on Plaque Accumulation, *J. Periodontol., 60,* 127, March, 1989.

McKenzie, W.T., Forgas, L., Vernino, A.R., Parker, D., and Limestall, J.D.: Comparison of a 0.12% Chlorhexidine Mouthrinse and

an Essential Oil Mouthrinse on Oral Health in Institutionalized, Mentally Handicapped Adults: One-year Results, *J. Periodontol., 63,* 187, March, 1992.

Moghadam, B.K.H., Drisko, C.L., and Gier, R.E.: Chlorhexidine Mouthwash-induced Fixed Drug Eruption. Case Report and Review of the Literature, *Oral Surg. Oral Med. Oral Pathol., 71,* 431, April, 1991.

Moran, J., Addy, M., and Roberts, S.: A Comparison of Natural Product, Triclosan, and Chlorhexidine Mouthrinses on 4-day Plaque Regrowth, *J. Clin. Periodontol., 19,* 578, September, 1992.

Netuschil, L., Reich, E., and Brecx, M.: Direct Measurement of the Bactericidal Effect of Chlorhexidine on Human Dental Plaque, *J. Clin. Periodontol., 16,* 484, September, 1989.

Newman, M.G., Sanz, M., Nachnani, S., Saltini, C., and Anderson, L.: Effect of 0.12% Chlorhexidine on Bacterial Recolonization Following Periodontal Surgery, *J. Periodontol., 60,* 577, October, 1989.

Nuuja, T.T., Murtomaa, H.T., Meurman, J.H., and Personen, T.J.: The Effect of an Experimental Chewable Antiplaque Preparation Containing Chlorhexidine on Plaque and Gingival Index Scores, *J. Dent. Res., 71,* 1156, May, 1992.

Persson, R.E., Truelove, E.L., LeResche, L., and Robinovitch, M.R.: Therapeutic Effects of Daily or Weekly Chlorhexidine Rinsing on Oral Health of a Geriatric Population, *Oral Surg. Oral Med. Oral Pathol., 72,* 184, August, 1991.

Pucher, J.J. and Daniel, J.C.: The Effects of Chlorhexidine Digluconate on Human Fibroblasts *In Vitro, J. Periodontol., 63,* 526, June, 1992.

Sanz, M., Newman, M.G., Anderson, L., Matoska, W., Otomo-Corgel, J., and Saltini, C.: Clinical Enhancement of Post-periodontal Surgical Therapy by a 0.12% Chlorhexidine Gluconate Mouthrinse, *J. Periodontol., 60,* 570, October, 1989.

Saravia, M.E., Svirsky, J.A., and Friedman, R.: Chlorhexidine as an Oral Hygiene Adjunct for Cyclosporine-induced Gingival Hyperplasia, *ASDC J. Dent. Child., 57,* 366, September-October, 1990.

Vaughan, M.E. and Garnick, J.J.: The Effect of a 0.125% Chlorhexidine Rinse on Inflammation After Periodontal Surgery, *J. Periodontol., 60,* 704, December, 1989.

Wade, W.G. and Addy, M.: *In Vitro* Activity of a Chlorhexidine-containing Mouthwash Against Subgingival Bacteria, *J. Periodontol., 60,* 521, September, 1989.

Peroxide and Bicarbonate

Amigoni, N.A., Johnson, G.K., and Kalkwarf, K.L.: The Use of Sodium Bicarbonate and Hydrogen Peroxide in Periodontal Therapy: A Review, *J. Am. Dent. Assoc., 114,* 217, February, 1987.

Bakdash, M.B., Wolff, L.F., Pihlstrom, B.L., Aeppli, D.M., and Bandt, C.L.: Salt and Peroxide Compared with Conventional Oral Hygiene, *J. Periodontol., 58,* 308, May, 1987.

Boyd, R.L.: Effects on Gingivitis of Daily Rinsing with 1.5% H_2O_2, *J. Clin. Periodontol., 16,* 557, October, 1989.

Cerra, M.B. and Killoy, W.J.: The Effect of Sodium Bicarbonate and Hydrogen Peroxide on the Microbial Flora of Periodontal Pockets. A Preliminary Report, *J. Periodontol., 53,* 599, October, 1982.

Etemadzadeh, H.: Plaque-growing Inhibiting Effect of Chewing Gum Containing Urea Hydrogen Peroxide, *J. Clin. Periodontol., 18,* 337, May, 1991.

Gold, S.I.: Early Origins of Hydrogen Peroxide Use in Oral Hygiene, *J. Periodontol., 54,* 247, April, 1983.

Gomes, B.C., Shakun, M.L., and Ripa, L.W.: Effect of Rinsing with a 1.5% Hydrogen Peroxide Solution (Peroxyl®) on Gingivitis and Plaque in Handicapped and Nonhandicapped Subjects, *Clin. Prev. Dent., 6,* 21, May-June, 1984.

Greenstein, G. and Rethman, M.: Hydrogen Peroxide and Salt Solutions: Are They Effective Antiplaque Agents? *Compendium, 8,* 348, May, 1987.

Harfst, S.: Baking Soda Revisited, *Dentalhygienistnews, 4,* 7, Fall, 1991.

Herrin, J.R., Rubright, W.C., Squier, C.A., Lawton, W.J., Osborn, M.O., Stumbo, P.J., and Grigsby, W.R.: Local and Systemic Effects of Orally Applied Sodium Salts, *J. Am. Dent. Assoc., 113,* 607, October, 1986.

Jones, C.M., Blinkhorn, A.S., and White, E.: Hydrogen Peroxide, the Effect on Plaque and Gingivitis When Used in an Oral Irrigator, *Clin. Prev. Dent., 12,* 15, December, 1990.

Kaminsky, S.B., Gillette, W.B., and O'Leary, T.J.: Sodium Absorption Associated with Oral Hygiene Procedures, *J. Am. Dent. Assoc., 114,* 644, May, 1987.

Lehne, R.K.: Abrasivity of Sodium Bicarbonate, *Clin. Prev. Dent., 5,* 17, January-February, 1983.

Lyne, S.M., Glasscock, N.D., and Allen, D.S.: Clinical Effectiveness of Hydrogen Peroxide-Sodium Bicarbonate Paste on Periodontitis Treated with and Without Scaling and Root Planing, *Dent. Hyg., 60,* 450, October, 1986.

Miyasaki, K.T., Genco, R.J., and Wilson, M.E.: Antimicrobial Properties of Hydrogen Peroxide and Sodium Bicarbonate Individually and in Combination Against Selected Oral, Gram-negative, Facultative Bacteria, *J. Dent. Res., 65,* 1142, September, 1986.

Newbrun, E., Hoover, C.I., and Ryder, M.I.: Bactericidal Action of Bicarbonate Ion on Selected Periodontal Pathogenic Microorganisms, *J. Periodontol., 55,* 658, November, 1984.

Pihlstrom, B.L., Wolff, L.F., Bakdash, M.B., Schaffer, E.M., Jensen, J. R., Aeppli, D.M., and Bandt, C.L.: Salt and Peroxide Compared with Conventional Oral Hygiene. I. Clinical Results, *J. Periodontol., 58,* 291, May, 1987.

Stindt, D.J. and Quenette, L.: An Overview of Gly-Oxide Liquid in Control and Prevention of Dental Disease, *Compendium, 10,* 514, September, 1989.

Tanzer, J.M., McMahon, T., and Grant, L.: Bicarbonate-based Powder and Paste Dentifrice Effects on Caries, *Clin. Prev. Dent., 12,* 18, April-May, 1990.

Wagner, M.J., Tvrdy, J.L., Barnes, G.P., Lyon, T.C., and Parker, W.A.: Sodium Retention from Mouthwashes, *Clin. Prev. Dent., 11,* 3, July-August, 1989.

Walsh, M.M. and Kaufman, N.: Subgingival Application of a Hydrogen Peroxide/Baking Soda Mixture with a Toothpick, *Clin. Prev. Dent., 7,* 21, March-April, 1985.

Weitzman, S.A., Weitberg, A.B., Niederman, R., and Stossel, T.P.: Chronic Treatment with Hydrogen Peroxide. Is It Safe?, *J. Periodontol., 55,* 510, September, 1984.

West, T.L. and King, W.J.: Toothbrushing with Hydrogen Peroxide-Sodium Bicarbonate Compared to Toothpowder and Water in Reducing Periodontal Pocket Suppuration and Darkfield Bacterial Counts, *J. Periodontol., 54,* 339, June, 1983.

Wolff, L.F., Pihlstrom, B.L., Bakdash, M.B., Schaffer, E.M., Jensen, J.R., Aeppli, D.M., and Bandt, C.L.: Salt and Peroxide Compared with Conventional Oral Hygiene. II. Microbial Results, *J. Periodontol., 58,* 301, May, 1987.

Triclosan Dentifrice

Addy, M., Jenkins, S., and Newcombe, R.: The Effect of Triclosan, Stannous Fluoride and Chlorhexidine Products on: (I) Plaque Regrowth Over a 4-day Period, *J. Clin. Periodontol., 17,* 693, November, 1990.

Cummins, D.: Zinc Citrate/Triclosan: A New Anti-plaque System for the Control of Plaque and the Prevention of Gingivitis: Short-term Clinical and Mode of Action Studies, *J. Clin. Periodontol., 18,* 455, July, 1991.

Gjermo, P.: Antibacterial Dentifrices. Clinical Data and Relevance with Emphasis on Zinc/Triclosan, *J. Clin. Periodontol., 18,* 468, July, 1991.

Jenkins, S., Addy, M., and Newcombe, R.: The Effects of 0.5% Chlorhexidine and 0.2% Triclosan Containing Toothpastes on Salivary Bacterial Counts, *J. Clin. Periodontol., 17,* 85, February, 1990.

Jenkins, S., Addy, M., and Newcombe, R.: The Effect of Triclosan, Stannous Fluoride and Chlorhexidine Products on (II) Salivary Bacterial Counts, *J. Clin. Periodontol., 17,* 698, November, 1990.

Jones, C.L., Saxton, C.A., and Ritchie, J.A.: Microbiological and Clinical Effects of a Dentifrice Containing Zinc Citrate and Triclosan in the Human Experimental Gingivitis Model, *J. Clin. Periodontol., 17,* 570, September, 1990.

Mankodi, S., Walker, C., Conforti, N., DeVizio, W., McCool, J.J., and Volpe, A.R.: Clinical Effect of a Triclosan-containing Dentifrice on Plaque and Gingivitis: A Six-month Study, *Clin. Prev. Dent., 14,* 4, November-December, 1992.

Stephan, K.W., Saxton, C.A., Jones, C.L., Ritchie, J.A., and Morrison, T.: Control of Gingivitis and Calculus by a Dentifrice Containing a Zinc Salt and Triclosan, *J. Periodontol., 61,* 674, November, 1990.

Svatun, B., Saxton, C.A., and Rölla, G.: Six-month Study of the Effect of a Dentifrice Containing Zinc Citrate and Triclosan on Plaque, Gingival Health, and Calculus, *Scand. J. Dent. Res., 98,* 301, August, 1990.

Wade, W.G. and Addy, M.: Antibacterial Activity of Some Triclosan-containing Toothpastes and Their Ingredients, *J. Periodontol., 63,* 280, April, 1992.

Sanguinaria

Balanyk, T.E.: Sanguinarine: Comparisons of Antiplaque/Antigingivitis Reports, *Clin. Prev. Dent., 12,* 18, August-September, 1990.

Gazi, M.I.: Photographic Assessment of the Antiplaque Properties of Sanguinarine and Chlorhexidine, *J. Clin. Periodontol., 15,* 106, February, 1988.

Hannah, J.J., Johnson, J.D., and Kuftinec, M.M.: Long-term Clinical Evaluation of Toothpaste and Oral Rinse Containing Sanguinaria Extract in Controlling Plaque, Gingival Inflammation, and Sulcular Bleeding During Orthodontic Treatment, *Am. J. Orthod. Dentofacial Orthop., 96,* 199, September, 1989.

Harper, D.S., Mueller, L.J., Fine, J.B., Gordon, J., and Laster, L.L.: Clinical Efficacy of a Dentifrice and Oral Rinse Containing Sanguinaria Extract and Zinc Chloride During 6 Months of Use, *J. Periodontol., 61,* 352, June, 1990.

Kopczyk, R.A., Abrams, H., Brown, A.T., Matheny, J.L., and Kaplan, A.L.: Clinical and Microbiological Effects of a Sanguinaria-containing Mouthrinse and Dentifrice With and Without Fluoride During 6 Months of Use, *J. Periodontol., 62,* 617, October, 1991.

Laster, L.L.: New Perspectives on Sanguinaria Clinicals: Individual Toothpaste and Oral Rinse Testing, *Can. Dent. Assoc. J., 56,* 19, July, Supplement, 1990.

Mauriello, S.M. and Bader, J.D.: Six-month Effects of a Sanguinarine Dentifrice on Plaque and Gingivitis, *J. Periodontol., 59,* 238, April, 1988.

Moran, J., Addy, M., and Newcombe, R.: A Clinical Trial to Assess the Efficacy of Sanguinarine-Zinc Mouthrinse (Veadent) Compared with Chlorhexidine Mouthrinse (Corsodyl), *J. Clin. Periodontol., 15,* 612, November, 1988.

Quirynen, M., Marechal, M., and van Steenberghe, D.: Comparative Antiplaque Activity of Sanguinarine and Chlorhexidine in Man, *J. Clin. Periodontol., 17,* 223, April, 1990.

24

Care of Dental Prostheses

Total cleanliness of the oral cavity for the health of the teeth and supporting structures involves specific procedures for the care of the natural teeth and all replacements, both fixed and removable. A *prosthesis* is an artificial replacement of a missing part of the body, and a dental prosthesis replaces one or more teeth. Other definitions may be studied in table 24–1. Additional definitions pertaining to orthodontic appliances are included in table 41–1.

The fit and function of a dental prosthesis depend to a large degree on the cooperation of the patient in daily cleaning of the prosthesis and bacterial plaque control for the remaining natural teeth. Likewise, orthodontic appliances must be kept clean and periodontal health maintained if the treatment is to have long-term success.

The patient's cooperation depends on the motivation, information, and sense of appreciation and concern imparted by the members of the dental team. For the natural teeth involved, instruction begins early, before construction of the partial denture or placement of orthodontic appliances. Instruction is supplemented when an appliance is inserted to demonstrate specific techniques for daily care. Continuing supervision and review of procedures at succeeding appointments and maintenance appointments are required.

A patient may have more than one prosthesis. For example, a complete maxillary denture may be accompanied by both fixed and removable partial dentures in the mandibular arch. For this patient, the regimen for personal care involves the natural teeth as well as the fixed and removable dentures. A program of instruction must be worked out for each patient, depending on individual needs. Examples of fixed and removable prostheses and appliances are listed in table 24–2.

ORTHODONTIC APPLIANCES

Without a strong and persistent preventive care program before, during, and following completion of orthodontic treatment, a high dental caries rate has been associated with orthodontic treatment. Gingival and periodontal infections during and following treatment are not unusual. An individualized preventive program that includes a specific plan of instruction, motivation, and supervision is essential for the patient with orthodontic appliances. The patient must understand that much more effort is required while in treatment than was required before the appliances were placed.

The patient may be under care with regular appointments for a long period, frequently over a few years. Periodic communication between the patient's referring dentist and dental hygienist is necessary to coordinate instruction along with other necessary dental and dental hygiene care.

I. COMPLICATING FACTORS
A. Age Group
Many orthodontic patients are in the preteen and teenage years, periods when the incidence of gingivitis is high. The incidence of periodontal infection increases from early childhood to late teenage years.

B. Gingivitis
Bacterial plaque retention by orthodontic appliances leads to gingivitis. The degree can vary from slight to severe with gingival enlargement, particularly of the interdental papillae. The tissue may greatly enlarge and cover the fixed appliance. The enlarged tissue with pockets provides additional plaque-retentive areas.

TABLE 24-1
KEY WORDS: DENTAL PROSTHESES*

Abutment (ah-but'ment): a tooth or implant used for the support or retention of a fixed or removable prosthesis.

Denture (den'chur): artificial substitute for missing natural teeth and adjacent tissues.

Complete denture: dental prosthesis that replaces the entire dentition and associated structures; may be a complete maxillary denture or a complete mandibular, or both.

Immediate denture: a complete or removable partial denture fabricated in advance for placement immediately following the removal of natural teeth.

Fixed partial denture: a replacement for one or more missing teeth that is securely retained to natural teeth, tooth roots, and/or dental implant abutments that furnish the primary support for the prosthesis; also called a fixed prosthesis.

Removable partial denture: a dental prosthesis that supplies teeth and/or associated structures in a partially edentulous jaw and can be removed and replaced at will.

Denture adhesive: a soft material used to adhere a denture to the underlying mucosa; also referred to as an adherent.

Hawley retainer: a removable plastic and wire appliance used to stabilize teeth; may be modified for special applications during or after orthodontic therapy.

Obturator (ob'tū-rā tor): a prosthesis used to close a congenital or acquired opening, such as for a cleft palate, an area lost because of trauma, or after surgery for removal of a diseased area.

Pontic (pon'tik): an artificial tooth on a partial denture that replaces a missing natural tooth, restores its function, and usually occupies the space previously filled by the natural crown.

Precision attachment: a type of connector that consists of a metal receptacle and a close-fitting part; the metal receptacle usually is included within the restoration of an abutment tooth, and the close-fitting part is attached to a pontic or removable partial denture framework.

Preventive orthodontics: dental services intended to prevent the development of a malocclusion by maintaining the integrity of an otherwise normally developing dentition.

Prosthesis (prös-thē'sïs): artificial replacement of an absent part of the body; may be a therapeutic device to improve or alter function; may be a device employed to aid in accomplishing a desired surgical result.

Rest: a rigid, stabilizing extension of a fixed or removable partial denture that contacts a remaining tooth or teeth; prevents movement toward the mucosa and transmits functional forces to the teeth.

Space maintainer: prosthetic replacement for prematurely lost primary teeth to prevent closure of the space before eruption of the permanent successors.

* Definitions in this chapter that pertain to prosthetic appliances are taken or adapted from and are in accord with the *Glossary of Prosthodontic Terms,* 6th ed., 1993, of the Academy of Prosthodontics Foundation.

Definitions pertaining to orthodontic appliances are taken or adapted from the Orthodontic Glossary of the American Society of Orthodontists.

TABLE 24-2
TYPES OF ORAL PROSTHESES AND APPLIANCES

FIXED
Orthodontic Appliance
Space Maintainer
Fixed Partial Denture
Periodontal Splint
Implant-supported Complete Denture

REMOVABLE
Removable Orthodontic Appliances
Removable Space Maintainer
Hawley Appliance
Removable Partial Denture
    Natural Teeth Supported
    Implant Supported
Complete Denture
Overdenture
Obturator

C. Position of Teeth

Teeth that are irregularly positioned are naturally more susceptible to the retention of bacterial deposits and are more difficult to clean. With the severe malocclusions presented by ortho-

dontic patients at the outset, this factor becomes even more significant.

D. Problems with Appliances

1. Orthodontic appliances retain plaque and debris.
2. Accidents may cause wires to bend adversely and become embedded in the gingiva. A loosened band may be forced under the gingiva.
3. Removable appliances or their clasps may press excessively against the gingiva.
4. Rubber bands used during therapy may slip under the gingiva and detach the junctional epithelium.

E. Self-care Is Difficult

Even the patient who tries to maintain oral cleanliness has difficulty because the appliances are in the way and interfere with the application of the toothbrush and other devices used for plaque control.

II. DISEASE CONTROL

A rigid program for dental caries and periodontal disease control is needed. The selection of plaque control procedures for an individual patient is determined by the anatomic features of the gingiva, the position of the teeth, and the type and position of the orthodontic appliance.

Many types of appliances are utilized for orthodontic treatment. Fixed orthodontic appliances may consist of brackets bonded directly to the tooth surfaces after an acid etch procedure, as shown in figure 41–1 (page 592). Other appliances are bands cemented around each tooth with brackets attached to the bands to support an arch wire. Figures 24–2 and 24–3 show teeth with complete bands.

A. General Instructions

1. Give instructions before appliances are placed. Every attempt must be made to have the oral tissues in health and the patient motivated to perform thorough daily plaque removal.
2. Perform brushing before a mirror so that brush application is accurate and brushing is thorough.
3. Use a disclosing solution rinse to assist in self-evaluation. Orthodontic patients may experience difficulty in chewing disclosing wafers without discomfort or pain.
4. Recommend an approved fluoride dentifrice to aid in dental caries control.
5. Place emphasis in brushing on sulcular brushing and cleaning the area between the orthodontic bands and brackets and the gingiva.

B. Toothbrushing

1. *Brush Selection*
   a. A soft brush with end-rounded filaments generally is recommended.
   b. A special bi-level orthodontic brush designed with spaced rows of soft nylon filaments and with a middle row that is shorter can be applied directly over the fixed appliance. It is used with a short horizontal stroke (figure 24–1).
2. *Brushing Procedure*
   a. A sulcular method is needed by most patients for cleaning the appliances and maintaining the gingiva.
   b. Special adaptation is required for facial surfaces. Place the brush with filament ends directed toward the occlusal surface Charters position, (figure 22–7) to clean over the wire and bracket (or under for mandibular arch); place in Stillman position for the opposite side (figure 24–2).
   c. To assure cleanliness, one should brush the appliances in any way that the filaments can be manipulated. Insert the brush from

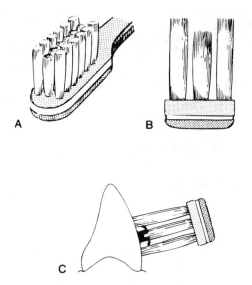

FIG. 24–1. **Orthodontic Bi-level Toothbrush. A.** Middle row of filaments trimmed shorter to fit over a fixed appliance. **B.** Cross section. **C.** Brush held over a bracket. Another bi-level shape is shown in figure 22–2, page 335.

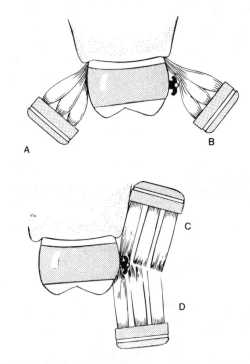

FIG. 24–2. **Toothbrushing for Orthodontic Appliance. A.** Sulcular brushing for periodontal tissues. **B.** Facial surface over bracket. **C.** Cleaning the bracket using brush in Charters brushing position for the gingival side. **D.** Brush in Stillman position for occlusal side of the bracket and arch wire.

below, over, and above the arch wire; rotate and vibrate to remove plaque and debris.
   d. Lingual approach to brushing is similar to the basic strokes used on the facial surfaces.

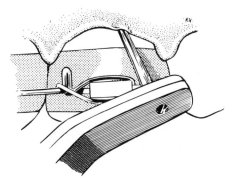

FIG. 24–3. Toothpick Holder for Orthodontic Patient. Moistened toothpick in holder can be applied for cleaning about appliances and in the subgingival area of the sulcus. Directions for use of the device are on page 360.

C. Additional Measures

1. *Interdental Aids*

   The previously described applications for the interdental tip and toothpick in holder (pages 359 and 360) also apply for care of the orthodontic patient (figure 24–3). A floss threader is needed for plaque removal from proximal tooth surfaces when the appliance prevents passage of floss from the occlusal aspect. Tufted dental floss or yarn used in the floss threader can remove plaque more efficiently than can regular dental floss.

   An interdental brush and a single-tuft brush can be particularly beneficial around individual teeth. The entire system should be kept as simple as possible.

2. *Oral Irrigation*[1]

   Most orthodontic patients can benefit from the regular use of an irrigator for removal of bacterial plaque and food debris and prevention of gingival inflammation.

III. CARE OF REMOVABLE APPLIANCE OR HAWLEY RETAINER (figure 24–4)

After fixed appliances have been removed, a retainer is worn to give support to the teeth while the bone and other supporting tissues are stabilizing.

A. Clean the appliance after each meal and before retiring. Instructions for cleaning procedures and agents for removable appliances are described with the care of the removable denture (pages 383 and 384).

B. Brush and rinse teeth and gingival tissue under the appliance each time the appliance is removed. Unless necessary as directed by the orthodontist, the health of the underlying tissues is best maintained when the appliance is not kept in the mouth continuously.

C. Brush the mucosa under the appliance. Methods are described on page 389.

D. Keep appliance in a container with water when it is out of the mouth.

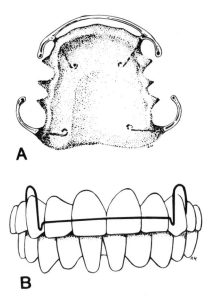

FIG. 24–4. Hawley Retainer. A. Removable acrylic retainer with labial retaining wire and clasps to be worn after removal of a fixed orthodontic appliance. **B.** Anterior view shows a Hawley appliance in position. The method for cleaning the appliance is similar to that for cleaning a removable denture (pages 383–384).

IV. SELF-APPLIED FLUORIDE

A patient with an orthodontic appliance has an increased risk of enamel demineralization and dental caries because of bacterial plaque retention. A daily fluoride program is mandatory to supplement mechanical daily plaque removal and periodic professional topical applications of fluoride solution or gel.

Self-applied fluorides are described on pages 449–453. A fluoride dentifrice is recommended, along with a daily mouthrinse, gel tray, or brush-on gel. Encouragement, repetition, reinforcement, and motivation are needed to achieve continuing interest and cooperation of an orthodontic patient in both the plaque control and the self-applied fluoride programs.

SPACE MAINTAINERS

When teeth are lost, the surrounding teeth tend to move toward the space. The loss of a permanent tooth is illustrated in figure 24–5. After the extraction of the mandibular first molar, the second and third molars inclined mesially and the maxillary first molar supererupted into the space. Prevention of such disruption of occlusion and function is a primary reason for the use of fixed or removable dental appliances described in the next sections in this chapter.

The premature loss of one or more primary molars disrupts the eruption pattern of the developing permanent teeth. The loss of a second primary molar creates a serious situation because the permanent molars begin

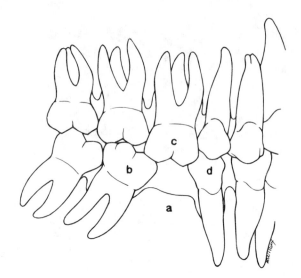

FIG. 24–5. Loss of Mandibular First Permanent Molar. Mandibular second (b) and third molars incline into the space from which the first molar was removed (a). Second premolar (d) drifts distally. Maxillary first molar (c) supererupts into the space. Occlusion and mastication are disabled, and predisposition to periodontal involvement around the irregularly positioned teeth is greatly increased.

to migrate mesially. The permanent premolars may be closed in and prevented from eruption, as shown in figure 24–6.

Many malocclusions result from early loss or prolonged retention of primary teeth. When a primary tooth cannot be saved through treatment and restoration, the space then must be held. The use of a space maintainer is a form of preventive orthodontics.

I. TYPES OF SPACE MAINTAINERS
The two general types of space maintainers are *fixed* and *removable*. An advantage of a fixed appliance is that the patient cannot lose or forget to wear the appliance. Some space maintainers may be designed for function during mastication, and others may have orthodontic attachments to move teeth.

II. FIXED SPACE MAINTAINER
A. Description
A fixed appliance is made of orthodontic arch wire soldered to a band or bands placed around natural teeth, usually around molars. A bilateral lingual appliance is shown in figure 24–7.

B. Personal Care Procedures
Bacterial plaque control can be accomplished by using many of the methods described for orthodontic appliances (pages 378 and 379). Adaptation of techniques is needed for cleaning the lingual arch wire and the lingual aspect of the molar bands for an appliance such as that shown in figure 24–7. A single-tuft brush with a bent

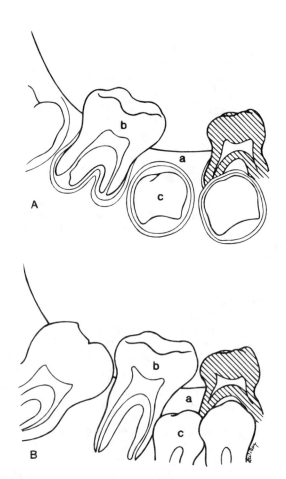

FIG. 24–6. Premature Loss of Second Primary Molar. **A.** Developing first permanent molar (b) inclines and drifts mesially into the space (a) from which the second primary molar was removed. Developing second premolar (c) is crowded. **B.** Space from which molar was removed (a) is nearly closed by the mesial drift and eruption of the first permanent molar (b). Developing second premolar (c) is closed in and prevented from eruption. Note that the second permanent molar has impacted against the first molar.

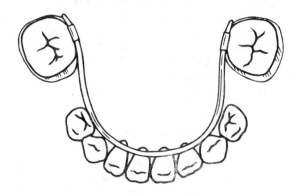

FIG. 24–7. Space Maintainer. Bilateral lingual mandibular space maintainer with orthodontic bands cemented around the permanent molars to hold the lingual arch wire. Space from which primary molar was removed is being maintained for eruption of the premolar.

shank may prove helpful (figure 23–9, page 359). Prevention of dental caries and gingivitis can be especially important during the ages of mixed dentition.

III. REMOVABLE SPACE MAINTAINER
A. Description
The removable appliance is constructed with an acrylic base and stainless steel wire formed into clasps. A lingual bar of stainless steel may be used for a mandibular appliance.

B. Personal Care Procedures
The removable space maintainer is similar to a removable partial denture, and the methods for denture hygiene described on pages 383 and 384 apply. Care of natural teeth, the abutments, and clasped teeth requires continuing demonstration and motivation for the young patient.

FIXED PARTIAL DENTURES

I. DESCRIPTION
Fixed partial dentures, formerly called dental "bridges," are composed of abutments, connectors, and pontics as defined in table 24–1 and shown in figure 24–8.

II. CHARACTERISTICS
A. Types of Fixed Partial Dentures
1. *Natural Teeth Supported*
   a. Bilateral. Supported by one or more natural teeth at each end (figure 24–8A).
   b. Cantilever. Supported by one or more teeth at one end only (figure 24–8B).
   c. Resin-bonded cast metal bridge. Uses resin-bonded retainer attached to etched enamel; characterized by little or no removal of tooth structure.
2. *Implant Supported* (figure 24–8C). Blade, cylinder, and screw types of implants used for abutments are shown in figure 25–5 (page 399).

B. Criteria for Fixed Partial Denture[2]
1. Harmonious with the teeth and surrounding periodontium.
2. All parts accessible for cleaning by the patient and the professional.
3. Must not interfere with the cleaning regimen for the remaining natural dentition.
4. Must not traumatize oral tissues.

CARE PROCEDURES

I. DEBRIS REMOVAL
When suggesting a procedure to follow for cleaning the oral cavity when a fixed partial denture is present, debris removal with an oral irrigator may be recommended as a first step. By removing food and debris, access of the toothbrush and other aids for plaque removal is facilitated. Procedure for use of an oral irrigator is described on pages 362 and 363.

II. PLAQUE REMOVAL FROM ABUTMENT TEETH
Nearly all the methods proposed for bacterial plaque control in the two previous chapters may be applicable to abutment teeth. The proximal surface and gingiva of an abutment tooth adjacent to a pontic usually require special attention.

A. Toothbrushing
Sulcular brushing is generally indicated. The area of the tooth surface adjacent to and beneath the gingival margin must be kept meticulously free of bacterial plaque.

B. Dentifrice Selection
A nonabrasive dentifrice is indicated to prevent the possibility of abrasion when pontic or crown facings are made of acrylic, when the gold of the partial denture is highly polished and could be scratched, and when areas of root exposure are on abutment teeth.

A fluoride-containing dentifrice is important for protection of remaining tooth surfaces, par-

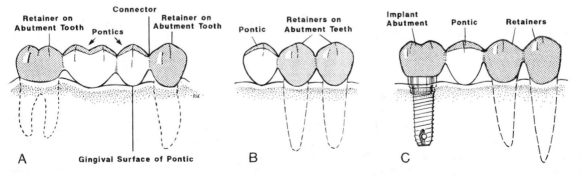

FIG. 24–8. Fixed Partial Dentures. A. Characteristic parts of mandibular four-unit fixed partial denture. Cast gold crowns on the abutment teeth serve as the retainers for this bridge. **B.** Cantilever bridge supported by double abutment. **C.** Fixed partial denture with natural teeth and implant abutments.

ticularly exposed cementum. Acidulated fluoride preparations are contraindicated for porcelain and composite restorations (pages 445 and 450).[3]

C. Additional Interdental Care

An interdental plaque removal method is indicated. This method is selected on the basis of the individual patient or the appliance. The interdental cleaning device is adapted specifically to the distal surface of the mesial abutment and the mesial surface of the distal abutment, and from both facial and lingual aspects. The same interdental cleaning procedure can usually be applied to the gingival surface of the fixed partial denture. Interdental cleaning methods and devices are described on pages 353–361.

III. THE PROSTHESIS

A. Areas Requiring Emphasis

The gingival surfaces of the pontics and beneath the connectors are particularly prone to plaque retention.

B. Toothbrushing

A toothbrush in the Charters position may be helpful for cleaning the gingival surface of the pontic from the facial aspect. The filaments can be directed under the pontic to clean the gingival surface. Charters brush position is described on page 342.

C. Dental Floss

1. Thread a 12- to 15-inch length into a floss threader. Several types are available (figure 24–9).
2. Apply threader between an abutment and pontic.
3. Draw the floss through, and using single or double thickness, remove loose debris (figure 24–10).
4. Apply dentifrice and a new section of the floss with moderate pressure to the undersurface (gingival surface) of the pontic and then to the proximal surfaces of each abutment tooth to remove bacterial plaque. Remove floss.

D. Knitting Yarn

Put length of yarn or tufted floss in floss threader and pull through under the appliance for a cleaning device that is thicker than floss alone (page 357).

E. Other Interdental Devices

A pipe cleaner, an interdental brush, a single-tuft brush, or an interdental tip should be recommended and demonstrated as indicated by the requirements of the individual appliance. These devices usually fit mesial and distal to the pontic, but not over the gingival surface of the pontic. Yarn or tufted loss with threader is essential.

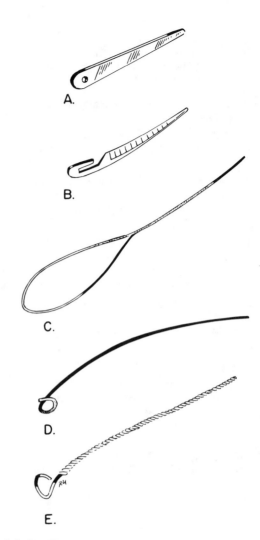

FIG. 24–9. Floss Threaders. A. Clear plastic with closed eye. **B.** Tinted plastic with open eye. **C.** Soft plastic loop. **D.** Flexible wire. **E.** Twisted wire.

REMOVABLE PARTIAL DENTURES

The removable partial denture replaces one or more, but less than all, of the natural teeth and associated structures, and can be removed from the mouth and replaced at will. Depending on the location and number of remaining natural teeth, a partial denture may receive all its support from the teeth, or it may be partly toothborne and partly tissueborne.

Self-care procedures for the patient with a removable appliance involve much more than cleaning the appliance. The abutment teeth, the gingival tissue, and the mucosa of edentulous areas require regular attention. Gingival health is unfavorably affected by removable partial dentures because bacterial plaque tends to accumulate more readily and in greater quantities. Bacterial plaque control is a major factor in the long-term effectiveness of a removable partial denture.

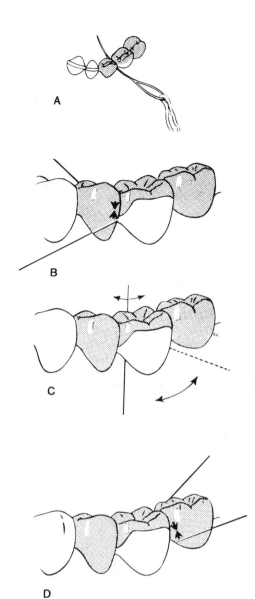

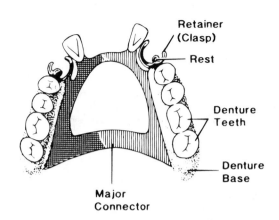

FIG. 24–11. Removable Partial Denture. Components of a removable partial denture shown for a maxillary prosthesis.

I. DESCRIPTION

The selection of cleansing agents and the procedures for cleaning are complicated by the intricacy of the metallic parts and their relation to the natural teeth, as well as by the dental materials used in construction.

The denture base rests on the oral mucosa and carries the artificial teeth. The base is most frequently made of plastic resin, but alloys of gold or chrome have also been used. The teeth may be made of porcelain, plastic resin, or metal.

The basic parts of a removable partial denture are shown in figure 24–11 and defined in table 24–1.

II. OBJECTIVES

A. The Prosthesis

Because natural teeth are adjacent to the appliance, objectives for cleaning the appliance take on added significance. The basic objectives are to remove irritants to the oral tissues (primarily bacterial plaque), prevent mouth odors, and improve appearance.

B. The Natural Teeth

The objective is to control plaque for the prevention of dental caries and periodontal infection.

CLEANING A REMOVABLE PROSTHESIS

Rinsing, immersion, and brushing methods, as well as the cleansing agents described for the complete denture on pages 386–388, apply alike to the partial appliance, with the few additions noted as follows.

I. RINSING

After each meal, the denture and the natural teeth should be brushed. When regular cleaning facilities are not available, rinsing is important for both the natural teeth and the removable appliance. While the appli-

FIG. 24–10. Use of Floss Threader. A. Use floss threader to draw the floss (or yarn or tufted floss) between abutment and a pontic. **B.** Apply floss to the distal surface of the mesial abutment; pull through 1 or 2 inches. **C.** Slide floss under pontic. Move back and forth several times, as shown by the arrows, to remove bacterial plaque from the gingival surface of the pontic. **D.** Apply new section of floss to the mesial surface of the distal abutment.

Procedures suggested here for care of the removable partial denture apply also to various other removable appliances. Examples of these are removable space maintainers; appliances for orthodontic purposes, such as a Hawley biteplate or retainer (figure 24–4); and obturators for closure of palatal openings, such as for cleft palate (page 621) or for replacement of tissue removal in the treatment of oral cancer.

ance is out, the tongue can be used to rub the sides of abutment teeth.

II. IMMERSION

Before immersion, the denture must be cleaned by rinsing and brushing to remove all bacterial plaque and debris. An agent known to discolor metal can be avoided. Procedures for immersion cleaning are described on page 387.

III. BRUSHING
A. Recommended Brushes

1. *Toothbrush.* One or more should be reserved for the natural teeth. The use of a regular toothbrush for care of a removable appliance is not recommended. When a patient chooses to do so, however, a separate brush is definitely indicated. Brushing the clasps and other metal parts can deform the filaments and make the brush ineffective for use on natural teeth.
2. *Power-assisted Brush.* A power-assisted toothbrush is sometimes appropriate for the natural teeth of the patient with a partial denture. The power-assisted brush, however, should not be used in and about the intricate clasps and other parts of a removable appliance because of the danger of catching the brush and damaging the appliance.
3. *Clasp Brush.* A specially designed narrow, tapered, cylindric brush about 2 to 3 inches long that can be adapted to the inner surfaces of clasps is recommended (figure 24–12). Clasps and their connectors are closely adapted to the supporting teeth, and the protected internal surfaces are prone to plaque accumulation. These difficult-to-clean areas require special care.
4. *Denture Brush.* A denture brush is shown in figure 24–14 and described on page 388. It

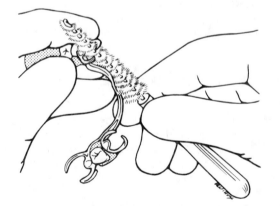

FIG. 24–12. Clasp Brush. A brush specially designed to remove bacterial plaque from the inside surfaces of clasps is available. The denture must be held carefully to avoid accidents.

is an excellent brush for cleaning all the smooth surfaces and the metal bars of the partial denture.

B. Precautions During Brushing

Too tight a grasp of a partial appliance can result in bending or fracture of clasps or bars. Filaments of a brush can inadvertently catch the appliance and cause it to drop. Partial filling of the sink with water or lining of the sink with a face cloth or towel is necessary to prevent accidents that cause breakage (page 388).

THE NATURAL TEETH

I. PLAQUE CONTROL

Toothbrushing and interdental cleaning methods selected for the particular needs of the patient must be followed meticulously. The longevity of the removable appliance depends on the health of the supporting teeth, and in turn, the health of the natural teeth depends on the cleanliness of the appliance.

II. DENTAL CARIES CONTROL

The topical application of fluoride, the use of a fluoride dentifrice and other self-applied fluoride measures, such as a daily mouthrinse or application of a gel, and the control of refined sugars in the diet must be definite parts of the complete program of oral care for the patient with a removable appliance.

The patient must be constantly alert to the control of plaque retention by the appliance and to the need for rinsing immediately after eating when brushing is not possible. For the patient who has been caries-susceptible and whose teeth are missing because of dental caries, a dietary analysis and specific dental caries control program may increase a patient's motivation.

COMPLETE DENTURES

One should not assume that the patient who is new to the dental office and is wearing dentures or a denture knows the proper techniques for caring for the appliances. During questioning for the patient history, information about the method and frequency of denture care is recorded. Later, the dentures are examined and the current method of care is reviewed. Alternate cleansing agents, devices, or procedures are recommended and demonstrated as needed.

Instruction may be given to the patient receiving a maxillary and mandibular denture for the first time, to the patient whose dentures have been remade or relined, or to the patient with a single denture that opposes natural teeth. Another patient may be receiving an immediate denture. Types of dentures and characteristics of the edentulous mouth are described on pages 646–649.

I. COMPONENTS OF A COMPLETE DENTURE (figure 24–13)

In an effort to understand the effects of various cleansing agents and devices, information about the structure and material of the parts of a denture is pertinent.

A. Denture Base

The part of a denture that rests on the oral mucosa and to which the teeth are attached is the denture base. Most denture bases are made of plastic resin. Others may be metal, for example, chrome-cobalt or gold in combination with a plastic resin.

B. Surfaces

1. *Impression Surface.* Also called the tissue or inner surface, the impression surface is the part that lies adjacent to the mucous membrane of the alveolar ridge and immediately associated parts; in the maxillary, the tissue surface is adjacent to the hard palate.
2. *Polished Surface.* The external or outer surface is highly polished. The occlusal surface is not polished.
3. *Occlusal Surface.* The portion of the surface of a denture that makes contact or near contact with the corresponding surface of the opposing denture or natural teeth is the occlusal surface.

C. Teeth

The denture teeth may be made of plastic resin or porcelain. Some posterior teeth have metal occlusal inserts. Anterior porcelain teeth have metal pins for retention.

II. PURPOSES FOR CLEANING

Inadequate oral tissue care and denture hygiene practices are major causes of oral lesions under dentures.

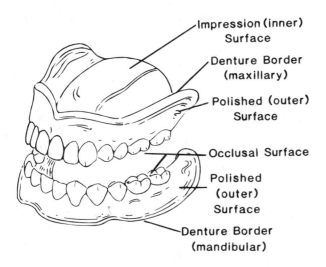

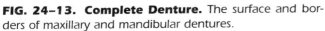

FIG. 24–13. Complete Denture. The surface and borders of maxillary and mandibular dentures.

A. Prevent Irritation to the Oral Tissues

1. *Mechanical Irritants.* Rough deposits of plaque, calculus, thick stains.
2. *Chemical Irritants.* Products of putrefaction of food debris and bacterial metabolic products.

B. Control Infection

Reactions to bacterial denture plaque and/or secondary infections by way of traumatic lesions may occur.

C. Prevent Mouth Odors

D. Maintain Appearance

III. DENTURE DEPOSITS

Accumulation of stains and deposits on dentures varies between individuals in a manner similar to that on natural teeth. The phases of deposit formation may be divided as follows:

A. Mucin and Food Debris on the Denture Surface

Readily removed by rinsing or brushing.

B. Denture Pellicle and Bacterial Plaque

Denture pellicle forms readily after a denture is cleaned. Denture plaque is composed predominantly of gram-positive cocci, rods, and filamentous forms of bacteria in an intermicrobial substance. Denture plaque also includes varying accumulations of *Candida albicans*, the yeast that causes candidiasis.

Plaque serves as a matrix for calculus formation and stain accumulation when the denture is not cleaned.

C. Calculus

Hard and fixed to the denture surface, calculus generally is located on the facial surfaces of the maxillary molars and the lingual surfaces of the mandibular anterior region.

CLEANING THE COMPLETE DENTURE

I. RINSING UNDER RUNNING WATER

Although a denture that could be kept clean only by this method would be unusual, the use of rinsing after meals when other methods are not possible is necessary.

II. BRUSHING

Brush with water, soap, or other mild cleansing agent. Coarse abrasives produce scratches.

III. IMMERSION

The denture is soaked in a solvent or detergent in which chemical action removes or loosens stains and deposits that can then be rinsed or brushed away.

IV. MECHANICAL DENTURE CLEANSERS

Commercially available devices include ultrasonic, sonic, magnetic, and agitating mechanisms that can be combined with an immersion agent. The action of the mechanical cleansing device seems to make the solution more efficient than a solution used alone. Ultrasonic cleaning during a professional appointment is described on page 572.

V. DENTURE CLEANSERS[4-7]

A. Requirements for a Denture Cleanser[4]

1. Easy for a patient to use.
2. Reasonably priced.
3. Effective removal of denture deposits (organic and inorganic) without abrasion of the denture surface.
4. Bactericidal and fungicidal action.
5. Nontoxic.
6. Harmless to the dental materials used for partial or complete dentures.

B. Chemical Solution Cleansers (Immersion)

1. *Alkaline Hypochlorite*
   a. Active ingredient. Dilute sodium hypochlorite with bleaching properties.
   b. Action. Loosens debris and light stains; bleaching; dissolves mucin; dissolves plaque matrix.
   c. Example. Household bleach.
   d. Disadvantage. Odor; tarnish; surface pitting; bleaching effect on soft lining materials and denture materials containing fibers.

2. *Alkaline Peroxide*
   a. Active ingredient. Alkaline detergent with an oxygen-liberating agent (sodium perborate or percarbonate).
   b. Action. Loosens debris and light stains by an oxygen-liberating mechanism. A preventive cleanser should be used regularly from the day a denture has been cleaned professionally to prevent accumulation of heavy deposits.
   c. Examples. Most proprietary cleansers are in the form of a powder or tablet that is dropped into water to create the alkaline solution of hydrogen peroxide.
   d. Disadvantage. Does not remove heavy stains or calculus.

3. *Dilute Acids*
   a. Active ingredient. Inorganic acids.
   b. Action. Dissolves inorganic components of denture deposits.
   c. Examples. 3% to 5% hydrochloric acid alone or with phosphoric acid; commercially prepared ultrasonic solutions. The strong acids (although in dilute forms) are not recommended for home use by the patient. Acetic acid (vinegar) has been used with some success when deposits were not old and hard.
   d. Disadvantage. Corrosion of metal parts of a denture.

4. *Enzymes.* The enzymes act to break down plaque proteins and polysaccharides. Enzyme agents have been incorporated into various immersion-type cleansers.

5. *Disinfectants.* A sanitary denture is necessary for the prevention of inflammation in the oral mucosa under the denture. Types of denture-induced lesions are described on pages 649 and 650. Regular daily maintenance procedures must be carried out.

   Patient instruction in disinfection of a denture is recommended. Disinfection can be accomplished by several EPA-registered products.[8]

   Full-strength commercially available sodium hypochlorite (household bleach) has been shown to be an antimicrobial agent. Before disinfection, preclean the denture under running water taking care not to splash and thus contaminate the area. To disinfect, immerse the denture for 5 minutes in full-strength bleach.[9] Because bleach can fade the color of a denture, immersion should be timed at 5 minutes, and the denture should be rinsed completely.

C. Abrasive Cleansers (Brushing)

1. *Denture Pastes and Powders, Toothpastes and Powders*
   a. Active ingredient. An abrasive, such as calcium carbonate (see Dentifrices, page 368).
   b. Action. Mechanical removal of bacterial plaque and stains by brushing.
   c. Examples. Various commercial products.
   d. Disadvantages. Can abrade the plastic resin denture base and acrylic teeth. A paste with low abrasiveness should be selected.

2. *Household Agents*
   a. Active ingredient. Detergent and/or abrasive agent.
   b. Examples. Salt and bicarbonate of soda are mildly abrasive; hand soap is cleansing and not particularly abrasive. Scouring powders or other excessively abrasive cleansers should not be used.

GENERAL CLEANING PROCEDURES

I. WHEN TO CLEAN

A. Regularly after each meal and before retiring.
B. Chemical immersion daily or twice weekly,

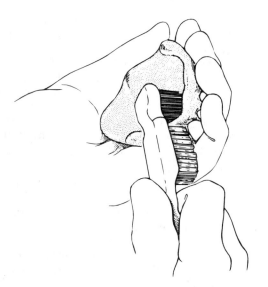

FIG. 24–14. Denture Brush. The denture is held securely, but without squeezing, in the palm of the nonworking hand. Place a face cloth in the bottom of the sink and partially fill with water. The specially designed brush is preferred because one group of tufts is arranged to provide access to the inner impression surface of the denture, as shown.

Prerequisite is that each area of each surface of the denture must be reached by the brush if bacterial plaque formation is to be controlled.

If a patient prefers to use an ordinary toothbrush, a multitufted soft nylon brush with end-rounded filaments should be acceptable if access to all the inner curvatures is possible without applying undue pressure on certain parts in the attempt to clean others. The patient who wears a single denture should keep separate brushes for the natural teeth and the denture to maintain the brush for the natural teeth in the best condition possible.

B. Procedure

1. Grasp denture in palm of hand securely, but without a squeezing pressure because dentures can be broken (figure 24–14).
2. Hold the denture low in a sink in which a towel, wash cloth, or rubber mat has been spread over the bottom to serve as a cushion should the denture be dropped. The sink should be partially filled with water.
3. Apply warm water, nonabrasive cleanser, and brush to all areas of the denture. Particular attention should be paid to the impression surfaces where configurations of the surface correspond with those of the oral topography. The anterior areas of the inner surfaces of both the maxillary and mandibular dentures require special adaptations of the brush.

4. Rinse denture and brush under running water. Use the brush to remove denture cleanser that may be retained in the grooves.
5. Visually check each area carefully for bacterial plaque. Teach the patient to run a finger over the surfaces to find "slippery" plaque areas.

C. Precautions Related to Brushing

1. Overzealous brushing with an abrasive cleansing agent on the impression surface could alter the fit of the denture.
2. Plastic resin can be abraded. Scratches make a rough surface; the denture may become more subject to the collection of debris and calculus.
3. Possibility of incomplete coverage during cleaning, particularly in the more inaccessible areas.
4. Possibility of cleaning with uneven pressure when the brush is applied more vigorously to accessible areas.
5. Danger of dropping and breaking the denture is increased when it is wet and, therefore, slippery.
6. Patient who requires eyeglasses should be advised to wear them when brushing to watch the procedure and to observe the cleanliness of the denture after brushing.

VI. ADDITIONAL INSTRUCTIONS

A. Care of Plastic Resin

An appliance made with plastic resin should be immersed in water or cleansing solution when it is not in the mouth.

B. Prevention of Denture Deposits

When the denture is kept clean by regular procedures from the time of insertion, accumulation of heavy stains and calculus can be prevented.

C. Professional Maintenance

A denture should never be scraped by the patient with a sharp instrument in the attempt to remove calculus deposits. When the cleaning methods recommended in this chapter do not remove deposits, the denture should be taken to the dental hygienist and dentist for professional cleaning. A regular maintenance plan is arranged.

D. Paste Cleaners

Paste cleansers (dentifrices or denture pastes) may cling and be difficult to rinse from the denture. Residual chemical agents, such as essential oils, may cause inflammatory or allergic reactions of the oral mucosa, and phenolic agents can have deleterious effects on plastic resin.

E. Soft Lining Materials

Temporary soft conditioning lining material may be sensitive to proprietary cleansers. Wash-

depending on the rate of formation of calculus and stain and the type of solution used.

1. May be at one of the daily cleanings.
2. Suggested while bathing.
3. Overnight when denture is removed as instructed by the dentist.

II. SELECTION OF PROCEDURE FOR CLEANING

Immersion, followed by brushing, is recommended. When unable to clean, rinsing after eating is advised.

III. PREPARATION FOR CLEANING

A. Rinse the denture thoroughly when it is taken from the mouth to remove saliva and loose debris.*
B. Remove denture-adhesive material.
   1. *Definition.* A denture adhesive is a commercially available paste or powder preparation. A patient may use it under the direction of the dentist for temporary stabilization. An occasional patient may use an adhesive indefinitely in an attempt to get along with ill-fitting dentures that should be adjusted or rebased.
   2. Method. Use a brush with light pressure to remove the adhesive.
   3. *Denture-bearing Mucosa.* Rinse and clean with a brush twice or more times daily (page 389).

IV. CLEANING BY IMMERSION

A. Advantages

1. The solution reaches all areas of the denture for a complete cleaning.
2. Minimizes the danger of dropping the appliance. Prevents need for handling, which is required during brushing.
3. Offers safe storage when dentures are out of the mouth.
4. Aids persons with limited ability to manage a brush.
5. When cleaning is distasteful, immersion involves the least handling and observation. This advantage is particularly attractive to a caregiver who must clean the denture of a helpless patient.

B. Procedure

1. Place denture in a plastic container with fitted cover that is maintained specifically for this purpose.
2. Use only warm water for rinsing and for mixing the solution. Warm water promotes the action of the cleanser. Hot water should never be used because it can distort plastic resin.
3. Follow manufacturer's specifications to as-

* Procedure for removal of a denture for a patient is described on page 572. It may be necessary to instruct a caregiver for a disabled patient.

sure correct dilution of cleanser.
4. Check that the denture is completel[y] merged in the solution; cover the con[tainer].
5. When the denture is removed, rinse [in] running water and remove loosened [debris] and chemicals before proceeding to cl[eaning by] brushing.
6. Empty and clean container daily. Mix [fresh] solution to prevent contamination [and] growth of microorganisms.[10]

C. Solutions

1. *Proprietary.* Available in powder or [tablet] form.
   a. Preparation. Add measured warm [water] as directed by the manufacturer.
   b. Length of immersion. Usually 10 [to 15] minutes or as suggested by the man[ufac]turer. Because the action depends o[n the] mechanical bubbling effect of rel[eased] oxygen, the solution has little value [after] the available oxygen has been relea[sed].
   c. Effect. The solutions are only effe[ctive] against loose debris; denture cleanl[iness] depends on regular daily immersion [sup]plemented by brushing.
2. *Hypochlorite Solution.* Household bleach [(5%] sodium hypochlorite) and Calgone. Calg[one] acts to improve the penetrating and [de]taching power of the bleach.
   a. Proportions

   1 tablespoon (15 ml) sodium hypochl[orite] (household bleach)
   2 teaspoons (8 ml) Calgone
   4 ounces (114 ml) water

   b. Length of immersion. Usually 10 to [30] minutes. When stains or calculus fo[rm,] the patient should be instructed to s[oak] the denture overnight provided there [are] no metal parts that can become corrod[ed.]

V. CLEANING BY BRUSHING

A. Type of Brush

1. *Denture Brush.* A good-quality denture bru[sh] with end-rounded filaments is reco[m]mended. The styles of denture brushes va[ry.] One type shown in figure 24–14 is design[ed] with two arrangements of filaments. O[ne] group in a large round arrangement of tu[fts] permits access to the inner, curved impre[s]sion surface of the denture. The secon[d] group of tufts is arranged to form a rectang[u]lar brush for convenient adaptation to th[e] polished and occlusal denture surfaces. An[other] design is shown in figure 50–9, pag[e] 696.
2. *Other Brushes.* A few patients prefer not t[o] have a denture brush for personal reason[s.] A hand brush can be used, provided the fila[ments are long enough to reach into th[e] deeper portions of the impression surface[s.]

The Patient with Oral Rehabilitation and Implants

Complete oral rehabilitation refers to the combined treatment of the teeth and periodontium to restore health, function, and physical form. As generally used, *oral rehabilitation* applies to involved extensive restorative procedures in a mouth that cannot be treated with routine dental care. It is also known as *mouth rehabilitation, occlusal rehabilitation, occluso-rehabilitation, complete reconstruction,* or *periodontal prosthesis.* Key words are defined in table 25–1. Other terms used in this chapter were defined in table 24–1, page 377, particularly the types and parts of dental prosthesis.

The term *periodontal prosthesis* is used to designate restorative and prosthetic treatment that is necessary for the treatment of advanced periodontal disease. The prosthesis used may be a splint for immobilization or stabilization of a group of teeth or an entire arch, maxillary or mandibular.

Periodontal, restorative, and prosthetic treatments are interdependent. The function and duration of all restorative and prosthetic treatments depend directly on the health of the periodontium, which provides the attachment and support necessary for the restored teeth. Periodontal health, in turn, is influenced by restorative and prosthetic treatment. Many predisposing factors that contribute to the initiation, development, and progress of periodontal infections are a direct result of untreated dental caries, incomplete or inadequate restorations, unreplaced missing teeth, and inadequate occlusal relationships built into restorations or prostheses.

I. OBJECTIVES OF COMPLETE REHABILITATION

Objectives for complete rehabilitation involve the same principles as for all oral care and include the need to

A. Restore optimal functional occlusion.
B. Maintain the health of the periodontium.
C. Produce biologically contoured restorations in harmony with normal oral physiology.
D. Replace missing teeth.
E. Provide support to teeth with advanced bone loss and marked mobility.
F. Provide desirable esthetics.
G. Establish acceptable phonetics.

II. COMPONENTS OF TREATMENT

Complete oral reconstruction means total mouth involvement, which brings in many phases of dentistry, often accomplished by individual specialists. The overall treatment plan may include some or all of the following:

A. Extensive periodontal therapy involving various surgical procedures.
B. Occlusal adjustment.
C. Endodontic therapy.
D. Correction of oral habits.
E. Orthodontic tooth movement.
F. Splinting of teeth temporarily or permanently.
G. Restorations involving individual teeth: crowns, inlays, onlays.
H. Replacement of teeth by fixed and/or removable prostheses.
I. Dental implants.

III. ACCOMPLISHMENT OF TREATMENT

Treatment may be long and involved for the patient who undergoes complete oral rehabilitation. It requires patience, persistence, and dedication of the patient, the dental hygienist, and the dentist.

The dental hygiene treatment plan overlaps every phase of the total treatment, beginning with the initial preparation of the patient's mouth. Maintenance and

393

TABLE 25–1
KEY WORDS: REHABILITATION AND IMPLANTS*

Crown: an artificial replacement that restores missing tooth structure by surrounding part or all of the remaining structure with a material, such as cast metal or porcelain, or a combination of materials, such as metal and porcelain fused (veneer crown).

Embrasure (em-brā'zhur): the space defined by proximal surfaces of adjacent teeth where those surfaces diverge apically, facially, lingually, or occlusally from an area of contact.

Furcation (fur-kā'shun) **invasion:** pathologic resorption of bone within a furcation; a periodontal bony defect.

Hydroxyapatite ceramic: a composition of calcium and phosphate to provide a dense, nonresorbable, biocompatible ceramic used for dental implants; metal implants may be coated with tricalcium phosphate or hydroxyapatite.

Implant: an alloplastic inert metal or plastic) material or device grafted or inserted surgically into intact tissues for diagnostic, prosthetic, therapeutic, or experimental purposes.

Inlay: a fixed restoration placed within tooth structure, prepared outside the mouth, and subsequently cemented into the tooth to restore intracoronal tooth structure; may be made of porcelain, composite resin, or cast gold.

Occlusal adjustment: treatment in which the occluding surfaces of teeth are reshaped by grinding to create harmonious contact relationships between maxillary and mandibular teeth; also known as occlusal equilibration or selective grinding.

Odontoplasty (ō-don'tō-plas'tē): the reshaping of a portion of a tooth; may be performed for therapeutic or esthetic purposes.

Onlay: a fixed restoration that is prepared outside the mouth and is subsequently cemented onto the tooth; it restores the occlusal surface, the mesial-distal or lingual-facial margins, and covers or replaces one or more cusps.

Osseous (os'ē-us) **integration:** the apparent direct attachment or connection of osseous tissue to an inert, alloplastic material without intervening connective tissue. Also called **osseointegration**

Peri-implantitis (ĭm-plan-tī'tĭs): inflammation of the tissue around a dental implant and/or its abutment.

Splint: an apparatus, appliance, or device used to prevent motion or displacement of fractured or movable parts.
 Dental splint: designed to immobilize and stabilize teeth in the same dental arch.

Supportive periodontal treatment: an extension of periodontal therapy; includes procedures performed at selected time intervals to review the general health history, reassess the status of periodontal health, and provide preventive oral hygiene care; also called **periodontal maintenance** or **preventive maintenance.**

Titanium: a uniquely biocompatible metal used for implants either in the commercially pure form or as an alloy.

Titanium alloy: the most common titanium alloy (Ti-6Al-4V) used for dental implants contains 6% aluminum to increase strength and decrease weight, and 4% vanadium to prevent corrosion.

Tomography: a radiographic technique that provides a distinct image of a selected plane through the body; the images of structures that lie above and below that plane are blurred.

Veneer: a layer of tooth-color material (composite or porcelain) that is bonded or cemented to a prepared tooth surface.

* Definitions in this chapter that pertain to prosthetic appliances are taken or adapted from and are in accord with the *Glossary of Prosthodontic Terms,* 6th ed., 1993, of the Academy of Prosthodontics Foundation.
Definitions that relate to periodontics are taken or adapted from the *Glossary of Periodontal Terms,* 3rd ed., 1992, of the American Academy of Periodontology.

supervision of the patient's self-care program are essential throughout restorative and prosthetic therapy and continuing into the maintenance phase.

Specific measures for self-care in terms of plaque removal and dental caries prevention must be selected and supervised. The patient is shown how to self-evaluate, so that minor deviations from normal can be recognized and called to the attention of the clinician.

CHARACTERISTICS OF THE REHABILITATED MOUTH

To select the appropriate methods for bacterial plaque control and dental caries prevention, one must assess existing conditions, such as contour and position of the gingiva, contour of restorations, and problem areas adjacent to fixed prostheses. When these are known,

the variety of possible techniques and devices for plaque removal can be reviewed and a plan for care outlined.

A patient who has undergone extensive periodontal therapy and restorative and prosthetic rehabilitation may have some or all of the characteristics listed here. Each condition may require specially selected or adapted plaque control measures. Fixed and removable appliances can provide many areas for bacterial plaque and debris retention.

I. PERIODONTAL FINDINGS
   A. Gingival recession.
   B. Exposed root surfaces.
   C. Exposed furcation areas.
   D. Alterations of gingival contour; the gingival margins may be rolled or rounded.
   E. Changes in size and shape of the gingival embrasures.

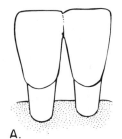

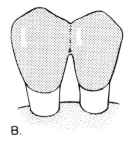

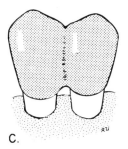

FIG. 25-1. Gingival Embrasures. A. Wide embrasure between two central incisors with missing interdental papilla and gingival recession. **B.** Double abutment with closed contact area with open embrasure provides access for plaque removal. **C.** Overcontoured crowns of a double abutment with a narrowed embrasure that provides limited access for bacterial plaque and debris removal.

1. Missing interdental papillae; wide embrasures with gingival recession and increased root exposure (figure 25–1).
2. Narrowed embrasures created by overcontoured restorations or variously shaped pontics (figure 25–2).

II. SINGLE TOOTH RESTORATIONS

A. The gingival margin around a crown restoration may appear bluish or bluish-red when the crown margin is below the gingival margin.

B. Various restorations may require selective cleaning agents.

III. FIXED PROSTHESIS

The parts of a fixed prosthesis are shown on page 381 in figure 24–8.

A patient may have

A. Fixed splinting around long segments of, or an entire, arch (figure 25–3).

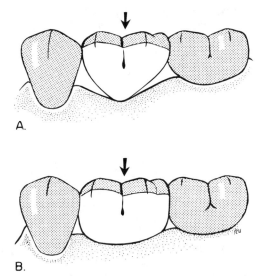

FIG. 25-2. Shape of Pontics. Mandibular three-unit fixed partial denture. **A.** "Bullet"-shaped pontic with wide embrasures for access for bacterial plaque removal. **B.** Improperly shaped pontic with closed embrasures and wide gingival surface for plaque retention. Arrows indicate pontics.

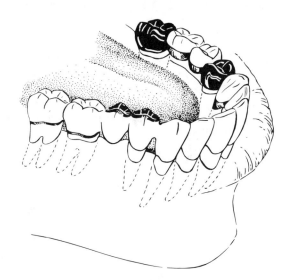

FIG. 25-3. Complete-Arch Fixed Splint. A continuous therapeutic fixed appliance stabilizes periodontally involved teeth and replaces missing components to provide appropriate occlusal relationships. Numerous problem areas for bacterial plaque removal exist.

B. Natural abutment teeth with difficult access areas adjacent to a pontic.

C. Implant abutment surfaces.

D. Closed contacts between teeth involved in a multitooth prosthesis.

E. Gingival surfaces of pontics.

F. Wide and triangular embrasures created by pontics or narrow, unnatural, nonself-cleansing areas created by improperly shaped pontics (figure 25–2B).

IV. REMOVABLE PROSTHESES

A. Complete denture may be used in one dental arch opposing natural teeth and partial dentures, fixed or removable.

B. Partial denture
1. Creation of potential areas of bacterial plaque and debris retention.
   a. Alteration of tooth form by clasp, rest, or precision attachment (defined in table 24–1, page 377).
   b. Improperly contoured edge of the partial denture at the junction of the partial denture and the abutment tooth.
2. Partial denture may impinge on the gingiva surrounding the abutment tooth.
3. Double abutment (two natural teeth with crowns that are soldered or cast together) has a closed contact requiring lateral (from facial or lingual aspects) access to the gingival embrasure (figure 25–1B and C).
4. The mucosa under the partial denture needs special care.

SELF-CARE FOR THE REHABILITATED MOUTH

These special patients require greater than average attention, patience, and teaching skill to obtain a favorable result that will assure continuing health of the patient's periodontal tissues. Total commitment on the part of the patient is necessary if the selected plan is to meet the requirements for daily care.

I. PLANNING THE DISEASE CONTROL PROGRAM

The control program should be planned as a concentrated effort to maintain gingival tissue, the exposed tooth structure, and, hence, the underlying supporting periodontium, as well as the restorations and prostheses. The instructions have three parts: first, before the surgical, restorative, and prosthodontic treatment; second, during therapy; and third, after reconstruction.

A. Part 1

Basic plaque control measures are learned and practiced by the patient during the preparatory phase. During these lessons, principles for self-evaluation can be presented.

B. Part 2

During therapy, adaptations are needed for applying techniques to temporary restorations. When the treatment extends over a long period, regular dental hygiene appointments for careful monitoring of the gingival health are essential.

C. Part 3

After therapy is completed, another set of self-care procedures is required to meet the needs

of the rehabilitated mouth. Special devices and techniques are selected and tried until the most efficient and thorough procedures are determined.

II. PLAQUE CONTROL: SELECTION OF METHODS[1]

Any of the methods and procedures described in Chapters 22, 23, and 24 may be needed in the care of the oral soft tissues, tooth surfaces, restorations, and fixed and removable prostheses. After assessment, methods selected must allow the patient to accomplish complete daily plaque removal from each area around every tooth or replacement. A summary of devices and methods is provided in table 25–2.

Most patients need a method for each of the following:

A. Debris removal, particularly from interproximal areas and around fixed prostheses.

B. Sulcular brushing procedure adapted to assure coverage for anatomic variations.

C. Interdental plaque removal
1. Proximal surfaces of natural and restored teeth, including exposed roots where access exists from the incisal or occlusal surfaces.
2. Proximal surfaces of abutment teeth under closed contact areas (figure 25–4).
3. Mesial and/or distal surfaces of teeth without proximal contact.

D. Removal of bacterial plaque around a fixed partial denture must include the gingival and proximal surfaces of pontics.

E. Cleaning the removable prosthesis and care of the supporting tissues.

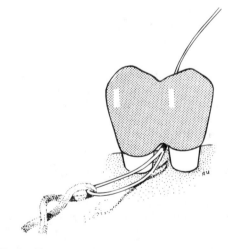

FIG. 25–4. Bacterial Plaque Removal from Embrasure. A floss threader is used with yarn or tufted floss to clean under a double abutment embrasure. Narrowed embrasure from overcontoured crown increases plaque and debris retention and makes cleaning difficult.

C. Oral Hygiene
The patient must demonstrate consistent and effective personal oral care.

II. INFORMATION FOR THE PATIENT
A. Explain procedures to be performed and the time schedule.
B. Explain possible complications.
C. Emphasize the role of personal oral care and the need for daily bacterial plaque control.
D. Obtain an informed consent statement and agreement of understanding.

III. SURGICAL STEPS
Acceptable bone integration has occurred with certain single-stage endosseous implants, but the more acceptable method is a two-stage procedure. The entire implant usually cannot be inserted in one step because forces of occlusion (chewing, biting) cause mobility and prevent bone healing. When the implant is first placed it must be stabilized. Movement of the implant may cause the formation of a fibrous tissue layer instead of osseointegration.

A. Instrumentation
The surgical procedure requires atraumatic placement of the implant into the bone. High-speed handpiece or other heat-producing methods cannot be used because they may cause bone damage.

B. Sterile Procedures
Whenever microorganisms are introduced during a surgical procedure, healing can be impaired. Manufacturers prepare implants in sterile packages.

IV. PROSTHETIC STEPS
Attention to ideal requirements for acceptable prostheses is necessary. Margins, embrasure shapes, crown contours, contact areas, and occlusal harmony must be designed to prevent bacterial plaque collection and permit thorough disease control procedures by the patient.

IMPLANT INTERFACES

An implant has an inner interface with the *bone* and a *soft tissue* interface where the terminal pin, abutment, post, or other protruding portion of the implant is surrounded by the mucosal or gingival tissue.

I. IMPLANT/BONE INTERFACE
Osseointegration refers to direct structural and functional union between the implant and healthy living bone. No discernible connective tissue is between the bone and the implant.

II. IMPLANT/SOFT TISSUE INTERFACE[9,10]
The external environment of an implant is the oral cavity, with saliva, bacterial plaque, and debris.

A. Biologic Seal (Permucosal Seal)
Between the implant or post and the soft tissue, a biologic seal must exist to prevent microorganisms and inflammation-producing agents from entering the tissues.

B. Soft Tissue Connection
Sulcular epithelium is in contact with the implant surface. The attachment appears similar to the epithelial attachment of the junctional epithelium of a natural tooth. Hemidesmosomes and basal lamina have been identified. The epithelium resembles a long junctional epithelium.

PERI-IMPLANT HYGIENE

A key requirement for implant success is the disease control program for the tissue surrounding the implant. Meticulous hygiene is a necessity for which repeated instruction may be needed.

I. BACTERIAL PLAQUE (IMPLANT PLAQUE)
Plaque microorganisms around implants with healthy permucosal tissue have been shown to be like the flora around natural teeth. Gram-positive, nonmotile coccoid and other forms predominate.[11,12]

The tissues around implant posts or abutments react to microorganisms and their toxic products in a manner similar to the gingiva surrounding natural teeth. When inflammation and pocket depths increase, the total numbers of microorganisms and numbers of spirochetes and motile rods increase also.[13]

II. PLANNING THE DISEASE CONTROL PROGRAM

A. Relation to Treatment
Supervision of a patient's oral hygiene must begin prior to the surgical phase for implant placement and carry on throughout the treatment phases.

B. Types of Prostheses
Implant-supported prostheses may be partial, complete, fixed, removable, or single-tooth replacements. Prostheses may be supported by natural teeth and/or implants. An individual may have a variety of areas and prostheses to care for.

III. SELECTION OF PLAQUE-REMOVAL METHODS
Any of the methods for plaque removal described in Chapters 22, 23, and 24 may be required in various combinations. Each patient needs an individually planned program so that each type of abutment and

prosthesis can be maintained in a plaque-free environment.

A. Conventional Prosthesis
Removable or fixed, partial or complete dentures made of conventional dental materials are to be cleaned by the usual methods described earlier. Suggestions provided here pertain primarily to the posts, abutments, or other protruding portions of implants.

B. Precautions
1. Prevent damage to implant materials. Care must be taken to use implements, dentifrices, or other cleaning agents that will not scratch or abrade the titanium or other material. Only smooth plastic or wooden implements should be used.
2. Each device should be checked before use. Toothbrush filaments must be smooth, soft, and end-rounded to prevent damage to the peri-implant tissue.

C. Subperiosteal Implant
The posts and surrounding tissue need to be cleaned completely around the circumference. Yarn or gauze strip can be used with a floss threader to position the material under the crossbar.

D. Endosseous Implant
1. *Abutments or Posts.* A floss threader can be used to position yarn or a gauze bandage strip around an abutment and under a fixed prosthesis. Tufted dental floss is also highly effective. Interdental brushes and single end-tuft brushes are adaptable. The end-tuft brush bent at the neck is particularly useful on lingual and palatal surfaces (figure 23-9, page 359).
2. *Undersurface of Fixed Prosthesis with Cantilever.* Several endosseous implants may be placed anterior to the mental foramen, and the complete overdenture may have a cantilevered portion distal to the terminal implant. Cleaning plaque from under the cantilever may be accomplished by using gauze strips.

IV. RINSING AND IRRIGATION
A. General Cleaning
Use of an irrigator can remove debris before specific cleaning with toothbrush and auxiliary aids.

B. Chemotherapy
1. Rinsing or daily irrigation with an approved antimicrobial can be recommended to help to minimize bacterial accumulation and inflammation. Specific directions for preparation of the solution and use of the irrigator must be demonstrated.

2. Chlorhexidine 0.12% has been shown to be effective. A cotton swab or interdental brush, dipped in the solution, can be applied directly to the gingival margins to help to prevent staining of oral tissues or tooth-color restorations.[14]

V. FLUORIDE MEASURES FOR DENTAL CARIES CONTROL
For the patient with natural teeth, daily fluoride self-application should be incorporated into the regime (pages 449-453). Titanium implants may be corroded by acidic fluoride preparations or preparations with a high fluoride concentration.[15,16] Low-concentration neutral sodium fluoride is recommended.

MAINTENANCE

I. BASIC CRITERIA FOR IMPLANT SUCCESS
The long-term success of an implant is assessed by routine, frequent examinations. A healthy implant shows the following:
A. No pain or discomfort reported by the patient.
B. No mobility.
C. No bleeding or increased probing depths on gentle probing.
D. No bone loss or peri-implant radiolucency in a radiograph.
E. No clinical signs of peri-implantitis (Table 11-2, page 188).

II. FREQUENCY OF APPOINTMENTS
The patient's daily oral plaque removal and regular supervision and monitoring through maintenance appointments directly influence the long-term success of an implant. When teeth were lost originally because of lack of daily plaque control by the patient, a more intense program of education and practice may be needed. Neglect may have been caused by lack of knowledge about, or appreciation for, preventive measures.

Each patient must have a personalized appointment interval, depending on individual needs. The first series of appointments following placement of the implant(s) should start within a week and be scheduled weekly until healing is completed and the patient has demonstrated the ability to control the bacterial plaque.

Maintenance appointments during the first year may be at 1- or 2-month intervals.

III. THE MAINTENANCE APPOINTMENT
Factors outlined for a maintenance appointment (pages 599 and 600) apply to a patient with an implant.

A. Health History Review; Vital Signs; Intraoral/Extraoral Examination
Basic review questions can reveal the present state of health, recent illnesses, changes in med-

ications, and other current information. Comparisons with previous records permit assessment of vital signs and extraoral/intraoral observations.

B. Selective Radiographs
A standard procedure must be used in order that comparisons can be made for bone level to determine status of implant stability. Special film placement devices have been developed.[17,18]

C. Periodontal Assessment
1. *Peri-implant Tissue.* Visual examination should show no signs of inflammation as evidenced by the usual criteria of changes in color, size, shape, and consistency.
2. *Probing.* Probe gently to determine bleeding tendency. A plastic probe must be used.
3. *Mobility Determination.*
4. *Deposits.* Bacterial plaque can be tested with a disclosing agent. The gingival surfaces of fixed prostheses should be checked carefully.

   Calculus is usually not extensive, hard, or firmly attached to implant abutments or other protruding parts, provided the patient has been faithful with daily procedures and professional maintenance appointments.

D. Review of Personal Bacterial Plaque Control Procedures
The patient demonstrates, and the clinician provides recommendations for improvements.

E. Instrumentation
Each type of implant requires attention to certain features. Manufacturer's instructions should be followed. Care must be taken not to scratch or alter in any way the surfaces of titanium and other materials making up the implant superstructures.
1. *Calculus Removal.* Plastic or wooden instruments are indicated for titanium. A porte polisher with wood point may be appropriate. Figure 25–8 shows various plastic instruments that have been developed for use on implants. In figure 25–9, adaptation of plastic instruments to implant abutments is illustrated.
2. *Prevention of Damage to the Implant Surface.* Severe abrasion can result from application of an ultrasonic scaler; an airbrasive can alter the hydroxylapatite coating on the implant.[19,20]
3. *Stain Removal.* Unless necessary for esthetics, stain removal is not included routinely. When selective stain removal is indicated, only a nonabrasive agent should be used and gently applied with a rubber cup.
4. *Professional Subgingival Irrigation.* The use of 0.12% chlorhexidine after professional instrumentation may be another treatment alternative when peri-implantitis has been present. Irrigation with chlorhexidine gluconate has been shown to be a safe procedure around implants.[21]

FACTORS TO TEACH THE PATIENT

I. IMPORTANCE OF DAILY CARE
The health of the periodontal tissues and the duration of the restorations and prostheses depend on daily self-care by the patient.

II. NEED FOR CONCENTRATION
More thought and concentration are required to maintain the mouth with advanced restorative dentistry, periodontal prostheses, or implants than are needed for an average mouth.

III. TIME REQUIREMENT
Cleaning a mouth with complex restorations takes longer. Time must be allotted in the daily schedule for complete cleaning and plaque removal once each day, supplemented by cleaning at least three times each day, or after each meal.

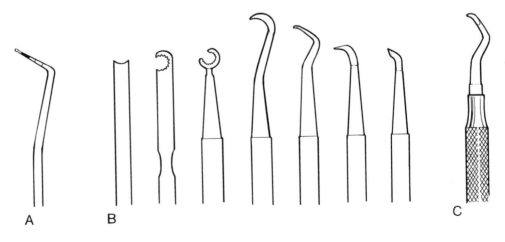

FIG. 25–8. Plastic Instrument Designs for Implants. A. Plastic probe with same markings as that in figure 19–1 (page 289). **B.** Scalers and curets. **C.** Exchangeable plastic curet tip fitted to metal handle for convenient sterilization and replacement. (*Implacare*, Hu-Friedy, used with permission.)

A   B   C

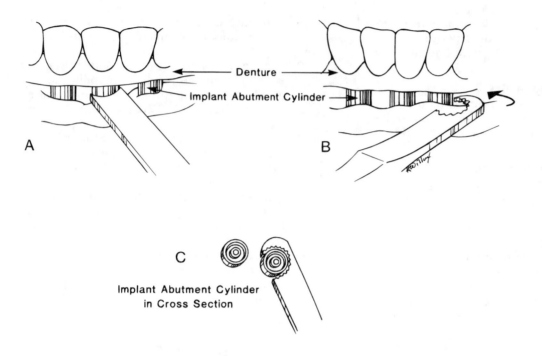

FIG. 25–9. Plastic Scaling and Cleaning Instrument. Specially designed double-ended plastic instrument for cleaning titanium abutment cylinders. **A.** One end is a crescent blade. **B.** The other end is a semicircular hook to apply around an abutment cylinder, shown in **C.** (Adapted from Balshi, T.J.: Hygiene Maintenance Procedures for Patients Treated with the Tissue Integrated Prosthesis (Osseointegration), *Quintessence Int., 17,* 95, February, 1986).

IV. DILIGENCE AND THOROUGHNESS

Do not go easy with the brush and other devices in the attempt to protect the restorations from breakage. *Protection* is for the gingival tissues and the preservation of the periodontium and is accomplished only by thorough bacterial plaque removal around every tooth.

V. IMPORTANCE OF MAINTENANCE

Frequent, regular appointments for professional supervision and cooperative care are necessary.

REFERENCES

1. **Bradbury,** E., Harvard University School of Dental Medicine, Boston, personal communication.
2. **American Dental Association,** Council on Dental Materials, Instruments, and Equipment and Council on Dental Therapeutics: Status Report: Effect of Acidulated Phosphate Fluoride on Porcelain and Composite Restorations, *J. Am. Dent. Assoc., 116,* 115, January, 1988.
3. **Lemons,** J.E.: Dental Implant Biomaterials, *J. Am. Dent. Assoc., 121,* 716, December, 1990.
4. **Albrektsson,** T., Zarb, G., Worthington, P., and Eriksson, A.R.: The Long-term Efficacy of Currently Used Dental Implants: A Review and Proposed Criteria of Success, *Int. J. Oral Maxillofac. Implants, 1,* 11, No. 1, 1986.
5. **Harris,** B.W.: A New Technique for the Subperiosteal Implant, *J. Am. Dent. Assoc., 121,* 422, September, 1990.
6. **Homoly,** P.A.: The Restorative and Surgical Technique for the Full Maxillary Subperiosteal Implant, *J. Am. Dent. Assoc., 121,* 404, September, 1990.
7. **Cranin,** A.N., Sher, J., and Schilb, T.P.: The Transosteal Implant: A 17-year Review and Report, *J. Prosthet. Dent., 55,* 709, June, 1986.
8. **Small,** I.A.: The Fixed Mandibular Implant: Its Use in Reconstructive Prosthetics, *J. Am. Dent. Assoc., 121,* 369, September, 1990.
9. **Meffert,** R.: Implant Therapy, in *Proceedings of the World Workshop in Clinical Periodontics.* Chicago, American Academy of Periodontology, 1989, pp. VIII-1 to VIII-4.
10. **Donley,** T.G. and Gillette, W.B.: Titanium Endosseous Implant-Soft Tissue Interface: A Literature Review, *J. Periodontol., 62,* 153, February, 1991.
11. **Mombelli,** A. and Mericske-Stern, R.: Microbiological Features of Stable Osseointegrated Implants Used as Abutments for Overdentures, *Clin. Oral Implants Res., 1,* 1, December, 1990.
12. **Quirynen,** M. and Listgarten, M.A.: The Distribution of Bacterial Morphotypes Around Natural Teeth and Titanium Implants Ad Modum Brånemark, *Clin Oral Implants Res., 1,* 8, December, 1990.
13. **Schou,** S., Holmstrup, P., Hjorting-Hansen, E., and Lang, N.P.: Plaque-induced Marginal Tissue Reactions of Osseointegrated Oral Implants: A Review of the Literature, *Clin. Oral Impl. Res., 3,* 149, December, 1992.
14. **Meffert,** R.M., Langer, B., and Fritz, M.E.: Dental Implants: A Review, *J. Periodontol., 63,* 859, November, 1992.
15. **Siirilä,** H.S. and Könönen, M.: The Effect of Oral Topical Fluorides on the Surface of Commercially Pure Titanium, *Int. J. Oral Maxillofac. Implants, 6,* 50, No. 1, 1991.
16. **Probster,** L., Lin, W., and Hüttemann, H.: Effect of Fluoride Prophylactic Agents on Titanium Surfaces, *Int. J. Oral Maxillofac. Implants, 7,* 390, Fall, 1992.
17. **Cox,** J.F. and Pharoah, M.: An Alternative Holder For Radiographic Evaluation of Tissue-integrated Prostheses, *J. Prosthet. Dent., 56,* 338, September, 1986.
18. **Meijer,** H.J.A., Steen, W.H.A., and Bosman, F.: Standardized Radiographs of the Alveolar Crest Around Implants in the Mandible, *J. Prosthet. Dent., 68,* 318, August, 1992.
19. **Thomson-Neal,** D., Evans, G.H., and Meffert, R.M.: Effects of Various Prophylactic Treatments on Titanium, Sapphire, and Hydroxyapatite-coated Implants: An SEM Study, *Int. J. Periodont. Restorative Dent., 9,* 301, No. 4, 1989.
20. **Rapley,** J.W., Swan, R.H., Hallmon, W.W., and Mills, M.P.: The Surface Characteristics Produced by Various Oral Hygiene In-

D. Involvement

With awareness and application to self, the response to action is forthcoming when attitude is influenced.

E. Action

Testing new knowledge and beginning of change in behavior may lead to an increased awareness that a real health goal is possible to attain.

F. Habit

Self-satisfaction in the comfort and value of sound teeth and healthy periodontal tissues helps to make certain practices become part of a daily routine. Ultimate motivation is finally reached.

INDIVIDUAL PATIENT PLANNING

Each patient has personal requirements for self-care, and objectives to fulfill these requirements must be related realistically to individual needs, interests, and ability level. If the patient is to participate effectively in the learning process, active involvement in setting goals is necessary.

The general objectives for disease control are for a reduced incidence of new dental carious lesions and for the elimination, control, and prevention of gingival and periodontal infections. The objectives for patient learning are selected with the patient to accomplish these objectives.

From the patient history, oral examination, radiographs, study casts, all other data collected during the initial evaluation, and the diagnosis, details of the self-care program are evolved.

I. FACTORS TO CONSIDER

A. The Gingiva

1. *Current Status of Gingival Health.* As evidenced by the color, size, contour, consistency, surface texture, tendency to bleed, probing depths, and severity of the periodontal condition.
2. *Treatment Plan.* Whether nonsurgical therapy will complete the professional treatment, or whether the condition will require more complicated periodontal therapy.
3. *Specific Anatomic Features*
   a. Open interdental areas or intact interdental gingiva.
   b. Recession with root exposure.
   c. Width of attached gingiva.

B. The Teeth

1. *Position*
   a. Malrelations, such as crowding, overbite, crossbite; malpositions of individual teeth; normal alignment.
   b. Teeth adjacent to edentulous areas.

2. *Abutment Teeth.*
3. *Dental Prostheses.* Fixed, removable, orthodontic.

C. General Health

1. *Chronic Disease.* Any systemic condition that may limit the ability to perform certain tasks or that may cause an exaggerated response of the gingiva to local irritants and require more intensive care.
2. *Capacity of Patient for Self-care.* Physical and mental handicaps that require that another person perform plaque control procedures.

D. Age

1. Young children require parental assistance.
2. Motivation varies with age.

E. Dexterity

1. Occupation that requires manual or digital dexterity may contribute to increased facility in the manipulation of oral care devices.
2. For most patients, unless a physical disability is apparent, dexterity cannot be detected until after instruction has begun.

F. Motivational Factors

1. *Immediate Evaluation.* Previous oral health habits can reveal attitudes and motivation, but frequently, a lack of oral cleanliness can be attributed to a lack of knowledge. Many people have had little or no instruction in how to care for their mouths.
2. *Long-range Motivation.* Prejudging a patient's motivation and willingness to carry out prescribed procedures is rarely possible. Some people show tremendous enthusiasm that may be short-lived; others reveal little interest at first, but prove to be highly conscientious.
3. *Motivation Related to Attitude.* Motivation can be directly related to the concern and enthusiasm of the members of the dental health team.

II. PROGRAM PLANNING

All of the aforementioned factors that apply to an individual patient are matched with the available bacterial plaque removal procedures. These include the selection of a toothbrush, toothbrushing method, interdental care devices and methods, dentifrice, and applied techniques for implants and fixed and removable dental prostheses.

With a clear definition of the needs of a patient, a recommended regimen or program can be outlined. The patient is shown the oral condition, changes and benefits that can be expected are explained, and cooperation is solicited. In this framework, the patient helps to formulate the goals that must be accomplished.

A. Immediate and Long-range Planning

Immediate and long-range programs are usually indicated. The immediate program is related to the treatment phase, whereas the long-range program is related to the maintenance phase of care.

The immediate program may be more complicated and intensified than the long-range program. It may seem more complicated to the patient because of the anxieties generally associated with learning new procedures and changing former habits.

The new habits and attitudes acquired during the immediate program phase may aid the transition to the long-range program. With continuing reinforcement of instruction and encouragement, plaque control measures become a part of the daily routine, and the health of the oral cavity can be maintained.

B. When to Teach

The initial instruction is best given *first*, before any clinical treatment. Reasons related to the educational aspects are as follows:

1. *Emphasis on Importance of Self-care.* Clinical professional services have only short-term effectiveness if the patient does not maintain tissue health through daily plaque removal. If considered first, and first in succeeding appointments, the degree of importance placed on self-care procedures by the dental team will become apparent to the patient.
2. *Teaching Is More Effective.* If instruction is delayed until after the clinical procedures in an appointment,
   a. Time may be limited.
   b. The gingival margin may be sensitive from instrumentation.
   c. Blood clots forming after scaling and root planing must not be disturbed so healing can progress favorably.
   d. Patient may be tired, anxious to leave, and less receptive to instruction.
3. *Plaque on Patient's Teeth.* With removal of tooth deposits during scaling, the opportunity to utilize the patient's existing plaque for demonstration is lost. With the use of a disclosing agent, a method of instruction is available that can clearly and dramatically show the patient what is to be accomplished. Bacterial plaque is not visible on most teeth without staining. Words fail to impress upon the patient that bacterial colonies exist on the teeth and that these multitudes of microorganisms are the responsible agents for dental and periodontal infections.

C. The Setting

Because of the need for the light and rinsing facilities during the demonstration, instruction may be given best at the dental chair. Without an extensive display of instruments and other equipment to distract the patient, and with the clinician seated beside the dental chair at the patient's eye level, an atmosphere conducive to learning can be created.

A specific area may be set aside and furnished for plaque control instruction in a dental office or clinic. Such an area should be planned with mirrors for the patient to use to observe the stained plaque on posterior teeth and distal surfaces. The patient also should be able to see placement of the toothbrush and floss in all areas of the mouth. Requirements for such a facility for a patient in a wheelchair are described on pages 683 and 684 and in figure 50–2.

PRESENTATION, DEMONSTRATION, PRACTICE

A suggested outline for conducting the plaque control program follows. Various adaptations will be needed to tailor the plan to individual patients.

Each of the "lessons" described in the following is meant to represent the opening few minutes of each of the treatment appointments. A plaque index or score (pages 291–295) and/or a bleeding index (page 300) is made at the start. The index or score is understood by the patient, and new and review instructions are provided as indicated. The scaling and root planing planned for that appointment are then started.

I. FIRST LESSON
A. Objective
Orientation to bacterial plaque removal.

B. Description
Describe the formation and composition of bacterial plaque, its relationship to oral disease, and specifically its relationship to the patient's present condition. Present an overview of the plaque control program, what it can accomplish, and its purposes in relation to professional treatment.

C. Illustration
Sketch on a pad of paper or use prepared materials. Show a tooth and gingiva and point out where the bacterial masses collect to form plaque. Explain how inflammation develops in the gingiva. The complete description should be divided over more than one instruction period. Too long a "lecture" with too many facts and details at one time may mean the patient cannot absorb any of them.

1. *Patient with Gingivitis.* Show and explain the formation of dental calculus and how periodontal disease can develop if gingivitis is left untreated.
2. *Patient with Periodontitis.* Introduce pocket formation and the reasons for pocket elimination.

3. *Patient Whose Most Severe Problem Is Dental Caries.* When a food diary for analysis is to be prepared, orientation to the preparation of the diary precludes discussion of plaque, sucrose, and dental caries, until the dietary record is obtained (pages 426–429).

D. Demonstration

1. While the patient observes in a hand mirror, a healthy area of gingiva and an inflamed area can be compared.
2. A probe is used to show a gingival sulcus and/or increased pocket depth related to periodontal involvement. Bleeding on probing is an important indicator of disease and should be recorded.
3. Remove a sample of plaque with a curet to demonstrate the thickness and consistency of plaque and to use for a phase microscope demonstration when available.

E. Application of a Disclosing Agent

1. *Explain Its Purpose.* Discoloration of plaque shows where the masses of bacteria accumulate.
2. *Apply Disclosing Agent.* Use a topical application, provide diluted concentrate for a rinse, or request the patient to chew a tablet, swish for approximately 1 minute, and rinse (page 409).
3. *Examine the Teeth with the Patient.* Point out the stained plaque and explain how these areas (generally the proximal surfaces and cervical third of the teeth) are adjacent to the gingiva, and therefore the bacteria must be removed to control inflammation.
4. *Record Plaque Score or Index* (pages 291–295). Explain the score to the patient and use it to compare at future evaluations.
5. *Observe Location.* Observation of the location of disclosed plaque guides the instruction for plaque removal.

F. Instruction

1. *Keep Instruction Simple.* It may be better not to teach both flossing and brushing during the first control lesson, depending on the patient's background and experience.
2. *Floss First*
   a. Review objective.
   b. Show manner of holding the floss, inserting proximally, pressing around the tooth, and activating for plaque removal (figure 23–1, page 355).
   c. Examine in mirror to observe proximal areas where plaque has been removed.
3. *Brush.* Give a soft brush and ask the patient to remove the stained plaque. No specific brushing instructions should be given at this time so that the patient can concentrate on the single objective related to plaque removal.

4. *After Brushing, Examine the Teeth with the Patient.* The patient will see where accessible plaque was removed.
5. *Explain.* The use of a toothbrush is the most effective means of plaque removal for facial and lingual surfaces. Dental floss and other interdental devices are needed for the proximal tooth surfaces.

G. Summary of Lesson I

1. Review the basic objectives of learning about plaque composition, occurrence, and relationship to oral disease and learning about the use of a disclosing agent to aid in plaque detection and removal.
2. At the first lesson, a specific toothbrushing method is not necessarily presented. The basic objectives should not be obscured by inclusion of excess information or diversion of the patient's thinking by concentration on details of brush position. The exceptions are:
   a. The patient who demonstrates an acceptable brushing technique and whose mouth has been kept reasonably clean and shows no signs of detrimental brushing may only need to be shown a few special adaptations for the difficult-to-reach areas or other improvements.
   b. The patient who demonstrates a brushing method that is detrimental, such as a vigorous horizontal stroke or a haphazard scrub-brush method, and whose teeth and/or gingiva show the effects of harmful brushing needs an introduction to a less destructive method.

H. Continuation of Appointment

Instruction and practice in plaque removal can occupy the first appointment. Clinical services may not be started until the gingival inflammatory clinical signs have been lessened and the patient shows good progress in learning self-care.

When calculus removal is initiated, the relation of clinical procedures to plaque control should be made clear to the patient. The satisfactory long-range outcome of scaling and other professional treatment depends on complete daily plaque removal.

I. Instruction at End of Appointment

1. Encourage use of disclosing agent at home; provide patient with tablets or instructions for purchasing. Suggest using a tablet for daily plaque checks.
2. Emphasize the need for cleaning regularly for complete daily bacterial plaque removal. Discuss carrying a toothbrush and dental floss for use when not at home.
3. When extra brushes cannot be supplied, explain that the toothbrush that has been used

that day will be kept in the office for use during future appointments. Write down the specific name (number) of the brush for the patient to purchase for home use.

J. Patient Records

Methods, procedures, and patient progress and problems should be recorded following each appointment. The documented record can be reviewed before each appointment as a guide to continuing instruction.

II. SECOND LESSON

A. Objectives

To evaluate patient's success to date and to review and expand the knowledge-content of the previous lesson.

B. Evaluation

1. *Examine the Gingival Tissue with the Patient.* Evaluate and compare with notes recorded from previous examination. Changes in color, size, and bleeding on probing should be noted and recorded.
2. *Apply the Disclosing Agent.* Evaluate the plaque as the patient self-evaluates, using a hand mirror. Chart plaque index or other record and compare, with the patient, with previous scores or indices.

C. Review and Extension of Knowledge

1. Invite questions from patient concerning plaque formation and gingival and periodontal infections to determine how clearly information from the previous lesson was understood and retained.
2. Discuss dentifrice recommendation when information from the dental history and the oral examination indicates the need for a change.
3. Explain why the patient needs a more scientific brushing method (or how a few alterations in the previous method can improve the oral condition).
4. Relate brushing to the treatment phase of oral care.

D. Demonstration

When not done previously, demonstrate the brushing technique of choice for this particular patient.

1. Show the basic stroke on the anterior teeth where the patient can observe brush position and activation. Explain each step. Demonstrate brush position for each quadrant.
2. Instruction is divided appropriately to permit the patient to learn at a comfortable pace. When a patient has a power-assisted brush, initial instruction should be given with the manual brush so that proficiency can be attained with both. The patient should be asked to bring the power-assisted brush to

the next appointment for demonstration and instruction.

E. Practice

1. Each position around each arch must be practiced because of the variations in grasp of brush and hand positions, the difficulty of access, and the individual tooth positions, particularly malpositions.
2. A recommended sequence for plaque removal that includes all areas and the tongue is discussed with the patient.

F. Instructions for Home Procedures

Use disclosing agent after flossing and brushing to test completeness of plaque removal. A mouth mirror for the patient to use at home can be helpful. Inexpensive plastic mirrors are available specifically for this purpose.

III. THIRD LESSON

A. Objectives

1. Patients with reasonable mastery of the flossing and brushing methods but who need auxiliary plaque control (interdental, dental prostheses, or other) begin the third phase of their instruction.
2. When a patient is not ready and the plaque score or index still shows a lack of reasonable skill and motivation, introduction of new material may be postponed and previous instruction reviewed and practiced.
3. Many dentists postpone therapy until the patient shows that an effective plaque control program can be carried out and an acceptable level of oral cleanliness can be maintained.

B. Evaluation and Review

1. *Evaluate Gingiva.* Inspect with the patient for color, size, bleeding, and other characteristics of disease. Review the features of normal gingiva and commend improvements. Quadrants that have been scaled can be compared with other quadrants so that the effect of healing can be shown.

   Question the patient about changes observed during the past week or since the previous appointment, such as less bleeding when brushing, better taste, and an overall feeling of cleanliness. Emphasize the role of self-care in accomplishing the improvements rather than the effects of professional treatment.
2. *Evaluate Plaque.* Apply disclosing agent and inspect for areas that need additional instruction. Relate areas of persistent gingival redness to areas inadequately flossed and brushed.
3. *Evaluate Brushing.* Patient demonstrates with emphasis on the areas missed as revealed by

Caries in the Primary Dentition, *Pediatr. Dent., 14,* 314, September/October, 1992.

Marthaler, T.M.: Changes in the Prevalence of Dental Caries: How Much Can be Attributed to Changes in Diet? *Caries Res., 24,* 3, Supplement 1, 1990.

Sundin, B., Granath, L., and Birkhed, D.: Variation of Posterior Approximal Caries Incidence with Consumption of Sweets with Regard to Other Caries-related Factors in 15–18-year-olds, *Community Dent. Oral Epidemiol., 20,* 76, April, 1992.

Counseling: Education

Chidyllo, S.A. and Chidyllo, R.: Nutritional Evaluation Prior to Oral and Maxillofacial Surgery, *N.Y. State Dent. J., 55,* 38, October, 1989.

Dreizen, S.: Dietary and Nutritional Counseling in the Prevention and Control of Oral Disease, *Compendium, 10,* 558, October, 1989.

Fuller, S.S. and Harding, M.: The Use of the Sugar Clock in Dental Health Education, *Br. Dent. J., 170,* 414, June 8, 1991.

Hölund, U.: Effect of a Nutrition Education Program, "Learning By Teaching" on Adolescents' Knowledge and Beliefs, *Community Dent. Oral Epidemiol., 18,* 61, April, 1990.

Thompson, G.W., Hargreaves, J.A., and Slusar, M.: Nutritional Assessment: A Computer-based Dietary Analysis, *Can. Dent. Assoc. J., 55,* 709, September, 1989.

Caries Activity Tests

Alaluusua, S., Savolainen, J., Tuompo, H., and Grönroos, L.: Slide-scoring Method for Estimation of *Streptococcus mutans* Levels in Saliva, *Scand. J. Dent. Res., 92,* 127, February, 1984.

Arnim, S.S. and Sweet, A.P.: Acid Production by Mouth Organisms. Use of Aqueous Methyl Red for Patient Education, *Dent. Radiogr. Photogr., 29,* 1, No. 1, 1956.

Bentley, C.D., Broderius, C.A., and Crawford, J.J.: Evaluation of Cariescreen SM Method for Enumeration of Salivary Mutans Streptococci, *Gen. Dent., 39,* 188, May-June, 1991.

Birkhed, D., Edwardsson, S., and Andersson, H.: Comparison among a Dip-slide Test (Dentocult), Plate Count, and Snyder Test for Estimating Number of Lactobacilli in Human Saliva, *J. Dent. Res., 60,* 1832, November, 1981.

Crossner, C.-G.: Salivary Lactobacillus Counts in the Prediction of Caries Activity, *Community Dent. Oral Epidemiol., 9,* 182, August, 1981.

El-Nadeef, M., Kalfas, S., Edwardsson, S., and Ericson, D.: Influence of Transient Salivary Flora on Assessment of Mutans Streptococci Level by the "Strip Mutans" Method, *Scand. J. Dent. Res., 100,* 149, June, 1992.

Grainger, R.M., Jarrett, M., and Honey, S.L.: Swab Test for Dental Caries Activity: An Epidemiological Study, *Can. Dent. Assoc. J., 31,* 515, August, 1965.

Harris, N.O. and Park, K.K.: Caries Activity Testing, in Harris, N.O. and Christen, A.G.: *Primary Preventive Dentistry,* 3rd ed. Norwalk, CT, Appleton & Lange, 1991, pp. 283–306.

Jensen, B. and Bratthall, D.: A New Method for the Estimation of Mutans Streptococci in Human Saliva, *J. Dent. Res., 68,* 468, March, 1989.

Köhler, B. and Emilson, C.-G.: Comparison Between a Micromethod and a Conventional Method for Estimation of Salivary *Streptococcus mutans, Scand. J. Dent. Res., 95,* 132, April, 1987.

Larmas, M.: Simple Tests for Caries Susceptibility, *Int. Dent. J., 35,* 109, June, 1985.

Newbrun, E.: *Cariology,* 3rd ed. Chicago, Quintessence, 1989, pp. 273–293.

Snyder, M.L.: A Simple Colorimetric Method for the Estimation of Relative Numbers of Lactobacilli in the Saliva, *J. Dent. Res., 19,* 349, August, 1940.

Takei, T., Ogawa, T., Alaluusua, S., Fujiwara, T., Morisaki, I., Ooshima, T., Sobue, S., and Hamada, S.: Latex Agglutination Test for Detection of Mutans Streptococci in Relation to Dental Caries in Children, *Arch. Oral Biol., 37,* 99, February, 1992.

Weinberger, S.J. and Wright, G.Z.. A Comparison of S. Mutans Clinical Assessment Methods, *Pediatr. Dent., 12,* 375, November/December, 1990.

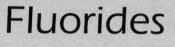

Fluorides

The use of fluorides provides the most effective method for dental caries prevention and control. Although historically associated primarily with dental caries, the action of fluoride on bacterial plaque also has important therapeutic and preventive effects on the control of periodontal infections and the maintenance of health after periodontal treatments.

Fluoride is important for optimum oral health at all ages. Fluoride is made available at the tooth surface by two general means: *systemically,* by way of the circulation to developing teeth, and *topically,* directly to the exposed surfaces of erupted teeth.

Fluoride as a systemic nutrient is available from the community drinking water, either naturally or by fluoridation, from prescribed dietary supplements, or in small amounts from certain foods. Key words associated with fluoride and fluoride therapy are defined in table 29–1.

FLUORIDE METABOLISM[1]

I. FLUORIDE INTAKE
Fluoride is taken in by way of fluoridated water, supplemental tablets, and, in small amounts, foods. Foods and beverages prepared at home or processed in industry using water containing fluoride are significant sources of fluoride.

II. ABSORPTION
A. Stomach and Small Intestine
Rapid absorption. Only 5% not absorbed is excreted in the feces.

B. Blood Stream
Maximum blood levels are reached within an hour of intake. The level fluctuates with intake. Normal plasma levels are very low. Fluoride in the saliva is lower than in the plasma.

III. DISTRIBUTION AND RETENTION
A. Young Child
About one half of the fluoride intake deposits in calcifying bones and teeth.

B. Adult
When the fluoride intake is continuous from daily use of fluoridated water, fluoride enters into the normal bone exchange and maintenance. Fluoride continues to accumulate in the skeleton throughout life.

C. Storage
Fluoride is stored in bone (95% of the body fluoride). The fluoride ion (F) is stored as an integral part of the crystal lattice of fluorapatite. The amount stored varies with the intake, the time of exposure, and the age and stage of the development of the individual. The teeth store small amounts, with highest levels on the tooth surface.

D. Fluoride in Soft Tissues
Some tissues have fluoride levels higher than that of the plasma. Fluoride concentration in human milk is low.

IV. EXCRETION
Most fluoride is excreted through the kidneys, with a small amount excreted by the sweat glands. Urinary

TABLE 29–1
KEY WORDS AND ABBREVIATIONS: FLUORIDES

Abrasive system: substances with cleaning and polishing properties utilized in the formulation of a dentifrice; must be compatible with fluoride compounds and other ingredients and not alter the tooth structure unfavorably.

Acidogenic (as'ĭ-dō-jen'ik): producing acid or acidity.

Apatite (ap'ah-tīt): a group of minerals of the general formula $Ca_{10}(PO_4)_6X_2$ wherein the X might include hydroxyl (OH), carbonate (CO), fluoride (F), or oxygen (O); crystalline mineral component of hard tissues (bones and teeth).

　Hydroxyapatite (hī-drok'sē-ap'ah-tīt): $Ca_{10}(PO_4)_6(OH)_2$; the form of apatite that is the principal mineral component of teeth, bones, and calculus.

　Fluorapatite (floor ap'ah-tīt): the form of hydroxyapatite in which fluoride ions have replaced some of the hydroxyl ions; with fluoride, the apatite is less soluble and therefore more resistant to the acids formed by plaque bacteria from carbohydrate intake.

　Fluorhydroxyapatite: apatite formed when low concentrations of fluoride react with tooth mineral; at higher concentrations, calcium fluoride is formed.

Cariogenic challenge: exposure of a tooth surface to an acid attack; acid is from the action of plaque bacteria and cariogenic food ingested.

Cariostatic (kār-ē-ō-sta'tĭk): exerting an inhibitory action on the progress of dental caries.

Defluoridation: lowering the amount of fluoride in fluoridated water to an optimum level for the prevention of dental caries and dental fluorosis.

Demineralization (dē-min'er-al-ĭ-zā'shun): excessive loss of mineral or inorganic salts from body tissues.

Enolase (ē'nō lās): enzyme involved in glycolysis and sugar transport.

Fluoride (floo'ō-rīd): a salt of hydrofluoric acid; occurs in many tissues and is stored primarily in bones and teeth.

Fluorosis (floo'-o-rō'sis): hypocalcification that results from excessive fluoride intake (over 2 ppm) during the development and mineralization of the teeth; depending on the length of exposure and the ppm of the fluoride, the fluorosed area may appear as a small white spot or as severe brown staining with pitting.

Gel: semisolid or solid phase of a colloidal solution.

Glass ionomer (ī'on'ō-mer): dental material used for restorations and for bases under composite or amalgam restorations; ionomers adhere to dentin and enamel, release fluoride, reduce microleakage, and prevent secondary (recurrent) dental caries.

Glycolysis (glī-kol'ĭ-sis): process by which sugar is metabolized by bacteria to produce acid.

Hypocalcification (hī'pō-kal'sĭ-fĭ-kā'shun): deficient calcification.

　Enamel hypocalcification: defect of enamel maturation caused by hereditary or systemic irregularities.

Maturation (mat-ū-rā'shun): stage or process of becoming mature or attaining maximal development; with respect to tooth development, maturation results from the continuous dynamic exchange of ions into the surface of the enamel from pellicle, bacterial plaque, and oral fluids.

ppm: parts per million; measure used to designate the amount of fluoride used for optimum level in fluoridated water, dentifrice, and other fluoride-containing preparations.

Remineralization (rē-min'er-al-ĭ-zā'shun): restoration of mineral elements; enhanced by presence of fluoride; remineralized lesions are more resistant to initiation of dental caries than is normal tooth structure.

Subsurface lesion: demineralized area below the surface of the enamel created by acid that has passed through micropores between enamel rods; is subject to remineralization by action of fluoride.

'White spot': term used to describe a small area on the surface of enamel that contrasts in appearance with the rest of the surface and may be visible only when the tooth is dried; two types of white spots can be differentiated, an area of demineralization and an area of fluorosis (also referred to as an "enamel opacity").

---

fluoride concentration is reached within 2 hours of intake of a single amount of fluoride, such as a fluoride tablet.

FLUORIDE AND TOOTH DEVELOPMENT

Fluoride is a nutrient essential to the formation of sound teeth and bones, as are calcium, phosphorus, and other elements obtained from food and water.

The teeth can acquire fluoride during three periods:

during the *mineralization stage* of tooth development, *after mineralization* and before eruption, and *after eruption*. At this point of study, a review of the histology of tooth development and mineralization can be a helpful supplement to the information included here.[2,3]

I. PRE-ERUPTIVE: MINERALIZATION STAGE
　A. Fluoride is deposited during the formation of the enamel, starting at the dentinoenamel junction, after the enamel matrix has been laid down by the ameloblasts (figure 29–1A).

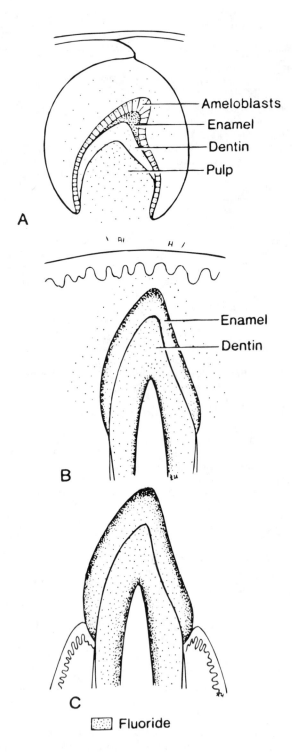

FIG. 29–1. Systemic Fluoride. Dots represent fluoride ions in the tissues and distributed throughout the tooth. **A.** Developing tooth during mineralization shows fluoride from water and from other systemic sources deposited in the enamel and dentin. **B.** Maturation stage prior to eruption when fluoride is taken up from tissue fluids around the crown. **C.** Erupted tooth continues to take up fluoride on the surface from external sources. Note concentrated fluoride deposition on the enamel surface.

B. Fluoride is incorporated as fluorapatite during mineralization. Table 14–2 (page 233) shows the weeks *in utero* when the hard tissue formation begins for the primary teeth. The first permanent molar begins to mineralize at birth (table 14–3, page 233).

C. Fluoride is available to the developing teeth by way of the blood stream to the tissues surrounding the tooth buds.

D. Sources of fluoride include drinking water and other ingested fluoride, such as that from tablets, drops, and foods.

E. During mineralization, when there is excess fluoride, the normal activity of the ameloblasts may be inhibited and a defective enamel matrix can form. This mechanism can lead to dental fluorosis. Dental fluorosis is a form of hypomineralization that results from ingestion of an excess amount of fluoride during tooth development.

II. PRE-ERUPTIVE: MATURATION STAGE

A. After mineralization is complete and before eruption, fluoride deposition continues in the surface of the enamel (figure 29–1B).

B. Fluoride is taken up from the nutrient tissue fluids surrounding the tooth crown. Much more fluoride is acquired by the outer surface during this period than in the underlying layers of enamel during mineralization. Children who are exposed to fluoride for the first time within the 2 years prior to eruption benefit from fluoride acquired during this pre-eruptive stage.

III. POSTERUPTIVE

A. After eruption and throughout the life span of the teeth, fluoride from the drinking water, dentifrice, mouthrinses, and other surface exposures acts to inhibit demineralization and enhance remineralization (Figure 29–2).

B. Uptake is rapid on the enamel surface during the first years after eruption. It is greater at high than at low levels of fluoride, especially from supplements used as chewable tablets or a swish-and-swallow liquid (page 442). Continuing intake of drinking water with fluoride provides a topical source as it washes over the teeth.

TOOTH SURFACE FLUORIDE

Fluoride concentration decreases inward from the enamel surface to the dentinoenamel junction.[4]

I. FLUORIDE UPTAKE

Uptake of fluoride depends on the amount of fluoride ingested and the length of time of exposure.

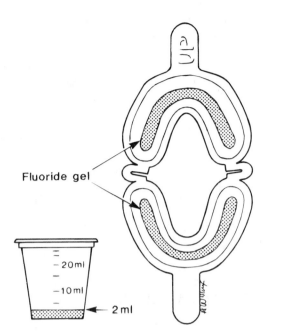

Fluoride gel

20ml

10ml

← 2 ml

FIG. 29–7. Measured Gel in Tray. No more than 2 ml gel should be placed in each tray for small children, and no more than 2.5 ml for larger patients with permanent teeth. A medicine cup can be used to measure the amount once, so that the correct level of gel in the tray can be determined. A minimum amount of gel is indicated to prevent ingestion by the patient.

placing it in the tray. This procedure may be tried for each tray size so that measuring is not necessary on a routine basis. Figure 29–7 shows the level of a measured 2 ml in a Styrofoam tray.

III. APPLICATION PROCEDURE

Table 29–5 summarizes the procedures recommended to reduce fluoride ingestion by the patient during the gel tray application.

A. Seat patient in upright position to prevent gel from passing into the throat.
B. Request patient to expectorate or swallow to clear the mouth.
C. Dry maxillary teeth for single tray insertion. When both trays will be placed simultaneously, dry mandibular teeth last (figure 29–5).
D. Insert tray or trays promptly, and place saliva ejector between trays. Start the time or note clock for 4-minute application.
E. Press tray against teeth starting over the occlusal surfaces and on the sides to force the gel between the teeth.
F. When appropriate, place a cotton roll between the trays over the premolar areas on each side to soften the pressure as the patient closes. The gentle pressure can aid in the adaptation of gel to tooth surfaces. It also prevents closure on the saliva ejector.
G. On completion, remove tray(s). Patient does not rinse, but can expectorate.

TABLE 29–5
PROCEDURES TO REDUCE FLUORIDE INGESTION DURING TOPICAL GEL-TRAY APPLICATION

Patient	Seat upright
	Instruct not to swallow
	Tilt head forward with trays; tilt away from side with cotton-roll holder
Trays	Custom-made or appropriate size with absorptive liners; post-dam; border rim
	Use minimum amount of gel: 2 ml per tray, less for small tray; no more than total of 5 ml for large trays
Isolation	Use saliva ejector with maximum efficiency suction
	Cotton-roll holder technique: position for security, stability; place saliva absorber in cheek
Attention	Do not leave patient unattended
Timing	Use a timer; do not estimate
Completion	Tilt head forward for removal of tray or cotton-roll holder
	Request patient to expectorate for several minutes; do not allow swallowing
	Wipe excess gel from teeth with gauze sponge
	Use high-power suction to draw out saliva and gel
	Instruct patient not to rinse, eat, drink, or brush teeth for at least 30 minutes

(Recommendations based on Oral Health Policies for Children: Protocol for Fluoride Therapy, American Academy of Pediatric Dentistry, 211 E. Chicago Avenue, Chicago, IL 60611.)

H. Immediately place the second tray when a two-step operation is preferred or necessary.
I. Do not allow the patient to rinse on removal of second tray.
 1. Wipe teeth with sponge to remove excess residual gel. Apply high-power suction.
 2. Request patient to expectorate for several minutes.
J. Instruct patient not to rinse, eat, drink, brush the teeth, or perform other activity that could disturb the fluoride action for at least 30 minutes, preferably longer.[45]

SELF-APPLIED FLUORIDES

I. METHODS

The three methods for self-application are by mouth tray, rinsing, and toothbrushing.

A. Mouth Tray

A fluoride gel is placed in a custom-made or disposable tray and is held in the mouth for 4 minutes.

B. Rinsing

The patient swishes for 1 minute with a measured amount of a fluoride rinse. Except when used as a rinse-supplement in a nonfluoridated community, the fluoride rinse is expectorated.

C. Toothbrushing

A gel or paste is used for regular brushing two or three times daily. In addition, a brush-on gel may be used after regular brushing to provide special benefits. Use interdental brush to apply fluoride to proximal surfaces or open furca.

II. INDICATIONS

Indications for use of mouth tray, rinsing, and/or toothbrushing depend on the individual patient problems. Patient needs are determined as a part of total treatment planning. Certain patients need multiple procedures combined with professional applications at the regular maintenance appointments. Special indications are suggested as each method is described in the following sections.

Frequent application using weak preparations of fluoride compounds is considered more beneficial than are infrequent high-concentration applications. Therefore, the daily applications are recommended when performed on an individual basis. Fluoridated water, described earlier in this chapter, provides another method of self-application.

TRAY TECHNIQUE: HOME APPLICATION[46]

The original gel tray studies using custom-fitted polyvinyl mouthpieces compared the use of 1.1% acidulated NaF with plain NaF gel. The gel was applied daily over a 2-year period by schoolchildren aged 11 to 14 years during the school years. Dental caries incidence was reduced up to 80%.[47]

I. INDICATIONS FOR USE

A. Rampant enamel or root caries in persons of any age.
B. Xerostomia of any cause, particularly loss of salivary gland function.
C. Exposure to radiation therapy (page 676).
D. Caries prevention under an overdenture (page 390).
E. Root surface hypersensitivity (page 557).

II. GEL USED

A. Concentrations

APF 0.5%; NaF 1.1%; SnF_2 0.4%.

B. Precautions

1. Do not dispense large quantities. Prescription of 24 to 30 ml of APF 0.5% in a dropper bottle that dispenses drops containing 0.1 ml F is suggested.
2. Do not use acidulated preparations on porcelain[41] or titanium restorations.

III. PROCEDURE: PATIENT INSTRUCTIONS

A. Brush and floss to remove thoroughly all bacterial plaque possible.
B. Prepare custom-made polyvinyl tray. A disposable tray can be used if the appropriate fit can be obtained. Load the tray by distributing no more than 5 drops of the gel around each tray. Each drop is equivalent to 0.1 ml.
C. Dry the mouth by swallowing several times.
D. Apply the tray(s) over the teeth and close gently. Hold head upright.
E. Time by a clock for 4 minutes. *Do not swallow.*
F. Expectorate several times when the trays are removed.
G. Do not eat or drink for 30 minutes. One application should be made just before retiring.

FLUORIDE MOUTHRINSES

Mouthrinsing is a practical and effective means for self-application of fluoride. The only persons excluded from the practice of this method are children under 6 years of age and those of any age who cannot rinse because of oral-facial musculature problems or other disability. Rinsing can be part of an individual treatment plan or can be included in a group program conducted during school attendance.

Mouthrinses containing fluoride are reviewed by the American Dental Association, Council on Dental Therapeutics. Approved products are listed annually and bear the seal of the Association (figure 23–15, page 370).

I. INDICATIONS

Mouthrinsing with a fluoride preparation may have particular meaning for the following:

A. General prevention of dental caries in
   1. Young persons during the high-risk preteen and adolescent years.
   2. Patients with areas of demineralization.
   3. Patients with root exposure following recession and periodontal therapy.
   4. Participants in a school health group program for all grades.
B. Patients with moderate to rampant dental caries who live in a fluoridated or nonfluoridated community.
C. Patients whose oral health care is complicated by plaque-retentive appliances, including orthodontics and partial dentures or space maintainers.
D. Patients with xerostomia from any cause, including head and neck radiation and saliva-depressing drug therapy.
E. Patients with hypersensitivity of exposed root surfaces.

II. PREPARATIONS

Rinse preparations are referred to as *low-potency/high-frequency rinses, high-potency/low-frequency rinses,* and *oral rinse supplements.*[48] Certain low-potency rinses may be purchased directly "over-the-counter" (OTC); all others are provided by prescription.

A. Over-the-counter: Sodium Fluoride 0.05%

1. *Fluoride Content.* 0.025% fluoride; 225 ppm.
2. *Specifications*
   a. Single container must contain no more than 264 mg NaF (120 mg fluoride) dispensed at 1 time. A 500-ml bottle of 0.05% NaF rinse contains 100 mg fluoride.
   b. Bottle must have child-proof cap.
   c. Label must state that the rinse is not to be used by children under 6 years of age or by children with a disability involving oral-facial musculature. Young children do not have sufficient control to expectorate, and they tend to swallow quickly.
   d. Label must indicate that the rinse is not to be swallowed.
3. *Procedure for Use*
   a. Rinse daily with 1 teaspoonful (5 ml) after brushing before retiring.
   b. Swish between teeth with lips tightly closed for 60 seconds; expectorate.
4. *Limitations*
   a. Alcohol content of commercial preparations is not advisable for children. Alcohol-containing preparations should never be recommended for a recovering alcoholic person.
   b. Motivation of patient and/or parent to carry out faithfully the recommended procedures. Daily rinse is better than weekly rinse when practiced on an individual home basis.

B. Prescription

1. *Oral Rinse Supplement: Acidulated NaF 0.04% (low potency).* Supplements were described and the recommendation listed on pages 442 and 443. They are swished and swallowed to provide daily systemic supplementation to inadequate fluoride in the drinking water. For rampant caries, hypersensitive teeth, or other conditions, the preparation may be used to provide local effect only by expectorating after 1 minute of swishing.
2. *Sodium Fluoride 0.2%*
   a. Fluoride content. .090% F; 900 ppm (high potency).
   b. Use. Weekly rinse using 5 ml (younger children) or 10 ml (older children) swished for 60 seconds and expectorated.

c. School group program. The use of the weekly rinse is the most common school-based program in the United States. Advantages are that it requires little time (about 5 minutes once weekly for an entire class); is inexpensive; is easy to learn and is well accepted by participants; and can be carried out by nondental personnel. Responsibility for providing the correctly mixed 0.2% solution and for locking the fluoride in an inaccessible place can be taken by school officials and a supervising dental hygienist.[48,49]

III. BENEFITS

Benefits from fluoride mouthrinsing have been documented many times since the original research using various percentages of various fluoride preparations.[50,51] Frequent rinsing with low concentrations of fluoride has the following effects:

A. A 30 to 40% average reduction in dental caries incidence.
B. Greater benefit for smooth surfaces, but some benefit to pits and fissures.
C. Greatest benefit to newly erupted teeth (thus, the program should be continued through the teenage years to benefit the second and third permanent molars).
D. Added benefits for a community with fluoridation.[52]
E. Increase in post-treatment benefits as the length of time of rinsing increases.[47,53]
F. Primary teeth present in school-age children benefit by as much as 42.5% average reduction in dental caries incidence.[54]

FLUORIDE DENTIFRICES

Historically dentifrices have been tried with various compounds, including stannous fluoride, sodium fluoride, sodium monofluorophosphate, and amine fluoride. The main research objective has been to find fluoride and abrasive systems that are compatible. Early dentifrices had problems of stability and fluoride availability for uptake by the tooth surface.

A dentifrice containing stannous fluoride 0.4% was the first fluoride-containing dentifrice to gain approval by the Council on Dental Therapeutics.[55] An excellent review by Stookey that describes the development of present formulations and the extensive research over past years is recommended for reading.[56] Guidelines for the acceptance of dentifrices by the Council are frequently updated and call for laboratory and clinical efficacy of each product.[57]

I. INDICATIONS

A. Dental Caries Prevention

A fluoride dentifrice approved by the American Dental Association should be recommended for each patient as part of the complete preventive program.

B. Caries-risk Patients

Patients with moderate to rampant dental caries should be advised to brush several times each day with a fluoride-containing dentifrice.

C. Desensitization

Certain dentifrices containing fluoride have desensitizing properties. These are included on pages 369 and 557.

II. PREPARATIONS

Fluoride dentifrices are available as gels or pastes. Sodium fluoride and sodium monofluorophosphate dentifrices are approved currently. Amine fluorides have not been developed and promoted in the United States.

A. Current Constituents

1. Sodium fluoride (NaF) 0.24% (1100 ppm).
2. Sodium monofluorophosphate (Na_2PO_3F) 0.76% (1000 ppm). An "extra-strength" Na_2PO_3F contains 1500 ppm.

B. Specifications from Guidelines for Acceptance[57]

To gain approval by the American Dental Association and to use the seal of acceptance (figure 23–15, page 370), a product must meet certain criteria, including the following:

1. The active fluoride (F) agent must be chemically free and available in both fresh and aged samples to the end of the specified expiration date.
2. The ability to deliver and incorporate levels of F into both sound and demineralized enamel must be demonstrated.
3. The product must promote or enhance remineralization of enamel.
4. The product must reduce the rate of demineralization.

III. PATIENT INSTRUCTION: RECOMMENDED PROCEDURES

Instruction in the selection of a dentifrice, the need for frequent use, the method for application to the tooth surfaces, and the effects of fluoride can help the patient appreciate the significant role of fluoride in oral health.

A. Select an approved fluoride-containing dentifrice.
B. Place a small amount of dentifrice on the toothbrush.
1. *Child.* Use only a small amount, the size of a pea (figure 29–8). Demonstrate this amount

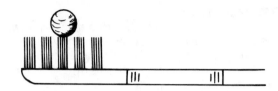

FIG. 29–8. Dentifrice for a Child. To prevent ingestion of an excess amount of dentifrice, a parent must be instructed to place only a small portion of dentifrice on the brush; the size can be compared to the size of a pea.

and explain that the child should not swallow excess amounts of dentifrice because that may cause white spots to develop in the enamel (pages 439 and 455).
2. *Older Children and Adults.* ½ inch or less.
C. Spread dentifrice over the teeth with a light touch of the brush.
D. Proceed with correct brushing for sulcular removal of bacterial plaque.
E. Keep dentifrice container out of reach of children.

IV. BENEFITS

Dentifrices are used often, at least once or twice each day as recommended. Caries-risk patients may use a dentifrice several times per day. The dentifrice is a continuing source of fluoride for the tooth surface in the control of demineralization and promotion of remineralization. Fluoride is deposited in demineralized white spots (figure 29–3).

Many research studies have shown that the incidence of dental caries can be reduced between 20 to 30% when NaF or Na_2PO_3F dentifrices are used regularly.

BRUSH-ON GEL

Brush-on gel has been used as an adjunct to the daily application of fluoride in a dentifrice and as a supplement to periodic professional applications. Although widely accepted, reviews of the research show limited and somewhat conflicting reports of the benefits.[58,59]

I. PREPARATIONS

A. Acidulated phosphate fluoride (APF) 0.5%.
B. Stannous fluoride (SnF_2) 0.4% in glycerin base.
C. Sodium fluoride (NaF) 1.1%.

II. PROCEDURE

A. Use once a day, preferably at night.
B. Complete toothbrushing and flossing.

C. Place about 2 mg of the gel over about one third of the brush head and spread over all teeth.
D. Brush 1 minute, then swish before expectorating.

III. PATIENT INSTRUCTION
A. APF gels are not for use on porcelain or composite.[41]
B. Gels of this category are not for use as dentifrices. Teeth are cleaned first with thorough brushing and flossing.
C. Regular use has been shown to help to control demineralization about orthodontic appliances,[60] and to provide protection against postirradiation caries in conjunction with other fluoride applications.[61]

COMBINED FLUORIDE PROGRAM

Most patients can benefit from more than one method of use of fluorides. When the preventive program is planned for an individual patient, the fluoride preparations and modes of application selected should provide the greatest possible protection against dental caries.

When self-administered methods are chosen, patient cooperation is a significant factor. Age and eruption pattern influence the method selected. Fluorides must be applied as soon after tooth eruption as possible and continued indefinitely to control demineralization.

Maintenance appointments can be scheduled for frequent topical applications and for continuing instruction and motivation. All methods are supplemented by the use of a dentifrice with fluoride.

FLUORIDE SAFETY

Fluoride preparations and fluoridated water have wide margins of safety. Fluoride is beneficial in small amounts, but can be injurious if used without attention to correct dosage and frequency. All dental personnel should be familiar with recommended approved procedures, know potentials for toxic effects, and be prepared to administer emergency measures should accidental overdosages occur.

I. SUMMARY OF FLUORIDE MANAGEMENT
A. Use and recommend for patient use only approved fluoride preparations. Products have approval from the Food and Drug Administration and the American Dental Association in the United States.
B. Use only researched, recommended amounts and methods for delivery.
C. Know potential toxicity of the various products and be prepared for administering emergency measures for treating an accidental toxic response.
D. Instruct patients in proper care of fluoride products.
1. Dentist prescribes no more than 264 mg of sodium fluoride at 1 time. Do not store large quantities in the home.
2. Request parental supervision of child's brushing or other fluoride administration. Rinses, for example, are not to be used by children under 6 years of age.
3. Fluoride products should have child-proof covers and should be kept out of reach of small children and other persons, such as the mentally or physically handicapped, who may not understand limitations.
4. In school health programs, dispensing of the fluoride product must be supervised by responsible adults. Containers must be stored under lock and key when not in active use.

II. ACUTE TOXICITY
Acute refers to rapid intake of an excess dose over a short time, whereas *chronic* applies to long-term ingestion of fluoride in amounts that exceed the approved therapeutic levels. An accidental ingestion of a concentrated fluoride preparation can lead to a toxic reaction. Acute fluoride poisoning is rare.[62]

A. Certainly Lethal Dose (CLD)[63]
A lethal dose is the amount of a drug likely to cause death if not intercepted by antidotal therapy.
1. *Adult CLD.* 5 to 10 g of sodium fluoride taken at 1 time. The fluoride ion equivalent is 32 to 64 milligrams fluoride per kilogram (mg F/kg) body weight (table 29–6A).
2. *Child.* Approximately 0.5 to 1.0 g variable with size and weight of the child.

B. Safely Tolerated Dose (STD): One Fourth of the CLD
1. *Adult STD.* 1.25 to 2.5 g of sodium fluoride (8 to 16 mg F/kg.)
2. *Child.* Table 29–6B shows STDs and CLDs for children. Weights given for each selected age are minimal, and calculations for the doses are conservative. As can be noted from the table, less than 1 g (1000 mg) may be fatal for children 12 years old and younger, and ½ g (500 mg) exceeds the STD for all ages

TABLE 29–6
LETHAL AND SAFE DOSES OF FLUORIDE

A. *Lethal and safe dosages of fluoride for a 70-kg adult.*

Certainly Lethal Dose (CLD)
5–10 g NaF
or
32–64 mg F/kg
Safely Tolerated Dose (STD) = ¼ CLD
1.25–2.5 g NaF
or
8–16 mg F/kg

B. *CLDs and STDs of fluoride for selected ages.*

Age (years)	Weight (lbs)	CLD (mg)	STD (mg)
2	22	320	80
4	29	422	106
6	37	538	135
8	45	655	164
10	53	771	193
12	64	931	233
14	83	1,206	301
16	92	1,338	334
18	95	1,382	346

(From Heifetz, S.B. and Horowitz, H.S.: The Amounts of Fluoride in Current Fluoride Therapies: Safety Considerations for Children, *ASDC J. Dent. Child., 51,* 257, July-August, 1984.)

shown. For children under 6 years of age, however, 500 mg would be lethal.[63]

III. SIGNS AND SYMPTOMS OF ACUTE TOXIC DOSE

Symptoms begin within 30 minutes of ingestion and may persist for as long as 24 hours.

A. Gastrointestinal Tract

Fluoride in the stomach is acted on by the hydrochloric acid to form hydrofluoric acid, an irritant to the stomach lining. Symptoms include
1. Nausea, vomiting, diarrhea.
2. Abdominal pain.
3. Increased salivation, thirst.

B. Systemic Involvement

1. *Blood.* Calcium may be bound by the circulating fluoride, thus causing symptoms of hypocalcemia.
2. *Central Nervous System.* Hyperreflexia, convulsions, paresthesias.
3. *Cardiovascular and Respiratory Depression.* If not treated, may lead to death in a few hours from cardiac failure or respiratory paralysis.

IV. EMERGENCY TREATMENT

A. Induce Vomiting (table 61–2, page 847)

1. *Mechanical.* Digital stimulation at back of tongue or in throat.
2. *Drug.* Ipecac syrup.

B. Second Person

Call emergency service; transport to hospital.

C. Administer Fluoride-binding Liquid when Patient Is Not Vomiting

1. Milk.
2. Lime water (CaOH₂ solution 0.15%).

D. Support Respiration and Circulation (Chapter 61, pages 835–837)

E. Additional Therapy Indicated at Emergency Room

1. Calcium gluconate for muscle tremors or tetany.
2. Gastric lavage.
3. Cardiac monitoring.
4. Endotracheal intubation.
5. Blood monitoring (calcium, magnesium, potassium, pH).
6. Intravenous feeding to restore blood volume, calcium.

V. CHRONIC TOXICITY

A. Skeletal Fluorosis[62]

Isolated instances of osteosclerosis result from chronic toxicity after long-term (20 or more years) use of water with 10 to 25 ppm fluoride or from industrial exposure.[62] Methods for defluoridation have been developed, as described on page 441.

B. Dental Fluorosis

Naturally occurring excess fluoride in the drinking water can produce visible fluorosis only when used during the years of development of the crowns of the teeth, namely, from birth until ages 8 or 9 or when the crowns of the second permanent molars are completed. No systemic effects result from the fluoride, and the individual has protection against dental caries. A classification of fluorosis is found in table 29–2, page 440.

C. Mild Fluorosis

1. *Clinical Evaluation.* In its mild and very mild forms, dental fluorosis appears as white opacities in the enamel surface. No esthetic or health problem is involved. Many such white spots are not visible except when scrutinized under a dental light and the surface

is dried. Because all white spots in the enamel are not related to fluoride intake, distinction must be made by reviewing the patient's dental and fluoride-intake history, by noting the location and distribution of the white spots, and by considering the sequence of tooth development.

2. *Relation to Fluoride Sources.* Mild fluorosis or white spots may result from inadvertent ingestion of excess fluoride by young children during topical procedures both self-applied and professional. No problem exists when care is taken to follow basic rules, such as those listed in table 29–5 for professional applications and shown in figure 29–8 for daily use of dentifrice the size of a pea. Mouthrinses are not indicated for children under 6 years of age.

Small amounts of dentifrice may be swallowed at each brushing. A child of 4 years who lives in a nonfluoridated community, uses a daily supplement (1 mg), and swallows 2 or 3 small amounts of dentifrice ingests far less than the STD of 106 mg shown in table 29–6B.

VI. HOW TO CALCULATE AMOUNTS OF FLUORIDE[63,64,65]

Figure 29–9 is a flowchart that shows the steps necessary to determine the amount of fluoride in a fluoride compound. By doing so, one then can calculate the amount ingested by the patient.

First, the percentage of fluoride ion in the compound is multiplied by the molecular weight conversion ratio, as shown in figure 29–9. The ratio was obtained by dividing the molecular weight of the compound by the atomic weight of fluoride. For example, the molecular weight of sodium fluoride is 42 (Na = 23, F = 19). When divided by 19, a 1 to 2.2 ratio results, as used in the example in figure 29–9.

TECHNICAL HINTS

I. ALTERNATE ISOLATION PROCEDURES FOR TOPICAL APPLICATION

The procedure described on page 447 is for isolation of one half of the dentition at one time. Objectives are to conserve time, to maintain as dry a field as possible, and to prevent the fluoride solution from being absorbed by cotton rolls or the saliva from contaminating or diluting the solution. Other systems that may be applied include:

A. Rubber Dam

1. *Use.* For application of fluoride following restorative procedures or sealant placement.
2. *Preparation.* When the rubber dam has not been fitted to include the entire quadrant, additional holes may be made in the dam with an explorer.
3. *Advantages*
   a. Better control of the patient during the application, particularly of a small child or disabled patient with special problems.
   b. Saves time. Dry teeth can be maintained.
   c. Helpful when general anesthesia is used, particularly for a hospitalized patient.
   d. Stannous fluoride solution is confined and the patient does not experience the unpleasant taste.

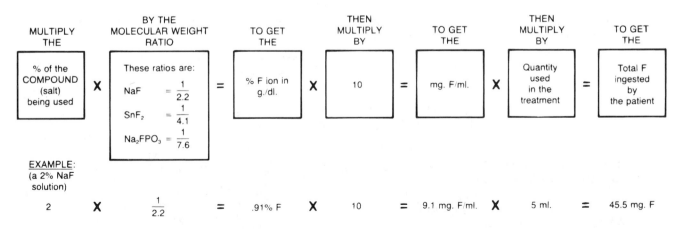

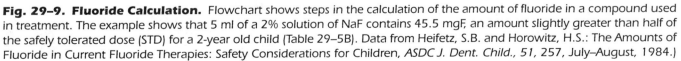

Fig. 29–9. Fluoride Calculation. Flowchart shows steps in the calculation of the amount of fluoride in a compound used in treatment. The example shows that 5 ml of a 2% solution of NaF contains 45.5 mgF, an amount slightly greater than half of the safely tolerated dose (STD) for a 2-year old child (Table 29–5B). Data from Heifetz, S.B. and Horowitz, H.S.: The Amounts of Fluoride in Current Fluoride Therapies: Safety Considerations for Children, *ASDC J. Dent. Child.*, 51, 257, July–August, 1984.)

4. *Disadvantage.* When root surface exposure needs fluoride, retraction of rubber dam may be difficult or impossible.

B. Single Quadrant

Each quadrant can be done separately by holding the cotton rolls with the fingers. In a very small mouth, a No. 1 continuous cotton roll may be held around the entire maxillary arch to make the entire application in 1 timing. This approach can be particularly useful for a small child.

II. FLUORIDE APPLICATION FOLLOWING POLISHING OF RESTORATIONS

Because abrasive stones and polishing agents remove a layer of surface enamel and polishing procedures extend over the margins of the restoration, a topical application of fluoride may be particularly important (page 589). The topical fluoride can help to promote remineralization.

III. COMMUNITIES WITH FLUORIDATION

Maintain list of communities. Update annually by contacting health department.

FACTORS TO TEACH THE PATIENT

I. PERSONAL USE OF FLUORIDES

A. Purposes, action, and expected benefits relative to the specific forms of fluoride treatment the patient will receive.

B. Specific instruction concerning self-applied techniques that will be performed at home. Prepared printed instruction materials can be especially useful.

II. NEED FOR PARENTAL SUPERVISION

A. Supervise daily care of child's teeth and mouth, including brushing of teeth using pea-sized quantity of dentifrice to prevent excess ingestion of fluoride.

B. Keep fluoride products out of reach of small children.

C. Brush teeth before using chewable dietary supplements. Avoid eating and drinking after use. Preferred time for use is just before going to bed.

III. DETERMINING NEED FOR FLUORIDE SUPPLEMENTS

A. Reference to list of communities with fluoride in the drinking water at optimum level.

B. Where to call to obtain information about fluoride in drinking water—health department, water department, or other community source.

C. Where to send private water source sample for fluoride analysis.

IV. PREPARATION FOR TOPICAL FLUORIDE APPLICATION

When the teeth are free from plaque and the gingival tissue is firm and healthy, uptake of fluoride by the teeth is greater and the possibility of a slight tissue reaction is lessened. When the gingiva is inflamed, the patient needs instruction to understand why the topical application must be postponed until the tissue has healed.

V. FLUORIDES ARE PART OF THE TOTAL PREVENTIVE PROGRAM

Control of cariogenic foods in the diet, particularly between meals, and professional care are still necessary to supplement fluoride treatment for caries control.

VI. FLUORIDATION

In a nonfluoridated community, information concerning the significance of fluoridation to the entire community and its benefits and operation should be available and disseminated.

VII. STANNOUS FLUORIDE

When stannous fluoride preparations are used, the patient (or parent) should be informed about the possibility of tooth staining.

REFERENCES

1. **Murray,** J.J., Rugg-Gunn, A.J., and Jenkins, G.N.: *Fluorides in Caries Prevention,* 3rd ed. Oxford, Wright, Butterworth-Heinemann, 1991, pp. 262–271.

2. **Bhaskar,** S.N., ed.: *Orban's Oral Histology and Embryology,* 11th ed. St. Louis, Mosby, 1990, pp. 28–48, 75–105.

3. **Melfi,** R.C.: *Permar's Oral Embryology and Microscopic Anatomy,* 8th ed. Philadelphia, Lea & Febiger, 1988, pp. 41–84.

4. **Brudevold,** F., Gardner, D.E., and Smith, F.A.: The Distribution of Fluoride in Human Enamel, *J. Dent. Res., 35,* 420, June, 1956.

5. **Brudevold,** F., Steadman, L.T., and Smith, F.A.: Inorganic and Organic Components of Tooth Structure, *Ann. N.Y. Acad. Sci., 85,* 110, March 29, 1960.

6. **Ekstrand,** J., Fejerskov, O., and Silverstone, L.M., eds.: *Fluoride in Dentistry.* Copenhagen, Munksgaard, 1988, pp. 44–50.

7. **Rolla,** G., Øgaard, B., and deAlmeida Cruz, R.: Topical Application of Fluorides on Teeth. New Concepts of Mechanisms of Interaction, *J. Clin. Periodontol., 20,* 105, February, 1993.

8. **Hamilton,** I. and Bowden, G.: Effect of Fluoride on Oral Microorganisms, in Ekstrand, J., Fejerskov, O., and Silverstone, L.M., eds.: *Fluoride in Dentistry.* Copenhagen, Munksgaard, 1988, pp. 77–101.

9. **Richards,** L.F., Westmoreland, W.W., Tashiro, M., McKay, C.H., and Morrison, J.T.: Determining Optimum Fluoride Levels for Community Water Supplies in Relation to Temperature, *J. Am. Dent. Assoc., 74,* 389, February, 1967.

10. **Striffler,** D.F., Young, W.O., and Burt, B.A.: *Dentistry, Dental Practice, and the Community,* 3rd ed. Philadelphia, W.B. Saunders Co., 1983, pp. 155–162.

11. **Herschfeld,** J.J.: Classics in Dental History. Frederick S. McKay and the "Colorado Brown Stain," *Bull. Hist. Dent., 26,* 118, October, 1978.

12. **McKay,** F.S.: The Relation of Mottled Enamel to Caries, *J. Am. Dent. Assoc., 15*, 1429, August, 1928.

13. **Churchill,** H.V.: Occurrence of Fluorides in Some Waters of United States, *J. Indust. Engin. Chem., 23*, 996, 1931.

14. **Dean,** H.T., Arnold, F.A., Jr., and Elvove, E.: Domestic Water and Dental Caries. V. Additional Studies of the Relation of Fluoride Domestic Waters to Dental Caries Experience in 4425 White Children, Aged 12 to 14 Years, of 13 Cities in 4 States, *Public Health Rep., 57*, 1155, August 7, 1942.

15. **United States Department of Health and Human Services,** Centers for Disease Control: *Fluoridation Census 1980.* Atlanta, GA, Centers for Disease Control, Dental Disease Prevention Activity, June, 1984, p. xi.

16. **Arnold,** F.A., Dean, H.T., Jay, P., and Knutson, J.W.: Effect of Fluoridated Public Water Supplies on Dental Caries Prevalence. Tenth Year of the Grand Rapids-Muskegon Study, *Public Health Rep., 71*, 652, July, 1956.

17. **Hayes,** R.L., Littleton, N.W., and White, C.L.: Posteruptive Effects of Fluoridation on First Permanent Molars of Children in Grand Rapids, Michigan, *Am. J. Public Health, 47*, 192, February, 1957.

18. **Russell,** A.L. and Hamilton, P.M.: Dental Caries in Permanent First Molars After Eight Years of Fluoridation, *Arch. Oral Biol., 6*, 50, July, 1961.

19. **Backer Dirks,** O., Houwink, B., and Kwant, G.W.: Some Special Features of the Caries Preventive Effect of Water Fluoridation, *Arch. Oral Biol., 4*, 187, August, 1961.

20. **Burt,** B.A., Ismail, A.I., and Eklund, S.A.: Root Caries in an Optimally Fluoridated and a High-fluoride Community, *J. Dent. Res., 65*, 1154, September, 1986.

21. **Stamm,** J.W., Banting, D.W., and Imrey, P.B.: Adult Root Caries Survey of Two Similar Communities with Contrasting Natural Water Fluoride Levels, *J. Am. Dent. Assoc., 120*, 143, February, 1990.

22. **Ast,** D.B. and Fitzgerald, B.: Effectiveness of Water Fluoridation, *J. Am. Dent. Assoc., 65*, 581, November, 1962.

23. **Salzmann,** J.A.: The Effects of Fluoride on the Prevalence of Malocclusion, *J. Am. Coll. Dent., 35*, 82, January, 1968.

24. **Russell,** A.L. and Elvove, E.: Domestic Water and Dental Caries. VII. A Study of the Fluoride-Dental Caries Relationship in an Adult Population, *Public Health Rep., 66*, 1389, October 26, 1951.

25. **Englander,** H.R. and Wallace, D.A.: Effects of Naturally Fluoridated Water on Dental Caries in Adults, *Public Health Rep., 77*, 887, October, 1962.

26. **Murray,** Rugg-Gunn, and Jenkins: op. cit., pp. 94–99.

27. **Horowitz,** H.S., Maier, F.J., and Law, F.E.: Partial Defluoridation of a Community Water Supply and Dental Fluorosis, *Public Health Rep., 82*, 965, November, 1967.

28. **Horowitz,** H.S. and Heifetz, S.B.: The Effect of Partial Defluoridation of a Water Supply on Dental Fluorosis—Final Result in Bartlett, Texas, after 17 Years, *Am. J. Public Health, 62*, 767, June 1972.

29. **Horowitz,** H.S.: Effectiveness of School Water Fluoridation and Dietary Fluoride Supplements in School-aged Children, *J. Public Health Dent., 49*, 290, Special Issue, 1989.

30. **Lemke,** C.W., Doherty, J.M., and Arra, M.C.: Controlled Fluoridation: The Dental Effects of Discontinuation in Antigo, Wisconsin, *J. Am. Dent. Assoc., 80*, 782, April, 1970.

31. **Ripa,** L.W.: A Half-century of Community Water Fluoridation in the United States: Review and Commentary, *J. Public Health Dent., 53*, 17, Winter, 1993.

32. **Ast,** D.B., Cons, N.C., Pollard, S.T., and Garfinkel, J.: Time and Cost Factors to Provide Regular, Periodic Dental Care for Children in a Fluoridated and Nonfluoridated Area: Final Report, *J. Am. Dent. Assoc., 80*, 770, April, 1970.

33. **American Dental Association,** Council on Dental Therapeutics. Chicago, American Dental Association, 1994.

34. **Aasenden,** R., DePaola, P.F., and Brudevold, F.: Effects of Daily Rinsing and Ingestion of Fluoride Solutions upon Dental Caries and Enamel Fluoride, *Arch. Oral Biol., 17*, 1705, December, 1972.

35. **Driscoll,** W.S., Heifetz, S.B., and Brunelle, J.A.: Treatment and Posttreatment Effects of Chewable Fluoride Tablets on Dental Caries: Findings after 7½ Years, *J. Am. Dent. Assoc., 99*, 817, November, 1979.

36. **Driscoll,** W.S., Heifetz, S.B., and Brunelle, J.A.: Caries-preventive Effects of Fluoride Tablets in Schoolchildren Four Years after Discontinuation of Treatments, *J. Am. Dent. Assoc., 103*, 878, December, 1981.

37. **Bibby,** B.G.: Use of Fluorine in the Prevention of Dental Caries. II. The Effects of Sodium Fluoride Applications, *J. Am. Dent. Assoc., 31*, 317, March 1, 1944.

38. **Knutson,** J.W.: Sodium Fluoride Solutions: Technique for Application to the Teeth, *J. Am. Dent. Assoc., 36*, 37, January, 1948.

39. **Galagan,** D.J. and Knutson, J.W.: The Effect of Topically Applied Fluorides on Dental Caries Experience. VI. Experiments with Sodium Fluoride and Calcium Chloride . . . Widely Spaced Applications . . . Use of Different Solution Concentrations, *Public Health Rep., 63*, 1215, September 17, 1948.

40. **Ripa,** L.W.: Professionally (Operator) Applied Topical Fluoride Therapy: A Critique, *Int. Dent. J., 31*, 105, June, 1981.

41. **American Dental Association,** Council on Dental Materials, Instruments, and Equipment and Council on Dental Therapeutics: Status Report: Effect of Acidulated Phosphate Fluoride on Porcelain and Composite Restorations, *J. Am. Dent. Assoc., 116*, 115, January, 1988.

42. **Ripa,** L.W.: Need for Prior Toothcleaning when Performing a Professional Topical Fluoride Application: Review and Recommendations for Change, *J. Am. Dent. Assoc., 109*, 281, August, 1984.

43. **Vrbic,** V., Brudevold, F., and McCann, H.G.: Acquisition of Fluoride by Enamel from Fluoride Pumice Pastes, *Helv. Odontol. Acta., 11*, 21, April, 1967.

44. **American Academy of Pediatric Dentistry:** Oral Health Policies for Children: Protocol for Fluoride Therapy, American Academy of Pediatric Dentistry, 211 E. Chicago Avenue, Chicago, IL 60611, May, 1992.

45. **Stookey,** G.K., Schemehorn, B.R., Drook, C.A., and Cheetham, B.L.: The Effect of Rinsing with Water Immediately after a Professional Fluoride Gel Application on Fluoride Uptake in Demineralized Enamel: An *In Vivo* Study, *Pediatr. Dent., 8*, 153, June, 1986.

46. **American Dental Association:** A Guide to the Use of Fluorides for the Prevention of Dental Caries, 2nd ed., *J. Am. Dent. Assoc., 113*, 558, September, 1986.

47. **Englander,** H.R., Keyes, P.H., and Gestwicki, M.: Clinical Anticaries Effect of Repeated Topical Sodium Fluoride Applications by Mouthpieces, *J. Am. Dent. Assoc., 75*, 638, September, 1967.

48. **Ripa,** L.W.: Fluoride Rinsing: What Dentists Should Know, *J. Am. Dent. Assoc., 102*, 477, April, 1981.

49. **Horowitz,** H.S. and Heifetz, S.B.: Topically Applied Fluorides, in Newbrun, E., ed.: *Fluorides and Dental Caries*, 3rd ed. Springfield, IL, Charles C Thomas, 1986, pp. 95–99.

50. **Torell,** P. and Ericsson, Y.: The Potential Benefits Derived from Fluoride Mouth Rinses, in Forrester, D.J. and Schulz, E.M., eds.: *International Workshop on Fluorides and Dental Caries Reductions.* Baltimore, University of Maryland School of Dentistry, 1974, pp. 114–176.

51. **Birkeland,** J.M. and Torell, P.: Caries-preventive Fluoride Mouthrinses, *Caries Res., 12*, 38, Supplement 1, 1978.

52. **Driscoll,** W.S., Swango, P.A., Horowitz, A.M., and Kingman, A.: Caries-preventive Effects of Daily and Weekly Fluoride

Mouthrinsing in a Fluoridated Community: Final Results after 30 Months, *J. Am. Dent. Assoc., 105,* 1010, December, 1982.

53. **Leske,** G.S., Ripa, L.W., and Green, E.: Posttreatment Benefits in a School-based Fluoride Mouthrinsing Program. Final Results after 7 Years of Rinsing by All Participants, *Clin. Prev. Dent., 8,* 19, September-October, 1986.

54. **Ripa,** L.W., Leske, G.S., and Varma, A.: Effect of Mouthrinsing with a 0.2 Percent Neutral NaF Solution on the Deciduous Dentition of First to Third Grade School Children, *Pediatr. Dent., 6,* 93, June, 1984.

55. **American Dental Association,** Council on Dental Therapeutics: Evaluation of Crest Toothpaste, *J. Am. Dent. Assoc., 61,* 272, August, 1960.

56. **Stookey,** G.K.: Are All Fluoride Dentifrices the Same? in Wei, S.H.Y., ed.: *Clinical Uses of Fluorides.* Philadelphia, Lea & Febiger, 1985, pp. 105–131.

57. **American Dental Association,** Council on Dental Therapeutics: Guidelines for the Acceptance of Fluoride-containing Dentifrices, *J. Am. Dent. Assoc., 110,* 545, April, 1985.

58. **Tolle,** S.L., Bauman, D.B., and Allen, D.S.: Effects of Fluoride Gels on Plaque and Gingival Health, *Dent. Hyg., 61,* 280, June, 1987.

59. **Naleway,** C.A.: Laboratory Methods of Assessing Fluoride Dentifrices and Other Topical Fluoride Agents, in Wei, S.H.Y., ed.: *Clinical Uses of Fluorides.* Philadelphia, Lea & Febiger, 1985, pp. 144–146.

60. **Stratemann,** M.W. and Shannon, I.L.: Control of Decalcification in Orthodontic Patients by Daily Self-administrated Application of a Water-free 0.4 Percent Stannous Fluoride Gel, *Am. J. Orthod., 66,* 273, September, 1974.

61. **Wescott,** W.B., Starcke, E.N., and Shannon, I.L.: Chemical Protection Against Postirradiation Dental Caries, *Oral Surg. Oral Med. Oral Pathol., 40,* 709, December, 1975.

62. **Hodge,** H.C. and Smith, F.A.: Fluoride Toxicology, in Newbrun, E., ed.: *Fluorides and Dental Caries,* 3rd ed. Springfield, IL, Charles C Thomas, 1986, pp. 199–220.

63. **Heifetz,** S.B. and Horowitz, H.S.: The Amounts of Fluoride in Current Fluoride Therapies: Safety Considerations for Children, *ASDC J. Dent. Child., 51,* 257, July–August, 1984.

64. **Bayless,** J.M. and Tinanoff, N.: Diagnosis and Treatment of Acute Fluoride Toxicity, *J. Am. Dent. Assoc., 110,* 209, February, 1985.

65. **Lyon,** T.C.: Topical Fluorides: How Much Are You Using? *Dent. Hyg., 59,* 58, February, 1985.

SUGGESTED READINGS

Banting, D.W.: The Future of Fluoride. An Update One Year after the National Toxicology Program Study, *J. Am. Dent. Assoc., 123,* 86, August, 1991.

Cirincione, U.K.: The Safe Use of Fluorides in Dental Hygiene Practice, *J. Dent. Hyg., 66,* 319, September, 1992.

DePaola, P.F.: Reaction Paper: The Use of Topical and Systemic Fluorides in the Present Era, *J. Public Health Dent., 51,* 48, Winter, 1991.

Hattab, F.N., Green, R.M., Pang, K.M., and Mok, Y.C.: Effect of Fluoride-containing Chewing Gum on Remineralization of Carious Lesions and on Fluoride Uptake in Man, *Clin. Prev. Dent., 11,* 6, November–December, 1989.

Jorgensen, J., Shariati, M., Shields, C.P., Durr, D.P., and Proskin, H.M.: Fluoride Uptake into Demineralized Primary Enamel from Fluoride-impregnated Dental Floss *In Vitro, Pediatr. Dent., 11,* 17, March, 1989.

Newbrun, E.: Preventing Dental Caries: Breaking the Chain of Transmission, *J. Am. Dent. Assoc., 123,* 55, June, 1992.

Newbrun, E.: Current Regulations and Recommendations Concerning Water Fluoridation, Fluoride Supplements, and Topical Fluoride Agents, *J. Dent. Res., 71,* 1255, May, 1992.

Reddy, J. and Grobler, S.R.: The Relationship of the Periodontal Status to Fluoride Levels of Alveolar Bone and Tooth Roots, *J. Clin. Periodontol., 15,* 217, April, 1988.

Tagomori, S. and Morioka, T.: Combined Effects of Laser and Fluoride on Acid Resistance of Human Dental Enamel, *Caries Res., 23,* 225, July–August, 1989.

Fluoride Action; Remineralization

Arends, J. and Christofferson, J.: Nature and Role of Loosely Bound Fluoride in Dental Caries, *J. Dent. Res., 69,* 601, February, 1990.

Barbakow, F., Imfeld, T., and Lutz, F.: Enamel Remineralization: How to Explain It to Patients, *Quintessence Int., 22,* 341, May, 1991.

Chow, L.C.: Tooth-bound Fluoride and Dental Caries, *J. Dent. Res., 69,* 595, February, 1990.

Dawes, C.: Fluorides: Mechanisms of Action and Recommendations for Use, *Can. Dent. Assoc. J., 55,* 721, September, 1989.

Dawes, C. and Weatherell, J.A.: Kinetics of Fluoride in the Oral Fluids, *J. Dent. Res., 69,* 638, February, 1990.

Frank, R.M.: Structural Events in the Caries Process in Enamel, Cementum, Dentin, *J. Dent. Res., 69,* 559, February, 1990.

Hargreaves, J.A.: The Level and Timing of Systemic Exposure to Fluoride with Respect to Caries Resistance, *J. Dent. Res., 71,* 1244, May, 1992.

Hayes, P.A. and Wefel, J.S.: *In Vivo* Remineralization of Enamel at the Buccal and Proximal Sites Using Two Fluoride Regimens, *Pediatr. Dent., 10,* 295, December, 1988.

Iijima, Y. and Koulourides, T.: Fluoride Incorporation into and Retention in Remineralized Enamel, *J. Dent. Res., 68,* 1289, August, 1989.

Lammers, P.C., Borggreven, J.M.P.M., and Driessens, F.C.M.: Influence of Fluoride on *In Vitro* Remineralization of Artificial Subsurface Lesions Determined with a Sandwich Technique, *Caries Res., 24,* 81, March–April, 1990.

Nakagaki, H., Weatherell, J.A., Strong, M., and Robinson, C.: Distribution of Fluoride in Human Cementum, *Arch. Oral Biol., 30,* 101, No. 2, 1985.

Niibu, I., Nakagaki, H., Kurosu, K., and Weatherell, J.A.: Distribution of Fluoride Across Human Primary Enamel, *Arch. Oral Biol., 36,* 603, No. 8, 1991.

Robinson, C. and Kirkham, J.: The Effect of Fluoride on the Developing Mineralized Tissues, *J. Dent. Res., 69,* 685, February, 1990.

Shern, R.J., Kennedy, J.B., and Roberts, M.W.: Fluoride Concentrations in Whole Saliva Following Use of Fluoride Tablets and a Rinse, *Pediatr. Dent., 11,* 307, December, 1989.

Sugihara, N., Nakagaki, H., Kunisaki, H., Ito, F., Noguchi, T., Weatherell, J.A., and Robinson, C.: Distribution of Fluoride in Sound and Periodontally Diseased Human Cementum, *Arch. Oral Biol., 36,* 383, No. 5, 1991.

Ten Cate, J.M.: *In Vitro* Studies on the Effects of Fluoride on De- and Remineralization, *J. Dent. Res., 69,* 614, February, 1990.

Ten Cate, J.M., Timmer, K., Shariati, M., and Featherstone, J.D.B.: Effect of Timing of Fluoride Treatment on Enamel De- and Remineralization *In Vitro:* A pH-cycling Study, *Caries Res., 22,* 20, January–February, 1988.

Thylstrup, A.: Clinical Evidence of the Role of Pre-eruptive Fluoride in Caries Prevention, *J. Dent. Res., 69,* 742, February, 1990.

White, D.J. and Nancollas, G.H.: Physical and Chemical Considerations in the Role of Firmly and Loosely Bound Fluoride in Caries Prevention, *J. Dent. Res., 69,* 587, February, 1990.

Whitford, G.M.: The Physiological and Toxicological Characteristics of Fluoride, *J. Dent. Res., 69*, 539, February, 1990.

Zero, D.T., Raubertas, R.F., Pedersen, A.M., Fu, J., Hayes, A.L., and Featherstone, J.D.B.: Studies of Fluoride Retention by Oral Soft Tissues after the Application of Home-use Topical Fluorides, *J. Dent. Res., 71*, 1546, September, 1992.

Fluoride and Bacterial Plaque

Bansal, G.S., Newman, H.N., and Wilson, M.: The Survival of Subgingival Plaque Bacteria in an Amine Fluoride-containing Gel, *J. Clin. Periodontol., 17*, 414, August, Part I, 1990.

Boyar, R.M., Thylstrup, A., Holmen, L., and Bowden, G.H.: The Microflora Associated with the Development of Initial Enamel Decalcification below Orthodontic Bands *In Vivo* in Children Living in a Fluoridated-water Area, *J. Dent. Res., 68*, 1734, December, 1989.

Eisenberg, A.D., Mundorff, S.A., Featherstone, J.D.B., Leverett, D.H., Adair, S.M., Billings, R.J., and Proskin, H.M.: Associations of Microbiological Factors and Plaque Index with Caries Prevalence and Water Fluoridation Status, *Oral Microbiol. Immunol., 6*, 139, June, 1991.

McHugh, W.D., Eisenberg, A.D., Leverett, D.H., and Jensen, Ø.E.: The Long-term Effects of Daily Rinsing with Stannous Fluoride or Sodium Fluoride on Bacteria in Dental Plaque, *Pediatr. Dent., 10*, 10, March, 1988.

Pearce, E.I.F.: Relationship Between Demineralization Events in Dental Enamel and the pH and Mineral Content of Plaque, *Proc. Finn. Dent. Soc., 87*, 527, No. 4, 1991.

Tatevossian, A.: Plaque Fluoride, *Proc. Finn. Dent. Soc., 87*, 501, No. 4, 1991.

Tatevossian, A.: Fluoride in Dental Plaque and Its Effects, *J. Dent. Res., 69*, 645, February, 1990.

Fluoridation

Ainamo, J. and Parviainen, K.: Influence of Increased Toothbrushing Frequency on Dental Health in Low, Optimal, and High Fluoride Areas in Finland, *Community Dent. Oral Epidemiol., 17*, 296, December, 1989.

Brossok, G.E., McTigue, D.J., and Kuthy, R.A.: The Use of a Colorimeter in Analyzing the Fluoride Content of Public Well Water, *Pediatr. Dent., 9*, 204, September, 1987.

Brown, M.D. and Aaron, G.: The Effect of Point-of-use Water Conditioning Systems on Community Fluoridated Water, *Pediatr. Dent., 13*, 35, January/February, 1991.

Brustman, B.A.: Impact of Exposure to Fluoride-adequate Water on Root Surface Caries in Elderly, *Gerodontics, 2*, 203, December, 1986.

Burt, B.A., Eklund, S.A., and Loesche, W.J.: Dental Benefits of Limited Exposure to Fluoridated Water in Childhood, *J. Dent. Res., 65*, 1322, November, 1986.

Edelstein, B.L., Cottrel, D., O'Sullivan, D., and Tinanoff, N.: Comparison of Colorimeter and Electrode Analysis of Water Fluoride, *Pediatr. Dent., 14*, 47, January/February, 1992.

Glass, R.G.: Water Purification Systems and Recommendations for Fluoride Supplementation, *ASDC J. Dent. Child., 58*, 405, September–October, 1991.

Grembowski, D., Fiset, L., and Spadafora, A.: How Fluoridation Affects Adult Dental Caries. Systemic and Topical Effects Are Explored, *J. Am. Dent. Assoc., 123*, 49, February, 1992.

Grembowski, D., Fiset, L., Spadafora, A., and Milgrom, P.: Fluoridation Effects on Periodontal Disease among Adults, *J. Periodont. Res., 28*, 166, May, 1993.

Grobler, S.R. and Louw, A.J.: Enamel-fluoride Levels in Deciduous and Permanent Teeth of Children in High, Medium and Low Fluoride Areas, *Arch. Oral Biol., 31*, 423, No. 7, 1986.

Horowitz, H.S.: Grand Rapids: The Public Health Story, *J. Public Health Dent., 49*, 62, Winter, 1989.

McGuire, S.: Fluoride Content of Bottled Water (Correspondence), *N. Engl. J. Med., 321*, 836, September 21, 1989.

Riordan, P.J.: Dental Caries and Fluoride Exposure in Western Australia, *J. Dent. Res., 70*, 1029, July, 1991.

Ripa, L.W.: A Half-century of Community Water Fluoridation in the United States: Review and Commentary, *J. Public Health Dent., 53*, 17, Winter, 1993.

Robinson, S.N., Davies, E.H., and Williams, B.: Domestic Water Treatment Appliances and the Fluoride Ion, *Br. Dent. J., 171*, 91, August, 1991.

Smith, K.G. and Christen, K.A.: A Fluoridation Campaign: The Phoenix Experience, *J. Public Health Dent., 50*, 319, Fall, 1990.

United States Centers for Disease Control: Public Health Focus: Fluoridation of Community Water Systems, *MMWR, 41*, 372, May 29, 1992.

Weinberger, S.J., Johnston, D.W., and Wright, G.Z.: A Comparison of Two Systems for Measuring Water Fluoride Ion Level, *Clin. Prev. Dent., 11*, 19, September–October, 1989.

Supplements

Driscoll, W.S.: What We Know and Don't Know about Dietary Fluoride Supplements—The Research Basis, *ASDC J. Dent. Child., 52*, 259, July–August, 1985.

Eldredge, J.B. and Levy, S.M.: The Dental Hygienist's Role in Recommending Dietary Fluoride Supplements, *Dent. Hyg., 62*, 385, September, 1988.

Horowitz, A.M.: Ways to Improve/Increase Appropriate Use of Dietary Fluorides, *ASDC J. Dent. Child., 52*, 269, July–August, 1985.

Levy, S.M. and Muchow, G.: Provider Compliance with Recommended Dietary Fluoride Supplement Protocol, *Am. J. Public Health, 82*, 281, February, 1992.

Levy, S.M. and Shavlik, D.A.: The Status of Water Fluoride Assay Programs and Implications for Prescribing of Dietary Fluoride Supplements, *ASDC J. Dent. Child., 58*, 23, January–February, 1991.

Pendrys, D.G. and Morse, D.E.: Use of Fluoride Supplementation by Children Living in Fluoridated Communities, *ASDC J. Dent. Child., 57*, 343, September–October, 1990.

Stannard, J., Rovero, J., Tsamtsouris, A., and Gavris, V.: Fluoride Content of Some Bottled Waters and Recommendations for Fluoride Supplementation, *J. Pedod., 14*, 103, No. 2, 1990.

Szpunar, S.M. and Burt, B.A.: Evaluation of Appropriate Use of Dietary Fluoride Supplements in the U.S., *Community Dent. Oral Epidemiol., 20*, 148, June, 1992.

Dental Fluorosis

Cutress, T.W. and Suckling, G.W.: Differential Diagnosis of Dental Fluorosis, *J. Dent. Res., 69*, 714, February, 1990.

Den Besten, P.K. and Thariani, H.: Biological Mechanisms of Fluorosis and Level and Timing of Systemic Exposure to Fluoride with Respect to Fluorosis, *J. Dent. Res., 71*, 1238, May, 1992.

Driscoll, W.S., Horowitz, H.S., Meyers, R.J., Heifetz, S.B., Kingman, A., and Zimmerman, E.R.: Prevalence of Dental Caries and Dental Fluorosis in Areas with Negligible, Optimal, and Above-optimal Fluoride Concentrations in Drinking Water, *J. Am. Dent. Assoc., 113*, 29, July, 1986.

Fejerskov, O., Manji, F., and Baelum, V.: The Nature and Mechanisms of Dental Fluorosis in Man, *J. Dent. Res., 69*, 692, February, 1990.

Haikel, Y., Cahen, P.M., Turlot, J.C., and Frank, R.M.: The Effects of Airborne Fluorides on Oral Conditions in Morocco, *J. Dent. Res., 68*, 1238, August, 1989.

Ishii, T. and Suckling, G.: The Severity of Dental Fluorosis in Children Exposed to Water with a High Fluoride Content for Various Periods of Time, *J. Dent. Res., 70*, 952, June, 1991.

Leverett, D.: Prevalence of Dental Fluorosis in Fluoridated and Nonfluoridated Communities—A Preliminary Investigation, *J. Public Health Dent.,* 46, 184, Fall, 1986.

Levy, S.M. and Zarei-M, Z.: Evaluation of Fluoride Exposures in Children, *ASDC J. Dent. Child.,* 58, 467, November–December, 1991.

Levy, S.M., Maurice, T.J., and Jakobsen, J.R.: Feeding Patterns, Water Sources and Fluoride Exposures of Infants and 1-year-olds, *J. Am. Dent. Assoc.,* 124, 65, April, 1993.

Lewis, H.A., Chikte, U.M.E., and Butchart, A.: Fluorosis and Dental Caries in Schoolchildren from Rural Areas with about 9 and 1 ppm F in the Water Supplies, *Community Dent. Oral Epidemiol.,* 20, 53, February, 1992.

Mason, J.O.: Too Much of a Good Thing? Questions about Fluorosis, *J. Am. Dent. Assoc.,* 122, 93, August, 1991.

McKnight-Hanes, M.C., Leverett, D.H., Adair, S.M., and Shields, C.P.: Fluoride Content of Infant Formulas: Soy-based Formulas as a Potential Factor in Dental Fluorosis, *Pediatr. Dent.,* 10, 189, September, 1988.

Pendrys, D.G. and Katz, R.V.: Risk of Enamel Fluorosis Associated with Fluoride Supplementation, Infant Formula, and Fluoride Dentifrice Use, *Am. J. Epidemiol.,* 130, 1199, December, 1989.

Pendrys, D.G. and Stamm, J.W.: Relationship of Total Fluoride Intake to Beneficial Effects and Enamel Fluorosis, *J. Dent. Res.,* 69, 529, February, 1990.

Riordan, P.J. and Banks, J.A.: Dental Fluorosis and Fluoride Exposure in Western Australia, *J. Dent. Res.,* 70, 1022, July, 1991.

Ripa, L.W.: A Critique of Topical Fluoride Methods (Dentifrices, Mouthrinses, Operator-, and Self-applied Gels) in an Era of Decreased Caries and Increased Fluorosis Prevalence, *J. Public Health Dent.,* 51, 23, Winter, 1991.

Tobin, E.A.: Dental Fluorosis in Children in the 1980s. A Review of the Literature, *Dent. Hyg.,* 62, 380, September, 1988.

Whitford, G.M.: Acute and Chronic Fluoride Toxicity, *J. Dent. Res.,* 71, 1249, May, 1992.

Williams, J.E. and Zwemer, J.D.: Community Water Fluoride Levels, Preschool Dietary Patterns, and the Occurrence of Fluoride Enamel Opacities, *J. Public Health Dent.,* 50, 276, Summer, 1990.

Wöltgens, J.H., Etty, E.J., Nieuwland, W.M.D., and Lyaruu, D.M.: Use of Fluoride by Young Children and Prevalence of Mottled Enamel, *Adv. Dent. Res.,* 3, 177, September, 1989.

Woolfolk, M.W., Faja, B.W., and Bagramian, R.A.: Relation of Sources of Systemic Fluoride to Prevalence of Dental Fluorosis, *J. Public Health Dent.,* 49, 78, Spring, 1989.

Root Caries

Burt, B.A., Ismail, A.I., and Eklund, S.A.: Root Caries in an Optimally Fluoridated and a High-fluoride Community, *J. Dent. Res.,* 65, 1154, September, 1986.

Eklund, S.A., Burt, B.A., Ismail, A.I., and Calderone, J.J.: High-fluoride Drinking Water, Fluorosis, and Dental Caries in Adults, *J. Am. Dent. Assoc.,* 114, 324, March, 1987.

Leverett, D.H.: Effectiveness of Mouthrinsing with Fluoride Solutions in Preventing Coronal and Root Caries, *J. Public Health Dent.,* 49, 310, No. 5, Special Issue, 1989.

Mitchell, T.L. and Forgay, M.G.E.: Root Surface Caries: Implications for Dental Hygienists, *Can. Dent. Hyg./Probe,* 21, 31, March, 1987.

Potter, D.E., Manwell, M.A., Dess, R., Levine, E., and Tinanoff, N.: SnF$_2$ as an Adjunct to Toothbrushing in an Elderly Institutionalized Population, *Spec. Care Dentist.,* 4, 216, September–October, 1984.

Schaeken, M.J.M., Keltjens, H.M.A.M., and van der Hoeven, J.S.: Effects of Fluoride and Chlorhexidine on the Microflora of Dental Root Surfaces and Progression of Root-surface Caries, *J. Dent. Res.,* 70, 150, February, 1991.

Topical Applications

Brewer, K.P., Retief, D.H., Wallace, M.C., and Bradley, E.L.: Cementum Fluoride Uptake from Topical Fluoride Agents, *Gerodontics,* 3, 212, October, 1987.

Brunn, C. and Givskov, H.: Formation of CaF$_2$ on Sound Enamel and in Caries-like Enamel Lesions after Different Forms of Fluoride Applications In Vitro, *Caries Res.,* 25, 96, March–April, 1991.

Cruz, R. and Rølla, G.: The Effect of Time of Exposure on Fluoride Uptake by Human Enamel from Acidulated Fluoride Solutions In Vitro, *Acta Odontol. Scand.,* 50, 51, February, 1992.

Hastreiter, R.J.: Is 0.4% Stannous Fluoride Gel an Effective Agent for the Prevention of Oral Diseases? *J. Am. Dent. Assoc.,* 118, 205, February, 1989.

Markitziu, A., Gedalia, I., Stabholz, A., and Shuval, J.: Prevention of Caries Progress in Xerostomic Patients by Topical Fluoride Applications; A Study *In Vivo* and *In Vitro, J. Dent.,* 10, 248, September, 1982.

Neuman, E. and Garcia-Godoy, F.: Effect of APF Gel on a Glass Ionomer Cement: An SEM Study, *ASDC J. Dent. Child.,* 59, 289, July–August, 1992.

Olivier, M., Brodeur, J.-M., and Simard, P.L.: Efficacy of APF Treatments Without Prior Toothcleaning Targeted to High-risk Children, *Community Dent. Oral Epidemiol.,* 20, 38, February, 1992.

Ostela, I. and Tenovuo, J.: Antibacterial Activity of Dental Gels Containing Combinations of Amine Fluoride, Stannous Fluoride, and Chlorhexidine Against Cariogenic Bacteria, *Scand. J. Dent. Res.,* 98, 1, February, 1990.

Ripa, L.W.: Review of the Anticaries Effectiveness of Professionally Applied and Self-applied Topical Fluoride Gels, *J. Public Health Dent.,* 49, 297, Special Issue, 1989.

Seppä, L. and Tolonen, T.: Caries Preventive Effect of Fluoride Varnish Applications Performed Two or Four Times a Year, *Scand. J. Dent. Res.,* 98, 102, April, 1990.

Sieck, B., Takagi, S., and Chow, L.C.: Assessment of Loosely-bound and Firmly-bound Fluoride Uptake by Tooth Enamel from Topically Applied Fluoride Treatments, *J. Dent. Res.,* 69, 1261, June, 1990.

Wei, S.H.Y. and Chik, F.F.: Fluoride Retention Following Topical Fluoride Foam and Gel Application, *Pediatr. Dent.,* 12, 368, November/December, 1990.

Wei, S.H.Y. and Hattab, F.N.: Enamel Fluoride Uptake from a New APF Foam, *Pediatr. Dent.,* 10, 111, June, 1988.

Wei, S.H.Y., Lau, E.W.S., and Hattab, F.N.: Time Dependence of Enamel Fluoride Acquisition from APF Gels. II. In Vivo Study, *Pediatr. Dent.,* 10, 173, September, 1988.

Dentifrices

Beltrán, E.D. and Szpunar, S.M.: Fluoride in Toothpastes for Children: Suggestion for Change, *Pediatr. Dent.,* 10, 185, September, 1988.

Duckworth, R.M., Knoop, D.T.M., and Stephen, K.W.: Effect of Mouthrinsing after Toothbrushing with a Fluoride Dentifrice on Human Salivary Fluoride Levels, *Caries Res.,* 25, 287, July–August, 1991.

Duckworth, R.M. and Morgan, S.N.: Oral Fluoride Retention after Use of Fluoride Dentifrices, *Caries Res.,* 25, 123, March–April, 1991.

Horowitz, H.S.: The Need for Toothpastes with Lower than Conventional Fluoride Concentrations for Preschool-aged Children, *J. Public Health Dent.,* 52, 216, Summer, 1992.

Jensen, M. and Kohout, F.: The Effect of a Fluoridated Dentifrice on Root and Coronal Caries in an Older Adult Population, *J. Am. Dent. Assoc.,* 117, 829, December, 1988.

Levy, S.M.: A Review of Fluoride Intake from Fluoride Dentifrice, *ASDC J. Dent. Child.,* 60, 115, March–April, 1993.

Moran, J., Addy, M., and Newcombe, R.: The Antibacterial Effect of Toothpastes on the Salivary Flora, *J. Clin. Periodontol.,* 15, 193, March, 1988.

Naccache, H., Simard, P.L., Trahan, L., Brodeur, J.-M., Demers, M., and Lachapelle, D.: Factors Affecting the Ingestion of Fluoride Dentifrice by Children, *J. Public Health Dent., 52,* 222, Summer, 1992.

Naccache, H., Simard, P.L., Trahan, L., Demers, M., Lapointe, C., and Brodeur, J.-M.: Variability in the Ingestion of Toothpaste by Preschool Children, *Caries Res., 24,* 359, September–October, 1990.

Page, D.J.: A Study of the Effect of Fluoride Delivered from Solution and Dentifrices on Enamel Demineralization, *Caries Res., 25,* 251, July–August, 1991.

Rolla, G., Øgaard, B., and deAlmeida Cruz, R.: Clinical Effect and Mechanism of Cariostatic Action of Fluoride-containing Toothpastes: A Review, *Int. Dent. J., 41,* 171, June, 1991.

Fluoride Programs

Doherty, N.J.G. and Martie, C.W.: Analysis of the Costs of School-based Mouthrinsing Programs, *Community Dent. Oral Epidemiol., 15,* 67, April, 1987.

Driscoll, W.S., Nowjack-Raymer, R., Selwitz, R.H., Li, S.-H., and Heifetz, S.B.: A Comparison of the Caries-preventive Effects of Fluoride Mouthrinsing, Fluoride Tablets, and Both Procedures Combined: Final Results after Eight Years, *J. Public Health Dent., 52,* 111, Winter, 1992.

Garcia, A.I.: Caries Incidence and Costs of Prevention Programs, *J. Public Health Dent., 49,* 259, Special Issue, 1989.

Haugejorden, O., Lervik, T., Birkeland, J.M., and Jorkjend, L.: An 11-year Follow-up Study of Dental Caries after Discontinuation of School-based Fluoride Programs, *Acta Odontol. Scand., 48,* 257, August, 1990.

Heidmann, J., Poulsen, S., Arnbjerg, D., Kirkegaard, E., and Laurberg, L.: Caries Development after Termination of a Fluoride Rinsing Program, *Community Dent. Oral Epidemiol., 20,* 118, June, 1992.

Horowitz, H.S., Meyers, R.J., Heifetz, S.B., Driscoll, W.S., and Li, S.-H.: Combined Fluoride, School-based Program in a Fluoride-deficient Area: Results of an 11-year Study, *J. Am. Dent. Assoc., 112* 621, May, 1986.

Ripa, L.W., Leske, G.S., and Forte, F.: The Combined Use of Pit and Fissure Sealants and Fluoride Mouthrinsing in Second and Third Grade Children: Final Clinical Results after Two Years, *Pediatr. Dent., 9,* 118, June, 1987.

Stephen, K.W., Kay, E.J., and Tullis, J.I.: Combined Fluoride Therapies. A 6-year Double-blind School-based Preventive Dentistry Study in Inverness, Scotland, *Community Dent. Oral Epidemiol., 18,* 244, October, 1990.

Sterritt, G.R., Frew, R.A., Rozier, R.G., and Brunelle, J.A.: Evaluation of a School-based Fluoride Mouthrinsing and Clinic-based Sealant Program on a Non-fluoridated Island, *Community Dent. Oral Epidemiol., 18,* 288, December, 1990.

Trubman, A., Silberman, S.L., and Meydrech, E.F.: Treatment Costs for Carious Primary Teeth Related to Fluoride Exposure, *ASDC J. Dent. Child., 58,* 69, January–February, 1991.

30

Sealants

As part of a complete preventive program, pit and fissure sealants are indicated for selected patients. Because topically or systemically applied fluorides protect smooth tooth surfaces more than occlusal surfaces, a method to reduce the incidence of occlusal dental caries is needed. The incidence of new pit and fissure caries can be lowered significantly by the application of adhesive sealants. Table 30–1 provides definitions and terminology relative to sealants and their application.

Other preventive measures used for and by the patient are necessary. Sealant application should be part of a complete prevention program, not an isolated procedure. As an isolated procedure, patient (and parent) may misunderstand the selected area of prevention that this measure represents. Other surfaces and other teeth still need other methods of preventive protection.

I. DEFINITION AND ACTION
A pit and fissure resin sealant is an organic polymer that bonds to the enamel surface mainly by mechanical retention. It acts as a physical barrier to prevent oral bacteria and their nutrients from collecting within a pit or fissure and creating the acid environment essential to the initiation of dental caries.

Before the sealant is applied, the enamel surface is treated with an acid etchant to increase the adhesion of the sealant. The acid etch creates micropores in the enamel. When the resin sealant is applied, it penetrates into the tiny pores and creates a bond or mechanical interlocking. Figure 30–1 is a diagram that shows irregularities created when an enamel surface is etched, and how the sealant resin penetrates into the tiny irregularities.

II. TYPES OF SEALANTS
Currently, most sealants in clinical use are made of Bis-GMA (a reaction product of bis-phenol A and glycidyl methacrylate). The techniques of application vary slightly among available products.

The American Dental Association Council on Dental Materials, Instruments, and Equipment has a program for evaluation and acceptance of pit and fissure sealants.[1] The three types of sealants currently available are filled, unfilled, and fluoride-releasing filled. Sealants are also identified by the method required for polymerization.

A. Chemical Cured or Autopolymerization
The product is available in two bottles. When the two liquids are mixed, polymerization begins. Placement, or working time, is limited, and the setting time after placement is usually short.

B. Visible Light Cured or Photopolymerization
Light-activated sealants harden when exposed to the special visible light for curing. The clinician has more working time, because polymerization does not start until the light is directed on to the sealant.

SELECTION OF TEETH FOR SEALANT APPLICATION

All caries-free pits and fissures are not necessarily indicated for sealant application. When assessment is made and the teeth that will receive a sealant are chosen selectively, several factors must be considered.

TABLE 30-1
KEY WORDS AND ABBREVIATIONS: PIT AND FISSURE SEALANTS

Acid etchant: in sealant placement, the enamel surface is prepared by the application of phosphoric acid, which etches the surface to provide mechanical retention for the sealant.

Autopolymerization (aw'tō-pol-ĭ-mer'ĭ-zā'shun): self-curing; a reaction in which a high-molecular-weight product is produced by successive additions of a simpler compound; hardening process of pit and fissure sealants.

Bibulous (bib'ū-lus): absorbent; a flat bibulous pad, placed in the cheek over the opening of Stensen's duct, is used to aid in maintaining a dry field while placing sealants.

BIS-GMA: Bisphenol A-glycidyl methacrylate; plastic material used for dental sealants.

Bonding (Mechanical): physical adherence of one substance to another; the adherence of a sealant to the enamel surface is accomplished by an acid etching technique that leaves microspaces between the enamel rods; the sealant becomes mechanically locked (bonded) in these microspaces.

Bond strength: expression of the degree of adherence between the tooth surface and the sealant.

Conditioner (kon-dish'un-er): a substance added to another substance to increase its usability; in sealant placement, the acid etchant is added to the enamel to prepare it for bonding with the sealant.

Polymer (pol'ĭ mer): a compound of high molecular weight formed by a combination of a chain of simpler molecules (monomers).

Sealant: organic polymer that bonds to an enamel surface by mechanical retention accommodated by projections of the sealant into micropores created in the enamel by etching; the two types of sealants, filled and unfilled, both are composed of BIS-GMA.

Filled sealant: contains, in addition to BIS-GMA, microparticles of glass, quartz, silica, and other fillers used in composite restorations; fillers make the sealant more resistant to abrasion.

I. LOCATION OF PITS AND FISSURES

Sealants are indicated for permanent and primary teeth that have pits and fissures. These include occlusal pits and fissures, facial pits (such as the buccal pits of the mandibular molars), palatal pits (such as at the cusps of Carabelli), and cingulum pits (such as the palatal of maxillary anterior teeth).

II. CONTOUR OF PITS AND FISSURES

Sealants are indicated especially for teeth with deep, narrow pits and fissures. Teeth with shallow and well-coalesced pits and fissures are less likely to become carious because they are more accessible for plaque removal.

III. RELATION TO ERUPTION

Applications should be made as soon as possible following eruption. When application is delayed, caries may start, and the surface no longer can be considered for sealant. When possible, sealant can be applied before full eruption, provided there is no tissue flap over the occlusal surface to interfere with application procedures.

IV. RELATION TO DENTAL CARIES HISTORY

Overall caries susceptibility is significant. When current carious lesions and previous restorations exist, newly erupted teeth should be treated with sealants promptly.

V. RADIOGRAPHIC PROXIMAL CARIES

Sealant is not indicated when proximal carious lesions in the same tooth require restoration.

VI. INCIPIENT DENTAL CARIES

Incipient pit and fissure caries is arrested by sealant placement.[2,3,4] Bacterial cultures under sealed lesions have been negative or insignificant because cariogenic bacteria cannot act to demineralize tooth structure without the presence of sucrose or other cariogenic substance (figure 28–2, page 425).

VII. AGE

The age of the patient may have particular significance. When teeth have been erupted several years and have not become carious, they are not necessarily less susceptible indefinitely. Habits may change. For example, application of a sealant to caries-free pits and fissures during early teenage years and during pregnancy, when caries rates are high, may prove beneficial to the individual.

CLINICAL PROCEDURES

Each quadrant should be treated separately. Isolation to prevent contamination and moisture can then be controlled. The precise technique is most effectively carried out when two dental team members work together.

The manufacturer's directions must be followed carefully for each specific product. Although the basic techniques are similar, characteristic steps are unique to each product.

General directions are described here in sequence, with brief explanations of the purposes of each step. The main steps are cleaning and drying the tooth surfaces, conditioning (enamel etching), applying the sealant, and polymerization. The success of treatment depends on precision in the techniques of application.

I. PREPARE THE TOOTH SURFACE

Although the rubber cup or bristle brush with plain pumice may have been used traditionally and is effec-

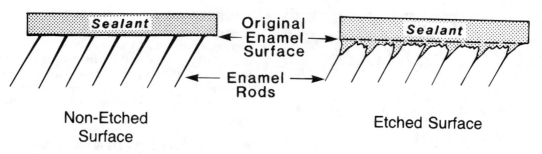

FIG. 30–1. Enamel-Sealant Interface. Diagram of enamel-sealant interface to compare nonetched surface with etched surface. Etching produces microscopic porosities in the enamel to increase the area of retention. The unpolymerized resin flows into the porosities and hardens in tag-like projections, as shown on the right. (Adapted from Buonocore, M.G., Matsui, A., and Gwinnett, A.J.: Penetration of Resin Dental Materials into Enamel Surfaces with Reference to Bonding, *Arch. Oral Biol., 13*, 61, 1968.)

tive, research also has shown successful sealant retention in pits and fissures when the surfaces had been prepared by the acid etch alone or with bristle brush and water.[5,6,7]

A. Purposes
1. Remove deposits and debris.
2. Permit maximum contact of the sealant with enamel surface.

B. Inspect the Surfaces
Usual instrumentation for removal of calculus and heavy stain is carried out first.

C. Patient with No Stain or Calculus
1. Request patient to brush; apply filaments vigorously to occlusal surfaces (figure 22–11, page 346).
2. Suction the pits and fissures with high-volume evacuator.
3. Use a sharp explorer (for example, No. 23 or other straight line to the tip) to dig out debris and bacteria from the pit or fissure.
4. Suction again to remove loosened material.
5. Additional cleaning is not necessary.

D. Cleansing Procedure
When indicated because of heavy dental stains or when believed necessary, cleaning can be accomplished by use of an airpolisher[8,9] or polishing brush in a slow-speed handpiece. Although cleansing pastes containing oils or fluoride traditionally are avoided, research suggests that such avoidance may not be necessary.[10,11]

II. ISOLATE THE TOOTH
A. Patient Position
The quadrant to be treated should be comfortably positioned for visibility and accessibility. The head is slightly tilted so saliva can flow to the opposite side of the mouth and not collect around the treatment area.

B. Purposes of Isolation
1. Keep the tooth clean and dry for optimal action and bonding of the sealant.
2. Eliminate possible contamination by saliva and moisture from the breath.
3. Keep the materials from contacting the oral tissues, being swallowed accidentally, or being unpleasant to the patient because of flavor.

C. Rubber Dam
1. Rubber dam application is the method of choice because the most complete isolation is obtained. This method is especially helpful when more than one tooth must be sealed.
2. Rubber dam is essential when profuse saliva flow and overactive tongue and oral muscles make retraction and consistent maintenance of a dry, clean field impossible.
3. Combined treatment should be planned. When a quadrant has a rubber dam and anesthesia for restoration of other teeth, teeth indicated for sealant may be treated.
4. Rubber dam is not possible when
   a. Application of the clamp could not be tolerated by the patient without anesthesia.
   b. Tooth is not fully erupted and may not hold a rubber dam clamp.

D. Cotton-Roll Isolation
Details for cotton-roll isolation and maintenance of a dry field are described on pages 446 and 447.
1. Request patient to expectorate and swallow.
2. Position cotton rolls (Garmer holder for mandibular arch, figure 29–4, page 446).
3. Place saliva ejector.
4. Apply triangular saliva absorber over the opening of the parotid gland in the cheek (bibulous pads: Dri-angle or Dri Aids).
5. Take great care to prevent the saliva from entering the etched area.

III. DRY THE TOOTH
A. Purposes
1. Prepare the tooth for the conditioner.
2. Prevent dilution and contamination of the conditioner.

B. Use Only Dry, Oil-free, Clean Air
Many syringes, particularly the multipurpose types, emit a combination of air and water spray. Some syringes may emit oil.
1. Clear the air by releasing the spray into a sink before directing it onto the tooth.
2. Test the air for water content by blowing on the back of the gloved hand or on a mirror surface.
3. Air dry for at least 10 seconds.

IV. APPLY CONDITIONER FOR ENAMEL ETCHING
A. Purposes
To increase the adherence of the sealant, the conditioner (either gel or solution) is used to
1. Create surface irregularities to increase the area for retention (figure 30–1).
2. Increase the size of the microspaces between enamel rods so they are accessible to the adhesive.
3. Remove bacterial plaque and pellicle.

B. Conditioner
1. Apply the phosphoric acid (35 to 50%) with a brush, cotton pellet, or plastic sponge over the surface where sealant is indicated.
2. Note the time or start timer. Total application time is 20 seconds.
3. Place gel over the surface and leave undisturbed.
4. For a solution, use a continuous dabbing, not a rubbing, motion. Gentle dabbing does not damage the fragile enamel latticework formed during the etching process.
5. If saliva contaminates the area, repeat procedure and apply conditioner for 20 seconds.

V. RINSE THOROUGHLY
A. Purposes
1. Remove all excess acid and complexes formed from the action of the minerals of the tooth and the acid.
2. Prevent saliva from reaching the etched surface. Saliva reduces the bonding strength of the sealant by depositing the salivary constituents on the surface.

B. Procedure
1. Do not permit the patient to rinse or expectorate. Contaminants must be kept from the etched area.
2. Clear the water in the tubing of the air/water syringe by releasing the water into a sink.

3. Hold wide aspirator tip between tooth and cotton. The tip should be maintained firmly against the tooth to collect the water as it flows across the occlusal surface.
4. Rinse thoroughly (10 to 15 seconds for solution; 30 seconds for a gel). Direct the water stream across the etched surfaces so that each portion of the surface is washed.
5. Evacuate excess water from the entire area immediately after rinsing.
6. Maintain dry area. When a rubber dam is not used, the cotton rolls are difficult to change. Two preferred procedures are suggested.
   a. Place one dry cotton roll over each wet cotton roll. Suction must be applied constantly. For some patients, the wet cotton roll can be slid out from under with great care and then can be removed in the direction of the opposite side of the mouth.
   b. Leave the wet cotton rolls in place, and suction excess moisture from the cotton rolls.
7. Should accidental contamination with saliva occur, wash, dry, and etch again for 10 seconds. Wash and dry to prepare for next step.

C. Examine the Surface
The etched surface should be a dull, chalky white. If not, repeat the application of the conditioner step-by-step. Primary teeth or older permanent teeth may require a repeat application.

VI. DRY THE TOOTH THOROUGHLY AGAIN
A. Purposes
1. Prepare the tooth for the sealant application.
2. Prevent moisture from reducing the affinity of the adhesive for the enamel surface, and thereby preventing penetration of the adhesive into the microspaces created by etching.

B. Procedure
1. Dry the tooth thoroughly for 15 to 30 seconds per tooth. Use only clean, dry, oil-free air (see previous section, ''Dry the Tooth'').
2. Do not blow saliva onto the etched surface.
3. Drying is continued while the assistant prepares the sealant resin.

VII. APPLY THE SEALANT
A. Follow Manufacturer's Instructions
Each type of sealant has specific timing, applicator, and details for manipulation. Autopolymerized sealants are measured by drops and mixed; photopolymerized sealants are not mixed, but are initiated to polymerization when the special light is placed on them.

B. Placement
1. Do the most posterior tooth first (when more than one sealant is to be placed in a quadrant).

2. Do only two teeth per mix (when more than two sealants are to be placed in one quadrant).

C. Application
1. Use disposable applicator (brush, sponge, or other) provided.
2. Flow the sealant first into the pit or fissure that has the maximum depth. Extend and thicken. Avoid marginal ridges, cusp tips.
3. Time by the instructions. After polymerization begins, the material should not be disturbed.

D. Photopolymerization
1. Connect special light in ample time before beginning the sealant preparation.
2. Wear protective amber eyewear to protect eyes from the light.
3. Apply sealant with special applicator.
4. Hold light tip 2 mm from sealant surface to prevent any contact during the first few seconds.
5. Polymerization time is 20 seconds. Make sure all parts of the sealant are equally exposed to the light. The most posterior portion may be the most difficult to reach.

VIII. FINAL STEPS
A. Observe Sealant
Before discontinuing the dry field, the sealant is examined. Voids may be filled, and portions may be added without re-etching. A fresh mix is needed.

B. Test for Retention
Run an explorer around the margin and try to pry the sealant away from the enamel. Sealants obtain optimum strength soon after polymerization, so they can be tested. Replacement can be made immediately using a 10-second re-etch.

C. Adjust the Occlusion[12,13]
Unfilled sealants may wear down readily. Filled sealants are more resistant because of their viscosity and flow.
1. *Effects of Premature Contacts.* Premature contacts are not only distracting and uncomfortable for the patient, but long-lasting prematurities can lead to occlusal and temporomandibular joint problems.
2. *Procedure*
   a. Dry the teeth; place articulating paper.
   b. Observe marks on the sealants; reshape using a low-speed handpiece with a round bur.

PENETRATION OF SEALANT

The penetration of a sealant depends on the configuration of the pit or fissure, the presence of deposits and debris within the pit or fissure, and the properties of the sealant itself.[14]

I. PIT AND FISSURE ANATOMY
A review of the anatomy of pits and fissures may be helpful in understanding the effects of sealants in the prevention of dental caries. The shape and depth of pits and fissures vary considerably even within one tooth.

Long narrow pits and grooves reach to, or nearly to, the dentinoenamel junction. Others are *wide V-shaped* or *narrow V-shaped*, whereas still others may have a *long constricted form with a bulbous terminal portion* (figure 30–2). The pit or fissure may take a wavy course; thus, it may not lead directly from the outer surface to the dentinoenamel junction.

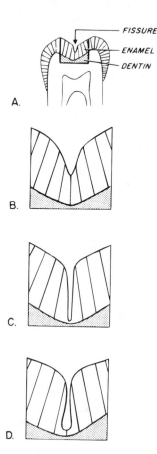

FIG. 30–2. Occlusal Fissures. Drawings made from microscopic slides show variations in shape and depth of fissures. **A.** Tooth with section enlarged for B, C, and D. **B.** Wide V-shaped fissure. **C.** Long narrow groove that reaches nearly to the dentinoenamel junction. **D.** Long constricted form with a bulbous terminal portion.

II. CONTENTS OF A PIT OR FISSURE

A pit or fissure contains bacterial plaque, pellicle, debris, and sometimes relatively intact remnants of tooth development.

III. EFFECT OF CLEANING

The narrow, long fissures are impossible to clean completely, and the condition cannot reach the deeper portions. Retained cleaning material can block the sealant from filling the fissure and can also become mixed with the sealant. Removal of pumice used for cleaning and thorough washing are necessary to the success of the sealant.

IV. AMOUNT OF PENETRATION

Wide V-shaped and shallow fissures are more apt to be filled by sealant (figure 30–3B). Although ideally the sealant should penetrate to the bottom of a pit or fissure, such penetration is frequently impossible because of the debris. Microscopic examination of pits

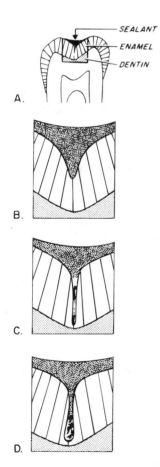

FIG. 30–3. Pit and Fissure Sealant in Fissures. Drawings made from microscopic slides show extent to which sealant fills a fissure. **A.** Tooth with section enlarged for B, C, and D. **B.** Sealant fills wide V-shaped fissure and extends a short way up the slopes of surrounding cusps. **C.** and **D.** Fissures partially filled as a result of narrow constriction of the groove and blockage by trapped debris.

and fissures after sealant application has shown that the sealant does not penetrate to the bottom because residual debris, cleansing agents, and trapped air prevent passage of the material (figure 30–3C and D).

RETENTION AND REPLACEMENT

Length of time of retention depends almost entirely on the precision of technique. Although surface sealant may be lost, sealant in the pits and fissures and sealant that penetrated into the microspaces of the enamel still remain and provide protection.[15]

I. FACTORS THAT INFLUENCE RETENTION TIME
A. Precision of Technique
Each step in the preparation of the tooth and the application of the sealant must be carefully performed. Improper technique is the major cause of early loss of sealant from the tooth surface.

B. Effect of Contamination
Any contact of the etched enamel surface, by saliva, water, or any other contaminant, before application of the sealant markedly decreases the effectiveness of the sealant.

II. RE-EXAMINATION
At each maintenance appointment, or at least every 6 months, the sealant should be examined for deficiencies that may have developed.

III. REPLACEMENT
Consult the manufacturer's instructions. Tooth preparation is the same as that for an original application.
   A. Removal of sections of retained sealant is not necessary.
   B. Re-etching of the tooth surface is always essential.

FLUORIDE AND SEALANT

I. TOPICAL APPLICATION IN CONJUNCTION WITH SEALANT
Topical fluoride application after placement of sealants is advisable to promote the remineralization of the tooth surface area that was etched but not covered with sealant.

II. COMBINED PREVENTIVE PROGRAM
Sealants are part of a total preventive program. Although sealant is applicable for occlusal surfaces, fluoride applications and other fluoride sources for self-administration are necessary for all other surfaces.

TECHNICAL HINTS

I. EYE PROTECTION
The patient must wear safety protective eyewear during the etching process. Phosphoric acid could cause loss of sight if a drop inadvertently falls into an eye.[16]

II. EQUIPMENT AND MATERIALS
A. Store materials without exposure to air, light, or heat.
B. Maintain equipment at high level of cleanliness and disinfection.[17]

III. MAINTENANCE
Avoid existing sealants when using an airpolisher during maintenance appointments. Sealant wear increases with the time of exposure to airpolisher abrasion.[18]

FACTORS TO TEACH THE PATIENT

I. Sealants are part of a total preventive program. Sealants are not substitutes for other preventive measures, including limitations of dietary sucrose, use of fluorides, and bacterial plaque control.
II. What a sealant is and why such a meticulous application procedure is required.
III. What can be expected from a sealant; how long it lasts, how it prevents dental caries.
IV. Need for examination of the sealant at frequent, scheduled appointments and need for replacement when indicated.

REFERENCES

1. **American Dental Association,** Council on Dental Health and Health Planning and Council on Dental Materials, Instruments, and Equipment: Pit and Fissure Sealants, *J. Am. Dent. Assoc., 114,* 671, May, 1987.
2. **Swift,** E.J.: The Effect of Sealants on Dental Caries: A Review, *J. Am. Dent. Assoc., 116,* 700, May, 1988.
3. **Handelman,** S.L.: Therapeutic Use of Sealants for Incipient or Early Carious Lesions in Children and Young Adults, *Proc. Finn. Dent. Soc., 87,* 463, No. 4, 1991.
4. **Weerheijm,** K.L., de Soet, J.J., van Amerongen, W.E., and de Graaff, J.: Sealing of Occlusal Hidden Caries Lesions: An Alternative for Curative Treatment? *ASDC J. Dent. Child., 59,* 263, July–August, 1992.
5. **Mertz-Fairhurst,** E.J., Fairhurst, C.W., Williams, J.E., Della-Giustina, V.E., and Brooks, J.D.: A Comparative Clinical Study of Two Pit and Fissure Sealants: 7-year Results in Augusta, GA, *J. Am. Dent. Assoc., 109,* 252, August, 1984.
6. **Simonsen,** R.J.: The Clinical Effectiveness of a Colored Pit and Fissure Sealant at 36 Months, *J. Am. Dent. Assoc., 102,* 323, March, 1981.
7. **Simonsen,** R.J.: Retention and Effectiveness of Dental Sealant after 15 years, *J. Am. Dent. Assoc., 122,* 34, October, 1991.
8. **Scott,** L., Brockmann, S., Houston, G., and Tira, D.: Retention of Dental Sealants Following the Use of Airpolishing and Traditional Cleaning, *Dent. Hyg., 62,* 402, September, 1988.
9. **Brockmann,** S.L., Scott, R.L., and Eick, J.D.: A Scanning Electron Microscopic Study of the Effect of Air Polishing on the Enamel-sealant Surface, *Quintessence Int., 21,* 201, March, 1990.
10. **Aboush,** Y.E.Y., Tareen, A., and Elderton, R.J.: Resin-to-Enamel Bonds: Effect of Cleaning the Enamel Surface with Prophylactic Pastes Containing Fluoride or Oil, *Br. Dent. J., 171,* 207, October 5, 1991.
11. **Bogert,** T.R. and Garcia-Godoy, F.: Effect of Prophylaxis Agents on the Shear Bond Strength of a Fissure Sealant, *Pediatr. Dent., 14,* 50, January/February, 1992.
12. **Tilliss,** T.S.I., Stach, D.J., Hatch, R.A., and Cross-Poline, G.N.: Occlusal Discrepancies after Sealant Therapy, *J. Prosthet. Dent., 68,* 223, August, 1992.
13. **Stach,** D.J., Hatch, R.A., Tilliss, T.S., and Cross-Poline, G.N.: Change in Occlusal Height Resulting from Placement of Pit and Fissure Sealants, *J. Prosthet. Dent., 68,* 750, November, 1992.
14. **Taylor,** C.L. and Gwinnett, A.J.: A Study of the Penetration of Sealants into Pits and Fissures, *J. Am. Dent. Assoc., 87,* 1181, November, 1973.
15. **Buonocore,** M.G.: Pit and Fissure Sealing, *Dent. Clin. North Am., 19,* 367, April, 1975.
16. **Colvin,** J.: Eye Injuries and the Dentist, *Aust. Dent. J., 23,* 453, December, 1978.
17. **Caughman,** G.B., Caughman, W.F., Napier, N., and Schuster, G.S.: Disinfection of Visible-light-curing Devices, *Oper. Dent., 14,* 2, Winter, 1989.
18. **Huennekens,** S.C., Daniel, S.J., and Bayne, S.C.: Effects of Air Polishing on the Abrasion of Occlusal Sealants, *Quintessence Int., 22,* 581, July, 1991.

SUGGESTED READINGS

Carstensen, W.: The Effects of Different Phosphoric Acid Concentrations on Surface Enamel, *Angle Orthod., 62,* 51, Spring, 1992.
Daniel, S.J., Grose, M.D., Scruggs, R.R., and Stoltz, R.F.: Examiner Reliability in Evaluating Dental Sealants, *Dent. Hyg., 61,* 410, September, 1987.
Daniel, S.J., Scruggs, R.R., and Grady, J.J.: The Accuracy of Student Self-evaluations of Dental Sealants, *J. Dent. Hyg., 64,* 339, September, 1990.
Dennison, J.B., Straffon, L.H., and More, F.G.: Evaluating Tooth Eruption on Sealant Efficacy, *J. Am. Dent. Assoc., 121,* 610, November, 1990.
Harris, N.O.: Pit and Fissure Sealants, in Harris, N.O. and Christen, A.G.: *Primary Preventive Dentistry,* 3rd ed. Norwalk, CT, Appleton & Lange, 1991, pp. 235–255.
Hitt, J.C. and Feigal, R.J.: Use of a Bonding Agent to Reduce Sealant Sensitivity to Moisture Contamination: An In Vitro Study, *Pediatr. Dent., 14,* 41, January/February, 1992.
Romberg, E., Cohen, L.A., and LaBelle, A.D.: Knowledge, Attitude, and Outlook Toward Dentistry: Their Affect on Sealant Use and Other Related Variables, *Clin. Prev. Dent., 11,* 3, September–October, 1989.
Selwitz, R.H., Colley, B.J., and Rozier, R.G.: Factors Associated with Parental Acceptance of Dental Sealants, *J. Public Health Dent., 52,* 137, Spring, 1992.

Clinical Procedures
Brockmann, S.L., Scott, R.L., and Eick, J.D.: The Effect of an Air-polishing Device on Tensile Bond Strength of a Dental Sealant, *Quintessence Int., 20,* 211, March, 1989.

Brownbill, J.W. and Setcos, J.C.: Treatment Selections for Fissured Grooves of Permanent Molar Teeth, *ASDC J. Dent. Child., 57,* 274, July–August, 1990.

Chosack, A. and Eidelman, E.: Effect of the Time from Application until Exposure to Light on the Tag Lengths of a Visible Light-polymerized Sealant, *Dent. Materials, 4,* 302, October, 1988.

DeCraene, G.P., Martens, C., and Dermaut, R.: The Invasive Pit-and-Fissure Sealing Technique in Pediatric Dentistry: An SEM Study of a Preventive Restoration, *ASDC J. Dent. Child., 55,* 34, January–February, 1988.

Eidelman, E., Shapira, J., and Houpt, M.: The Retention of Fissure Sealants Using Twenty-second Etching Time: Three-year Follow-up, *ASDC J. Dent. Child., 55,* 119, March–April, 1988.

Ellingson, P. and Nickerson, A.: Successful Sealant Placement. Discussion of One Technique, *J. Practical Hyg., 1,* 9, November/December, 1992.

Feigal, R.J., Hitt, J., and Splieth, C.: Retaining Sealant on Salivary Contaminated Enamel, *J. Am. Dent. Assoc., 124,* 88, March, 1993.

Kramer, P.F., Zelante, F., and Simionato, M.R.L.: The Immediate and Long-term Effects of Invasive and Non-invasive Pit and Fissure Sealing Techniques on the Microflora in Occlusal Fissures of Human Teeth, *Pediatr. Dent., 16,* 108, March/April, 1993.

Lehtinen, R. and Kuusilehto, A.: Absorption of UVA Light by Latex and Vinyl Gloves, *Scand. J. Dent. Res., 98,* 186, April, 1990.

Scott, L. and Greer, D.: The Effect of an Air Polishing Device on Sealant Bond Strength, *J. Prosthet. Dent., 58,* 384, September, 1987.

Tandon, S., Kumari, R., and Udupa, S.: The Effect of Etch-time on the Bond Strength of a Sealant and on the Etch-pattern in Primary and Permanent Enamel: An Evaluation, *ASDC J. Dent. Child., 56,* 186, May–June, 1989.

Wood, A.J., Saravia, M.E., and Farrington, F.H.: Cotton Roll Isolation Versus Vac-ejector Isolation, *ASDC J. Dent. Child., 56,* 438, November–December, 1989.

Wright, G.Z., Friedman, C.S., Plotzke, O., and Feasby, W.H.: A Comparison Between Autopolymerizing and Visible-light-activated Sealants, *Clin. Prev. Dent., 10,* 14, January–February, 1988.

Fluoride Releasing Sealants

Cooley, R.L., McCourt, J.W., Huddleston, A.M., and Casmedes, H.P.: Evaluation of a Fluoride-containing Sealant by SEM, Microleakage, and Fluoride Release, *Pediatr. Dent., 12,* 38, February, 1990.

Jensen, Ø.E., Billings, R.J., and Featherstone, J.D.B.: Clinical Evaluation of Fluroshield Pit and Fissure Sealant, *Clin. Prev. Dent., 12,* 24, October–November, 1990.

Tanaka, M., Ono, H., Kadoma, Y., and Imai, Y.: Incorporation into Human Enamel of Fluoride Slowly Released from a Sealant *In Vivo, J. Dent. Res., 66,* 1591, October, 1987.

Programs-Effectiveness

Brooks, J.D., Pruhs, R.J., Azhdari, S., and Ashrafi, M.H.: A Pilot Study of Three Tinted Unfilled Pit and Fissure Sealants: 23-month Results in Milwaukee, Wisconsin, *Clin. Prev. Dent., 10,* 18, January–February, 1988.

Rock, W.P., Weatherill, S., and Anderson, R.J.: Retention of Three Fissure Sealant Resins. The Effects of Etching Agent and Curing Method. Results over 3 Years, *Br. Dent. J., 168,* 323, April 21, 1990.

Romcke, R.G., Lewis, D.W., Maze, B.D., and Vickerson, R.A.: Retention and Maintenance of Fissure Sealants over 10 Years, *Can. Dent. Assoc. J., 56,* 235, March, 1990.

Sterritt, G.R., Frew, R.A., Rozier, R.G., and Brunelle, J.A.: Evaluation of a School-based Fluoride Mouthrinsing and Clinic-based Sealant Program on a Non-fluoridated Island, *Community Dent. Oral Epidemiol., 18,* 288, December, 1990.

Whyte, R.J., Leake, J.L., and Howley, T.P.: Two-year Follow-up of 11,000 Dental Sealants in First Permanent Molars in the Saskatchewan Health Dental Plan, *J. Public Health Dent., 47,* 177, Fall, 1987.

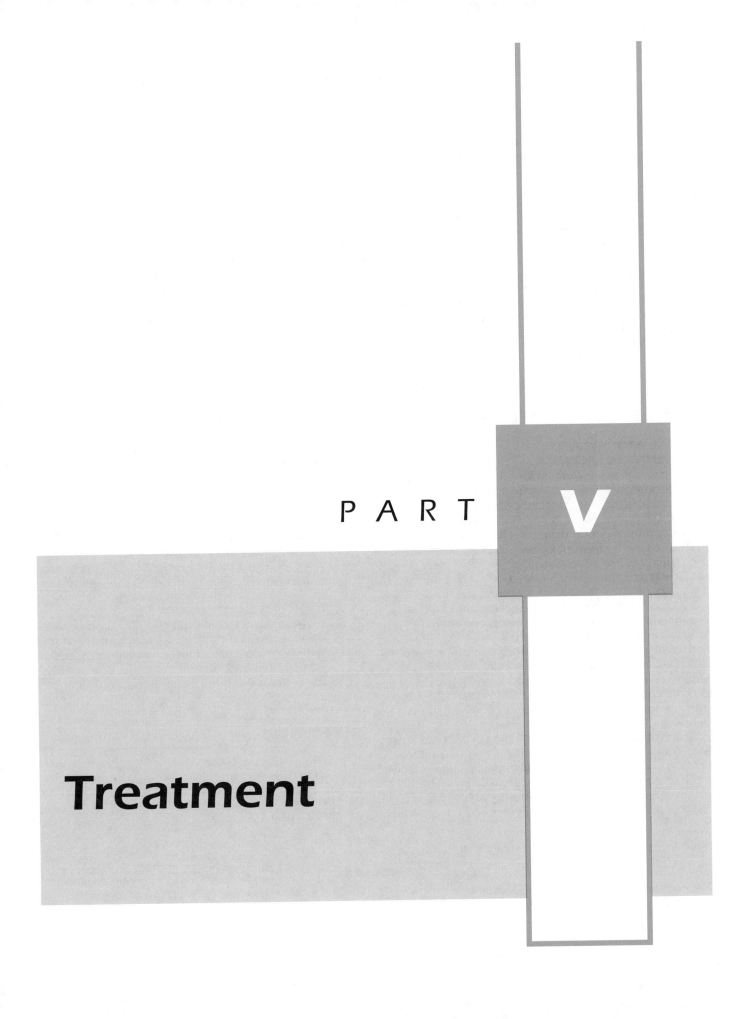

P A R T   **V**

Treatment

INTRODUCTION

Instrumentation for scaling, root planing, extrinsic stain removal, finishing amalgam restorations, debonding, and postoperative care are included in Part V. Postoperative procedures for placement and removal of dressings, removal of sutures, and treatment of hypersensitive teeth are outlined. Immediate evaluation of techniques and their effects, short-term follow-up, and maintenance evaluation are described. These procedures are all part of *nonsurgical periodontal therapy.*

The first objective of treatment is to create an environment in which the tissues can return to health. In the sequence of patient treatment, introduction to preventive measures occurs first, before professional instrumentation. After health has been attained, the patient's self-care on a daily basis is essential to keep the teeth and gingival tissues free from new or recurrent disease caused by the microorganisms of bacterial plaque. Professional instrumentation makes a limited contribution to arresting the progression of disease without daily plaque control measures performed by the patient.

I. ORAL PROPHYLAXIS: DEFINITION DILEMMA

The term *oral prophylaxis* means those specific treatment procedures aimed at removing local irritants to the gingiva, including complete calculus removal with bacterial debridement. A smooth tooth surface resists the retention of dental deposits. The oral prophylaxis performed with these objectives is truly a *preventive periodontal treatment procedure.*[1]

There is a definite need for clarification and new terminology for the various services performed under the title "oral prophylaxis." Through common usage, oral prophylaxis has taken on a variety of meanings.

Because *prophylaxis* means *prevention of disease*, then *oral prophylaxis*, as the *prevention of oral disease*, could include such preventive procedures as restoring individual teeth, replacing missing teeth, adjusting the occlusion, correcting faulty proximal contacts, and many other procedures, the basic purposes of which are preventive.[2]

Unfortunately, the term "oral prophylaxis" also is sometimes used to mean a superficial 5- to 10-minute application of a rubber polishing cup with an abrasive paste to the enamel surfaces that appear above the gingival margin. The term "oral prophylaxis" obviously must be carefully and specifically defined if it is to be applied to the comprehensive treatment services of a dental hygienist.

In the development of a meaningful concept of the oral prophylaxis upon which the procedures and anticipated outcomes described in this book could be based, the acceptable definition could only be based on the preventive aspects of periodontal infections.

II. OBJECTIVES OF TREATMENT

Specific objectives for each type of instrumentation are included in the chapter that describes the details of the technique. General objectives of dental hygiene instrumentation are to

A. Create an environment in which the tissues can return to health and then be maintained in health.
B. Eliminate or suppress periodontal pathogenic microorganisms and control reinfection.
C. Aid in the prevention and control of gingival and periodontal infections by removal of factors that predispose to the retention of bacterial plaque. Factors particularly implicated are dental calculus, irregular and overhanging restorations, and diseased, altered cementum.
D. Comprise the total treatment needed for certain patients with uncomplicated disease, and the initial preparatory phase of treatment for others with more advanced disease.
E. Assist in the maintenance phase of care to prevent recurrence of disease.
F. Provide the patient with smooth tooth surfaces, which are easier to clean and to keep plaque-free by daily self-care procedures.
G. Assist in instructing the patient in the appearance and feeling of a thoroughly clean mouth as a motivation toward the development of adequate habits of personal oral care.
H. Prepare the teeth and gingiva for dental procedures, including those performed by the restorative dentist, prosthodontist, orthodontist, pedodontist, and oral surgeon.
I. Improve oral esthetics and sanitation.

REFERENCES

1. *World Workshop in Periodontics.* Ann Arbor, University of Michigan, 1966, p. 450.
2. Bunting, R.W.: *Oral Hygiene,* 3rd ed. Philadelphia, Lea & Febiger, 1957, p. 233.

Principles for Instrumentation

Instrumentation begins with the identification of the various types of instruments for specific services to be performed and knowledge of the parts of those instruments. The requirements for putting the instruments into action to accomplish a particular task are stabilization by means of a correct grasp and finger rest, adaptation, angulation, lateral pressure, and stroke. Key words related to basic instrumentation are defined in table 31–1.

A study of oral and dental anatomy and histology necessarily accompanies learning instrumentation procedures and skills. Development of a thorough, efficient, and safe procedure depends on an understanding of the characteristics of the dental and periodontal tissues being influenced.

Knowledge of the specific morphology and topography of each tooth and the relationship to the other teeth in the permanent, mixed, and primary dentitions is essential to the understanding and use of the instruments. Recognition of the characteristic signs of health and disease of the periodontal tissues provides the basis for application of instruments for treatment.

A high degree of skill in the care and use of the fine instruments is required. Skill depends on knowledge and understanding of the goals of therapy and of how the goals can be reached through application of the fundamental principles of instrumentation.

INSTRUMENT IDENTIFICATION

I. RECOGNITION OF INSTRUMENTS

The instruments needed for examination and evaluation were described in Chapter 13, page 207, and instruments for scaling and related procedures are de-scribed in Chapter 32, page 488. Other instruments needed for various services may be found in other chapters.

Each instrument must be recognized by sight and distinguished at a glance by the profile of the instrument on the sterile tray. The clinician must be able to designate the names and numbers, and to associate each instrument promptly with the various phases of instrumentation. Such spot identification contributes to neatness of tray arrangement and efficiency of service rendered through prompt selection of the proper instrument for the service to be performed.

A. Classification by Purpose and Use
1. *Examination Instruments.* Probe, explorer.
2. *Treatment Instruments.* Curets, scalers (sickle, hoe, chisel).

B. Description on the Instrument Handle
1. *Design Name.* The school or individual responsible for the design or development.
2. *Design Number.* The traditional number used to identify the specific instrument. The same instrument may be made by various manufacturers using the same number.

II. INSTRUMENT BALANCE
A. Definition
The working end of a balanced instrument is centered in line with the long axis of the handle (figure 31–1).

B. Effect of Shank Length
The distance from the cutting edge (working end) of the blade to the junction of the shank and handle should not be greater than 35 to

TABLE 31–1
KEY WORDS: PRINCIPLES FOR INSTRUMENTATION

Adaptation: relationship between the working end of an instrument and the tooth surface being treated.

Angulation: the angle formed by the working end of an instrument with the surface to which the instrument is applied for treatment.

Blade: working end of an instrument with special design for a particular clinical treatment.

Finger rest: for an intraoral rest, the place on a tooth or teeth where the third or ring finger of the hand holding the instrument is placed to provide stabilization and control during activation of the instrument.

Fulcrum (ful'krum): the support upon which a lever rests while force intended to produce motion is exerted.

Lateral pressure: the minimal pressure that is required of an instrument against the tooth or soft tissue to accomplish the objective of the designated treatment.

Shank: the part of the instrument between the handle and the working end.

Lower or terminal shank: the part of the shank next to the blade.

Stroke: a single unbroken movement made by an instrument against a tooth surface during an examination or treatment procedure to accomplish a particular objective; the motion made for activation of an instrument.

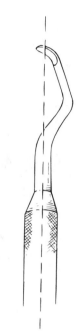

FIG. 31–1. Instrument Balance. The working end of a balanced instrument is centered in line with the long axis of the instrument handle.

40 mm (1½ inches). Too short a distance limits action; too long a distance may result in an unbalanced instrument.

INSTRUMENT PARTS

The three major parts are the *working end,* the *shank,* and the *handle* or shaft. The relationship of these parts is illustrated by the scaler in figure 31–2.

I. WORKING END

The working end refers to that part used to carry out the purpose and function of the instrument. Each working end is unique to the particular instrument.

A. Sharp Instruments

The working end of a sharp instrument is called a *blade.* The parts of a sharp blade are the

1. *Cutting Edge.* A very fine line where two surfaces meet. For example, the face and the lateral surfaces meet to form the sharp cutting edge of a curet (figure 32–1, page 489).
2. *Lateral Surfaces.* The lateral surfaces meet or are continuous (as in the round back of a curet) to form the back of the instrument.

B. Nonsharp Instruments

The working end of a nonsharp instrument is a dull blade, or a *nib.* Although the term nib is most frequently applied to instruments for restorative dentistry, such as a condenser or burnisher, it may also apply to nonsharp ends, such as the wood point at the end of the porte polisher (page 578) and the rubber cup of the prophylaxis angle (pages 568 and 569).

II. SHANK

The shank connects the working end with the handle, as shown in figure 31–2. The shape and rigidity of the

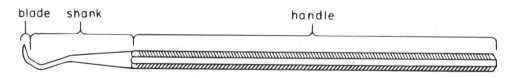

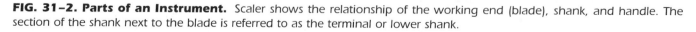

FIG. 31–2. Parts of an Instrument. *Scaler shows the relationship of the working end (blade), shank, and handle. The section of the shank next to the blade is referred to as the terminal or lower shank.*

shank govern the access of the working end to accomplish the intended purpose for which the instrument was designed.

A. Shape

1. *Straight.* For adaptation to tooth surfaces with unrestricted access, such as for anterior teeth. With many instruments, the straight shank is in line with the handle and together they aid in correct positioning for treatment.

2. *Angled.* For adaptation to tooth surfaces with restricted access, such as proximal surfaces of posterior teeth. In general, the more restricted the access, the more angular a shank must be and the sharper the bends of the angles. Examples are the Gracey curets nos. 11/12 and nos. 13/14, each of which has 3 bends. Because the *distal* surfaces of molars and premolars are much less accessible than are the mesial surfaces, the shank angles of the nos. 13/14 are designed with deeper bends to make access possible.

B. Lower or Terminal Shank

The section of the shank adjacent to the blade is called the lower or terminal shank.

1. *Instrument Positioning.* During positioning of a curet for treatment, the terminal shank is utilized to provide the clue to the appropriate blade adaptation and angulation for scaling and root planing.

2. *Elongated Terminal Shank.* Special instruments have been designed with terminal shanks longer than the traditional lengths. The purpose is to give better access to deep pockets.

C. Shank Flexibility

Instruments are made with shanks of varying degrees of thickness and rigidity that relate to the purpose for which they are used.

1. *Rigid, Thick Shank.* A thick shank is stronger and is able to withstand pressure without flexing when applied during instrumentation. Strong instruments are needed for removal of heavy calculus deposits. More rigid instruments may provide less tactile sensitivity.

2. *Less Rigid, More Flexible Shank.* A thinner shank may provide more tactile sensitivity and is used, for example, for removal of fine deposits of calculus and for root planing.

III. HANDLE

The handle is the part of the instrument that is held (grasped) during activation of the working end.

A. Overall Design

1. Single-end instrument has one working end.
2. Double-ended instrument may have paired (mirror image) or complementary working ends. Paired working ends are used for access

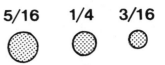

5/16   1/4   3/16

FIG. 31–3. Diameters of Instrument Handles. The most common diameters are ⁵⁄₁₆, ¼, and ³⁄₁₆ inch. For comfort and tactile sensitivity, the widest diameter in a lightweight, hollow handle is recommended.

to proximal surfaces from the facial or lingual aspects.

3. Cone socket handles are separable from the shank and working end. They permit instrument exchanges and replacements.

B. Weight

Hollow handles are lighter and are preferred to solid handles because the lighter weight enhances tactile sensitivity and lessens fatigue.

C. Diameter

In general, 3 diameters of instruments are available. As shown in figure 31–3, the most common diameters available from manufacturers are ⁵⁄₁₆, ¼, and ³⁄₁₆ inch.

The ideal instrument for comfort and best tactile sensitivity has a lightweight, serrated, hollow handle with a ⁵⁄₁₆-inch diameter.

D. Surface Texture: Serrations

Instrument handles may be smooth, ribbed, or knurled. For control and comfort without muscle fatigue, a smooth handle should be avoided.

INSTRUMENT GRASP

Stability is essential for effective, controlled action of an instrument. The correct use depends on maintaining *control* of the movement of the instrument through use of an effective *grasp* and the establishment and maintenance of an appropriate, firm, fulcrum *finger rest.*

I. FUNCTIONS OF THE INSTRUMENT GRASP

A. Dominant Hand

The right hand is the dominant hand for the right-handed clinician. A few rare people are completely ambidextrous, and others are partially dexterous with the nondominant hand, a useful accomplishment when carrying out dental and dental hygiene procedures. Exercises for developing dexterity are provided on pages 482 and 483.

The dominant hand is used to hold and activate the treatment instrument. The manner in which the instrument is held influences the entire procedure.

A rigid grasp, in which the instrument is gripped tightly, lessens the tactile sensitivity and, hence, the effectiveness of instrumentation. The appropriate grasp is firm, displays the confidence of the clinician in the work being done, and provides the following effects:

1. Increased fingertip tactile sensitivity.
2. Positive control of the instrument with balance and flexibility during motion.
3. Decreased hazard of trauma to the dental and periodontal tissues, which in turn results in less postoperative discomfort for the patient.
4. Prevention of fatigue to clinician's fingers, hand, and arm.

B. Nondominant Hand

The right-handed clinician uses the left hand and the left-handed clinician uses the right hand for essential supplementary functions to assist the dominant hand. Figure 31–4 shows the recommended modified pen grasp (described later) for each hand. The mouth mirror is frequently held by the nondominant hand. With the appropriate grasp and finger rest, the following effects can be provided:

1. Control of the position of the mirror for indirect vision, indirect lighting, and retraction.
2. Assistance in providing the dominant hand with an auxiliary finger rest.

II. TYPES

A. Modified Pen Grasp

1. *Description.* The modified pen grasp is a three-finger grasp with the tips of the thumb, index finger, and middle (second) finger all in contact with the instrument. The ring finger is the finger rest. The instrument is held by the thumb and index finger at the junction of the shank and handle. The middle (second) finger is placed on the shank to hold and guide the movement (figure 31–4).

2. *Role of Middle Finger.* The shank of the instrument is held against the pad of the middle finger. The instrument is not held across the nail or the side of the middle finger, as in a pen grasp usually used for writing. The specific position of the middle finger is extremely important to instrument control in preventing the instrument from slipping during adaptation and activation.

B. Palm Grasp

1. *Description.* The handle of the instrument is held in the palm by cupped index, middle, ring, and little fingers. The thumb is free to serve as the fulcrum (figure 31–5).

2. *Limitations of Use.* Instruments for scaling, planing, and gingival curettage are not used with a palm grasp. The possible exception is a chisel scaler when it is used to remove gross calculus by a push stroke (page 492). The palm grasp limits operation in that there is less tactile sensitivity and less flexibility of movement.

3. *Examples of Uses for Palm Grasp*
   a. Air syringe.

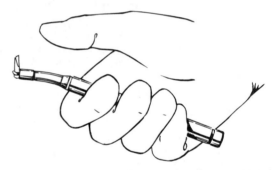

FIG. 31–5. Palm Grasp of Instrument. The instrument handle is held in the palm by cupped index, middle, ring, and little fingers. Thumb is free and serves as the finger rest.

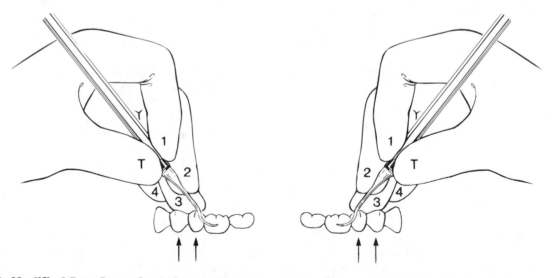

FIG. 31–4. Modified Pen Grasp for Left and Right Hands. An instrument is held by the thumb (T), index finger (1), and the second, or "middle," finger (2), which also provides support. The third, or "ring," finger (3) serves as the finger rest, and the fourth, or "little," finger (4) is positioned beside the ring finger to supplement the finger rest.

b. Rubber dam clamp holder.

c. Handpiece for instrument sharpening (figure 32–17, page 501, for holding the Nievert Whittler).

d. Porte polisher for facial surfaces. A porte polisher is shown in figure 31–5.

WRIST, ARM, ELBOW, SHOULDER: NEUTRAL POSITIONS

Neutral positions for the wrist, forearm, elbow, and shoulder are basic to efficient performance directed at the prevention of occupational pain risks, particularly for those risks related to cumulative trauma disorders. Clinical activities to prevent cumulative trauma disorders, particularly prevention of carpal tunnel syndrome, are considered later in this chapter (pages 483–486).

General clinician and dental chair positioning were described in Chapter 5. Principles of the 90°-90°-90° body position for the clinician were illustrated in figure 5–1 (page 72). Correct seating includes a right angle at each of the hips, knees, and ankles. In this section the neutral positions for the hand, wrist, elbow, and shoulder can be related directly to the grasp and finger rest for instrumentation.[1]

I. WRIST
The wrist is straight and the forearm and the hand are in the same horizontal plane when in the neutral position. Figure 31–6 illustrates the straight wrist and the effect of a bent wrist. Carpal tunnel syndrome, brought on by pressure on the median nerve in the carpal tunnel, is one of the nerve entrapment conditions that results from inappropriate work habits, such as working with a bent wrist (table 31–4, page 486).

II. ELBOW
The neutral elbow is at 90°, the forearm is positioned horizontally, and the hand is straight ahead.

III. SHOULDER
In neutral, both shoulders are level and relaxed to their lowest position. The arms are straight down.

FULCRUM: FINGER REST

A fulcrum must always be used when instruments are applied to the teeth and gingiva.

I. DEFINITION
A. Fulcrum
The support, or point of rest, on which a lever turns in moving a body.

B. Finger Rest
The support, or point of finger rest on the tooth surface, on which the hand turns in moving an instrument.

II. OBJECTIVES
An effective, well-established finger rest is essential to the following:

A. Stability
For controlled action of the instrument.

B. Unit Control
Provides a focal point from which the whole hand can move as a unit.

C. Prevention of Injury
Injury to the patient's oral tissues can result from irregular pressure and uncontrolled movement.

D. Comfort for the Patient
Confidence in clinician's ability, which results from the feeling of securely applied instruments.

E. Control of Length of Stroke
With instrument grasp, the finger rest limits the instrumentation to where it is needed.

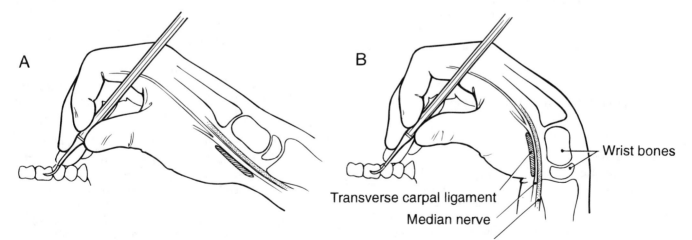

Transverse carpal ligament
Median nerve
Wrist bones

FIG. 31–6. Effect of Wrist Position. A. Wrist in neutral position in straight line with forearm. **B.** Bent wrist shows cramping of median nerve in the carpal tunnel of the wrist. Repeated pressure on the median nerve can cause carpal tunnel syndrome.

III. CONVENTIONAL INTRAORAL RESTS

The intraoral finger rest is essentially a total hand coordinated effort to provide stabilization. Figure 31–4 shows the fingers grouped together with the fulcrum where the ring finger (No. 3 in figure 31–4) maintains its position on a tooth near the tooth being treated.

A. Digits Used for Finger Rest

1. *Modified Pen Grasp*
    a. Ring finger. Little finger is held close beside ring finger (fingers Nos. 3 and 4 in figure 31–4).
    b. Supplementary. Pad of middle finger rests lightly on incisal or occlusal surface of tooth to which instrument is applied; ring finger maintains regular fulcrum position and middle finger maintains its grasp on instrument.
2. *Palm Grasp*. Thumb.

B. Location of Finger Rest

1. *Purposes.* The location of a finger rest is selected for the following reasons:
    a. Convenience to area of operation.
    b. Ease in instrument adaptation.
    c. Maintenance of an effective grasp.
    d. Application of the appropriate angulation.
    e. Stability and control of instrument during the activation (strokes).
    f. Safety of the clinician. A finger rest placed in line of the stroke direction could result in a rubber glove puncture and/or a finger stab if the patient moved suddenly or the instrument slipped for any reason.
2. *Principles*
    a. The first choice for a rest is usually the tooth adjacent to the tooth being treated.
    b. Maintain the rest on firm stable tooth or teeth. The patient's chin, lips, and cheeks are mobile and flexible and therefore less reliable for stability.
    c. Where possible, the rest should be on the same arch, maxillary or mandibular, as the instrumentation; also, where possible, the rest should be in the same quadrant.

IV. VARIATIONS OF FINGER REST

A basic fulcrum location cannot always be used or may require supplementation.

A. Problems

1. A patient's facial musculature, oral anatomic features, such as size of tongue or mouth opening (microstomia), arrangement of the teeth or malocclusions of individual teeth, or physical disability affecting the oral cavity indirectly may interfere with customary positioning for instrumentation.

2. Tenacious calculus in difficult-access areas may not be removed and root surfaces may not be planed by the usual procedures. Greater support and pressure to the instrument are required.
3. When the problem in instrumentation seems to be related to space and accessibility, the height and position of the patient's oral cavity should be checked. Also, a change in the clinician's working position may be necessary.

B. General Categories of Variations[2]

When a variation in finger rest is used, basic rules for stability and control are applied, and rests on movable tissues are avoided. Three types of variations are suggested here: *substitute, supplementary,* and *reinforced* finger rests. Any of these variations may require an external position.

1. *Substitute*
    a. Missing teeth where finger rest is usually applied. For an edentulous area, a cotton roll or gauze sponge may be packed into the area to provide a dry finger rest. Otherwise, a rest across the dental arch or in the opposite arch may be required to provide stability.
    b. Mobile teeth, or teeth with inadequate bony support. Avoid mobile teeth for finger rests or use only with minimal pressure for brief periods. Not only would the rest on a mobile tooth be unstable, but pressure, movement, and undue stress on the tooth could traumatize and tear the periodontal ligament fibers.
    c. Index finger of nondominant hand may be placed in the vestibule over a cotton roll. The usual finger rest can be placed on the index finger to aid retraction and visibility, particularly in the mouth of a small child.
2. *Supplementary.* Place the index finger of the nondominant hand on the occlusal surfaces of teeth adjacent to the working area. The finger rest can then be applied to the index finger. Such supplements are not useful for distal surfaces where the mouth mirror is essential for vision.
3. *Reinforced*
    a. In this type, a support is placed between the instrument handle and the working end to provide additional strength and force, particularly for hard, tenacious calculus in pockets. Greater control of the instrument can result and, when applied correctly, reduce the danger of instrument breakage. A definite rest for both hands is needed to distribute the pressure.

b. Index finger of nondominant hand can be rested on the tooth adjacent to the one being scaled while the thumb is placed on the instrument shank (or handle) for a reinforcement.

V. TOUCH OR PRESSURE APPLIED TO FINGER REST

A. Balance
The fulcrum finger maintains a firm hold with moderate pressure to balance the action of the instrument being applied.

B. Effects of Excess Pressure
1. Decreased stability.
2. Diminished control.
3. Overtightened grasp to accommodate.
4. Fatigue caused by use of mandibular fulcrums. Heavy pressure on the movable mandible can cause fatigue in the temporomandibular joint and related muscles, and thus discomfort for the patient.
5. Fatigue in clinician's fingers and hand.

ADAPTATION

With an appropriate grasp and finger rest, the instrument is next ready for application. The working end of the instrument is adapted to the surface of the tooth or tissue where instrumentation is to take place.

I. RELATION TO TOOTH SURFACE
The side of the tip or toe is maintained in close approximation to the surface being examined or treated. Figure 33–4 (page 512) shows the divisions of a curet blade.

II. CHARACTERISTICS OF A WELL-ADAPTED INSTRUMENT

A. Working End
1. The working end of the instrument is correctly positioned for the task to be accomplished. For example, when scaling, the angle formed by the face of the instrument and the tooth surface is crucial for effective calculus removal. Angulation is described in a following section.
2. The instrument is adapted for maximum usefulness of the working end. For example, 2 to 3 mm of the end of a curet may be adaptable when on a "flat" surface, whereas at a line angle or convex surface of a narrow root, less than 2 mm may be adaptable.
3. The working end is applied to conform to the contour of the tooth surface.
4. As the instrument is activated, it can be adjusted to changes required by variations in the surface topography.

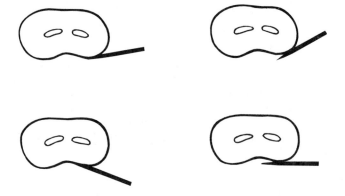

A   B

FIG. 31–7. Instrument Adaptation. Cross section of maxillary first permanent premolar to show adaptation of the tip of an explorer. **A.** Appropriate adaptation in which the tip of the explorer is maintained on the tooth surface in a series of strokes to explore around a line angle. **B.** Incorrect adaptation with the tip of the explorer extended away from the tooth surface.

B. Soft Tissue
A properly adapted instrument harms neither the tissue being treated nor the surrounding or adjacent tissues.

III. PROBLEM AREAS
Areas where instrument adaptation is most difficult and requires more attention, time, and careful application of skill include the following:

A. Line angles
All line angles require that the instrument be rolled between the fingers to turn the working end as the instrument is activated. At each change of direction around a line angle, the instrument must be rolled to keep it adapted to the surface Figure 31–7 shows the adaptation of an explorer tip to a line angle.

B. Convex and Rounded Surfaces
Particularly of narrow roots.

C. Cervical Area
Where the root is constricted.

D. Proximal Root Surfaces
Root surfaces may be concave, have longitudinal grooves, and have open furcations.

ANGULATION

A factor closely related to and directly influencing instrument adaptation is angulation. Angulation refers to the angle formed by a working end of an instrument with the surface to which the instrument is applied.

Each instrument is applied to a surface in a specific manner for optimum adaptation and angulation.

I. PROBE

The usual adaptation of a probe is to maintain the side of the working tip on the tooth, with the long axis of the working end nearly parallel with the tooth surface (page 214).

As used for a bleeding index, the tip is placed inside the pocket wall and pressed lightly on the wall as the probe is moved horizontally around the tooth (figure 19–9, page 302).

II. EXPLORER

An explorer is held with the tip at a right angle to the occlusal surface when detecting occlusal pit or fissure caries. On other surfaces, the side of the tip is kept on the tooth at all times. The angle is 5° or less. Figure 13–15, page 223, illustrates the use of the subgingival explorer.

III. SCALERS AND CURETS

Angulation for a scaler or a curet means the angle formed by the face of the instrument with the surface to which the instrument is applied. Figure 31–8 shows the various angles for curet adaptation. At zero angulation the curet face is flat against the tooth surface (figure 31–8A).

A. Scaling and Root Planing

An angle of less than 90° but of not less than 45° permits effective calculus removal. The preferred angulation is between 60° and 80° (figure 31–8B). Using a markedly closed angulation of less than 45° may result in burnishing the calculus to produce a smooth veneer.

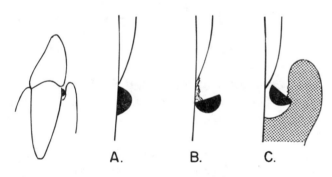

FIG. 31–8. Instrument Angulation. Enlargement of pocket area from the tooth on the left shows cross section of a curet blade in black. **A.** The curet is angulated at 0° with the tooth surface when used in an exploratory or insertion stroke. At 0° the face of the blade is flat against the tooth surface. **B.** Blade angulated at approximately 70° with the tooth surface for scaling and root planing. **C.** Open blade angulated toward the pocket wall in position for gingival curettage. The face of the blade forms an angle of approximately 70° with the soft tissue pocket wall.

B. Gingival Curettage

The face is turned toward the soft tissue wall of the pocket. The angle formed by the face of the curet blade and the soft tissue pocket wall being treated is less than 90° but more than 45° (figure 31–8C).

LATERAL PRESSURE

Lateral pressure means the pressure of the instrument against the tooth surface during activation. It is described as light, moderate, or heavy pressure.

I. DETECTION INSTRUMENTS

Explorers and probes are used with a light pressure to maximize the sense of touch in detecting irregularities.

II. TREATMENT INSTRUMENTS
A. Placement Stroke

A light but secure pressure applied as a curet is passed over the tooth surface to the edge of the calculus deposit or lower border of a rough root surface.

B. Scaling Stroke

A definite controlled moderate to heavy pressure for calculus removal.

C. Root Planing Stroke

A lighter pressure applied progressively as the root surface becomes smooth (page 516).

ACTIVATION: STROKE

A stroke is the action of an instrument in the performance of the task for which it was designed.

Strokes are usually identified by the instrumentation being performed. Examples are the "probing stroke," "scaling stroke," or "root planing stroke." Technique for each type is described in the chapters covering the specific procedures.

I. CHARACTERISTICS OF STROKES
A. Types

1. *Pull.* Example: scaler removing calculus.
2. *Placement.* Example: stroke when a curet is being positioned.
3. *Combined Push and Pull.* Example: explorer in a walking stroke, which is moving the instrument up and down with equal pressure on the surface (figure 13–15, page 223).
4. *Walking Stroke.* Example: probe is moved up and down, touching the coronal border of the periodontal attachment with each down stroke (figure 13–6, page 214).

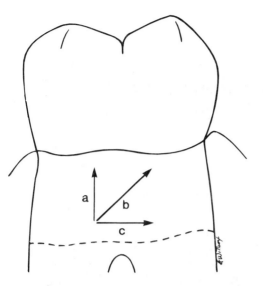

FIG. 31-9. Directions of Instrument Strokes. Arrows on root surface represent vertical stroke **(a),** diagonal or oblique stroke **(b),** and horizontal stroke **(c).**

B. Directions (figure 31-9)

1. *Vertical.* Strokes parallel with the long axis of the tooth being treated.
2. *Horizontal.* Strokes perpendicular to long axis of the tooth being treated. They are sometimes called circumferential, which should not be interpreted to mean that a stroke can be made to go around a tooth or large segment of a tooth. A horizontal stroke necessarily must be a short stroke because of the constant changes in the topography of the tooth surface.
3. *Diagonal or Oblique.* Stroke that is diagonal across the surface being treated.
4. *Circular.* Stroke used with a porte polisher. A small 1- to 2-mm-diameter circular stroke is used with pressure, for example, to apply desensitizing paste (pages 558 and 578).

II. FACTORS THAT INFLUENCE SELECTION OF STROKE

A. Size, contour, and position of gingiva.
B. Surface and section of surface where the instrument is used.
C. Probing depth.
D. Size and shape of instrument used.
E. Procedure objective, for example, nature of the deposit to be removed.

III. NATURE OF STROKE

A. Grasp

The grasp of a scaler or curet is light while the working end is positioned for the stroke, and then the instrument is held more firmly during movement. An explorer and a probe should be held lightly for tactile sensitivity at all times.

B. Hand Stability

During a stroke, the whole hand pivots or rotates on the fulcrum.

C. Motion

The motion for a stroke is generated by a unified action of the shoulder, arm, wrist, and hand.

D. Length

1. The length of the stroke is limited by the extent of calculus deposit and by the anatomic features of the area where the deposit is located.
2. The stroke is short, controlled, decisive, and directed to protect the tissues from trauma.
3. Instrumentation should be applied to the section of the tooth where treatment is indicated. This section is called the *instrumentation zone.* Strokes should not be long enough to pass over the whole crown when the calculus represents only a small area at the cervical third of the tooth.
4. The length of a stroke varies with each instrument and purpose. A description of strokes for each instrument is included in the respective chapters. The probe is described on pages 213 and 214; the explorer, page 222; scalers and curets, pages 512–516; and handpiece, pages 568 and 569.

VISIBILITY AND ACCESSIBILITY

I. EFFECTS OF ADEQUATE VISION AND ACCESSIBILITY

A. Instrumentation is more thorough with minimal trauma to the oral tissues.
B. Length of time required is lessened, thereby lessening fatigue for patient and clinician.
C. Patient cooperation is increased because of shortened treatment time and less discomfort.

II. CONTRIBUTING FACTORS

A. Patient and clinician positions (pages 71–73).
B. Efficient use of direct or reflected (by mouth mirror) illumination for each tooth surface.
C. Adequate, yet gentle, retraction of lips, cheeks, and tongue with consideration for the patient's comfort and clinician's convenience.

DEXTERITY DEVELOPMENT

The dental hygiene student and the dental hygienist returning to practice after a temporary leave of absence can appreciate the need for exercises to develop dexterity and strength for the efficient and effective use of instruments. In addition, all students, returning retirees, and dental hygienists continuing in practice need an understanding of preventive measures that can preserve the health of their hands, arms, shoulders, and all muscles and joints involved when undertaking patient care.

However generally dexterous a person may be, the use of new or unusual instruments requires different procedures for coordination. Control is essential, and guided strength contributes to control.

Proficiency during procedures comes from repeated correct use of the instruments. Exercises for the fingers, hands, and arms supplement experience. Directed exercises are needed for both hands, separately and together. A regular period of time each day during the training period should be set aside for exercises.

I. SQUEEZING THERAPY PUTTY OR A SOFT BALL
A. Purpose
To develop strength and control.

B. Procedure
1. Hold putty in palm of hand; grip with thumb and all fingers (figure 31–10A).
2. Tighten and release grip at regular intervals.
3. One hand rests while other is exercising.
4. Use one ball for each hand.

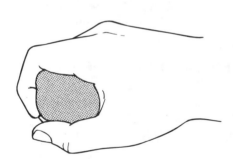

A

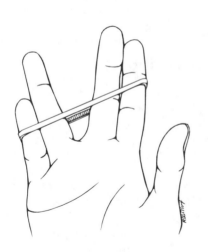

B

FIG. 31–10. Exercises for Dexterity Development.
A. Squeezing therapy putty can aid in developing strength and control. **B.** Stretching a rubber band can be applied at each group of finger and thumb joints.

II. STRETCHING
A. Purposes
1. To strengthen finger and hand muscles.
2. To develop control of finger movements.

B. Rubber Band on Finger Joints
1. Place band at joint between first phalanx and second phalanx.
2. Stretch band by separating middle and ring fingers (figure 31–10B).
3. Place band at joint between second phalanx and third phalanx and proceed as before.
4. Place bands on both hands and do exercises together.

C. Rubber Band on Finger Joints with Use of Fulcrum
1. Place band on joint between first phalanx and second phalanx.
2. Establish fulcrum (ring finger) on tabletop with little finger closely adjacent to it; elbow and forearm are free, as they are during instrumentation. Keep wrist straight, in same horizontal line as the forearm, hold elbow at 90°. Stretch band by separating middle and ring fingers.
3. Touch thumb and index and middle fingers to simulate a modified pen grasp for holding an instrument. Stretch band by separating middle and ring fingers.
4. Variations
   a. Hold instrument in modified pen grasp while doing the exercise.
   b. Do writing exercise with rubber band in place.
5. Rest one hand while other is being exercised.

III. WRITING
A. Purposes
1. To develop correct instrument modified pen grasp.
2. To propel instrument by activation from wrist and arm, without moving fingers.
3. To practice use of instruments when mouth mirror is required.
4. To develop control and precision.

B. Circles and Vertical Lines
1. Hold long, well-sharpened, wooden lead pencil with modified pen grasp.
2. Establish fulcrum (ring finger) on a piece of paper on tabletop. Keep wrist straight in line with forearm; elbow is at 90° and shoulder is in neutral position. Forearm and elbow are free.
3. Inscribe counterclockwise small circles and vertical lines on paper, rapidly and lightly at first, slowly and with more pressure later.

4. Accomplish writing by activation of the hand by the upper arm, without flexing or extending the thumb and fingers holding the pencil.

5. Practice each hand separately at first; then use a pencil in each hand at the same time, alternating writing action to simulate adaptation of the mirror first and then the explorer or scaler.

C. Using Mouth Mirror

1. Hold mouth mirror with modified pen grasp in nondominant hand close to pencil while practicing writing exercises (previous section) through the mirror. Reverse hands.

2. Using engineer's graph paper and modified pen grasp with fulcrum as described earlier, follow the lines of the small squares while looking in mirror held with opposite hand.

D. Everyday Penmanship

1. Use modified pen grasp whenever possible for writing.

2. Practice word writing with the left hand (with the right hand for left-handed person) to increase dexterity for handling instruments.

IV. MOUTH MIRROR, COTTON PLIERS, AND EXPLORER

A. Purposes

1. To develop ability to turn mouth mirror at various angles.

2. To develop dexterity in holding objects with cotton pliers.

3. To establish desired grasp of explorer to assure maximum touch sensitivity.

B. Mouth Mirror

1. Hold mouth mirror with modified pen grasp, ring finger on tabletop as fulcrum finger with little finger closely adjacent to it; elbow and forearm are free. The mirror is most frequently used in the nondominant hand.

2. Practice turning mirror with fingers, adjusting as to the several surfaces of the tooth.

3. Hold a small object in the dominant hand for viewing in mirror held in nondominant hand.

4. Practice crossing the mirror over fulcrum finger as in position for retracting lower lip while viewing lingual surfaces of mandibular anterior teeth in mouth mirror.

C. Cotton Pliers

1. Make small, tight cotton pellets with thumb and index and middle fingers of each hand; then make one in each hand simultaneously.

2. Hold cotton pliers with modified pen grasp and establish fulcrum finger on tabletop; elbow and forearm are free.

3. Practice picking up cotton pellets using mirror vision.

a. Use in wiping motion on tabletop or other object.
b. Move to different area to release pellet.

V. TACTILE SENSITIVITY

A. Explorer

1. Hold explorer with modified pen grasp and establish fulcrum finger on tabletop with upper arm and forearm free.

2. Mount small pieces of fine-grain sandpaper of varying abrasiveness. With eyes closed, compare roughness.

3. Use extracted teeth to feel with explorer tip until a light grasp permits maximum security of grasp and maximum sense of touch. Extracted teeth can be used to provide a contrast between exploring enamel, cementum, calculus, or other rough area of tooth surface (page 200).

B. Probe

1. Repeat exercises described for explorer.
2. Compare with explorer.

PREVENTION OF CUMULATIVE TRAUMA

Of the many types of cumulative trauma, carpal tunnel syndrome is most common and well known. Surveys have shown that as many as 6 to 7% of dental hygienists have been diagnosed with carpal tunnel syndrome, and many more have reported pain and other symptoms related to cumulative trauma.[3,4,5] Table 31–2 defines key words relating to cumulative trauma.

I. ANATOMY OF THE MEDIAN NERVE

The symptoms of carpal tunnel syndrome are caused by compression of the median nerve within the carpal tunnel. Figure 31–11 shows the anatomic parts of the wrist. The tunnel is formed by the concave arch of the carpal wrist bones and roofed over by the transverse carpal ligament.

The median nerve passes through the tunnel and emerges to send branches to the thumb, index, and second fingers, and to the medial aspect of the ring finger as illustrated in figure 31–12. Distribution of the ulnar and radial nerves is also shown. The ulnar and radial nerves do not pass through the carpal tunnel and are not subject to the pressures of compression that occur with the median nerve.

II. SYMPTOMS[5]

A. Pain in hand, wrist, shoulder, neck, lower back.
B. Nocturnal pain in hand(s) and forearm(s); pain in hand(s) while working.
C. Morning stiffness and numbness.
D. Daytime numbness and tingling in areas innervated by median nerve.

**TABLE 31–2
KEY WORDS: CUMULATIVE TRAUMA**

Carpal tunnel syndrome: the most common type of cumulative trauma; combination of symptoms that results from compression of the median nerve in the transverse carpal tunnel; also called compression neuropathy.

Cumulative trauma: refers to disorders of the musculoskeletal, autonomic, and peripheral nervous system caused by repeated stresses to tendons, muscles, or nerves. Repeated stresses include awkward postures, forceful grasps, as well as exposure to mechanical stresses, vibration, and cold temperatures.

Flexion (flek'shun): act of bending, such as the forearm bent at the elbow and raised toward shoulder.

Hypesthesia (hip'es-the'ze-ah): abnormally diminished sensitivity.

Median nerve: mixed nerve with both sensory and motor fibers; passes under the transverse carpal ligament at the wrist and branches to supply the thumb, first two fingers, and the medial aspect of the ring finger.

   Median nerve compression: nerve entrapment and compression within the carpal tunnel resulting from increased pressure from injury or inflammation.

Paresthesia (par'es-the'ze-ah): abnormal sensation, such as burning, prickling, or tingling.

Phelan's test (Fā'lanz): a test for carpal tunnel syndrome in which the hands are placed back to back with wrists flexed at 90° and held for 1 minute; if tingling or numbness occurs, the test is positive.

Tinel's sign (Tī nel'): nerve compression in the carpal tunnel can be diagnosed by tapping over the median nerve on the ventral side of the wrist; if the median nerve is compressed, tingling or electric shooting pain will result.

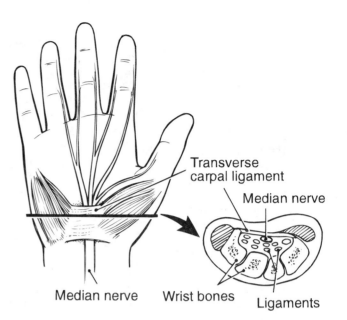

FIG. 31–11. Anatomy of the Wrist. Left, the median nerve passes through the transverse carpal tunnel of the wrist and branches to innervate the thumb, the index and middle fingers, and the medial aspect of the ring finger. **Right,** cross section of wrist shows the median nerve passing through the carpal tunnel. The tunnel is formed by the concave arch of the carpal (wrist) bones and roofed over by the transverse carpal ligament.

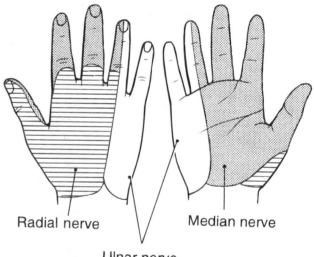

FIG. 31–12. Distribution of the Median Nerve Fibers. Back of hand on left and palm on right show distribution of radial, ulnar, and median nerves.

E. Loss of strength in hand(s); weakened grip.
F. Cold fingers.
G. Increased fatigue.

III. RISK FACTORS

Practicing clinical dental hygienists are at risk for problems of the hand, wrist, elbow, shoulder, and back.[5] Risk factors that are work related are listed in table 31–3.

IV. PREVENTION

As more information is learned about the effects of clinical practice habits on the development of carpal tunnel syndrome, detrimental habits can be prevented and corrected. New students will learn from the start how to prevent and control individual risk factors.

A. Clinical Procedures[5,6,7,8]

Table 31–4 provides a comprehensive list of recommendations for decreasing the incidence of cumulative trauma.

Each dental hygienist needs to analyze the daily clinical routine to identify the potential activities that can contribute to symptoms of cumulative trauma. By taking necessary precautions, later problems may be avoided.

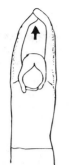

Clasp your fingers over your head and slightly back. Feel a stretch on your arms, shoulders and upper back. Hold for ten seconds.

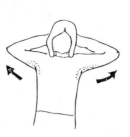

Lower your hands to behind your neck, keeping your elbows directly out to the side. Hold for ten to fifteen seconds. Feel a stretch in your chest and front shoulderss.

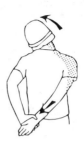

Seperate your legs. Tilt your head to your left shoulder, then look at your right arm down, across and behind your back with your left arm. Hold for ten seconds. Repeat on opposite side.

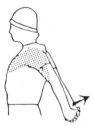

Clasp your hands gently behind your back. Lift your arms backward until you feel a gentle stretch in the arms, shoulders, or chest. Hold for five to fifteen seconds. Keep your chest out and chin in.

Lean your neck to your right shoulder. then rotate the neck slowly to the back, left shoulder and down across the chest. Feel a stretch on all sides of the neck. rotate slowly two to five times.

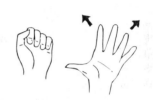

Gently open your hand, then open your fingers wide. Gently close and open them, three to five times periodically and between instrument retrieval.

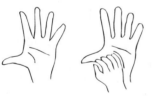

Open your right hand. Grasp the bulk of your thumb with your opposite hand. Gently move your thumb away from the palm of the hand. Feel a stretch on the base of your thumb, hold for ten seconds. Repeat periodically, especially after forceful or prolonged pinching.

Gently rotate your wrist in small circles clockwise. Perform slowly five times periodically and between procedures and patients.

FIG. 31–13. Stretching Exercises. *Several stretching exercises to benefit the back, neck, shoulders, arms, and hands are recommended to counteract the stress and repetitive body and hand positioning and movements of daily clinical practice. Stretching between patient appointments can be especially beneficial. (From Anderson, R.A. and Anderson, J.E.: Stretching. Bolinas, California, Shelter Publications, 1980. Used by permission.)*

B. Exercises

Stretching exercises for stress release, improvement of posture, and counteracting the repetitive movements used during patient care are shown in figure 31–13. Special exercises for the hand muscles can be important. A variety of exercises have been devised using therapy putty, as suggested in figure 31–10A.[7,8]

Stretching exercises performed between patients during working hours can contribute to less fatigue. One exercise to practice is shown in figure 31–14. Each time an instrument is re-

TABLE 31–3 RISK FACTORS FOR CUMULATIVE TRAUMA	
Repetition	Constant wrist and forearm flexion, extension, rotation Constant tight grasping with thumb and fingers
Force	Firm grasp on instrument handle during scaling and root planing Firm grasp on ultrasonic instrument
Awkward Posture	Back and shoulders rounded Arms elevated Elbows bent more than 90° Wrist flexed or deviated while fingers grasp
Static Posture	Maintaining same position for long period
Vibration	Cumulative use of instruments with vibration (ultrasonic and sonic handpieces)
Mechanical Stress	Instruments pressing on nerves or blood vessels in fingers
Cold Temperature	Hand washing with cold water Cold room temperature Cold constricts blood flow

(From Martha Sanders, Occupational and Sports Medicine Center, Meriden, CT. Used by permission.)

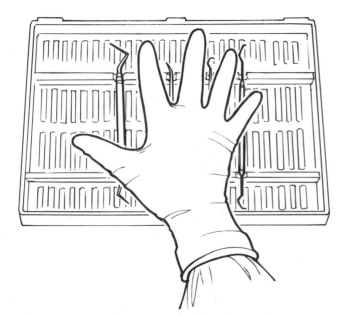

FIG. 31–14. Stretching Fingers Prior to Instrument Retrieval. One of the exercises that can be used during actual clinical practice.

TABLE 31–4 RECOMMENDATIONS TO DECREASE THE INCIDENCE OF CUMULATIVE TRAUMA	
Hand Use	Use proper instrumentation Keep wrist in neutral during forearm rotation Minimize extreme wrist flexion and extension Vary between intraoral and extraoral fulcrums Avoid thumb hypertension Wear proper-fitting gloves; avoid glove constriction at thumb joint
Instruments	Select balanced instruments Use wide-diameter handles Use instruments with handle serrations Keep instruments sharp Dampen vibration components (ultrasonic, sonic, handpieces) Minimize drag on hose; keep hose untangled
Posture	Use alternate work positions Keep neutral positions for shoulders, elbow, wrist Use properly adjusted clinician's stool with lumbar support Use indirect vision (mouth mirror) to avoid awkward, twisted positions Stretch forearm, neck, shoulders, and back periodically
Workplace Practices	Alternate scheduling of heavy- and light-calculus patients Allot adequate time per patient; haste tenses fingers and general posture Eliminate wasted motions; minimize reach distances Utilize selective polishing to minimize use of handpiece Add buffer time to schedule for relaxation and stretching
Body Signals	Pay attention to body signals, such as pain and fatigue

(Adapted from Atwood, M.J. and Michalak, C.: The Occurrence of Cumulative Trauma in Dental Hygienists, *WORK, 2,* 17, Summer, 1992.)

turned to the tray, fingers can be stretched before retrieval of the next instrument.

TECHNICAL HINTS

I. Time spent on exercises should be sufficient in any one period to cause moderate (but never severe) strain and fatigue of hand muscles.

II. To relax the muscles of the hands during a practice session, wash hands in warm water.

REFERENCES

1. **Meador,** H.L.: The Biocentric Technique: A Guide to Avoiding Occupational Pain, *J. Dent. Hyg., 67,* 38, January, 1993.

2. **Pattison,** A.M. and Pattison, G.L.: *Periodontal Instrumentation,* 2nd ed. Norwalk, CT, Appleton & Lange, 1992, pp. 166, 232, 371.

3. **MacDonald,** G., Robertson, M.M., and Erickson, J.A.: Carpal Tunnel Syndrome among California Dental Hygienists, *Dent. Hyg., 62,* 322, July/August, 1988.

4. **Osborn,** J.B., Newell, K.J., Rudney, J.D., and Stoltenberg, J.L.: Carpal Tunnel Syndrome among Minnesota Dental Hygienists, *J. Dent. Hyg., 64,* 79, February, 1990.

5. **Atwood,** M.J. and Michalak, C.: The Occurrence of Cumulative Trauma in Dental Hygienists, *WORK, 2,* 17, Summer, 1992.

6. **Dobias,** M.T.: Carpal Tunnel Syndrome: Can It Be Prevented? *Dentalhygienistnews, 5,* 1, Winter, 1992.

7. **Gerwatowski,** L.J., McFall, D.B., and Stach, D.J.: Carpal Tunnel Syndrome, Risk Factors and Preventive Strategies for the Dental Hygienist, *J. Dent. Hyg., 66,* 89, February, 1992.

8. **McFall,** D.B., Stach, D.J., and Gerwatowski, L.J.: Carpal Tunnel Syndrome: Treatment and Rehabilitation Therapy for the Dental Hygienist, *J. Dent. Hyg., 67,* 126, March–April, 1993.

SUGGESTED READINGS

Byrnes, J.M.: Reaching for Excellence: A Review of the Basics, *RDH, 5,* 10, June, 1985.

Hard, D.: Oral Prophylaxis, in Bunting, R.W.: *Oral Hygiene,* 3rd ed. Philadelphia, Lea & Febiger, 1957, pp. 249–258.

Hirschfeld, L.: Subgingival Curettage in Periodontal Treatment, *J. Am. Dent. Assoc., 44,* 301, March, 1952.

Kunovich, R.S., Rosenblum, R.H., and Beck, F.M.: The Effect of Training on Indirect Vision Skills, *J. Dent. Educ., 51,* 716, December, 1987.

MacDonald, G., Wilson, S.G., and Waldman, K.B.: Physical Characteristics of the Hand and Early Clinical Skill. Their Relationship in a Group of Dental Hygiene Students, *J. Dent. Hyg., 65,* 380, October, 1991.

Neumann, L.M.: A Simple Exercise for Teaching Mirror Vision Skills, *J. Dent. Educ., 52,* 170, March, 1988.

Nield, J.S. and Houseman, G.A.: *Fundamentals of Dental Hygiene Instrumentation,* 2nd ed. Philadelphia, Lea & Febiger, 1988, pp. 165–188.

Rosenblum, R.H., Hedge, T.K., Beck, F.M., and Kunovich, R.S.: Comparison of Three Intraoral Hand Mirror Positions, *J. Dent. Educ., 49,* 827, December, 1985.

Tondrowski, V.E.: Preclinical Procedures for the Dental Hygiene Student, J. Dent. Educ., 20, 321, November, 1956.

Cumulative Trauma Disorders

Bauer, M.E.: Carpal Tunnel Syndrome, An Occupational Risk to the Dental Hygienist, *Dent. Hyg., 59,* 218, May, 1985.

Conrad, J.C., Conrad, K.J., and Osborn, J.B.: Median Nerve Dysfunction Evaluated During Dental Hygiene Education and Practice (1986–1989), *J. Dent. Hyg., 65,* 283, July–August, 1991.

Conrad, J.C., Conrad, K.J., and Osborn, J.B.: A Short-term Epidemiological Study of Median Nerve Dysfunction in Practicing Dental Hygienists, *J. Dent. Hyg., 66,* 76, February, 1992.

Grossman, R.S.: CTS, *RDH, 10,* 12, January, 1990.

Huntley, D.E. and Shannon, S.A.: Carpal Tunnel Syndrome, A Review of the Literature, *Dent. Hyg., 62,* 316, July/August, 1988.

Osborn, J.B., Newell, K.J., Rudney, J.D., and Stoltenberg, J.L.: Musculoskeletal Pain among Minnesota Dental Hygienists, *J. Dent. Hyg., 64,* 132, March–April, 1990.

United States Centers for Disease Control and Prevention: Occupational Disease Surveillance: Carpal Tunnel Syndrome, *MMWR, 38,* 485, July 21, 1989.

Instruments and Sharpening

Knowledge and understanding of the purpose and use of each instrument and the development of dexterity in the effective manipulation of the instruments are basic to clinical dental hygiene practice. The clinical results obtained for the patient depend in part on the proficiency and thoroughness with which the instrumentation is accomplished. *The main purpose of instrumentation is to create an environment about the teeth in which the tissues can heal and be maintained in health.*

Key words related to the characteristics and sharpening of instruments are defined in table 32–1.

I. TYPES OF INSTRUMENTS

Each instrument is designed for a specific type of application during treatment procedures. An instrument first can be categorized by whether it is designed primarily for supragingival treatment procedures (scalers) or for subgingival treatment (curets). Scalers and curets are then subdivided by their blade anatomy into the following types:

A. Curets
1. Universal.
2. Area specific.

B. Scalers
1. Sickle scaler.
   a. Curved sickle scaler.
   b. Straight sickle scaler.
2. Hoe scaler.
3. Chisel scaler.
4. File scaler.

II. INSTRUMENT BLADE ANATOMY

The parts of the blade of a scaler or a curet are the *face* (inner surface), *lateral surfaces, back, tip* (scaler) or *toe*

(curet), and *cutting edges*. The cutting edges are formed by the junction of the face and the lateral surfaces.

Figure 32–1 shows a curet with each part labeled. The parts of a scaler are the same. The differences are the pointed tip and the V-shaped back, shown in figure 32–4. Each type of instrument is described in the next sections.

CURETS

I. CHARACTERISTICS
A. Blade
1. *Cutting Edges.* Two cutting edges on a curved blade (figure 32–1A). The two cutting edges curve around to meet at the toe. In reality, a curet has one continuous cutting edge because the two sides are united without interruption by the rounded toe.
2. *Face.* Flat in cross section (figure 32–1B) and curved lengthwise.
3. *Back or Undersurface.* Rounded.
4. *Cross Section of the Blade.* Shaped like a half circle.
5. *Internal Angles.* Angles of 70 to 80° are formed where the lateral surfaces meet the face. Figure 32–2 shows the cross section of a curet with the internal angles marked.

B. Shank
1. *Anterior Teeth.* Shank, blade, and handle may be in a relatively flat plane for curets primarily adaptable to anterior teeth.
2. *Posterior Teeth.* The shank is contra-angled for access to proximal surfaces.

TABLE 32–1
KEY WORDS: INSTRUMENTS AND SHARPENING

Arkansas stone: fine-grained sharpening stone quarried from natural mineral deposits.

Burnish: to smooth and polish; an effect that can result when a dull scaler or curet is passed over tenacious calculus in an attempt to remove the deposit.

Curet: a curved, rounded dental instrument utilized for scaling, root planing, and gingival curettage.

    Universal curet: a curet designed for use on any tooth surface where the adaptation, angulation, and other principles of instrument use can be correctly and effectively accomplished.

    Area-specific curet: a specialized instrument designed with specific angles in the shank for adaptation to a certain group of tooth surfaces.

Cutting edge: the fine line formed where the face and lateral surfaces of a scaler or curet meet when the instrument is sharp; when the instrument is dull, the line has thickness and may even reflect light.

Hone: a sharpening stone (noun).

    Honing: sharpening (verb).

Offset blade: the blade of an area-specific Gracey curet in which the lower shank is at a 70° angle to the face of the blade; contrasts with a universal curet blade, which is at a 90° angle with the lower shank (figure 32–3).

Rotary stone: a sharpening stone mounted on a metal mandrel for use in a dental handpiece.

Scaler: instrument with two cutting edges that meet at a point designed for supragingival **scaling** (the removal of calculus).

Sharpness: when a scaler or curet is sharp, the cutting edge is a fine line that does not reflect light.

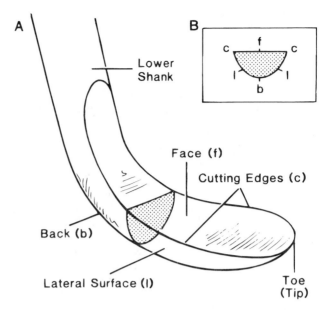

FIG. 32–1. Parts of a Curet. A. Curet with parts labeled. Lower shank is also called the terminal shank. The curet has a round toe, whereas the scaler has a pointed tip. **B.** Cross section of a curet labeled f (face), c (cutting edges), I (lateral surfaces), and b (back).

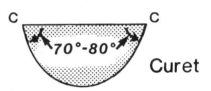

FIG. 32–2. Internal Angles of a Curet. Cross section of a curet shows the 70° to 80° internal angles at the cutting edges.

C. Universal Curet

A universal curet can be adapted for instrumentation on any tooth surface.

1. Designed with paired mirror-image working ends usually placed on a single handle.
2. The face of the blade is perpendicular (at a 90° angle) to the lower shank (figure 32–3A).
3. The cutting edge (continuous around the face), used on both sides, is sharpened on both sides and around the toe. Angulation and adaptation determine the side that is correct for the surface being treated.

D. Area-specific Curet

The Gracey curets are area specific, which means that each curet is designed for adaptation to specific surfaces.

1. Designed with paired mirror-image working ends usually placed on a single handle. The seven pairs are numbers 1–2, 3–4, 5–6, 7–8, 9–10, 11–12, and 13–14.
2. The face of the blade is "off-set" (at an angle of approximately 70°) in relation to the lower shank (figure 32–3B).

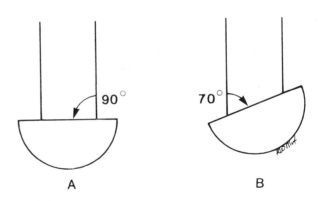

FIG. 32–3. Curet Design. A. A universal curet with the blade at a 90° angle to the lower shank. **B.** Offset blade of an area-specific curet at a 70° angle to the lower shank.

3. The cutting edge is continuous around the face.
4. Only the longer, outer cutting edge is used during instrumentation.
5. Variations of area-specific curets have been introduced to provide clinicians with greater opportunities to complete subgingival instrumentation with improved skills.
   a. Thinner and narrower blades for use with maintenance-level patients when the tissue is in a relatively healthy state and probing depths are minimal.
   b. Shorter-length blades for special adaptation to narrow anterior root surfaces and line angles otherwise difficult to access.
   c. Terminal (lower) shank elongated by a few millimeters to adapt in deeper pockets. The total length of the shank from blade to handle is not changed.

II. PURPOSES AND USES
A. Standard instrument for subgingival scaling and root planing (see also pages 513 and 514).
B. After ultrasonic scaling to complete the root planing.
C. Removal of supragingival calculus, especially the fine supragingival calculus close to the gingival margin. The rounded instrument is best adapted to the cervical area; round back does not traumatize the gingival margin.
D. Curettage of the lining of the gingival wall of the sulcus or pocket.
E. Useful for obtaining a sample of subgingival plaque to place on a glass slide for the phase microscope or for microbiologic tests.

III. APPLICATION
A. Angulation
Blade is applied to the tooth so that the face is at an angle of less than 90° but more than 45° with the tooth surface. The preferred angulation is between 60 and 80°.

B. Adaptation
The lower third of the cutting edge (the part nearest the toe) is maintained on the tooth surface at all times to minimize soft tissue trauma from extension of the toe away from the tooth in the narrow pocket. Changes in tooth surface contour require constant attention to accomplish proper contact. On line angles, only 1 or 2 mm near the toe may be used (figure 33–4 and 33–5, page 512).

C. Curet Selection
Universal curets are used for subgingival scaling for removal of as much of the calculus as possible, followed by area-specific curets for fine scaling and root planing.

D. Design
The design of the curet allows easy entrance into the sulcus, and the curved blade with rounded end permits access to the base of the sulcus or pocket. The slender shank permits entrance to the sulcus with minimal tissue distention.

E. Stroke
Pull stroke only; applied in vertical, horizontal, or oblique directions (figure 31–9, page 481).

SCALERS

I. SICKLE SCALER
By usual definition a sickle is considered curved. The shapes of sickle scalers vary, however, and in some forms the blade and cutting edges are straight. When reference is made to a specific instrument with either a curved or a straight blade, the types usually are called "curved sickle" or "straight sickle."

A. Curved Sickle Scaler
1. Two cutting edges on a curved blade (figure 32–4).
2. Face is flat in cross section and curved lengthwise.
3. The face converges with the two lateral surfaces to form the *tip* of the scaler, which is a sharp point.
4. In cross section, some blades are triangular (figure 32–4B), whereas others are trapezoidal.

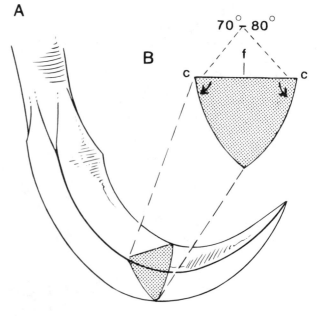

FIG. 32–4. Curved Sickle Scaler. A. The curved blade terminates in a point. **B.** Cross section shows the face (f) and the two cutting edges (c) formed where the lateral surfaces meet the face at 70- to 80-degree angles.

5. Internal angles of 70 to 80° are formed where the lateral surfaces meet the face at the cutting edges. Figure 32–5 shows the cross section of a scaler with the internal angles marked.

B. Straight Sickle Scaler
1. Two cutting edges on a straight blade (figure 32–6).
2. Face (between the cutting edges) is flat.
3. The face converges with the two lateral surfaces to form the tip of the scaler, which is a sharp point.
4. Cross section of the blade is triangular (figure 32–6B).
5. Internal angles of 70 to 80° are formed where the lateral surfaces meet the face at the cutting edges (figure 32–5).

C. Angulation of the Shank
Both curved and straight sickle scalers are available with angulated or straight shanks.

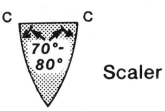

Scaler

FIG. 32–5. Internal Angles of a Scaler. *Cross section of a scaler shows the 70° to 80° internal angles. These angles are restored by sharpening techniques.*

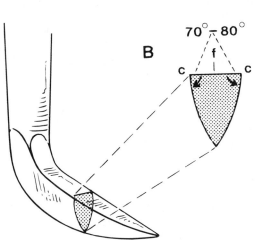

FIG. 32–6. Straight Sickle Scaler. A. *The straight blade converges to a point where the two cutting edges meet at the tip.* **B.** *Cross section of the scaler shows the face (f), the two cutting edges (c), and the 70° to 80° internal angles. This type of sickle scaler is also known as the Jacquette scaler.*

1. *Straight.* Single instrument in which the relationships of the shank, blade, and handle are in a flat plane; adaptable primarily for anterior teeth, although may be used for scaling premolars when the lips and cheeks permit retraction for correct angulation.
2. *Modified or Contra-angle.* Paired instruments that are mirror images of each other to provide access to the proximal surfaces of posterior teeth; one adapts from the facial and the other from the lingual and palatal aspects.

D. Purposes and Uses of Sickle Scalers
1. Principally for the removal of supragingival calculus.
2. May be useful for removal of gross calculus that is slightly below the gingival margin when the calculus is continuous with the supragingival calculus and when the gingival tissue is spongy and flexible to permit easy insertion of the instrument.
3. Contraindications for use of sickle scalers subgingivally:
   a. Cause undue trauma to the gingival tissue because of the large size, thickness, and length of the blade.
   b. Pointed tip and straight cutting edges cannot be adapted to the curved tooth surfaces. Possibility for grooving or scratching the cemental surface is greater.
   c. Tactile sensitivity decreased with larger, heavier blades.
4. Small sickle scalers can be useful for removal of fine supragingival deposits directly under contact areas and between overlapping teeth.

E. Application
1. *Angulation.* The face of the blade is adapted to the tooth surface at an angle of approximately 70°.
2. *Stroke.* Pull stroke only for this type of blade.

II. HOE SCALER
A. Characteristics
1. Single, straight cutting edge (figure 32–7).
2. Blade turned at a 99 to 100° angle to the shank.
3. Cutting edge beveled at a 45° angle to the end of the blade (figure 32–7B).
4. Shank variously angulated for adaptation of cutting edges to accessible tooth surfaces; some are paired.

B. Purposes and Uses of a Hoe Scaler
1. Removes supragingival calculus, particularly large, accessible, tenacious pieces.
2. May be useful to remove gross calculus 2 to 3 mm below the gingival margin provided the tissue is spongy, flexible, and easily displaced.

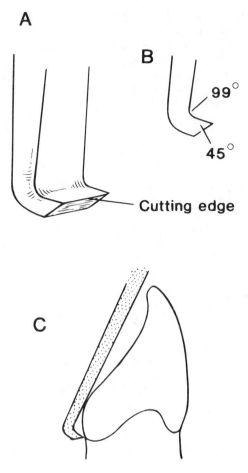

FIG. 32–7. Hoe Scaler. A. *The hoe has a single cutting edge.* **B.** *The blade is turned at an angle of 99° to the shank, and the cutting edge is beveled at a 45° angle.* **C.** *Adaptation to a tooth for removal of calculus is with a two-point contact where possible.*

3. Contraindications for use subgingivally
   a. Insertion of the thick-bladed instrument into the sulcus causes distention of the pocket wall.
   b. Lack of adaptability of the wide straight cutting edge to the curved root surface.
   c. Difficulty of use without gouging the cemental surface. The sharp "corners" should be rounded as shown in figure 32–20, page 503).
   d. Lack of sensitivity because of the bulk of the instrument and the marked angulation of the shanks of some hoes.
   e. Impossibility of reaching the bottom of the pocket without stretching and tearing the gingival pocket wall unnecessarily because of the size and shape of the blade.

C. Application
1. Full width of the cutting edge is in contact with the calculus, and when possible, a two-point contact is maintained with the tooth to

stabilize the instrument during the positioning and activation. Two-point contact means contact of the cutting edge and the side of the shank with the tooth (figure 32–7C).
2. Hoes are not generally applied to proximal surfaces except the surface adjacent to an edentulous area.
3. Pull stroke is used toward occlusal or incisal surfaces.

III. CHISEL SCALER
A. Characteristics
1. Single straight cutting edge (figure 32–8).
2. Blade is continuous with a slightly curved shank.
3. End of blade is flat and beveled at 45° (figure 32–8B).

B. Purposes and Uses of a Chisel Scaler
1. Useful for removal of supragingival calculus from exposed proximal surfaces of anterior teeth where interdental gingiva is missing.
2. Well suited for quick dislodgement of heavy calculus from the proximal areas of mandibular anterior teeth. When the calculus on the lingual surfaces forms a continuous bridge across several teeth, the chisel can be pushed horizontally from the facial aspect to break up the large masses of calculus.
3. Useful for proximal surfaces of premolars when flexibility of the lips and cheeks permits retraction for proper positioning of the cutting edge.

C. Application
1. Full width of cutting edge should be applied, as the sharp corners can nick and groove the tooth surface. The sharp "corners" should be rounded during sharpening (page 503).
2. Stroke is horizontal only, from facial to lingual on proximal surfaces of anterior, particularly mandibular teeth.

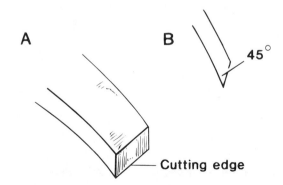

FIG. 32–8. Chisel Scaler. A. *A chisel scaler has a single cutting edge, and the blade is continuous with a slightly curved shank.* **B.** *A 45° bevel is at the cutting edge.*

A

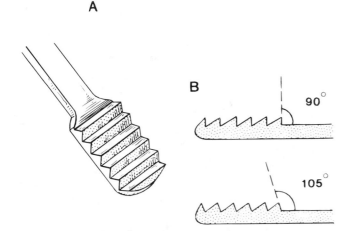

FIG. 32–9. File Scaler. A. A file has multiple cutting edges. **B.** Each blade is at a 90° or a 105° angle with the shank.

IV. FILE SCALER
A. Characteristics
1. Multiple cutting edges lined up as a series of miniature hoes on a round, oval, or rectangular base (figure 32–9A).
2. The multiple blades are at a 90 or 105° angle with the shank (figure 32–9B).
3. Shanks are variously angulated, similar to the hoes; some are paired instruments, others single.
4. Reduced tactile sensitivity because of the size and shape; files are wide, flat, and bulky.

B. Purposes and Uses of a File Scaler
In general, the file can be considered a supplementary instrument rather than a definitive instrument for routine use during scaling and root planing.

Although never used by some dental hygienists, the file is used by others for one or more of the following purposes:
1. Removal of calculus (accomplished by crushing or fragmentation).
2. Smoothing of the tooth at the cementoenamel junction.
3. Root planing, primarily the exposed root surface following periodontal surgery.
4. Smoothing down of overextended or rough amalgam restorations, particularly on proximal surfaces or in the cervical areas.

C. Application
1. The entire working surface is placed flat against the area to be treated.
2. Adaptation to the curved tooth surfaces is difficult. In certain relationships the file has only a tangential contact.

3. Pressure applied permits the cutting edges to grasp the surface.
4. Stroke is pull only.
5. When the file is used to assist in root planing, the file should be followed with a curet, because research has shown that a greater degree of smoothness can be attained with a curet.[1,2]

SPECIFICATIONS FOR INSTRUMENTS FOR SCALING AND ROOT PLANING

I. BASIC QUALITIES
Each instrument is designed for a specific purpose and is intended to be used for the purpose for which it was designed. Characteristics of instruments that influence their usefulness are as follows. An instrument should
A. Be effective and efficient for calculus removal and smoothing tooth surfaces with the least possible trauma to the gingival tissue or the tooth surface.
B. Provide comfort to the clinician without causing fatigue or muscle cramp. Hollow handles have a comfortably wide diameter and are lightweight.
C. Permit maximum use of tactile sensitivity.
D. Have balance (figure 31–1, page 474).
E. Have a blade of a size in keeping with
   1. Anatomy of the tooth; root curvatures.
   2. Location and extent of calculus deposits.
   3. Anatomy of the sulcus or pocket.
F. Be easy to care for when cleaning, sterilizing, sharpening.

II. SHARP CUTTING EDGES
Instruments must be sharp if scaling and root planing are to be completed efficiently with minimal trauma to the tissues. When the instrument blade is maintained with its original contour and sharp cutting edges, the following may be expected:
A. Greater precision of treatment, improved quality of results, and less working time involved.
B. Increased tactile sensitivity during instrumentation. A sharp instrument does not have to be gripped as firmly as a dull one.
C. Greater control of the instrument because of the lighter grasp needed; less pressure on the tooth being scaled or planed and decreased pressure on the finger rest are required.
D. Fewer strokes required.
E. Less possibility of burnishing rather than removing the calculus.
F. Prevention of unnecessary trauma to gingival tissues and, therefore, less discomfort experienced by the patient.
G. Decreased possibility of nicking, grooving, or scratching the tooth surfaces.
H. Less fatigue for the clinician.

INSTRUMENT SHARPENING

Objectives for techniques of sharpening emphasize the *preservation of the original shape* of the instrument while restoring a sharp cutting edge. Instruments designed for a particular purpose should continue to be used in the manner for which they were designed and should not be distorted by inaccurate sharpening techniques.

Sharpening procedures are not easy to learn and require skill and patience to accomplish. More instruments undoubtedly are worn out from sharpening than from use.

This chapter includes sharpening procedures for the curet, sickle, hoe, chisel, and explorer, using various sharpening stones and devices. The principles of sharpening that are outlined and illustrated here may be applied to various types of sharpening stones and instruments.

I. SHARPENING STONES
A. Materials and Their Sources
   1. *Natural Abrasive Stones.* Quarried from mineral deposits, the hard Arkansas stone is used for dental instruments because of its fine abrasive particle size.
   2. *Artificial Materials*
      a. Hard, nonmetallic substances impregnated with aluminum oxide, silicon carbide, or diamond particles; these are larger and coarser than particles of the Arkansas stone. Examples: ruby stone, carborundum stones, and the diamond hone.
      b. Ceramic aluminum oxide.
      c. Steel alloys are metals that are harder than most dental instrument steel and, therefore, are capable of sharpening the instrument. Example: tungsten carbide steel used in the Neivert Whittler.

B. Categories
Sharpening stones as they are manufactured for use may be classified into two general groups: those for manual (unmounted) sharpening and those for power-driven (mandrel mounted) sharpening. Examples of procedures using both unmounted and mounted stones are supplied in this chapter.
   1. *Unmounted*
      a. Stationary flat stones. Rectangular stones with square or rounded edges, or with one side grooved for the special adaptation of curved blades.
      b. Hand stones. Cylindrical (tapered or straight) or rectangular with rounded edges.
      c. Other types. Sharpening devices, such as the Neivert Whittler.
   2. *Mandrel Mounted.* Cylindrical (straight or tapered) small stones of various diameters designed to fit the various sizes of instrument blades.

II. FACILITIES FOR SHARPENING
The work area where instrument sharpening is accomplished should be arranged for convenience and comfort. Because sharpening is an everyday event, the procedure is planned so that available time can be utilized effectively without inconveniences.

A. Place
A definite place should be arranged where materials for sharpening can be kept together and work can be done from a seated position.

B. Lighting
A permanently fixed light that can be concentrated over the work area is needed; light must be shaded to protect the eyes.

C. Working Surface
The working surface should be firm and stationary. A bracket table or cervical tray is undesirable because of lack of stability.

D. Equipment
An adequate assortment of stones and the materials for their maintenance and cleanliness, a magnifying glass, and other incidental materials related to specific procedures should be available.

III. DYNAMICS OF SHARPENING
A. Sharpening Stone Surface
A sharpening stone acts as an abrasive to reshape a dulled blade by grinding the surface until the cutting edge is restored. The surface of the stone is made up of masses of minute crystals, which are the abrasive particles that accomplish the grinding of the instrument. A smaller particle size or a finer grain, as it is generally called, abrades or reduces more slowly and produces a finer cutting edge.

B. Cutting Edge
The cutting edge is a very fine *line* formed where the face and lateral surface meet at an angle. The edge is a line and, therefore, has length but no thickness. The edge becomes dull when pressed against a hard surface (the tooth), or it may be nicked when drawn over a rough surface. A dull edge is rounded and therefore has thickness. The object in sharpening is to reshape the cutting edge to a line.

C. Sharpening
Sharpening is accomplished by grinding the surface or surfaces that form the cutting edge.

IV. TESTS FOR INSTRUMENT SHARPNESS
A. Visual or Glare Test
   1. Examine the cutting edge under adequate light, preferably with a magnifying glass.

2. Because the sharp cutting edge is a fine *line*, it does not reflect light.

3. The dull cutting edge presents a rounded, shiny *surface*, which reflects light.

B. Plastic Testing Stick[3]

1. Use a plastic or acrylic ¼-inch rod, 3 inches long. The hardness and texture approximate a fingernail. A plastic disposable suction tip also may be useful for this purpose.

2. Apply the instrument blade to the plastic stick at the correct angle for scaling; press lightly but firmly.

3. The sharp cutting edge engages or grips the plastic and moves with resistance if an attempt is made to draw the cutting edge over the surface.

4. The dull cutting edge does not catch without undue pressure and slides easily over the surface of the stick.

5. Test each area along an entire cutting edge because the edge is not uniformly dulled during use.

SOME BASIC SHARPENING PRINCIPLES

I. SHARPENING BEFORE STERILIZATION

When sharpening before sterilization, the instruments must first be cleaned and disinfected. An ultrasonic cleaner is recommended for sanitization. As an alternate, the instruments may be scrubbed thoroughly with soap and water, provided heavy-duty household gloves are worn and other procedures are followed as described on pages 54 and 55.

After sharpening, the instruments are prepared for sterilization. When a dry stone is used, or when plain water is used on the stone, instruments and the stone are scrubbed thoroughly before packaging for sterilization.

When oil is used during sharpening, the instruments should be placed again in the ultrasonic cleaner or scrubbed thoroughly with soap and hot water to remove all the oil. Oil on the instruments or stone can protect microorganisms and thereby prevent complete sterilization. Rather than an oil, which is penetrating and difficult to remove, petroleum jelly may be preferred because it is water soluble and therefore readily removed before sterilizing.

II. STERILIZATION OF THE SHARPENING STONE

A sterile sharpening stone should be a part of the basic clinic set-up for a scaling appointment. Instruments then may be sharpened throughout the procedure as they show signs of dullness. Efficiency increases and the patient benefits from receiving a more thorough treatment in less time.

Sterilization of stones may be accomplished by any of the acceptable sterilization methods described in

Chapter 4 (pages 56–59). A limitation of the steam autoclave is that autoclaving may dry out an Arkansas stone and lead to chipping or breakage.

III. INSTRUMENT HANDLING

All instruments must be handled with care to preserve sharpness and prevent accidental damage to the cutting edges.

IV. PREPARATION OF STONE FOR SHARPENING
A. Lubricated Stone

Spread a thin layer of lubricant over the surface of the stone. A clear, fine sterile oil or petroleum jelly may be used. An excess amount of oil or petroleum jelly can obscure the view of the cutting edge being sharpened.

When sharpening is done during an appointment, a sterile swab is used to apply the lubricant to the sterile stone. The lubricant should be kept in a clinically clean covered jar or tube and set aside expressly for that purpose.

The lubricant can provide the following effects:

1. Facilitate the movement of the instrument blade over the stone and prevent scratching of the stone.

2. Suspend the metallic particles removed during sharpening and so help to prevent clogging of the pores of the stone (glazing).

B. Water on Stone

Ceramic stones require water.

C. Dry Stone

Because of the problems related to maintaining a sterile stone and preventing contamination when oil, tap water, or petroleum jelly is applied, the use of a dry stone provides a particular advantage.

A dry stone contributes to the following effects:

1. Sharpens the cutting edge without nicks in the blade; nicks can be created from particles of metal suspended in a lubricant.

2. Allows the stone to be completely sterilized without the problem of interference by the oil left in and on the stone.

V. SHARPENING
A. Objectives

The objectives during sharpening are to produce a sharp cutting edge and to preserve the original shape of the blade.

B. When to Sharpen

Sharpen at the first sign of dullness during an appointment. When instruments become grossly dulled, recontouring wastes the instrument. Restoration of the original contour while maintaining a strong blade is difficult to achieve.

C. Choice of Method

Select the sharpening method and sharpening stone or device consistent with the size and shape of the instrument being treated.

D. Angulation

Before starting to sharpen, analyze the cutting edge and establish the proper angle between the stone and the blade surface. Maintain the angle through the firm grasp, secure finger rest, moderate pressure, short stroke, and other features of the technique appropriate to the individual instrument.

E. Maintain Control

Maintain control so that the entire surface is reduced evenly. Care must be taken not to create a new bevel at the cutting edge.

F. Prevent Grooving

Prevent grooving of the sharpening stone by varying the areas for instrument placement. Cleaning and stain removal procedures are described on pages 503 and 504.

VI. AFTER SHARPENING

Gently hone or burnish the nonbeveled surface adjacent to the cutting edge.

A. Honing

Honing means sharpening, but in common usage, honing has been applied to the process whereby the "bur" or "wire edge" is removed from the side of the cutting edge that was not reduced.

B. How the Wire Edge Is Produced

During sharpening, some of the metal particles removed during grinding remain attached to the edge of the instrument and create the wire edge. If allowed to remain, the tiny particles may be removed when the instrument is applied to the tooth surface during treatment.

By sharpening into, toward, or against the cutting edge, the production of a wire edge is minimized.

C. Removal of Wire Edge

Using an even and light pressure, pass a sharpening stone along the side of the cutting edge. One or two strokes are usually sufficient. If heavy pressure is applied, the bevel of the cutting edge can be altered.

SHARPENING CURETS AND SICKLES

I. SELECTION OF CUTTING EDGE TO SHARPEN

Figure 32–10 shows the cutting edges to sharpen for a universal curet (2 sides), an area-specific curet (1 side), and a scaler (2 sides). These instruments were described on pages 488 to 491.

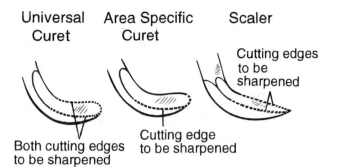

Universal Curet · Area Specific Curet · Scaler

Cutting edges to be sharpened

Both cutting edges to be sharpened

Cutting edge to be sharpened

FIG. 32–10. Selection of Cutting Edge to Sharpen. Both cutting edges and the rounded toe are sharpened for a universal curet (left). An area-specific curet is sharpened on the longer cutting edge and the rounded toe. A scaler is sharpened on the two sides and the tip is brought to a point.

To determine which side of an area-specific instrument to sharpen, hold the instrument upright with the back of the blade directed to the floor, and look into the face of the curet. In general, the cutting edge farthest from the handle (the one closest to the floor, the longest edge) is the correct edge to use for treatment and to sharpen.

II. SELECTION OF SHARPENING PROCEDURE

Sharpening of both the lateral surfaces and the face preserves the original contour of the blade. For both curets and sickles, the internal angle at the cutting edge is 70 to 80° (figures 32–2 and 32–5). To preserve this angle, sharpening stones must be placed and activated carefully.

Manual sharpening procedures are the methods of choice so that the blade is not reduced unnecessarily by a rapid-cutting mounted stone. Procedures in this section show the use of a flat stone for manual sharpening of lateral surfaces. When sharpening lateral surfaces, the flat stone may be used in one of two ways: the stone may be moved while the instrument is stationary, or the stone may be stationary while the instrument is moved.

MOVING FLAT STONE: STATIONARY INSTRUMENT

The side of the cutting edge formed by the lateral surface is reduced by this method. The technique described applies to both curets and sickles. Because the sickle has a pointed tip and the curet has a round toe end, a variation is necessary in the adaptation of the sharpening stone to that portion of the blade.

I. PREPARE THE STONE

Preparation of stones is described on page 495.

II. EXAMINE THE CUTTING EDGE TO BE SHARPENED

Test for sharpness to determine specific areas that are dull.

III. STABILIZE THE INSTRUMENT

A. Grasp the instrument in a palm grasp and hold the hand against the edge of an immovable workbench or table under adequate light (figure 32–11A). The instrument should be low enough to allow the clinician to see clearly the cutting edges and the angle formed by the instrument and the sharpening stone.

B. Turn the face of the instrument up and parallel with the floor. Point the toe toward the clinician to provide better access for moving the stone.

IV. APPLY SHARPENING STONE

A. Apply the stone in a vertical position to the lateral surface at the heel of the cutting edge. Figure 32–11B shows the position for one side of the blade, and figure 32–11C shows the position for the other side.

B. Adjust the angle at which the stone is held to maintain the internal 70 to 80° of the blade. The angle on the outside, between the instrument and the stone, is 100 to 110° (figure 32–12A and B).

V. ACTIVATE THE SHARPENING STONE

A. Keep the stone in contact with the blade and at the proper angle throughout the procedure. The broken line in figure 32–12 represents the flat surface of the sharpening stone.

B. Move the stone up and down with short rhythmic strokes about ½ to ¼ inch high. Put more pressure on the down stroke.

C. Follow the cutting edge from heel to toe, applying several strokes to each millimeter.

D. Do not change the angle of the stone with the face of the instrument. When the angle is varied, an irregularity is ground into the cutting edge.

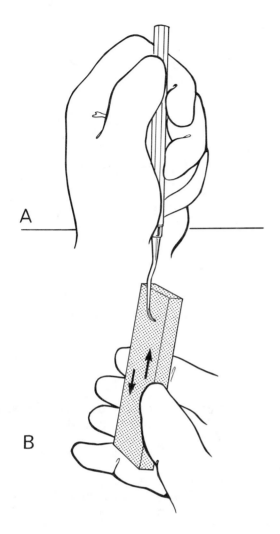

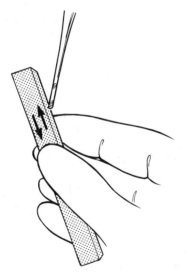

FIG. 32–11. Stationary Instrument—Moving Stone Technique. A. Grasp the instrument with the nondominant hand. Stabilize the hand on the edge of a stationary table or bench and provide good light on the instrument. **B.** The stone is angled with the face of the instrument at 100° to 110° (figure 32–12) to maintain the internal angle of the blade at 70 to 80°. **C.** Stone reversed to sharpen the opposite cutting edge of a universal curet.

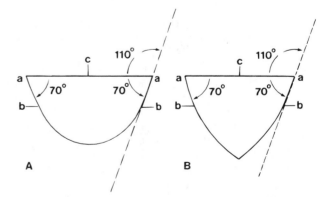

FIG. 32–12. Angulation for Sharpening. Cross sections of a curet **(A)** and a sickle scaler **(B)** show correct angulation of the face of the blade with the flat sharpening stone (broken line) to reproduce the internal angle of the instrument at 70°. Note the cutting edges (a) and the lateral surfaces (b).

E. Keep the wrist straight and use the whole arm to standardize the stroke and the adaptation of the stone to the instrument.

F. Variation at the toe end
1. For a sickle scaler, the stone is held straight as it nears the pointed tip.
2. For the curet, the position of the stone is adapted so that sharpening continues around the round toe. The same angle between the stone and the face is maintained.

G. Finish with a down stroke.

VI. TEST FOR SHARPNESS
Determine whether to repeat the first side before starting the second.

STATIONARY FLAT STONE: MOVING INSTRUMENT

I. CURET
A. Prepare the stone (page 495) and place it flat on a steady workbench or table.
B. Examine the cutting edges to be sharpened. Test for sharpness.
C. Hold the instrument in a modified pen grasp and establish a secure finger rest (figure 32–13A).
D. Apply the cutting edge to the stone. An angle of 110° is formed by the stone and face.
1. Because the curet is curved, only a small section of the cutting edge can be applied at one time.
2. Sharpening is performed in a *series* of applications of the cutting edge to the stone, each overlapping the previous, as the instrument is turned and drawn steadily along the stone.
3. The portion of the cutting edge nearest the shank is applied first (figure 32–13B, a).
E. Apply moderate to light but firm pressure while the instrument is activated.
F. Use a slow steady stroke to maintain control and to assure that each portion of the cutting edge receives equal treatment.
G. Move the blade forward into the cutting edge. Turn the instrument continuously until the center of the round end of the blade is reached (figure 32–13B, b).
H. Test for sharpness along the entire cutting edge; reapply to stone as necessary for ideal sharpness.
I. Turn the instrument to sharpen the second cutting edge. Overlap at the center of the round toe. Universal curets are sharpened on both sides and around the toe. Gracey curets are sharpened on one side only and around the toe (figure 32–10).
J. Use the hand sharpening cone (described in the next section) or the Neivert Whittler (pages 500 and 501) for sharpening the facial aspect.

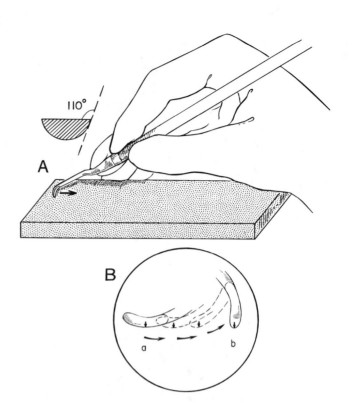

FIG. 32–13. Stationary Stone—Moving Instrument Technique. A. Stone placed flat with blade in position at the beginning of the sharpening stroke. With the finger rest stabilized on the edge of the stone, the cutting edge is maintained at the proper angulation (110°) as the instrument is drawn along the stone with an even moderate pressure. **B.** The movement of the blade is shown by the arrows, which indicate each portion of the cutting edge as the blade is turned on the stone from the beginning (a) to the completion (b) of the stroke at the center of the round toe of the curet. For a universal curet, the instrument is turned over and the opposite cutting edge is sharpened.

II. SICKLE SCALER
A. Prepare the stone (page 495) and place the stone flat on a firm table or bench top under adequate light. Do not tilt the stone while sharpening.
B. Examine cutting edges to be sharpened. Test for sharpness.
C. Hold the instrument with a firm pen grasp, using thumb, index, and middle (second) fingers to prevent the instrument from rotating or changing angles during sharpening (figure 32–14A).
D. Establish finger rest on side of stone using ring and little fingers.
E. Stabilize stone with fingers of opposite hand.
F. Apply cutting edge to be sharpened to the stone. Maintain 70 to 80° internal angle of the instrument (figure 32–12B). The portion of the cutting edge nearest the shank is applied first.

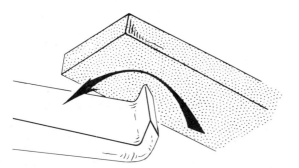

FIG. 32–20. Rounding a Hoe Scaler. To round the sharp corners of the hoe scaler, a flat stone is rubbed over the instrument with a gentle rolling motion.

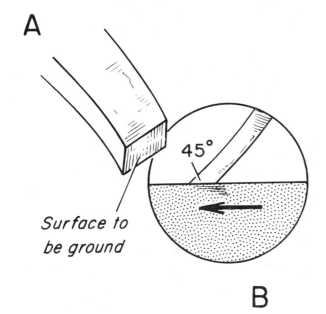

A

45°

Surface to be ground

B

FIG. 32–21. Sharpening a Chisel Scaler. A. Surface to be ground. **B.** Chisel is adapted to the surface of a stationary flat stone at the proper angle to maintain the original bevel of 45°. Arrow indicates direction of the sharpening stroke leading into the cutting edge.

SHARPENING THE CHISEL SCALER

Sharpening procedures for the chisel are similar to those for the hoe. Again, the surface is small, the angulation is difficult to visualize, and the use of a magnifying glass is recommended. Review the characteristics of the chisel scaler on page 492.

I. SURFACE TO BE GROUND
Examine surface to be ground (figure 32–21A). Test for sharpness.

II. SHARPENING PROCEDURE
A. Hold instrument with a modified pen grasp, establish finger rest, and apply the surface to be ground to the stone in the correct relationship to maintain the 45° bevel (figure 32–21B).
B. With moderate, steady pressure, push the instrument forward, toward the cutting edge, without changing the relationship with the stone.
C. After two or three applications, test for sharpness and reapply as necessary for an ideal cutting edge.
D. Hone the nonbeveled surface.

III. ROUND CORNERS
Round the corners at each end of the cutting edge. In a manner similar to that shown in figure 32–20 for the hoe scaler, rub the surface of the flat stone across each corner of the chisel with a gentle, even, rolling motion. Two or three applications are usually sufficient.

SHARPENING EXPLORERS

I. TESTS FOR SHARPNESS
A. Visual
When examined under concentrated light, a dull explorer tip appears rounded. The tip may reflect light.

B. Plastic Testing Stick
A sharp explorer grips the plastic tester on light pressure and moves with resistance when pulled over the surface. A dull explorer does not catch. It slides.

II. RECONTOUR
Small-nosed pliers can be used to straighten a bent tip.

III. SHARPENING PROCEDURE
A. Prepare flat stone.
B. Instrument is held with a modified pen grasp. Finger rest is established on side of stone.
C. Placement and movement of the tip over the stone resemble somewhat the procedure for the curet on the stone (figure 32–13, page 498).
   1. Place side of tip on stone at approximately a 15 to 20° angle of stone with shank of explorer.
   2. As tip is moved over the surface, the handle is rotated so that even pressure can be applied to each part of the tip.

CARE OF SHARPENING STONES

I. FLAT ARKANSAS STONE
A. Prepare for Sterilization
Submerge in ultrasonic cleaner or scrub with soap and hot water to remove oil, petroleum

jelly, and/or metal particles left from sharpening. Wrap and seal for sterilization.

B. Stain Removal

Periodically clean with ammonia, gasoline, or kerosene when stone becomes discolored. If the stone becomes "glazed" by metal particles ground into the surface, rub the stone over emery paper placed on a flat, solid surface.

C. Storage

Keep in sealed, sterilized package until needed for sharpening.

II. MOUNTED STONES
A. Arkansas Mounted Stones

Same basic procedures as those for the flat stone.

B. Ruby Stone

1. Clean by scrubbing with soap and water.
2. Maintain an ungrooved surface by frequently applying the stone to a Joe Dandy disc (figure 32–22). A sandpaper disc is too flexible for this purpose.
3. Sterilize in a sealed bag.

III. MANUFACTURER'S DIRECTIONS

Follow manufacturer's directions for all artificial stones.

TECHNICAL HINTS

I. Prevent unnecessary dulling of instruments by applying the following suggestions:
   A. When handling instruments for cleaning, sterilizing, or other reasons, keep blades from hooking, bumping, or pressing against each other, as cutting edges become dull from contact with hard metal surfaces. Thinner instruments, such as explorers and probes, are subject to bending and breaking.
   B. During instrumentation, utilize instruments at the appropriate angulation to the teeth. Avoid pressing instrument against hard surface of metallic restorations.
   C. Autoclave sterilization does not dull stainless steel instruments.

II. Discard instruments that have been reduced so much by frequent sharpening that even moderate to slight pressure flexes the blade. A tip could break off in a pocket or interproximally during instrumentation.

III. Sharpening of files has not been included in this chapter for several reasons. Because sharpening of files is a difficult procedure owing to the several parallel cutting edges, the amount of time consumed in sharpening with limited promise of effective results may not be justified. When sharpening of a file is required, a jeweler's tang file may be obtained for that purpose. Use of a professional sharpening service or return of the files to the manufacturer for sharpening is highly recommended.

REFERENCES

1. **Barnes,** J.E. and Schaffer, E.M.: Subgingival Root Planing: A Comparison Using Files, Hoes and Curettes, *J. Periodontol., 31,* 300, September, 1960.
2. **Green,** E. and Ramfjord, S.P.: Tooth Roughness after Subgingival Root Planing, *J. Periodontol., 37,* 396, September–October, 1966.
3. **Hu-Friedy Manufacturing Co.,** 3232 N. Rockwell Street, Chicago, IL 60618.

SUGGESTED READINGS

Biller, I.R. and Karlsson, U.L.: SEM of Curet Edges, *Dent. Hyg., 53,* 549, December, 1979.

Burns, S.: Partners in Practice, *RDH, 9,* 23, October, 1989.

Clark, S.M. and Ueno, H.: An Examination of Periodontal Curettes: An SEM Study, *Gen. Dent., 38,* 14, January–February, 1990.

Glenner, R.A.: The Scaler, *Bull. Hist. Dent., 38,* 31, April, 1990.

Long, B.A. and Singer, D.L.: A New Curet Series: The Gracey Curvettes, *RDH, 12,* 46, February, 1992.

McKechnie, L.B.: Instrumentation, Selection and Care, in Genco, R.J., Goldman, H.M., and Cohen, D.W., eds.: *Contemporary Periodontics.* St. Louis, Mosby, 1990, pp. 525–539.

Nield, J.S. and Houseman, G.A.: *Fundamentals of Dental Hygiene Instrumentation,* 2nd ed. Philadelphia, Lea & Febiger, 1988, pp. 229–335, 471–483.

Parker, M.E.: Recontouring Instruments to Prolong Life, *RDH, 3,* 44, July/August, 1983.

Parkes, R.B. and Kolstad, R.A.: Effects of Sterilization on Periodontal Instruments, *J. Periodontol., 53,* 434, July, 1982.

Pattison, A.M. and Pattison, G.L.: *Periodontal Instrumentation,* 2nd ed. Norwalk, CT, Appleton & Lange, 1992, pp. 288–300.

Rappold, A.P., Ripps, A.H., and Ireland, E.J.: Explorer Sharpness

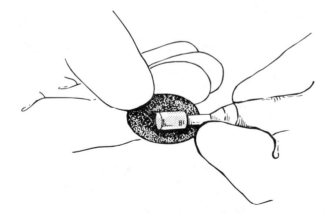

FIG. 32–22. Care of a Mounted Stone. A Joe Dandy disc is used to maintain a smooth surface on the stone. Repeated sharpenings tend to make grooves in a stone.

as Related to Margin Evaluations, *Oper. Dent., 17,* 2, January–February, 1992.

Sasse, J.: Cutting Edges of Curets. Effect of Repeated Sterilization, *Dent. Hyg., 61,* 14, January, 1987.

Tal, H., Kozlovsky, A., Green, E., and Gabbay, M.: Scanning Electron Microscope Evaluation of Wear of Stainless Steel and High Carbon Steel Curettes, *J. Periodontol., 60,* 320, June, 1989.

Sharpening Procedures

Bower, R.C.: An Aid for Sharpening Periodontal Instruments, *Aust. Dent. J., 28,* 212, August, 1983.

DeNucci, D.J. and Mader, C.L.: Scanning Electron Microscopic Evaluation of Several Resharpening Techniques, *J. Periodontol., 54,* 618, October, 1983.

Green, E. and Seyer, P.C.: *Sharpening Curets and Sickle Scalers,* 2nd ed. Berkeley, CA, Praxis Publishing Co., 1972, 40 pp.

Hoffman, L.A., Gross, K.B.W., Cobb, C.M., Pippin, D.J., Tira, D.E., and Overman, P.R.: Assessment of Curette Sharpness, *J. Dent. Hyg., 63,* 382, October, 1989.

Huntley, D.E.: Sharp-edged Tools Are Instrumental to Efficient Scaling and Root Planing, *RDH, 8,* 32, March, 1988.

Huntley, D.E.: A Fine Edge: Instrument Sharpening, Part I, *RDH, 2,* 15, July/August, 1982.

Huntley, D.E.: Honing Your Technique. Instrument Sharpening, Part II, *RDH, 2,* 51, September/October 1982.

Marquam, B.J.: Keep Eye on Sharpening Techniques to Prevent Disease Transmission, *RDH, 12,* 20, August, 1992.

Marquam, B.J.: Strategies to Improve Instrument Sharpening, *Dent. Hyg., 62,* 334, July/August, 1988.

Murray, G.H., Lubow, R.M., Mayhew, R.B., Summitt, J.B., and Usseglio, R.J.: The Effects of Two Sharpening Methods on the Strength of a Periodontal Scaling Instrument, *J. Periodontol., 55,* 410, July, 1984.

Schulze, M.B.: Instrument Sharpening—"The Flat Stone in Motion," *Dentalhygienistnews, 3,* 7, Summer, 1990.

Smith, B.A., Setter, M.S., Caffesse, R.G., and Bye, F.L.: The Effect of Sharpening Stones upon Curet Surface Roughness, *Quintessence Int., 18,* 603, September, 1987.

Wehmeyer, T.E.: Chairside Instrument Sharpening, *Quintessence Int., 18,* 615, September, 1987.

Zimmer, S.E.: Instrument Sharpening—Sickle Scalers and Curettes, *Dent. Hyg., 52,* 21, January, 1978.

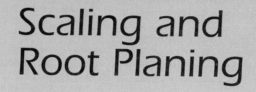

Scaling and Root Planing

Complete subgingival scaling and root planing are specific procedures in the treatment of inflammatory gingival and periodontal diseases. *Scaling* and *root planing* provide definitive or complete treatment for many patients with less advanced periodontal infections, and preparatory or initial therapy for those with more advanced disease.

In addition to the patient's personal daily plaque removal program, scaling and root planing are considered the first line of treatment in nonsurgical periodontal therapy. The ultimate goals are elimination of pathogenic microorganisms and health of the tissue. Terms related to scaling and root planing are defined in table 33–1.

The success of treatment depends on the control of bacterial plaque by the patient. Therefore, instruction and supervision in plaque control procedures precede, continue simultaneously with, and follow treatment instrumentation.

Development of ability, skill, and efficiency in the successful removal of calculus through positive scaling procedures requires more than the development of dexterity for applying instruments to the tooth surfaces. In these refined and exacting techniques, the dental hygienist must apply knowledge of the anatomic, histologic, and physiologic characteristics of the teeth and gingival tissues to the fullest advantage of the patient.

RATIONALE

Complete supragingival and subgingival scaling and root planing, accompanied by the patient's therapeutic bacterial plaque removal on a daily basis, are specific procedures for the treatment of inflammatory periodontal infections. The effects and benefits are listed here.

I. Interrupt or stop the progress of disease.
II. Induce positive changes in the quality and quantity of the subgingival bacterial flora.
   A. Before instrumentation, the predominant microorganisms are anaerobic, gram-negative, motile forms, with many spirochetes and rods, high counts of all types of microorganisms, and many leukocytes.
   B. After instrumentation, the composition of the bacterial flora shifts to a predominance of aerobic, gram-positive, nonmotile, coccoid forms, with lowered total counts and fewer leukocytes.
III. Create an environment that encourages the tissue to heal and the inflammation to be resolved.
   A. Convert pocket (disease) to sulcus (health).
   B. Shrink previously enlarged spongy tissue.
   C. Reduce probing depths.
   D. Eliminate bleeding on probing.
   E. Regenerate the gingival tissues to normal color, size, and contour (table 11–2, page 188).
   F. Change the quality of the tissues from spongy to firm.
   G. Improve the integrity of attachment.
IV. Increase the effectiveness of the patient's plaque control measures.
V. Provide initial preparation (tissue conditioning) for complicated periodontal therapy required for advanced disease.
   A. Reduce or eliminate etiologic and predisposing factors.
   B. Permit re-evaluation. Surgical procedures may be lessened in extent.

TABLE 33-1
KEY WORDS: SCALING AND ROOT PLANING

Analgesia (ăn′al-jē′zē-ah): insensibility to pain without loss of consciousness; usually induced by a drug, although trauma, a disease process, or a low temperature may produce a general or regional analgesia.

Anesthesia (ăn′ĕs-thē′zē-ah): loss of feeling or sensation, especially loss of tactile sensibility, with or without loss of consciousness.

  Block anesthesia: induced by injecting the anesthetic close to a nerve trunk; may be at some distance from the area to be treated.

  Infiltration: induced by injecting the anesthetic directly into or around the tissues to be anesthetized.

  Local anesthesia: loss of sensation in a circumscribed area without loss of consciousness; also called regional anesthesia.

  Topical anesthesia: a form of local anesthesia whereby free nerve endings in accessible structures are rendered incapable of stimulation by the application of an anesthetic drug directly to the surface of the area.

Bacteremia (bak′ter-ē′mē-ah): presence of bacteria in the blood.

Debridement (da-brēd′ment): a form of nonsurgical periodontal therapy accomplished by the mechanical removal of tooth surface irritants using manual and/or ultrasonic methods.

Endotoxin (en′dō-tok′sin): lipopolysaccharide (LPS) complex found in the cell wall of many gram-negative microorganisms; contained superficially within periodontally involved cementum.

Epinephrine (ĕp′ĭ-nĕf′rin): a hormone secreted by the adrenal medulla that, among many functions, causes vasodilation of blood vessels of skeletal muscles, vasoconstriction of arterioles of skin and mucous membranes, and stimulation of heart action; used in local anesthetics for its vasoconstrictive action.

Furcation (fur-kā′shun): anatomic area of a multirooted tooth where the roots diverge.

  Furcation invasion: pathologic resorption of bone within a furcation.

Instrumentation zone: area on tooth where instrumentation is confined; area where calculus and altered cementum are located and treatment is required.

Nonsurgical periodontal therapy: bacterial plaque removal and control, supra- and subgingival scaling, root planing, and adjunctive treatments, such as the use of chemotherapy, with the basic objectives to restore periodontal health, arrest or slow the progression of early periodontal disease, or, for more advanced disease, to prepare the tissues for more complex periodontal therapy

Root planing: a definitive treatment procedure designed to remove altered cementum or surface dentin that is rough, impregnated with calculus, or contaminated with toxins or microorganisms.

Scaling: instrumentation of the crown or root surfaces to remove bacterial plaque, calculus, and stains.

Sonic scaler: type of mechanical scaler that functions from energy delivered by a vibrating working tip in the frequency of 2500 to 7000 cycles per second; driven by compressed air, the handpiece connects directly to a conventional rotary handpiece tubing.

Ultrasonic scaler: mechanical scaling instrument that operates at a frequency range between 34,000 to 42,000 cycles per second to convert a high-frequency electrical current into mechanical vibrations via magnetostrictive or piezoelectric transducers.

VI. Prevent recurrence of disease through maintenance supervision and treatment.

PREPARATION FOR INSTRUMENTATION

I. REVIEW THE PATIENT'S RECORD
A. Study the data from the complete assessment.
B. Note special needs and plan accordingly.

II. CHECK PREMEDICATION REQUIREMENTS FOR RISK PATIENT
A. Bacteremia Following Instrumentation
Bacteremia means the presence of bacteria in the blood. A transient bacteremia can occur during and immediately after any type of oral surgery, periodontal therapy, scaling and root planing, or any treatment that may produce bleeding.[1,2,3]

B. Factors Affecting the Incidence of Bacteremia
1. Degree of trauma inflicted during instrumentation.[4]
2. Severity of gingival or periodontal infection present.[5,6] In one study, patients with clinically healthy gingiva had a 21.6% incidence of bacteremia, those with gingivitis a 29.0% incidence, and those with periodontitis a 51.2% incidence following scaling and root planing.[6]

C. Premedication
1. Certain risk patients who require antibiotic premedication are listed on pages 102 and 103.
2. Ask to make sure that the patient has taken the prescribed medication 1 hour before the scheduled appointment.

III. USE OF RADIOGRAPHS

The radiographic survey can be a useful adjunct during scaling appointments. Radiographic findings were outlined on pages 225–227.

A. Place the radiographs on a lighted viewbox before gloving.

B. Review findings applicable during instrumentation, such as
1. Anatomic features of roots, furcations, and bone level.
2. Overhanging restorations that must be removed (page 583).
3. Carious lesions that may "catch."

IV. PATIENT PREPARATION

Patient factors for the appointment were described on page 65. As the instrumentation for scaling and root planing is carried out, universal precautions must be followed.

A. Instruct patient to rinse with a germicidal mouthrinse to reduce the numbers of oral microorganisms and, hence, the contamination potential of aerosols.

B. Provide protective eyewear for the patient.

V. SUPRAGINGIVAL EXAMINATION

A. Visual

Gross and moderate deposits and surface irregularities can be seen directly. Fine, unstained, white or yellowish calculus is frequently invisible when wet with saliva. Dry calculus is seen more readily than is wet calculus. Procedures for calculus detection were described on page 275.

B. Tactile Method

Without deposits the enamel surface is smooth; an explorer passed over the surface slides freely, smoothly, and quietly. Calculus deposits are rough; the explorer does not slide freely, but meets with resistance and produces a scratchy sound.

VI. SUBGINGIVAL EXAMINATION

A. Determine the Need for Instrumentation

Prior to actual scaling and root planing, a probe and subgingival explorer must be used to locate calculus and areas of root roughness, thereby defining the extent of instrumentation that is required.

Scaling and root planing in shallow pockets (sulci) of fewer than 3 mm can lead to loss of periodontal attachment.[7,8,9] Research has shown that repeated use of a curet when no calculus is present can result in detachment of periodontal ligament fibers from the root cementum and that healing does not bring them back.[9]

B. Make a Direct Visual Examination

1. *Gingiva.* The following clinical appearance of the gingival tissues reveals or is highly suggestive of the presence of subgingival calculus.
   a. Gingival tissue that is soft, spongy, nonresilient, bluish-red, with enlargement of the marginal gingiva, a rolled edge that tends to be separated from the tooth surface, and a smooth shiny surface on which stippling is indistinct or missing.
   b. Dark-colored subgingival calculus that may sometimes be seen as a dark area beneath relatively translucent marginal gingiva.
2. *Subgingival Calculus.* A loose and resilient pocket wall can be separated from the tooth surface. Apply compressed air gently to the gingival margin, deflect the tissue, and look into the pocket. Dark subgingival calculus can be seen.

C. Note the Position and Anatomy of Teeth

1. Close, narrow contact areas where the insertion of a curet to the bottom of a pocket may be difficult or impossible.
2. Furcation variations. Figure 33–1 shows different anatomic features that may impede access for scaling and root planing.
3. Other contributing factors are listed in Chapter 12, pages 201–204.

D. Apply Probe and Explorer Findings

1. Use probing depth recordings from periodontal charting as a basic guide for scaling.
2. Perform additional probing during the immediate appointment.
   a. Anesthesia facilitates exact examination. When a patient is to receive anesthesia, the clinician can probe while the anesthetic is in effect.

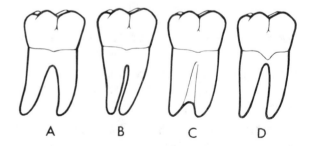

FIG. 33–1. Anatomic Variations of Furcations. A. Widely separated. **B.** Separated but close together. **C.** Fused roots separated only in the apical portion. **D.** Presence of an enamel projection that may be conducive to an early furcation involvement. (From Carranza, F.A.: *Glickman's Clinical Periodontology*, 7th ed. W.B. Saunders Co., 1990, page 862.)

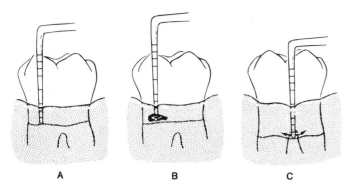

**FIG. 33-2. Subgingival Examination Using a Probe.
A.** Probe inserted to the bottom of a pocket for complete examination prior to subgingival scaling and root planing.
B. As the probe passes over the root surface, it may be intercepted by a hard mass of calculus. **C.** Using a horizontal probe stroke to examine the topography of a furcation area. Keep the side of the tip of the probe on the tooth surface and slide over one root, into the furcation, and across to the other root.

    b. Tissue may change between appointments. Patient's plaque control procedures often condition the tissue; bleeding is lessened, tissue may have tightened, and pockets may be more shallow.

    c. Figure 33–2 illustrates probing of irregularities of a tooth surface. A probe passing over the surface of the root may be intercepted by calculus (figure 33–2B).

    d. Tooth topography is evaluated. For example, the groove and furcation of a mandibular molar may be examined by using a horizontal stroke, as shown in figure 33–2C. A furcation probe should be used for examining Class II and III furcations (figure 13–8, page 216).

  3. Use explorer before, during, and at the completion of scaling and root planing to evaluate a tooth surface.

PROCEDURE FOR SCALING

I. CLINICAL APPROACH

Criteria for the determination of treatment sequence were described on page 323 in connection with treatment planning. Application of the concept of *tissue conditioning* by the patient in preparation for scaling and root planing contributes to more efficient treatment and more predictable and rapid postoperative healing. Tissue conditioning is described on page 325.

    Prerequisite to any selected procedure is the use of an efficient routine to minimize time. With respect to the use of individual instruments, one time-saver is the application of one instrument to all appropriate tooth surfaces within a quadrant or area being treated. Similar use of the next instrument follows. This procedure minimizes transfer to and from the tray. Each instrument may need supplemental sharpening during the treatment of the area.

    The advantages of a systematic procedure are

A. Thoroughness in the completion of treatment.
B. Ease and smoothness of procedure.
C. Increased efficiency through repeated routine.
D. Decrease in time required to complete the treatment.
E. Increase in patient comfort.
F. Increase in patient's confidence in the clinician.

II. OVERALL SYSTEM
A. Single Appointment

When a single appointment is expected to be sufficient to complete the scaling of the entire dentition and anesthesia is not indicated, a choice of sequences may be available. For example, one alternative is to remove supragingival deposits throughout the dentition first by manual or ultrasonic techniques. The finer scaling for each area can then be completed.

B. Planned Multiple Appointments

When extensive scaling and root planing must be accomplished because of generalized supra- and subgingival calculus, a series of appointments can be planned, as suggested on pages 325 and 326.

  1. *Quadrant Scaling and Root Planing Appointments*
    a. Appointments are scheduled at 1-week intervals to permit progressive healing.
    b. Use of local anesthesia for each quadrant may be indicated.*
    c. Bacterial plaque control procedures can be reviewed and supplemented before scaling at each appointment.

  2. *Complete a Selected Area*
    a. Scale one quadrant (or selected group of teeth) thoroughly before moving to the next. Do not move from area to area.
    b. When anesthesia is used, concentrate only on the anesthetized area.

C. Incomplete Scaling

One system that has been used by some clinicians involves an initial "gross scaling" or "prescaling." A series of appointments then is planned for deep scaling and root planing by quadrants or sextants. Before using this system, the following should be considered:

  1. *Potential for Abscess Formation.* Incomplete, superficial scaling of deep pockets can lead to

---

* Local anesthesia must be provided by the dentist in states where state practice acts have not been changed to allow the dental hygienist to administer the anesthesia.

abscess formation, especially when the pockets are deep and suppurating and/or extend into furcation areas or intrabony defects.

   a. With partial healing, the tissue at the gingival margin tightens, the pocket closes, bacteria multiply within, white blood cells are attracted until pus forms, and an abscess develops (page 542).

   b. Susceptibility to abscess formation is greater in persons susceptible to infection, such as those with uncontrolled diabetes or with an immunodeficiency disease, or those being medicated with an immunosuppressive drug.

2. *Healing at the Gingival Margin.* With tightening of the opening of the pocket at the gingival margin, insertion of curets for additional deep instrumentation can be difficult in chronically healed tissue.

3. *Tissue Conditioning.* At the initial appointment, the patient is instructed in the care of the mouth and the need for daily plaque removal. By teaching the patient about diseased tissue and letting the patient condition the tissues, many lessons are learned.

4. *Patient Instruction.* When supragingival calculus is removed all at once, the visual lesson is taken away. With complete treatment area by area, the patient can see and feel changes and improvements that contrast with non-treated areas.

5. *Roughened Calculus.* Calculus roughened by partial removal may be a source of great irritation to the gingiva because of its increased ability to hold a covering of bacterial plaque.

6. *Patient Misunderstanding.* For the patient with limited understanding of the seriousness and extent of periodontal infection, the mouth may "feel clean and look good" at the end of the gross scaling. Thus, the patient may not return for subsequent appointments because the personal objective has been fulfilled. When severe periodontitis, with continued loss of attachment, alveolar bone loss, and the signs of mobility, later develops, the patient may claim that incomplete treatment was given at earlier appointments. By receiving repeated information at each successive treatment, the patient may be able to understand and appreciate the necessity for multiple appointments.

III. CALCULUS REMOVAL

Calculus is removed by systematic scaling from tooth to tooth and section by section of the calculus deposit on each tooth surface. Each scaling stroke overlaps the previous stroke as the scaler is positioned progressively along the area of the deposit.

A. Location of Instrumentation

Figure 33–3 illustrates the location of instrumentation on the tooth surface. The type of pocket, location of calculus, position of the margin of the free gingiva, and level of periodontal tissue attachment all dictate the location of instrumentation and instrument selection for that instrumentation.

B. Effect of Mode of Calculus Attachment

Removal of calculus relates to the mode of attachment (page 276). Calculus removal from

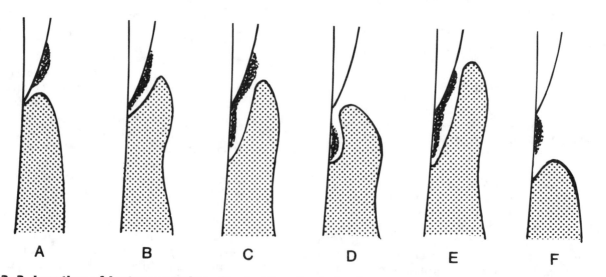

FIG. 33–3. Location of Instrumentation. The location of calculus deposits, level of periodontal attachment, depth of pocket, and position of the gingival margin determine the site of instrumentation. **A.** Supragingival calculus on the enamel. **B.** Gingival pocket with both supra- and subgingival calculus on enamel. **C.** Periodontal pocket with both supra- and subgingival calculus. **D.** Periodontal pocket with subgingival calculus only on cementum. **E.** Periodontal pocket with subgingival calculus only on both enamel and cementum. **F.** Calculus on cementum exposed by gingival recession.

TABLE 33-2
STEPS FOR SCALING AND ROOT PLANING

1. Explore to determine location of deposit and need for instrumentation.
2. Select correct instrument for area being treated.
3. Apply modified pen grasp.
4. Identify correct working end of instrument.
*5. Establish stable finger rest.
*6. Adapt blade to the surface to be treated.
7. Locate apical edge of calculus or tooth roughness (exploratory stroke).
8. Adjust working angulation (average at 70°).
9. Activate for the working stroke.
   a. Apply firm lateral pressure for scaling.
   b. Apply light lateral pressure for root planing.
   c. Control length and direction of stroke.
   d. Maintain continuous adaptation to the completion of the stroke.
10. Continue with channel scaling, overlapping strokes; repeat each step.
   a. Apply exploratory stroke to reposition blade for next stroke.
   b. Activate instrument circumferentially around line angles to treat the entire surfaces that require instrumentation.
11. Apply explorer to determine end point of treatment.

* For deep pockets associated with posterior teeth, steps 5 and 6 may be reversed to determine whether access can be attained best from an intraoral or extraoral rest.

enamel is different from the calculus removal and root planing required for cementum.

C. Steps

Scaling is not a shaving process in which layers are removed. Such a procedure tends to make the surface of the calculus smooth and burnished and sometimes indistinguishable from the tooth surface. The oldest calculus, that next to the tooth surface, is the hardest calculus.

The basic principles for the fundamental steps in the application of an instrument for calculus removal and root planing were described in Chapter 31, pages 475–481. In the sections following, the steps are described in detail for supragingival instrumentation and then are followed by additional adaptations required for subgingival instrumentation. Table 33–2 summarizes the steps for instrumentation.

SUPRAGINGIVAL SCALING

I. INSTRUMENTS
A. Scalers: Sickle, Hoe, Chisel

These instruments are designed for supragingival instrumentation. Sickles are sometimes used to remove gross calculus that may be 1 or 2 mm below the gingival margin, provided the tissue of the gingival pocket wall is loose and the instrument can be inserted without force.

B. Curet

A curet is for both supra- and subgingival instrumentation. It is recommended especially for supragingival scaling and planing in the following instances:

1. When a curved, rounded instrument is particularly adaptable for removing fine, hard deposits near the gingival margin.
2. When gingival recession has caused exposure of cementum, and root planing techniques are required.

II. STEPS FOR CALCULUS REMOVAL
A. Grasp the Instrument

1. Apply modified pen grasp (figure 31–4, page 476).
2. Use a light grasp while instrument is positioned and at the completion of the stroke; tighten grasp during the working stroke.

B. Establish the Finger Rest

1. Use ring and little fingers on firm tooth or teeth for the major rest; apply supplementary rests for increased stability when indicated (pages 477 and 478).
2. The fulcrum where the finger rest is applied must be dry for stability. Plaque and saliva make tooth surfaces slippery. Use a folded gauze sponge in the vestibular area with a corner over the fulcrum rest tooth; dry with compressed air or wipe with cotton, maintain retraction, and repeat the drying as needed for continued instrument control.
3. Finger rests are applied on the tooth adjacent to that being scaled, or as close as possible and convenient. Long stretches between the rest and the point of instrument application can decrease control.
4. Use light but firm pressure on the finger rest while the instrument is being positioned and at the end of the stroke.
5. During the working stroke, the pressure on the fulcrum increases slightly to balance the pressure of the instrument on the tooth being scaled.

C. Adaptation

The toe third of the curet blade is used primarily (figure 33–4). After the toe is adapted, as much of the blade as can be applied to the surface being scaled is used. Adaptation of the curet toe is shown in figure 33–5.

D. Angulation

1. *Sickle Scaler.* Blade is applied beneath the calculus deposit so that the angle formed by the face and the tooth surface is between 60 and 80° (less than 90° but at least 45°).

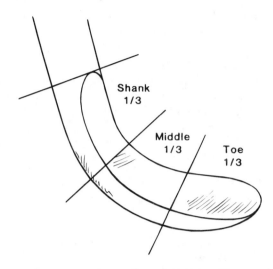

FIG. 33–4. Curet Divided Into Thirds. The toe third is kept in contact with the tooth surface during instrumentation. Because of tooth contours, most strokes for scaling and root planing are accomplished using the toe third. Adaptation of the toe third is shown in figure 33–5.

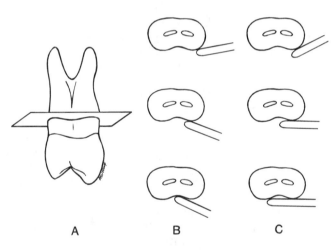

FIG. 33–5. Instrument Adaptation. A. Maxillary first premolar shows cross section of root drawn for **B.** and **C. B.** Diagram of three positions of a curet shows correct adaptation at a line angle and on the concave mesial surface with 2 mm. of the instrument maintained on the tooth as the instrument is adapted. **C.** Diagram shows incorrect adaptation with toe of curet extended away from the tooth surface.

    2. *Hoe Scaler.* The full width of the cutting edge is in contact with the calculus. The shank is adapted closely to the side of the tooth or is in contact with the crown of the tooth (figure 32–7, page 492).

    3. *Chisel Scaler.* The full width of the cutting edge is in contact with the calculus. The shank is adapted closely to the tooth, in position for scaling from the labial to the lingual surface.

    4. *Curet.* A curet is held at an angle formed by the face of the blade and the tooth surface between 60 and 80° (less than 90° but at least 45°).

E. Activate the Instrument: Working Stroke

    1. *Tighten the Grasp.* Move the instrument firmly and deliberately.

    2. *Maintain the Cutting Edge.* Maintain evenly on the tooth surface during the stroke. The side of the tip or toe should always stay adapted in contact with the tooth surface.

    3. *Direction of Strokes*
       a. Vertical pull strokes are used for sickle scalers and hoes; horizontal and oblique strokes may be used when away from the cervical region near the gingival margin.
       b. Vertical, horizontal, and oblique strokes may be used for the curet.
       c. Horizontal push strokes only are used for the chisel from the facial to the lingual surface at right angles with the long axis of anterior teeth.

    4. *Lateral Pressure of the Instrument* (on tooth surface). When the instrument is sharp, the minimum pressure applied allows the cutting edge to grip the calculus; a balance of pressure is maintained between the pressure of the instrument, the grasp of the instrument, and the pressure on the finger rest.

    5. *Control of Motion.* Without independent finger movement, the hand, wrist, and arm act as a continuum to activate the instrument.

    6. *Length of Stroke.* Short and smooth.
       a. Short strokes permit accommodation of the cutting edge to changes in the topography of the tooth surface.
       b. Short strokes assist in maintaining *control* and *precision.*
       c. Strokes are confined to the area of the deposit on the tooth surface known as the *instrumentation zone.*[10] Extending the instrument up the side of the tooth in unnecessarily long strokes is time-consuming, dulls the instrument, and decreases control by and concentration of the clinician.

F. Completion of Stroke

    1. Hold instrument in place momentarily, maintain the finger rest, lighten the grasp on the instrument, and then return the instrument to position for a repeat stroke.

    2. Repeat strokes until surface is smooth.

G. Continuation of Procedure

    1. Move instrument laterally on the tooth surface to adjacent undisturbed deposit; maintain the same finger rest.

    2. Overlap strokes in channels to ensure complete removal of deposit (figure 33–6). Roll

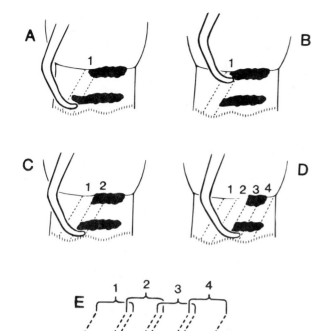

FIG. 33–6. Channel Scaling. A. Curet adapted in position for channel 1 stroke from the base of the pocket under the calculus deposit. **B.** Completion of stroke for channel 1. **C.** Using an exploratory stroke, the curet is lowered into the pocket and is positioned for calculus removal in channel 2. **D.** Curet positioned for channel 3. Several strokes in each channel may be needed to assure complete calculus removal. **E.** Strokes of each channel must overlap strokes of the previous channel. (Adapted from Parr, R.W., Green, E., Madsen, L., and Miller, S.: *Subgingival Scaling and Root Planing*. Berkeley, CA, Praxis Publishing Co., 1976.)

the handle between the fingers of the grasp to maintain adaptation at line angles and other variations of tooth anatomy.

3. Repeat strokes until the tooth surface has been completely scaled.
4. Examine surface with explorer assisted by compressed air; repeat scaling strokes as needed to produce a smooth surface that is free of calculus.

SUBGINGIVAL INSTRUMENTATION

Dexterity, deliberateness, and diligence are key words in perfecting the techniques for subgingival areas. *The principal objectives are to remove the calculus and to plane the root surface with a minimum of trauma to the gingival tissue.*

Root planing follows calculus removal. It is a continuation and an integral part of subgingival scaling. Not all root planing is subgingival, because when root surfaces are exposed as a result of recession or periodontal surgery, the cemental surface is supragingival (figure 33–3F).

I. COMPARISON OF SUPRAGINGIVAL AND SUBGINGIVAL INSTRUMENTATION

Although the basic techniques and steps described previously for removal of supragingival calculus are applied in the subgingival area, subgingival techniques are complicated by several factors.

A. Accessibility
Instrumentation is necessary in areas where access is difficult.

B. Invisible Working Area
Techniques depend almost entirely on tactile sensitivity. Location and removal of minute roughnesses of the tooth surface require a keenly developed tactile sensitivity.

C. Calculus Attachment
Attachment of calculus to the cementum is more tenacious than to the enamel. On the cementum, calculus attaches to minute irregularities and in areas of cemental resorption. Direct attachment of the calculus matrix to the root surface, which makes removal difficult, may also occur. Attachment to the enamel is primarily by means of the acquired pellicle, which makes calculus removal much easier (page 276).

D. Morphology of Calculus
Subgingival calculus is irregularly deposited and occurs in nodular, ledge or ring-like, smooth veneer, and in other forms (table 17–2, page 274).

E. Variations in Root Surface Topography
Although many variations can be expected as part of the normal tooth anatomy, some unusual variations complicate scaling primarily because of their invisibility. The roots and furcation areas shown in figure 33–1 are examples of differences that can be found.

F. Variations in Depth of Pockets
Pockets must be measured about each tooth because variations in depth can occur on a single surface. Instruments must be adapted to reach the bottom of the pocket around the entire periphery of each tooth.

G. Gingival Wall
The gingival wall is close to the tooth surface. Only a narrow area is available for manipulation of instruments. The width of the pocket varies; it narrows down at the base next to the attachment area.

II. INSTRUMENT SELECTION: CURETS
As mentioned previously, gross calculus just below the gingival margin may be removed during supragingival scaling, provided the tissue is loose and resilient

enough to permit easy access by the instruments without forcing them into the sulcus. The ultrasonic scaler may also be used to remove gross subgingival deposits (pages 517 and 518).

The curets are the instruments of choice deeper in the pocket and close to the root surface for several reasons:

A. Fine, thin instruments permit the increased tactile sensitivity that bulkier instruments cannot. Increased sensitivity is essential to thoroughness in areas with limited accessibility and visibility.

B. Root planing with curets produces smoother surfaces than does planing with other instruments.[11,12,13]

C. The curved, narrow, fine curets with rounded ends can be adapted to the anatomic features of the subgingival area with less trauma to the tooth surface and the gingival tissue. Supragingival sickles, hoes, and chisels have sharp points or corners and are thick, bulky, and straight.

D. The sulcus or pocket narrows in the deeper area close to the attachment. The smallest, smoothest instruments are best applied to this narrow area to prevent the need for excess stretching of the gingival wall, where a splitting of the attachment from the tooth can occur.

E. Because of the rounded toe end, a horizontal stroke can be used conservatively. The length of the horizontal stroke depends on variations in pocket depth. When used in position for a vertical stroke, the rounded back of the curet can be placed against the bottom of the pocket.

SUBGINGIVAL PROCEDURES

After root surface evaluation with probe and explorer, as described on pages 200 and 508, the same basic steps are followed for calculus removal as for supragingival scaling (table 33–2). Variations are listed in the following section.

A universal curet is used for convenience and efficiency to remove heavier subgingival calculus. The smaller, area-specific curets should be reserved and kept sharp for fine scaling and root planing, particularly in the narrow depth of the pocket.

I. GRASP THE INSTRUMENT
A modified pen grasp is used. The grasp is lightened as increased tactile sense is needed for refinement of the root surface with root planing.

II. ESTABLISH THE FINGER REST
A. A finger rest on dry, firm tooth structure as close to the tooth being treated as possible and convenient is considered first. Alternate rests were described on page 478.

B. Complete control is essential.

III. ADAPTATION
A. Position the toe third of the blade (figure 33–4) on the tooth surface near the gingival margin where the instrument will be inserted for subgingival scaling.

B. Ascertain whether the correct curet (of the mirror-image pair) is being applied. For a scaling or root planing stroke, the face of the instrument should be toward the tooth. Only the back of the blade is clearly seen. The wrong end is being used when the whole shiny face is clearly seen. This end is impossible to angulate correctly for scaling.

C. Make line angle adaptation (figure 33–5).

IV. ANGULATION
A. Hold at the appropriate angulation for scaling, that is, with the face at an angle between 60 and 80° with the tooth surface.

B. Note the relationship of the handle, finger rest, grasp, blade, and tooth so that after insertion the blade may be promptly reangulated for calculus removal.

V. INSERTION: PLACEMENT STROKE*
A. The exploratory stroke is a preliminary stroke in which the blade is applied lightly over the calculus until the base of the deposit is located. The blade then is positioned for the working stroke.

B. Direct the tip of the curet gingivally; maintain contact with the tooth surface.

C. With light grasp, insert the curet gently under the gingival margin (figure 33–7A).

D. Keep the instrument toe third in light contact with the tooth or calculus surface. The blade is closed toward the tooth surface and held at or near an angle of 0° during the placement stroke (figure 33–7B).

E. Pass the instrument over the surface of the deposit to the base of the pocket until tension of the soft tissue attachment is felt.

F. Adjust the blade to the correct angulation with the tooth surface (as determined before insertion) just below the calculus deposit (figure 33–7C). The side of the toe should be in contact with the tooth surface at all times.

VI. ACTIVATE THE INSTRUMENT: WORKING STROKE
A. Tighten the Grasp
Move the instrument firmly and deliberately (figure 33–7D).

---

* The placement stroke is sometimes referred to as the exploratory or preparatory stroke. When the term "exploratory" is used, it should be distinguished from the meaning of the word as it applies to the use of an explorer. The curet is not used as an explorer, and the calculus has been identified previously by using an explorer.

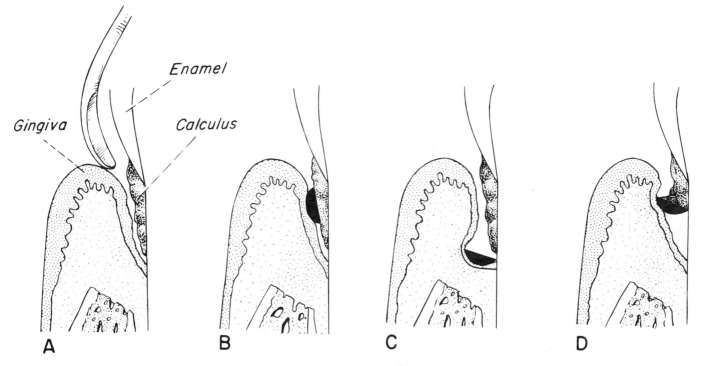

Fig. 33–7. Subgingival Scaling and Root Planing. A. The curet is inserted gently under the gingival margin. **B.** With a placement stroke, the blade is passed over the surface of the tooth or calculus. Note 0° angle of the face of the curet with the calculus. **C.** The curet is lowered to the base of the pocket until the tension of the soft tissue is felt with the rounded back of the curet. The curet then is positioned at an angle of 70 to 80° with the tooth surface beneath the calculus deposit. **D.** The blade is moved along the root surface in a scaling stroke to remove the calculus or in a planing stroke to smooth the surface.

B. Maintain the Cutting Edge

Maintain evenly on the tooth surface during the stroke and at the completion of the stroke.

C. Direction of Strokes

1. Vertical, oblique, or horizontal strokes may be applied (figure 31–9, page 481).
2. All strokes are limited in length by the constant adjustment needed to conform with the curved tooth surfaces and the varying depths of the sulcus or pocket around the tooth.
3. Horizontal strokes cannot be applied to the bottom of the sulcus or pocket except where the probe measurements show the depth is uniform; otherwise the curet would be dragged into the attachment at the higher areas.
4. Push-pull type of stroke is not used subgingivally as it would tend to push particles and bacteria deep into the sulcus and into the soft tissue.

D. Pressure of Instrument

A balance of pressure between the pressure of the instrument, the grasp of the instrument, and the finger rest must be maintained. Undue pressure decreases control and lessens tactile sensitivity. Uncontrolled, excessive pressure causes gouges in cementum and dentin.

E. Control of Motion

Without independent finger movement, the hand, wrist, and arm act as a continuum to activate the instrument.

F. Length of Stroke

1. Use short smooth decisive strokes, the length dependent on the height of the deposit (instrumentation zone, page 512).
2. Confine the strokes within the pocket to prevent the need for repeated removal and reinsertion of the instrument.
   a. To save time.
   b. To prevent trauma to the gingival margin.

G. Completion of Stroke

Maintain finger rest, lighten grasp, and repeat the placement stroke within the pocket. Reposition for a repeat or adjacent stroke. Several strokes are generally required for each area.

VII. CHANNEL STROKES
A. Calculus Removal

Calculus should not be shaved off in layers. With shaving, the remaining thin veneer of calculus may be smooth and indiscernible from the tooth surface, yet contain endotoxin and other substances that can keep the gingiva from healing.

B. Overlapping Strokes (figure 33–6)

1. Repeat strokes at each channel until the area is smooth.
2. Overlap each channel with the next.
3. Roll instrument between fingers to adapt to each part of the tooth surface as scaling continues around line angles and other anatomic features (figure 33–5).

C. Explorer

Use explorer to examine for completion of calculus removal. Some slight roughness of the cemental surface may be present. An enamel surface, however, should be smooth.

VIII. PLANE THE ROOT SURFACE

The technique for planing is basically the same as that for scaling. Instrument control, adaptation, directions for strokes, and other principles are not essentially different. Some clinicians prefer to close the angulation after the calculus is believed to be removed. The basic 70° angle may be closed a few degrees during root planing.

Specific differences in technique are related to touch and pressure. A lighter grasp must be used to increase tactile sensitivity. Because increased pressure is not needed, a lighter shaving-like stroke can be used for smoothing or finishing the root surface.

A. Check the Sharpness of the Curets

Generally, curets dulled during scaling should be resharpened, or a freshly sharpened set should be used for root planing.

B. Strokes

1. Light lateral pressure is applied for maximum sensitivity to minute irregularities of the surface.
2. Smooth strokes with even lateral pressure that systematically overlap and cross over each other are used. As the surface becomes smoother, longer strokes with reduced pressure help to remove small lines, scratches, or grooves without gouging the dentinal surface.
3. Vertical, then oblique, strokes are used. Then, when applicable at levels away from the attachment epithelium, horizontal strokes may be used (figure 33–8).
4. Many strokes usually are needed before a section of the root surface feels smooth.
5. Careful application is necessary to adapt the curet to the anatomic features of the roots. The convex rounded surfaces, the constricted cervical area, the concavities and grooves of proximal surfaces, and furcations all require precise adaptation.
6. As planing nears completion, a gradual change occurs in the sound of the instrument

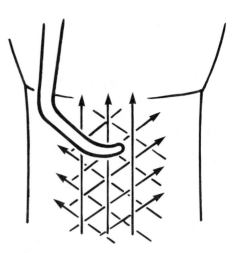

FIG. 33–8. Root Planing Strokes. The use of strokes in vertical and oblique directions with light lateral pressure can eliminate grooves left after scaling. A smooth, surface results. (Adapted from Parr, R.W., Green, E., Madsen, L., and Miller, S.: *Subgingival Scaling and Root Planing.* Berkeley, CA, Praxis Publishing Co., 1976, p. 42.)

on the root surface. At the completion, the instrument may be nearly as quiet as when used on polished enamel.

IX. POST-TREATMENT EVALUATION

A. Examine with a subgingival explorer to establish completion of instrumentation. Use explorer strokes in vertical, oblique, and horizontal directions (figure 33–8) to check for minute grooving of the cemental or dentinal surface.
B. Postcare procedures and supplemental and supportive measures are described in Chapter 34, page 526.

ULTRASONIC AND SONIC SCALING

Ultrasonic instrumentation and sonic instrumentation are adjuncts to, but not substitutes for, manual scaling. The American Dental Association, Council on Dental Materials, Instruments, and Equipment evaluates professional scaling devices. They are classified as Acceptable or Provisionally Acceptable, and use the seal shown in figure 23–16, page 370.[14]

The principle of the ultrasonic scaler is the use of very-high-frequency sound waves. The production of rapid vibrations at the tip of the instrument held on the surface of deposits, retained cement, or other substance to be removed causes breakup and removal.

Although the objectives of both manual and mechanical scaling procedures are similar, the techniques for use of the instruments bear little resemblance to each other. Study and practice are needed to learn the advanced skills required.

MODE OF ACTION[15,16]

The two types of ultrasonic instruments are magnetostrictive and piezoelectric. Sonic instruments are air turbine.

I. ULTRASONIC: MAGNETOSTRICTIVE
The ultrasonic unit consists of an electric generator, a handpiece assembly, a set of interchangeable prophylaxis inserts, and a foot control. The ultrasonic principle is based on the use of high-frequency sound waves.
  A. The ultrasonic machine converts high-frequency electrical energy into mechanical energy in the form of rapid vibrations.
  B. The instrument tip vibrations vary for different models, but may be, for example, 25,000 cycles per second (range 24,000 to 42,000) in an elliptical motion. The vibratory action fractures the deposit and causes its removal from the tooth.
  C. Ultrasonic waves are dissipated in the form of heat. The heat is reduced by keeping the handpiece cooled internally and the working end cooled by a constant flow of water, which is expelled through a metal tube or by means of an internal flow through the working end.
  D. The atomized water forms minute vacuum bubbles that collapse with release of tremendous local pressure; the effect is cleansing to the area. Because the instrument must be in contact with the deposit on the tooth surface if the deposit is to be removed, the bubbling cavitational action of the water has little, if any, actual influence on deposit removal.

II. ULTRASONIC: PIEZOELECTRIC
  A. A quartz or metal alloy crystal transducer converts electrical energy into ultrasonic vibrations.
  B. No magnetic field is present, and less heat is produced.
  C. Vibrations at the tip range from 29,000 to 50,000 cycles per second in a linear action.
  D. Water cooling is needed to cool the friction between the tip and the tooth surface.

III. SONIC
  A. Attached to conventional handpiece operated with clean, dry air (cannot attach to an oiled air line); advantage in small size and convenience of attachment without separate unit.
  B. Vibrations at the tip range from 2500 to 7000 cycles per second, a disadvantage because less power means less action for calculus removal. The tip revolves in an elliptical or an orbital path.

  C. Heat is not generated, but water cooling is indicated.
  D. Air turbine produces a high pitched sound.

PURPOSES AND USES

I. INDICATIONS FOR USE
  A. Supragingival removal of calculus deposits generalized throughout the dentition.
  B. Subgingival debridement.
  C. Initial debridement for a patient with necrotizing ulcerative gingivitis or other condition that can be relieved by removal of deposits, provided that loose debris, materia alba, and microorganisms are first removed by rinses, brushing, and flossing during patient instruction to prevent contaminated aerosol production.
  D. Prescaling for oral surgery, such as tooth removal (pages 655).
  E. Orthodontic cement removal; debonding.[17]
  F. Overhang removal of restorations.

II. CONTRAINDICATIONS AND PRECAUTIONS
  A. Patient with a known communicable disease that can be transmitted by aerosols.
  B. Compromised patient with a marked susceptibility to infection. Examples of conditions are immunosuppression from disease or medication, uncontrolled diabetes, debilitation, or renal and other organ transplant.
  C. Patient with a respiratory risk. Septic material and microorganisms from bacterial plaque and periodontal pockets can be aspirated into the lungs.[18]
    1. History of chronic pulmonary disease, including asthma, emphysema, or cystic fibrosis.
    2. History of cardiovascular disease with secondary pulmonary disease or breathing problem.
  D. Patient with a swallowing problem or who is prone to gagging.
  E. Patient with a cardiac pacemaker or other electronic life-support device. Some newer models have protective coverings. A consultation with the patient's cardiologist is necessary.
  F. Children.
    1. Young, growing, developing tissues are sensitive to ultrasonic vibrations.
    2. Primary and newly erupted permanent teeth have large pulp chambers. The vibrations and heat from the ultrasonic scaler may damage the pulp tissue.
  G. Characteristics of the teeth.
    1. *Demineralized Areas.* Ultrasonic vibrations can remove the delicate remineralizing cover of a white spot.

2. *Exposed Cemental Surfaces.* Tooth structure can be removed in excess. Mature calculus is harder than cementum.
3. *Restorative Materials.* Certain materials can be damaged or removed by ultrasonic instrumentation.
   a. Porcelain jacket crowns can be fractured by ultrasonic vibrations.[19]
   b. Composite resins; a laminate veneer can be removed.[20]
   c. Amalgam surface and margins can be altered.[21] Ultrasonic instruments can be used to reshape amalgam overhanging fillings, so margins can also be damaged.
   d. Titanium implant abutments can be damaged.[22,23]
4. *Patients with Sensitive Areas.* Ultrasonic instrumentation can aggravate existing sensitivity.

H. Subgingival areas where lack of visibility and narrow pockets can interfere with proper angulation. Overinstrumentation can result.

I. Maintenance-care patients who are oriented to daily bacterial plaque removal and have minimal amounts of calculus develop between appointments.

CLINICAL PROCEDURES[16,24]

The clinician and the assistant apply full barrier requirements with protective eyewear, mask, and gloves. Hair covering should also be used when possible.

I. UNIT PREPARATION

A. Minimize Water Contamination

Run water through the tubing of the ultrasonic unit for a full 2 minutes prior to use. Cultures of samples from water lines have shown high microbial counts, particularly in water left in the tubing overnight. The use of contaminated water provides a potential source for disease transmission. Such contaminated water forced into a pocket could produce bacteremia.[25]

B. Unit Adjustment

1. Tune according to the manufacturer's specifications. Use the lowest effective power setting.
2. Adjust water to a maximum mist about the working tip. Overheating must be prevented.

C. Working Tips

1. Sterilized tip is adapted to the handpiece after the unit water has cleared.
2. Instrument tips must be dull; if sharp, the tooth surface could be nicked or gouged.
3. Handle inserts with care to avoid damage to working ends or internal parts. Wrap individually for sterilization.

II. PATIENT PREPARATION

A. Review patient history and radiographs.
B. Check that risk patient has taken prescribed antibiotic medication. Prophylactic antibiotic premedication is indicated for risk patients. Bacteremia is produced in a high percentage of patients treated by ultrasonic, as well as by manual, instrumentation.[26]
C. Explain the procedure and the handpiece to the patient. Describe and demonstrate sound and spray, vibration, and the purpose for using the method. Hearing aid should be turned off.
D. Instruct the patient to use an antiseptic mouthrinse for 1 minute prior to ultrasonic scaling to lower the oral bacterial count and, hence, lower the bacterial count of the aerosols produced (page 64).
E. Use coverall and towel, and provide protective eyewear (patient should be requested to remove contact lenses).

III. INSTRUMENTATION

A. Place patient in supine position. In supine position, the airway is closed (figure 61–4, page 836). Help of an assistant is recommended for all patients, but is especially needed for
   1. Patients with deep suppurating periodontal pockets.[18]
   2. Patient with a respiratory disability.
B. Apply topical anesthetic or use local anesthetic as indicated and necessary.
C. Explore to review location of calculus.
D. Use high-velocity evacuation. When working solo, a saliva ejector must be in top running condition. Every effort must be made to prevent aspiration by the patient.
E. Plan systematic sequence. Finish one quadrant before starting another.
F. Use a modified pen grasp and apply finger rest on a tooth surface near the calculus to be removed.
G. Bring instrument to position before activating the water spray.
H. *Keep side of tip parallel with long axis of the tooth or at no more than a 15° angle with tooth surface.* Adaptation to variations in tooth topography is difficult but necessary. Maintenance of less than a 15° angle in all positions requires practice and concentration.
I. Stroke
   1. *Keep the tip in motion at all times.*
   2. Check to ensure that the water reaches the treatment area.
   3. Brush lightly over the deposit, moving in a vertical or diagonal direction. A maximum of six strokes should be applied at one spot. Do not press. Pressure can remove tooth structure.
   4. Move instrument with smooth, light, constant, and overlapping strokes.

5. Be sure the tip is not held perpendicular to the tooth surface.
6. Instrument may tend to bind when inserted interproximally, and the excess pressure stops the vibration. Remove and reactivate the instrument.
J. Release foot pedal switch at regular intervals to aid in water control. Stop periodically to evaluate the tooth surfaces with an explorer.
K. Complete the procedure with manual instruments directly following ultrasonic instrumentation.
   1. Check subgingival areas with a subgingival explorer.
   2. Remove remaining subgingival irregularities, and plane the surface smooth with curets.

IV. POSTOPERATIVE INSTRUCTIONS
A. Plaque control procedures should follow the usual pattern as recommended.
B. Use of fluoride dentifrice and mouthrinse is important for newly exposed tooth surfaces.
C. Counteract sensitivity to cold, hot, and condiments by avoiding extremes of temperature for a few days. If sensitivity persists, recommendations can be made at the next patient visit for use of special procedures or professional desensitization (pages 558).
D. When the gingiva is sensitive, rinsing with warm weak saline solution can be recommended (pages 526 and 527).

ADVANTAGES AND LIMITATIONS

I. ADVANTAGES
A. Calculus removal may be accomplished with less effort than by manual instrumentation. More time can be devoted to thorough, careful patient instruction.
B. Requires minimum tissue manipulation for hypersensitive tissues.
C. Water flushes out pockets. Too much water pressure into the pocket can force particles into the tissue, which is a disadvantage.
D. Treatment time is reduced for removal of heavy stains and calculus.
E. Equipment requires minimal care.

II. LIMITATIONS
A. Operational Factors
   1. Less tactile perception.
   2. Impeded visibility during instrumentation.
   3. Use of mirror not possible for vision and reflected light because of water spray.
   4. Patient and clinician have discomfort and in-

convenience of water spray and water accumulation when an assistant is not available.
5. Accessibility for instrument adaptation and angulation in posterior oral regions is difficult.

B. Heat Production
Potential damage to the pulp tissue should be kept in mind during instrumentation.[15,27] Constant motion of the instrument, correct angulation, and ample water for cooling are essential to operation.

C. Platelet Aggregation
Human platelets are susceptible to damage by forces associated with ultrasonic cavitation at the level used clinically. If such damage were to occur in the pulp chamber of a tooth, thrombosis could result. The effect would be unlikely in large arteries, but could happen in a tooth because of the close area of enclosure. Pulpal thrombosis could lead to pulp death.[28]

D. Aerosols
Aerosols produced by an ultrasonic scaler may contain high bacterial counts.[25,29,30,31] The ultrasonic scaler should not be used for a patient with a communicable disease or for one susceptible to infections.[32]

E. Hearing Shifts
Extended exposure to noises above a certain level, such as the noise of a high-speed handpiece or an ultrasonic scaler, may be potentially damaging. Temporary hearing shifts have been demonstrated for a group of patients.[33]

USE OF A TOPICAL ANESTHETIC

A topical or surface anesthetic is a drug applied to the mucous membrane to produce a loss of sensation. A topical anesthetic can be used with a degree of success for short-duration desensitization of the gingiva. As a soft tissue anesthetic, a topical agent does not influence sensations in the teeth and, therefore, is not a substitute for local anesthetic administered by injection.

Pain reaction varies from person to person and even in the same person, depending on emotional state and degree of fatigue. A person with a low reaction to pain, who is hyporeactive, is said to have a *high pain threshold.* The person with a high reaction is hyperreactive and has a *low pain threshold.*

In addition to emotional state and fatigue, other factors that influence pain threshold are age, sex, fear, and apprehension. Older individuals tend to have a pain threshold higher than that of younger individuals, and men tend to have a threshold higher than that of women. In fear or apprehension, however, the pain threshold for either sex at any age is lowered.

I. INDICATIONS FOR USE

A *local anesthetic* should be used when indicated by the extent of the procedure, by the patient's pain threshold, or by evidence of fear and apprehension. Although a local anesthetic would be indicated primarily for deep subgingival scaling and root planing, it may be indicated for any degree of scaling requirement.

Pain threshold can usually be detected during initial examination. A patient who hyperreacts to gentle, careful probing may indeed have a low pain threshold. A note should be made on the record to indicate possible need for anesthesia during clinical treatments.

A *topical anesthetic* can be used conservatively for many dental hygiene and dental services, including the following:
A. Prior to injection for local anesthesia.
B. Prevention of gagging in radiographic techniques and impression making.
C. Relief of pain from localized diseased areas, such as oral ulcers, wounds, or injuries.
D. During instrumentation for probing, exploring, scaling, and, sometimes, root planing. When root planing is deep and generalized, a local anesthetic is usually indicated.
E. Suture removal.
F. Replacement of a dressing after removal. When light pressure is needed for adaptation of the dressing, a topical application can provide relief.

II. ACTION OF A TOPICAL ANESTHETIC

The purpose of a topical anesthetic is to desensitize the mucous membrane by anesthetizing the terminal nerve endings. A superficial anesthesia is produced that is related to the amount of absorption of the drug by the tissue.

The absorption varies with the thickness of the stratified squamous epithelial covering and the degree of keratinization. The skin and lips are highly resistant; the attached gingiva and cheek and palatal mucosa absorb drugs slowly; and the tissues without keratinization absorb promptly.

III. REQUIREMENTS FOR AN ADEQUATE TOPICAL ANESTHETIC

A. Produces effective lasting anesthesia.
B. Is miscible and stable in vehicle used.
C. Anesthetizing agent readily released from the preparation when applied.
D. Is nonirritating to the tissues.
E. Does not induce hypersensitivity reaction or other toxic effect at the concentration required for anesthesia.
F. Does not delay healing.
G. Can be readily washed off with water.

IV. PREPARATIONS USED: CHARACTERISTICS

Several preparations have been used in the form of gels, ointments, solutions, troches, or sprays. The American Dental Association, Council on Dental Therapeutics evaluates and classifies topical anesthetics.[14]

General properties and characteristics of anesthetics for surface use follow.
A. Oils, alcohols, or glycols are used as the vehicle because most of the anesthetizing substances are only slightly soluble in water.
B. Most topical anesthetics are prepared in fairly concentrated form to allow for the resistance of the thick epithelial covering and viscid coating of saliva on the tissues. They are generally more concentrated than their counterparts used for local anesthesia. An example is lidocaine. For injection, a 2% solution is used, whereas for a topical preparation, the concentration is 5 or 10%.
C. The rate of absorption of a drug depends on solubility and the resistance of the mucous membrane.
D. Alcohols or glycols in concentrated solutions may be irritating to the sensitive mucous membranes and, therefore, are inferior vehicles (percent of alcohol or glycol should not be greater than 10%).
E. Carbowaxes used as vehicles for topical anesthetics are somewhat hygroscopic; thus, the jar in which the ointment is kept should be closed tightly.
F. Pressurized spray preparations must be used with caution because the amount of material expelled is difficult to control and the area of application is difficult to limit. Inhalation of the fine spray into the lungs can produce a toxic reaction. When the liquid flows into the throat (as may be possible with application of any type of preparation), coughing may be initiated.

V. AGENTS USED IN SURFACE ANESTHETIC PREPARATIONS

The six drugs most commonly contained in surface anesthetics for dental use are listed here with brief notes about their characteristics.[14,34]

A. Benzocaine (ester type)
1. Slow absorption; may be applied to abrasions or open lesions.
2. May produce localized allergic reactions after prolonged or repeated use.

B. Tetracaine (ester type)
1. Rapid absorption and high toxicity; not for use on open abraded tissue.
2. Use in small quantities; avoid spray media where quantity used cannot be controlled. Not recommended.

C. Butacaine (ester type)
1. Good action through mucous membrane.
2. Toxic; should be used cautiously.

D. Lidocaine (amide type)
1. Allergy is rare; aqueous form is more toxic than nonaqueous lidocaine base.
2. May be applied to lacerated or incompletely healed tissue.

E. Chlorbutanol (aliphatic compound)

1. Has both antiseptic and anesthetic properties.
2. Has been used in preparations for alleviation of pain from pulpitis in a near pulp exposure and in dressings for relief from postsurgical discomfort.

F. Dyclonine (ketone)

1. May be applied to lacerated or incompletely healed tissue because it is absorbed slowly.
2. Has low systemic toxicity; useful when other agents cannot be used.

VI. TECHNIQUE FOR APPLICATION OF A TOPICAL ANESTHETIC

A. Consult history and other records for pertinent information concerning a patient's previous experiences with anesthetics. A patient with an allergy to a local anesthetic may also be allergic to a surface anesthetic.
B. Explain purpose and anticipated effect to the patient.
C. Dry area with gauze sponge or cotton roll. Compressed air may be used, with consideration for sensitive tissues.
D. Apply anesthetic.
   1. Ointment
      a. A syringe with a bent blunt needle may be used to introduce an ointment into a sulcus or pocket.
      b. Apply a small amount to a limited area with a cotton pellet and rub into the proximal area.
   2. Liquid
      a. Use a cotton swab or pellet for application.
      b. Apply a small amount directly over the dry tissues.
E. Wait briefly for anesthetic to take effect before proceeding.

VII. ADVERSE REACTIONS
A. Causes and Symptoms

1. *Allergic Response*
   a. Cause. Ingredients of the preparation have high allergenicity (the ability to produce an allergic reaction). The ester-type drugs have a greater tendency to produce allergic reactions than do other anesthetics.
   b. Symptoms. Erythema or angioedema of mucous membranes and lips.
2. *Overdose*
   a. Cause. When a large quantity of the agent is spread over a large area and rapid absorption through the mucous membranes occurs, an immediate elevation of the anesthetic blood level results.
   b. Symptoms. Patient agitation, apprehension, excitement, speech irregularity, and tremors that progress to a mild convulsion. Pulse rate, blood pressure, and respiratory rate are elevated (table 61–2, pages 845 and 846).

B. Precautions and Prevention[35]

1. Use amide-type topical anesthetic.
2. Apply small amount to a limited area. For example, the anesthetic should not be spread over a whole quadrant for probing or scaling.
3. Use metered or measured dose forms, especially if a liquid spray is to be used. The metered-dose container has a dispenser that limits the amount that can be expelled.
4. Avoid areas of sepsis and open traumatized tissue unless the particular agent is specifically recommended for safe application on an open wound.
5. Prevent inspiration (inhalation) by avoiding spray preparations. A spray must never be directed toward the throat.

C. Adverse Reactions

1. Allergic-type reactions may occur. Such reactions are related to a topical anesthetic preparation that contains an ester-type agent.
2. Agents that are rapidly absorbed may cause an overdose reaction.

TECHNICAL HINTS

I. MAINTAIN SHARP INSTRUMENTS
Examine curets and scalers for sharpness at frequent intervals during instrumentation. Keep a sterile stone with each instrument set so that instruments can be sharpened during an appointment. Curets that are used most frequently may be packaged individually so a new package can be opened, or two curets of each type can be sterilized with the regular adult package.

II. REPLACE CURETS FREQUENTLY
While sharpening, examine for wear. Discard a curet with a thin weak blade to prevent breakage during a treatment.

III. BROKEN INSTRUMENT
The procedure to follow when an instrument blade tip breaks in a patient's mouth during treatment should be in accord with the dentist's own policy. Therefore, the procedure should be discussed and clarified before an accident happens.

The principal objective in the location of a broken instrument tip is to *know positively that the tip has been removed*. With this in mind, rinsing, use of suction or compressed air, or initiation of other procedures that could cause the removal of the tip unknowingly would be out of order. A general procedure is suggested here.

A. Cease procedure, retain retraction without moving the patient's head unnecessarily, and isolate with gauze or cotton roll.
B. Do not alarm patient by describing the accident.
C. Examine the immediate treatment area, the floor of the mouth, and the mucobuccal fold. Blot the gingival tissue dry with a cotton roll and examine around the tooth.
D. Apply transilluminator or mouth light when available.
E. The gingival sulcus can be gently examined using a curet in a spooning-like stroke, but take care not to push the tip into the base of the sulcus (should the tip be there).
F. Consult the dentist for assistance in accord with previously discussed policy.
G. When the tip is not removed by any means mentioned thus far, make a periapical radiograph of the area.

IV. SUMMARY: METHODS TO MINIMIZE PATIENT DISCOMFORT

A. Tissue Sensitivity

1. For gingival tissue, use topical anesthetic and/or local anesthetic as needed.
2. For exposed cementum or dentin, apply desensitizing agent (Chapter 37).
3. Protect lips and corners of mouth from irritation during instrumentation by application of petrolatum, cocoa butter, or other appropriate lubricant.
4. Use only *warm* water for rinsing.

B. Preventive Instrumentation

1. Use appropriate instrument, applied at the correct angulation, for each tooth surface.
2. Curets applied to base of sulcus or pocket must be small to prevent undue stretching of gingival wall and, hence, unnecessary detachment of the soft tissue attachment.
3. Instruments must be sharp, but the cementum can be scratched if sharp curets are not applied correctly and discriminately.
4. Maintain control of instrument at all times through effective grasp, appropriate finger rest, and correctly applied strokes to prevent accidental trauma to gingival tissue.
5. Apply minimum effective pressure on finger rest and of instrument on tooth to prevent patient from developing tired muscles and a stressed temporomandibular joint.
6. Finger rests on soft tissue give the patient a feeling of more pressure than do finger rests on the teeth and, consequently, may give the impression that the clinician is heavy-handed.

V. MAINTENANCE OF A CLEAR FIELD

A. Use of saliva ejector and evacuator as needed.
B. Use of rolled gauze sponge or cotton rolls.

1. A gauze sponge rolled in the long dimension and placed in the mucobuccal fold beneath the teeth being treated can assist by
   a. Retracting the cheek or lip.
   b. Keeping teeth dry for secure finger rest.
   c. Drying the individual area for better vision.
2. Aid in retraction of tongue and keeping field free from saliva by placing cotton roll under tongue.
C. Maintenance of clear field and/or control of bleeding.
   1. Application of pressure with cotton roll or pellet.
   2. Application of 3% hydrogen peroxide with cotton pellet, followed by patient rinsing and/or dry pellet applied with pressure.
   3. Use of compressed air to deflect tissue and remove debris.

FACTORS TO TEACH THE PATIENT

I. The nature, occurrence, and etiology of calculus.
II. The importance of the complete removal of calculus to the health of the oral tissues in the prevention of periodontal infections.
III. Relationship of the accumulation of bacterial plaque to the patient's personal oral hygiene procedures.
IV. Basic reasons for need and advantages of multiple appointments to complete the scaling and root planing.
V. Needed frequency of maintenance appointments in relation to oral health.

REFERENCES

1. **De Leo**, A.A., Schoenknecht, M.D., Anderson, M.W., and Peterson, J.C.: The Incidence of Bacteremia Following Oral Prophylaxis on Pediatric Patients, *Oral Surg., 37,* 36, January, 1974.
2. **Korn**, N.A. and Schaffer, E.M.: Comparison of the Postoperative Bacteremias Induced Following Different Periodontal Procedures, *J. Periodontol., 33,* 226, July, 1962.
3. **Royer**, R., Gaines, R., and Kruger, G.: Bacteremia Following Exodontia, Prophylaxis, and Gingivectomy, *J. Dent. Res., 43,* 877, September–October (Supplement), 1964.
4. **Bender**, I.B., Seltzer, S., Tashman, S., and Meloff, G.: Dental Procedures in Patients with Rheumatic Heart Disease, *Oral Surg., 16,* 466, April, 1963.
5. **Winslow**, M.B. and Kobernick, S.D.: Bacteremia after Prophylaxis, *J. Am. Dent. Assoc., 61,* 69, July, 1960.
6. **Connor**, H.D., Haberman, S., Collings, C.K., and Winford, T.E.: Bacteremias Following Periodontal Scaling in Patients with Healthy Appearing Gingiva, *J. Periodontol, 38,* 466, November–December, 1967.
7. **Knowles**, J.W., Burgett, F.G., Nissle, R.R., Shick, R.A., Morrison, E.C., and Ramfjord, S.P.: Results of Periodontal Treatment Related to Pocket Depth and Attachment Level. Eight Years, *J. Periodontol., 50,* 225, May, 1979.

8. **Badersten,** A., Nilvéus, R., and Egelberg, J.: Effect of Nonsurgical Periodontal Therapy. I. Moderately Advanced Periodontitis, *J. Clin. Periodontol., 8,* 57, February, 1981.

9. **Lindhe,** J., Nyman, S., and Karring, T.: Scaling and Root Planing in Shallow Pockets, *J. Clin. Periodontol., 9,* 415, September, 1982.

10. **Carranza,** F.A.: *Glickman's Clinical Periodontology,* 7th ed. Philadelphia, W.B. Saunders Co., 1990, p. 627.

11. **Barnes,** J.E. and Schaffer, E.M.: Subgingival Root Planing: A Comparison Using Files, Hoes and Curettes, *J. Periodontol., 31,* 300, September, 1960.

12. **Green,** E. and Ramfjord, S.P.: Tooth Roughness after Subgingival Root Planing, *J. Periodontol., 37,* 396, September–October, 1966.

13. **Walker,** S.L. and Ash, M.M.: A Study of Root Planing by Scanning Electron Microscopy, *Dent. Hyg., 50,* 109, March, 1976.

14. **American Dental Association,** Council on Dental Materials, Instruments and Equipment, and Council on Dental Therapeutics: *Clinical Products in Dentistry. A Desktop Reference.* Chicago, American Dental Association, published annually.

15. **American Dental Association,** Council on Dental Materials, Instruments, and Equipment: Status Report on Professional Scaling and Stain-removal Devices, *J. Am. Dent. Assoc., 111,* 801, November, 1985.

16. **Holbrook,** T.E. and Low, S.B.: Power-driven Scaling and Polishing Instruments, in Hardin, J.F., ed.: *Clark's Clinical Dentistry,* Revised edition—1989. Philadelphia, J.B. Lippincott Co., 1989, Section 5A, pp. 1–24.

17. **Krell,** K.V., Courey, J.M., and Bishara, S.E.: Orthodontic Bracket Removal Using Conventional and Ultrasonic Debonding Techniques, Enamel Loss, and Time Requirements, *Am. J. Orthod. Dentofacial Orthop., 103,* 258, March, 1993.

18. **Suzuki,** J.B. and Delisle, A.L.: Pulmonary Actinomycosis of Periodontal Origin, *J. Periodontol., 55,* 581, October, 1984.

19. **American Dental Association,** Council on Dental Materials, Instruments and Equipment: *Dentist's Desk Reference: Materials Instruments and Equipment,* 2nd ed. Chicago, American Dental Association, 1983, pp. 361–362.

20. **Carr,** E.H.: Laminate Veneers. Restoration Alternative Means Special Care, *RDH, 2,* 11, July–August, 1982.

21. **Rajstein,** J. and Tal, M.: The Effect of Ultrasonic Scaling on the Surface of Class V Amalgam Restorations—A Scanning Electron Microscopy Study, *J. Oral Rehabil., 11,* 299, May, 1984.

22. **Thomson-Neal,** D., Evans, G.H., and Meffert, R.M.: Effects of Various Prophylactic Treatments on Titanium, Sapphire and Hydroxy-coated Implants, *Int. J. Periodontics Restorative Dent., 9,* 301, No. 4, 1989.

23. **Rapley,** J.W., Swan, R.H., Hallmon, W.W., and Mills, M.P.: The Surface Characteristics Produced by Various Oral Hygiene Instruments and Materials on Titanium Implant Abutments, *Int. J. Oral Maxillofac. Implants, 5,* 47, No. 1, 1990.

24. **Clark,** S.M.: A Compact Guide to Ultrasonic Instrumentation, *Compendium, 12,* 760, October, 1991.

25. **Larato,** D.C., Ruskin, P.F., and Martin, A.: Effect of an Ultrasonic Scaler on Bacterial Counts in Air, *J. Periodontol., 38,* 550, November–December (Part 1), 1967.

26. **Bandt,** C.L., Korn, N.A., and Schaffer, E.M.: Bacteremias from Ultrasonic and Hand Instrumentation, *J. Periodontol., 35,* 214, May–June, 1964.

27. **Abrams,** H., Barkmeier, W.W., and Cooley, R.L.: Temperature Changes in the Pulp Chamber Produced by Ultrasonic Instrumentation, *Gen. Dent., 27,* 62, September–October, 1979.

28. **Williams,** A.R. and Chater, B.V.: Mammalian Platelet Damage *In Vitro* by an Ultrasonic Therapeutic Device, *Arch. Oral Biol., 25,* 175, No. 3, 1980.

29. **Holbrook,** W.P., Muir, K.F., MacPhee, I.T., and Ross, P.W.: Bacteriological Investigation of the Aerosol from Ultrasonic Scalers, *Br. Dent. J., 144,* 245, April 18, 1978.

30. **Muir,** K.F., Ross, P.W., MacPhee, I.T., Holbrook, W.P., and Kowolik, M.J.: Reduction of Microbial Contamination from Ultrasonic Scalers, *Br. Dent. J., 145,* 76, August 1, 1978.

31. **Gross,** K.B.W., Overman, P.R., Cobb, C., and Brockman, S.: Aerosol Generation by Two Ultrasonic Scalers and One Sonic Scaler. A Comparative Study, *J. Dent. Hyg., 66,* 314, September, 1992.

32. **Gross,** A., Devine, M.J., and Cutright, D.E.: Microbial Contamination of Dental Units and Ultrasonic Scalers, *J. Periodontol., 47,* 670, November, 1976.

33. **Möller,** P., Grevstad, A.O., and Kristoffersen, T.: Ultrasonic Scaling of Maxillary Teeth Causing Tinnitus and Temporary Hearing Shifts, *J. Clin. Periodontol., 3,* 123, May, 1976.

34. **Malamed,** S.F.: *Handbook of Local Anesthesia,* 3rd ed. St. Louis, Mosby, 1990, pp. 69–72, 103–104.

35. **Malamed,** S.F.: *Medical Emergencies in the Dental Office,* 4th ed. St. Louis, Mosby, 1993, pp. 319–320, 351.

SUGGESTED READINGS

Bader, H.I.: Scaling and Root Planing: Its Role in Contemporary Periodontal Therapy, *Compendium, 14,* 436, April, 1993.

Garrett, J.S.: Root Planing: A Perspective, *J. Periodontol., 48,* 553, September, 1977.

Parr, R.W., Green, E., Madsen, L., and Miller, S.: *Subgingival Scaling and Root Planing.* Berkeley, CA, Praxis Publishing Co., 1976, 90 pp.

Parr, R.W., John, R., and Ratcliff, P.A.: *Tooth Preparation.* Berkeley, CA, Praxis Publishing Co., 1974, 52 pp.

Pattison, A.M. and Pattison, G.L.: *Periodontal Instrumentation,* 2nd ed. Norwalk, CT, Appleton & Lange, 1992, pp. 127–285.

Schoen, D.H.: Instrument Effects on Smoothness Discrimination, *J. Dent. Educ., 56,* 741, November, 1992.

Singer, D.L., Long, B.A., Lozanoff, S., and Senthilselvan, A.: Evaluation of a New Periodontal Curet, An *In Vitro* Study, *J. Clin. Periodontol., 19,* 549, September, 1992.

Tal, H., Panno, J.M., and Vaidyanathan, T.K.: Scanning Electron Microscope Evaluation of Wear of Dental Curettes During Standardized Root Planing, *J. Periodontol., 56,* 532, September, 1985.

Walsh, M.M. and Robertson, P.B.: Professional Mechanical Oral Hygiene Practices in the Prevention and Control of Periodontal Diseases, *J. Dent. Hyg., 63,* 242, June, 1989.

Walsh, T.F., Figures, K.H., and Lamb, D.J.: *Clinical Dental Hygiene. A Handbook for the Dental Team.* Oxford, Wright, Butterworth-Heinemann, 1992, pp. 88–112.

Zappa, U., Rothlisberger, J.P., Simona, C., and Case, D.: In Vivo Scaling and Root Planing Forces in Molars, *J. Periodontol., 64,* 349, May, 1993.

Anatomic Features

Bower, R.C.: Furcation Morphology Relative to Periodontal Treatment. Furcation Entrance Architecture, *J. Periodontol., 50,* 23, January, 1979.

Bower, R.C.: Furcation Morphology Relative to Periodontal Treatment. Furcation Root Surface Anatomy, *J. Periodontol., 50,* 366, July, 1979.

Fox, S.C. and Bosworth, B.L.: A Morphological Survey of Proximal Root Concavities: A Consideration in Periodontal Therapy, *J. Am. Dent. Assoc., 114,* 811, June, 1987.

Gher, M.E. and Vernino, A.R.: Root Morphology—Clinical Significance in Pathogenesis and Treatment of Periodontal Disease, *J. Am. Dent. Assoc., 101,* 627, October, 1980.

Harris, J.H. and Overton, E.E.: Cementoenamel Defects in an Unusual Location, *J. Am. Dent. Assoc., 97,* 221, August, 1978.

Holton, W.L., Hancock, E.B., and Pelleu, G.B.: Prevalence and Distribution of Attached Cementicles on Human Root Surfaces, *J. Periodontol., 57,* 321, May, 1986.

Moskow, B.S. and Canut, P.M.: Studies on Root Enamel. (2) Enamel Pearls. A Review of Their Morphology, Localization, Nomenclature, Occurrence, Classification, Histogenesis and Incidence, *J. Clin. Periodontol., 17,* 275, May, 1990.

Ultrasonic Scaling

Dragoo, M.R.: A Clinical Evaluation of Hand and Ultrasonic Instruments on Subgingival Debridement. Part I. With Unmodified and Modified Ultrasonic Inserts, *Int. J. Periodontics Restorative Dent., 12,* 311, No. 4, 1992.

Mooney, M.K.: Ultrasonics Come of Age, *RDH, 12,* 25, April, 1992.

Nosal, G., Scheidt, M.J., O'Neal, R., and Van Dyke, T.E.: The Penetration of Lavage Solution into the Periodontal Pocket During Ultrasonic Instrumentation, *J. Periodontol., 62,* 554, September, 1991.

Oda, S. and Ishikawa, I.: *In Vitro* Effectiveness of a Newly-designed Ultrasonic Scaler Tip for Furcation Areas, *J. Periodontol., 60,* 634, November, 1989.

Reinhardt, R.A., Bolton, R.W., and Hlava, G.: Effect of Non-sterile Versus Sterile Water Irrigation With Ultrasonic Scaling on Postoperative Bacteremias, *J. Periodontol., 53,* 96, February, 1982.

Takacs, V.J., Lie, T., Perala, D.G., and Adams, D.F.: Efficacy of 5 Machining Instruments in Scaling of Molar Furcations, *J. Periodontol., 64,* 228, March, 1993.

Walmsley, A.D., Laird, W.R.E., and Williams, A.R.: Investigation into Patients' Hearing Following Ultrasonic Scaling, *Br. Dent. J., 162,* 221, March 21, 1987.

Walmsley, A.D., Laird, W.R.E., and Williams, A.R.: Intra-vascular Thrombosis Associated with Dental Ultrasound, *J. Oral Pathol., 16,* 256, May, 1987.

Walmsley, A.D.: Potential Hazards of the Dental Ultrasonic Descaler, *Ultrasound Med. Biol., 14,* 15, No. 1, 1988.

Wang, H.-L., Pappert, T.D., Burgett, F.G., and Somerman, M.J.: Evaluation of Root Instruments, *Compendium, 13,* 456, June, 1992.

Ultrasonics/Restorative Materials

Bjornson, E.J., Collins, D.E., and Engler, W.O.: Surface Alteration of Composite Resins after Curette, Ultrasonic, and Sonic Instrumentation: An *In Vitro* Study, *Quintessence Int., 21,* 381, May, 1990.

Gorfil, C., Nordenberg, D., Liberman, R., and Ben-Amar, A.: The Effect of Ultrasonic Cleaning and Air Polishing on the Marginal Integrity of Radicular Amalgam and Composite Resin Restorations. An *In Vitro* Study, *J. Clin. Periodontol., 16,* 137, March, 1989.

Sivers, J.E. and Johnson, G.K.: Comparison of Effects of Ultrasonic and Sonic Instrumentation on Amalgam Restorations, *Gen. Dent., 37,* 130, March–April, 1989.

Sonic Scaling

Gankerseer, E.J. and Walmsley, A.D.: Preliminary Investigation into the Performance of a Sonic Scaler, *J. Periodontol., 58,* 780, November, 1987.

Gellin, R.G., Miller, M.C., Javed, T., Engler, W.O., and Mishkin, D.J.: The Effectiveness of the Titan-S Sonic Scaler Versus Curettes in the Removal of Subgingival Calculus. A Human Surgical Evaluation, *J. Periodontol., 57,* 672, November, 1986.

Johnson, G.K., Reinhardt, R.A., Tussing, G.J., and Krejci, R.F.: Fiber Optic Probe Augmented Sonic Scaling Versus Conventional Sonic Scaling, *J. Periodontol., 60,* 131, March, 1989.

Jotikasthira, N.E., Lie, T., and Leknes, K.N.: Comparative *In Vitro* Studies of Sonic, Ultrasonic and Reciprocating Scaling Instruments, *J. Clin. Periodontol., 19,* 560, September, 1992.

Leknes, K.N. and Lie, T.: Influence of Polishing Procedures on Sonic Scaling Root Surface Roughness, *J. Periodontol., 62,* 659, November, 1991.

Lie, T. and Leknes, K.N.: Evaluation of the Effect on Root Surfaces of Air Turbine Scalers and Ultrasonic Instrumentation, *J. Periodontol., 56,* 522, September, 1985.

Loos, B., Kiger, R., and Egelberg, J.: An Evaluation of Basic Periodontal Therapy Using Sonic and Ultrasonic Scalers, *J. Clin. Periodontol., 14,* 29, January, 1987.

Patterson, M., Eick, J.D., Eberhart, A.B., Gross, K., and Killoy, W.J.: The Effectiveness of Two Sonic and Two Ultrasonic Scaler Tips in Furcations, *J. Periodontol., 60,* 325, June, 1989.

Reed, K.L.: Sonic Scalers: A Review, *Gen. Dent., 40,* 34, January–February, 1992.

Topical Anesthesia

Moore, P.A.: Preventing Local Anesthesia Toxicity, *J. Am. Dent. Assoc., 123,* 60, September, 1992.

Raab, F.J. and Young, L.L.: Episodic Factitious Gingival Injury Secondary to Topical Anesthesia. A Case Report, *J. Periodontol., 62,* 402, June, 1991.

Sisty-LePeau, N., Nielsen-Thompson, N., and Lutjen, D.: Use, Need, and Desire for Pain Control Procedures by Iowa Hygienists, *J. Dent. Hyg., 66,* 137, March–April, 1992.

Nonsurgical Periodontal Therapy: Postcare and Adjunctive Treatments

After scaling and root planing, as described in Chapter 33, an immediate evaluation is made, and instructions are provided for the patient to follow during personal therapeutic bacterial plaque control. Healing time depends on the severity of the gingival or periodontal infection at the outset, the depth of the pockets, and the extent of the required treatment. After health has been attained, it must be maintained. Planning for the short- and long-term maintenance program is described in Chapter 42, page 599.

Supplemental forms of treatment may be indicated. Gingival curettage and professional irrigation are described in this chapter. Table 34–1 defines terms related to postappointment care and adjunctive treatment.

IMMEDIATE EVALUATION

I. OBJECTIVES

A. Teeth

Observation and exploration reveal the immediate effects of instrumentation on the teeth. An objective has been to produce a smooth tooth surface, free from deposits and stains. The effect of specific instrumentation is to facilitate the patient's self-care by removing local factors, particularly calculus and overhanging fillings, that encourage plaque retention.

B. Gingiva

The gingival changes are not apparent immediately after instrumentation. Tissue regeneration and healing take approximately 1 week to 10 days for initial healing and even longer for maturation of connective tissue and keratinization of epithelium.

The objective at the treatment appointment is to *create an environment in which the gingival tissue can heal and be maintained in health by the patient.*

II. EXAMINATION

When scaling is accomplished over a series of appointments, each previously scaled quadrant or area is examined and rescaled as needed at each appointment. For the final evaluation, visual and tactile methods are applied carefully to each tooth surface. Instruments, methods, and procedures were described on page 508.

A. Visual

1. Compressed air should be used with a mouth mirror and adequate lighting to examine the supragingival areas and just below the gingival margins.
2. Transillumination methods are applied.
3. A disclosing agent can reveal small areas of remaining deposits.

B. Tactile

An evaluation by exploring immediately after completion of instrumentation is made to ascertain that the tooth surfaces are smooth and that all detectable calculus has been removed. The real evaluation, the true test of successful treatment, cannot be made until 1 to 2 weeks after the initial scaling and root planing. At that time, the response of the gingival tissue is apparent.

TABLE 34–1
KEY WORDS*: POSTCARE AND ADJUNCTIVE TREATMENTS

Antimicrobial therapy: use of specific chemical or pharmaceutical agents for the control or destruction of microorganisms, either systemically or at specific sites.

Attachment: with reference to the clinical attachment level of the gingival and periodontal tissues:

New attachment: the union of connective tissue or epithelium with a root surface that has been deprived of its original attachment apparatus; the new attachment may be epithelial adhesion and/or connective adaptation or attachment and may include new cementum.

Reattachment: the reunion of epithelial and connective tissues with root surfaces and bone such as occurs after an incision or injury.

Cannula (kan'ū-lah): tubular instrument placed in a cavity to introduce or withdraw fluid.

Chemotherapy (ke'mō-ther'ah-pē): treatment by means of chemical or pharmaceutical agents.

Controlled release: local delivery of a chemotherapeutic agent to a site-specific area; may be a patch to be worn on the skin or a polymeric fiber, such as that used to deliver an agent to a periodontal pocket.

Curettage (ku'rĕ-tahzh'): scraping or cleaning the walls of a cavity or surface using a curet.

Gingival curettage: process of debriding the soft tissue wall of a gingival or periodontal pocket.

Closed gingival curettage: removal of the diseased lining of a soft tissue pocket wall, including pocket and junctional epithelium and the underlying inflamed connective tissue; also called soft tissue curettage.

Open gingival curettage: a surgical flap procedure in which the diseased pocket epithelium and the underlying inflamed connective tissue are removed; also called surgical curettage, open-flap curettage, modified Widman flap, and excisional new attachment procedure (ENAP).

Healing (hēl'ing): restoration of structure and function of injured or diseased tissues; process of repair or regeneration of injured, lost, or surgically treated tissue.

First intention healing: primary union of a wound in which the incised tissue edges are approximated and held until union occurs.

Second intention healing: wound closure wherein the edges remain separated and the wound heals from the base and sides via the formation of granulation tissue.

Recolonization (rē kol'ŏ-nĭ-zā'shun): regrowth or multiplication of a particular bacterium or species; in periodontal therapy, the regrowth of the flora or a particular periodontal pathogen of a periodontal pocket after reduction or apparent elimination during therapy.

Repair: healing of a wound by tissue that does not fully restore the architecture or the function of the part.

Scaling: instrumentation of the crown and root surfaces to remove supra- and subgingival calculus, bacterial plaque, and stains.

Closed instrumentation: subgingival scaling accessed by way of the gingival sulcus or pocket covered by the pocket wall; dependent on tactile sensitivity.

Open instrumentation: access is provided by surgical flap to lay open to view the subgingival area, including furcations.

* Other definitions pertaining to irrigation may be found in table 23–1, page 353.

PATIENT INSTRUCTIONS AFTER SCALING AND ROOT PLANING

Personalized instructions are provided for each patient at the end of each dental hygiene and periodontal appointment. Printed general instructions help to give the patient a handy reference. An added personal note or underlining of significant parts of the printed material can let a patient sense the caring attitude of the professional team. Verbal instructions can be forgotten or misinterpreted by even the most conscientious patient.

Instruction pertaining to periodontal dressings is outlined in table 36–2 on pages 548 and 549. Many of the same principles can be applied for postoperative instruction when a dressing has not been applied.

Postoperative instruction is essential following scaling, particularly when the patient's gingiva has been hypersensitive or has hemorrhaged excessively, or when extensive subgingival instrumentation has been completed. Directions for postoperative care include suggestions for rinsing and toothbrushing. An explanation of what discomfort may be expected should also be given.

Dietary and nutritional factors may be discussed. The temporary use of bland foods lacking in strong, spicy seasonings, as well as continuing use of nutritional foods to promote healing, can be helpful.

I. RINSING

A warm solution is soothing to the tissues and improves the circulation, thereby helping healing. A suggested solution provides the appropriate concentration for osmotic balance of the salts of the solution with the salts of the oral tissue fluids.

A. Solutions Suggested for Use

1. *Hypertonic Salt Solution.* Level ½ teaspoonful of table salt in ½ cup (4 ounces) of warm water.

2. *Sodium Bicarbonate Solution.* Level ½ teaspoonful of baking soda in 1 cup (8 ounces) of warm water.

B. Directions for Rinsing

1. Every 2 hours; after eating; after toothbrushing; before retiring.
2. Use the rinse mouthful by mouthful, forcing the solution between the teeth.

II. TOOTHBRUSHING

The use of a soft brush is recommended after scaling and root planing. The patient must clearly understand the need for complete bacterial plaque removal.

EFFECTS OF SCALING AND ROOT PLANING

Scaling and root planing are basic to nonsurgical periodontal therapy. Clinically, they are aimed at the removal of extraneous calculus, microorganisms, and toxic materials so that, with adjunctive daily treatment by the patient, the gingival tissue may thrive in a healthy environment free of pathogenic microorganisms.

The outcomes and successes of treatment with scaling and root planing are influenced by many factors, including the severity of the periodontal infection at the outset, the instrumentation applied during treatment, and especially the motivation and compliance of the patient during the post-treatment period to minimize bacterial plaque accumulations.

Effects on the gingiva, pocket microorganisms, cementum, and endotoxin are summarized here.

I. EFFECT ON GINGIVA
A. Coincidental Curettage

Without intentional curettage during scaling and root planing, some debridement (coincidental inadvertent curettage) of the lining of the sulcus or pocket occurs.[1,2,3] In the research, this effect was noted particularly in the deeper aspects, where the pocket narrows toward the attachment area. The partial curettage that occurs results from the outer or unused side of the curet blade, even though a less-than-90° angulation of the face of the blade to the tooth surface is maintained.

The soft tissue attachment may be partially removed, depending on the severity of the inflammation, the size of the instrument, and the amount of trauma inflicted by the clinician. The objectives of curettage are described on page 528.

B. Healing

With scaling, root planing, and plaque control, the adjacent gingival tissue heals by resolution of the inflammation. Edema recedes, necrotic cells are cleared away, and the tissue regenerates.

Healing has been shown to start with beginning epithelial regeneration within 2 days of scaling. New attachment to the tooth surface has been demonstrated as early as 5 days, and complete regeneration occurs by approximately 2 weeks.[4,5] Healing time is generally related to the severity of the periodontal inflammation at the start of treatment.

After scaling and root planing, followed by bacterial plaque control by the patient, the formation of a long junctional epithelium can be expected.[6]

C. Clinical Changes

The objectives of scaling and root planing were outlined on page 506. The effects of treatment on the gingiva are the result of the removal of local infective agents, namely, bacterial plaque. In addition, the removal of plaque-retentive overhanging margins and rough calculus provides an environment for gingival healing.

Specific changes have been demonstrated in research, including reduced probing depths, reduced bleeding on probing, and gain of clinical attachment levels.[7,8,9]

II. EFFECT ON POCKET MICROORGANISMS[10,11,12,13]

The subgingival bacterial flora is changed after scaling and root planing as shown in table 34–2. Prior to instrumentation for treatment of periodontitis, the subgingival microorganisms are primarily anaerobic, gram-negative, motile forms, with bacterioides and spirochetes predominating.

After scaling and root planing, the total number of subgingival organisms decreases substantially. A shift to aerobic, gram-positive, nonmotile forms occurs. Spirochetes and bacterioides are reduced, and coccoid cells become more prominent.

With the conversion of the disease-producing gram-

TABLE 34–2
EFFECT OF INSTRUMENTATION ON POCKET MICROFLORA

Periodontal Infection Before Treatment	Periodontal Health After Treatment
Predominant flora is:	**Predominant flora is:**
Anaerobic	Aerobic
Gram-negative	Gram-positive
Motile	Nonmotile
Spirochetes, motile rods; pathogenic	Coccoid forms; nonpathogenic
Very high total count of all types of microorganisms	Much lower total counts of all types of microorganisms
Many leukocytes	Lower leukocyte counts

negative pocket microorganisms to a health-producing gram-positive flora, the gingiva reflects the changes. Gingival bleeding on probing is lessened, and the color, size, shape, and other characteristics assume a normal appearance.

Without personal daily plaque control, the microorganisms can return to pretreatment levels within an average of 42 days.[14] With plaque control, the repopulation of the pocket takes longer, even in susceptible patients. In many patients, nonsurgical periodontal therapy effects a gingival condition that can be maintained free from reinfection.

III. EFFECT ON TOOTH SURFACE AND ENDOTOXIN

Following subgingival scaling and root planing, some calculus frequently remains, particularly in deep pockets and in places in which instrumentation is anatomically difficult, such as furcations. Great skill is required to perform a thorough subgingival treatment where probing depths exceed 5 to 7 mm.[15,16,17]

For selected patients, small deposits of residual calculus appear not to present a serious healing problem. Re-evaluation after a short healing period following treatment can aid in recognizing when additional subgingival instrumentation is needed.

Endotoxin is a lipopolysaccharide (LPS) released from gram-negative bacterial cell walls. It occurs in the bacteria covering the cementum and superficially in the cementum itself. Endotoxin has been shown to be toxic to human cells.[18]

The removal of endotoxin was measured.[19] When tooth surfaces were scaled but not root planed, the endotoxin content of the surface was much greater than the content of healthy, unexposed root surfaces. After manual root planing, however, the exposed tooth surfaces were nearly as free of endotoxin as were the healthy, unexposed surfaces.[19]

Additional research has shown that endotoxin generally may be loosely attached to a root surface and may not penetrate as much as had been thought originally.[20,21] This and other studies have provided evidence that excessive root planing for the purpose of removing endotoxin apparently is not necessary.

GINGIVAL CURETTAGE

Gingival curettage is a selective procedure. When indicated, it is used to supplement the patient's disease control program (daily therapeutic plaque removal) and to enhance professional scaling and root planing.

I. PURPOSES OF GINGIVAL CURETTAGE
A. Overall Objectives

As a part of the treatment for the restoration of gingival health, with complete scaling and root planing and effective bacterial plaque control, curettage can contribute to

1. Reduction or elimination of inflammation.

2. Reduction or eradication of gingival or periodontal pockets.

B. Specific Objectives

Removal of the inflamed, ulcerated soft tissue of a pocket wall can

1. Allow inflammation to subside by establishing drainage for edema.
2. Cause shrinkage of the free gingiva and, hence, reduce pocket depth.
3. Remove area of soft tissue invaded by bacteria to discourage recolonization and disease redevelopment.
4. Promote fibrosis and healing.
5. Permit replacement of the diseased pocket lining with newly formed connective tissue and sulcular epithelium that can be maintained in health.
6. Contribute to a return of the gingiva to a normal contour.

II. SELECTION OF TREATMENT AREAS
A. Indications for Definitive Curettage

1. Gingival tissue with a soft, spongy consistency and other signs of inflammation (table 11–2, page 188).
2. Pockets that are relatively shallow (4 to 5 mm) and are suprabony.
3. Persistence of hyperemia, edema, and pocket depth after complete scaling and root planing.

B. Contraindications for Definitive Curettage

1. Gingival tissue with a firm, fibrous consistency contains fibrotic, collagenous elements that do not permit shrinkage of a pocket wall.
2. Thin, fragile pocket walls that could be punctured easily during instrumentation.
3. Acute periodontal inflammatory lesions, particularly necrotizing ulcerative gingivitis.
4. Periodontal conditions that require specific surgical treatment, such as
   a. Pockets that are deep and/or intrabony.
   b. Areas of narrow attached gingiva or mucogingival involvement.
   c. Furcation involvement.

C. Indications for Nondefinitive Curettage

1. As preparation for pocket elimination by surgical methods. Reduces inflammation and increases fibrosis.
2. As maintenance therapy. Aids in the control of recurrent infection.

III. PREPARATION FOR INSTRUMENTATION
A. Prerequisites

1. Adequate bacterial plaque removal must be performed daily. Otherwise, benefits from nonsurgical periodontal therapy are short-lived.

2. Complete scaling and root planing.
3. Removal of overhanging fillings.

B. Patient Preparation
1. *Explanation to Patient*
   a. Procedures.
   b. Possible postoperative discomforts.
   c. Expected results.
   d. Personal care responsibilities.
2. *Review of Patient's Medical History*
   a. Need for administration of antibiotic for prevention of bacteremia, or of other premedication, for certain risk patients.
   b. Limitations and special concerns.
3. *Anesthesia*
   a. Topical anesthesia. A topical application may be sufficient when the curettage is confined to an isolated area and when shallow pockets are present.
   b. Local anesthesia. Infiltration may be sufficient for certain patients and for limited areas. Block anesthesia is indicated for quadrant treatment of deep pockets.

C. Instruments
1. Root planing precedes curettage.
2. Curets for curettage should be kept separate from scaling and root planing curets. Marking tapes may prove helpful.
3. Curets must be very sharp for efficient instrumentation to prevent excess pressure and numbers of strokes.
4. When the same instruments are used for scaling and planing, they must be resharpened. A sterile stone for sharpening is part of every instrument set-up.

IV. STEPS FOR CLINICAL INSTRUMENTATION
A. Technique Objectives
The instrumentation is planned to remove
1. The diseased pocket lining epithelium and underlying inflamed connective tissue.
2. Tissue debris and chronic granulation tissue.
3. Particles of calcified debris not removed by irrigation and suction after scaling and planing.
4. Microorganisms embedded within the tissue.

B. Arrange Instruments and Equipment
Maintain aseptic field.

C. Isolate the Area
Use sterile sponges and adjust the saliva ejector.

D. Re-examine and Review
Use a probe to note pocket depths and pocket contour.

E. Select and Apply the Appropriate Curet
1. Use a modified pen grasp.
2. Establish a finger rest on a tooth near the area to be curetted. Fulcrum finger (ring finger supported by little finger) is applied and maintained.

F. Sequence
Begin with the most posterior tooth of the quadrant. For convenience of retraction and efficient continuity, work from posterior to anterior, facial surfaces, then lingual or palatal.

G. Angulation and Adaptation
1. Position the blade over the pocket to be treated. Blade is open and held at an angle of greater than 90°. For scaling and root planing, the blade is closed toward the tooth.
2. Note the relation of the handle, grasp, rest, and blade angle. By maintaining this relationship, one can promptly reposition the curet after insertion.
3. Insertion
   a. Direct the toe toward the opening of the pocket. Open the blade and slide under the margin.
   b. Move the curet to the base of the pocket. Use the round back to determine the base, where tension of the soft tissue can be felt.
4. Reposition the blade to correct angulation at approximately 70° between the face of the blade and the soft tissue pocket wall (figure 34–1).

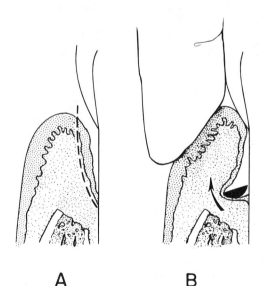

A   **B**

FIG. 34–1. Gingival Curettage. A. Broken line shows pocket tissue to be removed during gingival curettage, namely the pocket epithelium and the underlying inflamed connective tissue. **B.** Curet positioned at the bottom of the pocket with the cutting edge toward the gingival tissue wall. Pressure applied with a finger on the outside of the pocket provides support for the pressure of the curet as it is activated. The curet is angled for a vertical stroke as shown by the cross section of the blade and the arrow.

H. Strokes

1. *Maintain the Finger Rest.* Tighten the grasp slightly to permit definitive moderate pressure for removal of the pocket lining.
2. *Support the Pocket Wall*
   a. Facial and lingual or palatal surfaces. Apply a finger of the nonworking hand to the outer surface of the pocket wall to offset pressure of the curet and to produce effective cutting action (figure 34–1B).
   b. Interdental papilla. Press the curet toward the proximal surface of the adjacent tooth.
3. *Strokes.* Use even smooth strokes to minimize excess instrumentation.
   a. Vertical and oblique. Work toward the gingival margin to treat the walls of the pocket. Overlap deep strokes with those nearer the margin.
   b. Horizontal. Direct strokes circumferentially. Use a horizontal stroke to curet an entire facial or lingual surface.
      i. At the base of a pocket, keep the curet above the probing depth to prevent unnecessary detachment of attached connective tissue fibers under the epithelium.
      ii. A horizontal stroke is used near the gingival margin to finish off the ends of the vertical and oblique strokes.
   c. Removal of junctional epithelium. Research has shown that the attachment area is usually removed, or at least changed, during scaling and root planing when no deliberate strokes are applied to the attachment;[22] therefore, only conservative strokes need to be applied.
   d. Length of strokes
      i. Longer, continuous strokes produce clean areas of debrided pocket wall.
      ii. Length of strokes is governed by the tooth contour.
   e. Precaution. Evaluate the tissue. Do not pierce or tear the pocket wall.
4. *Proceed Systematically Around Each Tooth.* Overlap strokes at line angles.

I. Completion

1. *Determination.* An experienced sense of touch can distinguish the soft mushy granulation tissue from the underlying firm connective tissue. When the curet is sharp, only a few strokes are needed.
2. *Removal of Debris from Pocket.* Use suction.
3. *Test for Residual "Tags."* Use suction to pull "tags" of tissue out of the pocket. Remove with a sharp curet.

J. Irrigation

Irrigate with sterile water to limit the possibility of bacteremia.

K. Tissue Adaptation and Hemostasis

1. Press the area with a damp sponge to adapt the tissue closely and stop the bleeding.
2. Press to reduce the size of the blood clot. A thin clot is beneficial during healing.

L. Place a Dressing when Needed (page 545)

1. To hold detached papillary tissue over the interdental area; a suture may also be used.
2. To protect the healing tissue from trauma that might cause excess bleeding and thereby extend the healing period.
3. To minimize the size of the clot.

V. POSTOPERATIVE CARE

A. Postoperative Instructions

1. *Dressing Placed.* Printed instructions are advisable. Suggestions for care following dressing placement are found on page 548 (table 36–2).
2. *Without Dressing*
   a. Plaque removal is important. Use soft toothbrush with end-rounded filaments. Definite plaque removal with care taken not to traumatize the healing tissue is necessary.
   b. Rinse with warm weak saline solution (pages 526 and 527).

B. Follow-up

1. *Dressing Removal.* Dressing should be removed in approximately 1 week. Specific plaque removal instructions are given.
2. *Tooth Sensitivity.* Advise the patient that most sensitivity is transient. Toothbrushing with a fluoride dentifrice and daily use of a fluoride mouthrinse can be most effective. Desensitizing agents can be applied to persistent spots (page 558).
3. *Stain Removal.* Stain removal is not advised immediately following dressing removal because curettage leaves a wide healing area. An abrasive would be an irritant. Instruction for daily complete plaque removal by the patient is necessary to prevent reinfection.

HEALING FOLLOWING CURETTAGE

I. EFFECTS OF INSTRUMENTATION

Removal of the chronically inflamed ulcerated pocket lining and underlying inflamed connective tissue creates a surgical wound. Healing follows a pattern of epithelialization and collagenation and resolution of inflammation in the connective tissue. The effects are as follows:

A. Shrinkage of the gingival walls with fluid drainage.
B. Re-epithelialization with coverage of the exposed connective tissue.

C. Formation of a long junctional epithelium.

D. Formation of new connective tissue beneath the new epithelial lining of the sulcus and attachment.

E. Return to normal circulation.

II. STEPS IN HEALING

A. Formation of a blood clot immediately after curettage. The clot fills the pocket area, which is adapted against the tooth by pressure and a dressing.

B. Initial tissue reaction of inflammation as with any wound.

C. Proliferation of fibroblasts and new vessels to form granulation tissue.

D. Epithelial cells arise from the epithelium at the margin of the gingiva. The epithelium migrates in and over the granulation tissue by approximately 4 hours following the curettage.

E. New epithelium covers the sulcus lining within 5 to 6 days, and the new junctional epithelium begins to develop by 5 days.

F. Connective tissue healing proceeds and is well organized by 2 weeks.

G. Keratinization of oral (outer) epithelium may be observed by 2 weeks and reaches normal thickness by 28 to 40 days.

III. FACTORS AFFECTING HEALING

A. Residual and newly formed calculus. Repeated root planing is frequently necessary.

B. Plaque and other local irritants. Meticulous self-care must be supervised over several weeks following curettage.

C. Systemic factors may be involved when healing delay cannot be otherwise accounted for, but local factors must be rechecked first.

IV. CLINICAL APPEARANCE OF THE HEALED TISSUE

When healing is complete, the usual signs of healthy gingiva as outlined in table 11–2 on page 188 should be evident. Probe measurement in the sulcus should be minimal, the sulcus should be free from bleeding on probing, and the color, size, shape, and other characteristics should be normal.

PROFESSIONAL SUBGINGIVAL IRRIGATION

Professional subgingival irrigation is based on the premise that delivery of antimicrobial agents may enhance the effects of treatment by scaling and root planing. Irrigation into a pocket can disrupt the numbers of microorganisms left behind following instrumentation. Studies have shown that repopulation of the subgingival microflora can occur within weeks after treatment.[14] In addition, the reduction of the subgingival

flora depends on the ability of the clinician to remove subgingival plaque and calculus definitively; clearly, such removal is difficult in deep pockets. Residual calculus was reviewed on page 528.

Irrigation with an antimicrobial agent provides a supplemental therapeutic step and results in additional clinical benefits.[23]

I. DELIVERY METHOD

A presterilized disposable cannula, with a side port or end release (figure 34–2A), is used with one of the following:

A. Disposable hand syringe.

B. Specially designed jet irrigator.

C. Air-driven irrigation handpiece.

II. PROCEDURE

A. Prepare the cannula by bending it slightly as it is uncovered (figure 34–2B).

B. Insert the cannula subgingivally (figure 34–2C).

C. Allow the irrigant to fill the pocket.

D. Apply circumferentially, releasing solution at three points on the facial surface and three on the lingual surface.

E. Irrigate all teeth, quadrants, or specific selected sites as dictated by the patient's need.

III. RECOMMENDATIONS FOR USE
A. Preprocedural Delivery

An antimicrobial agent can aid in reducing the numbers of microorganisms to prevent aerosol contamination during instrumentation.

B. Preanesthesia Application

Used to reduce microorganisms before application of topical anesthetic in preparation for local anesthetic injection.

C. Maintenance Phase: Postprocedure Irrigation

1. Patient with site(s) not responding to traditional periodontal care.

2. Patient with gingivitis superimposed on periodontitis.

3. Patient with areas inaccessible to mechanical instrumentation because of root contour, furcations, or depth of pocket and in whom open scaling and root planing are not alternatives.

IV. ANTIMICROBIAL AGENTS

A variety of antimicrobial agents, saline solution, and water have been researched for professional irrigation with varying results. Products used include chlorhexidine gluconate and stannous fluoride.[23,24,25,26]

V. SPECIAL CONSIDERATIONS
A. Antibiotic Premedication

Professional irrigation requires premedication in patients susceptible to the effects of bacte-

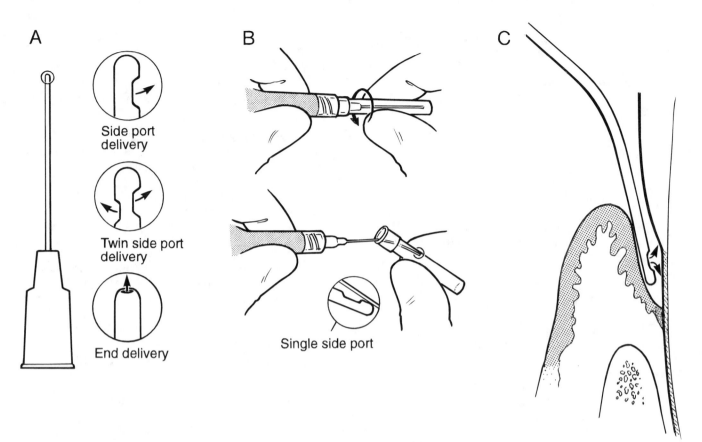

FIG. 34–2. Professional Irrigation. A. Types of cannula tips with side port or end delivery openings. **B.** Prepare the cannula for use by bending the sterile tip within the encasement to make the insertion easier. **C.** With knowledge of each probing depth, insert the cannula gently to near the bottom of a pocket. No force should be used.

remia. The usual procedure for all dental appointments should be followed.

B. Irrigation Pressure

Professional irrigation systems usually control the amount of pressure. Caution must be exercised, however, when irrigating with a disposable syringe because pressure may exceed the safety level for the oral tissues.

FACTORS TO TEACH THE PATIENT

I. Directions for posttreatment care.
II. Why pockets need to be treated; how curettage can contribute to pocket reduction or elimination.
III. Reasons for periodontal dressing placement.
IV. Postoperative care with and without a dressing. Care of teeth and gingiva not involved in the curettage.
V. Relationship of bacterial plaque and plaque control to healing.
VI. Desensitization, using proper toothbrushing

technique applied to cervical areas and a fluoride dentifrice and mouthrinse.

REFERENCES

1. **Ramfjord,** S. and Kiester, G.: The Gingival Sulcus and the Periodontal Pocket Immediately Following Scaling of Teeth, *J. Periodontol., 25,* 167, July, 1954.
2. **Moskow,** B.S.: Response of the Gingival Sulcus to Instrumentation: A Histological Investigation. I. The Scaling Procedure, *J. Periodontol., 33,* 282, July, 1962.
3. **Schaffer,** E.M., Stende, G., and King, D.: Healing of Periodontal Pocket Tissues Following Ultrasonic Scaling and Hand Planing, *J. Periodontol., 35,* 140, March-April, 1964.
4. **Stahl,** S.S., Weiner, J.M., Benjamin, S., and Yamada, L.: Soft Tissue Healing Following Curettage and Root Planing, *J. Periodontol., 42,* 678, November, 1971.
5. **Tagge,** D.L., O'Leary, T.J., and El-Kafrawy, A.H.: The Clinical and Histologic Response of Periodontal Pockets to Root Planing and Oral Hygiene, *J. Periodontol., 46,* 527, September, 1975.
6. **Caton,** J.G. and Zander, H.A.: The Attachment Between Tooth and Gingival Tissues after Periodic Root Planing and Soft Tissue Curettage, *J. Periodontol., 50,* 462, September, 1979.
7. **Pihlstrom,** B.L., McHugh, R.B., Oliphant, T.H., and Ortiz-Campos, C.: Comparison of Surgical and Nonsurgical Treatment

of Periodontal Disease. A Review of Current Studies and Additional Results after 6½ Years, *J. Clin. Periodontol., 10,* 524, September, 1983.

8. **Lindhe,** J., Westfelt, E., Nyman, S., Socransky, S.S., and Haffajee, A.D.: Long-term Effect of Surgical/Non-surgical Treatment of Periodontal Disease, *J. Clin. Periodontol., 11,* 448, August, 1984.

9. **Ramfjord,** S.P., Caffesse, R.G., Morrison, E.C., Hill, R.W., Kerry, G.J., Appleberry, E.A., Nissle, R.R., and Stults, D.L.: 4 Modalities of Periodontal Treatment Compared Over 5 Years, *J. Clin. Periodontol., 14,* 445, September, 1987.

10. **Listgarten,** M.A. and Helldén, L.: Relative Distribution of Bacteria at Clinically Healthy and Periodontally Diseased Sites in Humans, *J. Clin. Periodontol., 5,* 115, May, 1978.

11. **Slots,** J., Mashimo, P., Levine, M.J., and Genco, R.J.: Periodontal Therapy in Humans. I. Microbiologic and Clinical Effects of a Single Course of Periodontal Scaling and Root Planing, and of Adjunctive Tetracycline Therapy, *J. Periodontol., 50,* 495, October, 1979.

12. **van Winkelhoff,** A.J., van der Velden, U., and deGraaff, J.: Microbial Succession in Recolonizing Deep Periodontal Pockets after a Single Course of Supra- and Subgingival Debridement, *J. Clin. Periodontol., 15,* 116, February, 1988.

13. **Sbordone,** L., Ramaglia, L., Gulletta, E., and Iacono, V.: Recolonization of the Subgingival Microflora after Scaling and Root Planing in Human Periodontitis, *J. Periodontol., 61,* 579, September, 1990.

14. **Mousquès,** T., Listgarten, M.A., and Phillips, R.W.: Effect of Scaling and Root Planing on the Composition of the Human Subgingival Microbial Flora, *J. Periodont. Res., 15,* 144, March, 1980.

15. **Waerhaug,** J.: Healing of the Dento-epithelial Junction Following Subgingival Plaque Control. II. As Observed on Extracted Teeth, *J. Periodontol., 49,* 119, March, 1978.

16. **Rabbani,** G.M., Ash, M.M., and Caffesse, R.G.: The Effectiveness of Subgingival Scaling and Root Planing in Calculus Removal, *J. Periodontol., 52,* 119, March, 1981.

17. **Sherman,** P.R., Hutchens, L.H., Jewson, L.G., Moriarty, J.M., Greco, G.W., and McFall, W.T.: The Effectiveness of Subgingival Scaling and Root Planing. I. Clinical Detection of Residual Calculus, *J. Periodontol., 61,* 3, January, 1990.

18. **Aleo,** J.J., DeRenzis, F.A., Farber, P.A., and Varboncoeur, A.P.: The Presence and Biologic Activity of Cementum-bound Endotoxin, *J. Periodontol., 45,* 672, September, 1974.

19. **Jones,** W.A. and O'Leary, T.J.: The Effectiveness of *In Vivo* Root Planing in Removing Bacterial Endotoxin from the Roots of Periodontally Involved Teeth, *J. Periodontol., 49,* 337, July, 1978.

20. **Nakib,** N.M., Bissada, N.F., Simmelink, J.W., and Goldstine, S.N.: Endotoxin Penetration into Root Cementum of Periodontally Healthy and Diseased Human Teeth, *J. Periodontol., 53,* 368, June, 1982.

21. **Moore,** J., Wilson, M., and Kieser, J.B.: The Distribution of Bacterial Lipopolysaccharide (Endotoxin) in Relation to Periodontally Involved Root Surfaces, *J. Clin. Periodontol., 13,* 748, September, 1986.

22. **Ramfjord,** S. and Kiester, G.: The Gingival Sulcus and the Periodontal Pocket Immediately Following Scaling of Teeth, *J. Periodontol., 25,* 167, July, 1954.

23. **Southard,** S.R., Drisko, C.L., Killoy, W.J., Cobb, C.M., and Tira, D.E.: The Effect of 2% Chlorhexidine Digluconate Irrigation on Clinical Parameters and the Level of *Bacteroides gingivalis* in Periodontal Pockets, *J. Periodontol., 60,* 302, June, 1989.

24. **Schmid,** E., Kornman, K.S., and Tinanoff, N.: Changes of Subgingival Total Colony Forming Units and Black Pigmented Bacteroides after a Single Irrigation of Periodontal Pockets with 1.64% SnF$_2$, *J. Periodontol., 56,* 330, June, 1985.

25. **Mazza,** J.E., Newman, M.G., and Sims, T.N.: Clinical and Antimicrobial Effect of Stannous Fluoride on Periodontitis, *J. Clin. Periodontol., 8,* 203, June, 1981.

26. **Schlagenhauf,** U., Stellwag, P., and Fiedler, A.: Subgingival Irrigation in the Maintenance Phase of Periodontal Therapy, *J. Clin. Periodontol., 17,* 650, October, 1990.

SUGGESTED READINGS

Coldiron, N.B., Yukna, R.A., Weir, J., and Caudill, R.F.: A Quantitative Study of Cementum Removal with Hand Curettes, *J. Periodontol., 61,* 293, May, 1990.

Corbet, E.F., Vaughan, A.J., and Kieser, J.B.: The Periodontally-involved Root Surface, *J. Clin. Periodontol., 20,* 402, July, 1993.

Gantes, B.G., Nilvéus, R., Lie, T., and Leknes, K.N.: The Effect of Hygiene Instruments on Dentin Surfaces: Scanning Electron Microscopic Observations, *J. Periodontol., 63,* 151, March, 1992.

Greenstein, G.: Periodontal Response to Mechanical Non-surgical Therapy: A Review, *J. Periodontol., 63,* 118, February, 1992.

Kaldahl, W.B., Kalkwarf, K.L., Patil, K.D., and Molvar, M.P.: Evaluation of Gingival Suppuration and Supragingival Plaque Following 4 Modalities of Periodontal Therapy, *J. Clin. Periodontol., 17,* 642, October, 1990.

Kaldahl, W.B., Kalkwarf, K.L., Patil, K.D., and Molvar, M.P.: Responses of Four Tooth and Site Groupings to Periodontal Therapy, *J. Periodontol., 61,* 173, March, 1990.

Kepic, T.J., O'Leary, T.J., and Kafrawy, A.H.: Total Calculus Removal: An Attainable Objective? *J. Periodontol., 61,* 16, January, 1990.

Khatiblou, F.A. and Ghodssi, A.: Root Surface Smoothness or Roughness in Periodontal Treatment, *J. Periodontol., 54,* 365, June, 1983.

Loos, B., Nylund, K., Claffey, N., and Egelberg, J.: Clinical Effects of Root Debridement in Molar and Nonmolar Teeth. A 2-year Follow-up, *J. Clin. Periodontol., 16,* 498, September, 1989.

Nyman, S., Westfelt, E., Sarhed, G., and Karring, T.: Role of "Diseased" Root Cementum in Healing Following Treatment of Periodontal Disease. A Clinical Study, *J. Clin. Periodontol., 15,* 464, August, 1988.

O'Leary, T.J.: The Impact of Research on Scaling and Root Planing, *J. Periodontol., 57,* 69, February, 1986.

O'Leary, T.J. and Kafrawy, A.H.: Total Cementum Removal: A Realistic Objective? *J. Periodontol., 54,* 221, April, 1983.

Rateitschak-Plüss, E.M., Schwarz, J.-P., Guggenheim, R., Düggelin, M., and Rateitschak, K.H.: Non-surgical Periodontal Treatment: Where Are the Limits? *J. Clin. Periodontol., 19,* 240, April, 1990.

Ritz, L., Hefti, A.F., and Rateitschak, K.H.: An *In Vitro* Investigation on the Loss of Root Substance in Scaling with Various Instruments, *J. Clin. Periodontol., 18,* 643, October, 1991.

Robertson, P.B.: The Residual Calculus Paradox [Editorial], *J. Periodontol., 61,* 65, January, 1990.

Vanooteghem, R., Hutchens, L.H., Bowers, G., Kramer, G., Schallhorn, R., Kiger, R., Crigger, M., and Egelberg, J.: Subjective Criteria and Probing Attachment Loss to Evaluate the Effects of Plaque Control and Root Debridement, *J. Clin. Periodontol., 17,* 580, September, 1990.

Walsh, T.F. and Walmsley, A.D.: A New Method to Assess Damaging Effects on the Gingival Tissues of Non-surgical Instrumentation, *J. Clin. Periodontol., 18,* 785, November, 1991.

Wong, R., Hirsch, R.S., and Clarke, N.G.: Endodontic Effects of Root Planing in Humans, *Endo. Dent. Traumatol., 5,* 193, August, 1989.

Zappa, U., Smith, B., Simona, C., Graf, H., Case, D., and Kim, W.: Root Substance Removal by Scaling and Root Planing, *J. Periodontol., 62,* 750, December, 1991.

Zappa, U.E.: Factors Determining the Outcome of Scaling and Root Planing, *Can. Dent. Hyg./Probe, 26,* 152, Winter, 1992.

Effects on Pocket Flora

Ali, R.W., Lie, T., and Skaug, N.: Early Effects of Periodontal Therapy on the Detection Frequency of Four Putative Periodontal Pathogens in Adults, *J. Periodontol., 63,* 540, June, 1992.

Baehni, P., Thilo, B., Chapuis, B., and Pernet, D.: Effects of Ultrasonic and Sonic Scalers on Dental Plaque Microflora *In Vitro* and *In Vivo, J. Clin. Periodontol., 19,* 455, August, 1992.

Drisko, C.L. and Killoy, W.J.: Scaling and Root Planing: Removal of Calculus and Subgingival Organisms, *Curr. Opin. Dent., 1,* 74, February, 1991.

Garnick, J.J. and Dent, J.: A Scanning Electron Micrographical Study of Root Surfaces and Subgingival Bacteria after Hand and Ultrasonic Instrumentation, *J. Periodontol., 60,* 441, August, 1989.

Hinrichs, J.E., Wolff, L.F., Pihlstrom, B.L., Schaffer, E.M., Liljemark, W.F., and Bandt, C.L.: Effects of Scaling and Root Planing on Subgingival Microbial Proportions Standardized in Terms of Their Naturally Occurring Distribution, *J. Periodontol., 56,* 187, April, 1985.

Loos, B., Claffey, N., and Egelberg, J.: Clinical and Microbiological Effects of Root Debridement in Periodontal Furcation Pockets, *J. Clin. Periodontol., 15,* 453, August, 1988.

Renvert, S., Wikström, M., Dahlén, G., Slots, J., and Egelberg, J.: Effect of Root Debridement on the Elimination of *Actinobacillus actinomycetemcomitans* and *Bacteroides gingivalis* from Periodontal Pockets, *J. Clin. Periodontol., 17,* 345, July, 1990.

Renvert, S., Wikström, M., Dahlén, G., Slots, J., and Egelberg, J.: On the Inability of Root Debridement and Periodontal Surgery to Eliminate *Actinobacillus actinomycetemcomitans* from Periodontal Pockets, *J. Clin. Periodontol., 17,* 351, July, 1990.

Sato, K., Yoneyama, T., Okamoto, H., Dahlén, G., and Lindhe, J.: The Effect of Subgingival Debridement on Periodontal Disease Parameters and the Subgingival Microbiota, *J. Clin. Periodontol., 20,* 359, May, 1993.

Slots, J., Emrich, L.J., Genco, R.J., and Rosling, B.G.: Relationship Between Some Subgingival Bacteria and Periodontal Pocket Depth and Gain or Loss of Periodontal Attachment after Treatment of Adult Periodontitis, *J. Clin. Periodontol., 12,* 540, August, 1985.

Endotoxin

Cheetham, W.A., Wilson, M., and Kieser, J.B.: Root Surface Debridement—An *In Vitro* Assessment, *J. Clin. Periodontol., 15,* 288, May, 1988.

Chiew, S.Y.T., Wilson, M., Davies, E.H., and Kieser, J.B.: Assessment of Ultrasonic Debridement of Calculus-associated Periodontally-involved Root Surfaces by Limulus Amoebocyte Lysate Assay. An *In Vitro* Study, *J. Clin. Periodontol., 18,* 240, April, 1991.

Daly, C.G., Seymour, G.J., Kieser, J.B., and Corbet, E.F.: Histological Assessment of Periodontally Involved Cementum, *J. Clin. Periodontol., 9,* 266, May, 1982.

Smart, G.J., Wilson, M., Davies, E.H., and Kieser, J.B.: The Assessment of Ultrasonic Root Surface Debridement by Determination of Residual Endotoxin Levels, *J. Clin. Periodontol., 17,* 174, March, 1990.

Wilson, W.M., Moore, J., and Kieser, J.B.: Identity of Limulus Amoebocyte Lysate-active Root Surface Materials from Periodontally Involved Teeth, *J. Clin. Periodontol., 13,* 743, September, 1986.

Open Vs. Closed Root Planing

Brayer, W.K., Mellonig, J.T., Dunlap, R.M., Marinak, K.W., and Carson, R.E.: Scaling and Root Planing Effectiveness: The Effect of Root Surface Access and Operator Experience, *J. Periodontol., 60,* 67, January, 1989.

Buchanan, S.A. and Robertson, P.B.: Calculus Removal by Scaling/Root Planing With and Without Surgical Access, *J. Periodontol., 58,* 159, March, 1987.

Caffesse, R.G., Sweeney, P.L., and Smith, B.A.: Scaling and Root Planing With and Without Periodontal Flap Surgery, *J. Clin. Periodontol., 13,* 205, March, 1986.

Eaton, K.A., Kieser, J.B., and Davies, R.M.: The Removal of Root Surface Deposits, *J. Clin. Periodontol., 12,* 141, February, 1985.

Johnson, G.K., Reinhardt, R.A., and DuBois, L.M.: Comparison of Closed and Fiber-optic-augmented Sonic Scaling Performed by General Dentists, *Gen. Dent., 39,* 333, September-October, 1991.

Parashis, A.O., Anagnou-Vareltzides, A., and Demetriou, N.: Calculus Removal from Multirooted Teeth With and Without Surgical Access. (1) Efficacy on External and Furcation Surfaces in Relation to Probing Depth, *J. Clin. Periodontol., 20,* 63, January, 1993.

Parashis, A.O., Anagnou-Vareltzides, A., and Demetriou, N.: Calculus Removal from Multirooted Teeth With and Without Surgical Access. (II). Comparison Between External and Furcation Surfaces and Effect of Furcation Entrance Width, *J. Clin. Periodontol., 20,* 294, April, 1993.

Pedrazzoli, V., Kilian, M., Karring, T., and Kirkegaard, E.: Effect of Surgical and Non-surgical Periodontal Treatment on Periodontal Status and Subgingival Microbiota, *J. Clin. Periodontol., 18,* 598, September, 1991.

Reinhardt, R.A., Johnson, G.K., and Dubois, L.M.: Clinical Effects of Closed Root Planing Compared to Papilla Reflection and Fiber Optic Augmentation, *J. Periodontol., 62,* 317, May, 1991.

Schwarz, J.-P., Rateitschak-Plüss, E.M., Guggenheim, R., Düggelin, M., and Rateitschak, K.H.: Effectiveness of Open Flap Root Debridement with Rubber Cups, Interdental Plastic Tips and Prophy Paste, An SEM Study, *J. Clin. Periodontol., 20,* 1, January, 1993.

Instrumentation in Shallow Pockets

Knowles, J., Burgett, F., Morrison, E., Nissle, R., and Ramfjord, S.: Comparison of Results Following Three Modalities of Periodontal Therapy Related to Tooth Type and Initial Pocket Depth, *J. Clin. Periodontol., 7,* 32, February, 1980.

Lindhe, J., Westfelt, E., Nyman, S., Socransky, S.S., Heijl, L., and Bratthall, G.: Healing Following Surgical/Non-surgical Treatment of Periodontal Disease. A Clinical Study, *J. Clin. Periodontol., 9,* 115, March, 1982.

Linde, J., Socransky, S.S., Nyman, S., Haffajee, A., and Westfelt, E.: "Critical Probing Depths" in Periodontal Therapy, *J. Clin. Periodontol., 9,* 323, July, 1982.

Pihlstrom, B.L., Ortiz-Campos, C., and McHugh, R.B.: A Randomized Four-year Study of Periodontal Therapy, *J. Periodontol., 52,* 227, May, 1981.

Curettage

Buethe, C.G., Kalkwarf, S.R., Kalkwarf, K.L., and Tussing, G.J.: Gingival Curettage. Is It a Viable Therapy Alternative? *Dent. Hyg., 60,* 24, January, 1986.

Carranza, F.A. and Perry, D.A.: *Clinical Periodontology for the Dental Hygienist.* Philadelphia, W.B. Saunders Co., 1986, pp. 221–224.

Echeverria, J.J. and Caffesse, R.G.: Effects of Gingival Curettage when Performed 1 Month after Root Instrumentation, A Biometric Evaluation, *J. Clin. Periodontol., 10,* 277, May, 1983.

Fedi, P.F., ed.: *The Periodontic Syllabus,* 2nd ed. Philadelphia, Lea & Febiger, 1989, pp. 126–131.

Grant, D.A., Stern, I.B., and Listgarten, M.A., eds.: *Periodontics,* 6th ed. St. Louis, Mosby, 1988, pp. 740–760, 823–837.

Hirschfeld, L.: Subgingival Curettage in Periodontal Treatment, *J. Am. Dent. Assoc., 44,* 301, March, 1952.

Hoag, P.M. and Pawlak, E.A.: *Essentials of Periodontics,* 4th ed. St. Louis, Mosby, 1990, pp. 208–209.

Knowles, J., Burgett, F., Morrison, E., Nissle, R., and Ramfjord, S.: Comparison of Results Following Three Modalities of Periodontal Therapy Related to Tooth Type and Initial Pocket Depth, *J. Clin. Periodontol., 7,* 32, February, 1980.

Pattison, A.M. and Pattison, G.L.: *Periodontal Instrumentation,* 2nd ed. Norwalk, CT, Appleton & Lange, 1992, pp. 426–437.

Pollack, R.P.: Curettage: A New Look at an Old Technique, *Int. J. Periodontics Restorative Dent., 4,* 24, No. 5, 1984.

Smith, B.A. and Echeverri, M.: The Removal of Pocket Epithelium: A Review, *J. West. Soc. Periodont./Periodont. Abstr., 32,* 45, No. 2, 1984.

Chemical Curettage

Adcock, J.E., Berry, W.C., and Kalkwarf, K.L.: Effect of Sodium Hypochlorite Solution on the Subgingival Microflora of Juvenile Periodontitis Lesions, *Pediatr. Dent., 5,* 190, September, 1983.

Forgas, L.: Soft Tissue Curettage. Literature Review, *Dent. Hyg., 60,* 402, September, 1986.

Forgas, L.B. and Gound, S.: The Effects of Antiformin-Citric Acid Chemical Curettage on the Microbial Flora of the Periodontal Pocket, *J. Periodontol., 58,* 153, March, 1987.

Kalkwarf, K.L., Tussing, G.J., and Davis, M.J.: Histologic Evaluation of Gingival Curettage Facilitated by Sodium Hypochlorite Solution, *J. Periodontol., 53,* 63, February, 1982.

Vieira, E.M., O'Leary, T.J., and Kafrawy, A.H.: The Effect of Sodium Hypochlorite and Citric Acid Solutions on Healing of Periodontal Pockets, *J. Periodontol., 53,* 71, February, 1982.

Professional Irrigation

Chapple, I.L.C., Walmsley, A.D., Saxby, M.S., and Moscrop, H.: Effect of Subgingival Irrigation with Chlorhexidine During Ultrasonic Scaling, *J. Periodontol., 63,* 812, October, 1992.

Greenstein, G.: The Ability of Subgingival Irrigation to Enhance Periodontal Health, *Compendium, 9,* 327, April, 1988.

Lofthus, J.E., Waki, M.Y., Jolkovsky, D.L., Otomo-Corgel, J., Newman, M.G., Flemmig, T., and Nachnani, S.: Bacteremia Following Subgingival Irrigation and Scaling and Root Planing, *J. Periodontol., 62,* 602, October, 1991.

Oosterwaal, P.J.M., Matee, M.I., Mikx, F.H.M., van't Hof, M.A., and Renggli, H.H.: The Effect of Subgingival Debridement with Hand and Ultrasonic Instruments on the Subgingival Microflora, *J. Clin. Periodontol., 14,* 528, October, 1987.

Oosterwaal, P.J.M., Mikx, F.H.M., van't Hof, M.A., and Renggli, H.H.: Comparison of the Antimicrobial Effect of the Application of Chlorhexidine Gel, Amine Fluoride Gel and Stannous Fluoride Gel in Debrided Periodontal Pockets, *J. Clin. Periodontol., 18,* 245, April, 1991.

Reynolds, M.A., Lavigne, C.K., Minah, G.E., and Suzuki, J.B.: Clinical Effects of Simultaneous Ultrasonic Scaling and Subgingival Irrigation with Chlorhexidine. Mediating Influence of Periodontal Probing Depth, *J. Clin. Periodontol., 19,* 595, September, 1992.

Taggart, J.A., Palmer, R.M., and Wilson, R.F.: A Clinical and Microbiological Comparison of the Effects of Water and 0.02% Chlorhexidine as Coolants During Ultrasonic Scaling and Root Planing, *J. Clin. Periodontol., 17,* 32, January, 1990.

Wikesjo, U.M.E., Reynolds, H.S., Christersson, L.A., Zambon, J.J., and Genco, R.J.: Effects of Subgingival Irrigation on *A. actinomycetemcomitans, J. Clin. Periodontol., 16,* 116, February, 1989.

35

Acute Gingival Conditions

The dental hygienist frequently participates in clinical treatment procedures for acute gingival lesions. Key words for acute conditions are defined in table 35–1.

NECROTIZING ULCERATIVE GINGIVITIS/PERIODONTITIS

Necrotizing ulcerative gingivitis (NUG) or necrotizing ulcerative periodontitis (NUP) are acute, inflammatory, destructive diseases of the periodontium. Other names that have been used include necrotizing gingivitis (NG), acute necrotizing ulcerative gingivitis (ANUG), trench mouth, Vincent's infection, Vincent's disease, and ulceromembranous gingivitis.

The condition may be superimposed over existing periodontitis. With recurrent attacks of the gingival infection, bone loss and other symptoms of periodontitis can develop. The condition is then called necrotizing ulcerative periodontitis (NUP) or necrotizing periodontitis (NP).

Although NUG may occur at any age, it is usually seen among young people between ages 15 and 30. It is rare in children under 10 years of age in the United States, but is not uncommon in young children from low socioeconomic groups studied in South America and in some developing countries.[1,2] Malnutrition and lowered resistance to infection are significant predisposing factors. Individuals with Down's syndrome have been shown to have an increased incidence of NUG, as described on page 754.

An increased incidence of NUG/NUP has been diagnosed in HIV-positive individuals.[3] Destructive rapid progressive periodontitis has many of the signs of NUP and is related to a lowered immune system.

CLINICAL RECOGNITION

I. INITIAL SIGNS AND SYMPTOMS
The patient reports
  A. Sudden onset.
  B. Pain and soreness caused by slight pressure, such as during chewing and toothbrushing; may be intensified by hot or highly seasoned foods. Gentle probing may produce an exaggerated pain response.
  C. Bleeding that occurs spontaneously or on slight pressure.
  D. Poor appetite.
  E. Metallic or other unpleasant taste.

II. CHARACTERISTIC CLINICAL FINDINGS
  A. Interdental necrosis with ulceration of the papillae produces crater-like defects in the col area. In early disease, only the tips of papillae are involved, followed by progressive destruction of the entire papillae and extension to the marginal gingiva facially and lingually (figure 35–1).
  B. A pseudomembrane may form over the necrotic area. It is a gray, loose, necrotic slough that, when wiped off, exposes a red and shiny hemorrhagic gingiva.
  C. The membranous ulceration may be seen locally, that is, between two or three teeth, or it may be generalized throughout both maxillary and mandibular arches.
  D. Other clinical findings that usually accompany the characteristic signs and symptoms are
    1. Debris, materia alba, and plaque that collect

TABLE 35–1
KEY WORDS: ACUTE GINGIVAL CONDITIONS

Abscess (ab′ses): localized collection of pus in a circumscribed or walled-off area formed by the disintegration of tissues.

  Acute: runs a relatively short course; produces pain and local inflammation.

  Chronic: slow development with little evidence of inflammation; usually an intermittent pus discharge; may follow an acute abscess.

  Periodontal: localized in the periodontal tissues; also called **lateral** or **parietal.**

Fetor oris (fe′tor ŏ′ris): foul, offensive odor from the mouth; halitosis.

Fistula (fis′tū-lah): a pathologic sinus or abnormal passage that leads from an abscess to the surface of the gingiva or mucosa.

Malaise (mal āz′): feeling of general indisposition, uneasiness, discomfort; may be early indication of illness.

Necrosis (nĕ-krō′sĭs): death of tissue; morphologic changes indicative of cell death caused by enzymatic degradation.

Necrotizing ulcerative periodontitis (NUP): Severe and rapidly progressive disease that has a distinctive erythema of the free gingiva, attached gingiva, and the alveolar mucosa; extensive soft tissue necrosis that usually starts with the interdental papillae; marked loss of periodontal attachment; deep probing depths may not be evident because of marked recession.

Parenteral (pah-ren′ter-al): not administered by way of the alimentary canal, but, for example, subcutaneous, intramuscular, or intravenous.

Pseudomembrane (soo′dō-mem′brān): false membrane; false layer of tissue that covers a surface.

Purulent (pu′roo-lent): accompanied by or containing pus.

Sinus tract (sī′nus): a channel that connects with an abscess or suppurating area.

Ulceration (ul′sĕ-rā′shun): formation or development of an ulcer with loss of epithelial surface and sloughing of necrotic inflammatory tissue.

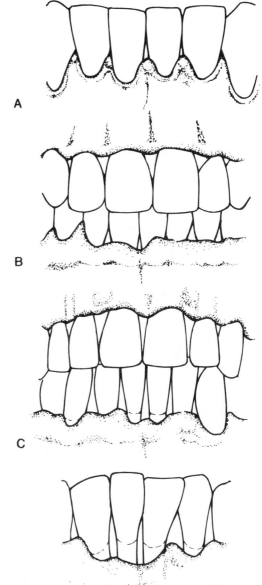

FIG. 35–1. Necrotizing Ulcerative Gingivitis/Periodontitis. A. Early lesion with blunted papillae and interdental necrosis. **B.** Increased destruction with loss of interdental tissue; rolled margins of the gingiva. **C.** More advanced destruction with recession and interdental cratering. **D.** Very advanced lesions, with loss of attached gingiva, recession, and tooth mobility.

profusely because the patient avoids brushing the sensitive teeth and gingiva.

  2. Fetor oris (bad breath) that is often severe. It is caused by necrotic tissue, stagnant saliva, and breakdown products of blood and debris.

  3. Increased salivation.

E. A few patients have signs of systemic involvement. Examination should always be made to detect the presence of the following:

  1. Malaise.

  2. Lymphadenopathy of submaxillary and cervical nodes.

  3. Possible slight elevation of body temperature.

III. PREDISPOSING FACTORS

NUG is an infectious disease caused by a fusospirochetal complex of microbes that develops and increases in association with predisposing factors that have lowered the body's defenses. Other major predisposing factors are stress, very poor oral hygiene, inadequate diet, and tobacco smoking.

A. Local Factors

NUG is rarely, if ever, seen in a clean, healthy, cared-for, and professionally supervised mouth. Many of the factors that can be considered predisposing are the same as those that predispose to chronic marginal gingivitis.

Predisposing factors include

1. Pre-existing gingivitis and/or periodontitis.
2. Inadequate personal oral care with general neglect.
3. Tobacco use.
4. Factors related to retention of microorganisms and deposits.
   a. Calculus as a retainer for plaque and debris.
   b. Open contacts, which encourage food impaction and stagnation.
   c. Oral habits, for example, mouth breathing.
   d. Periodontal pockets, which retain microorganisms and debris.
   e. Malposition of teeth; overcrowding.
   f. Iatrogenic causes, such as overhanging fillings.
   g. Tissue flap, for example, over a partially erupted third mandibular molar.
   h. Open carious lesions.

B. Stress Factors

1. Acute anxiety related to life situations is a common characteristic of patients with NUG. In susceptible people, the condition has been found to occur or recur during periods of stress. Examples include students during examination periods, military men in combat, and people during important decision-making times.
2. Emotional stress is frequently accompanied by poor oral care, improper diet, excessive smoking, overexertion, interrupted sleep, and other deviations in health habits.

C. Systemic: Disease-resistance Factors

1. Dietary and nutritional inadequacies; vitamin deficiencies.
2. Recent illnesses; frequent upper respiratory infections; debilitating diseases, such as infectious mononucleosis, pernicious anemia, hepatitis or human immunodeficiency virus (HIV) infection.
3. Side effects of chemotherapy and radiation.
4. Fatigue; insufficient sleep.

IV. ETIOLOGY

Bacteriologic and immunologic factors are implicated. For many years, bacteriologic smears were made from the NUG lesion and examined by microscope for the presence of fusiform bacilli and spirochetes. The smear test is no longer considered significant for making a diagnosis.

NUG has not been identified as a communicable disease. Research has shown that a transfer of organisms from an infected patient does not produce the typical disease.

A. Microbiologic Factors[4,5]

Of the many types of organisms found in NUG lesions, fusiform bacilli and medium-sized spirochetes predominate. The constant flora has been shown to include *Treponema* and *Selenomonas* species, *Prevotella intermedia*, *Porphyromonas gingivalis*, and *Fusobacterium* species.

B. Immune Factors[6,7]

Patients with NUG may have depressed polymorphonuclear leukocyte (PMN) responsiveness in chemotaxis and phagocytosis, as well as other signs of altered host response. A high incidence of NUG has been shown in patients with acquired immune deficiency syndrome (AIDS).[3] Such an altered immune response permits opportunistic microorganisms to flourish and destructive periodontal infections to develop.

V. COURSE OF DEVELOPMENT
A. Description of the Lesion

1. NUG is superimposed on gingivitis or periodontitis.
2. Ulceration and necrosis begin in the col area.
3. Both epithelial tissue and connective tissue are involved.
4. The disease process progresses to involve the entire papilla, and eventually, to the marginal gingiva on the facial and lingual surfaces.
5. The pseudomembrane covering the lesion is a necrotic slough of the surface epithelium. It contains leukocytes, bacteria, epithelial cells, and fibrin.
6. Connective tissue shows the signs of acute inflammation. It is hyperemic and filled with leukocytes, and its capillaries are engorged. When the pseudomembrane is lifted, the red inflamed connective tissue can be seen.

B. Microscopic Examination

The four layers in the lesion have been described from observations made by electron microscopy.[8] All layers contain spirochetes.

1. *Bacterial Zone.* The most superficial zone consists primarily of a mass of varied bacteria, including a few spirochetes.
2. *Neutrophil-rich Zone.* Under the bacterial zone is a layer of leukocytes, predominantly neutrophils. Microorganisms, including many spirochetes, are found among the leukocytes.
3. *Necrotic Zone.* This zone contains disintegrating tissue cells, many spirochetes, and other bacteria.
4. *Spirochetal Infiltration Zone.* In this nonnecrotized layer where tissue components are still

E. Dental Caries

A diseased pulp leading to a periapical abscess is caused by either trauma to the tooth or dental caries extending inward until the pulp becomes infected. A carious lesion may also be present with a periodontal abscess and may complicate the differential diagnosis.

F. Radiographic Examination

Early stages of either a periapical or a periodontal abscess are not evident in a radiograph. A widening of the periodontal ligament space may appear.

V. TREATMENT

Two phases of treatment are used for the patient with a periodontal abscess. The first is for immediate relief of acute symptoms, and the second is the definitive treatment followed by preventive maintenance. The entire plan should be explained to the patient at the outset.

A. Objectives of Emergency Treatment

1. Relieve pain.
2. Establish drainage.
3. Determine need for systemic antibiotic therapy.

B. Review Medical History

Determine necessary preappointment precautions, such as the need for antibiotic premedication (pages 102 and 103).

C. Examination for Systemic Involvement

Antibiotic medication is frequently prescribed by the dentist when systemic involvement is definite.

1. Determine and record the patient's body temperature (pages 106 and 107).
2. Examine submaxillary and neck nodes for lymphadenopathy (page 119).

D. Provide Anesthesia

When the abscess is confined to the gingival area, and the drainage may be expected to cause little if any discomfort, a topical anesthetic may suffice. Usually, block anesthesia is indicated.

E. Methods for Drainage[12,13,14]

1. *Via Pocket or Sulcus Opening.* Isolate the area, swab with a topical antiseptic, and use a probe to gain admission into the sulcus or pocket. Gently probe circumferentially until an opening into the abscess is found. Drainage usually begins promptly.

   Use a curet to open the area, and locate and remove a foreign body irritant when it is known to be present from the history obtained from the patient. Scaling and root planing are performed as needed.

2. *Direct Incision.* The type of incision varies. A horizontal or semilunar incision may be made directly over the abscess. A drain may be needed to keep the incision open long enough to drain completely. A piece of rubber dam or iodophor gauze may be used.

   All incisions should be avoided, if possible, to prevent gingival recession from a vertical incision, unsightly scars from any type of incision, or complications during healing.

F. Postoperative Instructions

Rinsing with hot saline solution every 2 hours is advised. The patient should return for observation in 24 to 48 hours. Relief from pain and discomfort can be expected and appointments for definitive treatment planned. Plaque control instruction is initiated or continued, and scaling and root planing are completed.

G. Anticipated Results

1. Acute symptoms are resolved.
2. Pain relief occurs within a short time following the initiation of drainage, because the pressure is released from within the abscessed area.
3. Extruded tooth returns to its normal position.
4. Swelling is reduced.
5. Temporary comfort is obtained for the patient; the lesion is reduced to a standard chronic lesion that requires additional treatment.
6. If drainage is not complete, an acute lesion may develop into a lesion with a chronic sinus.

VI. DEFINITIVE THERAPY

Whatever pocket elimination procedures are indicated should be completed within a reasonable time to prevent further complications. Careful and regular bacterial plaque control with scaling and root planing are usually needed.

TECHNICAL HINTS

I. Provide explicit directions concerning rinsing when hydrogen peroxide is prescribed. Extended use of oxygenating drugs can cause tissue changes.

II. Instructions for patients can be printed or written. Because instructions change each day during the acute phase, individual slips should be prepared, using paper of different colors. Printed instructions can be personalized with added written notations.

FACTORS TO TEACH THE PATIENT

I. Premature discontinuation of treatment for NUG because acute signs have subsided can lead to recurrence of the infection.

II. The role of diet, rest, and bacterial plaque control in the prevention of NUG.

III. The avoidance of an oral irrigating device in the presence of acute inflammatory conditions. Microorganisms may be forced into the tissues beneath a pocket, and bacteremia can be produced.

REFERENCES

1. **Jimenez** L., M. and Baer, P.N.: Necrotizing Ulcerative Gingivitis in Children: A 9 Year Clinical Study, *J. Periodontol., 46,* 715, December, 1975.

2. **Enwonwu,** C.O.: Infectious Oral Necrosis (cancrum oris) in Nigerian Children: A Review, *Community Dent. Oral Epidemiol., 13,* 190, June, 1985.

3. **Greenspan,** D., Greenspan, J.S., Schiødt, M., and Pindborg, J.J.: *AIDS and the Mouth. Diagnosis and Management of Oral Lesions.* Copenhagen, Munksgaard, 1990, pp. 104–108.

4. **Loesche,** W.J., Syed, S.A., Laughon, B.E., and Stoll, J.: The Bacteriology of Acute Necrotizing Ulcerative Gingivitis, *J. Periodontol., 53,* 223, April, 1982.

5. **Falkler,** W.A., Martin, S.A., Vincent, J.W., Tall, B.D., Nauman, R.K., and Suzuki, J.B.: A Clinical, Demographic and Microbiologic Study of ANUG Patients in an Urban Dental School, *J. Clin. Periodontol., 14,* 307, July, 1987.

6. **Dennison,** D.K., Smith, B., and Newland, J.R.: Immune Responsiveness and ANUG, *J. Dent. Res., 64,* 197, Abstract 204, March, 1985.

7. **Rowland,** R.W., Mestecky, J., Gunsolley, J.C., and Cogen, R.B.: Serum IgG and IgM Levels to Bacterial Antigens in Necrotizing Ulcerative Gingivitis, *J. Periodontol., 64,* 195, March, 1993.

8. **Listgarten,** M.A.: Electron Microscopic Observations on the Bacterial Flora of Acute Necrotizing Ulcerative Gingivitis, *J. Periodontol., 36,* 328, July-August, 1965.

9. **Nizel,** A.E.: *Nutrition in Preventive Dentistry: Science and Practice,* 2nd ed. Philadelphia, W.B. Saunders Co., 1981, pp. 485–488.

10. **Armitage,** G.C.: *Biologic Basis of Periodontal Maintenance Therapy.* Berkeley, CA, Praxis Publishing Co., 1980, pp. 154–159.

11. **Gillette,** W.B. and Van House, R.L.: Ill Effects of Improper Oral Hygiene Procedures, *J. Am. Dent. Assoc., 101,* 476, September, 1980.

12. **Carranza,** F.A.: *Glickman's Clinical Periodontology,* 7th ed. Philadelphia, W.B. Saunders Co., 1990, pp. 668–672.

13. **Grant,** D.A., Stern, I.B., and Listgarten, M.A., eds.: *Periodontics,* 6th ed. St. Louis, Mosby, 1988, pp. 429–431.

14. **Fedi,** P.F., ed.: *The Periodontic Syllabus,* 2nd ed. Philadelphia, Lea & Febiger, 1989, pp. 188–190.

SUGGESTED READING

Necrotizing Ulcerative Gingivitis

Carranza, F.A.: *Glickman's Clinical Periodontology,* 7th ed. Philadelphia, W.B. Saunders Co., 1990, pp. 149–159, 657–664.

Cogen, R.B., Stevens, A.W., Jr., Cohen-Cole, S., Kirk, K., and Freeman, A.: Leukocyte Function in the Etiology of Acute Necrotizing Ulcerative Gingivitis, *J. Periodontol., 54,* 402, July, 1983.

Deasy, M.J., Sullivan, A.J., and Rosenblatt, G.: Acute Necrotizing Ulcerative Gingivitis Associated with Von Willebrand's Disease: A Case Report, *Compendium, 11,* 652, November, 1990.

Fedi, P.F., ed.: *The Periodontic Syllabus,* 2nd ed. Philadelphia, Lea & Febiger, 1989, pp. 190–197.

Grant, D.A., Stern, I.B., and Listgarten, M.A., eds.: *Periodontics,* 6th ed. St. Louis, Mosby, 1988, pp. 398–412.

Haroian, A. and Vissichelli, V.P.: A Patient Instruction Guide Used in Treating ANUG, *Gen. Dent., 39,* 40, January-February, 1991.

Hartnett, A.C. and Shiloah, J.: The Treatment of Acute Necrotizing Ulcerative Gingivitis, *Quintessence Int., 22,* 95, February, 1991.

MacCarthy, D. and Claffey, N.: Acute Necrotizing Ulcerative Gingivitis Is Associated with Attachment Loss, *J. Clin. Periodontol., 18,* 776, November, 1991.

O'Hehir, T.E.: ANUG Data Needs Study, *RDH, 11,* 30, October, 1991.

Riviere, G.R., Weisz, K.S., Simonson, L.G., and Lukehart, S.A.: Pathogen-related Spirochetes Identified Within Gingival Tissue from Patients with Acute Necrotizing Ulcerative Gingivitis, *Infect. Immun., 59,* 2653, August, 1991.

Periodontal Abscess

Ahl, D.R., Hilgeman, J.L., and Snyder, J.D.: Periodontal Emergencies, *Dent. Clin. North Am., 30,* 459, July, 1986.

Dello Russo, N.M.: The Post-prophylaxis Periodontal Abscess: Etiology and Treatment, *Int. J. Periodontics Restorative Dent., 5,* 28, No. 1, 1985.

Flood, T.R., Samaranayake, L.P., MacFarlane, T.W., McLennan, A., MacKenzie, D., and Carmichael, F.: Bacteremia Following Incision and Drainage of Dento-alveolar Abscesses, *Br. Dent. J., 169,* 51, July 21, 1990.

Killoy, W.J.: Treatment of Periodontal Abscesses, in Genco, R.J., Goldman, H.M., and Cohen, D.W., eds.: *Contemporary Periodontics.* St. Louis, Mosby, 1990, pp. 475–482.

Kryshtalskyj, E.: Management of the Periodontal Abscess, *Can. Dent. Assoc. J., 53,* 519, July, 1987.

Smith, R.G. and Davies, R.M.: Acute Lateral Periodontal Abscesses, *Br. Dent. J., 161,* 176, September 6, 1986.

Topoll, H.H., Lange, D.E., and Müller, R.F.: Multiple Periodontal Abscesses after Systemic Antibiotic Therapy, *J. Clin. Periodontol., 17,* 268, April, 1990.

Dressings and Sutures

A dressing may be placed over the surgical wound following periodontal surgery. Dressings are used for all surgical procedures by some clinicians, used occasionally by others, and used rarely by still others. Some key words related to the use of dressings and sutures are described in table 36–1.

I. PURPOSES AND USES

A. Provide protection for the surgical wound against external irritation or trauma.
B. Help to prevent postoperative bleeding by maintaining the initial clot in place.
C. Support mobile teeth during healing.
D. Assist in shaping or molding the newly formed tissues; aid in holding a flap in place or immobilizing a graft.
E. Retain site-specific fibers for slow-release chemotherapy in pockets.

II. CHARACTERISTICS OF ACCEPTABLE DRESSING MATERIAL

An acceptable periodontal dressing should have the following characteristics:

A. Be conveniently prepared, placed, and removed with minimal discomfort for the patient.
B. Be adhesive to itself, the teeth, and adjacent tissues, and maintain retention in interdental areas.
C. Provide stability and flexibility to withstand distortion and displacement without fracturing.
D. Be nontoxic and nonirritating to the oral tissues.
E. Have a smooth surface that resists accumulation of bacterial plaque.
F. Not damage or stain the teeth or restorative materials.
G. Be esthetically acceptable.

TYPES OF DRESSINGS

Traditionally, dressings were classified into two groups: those that contained eugenol and those that did not contain eugenol. With the development of new products, the "noneugenol-containing" dressings have been reclassified into chemical-cure and visible-light-cure systems. They may be available as ready-mix, paste-paste, or paste-gel.

Products are reviewed by the American Dental Association, Council on Dental Therapeutics. Approved products use the ADA CDT Seal (figure 23–15, page 370) and are listed in *Clinical Products in Dentistry*, published annually.

I. ZINC OXIDE WITH EUGENOL DRESSING
A. Basic Ingredients

1. *Powder.* Zinc oxide, powdered rosin, and tannic acid. Formerly, asbestos fiber was used as a binder in some formulas. Because airborne asbestos is a recognized pulmonary health hazard, dental team members responsible for mixing periodontal dressings frequently and in quantity may become overexposed. Asbestos fiber is no longer an acceptable ingredient of dressings.
2. *Liquid.* Eugenol, with an oil, such as peanut or cottonseed, and thymol.

545

TABLE 36–1
KEY WORDS: DRESSINGS AND SUTURES

Border mold: the shaping of the peripheries of a dressing by manual manipulation of the tissue adjacent to the borders (for example, lips, cheeks) to duplicate the contour and size of the vestibule.

Catgut suture: an absorbable suture prepared from submucous connective tissue of the small intestine of healthy sheep.

Chemical cure (kem´ĭ-kal): mode of self-cure or setting of a dressing in which the ingredients unite in a chemical process that starts as soon as the blending is complete; the setting time is influenced by warm temperature and the addition of an accelerator.

Coapt (kō´apt): to approximate, as the edges of a wound; bring edge to edge with no overlap.

Dressing (dres´ing): any of various materials used for covering and protecting a wound; in dentistry may sometimes be called a pack.

   Pressure dressing: for maintaining pressure to control bleeding or to hold a particular flap or graft in position.

   Protective dressing: to shield the area from injury or trauma.

Eugenol (ū´jĕn-ol): constituent of clove oil; used in early periodontal dressings with zinc oxide for its alleged antiseptic and anodyne properties; more recently found to be toxic, to elicit allergic reactions, and to hinder, more than promote, healing.

Suture (su´chur): a stitch or series of stitches made to secure apposition of the edges of a surgical or traumatic wound.

   Absorbable suture: becomes dissolved in body fluids and disappears, for example, catgut and tendon.

   Interrupted suture: one in which each stitch is made with a separate piece of material; in contrast with a **continuous suture** made with an uninterrupted length that connects each stitch with the previous one.

Swage (swāj): to fuse, as suture material to the end of a suture needle.

Visible-light cure: light activation using a photocure system; shorter curing time than self-cure (chemical cure); does not start setting until the light is activated, thereby allowing longer working time for adapting the dressing material.

B. Examples

Well-known dressings are Ward's (Wonderpack); and Kirkland Periodontal Pack.

C. Advantages

1. *Consistency.* Firm and heavy; provides support for tissues and flaps.
2. *Slow Setting.* Good working time.
3. *Preparation and Storage.* Can be prepared in quantity and stored (frozen) in work-size pieces.

D. Disadvantages

1. *Taste.* Sharp, unpleasant taste.
2. *Tissue Reaction.* Irritating to membranes; sensitivity reactions can occur.
3. *Consistency.* Dressing is hard, brittle, and breaks easily. Rough surface encourages bacterial plaque retention.

II. CHEMICAL-CURED DRESSING

The ingredients of commercial products are trade secrets, but some general information about available dressings can be found. Two examples of chemical-cured dressings are PerioCare and Coe-Pak.

A. Basic Ingredients[1]

1. *PerioCare.* Paste-gel.
   a. Paste. Zinc oxide, magnesium oxide, calcium hydroxide, vegetable oils.
   b. Gel. Resins, fatty acids, ethyl cellulose, lanolin, calcium hydroxide.
2. *Coe-pak.* Paste-paste.
   a. Base. Rosin, cellulose, natural gums and waxes, fatty acid, chlorothymol, zinc acetate, alcohol.
   b. Accelerator. Zinc oxide, vegetable oil, chlorothymol, magnesium oxide, silica, synthetic resin, coumarin.

B. Advantages

1. *Consistency.* Pliable, easy to place with light pressure.
2. *Smooth Surface.* Comfortable to patient; resists plaque and debris deposits.
3. *Taste.* Acceptable.
4. *Removal.* Easy, often comes off in one piece.

III. VISIBLE-LIGHT-CURED DRESSING

Visible-light-cured (VLC) dressing (Barricaid) is available in a syringe for direct application when appropriate, or from a mixing pad for indirect application. The same light-curing unit is used that is available in most dental practices for composite restorations and sealants.

A. Basic Ingredients[1]

Gel ingredients include polyether urethane dimethacrylate resin, silanated silica, visible-light-cure photo-initiator and accelerator, stabilizer, and colorant.

B. Advantages

1. *Color.* More like gingiva than are most other dressings.
2. *Setting.* Does not start until activated by the light-curing unit. (Exposure before placement should be limited because daylight in a room can activate it slightly.)
3. *Removal.* Easy, often comes off in one piece.

6. **Grant,** Stern, and Listgarten: op. cit., pp. 638–641.
7. **Pashley,** D.H.: Mechanisms of Dentin Sensitivity, *Dent. Clin. North Am., 34,* 449, July, 1990.
8. **Brännström,** M., Lindén, L.Å., and Åström, A.: The Hydrodynamics of the Dental Tubule and of Pulp Fluid. A Discussion of Its Significance in Relation to Dentinal Sensitivity, *Caries Res., 1,* 310, No. 4, 1967.
9. **Greenhill,** J.D. and Pashley, D.H.: The Effects of Desensitizing Agents on the Hydraulic Conductance of Human Dentin *In Vitro, J. Dent. Res., 60,* 686, March, 1981.
10. **Addy,** M. and Dowell, P.: Dentine Hypersensitivity—A Review. Clinical and *In Vitro* Evaluation of Treatment Agents, *J. Clin. Periodontol., 10,* 351, July, 1983.
11. **Dowell,** P. and Addy, M.: Dentine Hypersensitivity—A Review. I. Aetiology, Symptoms and Theories of Pain Production, *J. Clin. Periodontol., 10,* 341, July, 1983.
12. **Ong,** G.: Desensitizing Agents. A Review, *Clin. Prev. Dent., 8,* 14, May-June, 1986.
13. **Trowbridge,** H.O. and Silver, D.R.: A Review of Current Approaches to In-office Management of Tooth Hypersensitivity, *Dent. Clin. North Am., 34,* 561, July, 1990.
14. **Collaert,** B. and Fischer, C.: Dentine Hypersensitivity: A Review, *Endod. Dent. Traumatol., 7,* 145, August, 1991.
15. **Grossman,** L.I.: A Systematic Method for the Treatment of Hypersensitive Dentin, *J. Am. Dent. Assoc., 22,* 592, April, 1935.
16. **Colaneri,** J.N.: A Simple Treatment of Hypersensitive Cervical Dentin, *Oral Surg. Oral Med. Oral Pathol., 5,* 276, March, 1952.
17. **Meffert,** R.M. and Hoskins, S.W.: Effect of a Strontium Chloride Dentifrice in Relieving Dental Hypersensitivity, *J. Periodontol., 35,* 232, May-June, 1964.
18. **Minkoff,** S. and Axelrod, S.: Efficacy of Strontium Chloride in Dental Hypersensitivity, *J. Periodontol., 58,* 470, July, 1987.
19. **Hodosh,** M.: A Superior Desensitizer—Potassium Nitrate, *J. Am. Dent. Assoc., 88,* 831, April, 1974.
20. **Green,** B.L., Green, M.L., and McFall, W.T.: Calcium Hydroxide and Potassium Nitrate as Desensitizing Agents for Hypersensitive Root Surfaces, *J. Periodontol., 48,* 667, October, 1977.
21. **Tarbet,** W.J., Silverman, G., Stolman, J.M., and Fratarcangelo, P.A.: Clinical Evaluation of a New Treatment for Dentinal Hypersensitivity, *J. Periodontol., 51,* 535, September, 1980.
22. **Hiatt,** W.H. and Johansen, E.: Root Preparation. I. Obturation of Dentinal Tubules in Treatment of Root Hypersensitivity, *J. Periodontol., 43,* 373, June, 1972.
23. **Pashley,** D.H., Kalathoor, S., and Burnham, D.: The Effects of Calcium Hydroxide on Dentin Permeability, *J. Dent. Res., 65,* 417, March, 1986.
24. **Lukomsky,** E.H.: Fluorine Therapy for Exposed Dentin and Alveolar Atrophy, *J. Dent. Res., 20,* 649, December, 1941.
25. **Hoyt,** W.H. and Bibby, B.G.: Use of Sodium Fluoride for Desensitizing Dentin, *J. Am. Dent. Assoc., 30,* 1372, September 1, 1943.
26. **Minkov,** B., Marmari, I., Gedalia, I., and Garfunkel, A.: The Effectiveness of Sodium Fluoride Treatment With and Without Iontophoresis on the Reduction of Hypersensitive Dentin, *J. Periodontol., 46,* 246, April, 1975.
27. **Miller,** J.T., Shannon, I.L., Kilgore, W.G., and Bookman, J.E.: Use of a Water-free Stannous Fluoride-containing Gel in the Control of Dental Hypersensitivity, *J. Periodontol., 40,* 490, August, 1969.
28. **Blong,** M.A., Volding, B., Thrash, W.J., and Jones, D.L.: Effects of a Gel Containing 0.4 Percent Stannous Fluoride on Dentinal Hypersensitivity, *Dent. Hyg., 59,* 489, November, 1985.
29. **Zinner,** D.D., Duany, L.F., and Lutz, H.J.: A New Desensitizing Dentifrice: Preliminary Report, *J. Am. Dent. Assoc., 95,* 982, November, 1977.
30. **Muzzin,** K.B. and Johnson, R.: Effects of Potassium Oxalate on Dentin Hypersensitivity *In Vivo, J. Periodontol., 60,* 151, March, 1989.
31. **Javid,** B., Barkhordar, R.A., and Bhinda, S.V.: Cyanoacrylate—A New Treatment for Hypersensitive Dentin and Cementum, *J. Am. Dent. Assoc., 114,* 486, April, 1987.
32. **Brännström,** M., Johnson, G., and Nordenvall, K.-J.: Transmission and Control of Dentinal Pain: Resin Impregnation for the Desensitization of Dentin, *J. Am. Dent. Assoc., 99,* 612, October, 1979.
33. **American Dental Association,** Ad Hoc Advisory Committee on Dentinal Hypersensitivity, Council on Dental Therapeutics: Recommendations for Evaluating Agents for the Reduction of Dentinal Hypersensitivity, *J. Am. Dent. Assoc., 112,* 709, May, 1986.
34. **Renton-Harper,** P. and Midda, M.: NdYAG Laser Treatment of Dentinal Hypersensitivity, *Br. Dent. J., 172,* 13, January 11, 1992.
35. **Starr,** C.B., Mayhew, R.B., and Pierson, W.P.: The Efficacy of Hypnosis in the Treatment of Dentin Hypersensitivity, *Gen. Dent., 37,* 13, January-February, 1989.
36. **Gillam,** D.G. and Newman, H.N.: Iontophoresis in the Treatment of Cervical Dentinal Sensitivity—A Review, *J. West. Soc. Periodont./Periodont. Abstr., 38,* 129, No. 4, 1990.
37. **McBride,** M.A. Gilpatrick, R.O., and Fowler, W.L.: The Effectiveness of Sodium Fluoride Iontophoresis in Patients with Sensitive Teeth, *Quintessence Int., 22,* 637, August, 1991.

SUGGESTED READINGS

Absi, E.G., Addy, M., and Adams, D.: Dentine Hypersensitivity. A Study of the Patency of Dentinal Tubules in Sensitive and Nonsensitive Cervical Dentine, *J. Clin. Periodontol., 14,* 280, May, 1987.

Addy, M., Mostafa, P., and Newcombe, R.G.: Dentine Hypersensitivity: The Distribution of Recession, Sensitivity and Plaque, *J. Dent., 15,* 242, December, 1987.

Cuenin, M.F., Scheidt, M.J., O'Neal, R.B., Strong, S.L., Pashley, D.H., Horner, J.A., and Van Dyke, T.E.: An *In Vivo* Study of Dentin Sensitivity: The Relation of Dentin Sensitivity and the Patency of Dentin Tubules, *J. Periodontol., 62,* 668, November, 1991.

Fusayama, T.: Etiology and Treatment of Sensitive Teeth, *Quintessence Int., 19,* 921, December, 1988.

Haugen, E. and Johansen, J.R.: Tooth Hypersensitivity after Periodontal Treatment. A Case Report Including SEM Studies, *J. Clin. Periodontol., 15,* 399, July, 1988.

Kerns, D.G., Scheidt, M.J., Pashley, D.H., Horner, J.A., Strong, S.L., and Van Dyke, T.E.: Dentinal Tubule Occlusion and Root Hypersensitivity, *J. Periodontol., 62,* 421, July, 1991.

Knight, N.N., Lie, T., Clark, S.M., and Adams, D.F.: Hypersensitive Dentin: Testing of Procedures for Mechanical and Chemical Obliteration of Dentinal Tubuli, *J. Periodontol., 64,* 366, May, 1993.

Orchardson, R. and Collins, W.J.N.: Clinical Features of Hypersensitive Teeth, *Br. Dent. J., 162,* 253, April 11, 1987.

Oyama, T. and Matsumoto, K.: A Clinical and Morphological Study of Cervical Hypersensitivity, *J. Endod., 17,* 500, October, 1991.

Reinhart, T.C., Killoy, W.J., Love, J., Overman, P.R., and Sakumura, J.S.: The Effectiveness of a Patient-applied Tooth Desensitizing Gel. A Pilot Study, *J. Clin. Periodontol., 17,* 123, February, 1990.

Yoshiyama, M., Noiri, Y., Ozaki, K., Uchida, A., Ishikawa, Y., and Ishida, H.: Transmission Electron Microscopic Characterization of Hypersensitive Human Radicular Dentin, *J. Dent. Res., 69,* 1293, June, 1990.

Treatment Agents
Addy, M., Loyn, T., and Adams, D.: Dentine Hypersensitivity—Effects of Some Proprietary Mouthwashes on the Dentine Smear Layer: A SEM Study, *J. Dent., 19,* 148, June, 1991.

Cooley, R.L. and Sandoval, V.A.: Effectiveness of Potassium Oxalate Treatment on Dentin Hypersensitivity, *Gen. Dent., 37,* 330, July-August, 1989.

Lawson, K., Gross, K.B.W., Overman, P.R., and Anderson, D.: Effectiveness of Chlorhexidine and Sodium Fluoride in Reducing Dentin Hypersensitivity, *J. Dent. Hyg., 65,* 340, September, 1991.

Liu, G.-H. and Morimoto, M.: Magnesium Sulphate as a New Desensitizing Agent, *J. Oral Rehabil., 18,* 363, July, 1991.

Mazor, Z., Brayer, L., Friedman, M., and Steinberg, D.: Topical Varnish Containing Strontium in a Sustained-release Device as Treatment for Dentin Hypersensitivity, *Clin. Prev. Dent., 13,* 21, May-June, 1991.

Overman, P.R.: Calcium Hypophosphate as a Root Desensitizing Agent, *Dent. Hyg., 57,* 30, August, 1983.

Pashley, D.H., Leibach, J.G., and Horner, J.A.: The Effects of Burnishing NaF/Kaolin/Glycerin Paste on Dentin Permeability, *J. Periodontol., 58,* 19, January, 1987.

Dentifrices

Addy, M., Mostafa, P., and Newcombe, R.G.: Effect on Plaque of Five Toothpastes Used in the Treatment of Dentin Hypersensitivity, *Clin. Prev. Dent., 12,* 28, October-November, 1990.

Clark, D.C., Al-Joburi, W., and Chan, E.C.S.: The Efficacy of a New Dentifrice in Treating Dentin Sensitivity: Effects of Sodium Citrate and Sodium Fluoride as Active Ingredients, *J. Periodont. Res., 22,* 89, March, 1987.

Gillam, D.G., Newman, H.N., Bulman, J.S., and Davies, E.H.: Dentifrice Abrasivity and Cervical Dentinal Hypersensitivity. Results 12 Weeks Following Cessation of 8 Weeks' Supervised Use, *J. Periodontol., 63,* 7, January, 1992.

Gillam, D.G., Newman, H.N., Davies, E.H., and Bulman, J.S.: Clinical Efficacy of a Low Abrasive Dentifrice for the Relief of Cervical Dentinal Hypersensitivity, *J. Clin. Periodontol., 19,* 197, March, 1992.

Kanapka, J.A.: Over-the-counter Dentifrices in the Treatment of Tooth Hypersensitivity, *Dent. Clin. North Am., 34,* 545, July, 1990.

Martens, L.C. and Surmont, P.A.: Effect of Anti-sensitive Toothpastes on Opened Dentinal Tubules and on Two Dentin-bonded Resins, *Clin. Prev. Dent., 13,* 23, March-April, 1991.

Mason, S., Levan, A., Crawford, R., Fisher, S., and Gaffar, A.: Evaluation of Tartar Control Dentifrices *In Vitro* Models of Dentin Sensitivity, *Clin. Prev. Dent., 13,* 6, January, 1991.

Ong, G. and Strahan, J.D.: Effect of a Desensitizing Dentifrice on Dentinal Hypersensitivity, *Endod. Dent. Traumatol., 5,* 213, October, 1989.

Iontophoresis

Gangarosa, L.P., Buettner, A.L., Baker, W.P., Buettner, B.K., and Thompson, W.O.: Double-blind Evaluation of Duration of Dentin Sensitivity Reduction by Fluoride Iontophoresis, *Gen. Dent., 37,* 316, July-August, 1989.

Kern, D.A., McQuade, M.J., Scheidt, M.J., Hanson, B., and Van Dyke, T.E.: Effectiveness of Sodium Fluoride on Tooth Hypersensitivity With and Without Iontophoresis, *J. Periodontol., 60,* 386, July, 1989.

Parr, O.D. and Brokaw, W.C.: Economical Iontophoresis for Dentistry, *Quintessence Int., 20,* 841, November, 1989.

Wilson, J.M., Fry, B.W., Walton, R.E., and Gangarosa, L.P.: Fluoride Levels in Dentin after Iontophoresis of 2% NaF, *J. Dent. Res., 63,* 897, June, 1984.

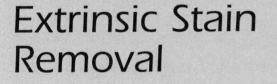

Extrinsic Stain Removal

38

After treatment by scaling, root planing, and other periodontal therapy, the teeth are assessed for the presence of stains. The use of polishing agents for stain removal is a selective procedure that not every patient needs, especially on a routine basis.

Stains on the teeth are not etiologic factors for any disease or destructive process. Therefore, the removal of stains is for esthetic, not for health, reasons. The need to remove stains by polishing should be evaluated after the plaque is under control, because some stains are incorporated in plaque and can be removed during brushing and flossing by the patient.

The objectives for stain removal may need to be clarified, because polishing has been a routine procedure in many offices and clinics. Information should be provided for each patient concerning individual needs.

When the assessment is made, several factors must be taken into consideration. These factors are described in this chapter. Key words related to stain removal, instruments, coronal polishing, and air-polishing are defined in table 38–1.

EFFECTS OF POLISHING

Because of the potentially detrimental effects, the needs of an individual patient must be reviewed before stain removal. *Professional judgment based on patient need decides when a service is to be included in a treatment plan.*

I. BACTEREMIA
Because bacteremia can be created during the use of power-driven stain removal instruments, the *medical history* must be recorded initially and then reviewed and updated at succeeding appointments.

Bacteremias result from manipulation of the gingival tissues. In one research study, 11 of 39 children (mean age, 9 years) developed bacteremia following application of a rubber cup with a prophylaxis paste.[1] It is recommended that use of a rubber cup be withheld until the plaque is under control and the gingiva do not bleed when the patient brushes.

For patients at risk, particularly those with damaged or abnormal heart valves, prosthetic valves, joint replacements, rheumatic heart disease, and other conditions listed on pages 102 and 103, antibiotic prophylaxis as outlined by the American Heart Association is needed.

II. ENVIRONMENTAL FACTORS
A. Aerosol Production
Aerosols are created during use of all rotary instruments, including a prophylaxis handpiece with a polishing paste and the air and water sprays used during rinsing.[2] The biologic contaminants of aerosols stay suspended for long periods and provide a potential means for disease transmission to dental personnel, as well as to succeeding patients (pages 14 and 15).

The use of rotary instruments should be limited when a patient is known to have a communicable disease. Precautions for hepatitis B and other diseases were described on page 65.

B. Spatter
Protective eyewear is needed for all dental team members and for the patient. Serious eye damage has occurred as a result of spatter in the eye from a polishing paste or from instruments. Constituents of commercial prophylaxis pastes may include various chemicals, such as oils, that can aggravate a severe inflammatory response.[3]

TABLE 38–1 **KEY WORDS AND ABBREVIATIONS: EXTRINSIC STAIN REMOVAL**
Abrasion (ah-bra'zhun): wearing away of surface material by friction. **Abrasive** (ah-bra'siv): a material composed of particles of sufficient hardness and sharpness to cut or scratch a softer material when drawn across its surface; available in various particle sizes. **Airbrasive:** air-powered device using air and water pressure to deliver a controlled stream of a specially processed sodium bicarbonate in a slurry through the handpiece nozzle; also called airabrasive, air-polishing, air-powder abrasive, or air-powered slurry. **Binder:** substance used to hold abrasive particles together; examples are ceramic bonding used for mounted abrasive points, electroplating for binding diamond chips for rotary instruments, and rubber or shellac for soft discs. **Coronal polishing:** polishing of the anatomic crowns of the teeth to remove bacterial plaque and extrinsic stains; does not involve calculus removal. **Glycerin** (glis'er-in): clear, colorless, syrupy fluid used as a vehicle and sweetening agent for drugs and as a solvent and vehicle for abrasive agents. **Grit:** with reference to abrasive agents, grit is the particle size. **Polishing:** the production, especially by friction, of a smooth, glossy, mirror-like surface that reflects light; a very fine agent is used for polishing after a coarser agent is used for cleaning. **p.s.i.:** pounds per square inch. **r.p.m.:** revolutions per minute. **Slurry:** thin, semifluid suspension of a solid in a liquid.

III. EFFECT ON TEETH

A. Removal of Tooth Structure

Polishing for 30 seconds with a pumice paste may remove as much as 4 μm of the outer enamel.[4] Performed repeatedly over the years, the tooth loss could be substantial. The effect has particular significance for children because the surfaces of young, newly erupted teeth are incompletely mineralized.

Cementum and dentin are softer and more porous, so greater amounts of these can be removed during polishing than of the enamel.[5,6] When cementum is exposed because of gingival recession, polishing of the exposed surfaces should be avoided. Also to be avoided are areas of demineralization. Nearly three times more surface enamel is lost from abrasive polishing over demineralized white spots than over intact enamel.[7]

B. Increased Roughness

A coarse abrasive may create a rougher tooth surface than existed before polishing. Grooves and scratches created by an abrasive applied with a rubber cup have been studied microscopically.[8,9]

C. Areas of Thin Enamel

Certain patients have teeth with thin enamel, such as those with amelogenesis imperfecta (page 284) or those over a demineralized area (figure 29–3, page 438).

Removal of tooth structure in the cervical portion of the tooth, where enamel is thin and cementum is exposed, can create unnecessary sensitivity. Special treatment problems may follow. These areas should not be polished with an abrasive because dentinal tubules can be exposed.

D. Removal of Fluoride-rich Surface

More important than the amount of enamel lost during polishing is that the outermost layer of tooth structure contains the greatest amounts of fluoride.[10] The surface fluoride protects against dental caries. The concentration of fluoride drops quickly inward toward the dentin, so that, if the surface layer is polished away, the protection is greatly diminished.

The *fluoride-rich surface* is important and should not be removed. Certain conditions increase caries susceptibility and therefore preclude the removal of this surface through polishing. Patients with *xerostomia* from any cause, for example drug or radiation therapy, cannot afford to have the enamel surface weakened by polishing. In contrast, their therapy must include daily addition of concentrated fluoride, usually through self-applied methods, such as rinsing or gel tray.

When upon assessment stain removal is shown to be required and therefore loss of the fluoride-rich surface is unavoidable, topical fluoride (gel or solution) must be applied in an attempt to replace the lost protection.[11] Fluoride uptake is minimal from prophylaxis pastes as compared with that from topical solutions or gels; therefore, a paste is not a substitute. In addition to topical application, daily self-applied fluoride should be recommended and prescribed. All patients need a fluoride-containing dentifrice, and in addition, a rinse, chewable tablet, or gel tray can be used, depending on the patient's age and caries susceptibility.

E. Heat Production

Steady pressure with a rapidly revolving rubber cup or bristle brush and a minimum of wet abrasive agent can create sufficient heat to cause pain and discomfort for the patient. Damage to the pulp by the heat has not been documented, but the pulps of young people are large and may be more susceptible to heat. The rule is light pressure, a slow-motion instrument, and plenty of moisture mixed with the abrasive agent.

Serio, F.G., Strassler, H.E., Litkowski, L.J., Moffitt, W.C., and Krupa, C.M.: The Effect of Polishing Pastes on Composite Resin Surfaces. A SEM Study, *J. Periodontol., 59,* 837, December, 1988.

Stoddard, J.W. and Johnson, G.H.: An Evaluation of Polishing Agents for Composite Resins, *J. Prosthet. Dent., 65,* 491, April, 1991.

Wilson, F., Heath, J.R., and Watts, D.C.: Finishing Composite Restorative Materials, *J. Oral Rehabil., 17,* 79, January, 1990.

Tooth Whitening

Berry, J.H.: What About Whiteners? Safety Concerns Explored, *J. Am. Dent. Assoc., 121,* 223, August, 1990.

Croll, T.P.: Enamel Microabrasion for Removal of Superficial Dysmineralization and Decalcification Defects, *J. Am. Dent. Assoc., 120,* 411, April, 1990.

Gegauff, A.G., Rosenstiel, S.F., Langhout, K.J., and Johnston, W.M.: Evaluating Tooth Color Change from Carbamide Peroxide Gel, *J. Am. Dent. Assoc., 124,* 65, June, 1993.

Howard, W.R.: Patient-applied Tooth Whiteners, *J. Am. Dent. Assoc., 123,* 57, February, 1992.

Tong, L.S.M., Pang, M.K.M., Mok, N.Y.C., King, N.M., and Wei, S.H.Y.: The Effects of Etching, Micro-abrasion, and Bleaching on Surface Enamel, *J. Dent. Res., 72,* 67, January, 1993.

39

The Porte Polisher

The porte polisher is a prophylactic hand instrument constructed to hold a wood polishing point at a contra-angle. Figure 39–1A shows an assembled porte polisher.

Manual stain removal is accomplished by applying pressure with the wood point on the tooth surfaces as a moist abrasive is applied. The firm, carefully directed, rhythmic strokes impart a vigorous massage to the periodontal tissues. This is considered beneficial to the periodontal ligament because the periodontal fibers serve as a cushion for the slight movement of the tooth that occurs with the pressure of the instrument. Fones described the beneficial effects to the gingival margin.[1] He suggested that the gentle bumping of the wood point on the tissue causes a light pressure and release that have a massaging effect in producing a stimulation of the peripheral circulation.

I. PURPOSES AND USES

The entire stain removal procedure may be accomplished with the porte polisher, although such an approach is unusual in routine practice because of the time factor. The porte polisher and the prophylaxis angle are compared in table 39–1.

Patients can be highly appreciative of smooth, quiet, manual instrumentation. For certain patients, under particular circumstances and for selected procedures, porte polishing is specifically indicated. Functions, purposes, and uses of the porte polisher are suggested as follows:

A. Removes stains from the natural and restored surfaces of the teeth.
B. Effective for cervical areas and exposed cementum or dentin of teeth that are hypersensitive to the heat produced by even a slowly revolving rubber polishing cup. A superfine, unflavored abrasive mixed with water only is appreciated by the patient and causes less abrasion of tooth structure.
C. Effective for care of titanium implant abutments.
D. Adapts to tooth surfaces that are inaccessible to a prophylaxis angle, such as the following:
   1. Exposed proximal surfaces of the teeth of patients who have undergone periodontal surgery.
   2. Lingual surfaces of lingually inclined mandibular molars, or distal surfaces of maxillary third permanent molars.
E. Indicated for a patient with an infectious disease to prevent aerosol production and hence disease dissemination.
F. Instrument of choice for application of certain desensitizing agents for exposed cementum and dentin (page 558).
G. Useful for the homebound or bedridden patient when portable power-driven equipment is not available.
H. Helpful for orientation of small children, disabled patients, or other patients apprehensive of power-driven equipment.

II. CHARACTERISTICS OF A PORTE POLISHER

Several types of porte polishers are available for use. Practical features that influence selection follow.

A. Can be taken apart conveniently for cleaning and sterilization (figure 39–1B).
B. Does not rust or discolor when given ordinary care.
C. Has convenient adjustment for attachment of wood points of various widths.
D. Is lightweight for comfort of the clinician during use.

576

TABLE 40-1
KEY WORDS: AMALGAM RESTORATIONS

Amalgam: an alloy of one or more metals in combination with mercury. A dental amalgam contains silver, copper, tin, and other metals.

Burnishing: process of smoothing a surface by rubbing.

Cavosurface junction: the junction of any wall of a cavity preparation with the unprepared tooth structure; encircles the preparation.

Corrosion (kŏ-rō′zhun): chemical deterioration on the surface of an amalgam restoration that usually begins as a tarnish.

Ditching: formation of a gap or groove between the cavity preparation margin and the amalgam.

Finishing: process that involves removing marginal irregularities, defining anatomic contours, and smoothing away surface roughness of a restoration.

Flash: type of overhang in which a thin layer of amalgam extends beyond the cavosurface junction; also called a feather ledge.

Margination: process of removing excess restorative material to establish a smooth cavosurface margin, to smooth the surfaces of the restorative material, and to recontour functional tooth anatomy.

Overcontour: an excess of amalgam such that the normal anatomic form is altered.

Overhang: area of a restoration where the restorative material extends outward past the cavosurface margin of the cavity preparation.

Polishing: process carried out after placement of a restoration to remove minute scratches from the surface of a restoration and obtain a smooth, shiny luster.

Recontour: instrumentation to reshape and remove marginal excess and to restore the natural anatomic form.

Tarnish: a discoloration of the surface of a metal restoration.

A. Design of the cavity preparation.
B. Mix and manipulation of the dental material.
C. Condensation during placement of the restoration.
D. Prevention of contamination and moisture.
E. Finishing and polishing.
F. Care of the completed restoration by a daily preventive program of bacterial plaque control, low cariogenic diet, and fluoride application daily, combined with maintenance supervision at professional appointments.

II. AMALGAM PROPERTIES AND AGE CHANGES
A. Surface Changes

1. *Tarnish.* Tarnish is principally a sulfide. It is usually caused by lack of oral cleanliness, with resultant plaque collection, and by certain foods, especially foods containing sulfur. Tarnish is less frequently found on properly finished and polished restorations.

2. *Corrosion.* Corrosion is caused by environmental factors, such as air, moisture, acid or alkaline solutions, and other chemicals.[4] Polished amalgam resists corrosion.

   Corrosion at the margin of a restoration can cause deterioration and fracture of the margin. An open gap where plaque can collect is the usual result. The products of corrosion may be carried into the dentinal tubules, and the entire area around the restoration may appear bluish-black.

B. Dimensional Changes[1,2]

Expansion can occur as a result of incomplete trituration and condensation or contamination from moisture entering the amalgam during the mixing and placing of the restoration. When expansion occurs in excess, the filling appears extruded above the cavosurface margin. Expansion can also produce postoperative pain or tooth sensitivity because of pressure on the pulp.

When contraction occurs, the amalgam may pull away from the cavosurface margin. Contraction is one of the causes of "ditching," a term used to describe a space between the filling material and the tooth structure, as described on page 583.

C. Amalgam Strength

Fractures are a result of insufficient strength. A fracture may be seen as a gross irregularity, a crack line across an entire restoration, or a marginal chip. Several factors can be involved in amalgam fractures, including the following:

1. *Manipulation of the Filling Material.* Undertrituration of amalgam results in low strength.

2. *Overload of Pressure on a Restoration Before Setting is Complete.* Strength of the amalgam is low during the first few hours after placement. After carving, the occlusal relationship should be checked for high contact spots, which, if subjected to masticatory stress, can lead to fracture.

3. *Inadequate Strength of Surrounding Tooth Structure.* Strength and support for an amalgam restoration depend in part on the strength of the surrounding tooth structure. When dental caries requires wide extension of the cavity preparation, the tooth walls may be subject to fracture. Both the amalgam and the tooth may fracture together.

4. *Improper Carving of the Restoration.* Marginal strength can be compromised when a thin excess of amalgam is left to extend over the cavosurface margin. If the small overhang (flash) breaks off, a part of the margin of the restoration may also break off with the flash (figure 40-1). The fracture may be caused by occlusal pressures or finishing procedures.

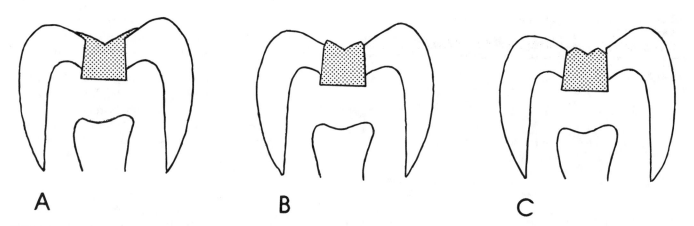

FIG. 40–1. Amalgam Irregularities. A. *Flash on the occlusal surface related to a Class 1 restoration. Flash refers to a thin layer of amalgam that extends over the margin of the cavity preparation.* **B.** *Irregular margin results when the flash breaks off.* **C.** *Ditching that results from broken off flash.*

MARGINAL IRREGULARITIES

When an amalgam restoration is to be finished and polished, it is first examined by moving an explorer over the surfaces and margins. A variety of irregularities or defects may be found. The defects represent excesses or deficiencies of amalgam.

The finished functional restoration follows the normal contours of the tooth. All cavosurface junctions should feel smooth to an explorer.

Excesses and deficiencies must be recognized and differentiated, so that finishing and polishing procedures can be carried out effectively. When deficiencies of amalgam occur, correction by finishing techniques may require removal of excess tooth structure. Usually, deficiencies must be corrected by replacement of the restoration.

The common irregularities and defects of amalgam restorations are defined and described in the following section.

I. OVERHANGING MARGIN

An amalgam overhang is illustrated in figure 40–2A. Proximal overhangs result primarily from improper placement of the matrix band and wedge. Overhangs may occur on any tooth surface, supra- or subgingivally, in any class of cavity. They may be caused by errors of manipulation, carving, and/or finishing.

II. FLASH
A. Occlusal
Figure 40–1A illustrates a feather ledge or flash that was left during carving. When performed correctly, carving brings the cavosurface margin into view and makes the filling material flush with the enamel.

B. Proximal-Gingival
A flash-type overhang can result when an amalgam is packed between a matrix band and the

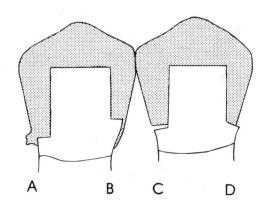

FIG. 40–2. Irregularities of Amalgam Margins. A. *Overhang.* **B.** *Flash on a proximal surface.* **C.** *Open or deficient margin.* **D.** *Undercontoured margin that can result from an improperly placed matrix band or misdirected carving.*

tooth surface below the cavity preparation (figure 40–2B). The irregularity can occur when a proximal wedge is not used or not positioned to adapt the matrix tightly against the tooth surface. A tooth with a concave proximal surface is most vulnerable to flash.

III. OPEN MARGIN
An open margin is found when a distinct space is between the amalgam and the wall of the cavity preparation (figure 40–2C). The causes include the following:
  A. Too much time elapses after trituration before condensation. The amalgam material begins to set and becomes difficult to condense properly.
  B. Too large an amount of the amalgam mix is inserted into the cavity preparation at one time.

IV. UNDERCONTOURED
The opposite of an overhang is a deficiency of amalgam between the margin of the amalgam and the cavity wall, as shown in figure 40–2D. On the proximal sur-

face, causes may be related to improper placement of the matrix or wedge, or both, or to misdirected carving with poorly selected instruments.

Undercontouring is exemplified also by missing contact areas, flattened cervical ridges, incomplete marginal ridges, and incomplete filling of the cavity preparation.

V. OVERCONTOURED

An overcontoured restoration has an excess of amalgam in such a position as to change the normal anatomic form of the restoration. Interproximally overcontoured surfaces may widen the contact area or narrow the embrasure. When the crown is overcontoured, the effect can be plaque retention and pressure on the gingival margin.

In figure 25–1C, on page 395, overcontoured crowns of a double abutment have narrowed the embrasure. Problems of plaque control for the overcontoured crowns are illustrated in figure 25–4 on page 396.

VI. DITCH OR GROOVE

Figure 40–1C shows the gap on the occlusal surface, where either the flash broke off or contraction of the amalgam caused the restoration to pull away from the tooth structure. Plaque retention can lead to recurrent caries in such an area.

OVERHANGING RESTORATIONS

Recontouring overhanging restorations is an essential part of dental and periodontal treatment. Treatment planning for initial therapy, or Phase I periodontal therapy, must include the correction of overhangs if inflammation is to be controlled.[5]

I. DESCRIPTION

An overhang is identified by its relation to the gingival margin, location on a specific tooth surface, and size or extent. From these data, the required finishing procedures can be selected for a specific treatment plan.

A. Relation to Gingival Margin
1. Supragingival.
2. Subgingival.

B. Location on Tooth Surface
1. Occlusal, mesial, distal, facial, lingual, palatal, or combination.
2. Tooth surface margin
   a. Enamel only.
   b. Enamel and cementum.
   c. Cementum only.

C. Size Determined by Visual and Tactile Examination[6]
Overhangs are found by running a sharp explorer back and forth over the junction between the tooth and the amalgam.

1. *Type I.* Small overhang; slight catch with explorer in at least one section.
2. *Type II.* Moderately large overhang with definite catch with explorer, usually involving more than one side of the restoration.
2. *Type III.* Large, gross overhang clearly apparent by exploration and often visually apparent on direct observation.

II. RADIOGRAPHIC EXAMINATION

Overhangs on surfaces other than proximal are rarely visible on radiographic examination. Visibility of proximal surface overhangs depends on angulation of the x ray. In other words, radiographic examination for overhangs should be a supplementary procedure to examination using an explorer. The entire outline of each restoration can be explored.

A magnifying glass is recommended for examining radiographs for small type I overhangs. Adjacent and undermining carious lesions are more definitively seen when magnification is used.

III. EFFECTS OF OVERHANGS
A. Relation to Periodontal Disease
Because overhanging restorations harbor plaque and hinder plaque removal by the patient, they are considered significant iatrogenic contributing factors in periodontal disease development. In the presence of overhangs, plaque collects in greater amounts and inflammation is more severe than in teeth that do not have overhangs.[7,8,9] Increased bone loss adjacent to overhangs has been demonstrated.[7,10]

Removal of overhangs is beneficial to the periodontal tissues. Combined with scaling and plaque control, a marked improvement in the periodontal condition has been shown after overhang removal.[8,11]

B. Problems of Bacterial Plaque Control
1. Irregular margins of overhangs catch and tear dental floss.
2. Inaccessible areas
   a. Area under the ledge of the overhang, particularly a proximal overhang, is inaccessible for the direct application of a toothbrush and other plaque removal aids.
   b. Gingival enlargement can result from inflammation caused by bacterial plaque held by the overhang and may cover a portion of the overhang. After shrinkage of the soft tissue pocket wall and removal of the overhang, the restoration may be wholly supragingival and, therefore, accessible for maintenance.
3. Debris retention contributes to a general lack of oral sanitation and to halitosis from breakdown products in bacterial plaque and food debris held by the overhang.

C. Dental Caries

Marginal irregularities harbor microorganisms and sucrose in an environment conducive to the formation of secondary caries. The caries process is described on page 267.

IV. INDICATIONS AND CONTRAINDICATIONS FOR REMOVAL OF OVERHANGS

All overhanging restorations should be corrected or removed and replaced for the health of the periodontium. Large overhangs cannot usually be treated by finishing procedures and are, therefore, an indication for total replacement of the restoration. If replacement will be delayed, the gross overhang should be reshaped and smoothed to make plaque control possible. The periodontal tissues can recover, inflammation can be reduced, and continuing treatment can be more satisfactory.

Whether a certain overhang can be removed by finishing procedures or whether it must be replaced with a new restoration is the professional decision that must be made. Guidelines for selection of the correct procedure are suggested here. Contraindications for finishing procedures apply to all restorations of any size or location.

A. Indications for Finishing

1. Tooth anatomy can be maintained or improved to conform with normal contour.
2. The overhang is small or moderate in size.
3. Proximal contact is intact.
4. No adjacent secondary dental caries is present.
5. There are no fractures of the cavity margin either of the tooth or of the filling and no large fractures of the bulk of the restoration.
6. The overhang is accessible for the instrumentation necessary for finishing and polishing without damaging the adjacent tooth structure or unduly traumatizing the gingival tissues.

B. Indications for Removal and Restoration

1. The overhang is extensive and would require an excessively long time to recontour completely.
2. Secondary marginal or undermining dental caries is present.
3. The contact area must be restored.
4. Fractures, chips, cracks, or broken margins are apparent that cannot be corrected by finishing and polishing procedures.

CLINICAL MANAGEMENT: MERCURY HYGIENE

The mercury vapor level in a dental treatment room can be higher than that in the normal atmosphere when many amalgam restorations are completed during each day. Although members of the dental team rarely exhibit symptoms of toxicity, the potential danger exists, and certain precautions are necessary.

I. MERCURY POLLUTION OF ENVIRONMENT

Sources of mercury include the following:
A. Direct contact or handling of mercury.
B. Inhalation of vapors from mercury.
C. Exposure to accidental spills and leaky or contaminated amalgamator capsules and amalgamators.
D. Vaporization of mercury from contaminated instruments in sterilizers.
E. Amalgam condensation, especially with ultrasonic compactors.
F. Milling old amalgam restorations.

II. MERCURY HYGIENE PRACTICES

Recommendations include the following:
A. Work in well-ventilated areas.
B. Wear mask, protective eyewear, and gloves for protection from mercury vapor and amalgam dust.
C. Avoid carpeting or porous materials for treatment room floors.
D. Monitor the office or clinic periodically for atmospheric mercury.
E. Provide yearly urinalysis for mercury for all personnel who request it.
F. Store mercury in unbreakable, tightly sealed containers away from heat sources.
G. Keep amalgam scrap in a tightly sealed container.
H. Handle amalgam with caution and without direct contact; clean up spilled mercury immediately.
I. Use water stream and high-volume evacuation when removing or finishing amalgam restorations.
J. Avoid heating mercury, amalgam, or mercury-containing solutions.
K. Do not eat, drink, or smoke in treatment rooms.

FINISHING PROCEDURES

I. DEFINITIONS

A. Carving

Carving is the removal of excess filling material, using specially designed instruments, immediately after condensation of the amalgam in the cavity preparation. The goal of carving is to produce accurate anatomic contours to restore the form and function of the particular tooth.

B. Contouring

Contouring includes procedures to reproduce the size, shape, grooves, and other details of tooth form in the restoration. The term *contouring* is usually used when a new restoration is

c. Keep the brush or cup in constant motion with light, intermittent strokes to prevent heat generation. Replenish slurry often.

d. Apply polishing agent to proximal surfaces with waxed dental tape. Avoid the contact area. Curve the tape around the tooth to prevent damage to the interdental gingival tissue.

4. *Examination.* Rinse and inspect frequently to prevent overpolishing.

B. Fine Finish

1. *Agent.* Apply tin oxide in a thin, wet slurry with water.
2. *Selection of Polisher.* Use a new rubber cup or brush to prevent mixing the agents.
3. *Application.* Apply with light, intermittent strokes.
4. *Examination.* Rinse and inspect to prevent overpolishing.

IV. FINAL EVALUATION

The finished and polished restoration has the characteristics described in Technique Objectives, page 585.

FLUORIDE APPLICATION

The use of abrasive stones and polishing agents at the margin of a restoration removes a layer of the surface enamel and, with it, the concentration of fluoride that is protective against dental caries. Commercially prepared paste containing fluoride may restore in part the lost fluoride (page 567) and can be used during the polishing procedure.

After polishing, a topical application of fluoride should be made, followed by periodic applications at succeeding maintenance appointments, depending on individual needs. Self-application on a daily basis, using a mouthrinse, custom tray, or brush-on gel, may also be recommended to supplement fluoride derived from the use of a dentifrice.

FACTORS TO TEACH THE PATIENT

I. Advantages of having restorations smooth and well finished.

II. Reasons for having to wait 24 to 48 hours to have finishing procedures completed for the newly placed restoration.

III. The importance of having inadequate contact areas restored rather than using floss repeatedly to alleviate the discomforts of food impaction.

IV. The need for daily and professional applications of fluoride to promote remineralization around each restoration. Daily mouthrinse, brush-on gel, gel in a tray, or other form of fluoride is advised.

V. Advantages of maintaining all restorations by daily plaque control measures, limiting cariogenic foods, and all possible preventive procedures.

REFERENCES

1. **Phillips,** R.W.: *Skinner's Science of Dental Materials,* 9th ed. Philadelphia, W.B. Saunders Co., 1991, pp. 303–347.
2. **Craig,** R.G., ed.: *Restorative Dental Materials,* 8th ed. St. Louis, Mosby, 1989, pp. 227–254.
3. **Leinfelder,** K.F. and Lemons, J.E.: *Clinical Restorative Materials and Techniques.* Philadelphia, Lea & Febiger, 1988, pp. 1–48, 197.
4. **Phillips:** op. cit., pp. 291–302.
5. **Carranza,** F.A.: *Glickman's Clinical Periodontology,* 7th ed. Philadelphia, W.B. Saunders Co., 1990, pp. 677–680.
6. **Langslet,** J.: *Margination—Rationale and Technique.* Seattle, WA, Department of Dental Hygiene, University of Washington, 1976, 28 pp.
7. **Gilmore,** N. and Sheiham, A.: Overhanging Dental Restorations and Periodontal Disease, *J. Periodontol.,* 42, 8, January, 1971.
8. **Highfield,** J.E. and Powell, R.N.: Effects of Removal of Posterior Overhanging Metallic Margins of Restorations upon the Periodontal Tissues, *J. Clin. Periodontol.,* 5, 169, August, 1978.
9. **Gorzo,** I., Newman, H.N., and Strahan, J.D.: Amalgam Restorations, Plaque Removal and Periodontal Health, *J. Clin. Periodontol.,* 6, 98, April, 1979.
10. **Jeffcoat,** M.K. and Howell, T.H.: Alveolar Bone Destruction Due to Overhanging Amalgam in Periodontal Disease, *J. Periodontol.,* 51, 599, October, 1980.
11. **Rodriguez-Ferrer,** H.J., Strahan, J.D., and Newman, H.N.: Effect on Gingival Health of Removing Overhanging Margins of Interproximal Subgingival Amalgam Restorations, *J. Clin. Periodontol.,* 7, 457, December, 1980.

SUGGESTED READINGS

Chen, J.J., Burch, J.G., Beck, F.M., and Horton, J.E.: Periodontal Attachment Loss Associated with Proximal Tooth Restorations, *J. Prosthet. Dent.,* 57, 416, April, 1987.

Eid, M.: Relationship Between Overhanging Amalgam Restorations and Periodontal Disease, *Quintessence Int.,* 18, 775, November, 1987.

Fayyad, M.A. and Ball, P.C.: Bacterial Penetration Around Amalgam Restorations, *J. Prosthet. Dent.,* 57, 571, May, 1987.

Goldstein, G.R. and Waknine, S.: Surface Roughness Evaluation of Composite Resin Polishing Techniques, *Quintessence Int.,* 20, 199, March, 1989.

Holmstrup, P.: Reactions of the Oral Mucosa Related to Silver Amalgam, *J. Oral Pathol. Med.,* 20, 1, January, 1991.

Margination

Biller-Karlsson, I. and Sheaffer, J.K.: Class II Amalgam Overhangs—Prevalence, Significance, and Removal Techniques, *Dent. Hyg., 62,* 180, April, 1988.

deVries, J., deWet, F.A., and Eick, J.D.: Polishing Dental Amalgam Restorations, *J. Prosthet. Dent., 58,* 148, August, 1987.

Eide, R. and Tveit, A.B.: A Comparison of Different Techniques for Finishing and Polishing Amalgam, *Acta Odontol. Scand., 45,* 147, No. 3, 1987.

Geiger, F., Reller, U., and Lutz, F.: Burnishing, Finishing, and Polishing Amalgam Restorations: A Quantitative Scanning Electron Microscopic Study, *Quintessence Int., 20,* 461, July, 1989.

LaBrie, M.: Finishing and Polishing Amalgam Restorations: A Review, *Dentalhygienistnews, 2,* 10, Fall, 1989.

Latcham, N.: Quadrant Iatrodontics: A Technique for Removing Overhangs, *Quintessence Int., 21,* 345, May, 1990.

Paarmann, C.: Finishing, Recontouring, and Polishing Amalgam Restorations, *Practical Hygiene, 2,* 9, January/February, 1993.

Pack, A.R.C.: The Amalgam Overhang Dilemma: A Review of Causes and Effects, Prevention and Removal, *N.Z. Dent. J., 85,* 55, April, 1989.

Project Acorde, United States Department of Health, Education, and Welfare: *Recontouring, Finishing, and Polishing.* Castro Valley, CA, Quercus, 1976, 85 pp.

can be damaged can help the clinician avoid unnecessary trauma during the various procedures.

I. ENAMEL LOSS
Total enamel loss from etching, bracket removal, residual resin removal, surface finishing, and application of pumice averages approximately 55 to 80 μm.[10,22] Enamel loss is greater when filled resins (composites) are used for bonding than when unfilled resins are used. The loss is also greater when a rotating bristle brush rather than a rubber cup is used with the abrasive for finishing.

The outer layer of enamel is the most significant. The fluoride-rich surface enamel is approximately 50 μm deep. Therefore, the entire protective layer can be removed. When multiple bonding and debonding procedures are done, such as when a bracket becomes detached, the enamel loss is compounded. As much as 72 μm of enamel may be lost during a complete multiple procedure.[23]

The need for careful selection of instruments and abrasives, along with minimal instrumentation, to prevent unnecessary enamel loss is apparent.

II. WHITE SPOTS (DEMINERALIZATION)
White spots or dental caries have been relatively common findings after orthodontic treatment. Patients with teeth that have been banded or bonded tend to develop the spots significantly more often than do patients who have not had orthodontic therapy.

Bacterial plaque retention by the appliances and the resin, along with the difficulty of plaque removal by the patient, contributes to demineralization and dental caries.

III. ETCHED ENAMEL NOT COVERED BY ADHESIVE
Surface areas etched but not covered with adhesive resin become remineralized when the fluoride contact is high through personal and professional applications. Etched enamel has a high fluoride uptake.

POSTDEBONDING PREVENTIVE CARE

I. PERIODONTAL EVALUATION
A complete examination with careful probing and charting is necessary, because many changes take place during treatment. Calculus removal should be completed as needed.

II. DENTAL CARIES
Examination for demineralization (white spots) and dental caries is essential. Bacterial plaque retention by orthodontic appliances can be extensive. The configurations of the appliances make plaque control efforts by the patient extremely difficult. Plaque collects on brackets and some resins even when the patient's oral hygiene is generally good.[4]

Composite resin may be left on the tooth surface around the bracket. The surface of resins is difficult to make smooth; thus, plaque collects. The bacteria of the plaque, not the rough surface, cause the gingival inflammatory response and the white spots, or demineralization.

After debonding, the use of a retainer provides another source for retention of bacterial plaque. Special instruction for cleaning the retainer is needed (pages 379 and 383).

III. FLUORIDE THERAPY[24]
A complete program of fluoride treatments, professionally at frequent maintenance appointments and by the patient on a daily basis, is prerequisite. With the loss of the fluoride-rich enamel surface during bonding and debonding procedures, the need for remineralization and replenishment of fluoride is clear.

TECHNICAL HINTS

I. Document any irregularities of the patient's teeth, such as white spots or cracks, before orthodontic treatment begins and appliances are affixed, to prevent misunderstanding by the patient after debonding.[25]
II. Take periodic photographs to compare gingival tissue changes and teeth before and after disclosing agent application for documentation and patient instruction.

FACTORS TO TEACH THE PATIENT

I. The significance of plaque around orthodontic appliances and the teeth.
II. How to apply the toothbrush and auxiliary devices to remove plaque from the bracket, the arch wire, and the teeth (Chapters 23 and 24).
III. How, when, and why to use fluoride rinse, toothpaste, and brush-on gel.
IV. The frequency of follow-up after debonding.

REFERENCES

1. **Zachrisson,** B.U: Bonding in Orthodontics, in Graber, T.M. and Swain, B.F.: *Orthodontics, Current Principles and Techniques.* St. Louis, Mosby, 1985, pp. 485–487.
2. **American Dental Association,** Council on Dental Materials, Instruments, and Equipment: Ceramic Orthodontic Brackets: How and When to Use Them, *J. Am. Dent. Assoc., 123,* 243, July, 1992.
3. **Flores,** D.A., Caruso, J.M., Scott, G.E., and Jeiroudi, M.T.: The Fracture Strength of Ceramic Brackets: A Comparative Study, *Angle Orthod., 60,* 269, Winter, 1990.
4. **Gwinnett,** A.J. and Ceen, R.F.: Plaque Distribution on Bonded

Brackets: A Scanning Microscopic Study, *Am. J. Orthod., 75,* 667, June, 1979.

5. **Zachrisson,** B.U. and Brobakken, B.O.: Clinical Comparison of Direct Versus Indirect Bonding With Different Bracket Types and Adhesives, *Am. J. Orthod., 74,* 62, July, 1978.

6. **Proffit,** W.R.: *Contemporary Orthodontics,* 2nd ed. St. Louis, Mosby, 1993, pp. 353–357.

7. **Gwinnett,** A.J. for the American Dental Association, Council on Dental Materials, Instruments, and Equipment: State of the Art and Science of Bonding in Orthodontic Treatment, *J. Am. Dent. Assoc., 105,* 844, November, 1982.

8. **Buonocore,** M.G., Matsui, A., and Gwinnett, A.J.: Penetration of Resin Dental Materials into Enamel Surfaces with Reference to Bonding, *Arch. Oral Biol., 13,* 61, January, 1968.

9. **Retief,** D.H.: Effect of Conditioning the Enamel Surface with Phosphoric Acid, *J. Dent. Res., 52,* 333, March-April, 1973.

10. **Diedrich,** P.: Enamel Alterations from Bracket Bonding and Debonding: A Study with the Scanning Electron Microscope, *Am. J. Orthod., 79,* 500, May, 1981.

11. **Sonis,** A.L. and Snell, W.: An Evaluation of a Fluoride-releasing, Visible Light-activated Bonding System for Orthodontic Bracket Placement, *Am. J. Orthod. Dentofacial Orthop., 95,* 306, April, 1989.

12. **Chan,** D.C.N., Swift, E.J., and Bishara, S.E.: *In Vitro* Evaluation of a Fluoride-releasing Orthodontic Resin, *J. Dent. Res., 69,* 1576, September, 1990.

13. **Bishara,** S.E., Swift, E.J., and Chan, D.C.N.: Evaluation of Fluoride Release from an Orthodontic Bonding System, *Am. J. Orthod. Dentofacial Orthop., 100,* 106, August, 1991.

14. **Everett,** M.S.: Debonding Orthodontic Adhesives, *Dent. Hyg., 59,* 364, August, 1985.

15. **Bishara,** S.E. and Trulove, T.S.: Comparisons of Different Debonding Techniques for Ceramic Brackets: An *In Vitro* Study, Part I. Background and Methods, *Am. J. Orthod. Dentofacial Orthop., 98,* 145, August, 1990.

16. **Bishara,** S.E. and Trulove, T.S.: Comparisons of Different Debonding Techniques for Ceramic Brackets: An *In Vitro* Study. Part II. Findings and Clinical Implications, *Am. J. Orthod. Dentofacial Orthop., 98,* 263, September, 1990.

17. **Bennett,** C.G., Shen, C., and Waldron, J.M.: The Effects of Debonding on the Enamel Surface, *J. Clin. Orthod., 18,* 330, May, 1984.

18. **Gwinnett,** A.J. and Gorelik, L.: Microscopic Evaluation of Enamel after Debonding: Clinical Application, *Am. J. Orthod., 71,* 651, June, 1977.

19. **Retief,** D.H. and Denys, F.R.: Finishing of Enamel Surfaces after Debonding of Orthodontic Attachments, *Angle Orthod., 49,* 1, January, 1979.

20. **Rouleau,** B.D., Marshall, G.W., and Cooley, R.O.: Enamel Surface Evaluations after Clinical Treatment and Removal of Orthodontic Brackets, *Am. J. Orthod., 81,* 423, May, 1982.

21. **Andreasen,** G.F. and Chan, K.C.: A Hazard in Direct Bonding Bracket—A Case Report, *Quintessence Int., 12,* 569, June, 1981.

22. **Pus,** M.D. and Way, D.C.: Enamel Loss Due to Orthodontic Bonding with Filled and Unfilled Resins Using Various Cleanup Techniques, *Am. J. Orthod., 77,* 269, March, 1980.

23. **Thompson,** R.E. and Way, D.C.: Enamel Loss Due to Prophylaxis and Multiple Bonding/Debonding of Orthodontic Attachments, *Am. J. Orthod., 79,* 282, March, 1981.

24. **Boyd,** R.L.: Comparison of Three Self-applied Topical Fluoride Preparations for Control of Decalcification, *Angle Orthod., 63,* 25, Spring, 1993.

25. **Zachrisson,** B.U., Skogan, Ö., and Höymyhr, S.: Enamel Cracks in Debonded, Debanded, and Orthodontically Untreated Teeth, *Am. J. Orthod., 77,* 307, March, 1980.

SUGGESTED READINGS

Barcroft, B.D., Childers, K.R., and Harris, E.F.: Effects of Acidulated and Neutral NaF Solutions on Bond Strengths, *Pediatr. Dent., 12,* 180, May–June, 1990.

Boyd, R.L. and Baumrind, S.: Periodontal Considerations in the Use of Bonds or Bands on Molars in Adolescents and Adults, *Angle Orthod., 62,* 117, Summer, 1992.

Carstensen, W.: Direct Bonding with Reduced Acid Etchant Concentrations, *J. Clin. Orthod., 27,* 23, January, 1993.

Garcia-Godoy, F., Perez, R., and Hubbard, G.W.: Effect of Prophylaxis Pastes on Shear Bond Strength, *J. Clin. Orthod., 25,* 571, September, 1991.

Kao, E.C. and Johnston, W.M.: Fracture Incidence on Debonding of Orthodontic Brackets from Porcelain Veneer Laminates, *J. Prosthet. Dent., 66,* 631, November, 1991.

Ødegaard, J. and Segner, D.: The Use of Visible Light-curing Composites in Bonding Ceramic Brackets, *Am. J. Orthod. Dentofacial Orthop., 97,* 188, March, 1990.

Øgaard, B., Rezk-Lega, F., Ruben, J., and Arends, J.: Cariostatic Effect and Fluoride Release from a Visible Light-curing Adhesive for Bonding of Orthodontic Brackets, *Am. J. Orthod. Dentofacial Orthop., 101,* 303, April, 1992.

Øgaard, B., Rølla, G., and Arends, J.: Orthodontic Appliances and Enamel Demineralization. Part I. Lesion Development, *Am. J. Orthod. Dentofacial Orthop., 94,* 68, July, 1988.

Scott, G.E.: Fracture Toughness and Surface Cracks—The Key to Understanding Ceramic Brackets, *Angle Orthod., 58,* 5, January, 1988.

Staggers, J.A. and Margeson, D.: The Effects of Sterilization on the Tensile Strength of Orthodontic Wires, *Angle Orthod., 63,* 141, Summer, 1993.

Valk, J.W.P. and Davidson, C.L.: The Relevance of Controlled Fluoride Release with Bonded Orthodontic Appliances, *J. Dent., 15,* 257, December, 1987.

Debonding Procedures

Bishara, S.E. and Fehr, D.E.: Comparisons of the Effectiveness of Pliers with Narrow and Wide Blades in Debonding Ceramic Brackets, *Am. J. Orthod. Dentofacial Orthop., 103,* 253, March, 1993.

Bishara, S.E., Thunyaudom, T., and Chan, D.: The Effect of Temperature Change of Composites on the Bonding Strength of Orthodontic Brackets, *Am. J. Orthod. Dentofacial Orthop., 94,* 440, November, 1988.

Chate, R.A.C.: Safer Orthodontic Debonding with Rubber Dam, *Am. J. Orthod. Dentofacial Orthop., 103,* 171, February, 1993.

Gorbach, N.R.: Heat Removal of Ceramic Brackets, *J. Clin. Orthod., 25,* 247, April, 1991.

Krell, K.V., Courey, J.M., and Bishara, S.E.: Orthodontic Bracket Removal Using Conventional and Ultrasonic Debonding Techniques, Enamel Loss, and Time Requirements, *Am. J. Orthod. Dentofacial Orthop., 103,* 258, March, 1993.

Oliver, R.G. and Griffiths, J.: Different Techniques of Residual Composite Removal Following Debonding—Time Taken and Surface Enamel Appearance, *Br. J. Orthod., 19,* 131, May, 1992.

Redd, T.B. and Shivapuja, P.K.: Debonding Ceramic Brackets: Effects on Enamel, *J. Clin. Orthod., 25,* 475, August, 1991.

Strobl, K., Bahns, T.L., Willham, L., Bishara, S.E., and Stwalley, W.C.: Laser-aided Debonding of Orthodontic Ceramic Brackets, *Am. J. Orthod. Dentofacial Orthop., 101,* 152, February, 1992.

Sylvester, E.: Thermal Debonding of Ceramic Brackets, *J. Clin. Orthod., 25,* 748, December, 1991.

Tocchio, R.M., Williams, P.T., Mayer, F.J., and Standing, K.G.: Laser Debonding of Ceramic Orthodontic Brackets, *Am. J. Orthod. Dentofacial Orthop., 103,* 155, February, 1993.

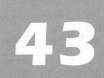

The Pregnant Patient and the Infant/Toddler

During pregnancy, attention is focused on good health practices for the mother. She is concerned for the health of her baby and for herself. This alertness to total health, of which oral health is an important part, provides an unusual opportunity to help the patient learn principles that may be applied to the future care of the child.

The term *prenatal care* refers to the supervised preparation for childbirth that helps the mother enjoy optimum health during and after pregnancy and provides the maximum chance for the baby to be born healthy. Such a program involves the combined efforts of the obstetrician and/or midwife, nurse practitioner, dentist, dental hygienist, and the expectant parents. Key words for study with this chapter are defined in table 43–1.

Certain women who do not receive routine dental care may appear for emergency dental services and may be receptive to a program of care and instruction to prevent further emergencies. The dental hygienist in public health participates in community educational programs with public health nurses, whereby some less informed women may learn of the need for professional dental care and advice during pregnancy.

Obstetricians should recommend dental examination early in pregnancy. This brings to the dental office or clinic many women who previously would not have had a regular plan for obtaining professional service. Many of these women have not known the advantages of personal habits of daily care and diet related to the health of the oral tissues. Numerous misconceptions must be counteracted when providing up-to-date information about the relationship of pregnancy and oral health.

FETAL DEVELOPMENT

Pregnancy is arbitrarily divided into 3 periods of 3 months each called the first, second, and third trimesters. Normal pregnancy, or period of *gestation*, is approximately 40 weeks. *Premature birth* refers to a birth before 37 weeks' gestation.

Physiologic changes in the mother are related to nearly every bodily system. Early development of the embryo is greatly influenced by heredity, infections, and drug intake.

I. FIRST TRIMESTER
During the first trimester, the embryo is highly susceptible to injuries and malformations. Teratogenic effects can be produced by many sources, including infections and drugs.

All organ systems are formed (organogenesis) during the first trimester. By 12 weeks, the fetus moves and swallows. In the oral cavity, the following occurs:

A. Teeth
1. Tooth buds develop between the fourth and fifth week.
2. Initial mineralization occurs from the ninth to the twelfth week.

B. Lips and Palate
1. Lips form during the fourth to the seventh week.
2. Palate forms between the eighth and the twelfth week.
3. Cleft lip is apparent by the eighth week; cleft palate, by the twelfth week (page 617).

TABLE 43–1
KEY WORDS: PREGNANCY, INFANTS, AND TODDLERS

Amniocentesis (am′nē-ō-sen-tē′sĭs): a testing procedure on fluid aspirated from the amniotic sac to detect chromosomal abnormalities and metabolic disorders.

Amniotic sac (am′nē-ot′ik): the innermost of the membranes enveloping the embryo *in utero;* **amniotic fluid** fills the sac in which the embryo is free to move and is protected against mechanical injury.

Cesarean section (sĕ-sa′rē-an): delivery of a fetus by incision through the abdominal wall and uterus.

Embryo: developing organism from conception to approximately the end of the second month.

Epulis: nonspecific term referring to a growth on the gingiva.

Estradiol: the most potent natural estrogen in humans; the circulating blood level of estradiol rises during the follicular phase of the reproductive cycle and drops when ovulation occurs (figure 45–1, page 628).

Fetus: developing organism from the second month after conception to birth.

Gestation: the period of pregnancy.

Granuloma: nonspecific term applied to a nodular inflammatory lesion containing macrophages and surrounded by lymphocytes.

"Pyogenic" granuloma: a misnomer because it does not contain pus, but contains blood vessels and inflammatory cells.

In utero: within the womb; not yet born.

Infant: child younger than 1 year of age.

Intrapartum: occurring during childbirth.

Midwife: a person who attends a woman during delivery.

Nurse-midwife: a registered nurse specializing in midwifery; requires additional education and special licensure in certain states and countries.

Neonate (ne′ō-nāt): newborn.

Neonatal: refers to the period immediately following birth and continuing through the first month of life.

Non-nutritive sucking: sucking fingers, pacifiers, or other objects.

Obstetrics: the branch of medicine that has to do with the care of the pregnant woman during pregnancy and parturition.

Obstetrician: physician who practices obstetrics.

Parturition (par′tu-rish′un): childbirth; labor; giving birth.

Postpartum: pertaining to the period following childbirth or delivery.

Premature birth: birth that occurs before the expected delivery date; denotes an infant born prior to 37 weeks of gestation.

Teratogen (ter′ah-tō-jen): nongenetic factors that cause malformations and disease syndromes *in utero.*

Teratogenic agent: any drug, virus, or irradiation the exposure to which can cause malformation of the fetus.

Tippy cup: a special cup designed to teach a young child to drink.

Toddler: child from age 1 year to approximately 3 years of age.

Trimester: a period of 3 months; one third of a pregnancy.

Wean: to discontinue breast-feeding; to nourish the infant with other food.

II. SECOND AND THIRD TRIMESTERS

The organs are completed, and growth and maturation continue. Fetal weight changes from 1 ounce at 3 months to an average of 7.5 pounds at birth.

III. FACTORS THAT CAN HARM THE FETUS
A. Infections

Protection from infectious diseases is necessary because damage to and infection of the fetus can result. Women of childbearing age should avail themselves of all available vaccines prior to conception.

Defects, deformities, and life-threatening infections can result from infection acquired during pregnancy or during delivery and after birth. Rubella (German measles), rubeola, varicella, herpesviruses, hepatitis B (page 22), human immunodeficiency virus (HIV) infection (page 32), syphilis (congenital syphilis), and gonorrhea all can have serious effects on the fetus.

B. Drugs

Ideally no medications or other drugs should be used during pregnancy. Nearly all drugs can pass across the placenta to enter the circulation of the developing fetus. Many drugs have teratogenic effects.[1,2] Table 43–2 lists selected drugs with examples of their possible effects on the fetus.

1. *Effect of Tetracycline.* Tetracycline is well known for intrinsic staining of tooth structure. The effect occurs during mineralization of the primary teeth beginning at about 4 months of gestation and of the permanent teeth near and after birth (page 284). When an antibiotic is required during pregnancy, a choice other than tetracycline can be made.

2. *Effect of Medication for HIV Infection.* Zidovudine has been shown to be well tolerated by pregnant women with HIV infection. Although no associated malformations in newborns, premature birth, or fetal distress have been noted, the occasional anemia and

TABLE 43–2
DRUGS CONTRAINDICATED DURING PREGNANCY AND BREAST FEEDING

Classification	Drugs Prescribed for Treatment	Possible Adverse Effects on Fetus and Infant
Anticoagulant	Warfarin (Coumadin) (D)* Dicumarol (D)	Hemorrhagic; fetal death Birth malformations
Anticonvulsant	Barbiturates (phenobarbital) (D) Phenytoin sodium (D) Trimethadione (D) Valproate sodium (D)	Congenital malformations (page 744) Developmental delays Fetal phenobarbital syndrome Fetal hydantoin syndrome Fetal trimethadione syndrome Fetal valproate syndrome
Antimicrobial	Streptomycin (B) Tetracycline (D)	Toxic action on ear: 8th cranial nerve damage Bone growth inhibition; intrinsic dental stain
Antineoplastic	Cyclophosphamide (Cytoxan) (D) Mercaptopurine (D) Methotrexate (D)	Multiple anomalies; fetal death

Hormones	Clomiphene (Clomid) (X)
	 Estrogenic substances (X)
	    Diethylstilbestrol (X)
	 Prednisone (C)
	 Progesterone (X)
		Increased anomalies; neural tube defects
		 Cancer of the vagina and cervix; genital tract
		    anomalies; congenital heart defects

Psychotrophic	Antianxiety
	    Chlordiazepoxide (Librium) (D)
	    Diazepam (Valium) (D)
	    Meprobamate (Miltown) (D)
	 Antimanic
	    Lithium carbonate (D)
		Low heart rate, muscle tone, respiration, poor
		    sucking reflex
		 Birth defects
		
		 Lethargy, cyanosis, teratogenic (dose related)

Drugs of Abuse	*Alcohol*	Fetal alcohol syndrome (page 778) Spontaneous abortion; low birth rate Mental retardation
	Cocaine Prenatal exposure Inhale free-base vapors (postpartum)	Decreased birth weight; prematurity Fetal growth retardation; microcephaly Teratogenic effects Increased rate of seizures

	Narcotics
	    Heroin
	    Methadone
		Decreased birth weight
		 Withdrawal symptoms
		 Convulsions; sudden infant death

	Tobacco
	    Cigarette smoking
	
	    Involuntary smoking
	
	      Environmental
	
	      Second-hand
		Low birth weight; prematurity; miscarriage; still
		    birth; infant mortality
		 Sudden infant death syndrome
		 Children: increased respiratory infections and
		    symptoms
		 Deficiencies in physical growth, intellectual
		    development
		 Higher Incidence in mortality rate of infant and
		    child

* United States Food and Drug Administration (FDA) categorizes drugs and their relation to pregnancy as: **A.** No risk demonstrated to fetus in any trimester. **B.** No adverse effects in animals; no human studies available. **C.** Only given after risks to fetus are considered; animal studies have shown no adverse reactions, no human studies available. **D.** Definite fetal risks; may be given in spite of risks if needed in life-threatening conditions. **X.** Absolute fetal abnormalities; not to be used at any time in pregnancy.

growth retardation may be related to maternal zidovudine.[3]

ORAL FINDINGS DURING PREGNANCY

The condition of the gingiva may be the result of an exaggerated response of the tissues to bacterial plaque. When the mouth is in good health and the patient uses adequate personal oral care measures for plaque control, no adverse gingival changes may be expected.

For some patients, the hormones of pregnancy tend to aggravate existing gingival conditions and, therefore, act as secondary or conditioning factors. The gingival reaction in pregnancy is usually seen by the second month and continues to a maximum by the eighth month, when the hormone levels rise.

Exaggerated symptoms abate after the birth of the child, but a completely healthy condition does not necessarily result. A patient with a gingival disturbance during pregnancy continues to have the disturbance, even if to a somewhat lessened degree, after the birth.

I. GENERALIZED GINGIVAL ENLARGEMENT[4,5,6]

A. Clinical Appearance

The appearance varies and shows characteristics of inflamed tissues, including enlargement, shiny surface, bleeding readily on probing, and color changes.

B. Predisposing Factors

1. Local irritation because of an unhygienic oral condition and bacterial plaque on the teeth and gingiva.
2. Hormonal changes during pregnancy that may alter the tissue reaction.

C. Microbiology[7]

Increased proportions of *Prevotella intermedia* may be found with an increase in gingivitis and elevated serum levels of the hormones of pregnancy (estrogen and progesterone).

II. ISOLATED GINGIVAL ENLARGEMENT

An isolated or discrete gingival enlargement, which has been called a "pregnancy tumor," may occur. The use of the word tumor is misleading, because the lesion is not a tumor but a hyperplasia and also occurs in men and nonpregnant women. It has also been called an epulis gravidarum, pregnancy granuloma,[8] or pyogenic granuloma.[9]

A. Clinical Appearance

The enlargement is located superficially on the free gingiva, usually associated with an interdental papilla. It forms in a mushroom-like flat-tened mass, with a smooth, glistening surface.

The color depends on the vascularity and may be purplish-red, magenta, or deep blue, sometimes dotted with red.

B. Symptoms

1. Bleeds readily with slight trauma.
2. Painless unless it becomes large enough to interfere with occlusion and mastication.

III. ENAMEL EROSION

Morning sickness with vomiting over an extended period can lead to demineralization and acid erosion primarily of the palatal surfaces. Nausea associated with early pregnancy can be relieved by frequent eating of small amounts of food. Careful selection of nutritious yet noncariogenic foods is necessary to avoid dental caries.

ASPECTS OF PATIENT CARE

The first few months may be challenging for the mother-to-be, because pregnancy provides an emotional experience with many adjustments that must be made.

I. ORAL EXAMINATION AND TREATMENT PLANNING

The patient should be seen as early in her pregnancy as possible. Consultation with the patient's physician is particularly important to integrate total prenatal care.

Generally, all reasonable treatment is acceptable unless the patient's obstetrician advises otherwise.[10] The second trimester, after the vital organ development period of the first 3 months, is considered the safest period for routine care.

II. RADIOGRAPHY

Radiographs are not made for any patient unless necessary. When they are required during pregnancy, the patient is covered with a lead apron, a thyroid collar, and a second apron for the back to prevent secondary radiation from reaching the abdomen. As always, all current methods for radiation safety and protection are applied, including optimum filtration, collimation, use of the fastest film, and extended target film distance.

Determine the minimum number of film exposures that will produce the required diagnostic information. The use of a paralleling technique does not require angulation directed toward the patient's abdomen. Careful and skillful film placement, angulation, processing, and all phases of technique prevent the need for remaking radiographs that are not acceptable for diagnosis.

III. PERIODONTAL TREATMENT

Areas of food impaction should be corrected and all overhanging restorations reshaped or replaced. All scaling and root planing procedures should be carefully and thoroughly completed. Elective complicated periodontal treatment should be deferred until after delivery.

IV. RESTORATIVE DENTISTRY

Restorations should be completed with permanent restorative materials. One important contraindication for the use of temporary restorations is that, after the baby is born, the mother may be too busy to attend to appointments because of added family responsibilities and/or a return to career employment.

DENTAL HYGIENE CARE

The dental hygienist must be well informed about dental care to motivate the patient and alleviate fears related to certain services. The patient often consults with the dental hygienist for reassurance and interpretation of the dentist's recommendations and procedures.

Gingival disease need not be expected when the patient is motivated to practice conscientious self-care procedures for oral cleanliness and plaque control. This calls for a specific appointment plan for scaling and disease control instruction.

A concentrated plan for dental caries control is indicated. A multiple fluoride program and limitation of cariogenic foods are basic to the preventive efforts.

I. APPOINTMENT PLANNING
A. Frequency
Monthly appointments or appointments 3 times during the 9-month period may be required, depending on the patient's needs as well as ability and motivation to maintain a healthy oral environment.

B. Length of Individual Appointments
An appointment should be short, for patient comfort. A series of appointments is indicated when calculus deposits are heavy.

C. Postpartum Maintenance Appointments
For the patient who has not been on a regular maintenance plan prior to pregnancy, emphasis must be placed on motivating the patient to continue regular appointments for dental hygiene and dental care after the baby is born.

II. APPOINTMENT PROCEDURES
A. Patient History
The medical history must be reviewed carefully at each appointment to identify changes and adapt procedures accordingly. The prenatal patient may require applied techniques for conditions other than pregnancy. For example, diabetes or cardiovascular diseases can involve serious complications.

When the expectant mother is an adolescent, consideration for her own health takes on a different perspective than that for the mature woman. Aspects of adolescent development and psychology are described on pages 624–626.

B. Consultation with Physician
The dentist and the physician benefit mutually through discussion of the patient's treatment plan with the consent of the patient. The need for particular precautions before, during, or after treatment becomes evident.

When a patient seeks dental and dental hygiene care and is not under the care of a physician, she should be urged to obtain medical supervision, have examinations, and thereby improve her health, as well as that of the baby.

III. CLINICAL ASPECTS
It is not within the scope of this book to review all the physiologic changes that occur during pregnancy. Common physical changes should be identified because they can affect appointment procedures. Nearly every woman is bothered by one or more minor complaints at some time during her pregnancy.

Attention to details provides the patient with comfort and motivates her to continue oral care. Table 43–3 lists the more common physical changes of pregnancy and suggests a few appointment considerations.

A. Instrumentation
When a patient has gingival enlargement and inflammation, a good part of the first appointment should be spent on instruction in plaque control and other preventive measures. At the second appointment, evaluation is made and instruction continued.

Careful instrumentation for scaling and planing is indicated. Bleeding may be excessive. If stain removal is indicated, the use of an abrasive cleaning paste should be postponed until the tissue has responded to the plaque control measures.

B. Fluoride Program
1. *Professional Topical Application.* All patients can benefit from a topical application of fluoride solution or gel after scaling and root planing. Applications can be indicated, especially for patients with a tendency toward rampant caries and who have numer-

TABLE 43–3
APPOINTMENT ADAPTATIONS FOR THE PRENATAL PATIENT

Characteristic	Dental Hygiene Implication
Fatigues easily, may even fall asleep	Short appointments; several in series, as needed Work with an assistant to accomplish more at each appointment
Discomfort of remaining in one position too long	Interrupt in middle of appointment to change chair position Assistance with evacuation during intraoral instrumentation can shorten appointment time
Backache	Adjust chair appropriately for comfort
Frequent urination	Allow sufficient appointment time for interruptions Suggest at beginning of appointment that patient mention need for interruption
General awkwardness because of new shape and weight gain	Attend to details, such as gently lowering and straightening chair for patient Make sure rinsing facilities are convenient; or preferably, an assistant attends to evacuation
Dyspnea (aggravated by supine chair position)	Adapt chair for patient comfort
Faintness and dizziness	Be prepared for emergency (table 61–3, pages 842–848). Place the patient on her *side* and not in supine or Trendelenburg position because pressure from the enlarged uterus and the abdominal organs on the inferior vena cava can interfere with venous return; placental separation could result

Nausea and vomiting (first trimester)
  a. Unpleasant taste in mouth
  b. Gagging
 	
  c. Exaggerated reactions to odors and flavors of medicaments and other office materials
 	
  d. Physician's recommendations for alleviation of symptoms: frequent eating of small amounts of foods
	Suggest toothbrushing or rinsing at frequent intervals.
	Recommend a small toothbrush.
	Turn head down over sink while brushing; helps to relax throat and allow saliva to flow out
	Take care in instrument and radiographic film placement
	Determine particularly obnoxious odors for an individual patient and remove them
	Pay attention to cleanliness of cuspidor
	Encourage use of noncariogenic foods

Unusual food cravings	If cravings are for sweets, clearly define relationship of frequent nibbling of cariogenic foods to dental caries Provide list of nutritious noncariogenic snacks

ous restorations. The fluoride agents and techniques are described in Chapter 29, pages 443–449.

2. *Self-application.* A fluoride dentifrice is recommended for all patients. A daily non-alcohol-containing mouthrinse, gel tray, or other mode of application is essential, depending on the individual evaluation. A concentrated fluoride effort can be particularly important to the teeth of the adolescent mother-to-be.

PATIENT INSTRUCTION

The emphasis on general health during pregnancy provides the ideal setting for instruction relative to many aspects of oral health for the mother and her expected child, as well as for other members of the family. New developments in disease prevention and control should be explained.

Printed materials concerning the prevention of periodontal infections and dental caries and the development and care of children's teeth are available from the American Dental Association.* Reading material to supplement personal discussions can contribute to patient understanding and cooperation.

I. BACTERIAL PLAQUE CONTROL

A rigid schedule for self-care must be demonstrated and supervised. A series of instructional periods is usually needed.

Emphasis should not be placed on the hormonal changes of pregnancy as influential in producing gingival changes. The patient may be all too willing to use the systemic factor as an excuse for her lack of attention to adequate self-care.

II. DIET

Instruction must be provided in prevention of dental caries and maintenance of the health of the supporting structures of the teeth. The use of a varied diet containing the essential protective food groups, with a minimum of cariogenic foods, is necessary. The Food Guide Pyramid is shown on page 424.

A. Purposes of Adequate Diet During Pregnancy
1. To maintain daily strength and feeling of well-being.
2. To provide the essential building materials for the developing fetus.
3. To protect and promote the health of the oral tissues of the mother.
4. To minimize any postpartum problems.

B. Dietary Needs During Pregnancy
The *Recommended Dietary Allowances* of the Food and Nutrition Board of the National Research Council specifies the increased allowances during pregnancy and lactation.[11] Because the embryo or fetus is a parasite and thrives at the mother's expense, the mother's diet must be adequate to maintain her own nutritional status and to meet the needs of the fetus.

The particular needs of the fetus are
1. Proteins, for general tissue construction.
2. Minerals, especially calcium and phosphorus, for bone and tooth mineralization; iron for blood corpuscles.
3. Vitamins.

C. Dietary Adjustments[12]
A quart of milk or its equivalent in milk products is sufficient to meet the needs for calcium, phosphorus, and riboflavin, except for the teenage mother, who needs a quart and one half if her

own maturing body requirements are to be met.

An added citrus fruit or other good source of vitamin C, a dark green or deep yellow vegetable daily for vitamin A, and sources for iron, thiamine, and vitamin D are indicated. Proteins of high physiologic value are important, that is, proteins from meat, eggs, fish, and fowl rather than of vegetable origin only.

Calories may be adjusted in accord with exercise and tendency for weight gain. A decreased use of cariogenic foods is important for general nutrition and weight problems, as well as for the prevention of dental caries.

III. DENTAL CARIES CONTROL
A. Incidence During Pregnancy
Some patients believe that they have more dental caries during and because of pregnancy. Research has shown that this is not true, and that any relationship is indirect. Factors that result in dental caries formation are the same during pregnancy as at other times (pages 267 and 268).

B. Factors that May Contribute to Apparent Increase in Dental Caries Rate
1. *Previous Neglect.* A patient may not have kept a regular appointment plan, so that the existing dental caries during pregnancy represents an accumulation, possibly even of years.
2. *Diet During Pregnancy.* Possible increase in intake of fermentable carbohydrates.
   a. Unusual cravings may be for sweet foods.
   b. Frequency of eating; patient may be eating every few hours for prevention of nausea and these foods may be cariogenic.
3. *Neglect of Personal Oral Care Procedures.* Lack of interest or laxity in daily bacterial plaque removal or rinsing immediately following intake of a cariogenic food.

C. Calcium and the Mother's Teeth
The misconception concerning the withdrawal of calcium from the mother's teeth and its relationship to dental caries is widespread. It is important to review the known facts, because the patient's beliefs may need clarification. In discussing the problem with the patient, a summary of the process of dental caries initiation can be helpful (pages 267 and 268).
1. Minerals contained in the erupted tooth enamel and dentin are not available, and no removal of minerals can occur by way of the pulp.

---

* An American Dental Association catalog for the current year may be obtained by writing the Department of Salable Materials, 211 East Chicago Avenue, Chicago, IL 60611.

2. Minerals contained within the alveolar bone are available as they are from other bones of the body. When the mother's diet does not contain sufficient calcium and phosphorus, her own reserve is utilized.

3. Most calcium and phosphorus of bones and teeth is added to the fetus during the third trimester. The incidence of dental caries in the mother is not different during that period, although the carious lesions may be larger if the teeth have been neglected throughout the pregnancy.

4. The teeth of the fetus tend to develop and mineralize normally in spite of the diet of the mother, because the reserve in her bones is used.

D. Relationship of Fluoride

No direct evidence shows that prenatal fluoride intake influences the rate of dental caries in the child.[13,14,15] When the community water supply is not fluoridated, dietary fluoride by prescription brings the fluoride intake to the optimum level and provides some benefit for the mother.

INFANT AND TODDLER ORAL HEALTH

The goal is a child free of dental caries with optimum gingival health. Parents need to understand the importance of the oral health of the newborn and how habits practiced during the early years of life can influence future health.

Counseling for parents starts before and continues after the birth of the baby. Before birth, the parents are looking ahead and planning for the very best care for their baby. They are most receptive to meaningful recommendations.

Through early guidance, parents can be aware of the infant's needs for oral health and anticipate the kind of attention that will be required. Anticipatory guidance is the term that has been applied to teaching ahead of time so that untoward, unfavorable conditions can be prevented.[16]

I. PRENATAL ANTICIPATORY GUIDANCE, BIRTH THROUGH 6 MONTHS (TABLE 43-4)

A. Help the parent understand that infants and toddlers can have dental caries and infections of the oral mucosa.

B. Suggest procedures for the parent's own oral health. The oral flora of the infant reflects the oral flora of the parents. *Mutans streptococci* are transmitted from the parents to the infant.

C. Fluoride must be in the infant's daily diet soon after birth for proper mineralization of the bones and teeth.

1. Determine the fluoride content of the water used at home (page 442).

2. Analyze the need for prescription of fluoride supplements.

3. Totally breastfed infants after 6 months of age need .25 mg NaF daily supplement (drops).

4. After the infant is weaned, continue fluoride supplement when fluoride is not in the water supply (page 443).

5. Bottle-fed infants receive formula made with fluoridated water; a supplement is prescribed when the water is not fluoridated.

D. Plan ahead for the infant's first dental hygiene visit.

II. FIRST DENTAL/DENTAL HYGIENE VISIT

A. Age

The first appointment should be planned between ages 6 and 12 months, but within 6 months of the eruption of the first tooth.[17]

B. Purposes

The early appointments are planned for prevention, introduction to dentistry, and oral assessment.[18]

1. Discover, intercept, and change any practices applied by the parents that may be detrimental to the infant's oral health.

2. Initiate positive preventive measures, such as fluoride, feeding practices, and bacterial plaque removal.

3. Develop rapport with the baby and the family.

C. Record Medical, Dental, and Feeding History[18]

The forms for the histories may be best filled out before the appointment. They can be mailed to the parents prior to the first appointment.

D. Appointment Procedures

1. *Patient Position During Oral Examination.* Clinician and parent sit knee-to-knee with infant positioned on their laps. The clinician cradles the head; the parent gently holds the baby's hands, and may stabilize the legs with the elbows (figure 43–1).

2. *Extra- and Intraoral Examination*
   a. Follow routine in table 8–2 (pages 120 and 121) and table 11–2 (page 188).
   b. Proceed calmly with soft talk. Anticipate that many infants will fuss and cry; reassure parent.
   c. Watch for physical signs of child abuse (pages 127 and 128).

3. *Instruction for Bacterial Plaque Removal*
   a. Clinician demonstrates cleaning the teeth with a soft toothbrush; patient is held as described for the oral examination.

TABLE 43–4
ANTICIPATORY GUIDANCE: INFANTS AND TODDLERS

Area of Concern	Birth to 6 Months	6 to 12 Months	18 Months
Developmental Milestone	Eruption of first tooth Pattern of eruption	Pattern of eruption Expected new teeth	Check tooth contacts Close contacts: teach to floss
Nutrition and Feeding	Appropriate use of nursing bottle Use of only tap water Causes of nursing caries Discourage parent sleeping with child	Discontinue bottle feeding Use Tippy Cup Discuss sugar use, sugar retention, and caries initiation	Nutrition, snacking based on child's diet Snacking safety (aspiration)
Oral Hygiene and Caries Prevention	Clean teeth after each feeding (wash cloth, soft brush)	Use of brush Position of infant for brushing	Disclose for bacterial plaque Review brushing
Fluoride Information	Need for fluoride (F) Provide systemic F Check water supply for existing F Prescribe supplements when deficient	Review fluoride used Discuss compliance Review manner of storage	Update fluoride status Use of pea-size fluoride dentifrice on brush
Trauma Prevention		Trauma-proofing Confirm emergency access to dental provider	Discuss oral electrical burns and child-proofing home
Habits/Function Behaviors	Discuss teething, nonnutritive sucking, and *Streptococcus mutans* transmission	Discuss oral signs of child abuse	Home preparation for dental hygiene visit
Dental/Dental Hygiene Visit	What happens at baby's dental visit	First visit within 6 months of eruption first tooth	Frequency depends on parent compliance with home preventive measures

(Adapted from Casamassimo, P.S., Griffiths, P., and Nowak, A.: Anticipatory Guidance in Dentistry, *Dentalhygienistnews, 5,* 19, Fall, 1992.)

Flossing is needed when teeth are in close contact.
  b. Parent demonstrates the cleaning procedure; the baby is turned around so that the clinician holds the hands and stabilizes the legs with the elbows.
4. *Counseling* (table 43–4)
All aspects of significance for the particular child are discussed with the parents: fluoride, diet and feeding, daily oral care. Reading materials are provided for review and discussion with the parents.

III. DAILY BACTERIAL PLAQUE REMOVAL
A. Planned Time
Parents need a routine for cleaning the infant's mouth. They must continue to care for the mouth until the child is old enough to care for all personal bathing and health care habits.
1. Until the infant's first tooth erupts, place a clean damp cloth over finger and wipe over oral tissues and gingiva after each feeding.

2. After first tooth erupts, use a soft small toothbrush.

B. Position of Infant
Two family members can work together to make this experience pleasant and easy. Sit opposite each other with the infant between (figure 43–1). For other positions, see figure 50–10, page 697.

IV. DIET AND FEEDING
A. Prevention of Nursing Caries
1. Describe nursing caries, how it is caused, and which teeth are most frequently involved (page 234).[19,20]
2. Nap or nighttime bottle
   a. It is best never to start giving a bottle for bedtime use.
   b. If a bottle is used, avoid sweet juices or milk and use only plain tap water.
   c. Recommend discontinuance of bottle

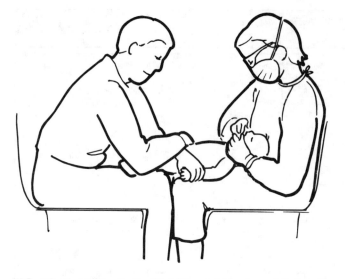

FIG. 43–1. Infant's Dental/Dental Hygiene Visits. Clinician and parent sit knee-to-knee with the child across their laps. Parent stabilizes the infant's legs and holds the hands in a position that allows a good view of the patient's oral cavity for watching and learning. The clinician makes the oral examination, discusses any oral problems, and shows the parent oral care.

feeding at least by the age of 12 months and teach the child to use a cup.[21]

3. Avoid "on-demand" breast-feeding practices. When the infant falls asleep, milk collects around the teeth. Demineralization begins, and dental caries can result.

B. Snacks

Nonsucrose-containing snacks must be used. *Frequency* and *consistency* of snack foods are most significant.

C. Medications and Nutritional Supplements

Many medications and other products for child consumption are made with a sugar or syrupy base to disguise the bad flavor of the drug.[22,23] For counteractivity, rinse and brush the child's mouth with clear water immediately after the medication is given.

V. MAINTENANCE

Certain risk factors need consideration when frequency of appointments is determined.[24] The history and record of assessment contain most of the basic information needed. Infants with a high risk for dental caries need frequent preventive maintenance appointments. As the child grows older, attention must be paid to risks related to gingival conditions.

A. Low Risk

1. Family members oriented to oral health care; family with no history of needing extensive

professional care.

2. Infant has received systemic fluoride from birth through fluoridation or fluoride supplements.

3. A normal general health history.

B. High Risk

1. Family members with history of irregular professional care in whom moderate to severe dental and periodontal treatment has been needed.

2. Residence in nonfluoridated community; systemic supplements not provided.

3. Presence of congenital or hereditary defect or developmental disability.

4. Administration of medications with potentially high sucrose base is required.

5. Dental examination that shows early eruption pattern, areas of demineralization, and notable bacterial plaque build-up.

6. Need for parental supervision and reminders for maintenance of daily routine of oral hygiene, weaning from nursing bottle, and general compliance with the plan for prevention.

REFERENCES

1. **Fiese,** R. and Herzog, S.: Issues in Dental and Surgical Management of the Pregnant Patient, *Oral Surg. Oral Med. Oral Pathol., 65,* 292, March, 1988.

2. **Gier,** R.E. and Janes, D.R.: Dental Management of the Pregnant Patient, *Dent. Clin. North Am., 27,* 419, April, 1983.

3. **Sperling,** R.S., Stratton, P., O'Sullivan, M.J., Boyer, P., Watts, D.H., Lambert, J.S., Hammill, H., Livingston, E.G., Gloeb, D.J., Minkoff, H., and Fox, H.E.: A Survey of Zidovudine Use in Pregnant Women with Human Immunodeficiency Virus Infection, *N. Engl. J. Med., 326,* 857, March 26, 1992.

4. **Carranza,** F.A.: *Glickman's Clinical Periodontology,* 7th ed. Philadelphia, W.B. Saunders Co., 1990, pp. 136–138, 364, 452-455, 576.

5. **Rose,** L.F.: Sex Hormonal Imbalances, Oral Manifestations, and Dental Treatment, in Genco, R.J., Goldman, H.M., and Cohen, D.W., eds.: *Contemporary Periodontics.* St. Louis, Mosby, 1990, pp. 221–224.

6. **Hoag,** P.M. and Pawlak, E.A.: *Essentials of Periodontics,* 4th ed. St. Louis, Mosby, 1990, pp. 47–49.

7. **Kornman,** K.S. and Loesche, W.J.: The Subgingival Microbial Flora During Pregnancy, *J. Periodont. Res., 15,* 111, March, 1980.

8. **Pindborg,** J.J.: *Atlas of Diseases of the Oral Mucosa,* 5th ed. Philadelphia, W.B. Saunders Co., 1992, pp. 286–288.

9. **Shafer,** W.G., Hine, M.K., and Levy, B.M.: *A Textbook of Oral Pathology,* 4th ed. Philadelphia, W.B. Saunders Co., 1983, p. 359.

10. **Shrout,** M.K., Comer, R.W., Powell, B.J., and McCoy, B.P.: Treating the Pregnant Dental Patient: Four Basic Rules Addressed, *J. Am Dent. Assoc., 123,* 75, May, 1992.

11. **National Research Council,** Committee on Dietary Allowances, Food and Nutrition Board: *Recommended Dietary Allowances,* 10th ed. Washington, D.C., National Academy of Sciences, Office of Publications, 1989.

12. **Worthington-Roberts,** B.S.: Nutrition During Pregnancy and

Lactation, in Mahan, L.K. and Arlin, M.T.: *Krause's Food, Nutrition & Diet Therapy,* 8th ed. Philadelphia, W.B. Saunders Co., 1992, pp. 151–167.

13. **Driscoll,** W.S.: A Review of Clinical Research on the Use of Prenatal Fluoride Administration for Prevention of Dental Caries, *ASDC J. Dent. Child., 48,* 109, March-April, 1981.

14. **Thylstrup,** A.: Is There a Biologic Rationale for Prenatal Fluoride Administration? *ASDC J. Dent. Child., 48,* 103, March-April, 1981.

15. **Bawden,** J.W., ed.: Changing Patterns of Fluoride Intake, Workshop Report—Group III, *J. Dent. Res., 71,* 1224, Special Issue, May, 1992.

16. **Casamassimo,** P.S., Griffiths, P., and Nowak, A.: Anticipatory Guidance in Dentistry, *Dentalhygienistnews, 5,* 19, Fall, 1992.

17. **American Academy of Pediatric Dentistry:** A.A.P.D. Oral Health Policies, Guidelines, and Quality Assurance Documents, Reference Manual 1993–94, *Pediatr. Dent., 15,* 30, Special Issue, No. 7, 1993.

18. **Goepferd,** S.: Examination of the Infant and Toddler, in Pinkham, J.R., ed.: *Pediatric Dentistry: Infancy Through Adolescence,* 2nd ed. Philadelphia, W.B. Saunders Co., 1994, pp. 181–191.

19. **Yasin-Harnekar,** S.: Nursing Caries. A Review. *Clin Prev. Dent., 10,* 3, March-April, 1988.

20. **Steiner,** J.F.: Baby Bottle Tooth Decay: Recognition, Intervention, and Prevention, in American Academy of Pediatric Dentistry: *Pediatric Dental Care. An Update for the 90s.* Evansville, IN, Bristol-Myers Squibb Co., 1991, pp. 21–22.

21. **American Academy of Pediatric Dentistry:** A.A.P.D. Oral Health Policies, Guidelines, and Quality Assurance Documents, Reference Manual 1993–94, *Pediatr. Dent., 15,* 27, Special Issue, No. 7, 1993.

22. **Gehrke,** P.S. and Johnsen, D.S.: Bottle Caries Associated with Anti-HIV Therapy, *Pediatr. Dent., 13,* 73, January/February, 1991.

23. **Howell,** R.B. and Houpt, M.: More Than One Factor Can Influence Caries Development in HIV-Positive Children, *Pediatr. Dent., 13,* 247, July/August, 1991.

24. **Nowak,** A. and Crall, J.: Prevention of Dental Disease, in Pinkham, J.R., ed.: *Pediatric Dentistry: Infancy Through Adolescence,* 2nd ed. Philadelphia, W.B. Saunders Co., 1994, pp. 192–194.

SUGGESTED READINGS

Daley, T.D., Nartey, N.O., and Wysocki, G.P.: Pregnancy Tumor: An Analysis, *Oral Surg. Oral Med. Oral Pathol., 72,* 196, August, 1991.

Kay, E.J., and McGuiness, J.: Pregnant Women's Dental Health Knowledge, *Dental Health, 29,* 3, No. 2, 1990.

Lynch-Salamon, D.I. and Combs, C.A.: Hepatitis C in Obstetrics and Gynecology, *Obstet. Gynecol., 79,* 621, April, 1992.

Miyazaki, H., Yamashita, Y., Shirahama, R., Goto-Kimura, K., Shimada, N., Sogame, A., and Takehara, T.: Periodontal Condition of Pregnant Women Assessed by CPITN, *J. Clin. Periodontol., 18,* 751, November, 1991.

Ojanotko-Harri, A.O., Harri, M.-P., Hurttia, H.M., and Sewón, L.A.: Altered Tissue Metabolism of Progesterone in Pregnancy Gingivitis and Granuloma, *J. Clin. Periodontol., 18,* 262, April, 1991.

Ringdahl, E.N.: The Role of the Family Physician in Preventing Teenage Pregnancy, *Am. Fam. Physician, 45,* 2215, May, 1992.

Soorlyamoorthy, M. and Gower, D.B.: Hormonal Influences on Gingival Tissue: Relationship to Periodontal Disease, *J. Clin. Periodontol., 16,* 201, April, 1989.

Tolle-Watts, L.: The Pregnant Patient, *Dentalhygienistnews, 3,* 4, Summer, 1990.

Whitehead, R.G.: Pregnancy and Lactation, in Shils, M.E. and Young, V.R., eds.: *Modern Nutrition in Health and Disease,* 7th ed. Philadelphia, Lea & Febiger, 1988, pp. 931–943.

Zachariasen, R.D.: Ovarian Hormones and Oral Health: Pregnancy Gingivitis, *Compendium, 10,* 508, September, 1989.

Drugs, Smoking

Fingerhut, L.A., Kleinman, J.C., and Kendrick, J.S.: Smoking Before, During, and After Pregnancy, *Am. J. Public Health, 80,* 541, May, 1990.

Jauniaux, E. and Burton, G.J.: The Effect of Smoking in Pregnancy on Early Placental Morphology, *Obstet. Gynecol., 79,* 645, May, 1992.

Kleinman, J.C. and Madans, J.H.: The Effects of Maternal Smoking, Physical Stature, and Educational Attainment on the Incidence of Low Birth Weight, *Am. J. Epidemiol., 121,* 843, No. 6, 1985.

Kleinman, J.C., Pierre, M.B., Madans, J.H., Land, G.H., and Schramm, W.F.: The Effects of Maternal Smoking on Fetal and Infant Mortality, *Am. J. Epidemiol., 127,* 274, February, 1988.

Mennella, J.A. and Beauchamp, G.K.: The Transfer of Alcohol to Human Milk, *N. Engl. J. Med., 325,* 982, October 3, 1991.

Rosenberg, N.M., Meert, K.L., Knazik, S.R., Yee, H., and Kauffman, R.E.: Occult Cocaine Exposure in Children, *Am. J. Dis. Child., 145,* 1430, Decemmber, 1991.

Schoendorf, K.C. and Kiely, J.L.: Relationship of Sudden Infant Death Syndrome to Maternal Smoking During and after Pregnancy, *Pediatrics, 90,* 905, December, 1992.

Slutsker, L.: Risks Associated with Cocaine Use During Pregnancy, *Obstet. Gynecol., 79,* 778, May, 1992.

United States Centers for Disease Control: Cigarette Smoking among Reproductive-aged Women—Behavioral Risk Factor Surveillance System, 1989, *MMWR, 40,* 719, October 25, 1991.

Volpe, J.J.: Effect of Cocaine Use on the Fetus, *N. Engl. J. Med., 327,* 399, August 6, 1992.

Wen, S.W., Goldenburg, R.L., Cutter, G.R., Hoffman, H.J., Cliver, S.P., Davis, R.O., and DuBard, M.B.: Smoking, Maternal Age, Fetal Growth, and Gestational Age at Delivery, *Am. J. Obstet. Gynecol., 162,* 53, January, 1990.

Infant/Toddler

Acs, G., Lodolini, G., Kaminsky, S., and Cisneros, G.J.: Effect of Nursing Caries on Body Weight in a Pediatric Population, *Pediatr. Dent., 14,* 302, September/October, 1992.

American Academy of Pediatric Dentistry: *Pediatric Dental Care: An Update for the 90s.* Evansville, IN, Bristol-Myers Squibb, 1991.

Berkowitz, R.J. and Jones, P.: Mouth-to-mouth Transmission of the Bacterium *Streptococcus mutans* Between Mother and Child, *Arch. Oral Biol., 30,* 377, No. 4, 1985.

Bishara, S.E., Nowak, A.J., Kohout, F.J., Heckert, D.A., and Hogan, M.M.: Influence of Feeding and Non-nutritive Sucking Methods on the Development of the Dental Arches: Longitudinal Study of the First 18 Months of Life, *Pediatr. Dent., 9,* 13, March, 1987.

Frazier, P.J. and Horowitz, A.M.: Oral Health Education and Promotion in Maternal and Child Health: A Position Paper, *J. Public Health Dent., 50,* 391, Special Issue, 1990.

Goepferd, S.J.: An Infant Oral Health Program: The First 18 Months, *Pediatr. Dent., 9,* 8, March, 1987.

Haddad, R.Y.: An Unusual Hazard of Toothbrushing, *Br. Dent. J., 168,* 296, April 7, 1990.

Holm, A.-K.: Education and Diet in the Prevention of Caries in the Preschool Child, *J. Dent., 18,* 308, December, 1990.

Holm, A.-K.: Caries in the Preschool Child: International Trends, *J. Dent., 18,* 291, December, 1990.

McIlveen, L.P.: Pediatric Behavior Management: The Dental Assistant's Role, *Dent. Assist., 60,* 11, March/April, 1991.

Nowjack-Raymer, R. and Gift, H.C: Contributing Factors to Maternal and Child Oral Health, *J. Public Health Dent., 50,* 370, Special Issue, 1990.

Reilly, S., Wolke, D., and Skuse, D.: Tooth Eruption in Failure-to-thrive Infants, *ASDC J. Dent. Child., 59,* 350, September-October, 1992.

Wilson, A.A.: Standards in Maternal and Child Oral Health, *J. Public Health Dent., 50,* 432, Special Issue, 1990.

Wright, F.A.C., McMurray, N.E., and Giebartowski, J.: Strategies Used by Dentists in Victoria, Australia, to Manage Children with Anxiety or Behavior Problems, *ASDC J. Dent. Child., 58,* 223, May-June, 1991.

The Patient with a Cleft Lip and/or Palate

The patient with a cleft lip and/or cleft palate may be a dental cripple unless extensive rehabilitative supervision is available. Treatment and care require the united efforts of nearly all the dental specialists, as well as of the family physician, plastic surgeon, speech therapist, psychologist, otolaryngologist, audiologist, social worker, and vocational counselor. The dental hygienist is an important member of the team responsible for oral care.

Speaking ability and appearance are among the first factors considered when the long-range treatment program is planned, because the objective is to help the patient lead a normal life. Dental personnel need to maintain a current list of the health agencies, clinics, and other community resources where the patient and family may obtain assistance for the various phases of treatment and habilitation.

Key words relating to cleft lip and/or palate are defined in table 44–1.

CLASSIFICATION OF CLEFTS

The classification is based on disturbances in the embryologic formation of the palate as it develops from the premaxillary region toward the uvula in a definite pattern. Interference with normal development of the palate may occur at one age level of the embryo, and the normal pattern may be re-established at a later age. Such interferences would modify the classification suggested in this chapter.

All degrees are found, from an insignificant notch in the mucous membrane of the lip or uvula, which produces no functional disability, to the complete cleft defined by Class 6 of this classification. The first six classes are illustrated in figure 44–1.

Class 1. Cleft of the tip of the uvula.
Class 2. Cleft of the uvula (bifid uvula).
Class 3. Cleft of the soft palate.
Class 4. Cleft of the soft and hard palates.
Class 5. Cleft of the soft and hard palates that continues through the alveolar ridge on one side of the premaxilla; usually associated with cleft lip of the same side.
Class 6. Cleft of the soft and hard palates that continues through the alveolar ridge on both sides, leaving a free premaxilla; usually associated with bilateral cleft lip.
Class 7. Submucous cleft in which the muscle union is imperfect across the soft palate. The palate is short; the uvula is often bifid; a groove is situated at the midline of the soft palate; and the closure to the pharynx is incompetent.

ETIOLOGY

I. EMBRYOLOGY[1,2]

Cleft lip and palate represent a failure of normal fusion of embryonic processes during development in the first trimester of pregnancy. Figure 44–2 shows the locations of the globular process and the right and left maxillary processes. These fuse normally and no cleft of the lip results.

Formation of the lip occurs between the fourth and seventh week in utero. The development of the palate takes place during the eighth to twelfth week. Fusion begins in the premaxillary region and continues backward toward the uvula.

617

TABLE 44-1
KEY WORDS: CLEFT LIP AND/OR PALATE

Bifid uvula (bī'fĭd ū'vū-lah): cleft of the uvula of the soft palate into two parts (figure 44–1).

Cleft lip: a unilateral or bilateral congenital fissure in the upper lip usually lateral to the midline; can extend into the nares and may involve the alveolar process; caused by defect in the fusion of the maxillary and medial nasal processes.

Cleft palate: a congenital fissure in the palate caused by failure of the palatal shelves to fuse; may extend to connect with unilateral or bilateral cleft lip.

Congenital (kon-jen'ĭ tal): present at and existing from the time of birth.

Heredity (hĕ-red'ĭ-tē): genetic transmission of traits from parents to offspring; the hereditary material, chromosomes, is contained within the ovum and the sperm (23 chromosomes each), which unite when the sperm penetrates the ovum.

Obturator (ob'tu-rā'tor): a prosthesis designed to close a congenital or acquired opening, such as a cleft of the hard palate.

Prosthesis (pros-thē'sĭs): an artificial replacement of an absent part of the human body; a therapeutic device to improve or alter function.

Rehabilitation (rē'hah-bil'ĭ-tā'shun): the process of restoring a person's ability to live and work as normally as possible after a disabling injury or illness; aims to help the individual to achieve maximum possible physical and psychologic fitness and to regain ability to carry out personal care.

   Habilitation: the same goals and objectives, but for a person with a congenitally acquired disability for whom the ability to achieve maximum physical and psychologic fitness is acquired for the first time.

Speech aid prosthesis: a prosthetic device with a posterior section to assist with palatopharyngeal closure; also called bulb, speech bulb, or prosthetic speech appliance.

   Pediatric speech aid prosthesis: a temporary or interim prosthesis used to close a defect in the hard and/or soft palate; may replace tissue lost as a result of developmental or surgical alterations; necessary for intelligible speech.

   Adult speech aid prosthesis: a definitive prosthesis to improve speech by obturating (sealing off) a palatal cleft or occasionally assisting an incompetent soft palate.

Syndrome (sin'drōm): a combination of symptoms either resulting from a single cause or occurring so commonly together as to constitute a distinct clinical picture.

Velopharyngeal insufficiency (vel'-ō-fah-rin'jē-al): anatomic or functional deficiency in the soft palate or the muscle affecting closure of the opening between mouth and nose in speech; results in a nasal speech quality.

Velum (vē'lum): covering structure or veil.

   Palatine velum (or velum palatinum): soft palate.

A cleft lip becomes apparent by the end of the second month. A cleft palate is evident by the end of the third month *in utero*.

II. PREDISPOSING FACTORS

Genetic and environmental factors are significant. The most critical period is prior to the fifth week. Infectious diseases, nutritional deficiencies, drugs (for example, alcohol, steroids, anticonvulsant medications), substance abuse, and cigarette smoking have all been implicated. Lack of prenatal care is also considered a risk factor.

ORAL CHARACTERISTICS

I. TOOTH DEVELOPMENT

Disturbances in the normal development of the tooth buds occur more frequently in patients with clefts than in the general population. There is a higher incidence of missing and supernumerary teeth, as well as of abnormalities of tooth form.

II. MALOCCLUSION

A high percentage of patients with cleft lip and palate require orthodontic care.

III. OPEN PALATE

Before surgical correction, an open palate provides direct communication with the nasal cavity.

IV. MUSCLE COORDINATION

A lack of coordinate movements of lips, tongue, cheeks, floor of mouth, and throat may exist and lead to compensatory habits formed in the attempt to produce normal sounds while speaking.

V. GINGIVAL DISTURBANCES

These are created by effects of bacterial plaque accumulation influenced by irregularly positioned teeth, displaced teeth, inability to keep lips closed, mouth breathing, and difficulties in accomplishing adequate personal oral care. Early periodontal disease with loss of bone and attachment at cleft sites is common in adolescents.[3]

VI. DENTAL CARIES

The incidence of dental caries should be no different from that in noncleft patients, except that predisposing factors, such as irregularly positioned teeth, problems of mastication, and dietary selection factors, may be intensified.

VII. TREATED PATIENT

   A. Suture lines from surgical correction may be evident.

   B. Patient may have a prosthesis, obturator, or speech aid.

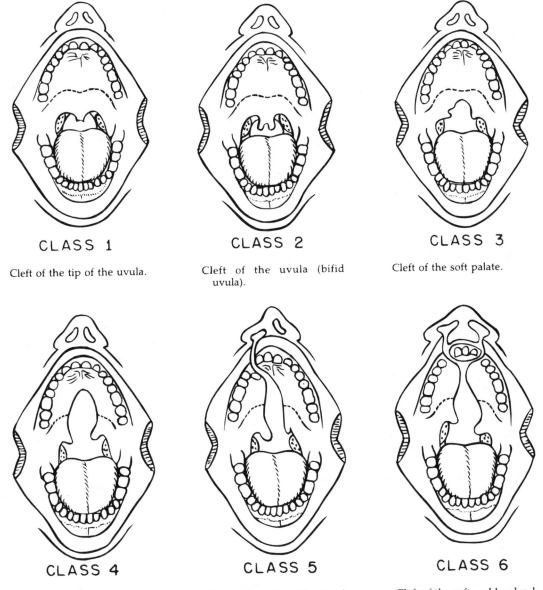

CLASS 1

Cleft of the tip of the uvula.

CLASS 2

Cleft of the uvula (bifid uvula).

CLASS 3

Cleft of the soft palate.

CLASS 4

Cleft of the soft and hard palates.

CLASS 5

Cleft of the soft and hard palates that continues through the alveolar ridge on one side of the premaxilla. Usually associated with cleft lip of the same side.

CLASS 6

Cleft of the soft and hard palates that continues through the alveolar ridge on both sides, leaving a free premaxilla. Usually associated with bilateral cleft lip.

FIG. 44–1. Classification of Cleft Lip and Cleft Palate. (Courtesy of O.E. Beder.)

GENERAL PHYSICAL CHARACTERISTICS

I. OTHER CONGENITAL ANOMALIES

Incidence is higher than that in noncleft people. In more than 300 disorders, cleft lip, cleft palate, or both represent 1 feature of a syndrome.[4]

II. FACIAL DEFORMITY

Facial deformities may include depression of the nostril on the side with the cleft lip; deficiency of upper lip, which may be short or retroposed; and overprominent lower lip.

III. INFECTIONS

Predisposition to upper respiratory and middle ear infections is common.

IV. HEARING LOSS

The incidence of hearing loss is significantly higher in individuals with cleft palate than in the noncleft population.

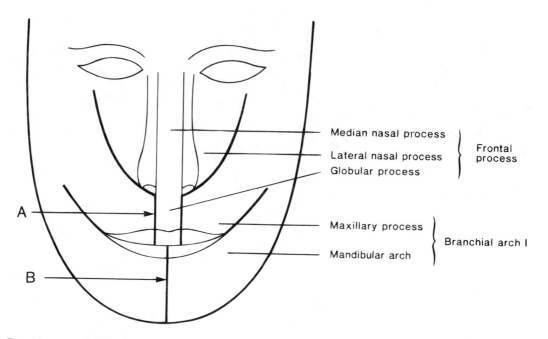

FIG. 44–2. Developmental Processes of the Face. The derivations of parts of the face from the frontal process and the branchial arch. **A.** Location of cleft lip when fusion of the globular process and a maxillary process fails. **B.** Cleft of the mandible can occur at the midline. (Redrawn from Melfi, R.C.: *Permar's Oral Embryology and Microscopic Anatomy,* 8th ed. Philadelphia, Lea & Febiger, 1988.)

V. SPEECH
Patients with cleft lip and/or cleft palate have difficulty in making certain sounds and may produce nasal tones. Anatomic structure is not considered the only contributing factor to the speech problem. It may be related to the hearing loss or to psychologic factors related to inferior feelings or parental attitude.

VI. UNDERNOURISHMENT
Undernourishment may result when feeding problems continue for a long period.

PERSONAL FACTORS

Most patients with a cleft lip or palate do not have personality problems, but realization of the social effects of speech and appearance makes it possible to understand why some of these patients exhibit evidences of maladjustment. The ridicule of contemporaries soon leads even young children to think they are "different." Parental acceptance or rejection no doubt can be a strong influence in adjustment. A few possible characteristics are suggested here.

I. SELF-CONSCIOUSNESS
Hypersensitivity to taunts or obvious pity.

II. FEELINGS OF INFERIORITY
The result may be a person who is quiet, unresponsive, and withdrawn, or one who is openly brash or rebellious until rapport is established.

TREATMENT

Treatment is coordinated by a team of specialists and is based on the patient's progress at each age period. Several reviews provide overviews of the types of treatment and the objectives of each.[5,6]

I. CLEFT LIP
Surgical union of the cleft lip is made early, for example when the child weighs 10 pounds and is 10 weeks old. The infant's general health is a determining factor, and some surgeons wait until the birth weight is regained or the weight has reached 12 pounds. Another timetable is to repair the cleft lip within 48 hours after birth and the cleft palate by 16 weeks.[5,7]

The closure aids in feeding, development of the premaxilla, and growth of the lip, and may also help to partially close the palatal cleft. The operation has a favorable effect on parents and family members in that it helps to lessen their apprehension and concern.

At the time of lip surgery, an obturator may be made for the palate to make feeding easier and provide support for the lip and premaxilla. It is remade periodically to accommodate for the growth and development of the child. For each step in treatment, the parents or caregiver need instruction for the daily care of the patient's oral cavity and the frequent, meticulous cleaning and care of the appliance.

II. CLEFT PALATE

Repair of the palate should be undertaken between ages 1 and 2 years. Occlusion has a strong influence on the development of palatal dimensions, and growth is rapid during this period. Surgical intervention too early could interfere with normal growth. The combined efforts of many specialists are required.

A. Purposes for Early Treatment
1. Improve child's appearance.
2. Aid child's mental development.
3. Prevent malnourishment by improving the feeding apparatus.
4. Aid in development of the speech pattern.
5. Reduce possibilities of repeated infections of the nasopharyngeal region.

B. Maxillofacial Surgery
Closure of the palate is accomplished by surgery or prosthodontics or both. Surgery provides direct union of the existing tissue that has been moved to a more desirable position for function.

III. PROSTHODONTICS
A. Types of Appliances
A removable prosthesis is designed to provide closure of the palatal opening (obturator) and/or to complete the palatopharyngeal valving required for speech (speech aid prosthesis).

B. Purposes and Functions of the Prosthesis
The prosthesis may be designed to accomplish one or all of the following factors:
1. Closure of the palate.
2. Replacement of missing teeth.
3. Scaffolding to fill out the upper lip.
4. Masticatory function.
5. Restoration of vertical dimension.
6. Postorthodontic retainer.

IV. ORTHODONTICS
Treatment may be initiated as early as 3 years of age, depending on the problems of dentofacial development.

V. SPEECH THERAPY
Training may be started with very young children and is particularly emphasized after the surgical or prosthodontic treatment has been accomplished.

VI. RESTORATIVE DENTISTRY (PEDIATRIC DENTIST OR GENERAL DENTAL PRACTITIONER)
A major problem can be dental caries, leading to tooth loss. With missing teeth, major difficulties arise related to all phases of treatment, particularly the retention of a prosthesis. Preservation of the primary teeth is very important.

DENTAL HYGIENE CARE

Preventive measures for preservation of the teeth and their supporting structures are essential to the success of the special care needed for the rehabilitation of the cleft palate patient. Each phase of dental hygiene care and instruction, important for all patients, takes on even greater significance in the light of the magnified problems of the patient with a cleft lip and/or cleft palate.

Every attempt should be made to avoid the need for removal of teeth because the patient has enough oral problems without also being edentulous. Primary and permanent teeth are needed for the stabilization of a speech aid or obturator and for the success of all treatment procedures. Understanding by the patient and the parents of the value of preventive procedures is accomplished through explanation and instruction.

When the patient has not had specialized care, the dental team has a responsibility to arrange referral to an available agency, clinic, or private practice specialist.

I. OBJECTIVES FOR APPOINTMENT PLANNING
Frequent appointments, scheduled every 3 or 4 months, are usually needed during the maintenance phase of the patient's care.
A. To review plaque control measures and provide encouragement for the patient in maintaining the health of the supporting structures and the cleanliness of the obturator or speech aid.
B. To remove all calculus and smooth the tooth surfaces as a supplement to the patient's personal daily care procedures.
C. To provide topical fluoride applications at proper intervals for both primary and permanent dentitions, and to supervise self-application of daily fluoride.

II. APPOINTMENT CONSIDERATIONS
A. A patient who has often been in a hospital for oral surgery may be very apprehensive about dental and dental hygiene care.
B. Speech may be almost unintelligible, although with repeated contact, understanding can be developed.
   1. Avoid embarrassment produced by constantly asking the patient to repeat what has been said.
   2. Provide pencil and paper for the older child to write requests or comments.
   3. Let parent or other person accompanying small child interpret.
C. Depending on the severity of hearing loss, the approach is similar to that for speech difficulties. Suggestions for care of patients with hearing problems are described on pages 734–740.

D. Avoid solicitousness or obvious pity. Approach as a normal patient.

E. Provide motivations for quiet unresponsive or bold rebellious types that help them gain an objective approach to the care of their mouths.

III. INFECTION CONTROL

Although procedures for asepsis should be the same for all patients, one should remember that the open fissure lines make the patient with a cleft palate particularly susceptible to infections.

IV. INSTRUMENTATION

Techniques are adapted to the oral characteristics. All objectives of scaling and other instrumentation have particular implications for the patient with a cleft palate.

A. Malaligned Teeth

Adjust scaling and root planing procedures.

B. Free Premaxilla (Unoperated Older Patient)

Related to bilateral cleft of alveolar ridge; avoid undue pressure with finger rests or instrument to prevent movement of the part.

C. Area of Recent Surgery

Avoid pressure.

D. Sensitive, Enlarged Gingival Tissue that Bleeds Readily

1. Begin plaque control instruction before any instrumentation.
2. Continue plaque control instruction as small sections of scaling are done over several appointments.
3. Arrange follow-up appointments to check response of tissue.

E. Open Fissures

Prevent debris or pieces of calculus from passing into or being retained in the clefts. Whenever possible, use rubber dam for indicated procedures.

F. Lack of Coordinated Movements

Young children especially may need instruction in how to rinse when this procedure is new for them.

G. Prosthesis or Speech Aid

Use same procedures and precautions as for cleaning a removable denture (pages 383).

V. TOPICAL APPLICATION OF FLUORIDE

Free premaxilla or short upper lip may complicate cotton-roll or tray placement.

VI. PATIENT INSTRUCTION

A. Personal Oral Care Procedures

The self-conscious patient may actually fear or exhibit rejection toward the oral cavity. With a small child, the parents may be afraid of damaging the deformed areas or hurting the child if cleaning methods are employed. An empathetic and sympathetic approach and plan for continued instruction over a long period of time is needed.

1. *Teeth and Gingiva*
   a. Select toothbrush, brushing method, and auxiliary aids according to the individual needs.
   b. Adapt techniques for patient with free premaxilla to prevent its movement. A soft nylon brush with end-rounded filaments is indicated.
   c. Instigate daily self-application of fluoride by way of mouthrinse, fluoride dentifrice, and diet supplements for a young child in a nonfluoridated community (pages 449–453).

2. *Prosthesis or Speech Aid*. Halitosis may be a real problem when the prosthesis forms the soft palate and the floor of the nasal cavity because of the accumulation of mucus secreted by the nasal cavity surfaces.
   a. Instruct patient in the need for frequent removal of appliance for cleaning, particularly following eating.
   b. Method for cleaning the prosthesis is the same as that for a removable partial denture (pages 383 and 384).

B. Diet

1. *Need for a Varied Diet*. Should include adequate proportions of all essential food groups (figure 28–1, page 424).
2. *Need for Prevention of Dental Caries*. Limitation of cariogenic foods, particularly for between-meal snacks.

VII. DENTAL HYGIENE CARE RELATED TO ORAL SURGERY

A. Presurgery (pages 657–659)

Objectives have particular significance because the patient with a cleft palate is unusually susceptible to infections of the upper respiratory area and middle ear. Every precaution should be taken to prevent complications.

B. Postsurgery Personal Oral Care

In certain of the palate operations, arm restraints are applied to prevent accidental damage to the repaired region. After each feeding (liquid diet for several days, soft diet for the next week), the mouth must be rinsed carefully. Brushing must be accomplished with great care, usually by the parent or caregiver, to avoid damage to the healing suture lines. In some cases, a toothbrush with suction attachment may be useful (page 708).

REFERENCES

1. **Melfi,** R.C.: *Permar's Oral Embryology and Microscopic Anatomy,* 9th ed. Philadelphia, Lea & Febiger, 1994, pp. 25–41.
2. **Avery,** J.K. and Steele, P.F.: *Essentials of Oral Histology and Embryology.* St. Louis, Mosby, 1992, pp. 39–50.
3. **Brägger,** U., Schürch, E., Gusberti, F.A., and Lang, N.P.: Periodontal Conditions in Adolescents with Cleft Lip, Alveolus and Palate Following Treatment in a Co-ordinated Team Approach, *J. Clin. Periodontol., 12,* 494, July, 1985.
4. **Cohen,** M.M., Jr. and Bankier, A.: Syndrome Delineation Involving Orofacial Clefting, *Cleft Palate Craniofac. J., 28,* 119, January, 1991.
5. **Bell,** W.T. and Wright, J.T.: The Cleft Lip and Palate Patient, in Thornton, J.B. and Wright, J.T., eds.: *Special and Medically Compromised Patients in Dentistry.* Littleton, MA, PSG Publishing Co., Inc., 1989, pp. 272–293.
6. **Kaufman,** F.L.: Managing the Cleft Lip and Palate Patient, *Pediatr. Clin. North Am., 38,* 1127, October, 1991.
7. **Desai,** S.N.: Early Cleft Palate Repair Completed Before the Age of 16 Weeks: Observations on a Personal Series of 100 Children, *Br. J. Plast. Surg., 36,* 300, July, 1983.

SUGGESTED READINGS

Brägger, U., Nyman, S., Lang, N.P., von Wyttenbach, Th., Salvi, G., and Schürch, E.: The Significance of Alveolar Bone in Periodontal Disease. A Long-term Observation in Patients with Cleft Lip, Alveolus and Palate, *J. Clin. Periodontol., 17,* 379, July, 1990.

Farnan, S.: Cleft Lip/Palate and Craniofacial Anomalies, in Ekvall, S.W., ed.: *Pediatric Nutrition in Chronic Diseases and Developmental Disorders.* New York, Oxford University Press, 1993, pp. 219–223.

Freni, S.C. and Zapisek, W.F.: Biologic Basis for a Risk Assessment Model for Cleft Palate, *Cleft Palate Craniofac. J., 28,* 338, October, 1991.

Gould, H.J.: Hearing Loss and Cleft Palate: The Perspective of Time, *Cleft Palate J., 27,* 36, January, 1990.

Khoury, M.J., Gomez-Farias, M., and Mulinare, J.: Does Maternal Cigarette Smoking During Pregnancy Cause Cleft Lip and Palate in Offspring? *Am. J. Dis. Child., 143,* 333, March, 1989.

Leonard, B.J., Brust, J.D., Abrahams, G., and Sielaff, B.: Self-concept of Children and Adolescents with Cleft Lip and/or Palate, *Cleft Palate Craniofac. J., 28,* 347, October, 1991.

Markus, A.F., Delaire, J., and Smith, W.P.: Facial Balance in Cleft Lip and Palate. I. Normal Development and Cleft Palate, *Br. J. Oral Maxillofac. Surg., 30,* 287, October, 1992.

Markus, A.F., Delaire, J., and Smith, W.P.: Facial Balance in Cleft Lip and Palate. II. Cleft Lip and Palate and Secondary Deformities, *Br. J. Oral Maxillofac. Surg., 30,* 296, October, 1992.

Minsley, G.E., Warren, D.W., and Hairfield, W.M.: The Effect of Cleft Palate Speech Aid Prostheses on the Nasopharyngeal Airway and Breathing, *J. Prosthet. Dent., 65,* 122, January, 1991.

Noar, J.H.: Questionnaire Survey of Attitudes and Concerns of Patients with Cleft Lip and Palate and Their Parents, *Cleft Palate Craniofac. J., 28,* 279, July, 1991.

Paynter, E.T., Edmonson, T.W., and Jordan, W.J.: Accuracy of Information Reported by Parents and Children Evaluated by a Cleft Palate Team, *Cleft Palate Craniofac. J., 28,* 329, October, 1991.

Philip, C.: Orthodontic Management of the Congenital Cleft Palate Patient, *Dent. Clin. North Am., 34,* 343, April, 1990.

Ramstad, T.: Periodontal Condition in Adult Patients with Unilateral Complete Cleft Lip and Palate, *Cleft Palate J., 26,* 14, January, 1989.

Ranta, R.: Orthodontic Treatment in Adults with Cleft Lip and Palate, *J. Craniomaxillofac. Surg., 17,* 42, Supplement 1, December, 1989.

Sauter, S.K.: Cleft Lips and Palates. Types, Repairs, Nursing Care, *Am. Oper. Room Nurse J., 50,* 813, October, 1989.

Slavkin, H.C.: Incidence of Cleft Lips, Palates Rising, *J. Am. Dent. Assoc., 123,* 61, November, 1992.

Strauss, R.P. and Davis, J.U.: Prenatal Detection and Fetal Surgery of Clefts and Craniofacial Abnormalities in Humans: Social and Ethical Issues, *Cleft Palate J., 27,* 176, April, 1990.

Verdi, F.J., Lanzi, G.L., Cohen, S.R., and Powell, R.: Use of the Branemark Implant in the Cleft Palate Patient, *Cleft Palate Craniofac. J., 28,* 301, July, 1991.

Werler, M.M., Lammer, E.J., Rosenberg, L., and Mitchell, A.A.: Maternal Cigarette Smoking During Pregnancy in Relation to Oral Clefts, *Am. J. Epidemiol., 132,* 926, November, 1990.

Wirt, A., Wyatt, R., Sell, D.A., Grunwell, P., and Mars, M.: Training Assistants in Cleft Palate Speech Therapy in the Developing World: A Report, *Cleft Palate J., 27,* 169, April, 1990.

Wyse, R.K., Mars, M., Al-Mahdawi, S., Russell-Eggitt, I.M., and Blake, K.D.: Congenital Heart Anomalies in Patients with Clefts of the Lip and/or Palate, *Cleft Palate J., 27,* 258, July, 1990.

Yetter, J.F.: Cleft Lip and Cleft Palate, *Am. Fam. Physician, 46,* 1211, October, 1992.

Infants/Children

Chapman, K.L.: Vocalization of Toddlers with Cleft Lip and Palate, *Cleft Palate Craniofac. J., 28,* 172, April, 1991.

Copeland, M.: The Effects of Very Early Palatal Repair on Speech, *Br. J. Plast. Surg., 43,* 676, November, 1990.

Dahllöf, G., Ussisoo-Joandi, R., Ideberg, M., and Modeer, T.: Caries, Gingivitis, and Dental Abnormalities in Preschool Children with Cleft Lip and/or Palate, *Cleft Palate J., 26,* 233, July, 1989.

Goldberg, W.B., Ferguson, F.S., and Miles, R.J.: Successful Use of a Feeding Obturator for an Infant with a Cleft Palate, *Spec. Care Dentist., 8,* 86, March/April, 1988.

Idelberg, J.: The Needs of a Cleft Lip and Cleft Palate Child, *Dentalhygienistnews, 4,* 8, Winter, 1991.

Lipp, M.J. and Lubit, E.C.: An Impression Procedure for the Neonatal Patient with a Cleft Palate, *Spec. Care Dentist., 8,* 224, September/October, 1988.

Moss, A.L.H., Jones, K., and Pigott, R.W.: Submucous Cleft Palate in the Differential Diagnosis of Feeding Difficulties, *Arch. Dis. Child., 65,* 182, February, 1990.

Mueller, A.P.: The Cleft Lip and Cleft Palate Child: An Overview, *Dent. Assist., 59,* 19, March/April, 1990.

Saunders, I.D., Geary, L., Fleming, P., and Gregg, T.A.: A Simplified Feeding Appliance for the Infant with a Cleft Lip and Palate, *Quintessence Int., 20,* 907, December, 1989.

Preadolescent to Postmenopausal Patients

The endocrine glands are glands of internal secretion. They secrete highly specialized substances—the hormones—which, with the nervous system, maintain body homeostasis.

Hormones are transported by the blood or lymph. They may act directly on body cells or may act to control the hormones of other glands. Their complex and unified action augments and regulates many vital functions, including growth and development, energy production, food metabolism, reproductive processes, and the responses of the body to stress.

The major endocrine glands are the pituitary, thyroid, parathyroids, pancreas, adrenals, and gonads. The anterior pituitary is called the master gland, because it regulates the output of hormones by other glands. In turn, the pituitary itself is regulated by the hormones of the other glands.

Both hyposecretion and hypersecretion of a hormone can cause physical and mental disturbances. Regulation of hormonal secretion is complex, and the mechanisms are not fully known. Normally, hormones are secreted when needed. The external temperature, for example, can influence the production of thyroxin by the thyroid gland. The calcium level of the blood affects parathyroid activity.

Hormones of the reproductive system have an effect on the development and function of the individual. Some of the influences on oral health and patient care are described in this chapter. Key words are defined in table 45–1.

PUBERTY AND ADOLESCENCE[1,2]

I. PUBERTAL CHANGES

Chronologic age is an unreliable indicator, because puberty may begin normally in either sex between 9 and 17 years or age, depending on such factors as race, heredity, and nutritional status. Generally, the secondary sex characteristics begin to appear between 10 and 13 years of age in girls; changes appear later in boys, starting at about 13 or 14 years. The major changes are usually complete in 3 to 4 years.

A. Hormonal Influences

Pituitary hormones control the hormones produced by the ovaries and the testes. The several hormones produced by the ovaries are known collectively as *estrogens,* and those produced by the testes are called *androgens.* They are responsible for the development of the sex organs, the accessory sex organs, and the secondary sex characteristics, and have strong physical, mental, and emotional influences throughout the body.

B. Female Development

1. Accelerated growth spurt.
2. Development of the sex organs: fallopian tubes, uterus, vagina, and breasts.
3. Appearance of secondary sex characteristics.
   a. Growth of pubic and axillary hair.
   b. Skeletal development, especially enlargement of the pelvis.
   c. Fat deposition on the hips.
   d. Voice drops one or two tones.
4. Beginning of menstruation and ovulation. Menstruation may precede the first ovulation.

C. Male Development

1. Increase in size of testes and scrotum and beginning of spermatogenesis.

**TABLE 45–1
KEY WORDS: PREADOLESCENT TO
POSTMENOPAUSAL PATIENTS**

Acne vulgaris (ak′nē vul-ga′rĭs): a chronic skin disorder with increased production of oil from the sebaceous glands and the formation of blackheads that plug the pores; may be inflammatory or noninflammatory; appears on the face, back, and chest, primarily in adolescents and young adults.

Adolescence: the period extending from the time the secondary sex characteristics appear to the end of somatic growth, when the individual is psychologically mature.

Amenorrhea: absence of spontaneous menstrual periods in a female of reproductive age.

Circumpubertal: on or around the age of puberty.

Climacteric: the phase in the aging of a woman that marks the transition from the reproductive to the nonreproductive stage.

Coitus: sexual union; copulation; intercourse.

Dysmenorrhea: difficult and painful menstruation.

Gynecologist (gĭ′nĕ-kol′ō-jist): physician who specializes in the conditions peculiar to women, particularly of the genital tract, female endocrinology, and reproductive physiology.

Homeostasis (hō′mē-ō-sta′sĭs): the tendency of biologic systems to maintain stability while continually adjusting to conditions that are optimal for survival.

Hormonal replacement therapy: prescription of a purified or synthetic hormone to correct or prevent undesirable symptoms resulting from the surgical removal or degeneration of the hormone-producing organ.

Hormone: a chemical product of an organ or of certain cells within the organ that has a specific regulatory effect upon cells remote from its origin.

Mastalgia: fullness, soreness, or pain in the breast.

Maturity: state of complete growth.

Menarche: onset of menstruation; may occur from ages 9 to 17 years.

Menopause (men′ō-pawz): the time of life when a woman ceases menstruation; clinically a period of 6 to 12 months of amenorrhea in a woman older than 45 years.

Menses: menstruation.

Oligomenorrhea: menstrual intervals of greater than 45 days.

Premenstrual syndrome: a cluster of behavioral, somatic, affective, and cognitive disorders that appears in the premenstrual (luteal) phase of the menstrual cycle and that resolve rapidly with the onset of menses.

Puberty (pu′ber-tē): period in which the gonads mature and begin to function.

Pubescence (pu-bes′ens): coming to the age of puberty or sexual maturity.

2. Development of the sex organs: vas deferens, seminal vesicles, prostate, and penis.
3. Appearance of secondary sex characteristics.
   a. Growth of facial, pubic, and axillary hair.
   b. Voice deepens.

II. CHARACTERISTICS OF ADOLESCENCE
A. Growth Spurt
1. Varies in age of occurrence, extent, and duration; usually occurs in boys between 12 and 16, girls 11 to 14.
2. Marked by rapid, extensive growth in height, weight, and muscle mass.
3. Overeating with underexercise, along with psychologic problems, makes obesity a difficult and serious problem.
4. Poor coordination and awkwardness in young adolescents may result from irregular, uneven stages of growth.

B. Nutritional Requirements
1. Highest of any time in life for boys; will be exceeded only during pregnancy for girls.
2. Undernutrition is common; in boys, because of overactivity and poor food selection; in girls, because of voluntary diet restrictions with poor food selection and fad diets in the attempt to keep slim.
3. Iron-deficiency anemia is not uncommon among teenage girls, particularly after the onset of menstruation.

C. Skin Disorders
Acne vulgaris commonly results from overactivity of the sebaceous glands. Usually, relief occurs when adolescence is completed, although the condition may persist longer.

III. PERSONAL FACTORS
Adolescents are no longer children, and yet they have not reached adulthood. They may respond and wish to be treated as adults or as children at different times. They are learning to adapt to body changes, sexual impulses, and secondary sex characteristics.

The most likely causes of anxiety in adolescents are sex, performance in school, family relationships, peer pressures, substance abuse, confusion over their beliefs, and concern about their futures. Younger, less healthy teenagers tend to show greater health concerns.

No fixed picture can be described, but characteristics listed here are exhibited to one degree or another by many adolescents.

A. Increased Self-interest
1. Adolescents have a great deal of concern for themselves and respond best to those who show concern for them.
2. They want attention and tend to reject those who do not listen.

B. Growing Independence
1. Adolescence is a period of rapidly growing independence of thought and action with conflicts between feelings of dependence and independence.
2. Childhood dependence on parents is gradually given up; the idea of infallibility of par-

ents is lost; teachers and others in authority are questioned.

3. Personal identity is sought; adolescents are uncertain about their place and role in society.

4. Independence from parents frequently means increased confidence in and respect for other adults outside the family.

C. Concern over Physical Characteristics

1. Girls mature earlier than boys, and young female adolescents are usually taller than their male counterparts, which may present social problems.

2. Increased interest in personal appearance; adolescents want to dress and be like their peers.

3. Such problems as delayed growth and sexual development and obesity can be extremely important.

ORAL CONDITIONS

I. DENTAL CARIES

The incidence of dental caries is often higher during adolescence than in other age groups in communities without fluoridation. This can be related to the dietary and eating habits of most adolescents. Appetite becomes intensified by the demands of rapid growth, as well as by the emotional problems confronted, thus leading to frequent eating. Many cariogenic foods are eaten, particularly between meals and in social settings.

II. PERIODONTAL INFECTIONS

Adolescents are subject to all categories of periodontal infections (table 12–3, page 198). Gingivitis is common in this age group.

A. Gingivitis

1. *Contributing and Predisposing Factors.* Many of the factors described on pages 201–204 in Chapter 12 can be applied when considering the periodontal conditions of adolescents. Orthodontic appliances, dietary habits, and compliance for bacterial plaque removal seem to be special problems for this age group. Some teenagers have systemic conditions, such as diabetes mellitus, that may have gingival manifestations, or the medications required for the treatment of a systemic condition, such as an antiseizure drug, may produce a gingival reaction.

2. *"Puberty" Gingivitis.* An exaggerated response to local irritants sometimes occurs during puberty and is believed to be related to hormonal changes. The gingiva enlarge, particularly the papillae; the tissue appears

a bluish-red color and bulbous in shape.[3,4] The presence of bacterial plaque is always necessary.

B. Early-onset Periodontitis

Loss of periodontal attachment and supporting bone is evident in from 5 to 47% of adolescents around the world.[5,6,7,8,9] Careful probing and study of radiographs are indicated for each patient so that emphasis can be placed on preventive measures, early recognition, early treatment, and regular maintenance appointments.

C. Juvenile Periodontitis[10]

A specific category of early-onset periodontitis is juvenile periodontitis. The two distinct disease categories are localized (LJP) and generalized (GJP). Both types have a familial tendency.

1. *Localized Juvenile Periodontitis.* LJP is characterized by severe bone loss about the first permanent molars and the incisors. It is usually first diagnosed during the circumpubertal years. The pathogenic microorganism of etiologic importance is the *Actinobacillus actinomycetemcomitans* (table 16–4, page 264). *A. actinomycetemcomitans* is a powerful microorganism that can invade tissue and destroy white blood cells. The patient usually has a neutrophil dysfunction with a slowed immune response.

2. *Generalized Juvenile Periodontitis.* GJP is characterized by generalized alveolar bone loss. It occurs in the older adolescent and young adult. The microflora found in pockets of GJP has similarities to the microflora of adult periodontitis. A neutrophil disturbance is also noted in this type of juvenile periodontitis.

D. Necrotizing Ulcerative Gingivitis/Periodontitis

Although found infrequently in children, necrotizing ulcerative gingivitis has its highest frequency in older adolescents and young adults. Stress, undernutrition, lack of bacterial plaque control, neglect of oral health, depressed immune reactions, and psychosomatic factors are implicated as predisposing influences in its development (pages 537 and 538).

DENTAL HYGIENE CARE

Dental and dental hygiene care during adolescence can impact oral health throughout the patient's lifetime. The knowledge, attitudes, and practices acquired and developed by adolescents can have wide-reaching significance as they become the parents and community participants of the future.

I. PATIENT APPROACH

Adolescence is a period of transition. Working with adolescents offers a real challenge, and each situation requires its own approach. Some of the physical and psychologic characteristics have been listed in this chapter to provide a framework for what may be expected. A few basic suggestions for approach include the following:

A. Treat adolescents as adults. Physically many of them are mature, although their emotional development varies.

B. Set the stage to let them know of your interest in them and their problems. Encourage them to talk, and then listen attentively.

C. Suggest and advise, but do not become impatient or take offense when they choose to make their own decisions.

D. They are usually interested in health matters and details about their physical condition, although they may appear indifferent. Cleanliness and attractiveness are important to teenage patients.

E. Health, including oral health, may be a real concern. Adolescents need to be well informed about their oral conditions, and explanations on a scientific basis are generally appreciated.

II. PATIENT HISTORY

Adolescents should provide their own information for the medical and dental histories. A consult with the parents for additional details should be made, but not in the same interview with the patient and not without the patient's knowledge.

Adolescents need to take increasing responsibility for their own health. Although the initial dental visit may be at the insistence of the parents, every effort should be to focus on the patient, not the parents.

The adolescent patient may have other health problems. The patient with diabetes, heart disease, a mental, physical, or sensory disability, or other systemic involvement requires special methods for approach as described in the various chapters of this book. Medical clearance by parent or legal guardian is necessary for conditions requiring antibiotic coverage or other medication for a patient under legal age. Approval of the treatment plan by parent or legal guardian is necessary.

III. ORAL HEALTH PROBLEMS IN ADOLESCENCE[11]

Dental caries and periodontal infections of the adolescent years have been described. Some examples of other oral problems related to adolescent development and behavior characteristics are listed here.

A. Oral manifestations of sexually transmitted infections (STI).

B. Effects of tobacco use, such as leukoplakia and periodontal damage from smokeless tobacco products.

C. Potential effects of oral contraceptives on periodontal tissues (page 629).

D. Oral findings of anorexia nervosa or bulimia (pages 769–771).

E. Traumatic injury to teeth and oral structures from athletic activities, as well as from automobile, motorcycle, and other motorized vehicle accidents.

IV. BACTERIAL PLAQUE CONTROL

A clear explanation of the causes of dental caries and periodontal conditions, with the methods for their prevention, is basic. Adolescents need to understand the effects of the accumulation of bacterial plaque, the purposes of professional calculus removal, and the relation of the daily self-care plaque control program to the health status of the gingiva.

For dental caries prevention, adolescents must appreciate the effects of fluoride and the need to restrict cariogenic foods. The program is outlined and conducted on the basis of these clearcut preventive measures.

A. Instruction in self-care procedures.

B. Continuing reassessment over a series of appointments to develop daily practices that can be carried over into adult life.

V. INSTRUMENTATION

A series of appointments frequently may be required, depending on probing depth and extent of calculus deposits. Careful and complete scaling and root planing and removal of all local irregularities, such as inadequate margins of restorations, are the basic treatment procedures.

VI. FLUORIDE TREATMENT PROGRAM

A combined fluoride program is indicated for most adolescent patients, particularly for those who have not lived in a community with a fluoridated water supply. In addition to the topical applications made in conjunction with dental hygiene professional appointments, self-administered methods should include a fluoride dentifrice and a daily fluoride mouthrinse. A daily application of a fluoride gel in a custom-made tray may be necessary for remineralization in selected cases (pages 449 and 450). The methods are described in Chapter 29.

VII. DIET CONTROL

A. Dietary Analysis (pages 425–429)

A study of the patient's diet and counseling relative to general nutrition and dental caries control can provide important learning experiences for many adolescents. The parent or other person who is in charge of shopping and food preparation must be included so that appropriate foods are available. As much responsibility as possible should be placed on the patient.

B. Instruction Suggestions

1. *Advise Foods from the Food Guide Pyramid* (page 424). For growth, energy, clear complexion, and prevention of illness.

2. *Emphasize a Good Breakfast.* Teenagers tend to slight or omit breakfast, particularly if they have to prepare it for themselves.

3. *Snack Selection.* From the nutritious foods, with recognition of cariogenic foods. Snacks suggested can include raw fruits and vegetables, nuts, nonsweetened milk, use of sugar-free foods when possible, and sugarless chewing gum if gum is used.

MENSTRUATION

The menstrual cycle refers to the cyclic structural changes in the uterus, instigated by hormones, which represent periodic preparation of the lining of the uterus for fertilization of the ovum and pregnancy (figure 45–1). When fertilization does not take place, changes in the mucous membrane lining the uterus (the endometrium) lead to the menstrual discharge.

The fluid discharged is composed primarily of blood with fragments of the disintegrated endometrium.

I. CHARACTERISTICS

A. Occurrence
The cyclic changes occur from puberty to menopause except during pregnancy and part of breast-feeding. Although the average cycle is complete in about 28 days, the normal range is from 22 to 34 days.

B. Menarche
Menstruation may begin at any time from ages 9 to 17. The mean age in the United States is between 12 and 13 years.

Menarche frequently occurs before the first ovulation, that is, before the pituitary and ovarian hormones are synchronized and ovulation becomes a part of the menstrual cycle. Timing and extent of flow may be irregular for several months or years after the onset of menstruation.

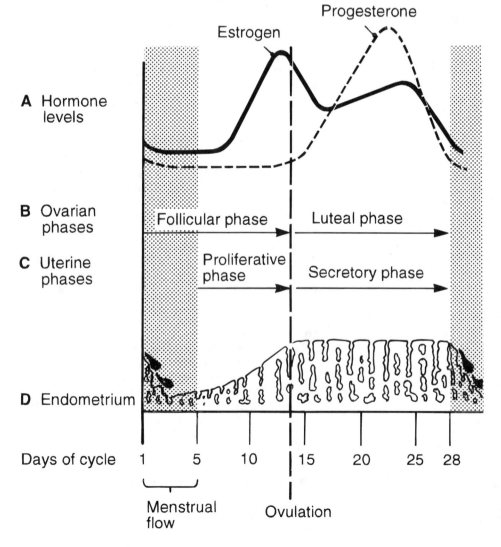

FIG. 45–1. Changes During the Menstrual Cycle. The 28 days of a normal cycle are shown with ovulation between days 12 and 15 and the menstrual flow between days 1 to 5 and again at day 28. **A.** Hormonal levels show the estrogen peak shortly before ovulation during the follicular phase of the ovary **(B)** and the proliferative phase of the uterus **(C). D.** The endometrium builds up from the end of one menstrual flow in preparation for possible implantation of a fertilized ovum.

II. IRREGULARITIES

Although variations in the menstrual cycle are common, many females never have any problems or discomforts. The pattern of the cycle may be upset by factors such as changes in climate, changes in work schedule, emotional trauma, acute or chronic illnesses, weight loss, and excessive exercise.

Menstruation may have strong emotional impact, and associated disturbances may have psychologic bases. Intense emotional conflicts may be related to the inability to accept the feminine role and assume the responsibilities of womanhood. The symptoms of premenstrual tension and dysmenorrhea described in the following can continue beyond adolescence and even through menopause.

A. Premenstrual Syndrome

This condition is associated with fluid retention in the body and psychologic depression occurring within 10 days prior to menstruation.

1. *Physical Symptoms.* The most frequent symptoms are fatigue, headache, abdominal bloating, mastalgia, joint pain, increased appetite, and incoordination.
2. *Affective Symptoms.* Depression, anxiety, irritability, and hostility can be noted.
3. *Management.* Severe symptoms require medical care and supervision. Self-help methods include daily exercise; diet modification to eliminate caffeine, salt, alcohol, and simple carbohydrates; and rest.

B. Dysmenorrhea

Difficult or painful menstruation may be primary or secondary. With primary or functional dysmenorrhea, the organs are normal and there are symptoms of hyperactivity and contractions. Secondary or acquired dysmenorrhea is associated with organ disorders, such as endometriosis or pelvic inflammatory disease.

Dysmenorrhea in the adolescent can be related to physiologic or psychologic factors. It may indicate emotional status, may be a result of poor preparation for the arrival of puberty and menstruation, or can result from parental example.

Although most women have little or no discomfort, a small percentage suffers severe pain with "cramps," sometimes accompanied by nausea and vomiting.

III. DENTAL HYGIENE CARE
A. Patient History

Menstruation is a normal process and should not be referred to as a "sick period" or a "monthly illness." When presenting questions for the patient history, use of terms such as the "period" or "monthly period" is preferable. A question about the regularity of menstruation should be included in each medical history review.

The menstrual history may provide indications of a woman's general health. Regularly excessive menstrual flow may be related to an anemic state, and medical examination and treatment are indicated.

B. Oral Findings[4]

No specific gingival changes are related to the menstrual cycle. An exaggerated response to local irritants or unusual gingival bleeding during or following scaling may be noted in an occasional patient. With control of local irritants through bacterial plaque control, self-care measures, and removal of calculus at regular maintenance appointments, bleeding usually can be controlled.

HORMONAL CONTRACEPTIVES

Birth control pills are recognized as the most effective method of contraception when they are taken as prescribed. Because of their convenience, they are used by millions of women worldwide.

I. TYPES[12]
A. Combination Preparations

1. *Estrogen and Progestin.* The combination of the synthetically produced hormones estrogen and progestin is nearly 100% effective in preventing ovulation. Estrogen inhibits the secretion of follicle-stimulating hormone (FSH) and progestin inhibits the release of luteinizing hormone (LH) by the anterior pituitary gland. Without the hormones FSH and LH, the ovum cannot be released from the ovary.
2. *Schedule of Administration.* One pill is taken each day for 20 or 21 days starting 5 days after the onset of the menstrual flow. Then, for a period of 7 days, no pill is taken. The routine is followed regardless of when menstruation starts or stops.

B. Single Preparations: Minipill

Progestin alone has been used when the effects of estrogen are contraindicated. Pregnancy rate is increased with this pill. When this type of pill is used, menstrual cycles tend to be more irregular and side effects more frequent.

II. CONTRAINDICATIONS[12]

Contraceptives containing hormones should not be taken when the woman has a history of the following:
A. Thromboembolic disorders.
B. Cerebrovascular disease.
C. Severe hypertension.
D. Impaired liver function.
E. Known or suspected cancer of the breast or other estrogen-dependent neoplasia.

F. Undiagnosed uterine bleeding.
G. Smoking.
H. Pregnancy.

III. SIDE EFFECTS[12]

Side effects sometimes may be related more to incorrect use of the drug than to hormonal effects. Visual problems, mental depression, rashes, and bleeding irregularities occur in some women. The most significant effects are the following:

A. Cardiovascular (including increased blood pressure).
B. Weight gain.
C. Decreased effectiveness of the contraceptive when certain drugs are used, including the following:
   1. Antibiotics.[13,14]
   2. Anticonvulsants.
   3. Rifampin (used in treatment of tuberculosis).

IV. EFFECT ON THE GINGIVA

An exaggerated response to bacterial plaque and other local irritants has been noted, especially when the personal oral hygiene is less than adequate. The gingivitis is similar to that described for pregnancy (page 608). There appears to be an increase in the extent of gingival reaction associated with extended use of the contraceptive over several years.[15]

V. APPOINTMENT CONSIDERATIONS
A. Medical History

A record of the use of oral contraceptives should be updated with each history review.

B. Patient Information

1. Explain the need for exceptional personal oral care and regular professional maintenance appointments to prevent complications from gingivitis.
2. Explain the need for additional contraception when antibiotic premedication or other use of antibiotics is indicated.
3. Alert patient to side effects and advise medical evaluation if side effects become troublesome.

MENOPAUSE AND CLIMACTERIC

Menopause is the cessation of menstruation. It occurs normally between the ages of 42 and 55 years, with the average of approximately 50 years. It may be induced by surgical removal of the ovaries or by radiation therapy.

The female *climacteric* is that period of change during the gradual decline of ovarian efficiency when ovulation is less regular and finally ends, through the menopause, and including the period after menopause when the body is adjusting to endocrine and other changes. While adolescence is considered the transitional period from childhood into maturity, the climacteric has been described as the transitional period from maturity into senescence.

I. CHARACTERISTICS

Prior to menopause, menstruation decreases in frequency, duration, and amount of flow over a period of about 12 to 24 months. Although many women may experience minor symptoms, only about 10% have any pronounced effects from menopause.

A. General Symptoms

As ovarian function declines with diminishing estrogen, physiologic changes in body function take place.

1. *Vasomotor Reactions.* Vasomotor instability in the form of hot flashes, in which sudden, periodic surges of heat involving the whole body and accompanied by drenching sweats, may occur during the day or night. Although a strict distinction is not always made between flush and flash, the term hot flush may be used to mean a reaction of lesser degree in which a wave of warmth is felt over the face, neck, and upper thorax. Headaches, heart palpitations, and sleeplessness may occur.
2. *Emotional Disturbances.* Emotional problems are not caused specifically by estrogen deficiencies but are frequently related to personal and family circumstances and concern over growing old. Anxiety, tension, and irritability, with depression and feelings of uselessness, may appear.

B. Postmenopausal Effects

1. Reproductive organs atrophy.
2. Changes in bones may lead to osteoporosis. This condition is less frequent among women who have used drinking water containing fluoride over the years.
3. Skin and mucous membranes decrease in thickness and keratinization.
4. Predisposition to conditions including atherosclerosis, diabetes, and hypothyroidism.

II. ORAL FINDINGS

Oral disturbances that can be related to the menopause are relatively uncommon. Findings are nonspecific.

A. Gingiva

Gingival changes associated with menopause usually represent an exaggerated response to bacterial plaque, which reflects the conditioning influence of the hormonal changes taking place. When local factors are controlled through preventive dental hygiene appointments for maintenance to supplement daily personal oral care, unusual gingival changes are uncommon.

Rarely, a condition that has been called menopausal gingivostomatitis may develop.[16] It may also occur after removal of, or radiation therapy to, the ovaries.

B. Mucous Membranes and Tongue

1. Dryness with burning or unusual taste sensations may be present.
2. Epithelium may become thin and atrophic with decreased keratinization; tolerance for removable prostheses may lessen.
3. Inadequate diet and eating habits may contribute to the adverse changes of the mucosal tissues. The appearance and symptoms frequently resemble those associated with vitamin deficiencies, particularly B vitamins.

III. DENTAL HYGIENE CARE

In the approach to the patient, a specific relationship of oral conditions to menopause should not be made, because the patient may tend to overemphasize such a relationship and de-emphasize the need for self-care measures. Because of the importance of local factors, attention should be directed to the need for regular and frequent professional care, as well as to increased efforts for daily plaque control.

A. Appointment Suggestions

The symptoms of physical and emotional changes should be kept in mind when planning and conducting the appointment. The patient's possible tenseness and irritability can be anticipated. Rapport begins with the clinician's courtesy, personal attention, and friendly, unhurried manner.

Attention to details, such as not keeping the patient waiting unduly and handling materials and instruments with calm assurance and maintaining conservativeness in conversation to prevent annoyances may be significant.

B. Instruction of Patient

Preservation of oral health is particularly important to the woman who has her natural teeth. Because of the possible difficulties and discomforts of wearing prostheses, every effort should be made to prevent the need for tooth removal. A saliva substitute may provide a degree of relief from xerostomia (pages 204 and 205).

Measures for the prevention of periodontal infections should be carefully explained, and emphasis should be placed on reasons for frequent calculus removal to supplement meticulous daily care. Because good general health practices are very important to this age group, the relationship of general and oral health can be emphasized.

C. Diet

A dietary survey may prove to be a helpful teaching-learning experience (pages 425–431) by helping the patient to identify and correct inadequately balanced food selection. Dental caries prevention through selection of nutritious and noncariogenic foods is especially important for the patient who tends to indulge in between-meal eating.

D. Fluoride Therapy

A fluoride-containing dentifrice and a brush-on gel applied before retiring are necessary for nearly all patients in this age group (pages 449–453).

REFERENCES

1. **Garn,** S.M.: Physical Growth and Development, in Friedman, S.B., Fisher, M., and Schonberg, S.K., eds.: *Comprehensive Adolescent Health Care.* St. Louis, Quality Medical Publishing, Inc., 1992, pp. 18–23.
2. **Marlow,** D.R. and Redding, B.A.: *Textbook of Pediatric Nursing,* 6th ed. Philadelphia, W.B. Saunders Co., 1988, pp. 1114–1142.
3. **Hoag,** P.M. and Pawlak, E.A.: *Essentials of Periodontics,* 4th ed. St. Louis, Mosby, 1990, pp. 35, 46–47.
4. **Carranza,** F.A.: *Glickman's Clinical Periodontology,* 7th ed. Philadelphia, W.B. Saunders Co., 1990, pp. 138, 451–452.
5. **MacGregor,** I.D.M.: Radiographic Survey of Periodontal Disease in 264 Adolescent Schoolboys in Lagos, Nigeria, *Community Dent. Oral Epidemiol., 8,* 56, February, 1980.
6. **Latcham,** N.L., Powell, R.N., Jago, J.D., and Seymour, G.J.: A Radiographic Study of Chronic Periodontitis in 15 Year Old Queensland Children, *J. Clin. Periodontol., 10,* 37, January, 1983.
7. **Gjermo,** P., Bellini, H.T., Santos, V.P., Martins, J.G., and Ferracyoli, J.R.: Prevalence of Bone Loss in a Group of Brazilian Teenagers Assessed on Bite-wing Radiographs, *J. Clin. Periodontol., 11,* 104, February, 1984.
8. **Wolfe,** M.D. and Carlos, J.P.: Periodontal Disease in Adolescents: Epidemiologic Findings in Navajo Indians, *Community Dent. Oral Epidemiol., 15,* 33, February, 1987.
9. **Aass,** A.M., Albandar, J., Aasenden, R., Tollefsen, T., and Gjermo, P.: Variation in Prevalence of Radiographic Alveolar Bone Loss in Subgroups of 14-year-old Schoolchildren in Oslo, *J. Clin. Periodontol., 15,* 130, February, 1988.
10. **American Academy Periodontology:** Position Paper: *Periodontal Diseases of Children and Adolescents.* Chicago, A.A.P., 737 North Michigan Avenue, Chicago, IL 60611, 1991.
11. **Machen,** J.B.: Guidelines for Dental Health of the Adolescent—May, 1986, 1985–86 AAPD Clinical Affairs Committee, *Pediatr. Dent., 9,* 247, September, 1987.
12. **Greydanus,** D.E. and Patel, D.R.: Contraception, in McAnarney, E.R., Kreipe, R.E., Orr, D.P., and Comerci, G.D.: *Textbook of Adolescent Medicine.* Philadelphia, W.B. Saunders Co., 1992, pp. 676–685.
13. **Zachariasen,** R.D.: Effect of Antibiotics on Oral Contraceptive Efficacy, *J. Dent. Hyg., 65,* 334, September, 1991.
14. **American Dental Association,** Health Foundation Research Institute, Department of Toxicology: Antibiotic Interference with Oral Contraceptives, *J. Am. Dent. Assoc., 122,* 79, December, 1991.

15. **Pankhurst,** C.L., Waite, I.M., Hicks, K.A., Allen, Y., and Harkness, R.D.: The Influence of Oral Contraceptive Therapy on the Periodontium—Duration of Drug Therapy, *J. Periodontol., 52,* 617, October, 1981.

16. **Carranza:** op. cit., p. 455.

SUGGESTED READINGS

Cowan, B.D. and Morrison, J.C.: Management of Abnormal Genital Bleeding in Girls and Women, *N. Engl. J. Med., 324,* 1710, June 13, 1991.

Folkers, S.A., Weine, F.S., and Weissman, D.P.: Periodontal Disease in the Life Stages of Women, *Compendium, 13,* 52, October, 1992.

Morishita, M., Aoyama, H., Tokumoto, K., and Iwamoto, Y.: The Concentration of Salivary Hormones and the Prevalence of Gingivitis at Puberty, *Adv. Dent. Res., 2,* 397, November, 1988.

Reid, R.L.: Premenstrual Syndrome (Editorial), *N. Engl. J. Med., 324,* 1208, April 25, 1991.

Rowland, A.S., Baird, D.D., Weinberg, C.R., Shore, D.L., Shy, C.M., and Wilcox, A.J.: Reduced Fertility Among Women Employed as Dental Assistants Exposed to High Levels of Nitrous Oxide, *N. Engl. J. Med., 327,* 993, October 1, 1992.

Sooriyamoorthy, M. and Gower, D.B.: Hormonal Influences on Gingival Tissue: Relationship to Periodontal Disease, *J. Clin. Periodontol., 16,* 201, April, 1989.

United States Centers for Disease Control and Prevention: Premarital Sexual Experience among Adolescent Women—United States 1970–1988, *MMWR, 39,* 929, January 4, 1991.

Adolescence

Bailey, S.L.: Adolescents' Multisubstance Use Patterns: The Role of Heavy Alcohol and Cigarette Use, *Am. J. Public Health, 82,* 1220, September, 1992.

Chiodo, G.T. and Tolle, S.W.: Doctor-patient Confidentiality and the Adolescent Patient, *J. Am. Dent. Assoc., 120,* 126, February, 1990.

Cucalon, A. and Smith, R.J.: Relationship Between Compliance by Adolescent Orthodontic Patients and Performance on Psychological Tests, *Angle Orthod., 60,* 107, Summer, 1990.

DuRant, R.H., Rickert, V.I., Ashworth, C.S., Newman, C., and Slavens, G.: Use of Multiple Drugs among Adolescents Who Use Anabolic Steroids, *N. Engl. J. Med., 328,* 922, April 1, 1993.

Gayle, H.D. and D'Angelo, L.J.: Epidemiology of Acquired Immunodeficiency Syndrome and Human Immunodeficiency Virus Infection in Adolescents, *Pediatr. Infect. Dis. J., 10,* 322, April, 1991.

Irwin, C.E. and Shafer, M.-A.: Adolescent Medicine, *JAMA, 268,* 333, July 15, 1992.

Offer, D. and Schonert-Reichl, K.A.: Debunking the Myths of Adolescence: Findings from Recent Research, *J. Am. Acad. Child Adolesc. Psychiatry, 31,* 1003, November, 1992.

Ringdahl, E.N.: The Role of the Family Physician in Preventing Teenage Pregnancy, *Am. Fam. Physician, 45,* 2215, May, 1992.

Roszkowski, M.J.: Temporomandibular Disorders in Adolescents, *Dentalhygienistnews, 5,* 13, Spring, 1992.

Seppä, L., Hausen, H., Pöllänen, L., Kärkkäinen, S., and Helasharjw, K.: Effect of Intensified Caries Prevention on Approximal Caries in Adolescents with High Caries Risk, *Caries Res., 25,* 392, September-October, 1991.

United States Centers for Disease Control and Prevention: Results from the National Adolescent Student Health Survey, *MMWR, 38,* 147, March 10, 1989.

Adolescents: Periodontitis

Aass, A.M., Preus, H.R., and Gjermo, P.: Association Between Detection of Oral *Actinobacillus actinomycetemcomitans* and Radiographic Bone Loss in Teenagers. A 4-Year Longitudinal Study, *J. Periodontol., 63,* 682, August, 1992.

Albandar, J.M., Baghdady, V.S., and Ghose, L.J.: Periodontal Disease Progression in Teenagers with No Preventive Dental Care Provisions, *J. Clin. Periodontol., 18,* 300, May, 1991.

Albandar, J.M., Buischi, Y.A.P., and Barbosa, M.F.Z.: Destructive Forms of Periodontal Disease in Adolescents. A 3-Year Longitudinal Study, *J. Periodontol., 62,* 370, June, 1991.

Asikainen, S., Alahuusua, S., and Kleemola-Kujala, E.: A 2-Year Follow-up on the Clinical and Microbiological Conditions of Periodontium in Teenagers, *J. Clin. Periodontol., 18,* 16, January, 1991.

D'Angelo, M., Margiotta, V., Ammatuna, P., and Sammartano, F.: Treatment of Prepubertal Periodontitis, *J. Clin. Periodontol., 19,* 214, March, 1992.

Greenstein, G.: Juvenile Periodontitis, *Dentalhygienistnews, 5,* 3, Fall, 1992.

Gusberti, F.A., Mombelli, A., Lang, N.P., and Minder, Ch.E.: Changes in Subgingival Microbiota During Puberty, *J. Clin. Periodontol., 17,* 685, November, 1990.

Jenkins, S.M., Dummer, P.M.H., and Addy, M.: Radiographic Evaluation of Early Periodontal Bone Loss in Adolescents, an Overview, *J. Clin. Periodontol., 19,* 363, July, 1992.

Källestål, C. and Matsson, L.: Criteria for Assessment of Interproximal Bone Loss on Bite-wing Radiographs in Adolescents, *J. Clin. Periodontol., 16,* 300, May, 1989.

Källestål, C., Matsson, L., and Holm, A.-K.: Periodontal Conditions in a Group of Swedish Adolescents. (1) A Descriptive Epidemiologic Study, *J. Clin. Periodontol., 17,* 601, October, 1990.

Källestål, C., Matsson, L., and Persson, S.: Proximal Attachment Loss in Swedish Adolescents, *J. Clin. Periodontol., 18,* 760, November, 1991.

Källestål, C. and Matsson, L.: Marginal Bone Loss in 16-year-old Swedish Adolescents in 1975 and 1988, *J. Clin. Periodontol., 18,* 740, November, 1991.

Löe, H. and Morrison, E.: Periodontal Health and Disease in Young People: Screening for Priority Care, *Int. Dent. J., 36,* 162, September, 1986.

Modéer, T., Dahllöf, G., Axiö, E., and Sundquist, K.-G.: Subpopulations of Lymphocytes in Connective Tissue from Adolescents with Periodontal Disease, *Acta Odontol. Scand., 48,* 153, June, 1990.

Mombelli, A., Gusberti, F.A., van Oosten, M.A.C., and Lang, N.P.: Gingival Health and Gingivitis Development During Puberty, *J. Clin. Periodontol., 16,* 451, August, 1989.

Mombelli, A., Lang, N.P., Bürgin, W.B., and Gusberti, F.A.: Microbial Changes Associated with the Development of Puberty Gingivitis, *J. Periodont. Res., 25,* 331, November, 1990.

Neely, A.L.: Prevalence of Juvenile Periodontitis in a Circumpubertal Population, *J. Clin. Periodontol., 19,* 367, July, 1992.

Perry, D.A. and Newman, M.G.: Occurrence of Periodontitis in an Urban Adolescent Population, *J. Periodontol., 61,* 185, March, 1990.

Sbordone, L., Ramaglia, L., and Bucci, E.: Generalized Juvenile Periodontitis: Report of a Familial Case Followed for 5 Years, *J. Periodontol., 61,* 590, September, 1990.

Sjödin, B., Crossner, C.-G., Unell, L., and Ostlund, P.: A Retrospective Radiographic Study of Alveolar Bone Loss in the Primary Dentition in Patients with Localized Juvenile Periodontitis, *J. Clin. Periodontol., 16,* 124, February, 1989.

Oral Contraceptives

Baird, D.T. and Glasier, A.F.: Hormonal Contraception, *N. Engl. J. Med., 328,* 1543, May 27, 1993.

Donley, T.G., Smith, R.F., and Roy, B.: Reduced Oral Contraceptive Effectiveness with Concurrent Antibiotic Use: A Protocol for Prescribing Antibiotics to Women of Childbearing Age, *Compendium, 11,* 392, June, 1990.

Mishell, D.R.: Contraception, *N. Engl. J. Med., 320,* 777, March 23, 1989.

Monier, M. and Laird, M.: Contraceptives: A Look at the Future, *Am. J. Nurs., 89,* 496, April, 1989.

Zachariasen, R.D.: Ovarian Hormones and Gingivitis, *J. Dent. Hyg., 65,* 146, March-April, 1991.

Menopause

Forabosco, A., Criscuolo, M., Coukos, G., Uccelli, E., Weinstein, R., Spinato, S., Botticelli, A., and Volpe, A.: Efficacy of Hormone Replacement Therapy in Postmenopausal Women with Oral Discomfort, *Oral Surg. Oral Med. Oral Pathol., 73,* 570, May, 1992.

Ship, J.A., Patton, L.L., and Tylenda, C.A.: An Assessment of Salivary Function in Healthy Premenopausal and Postmenopausal Females, *J. Gerontol., 46,* M11-5, January, 1991.

Wardrop, R.W., Hailes, J., Burger, H., and Reade, P.C.: Oral Discomfort at Menopause, *Oral Surg. Oral Med. Oral Pathol., 67,* 535, May, 1989.

46

The Gerodontic Patient

Preventive measures for the aging population through care and instruction require greater emphasis as the number of people involved in this group increases steadily. By the year 2000, the population over age 65 is expected to represent nearly 13% of the total population of the United States, and by the year 2030, it will have increased to nearly 21%.[1]

Only 5% of persons 65 or older are in institutions, such as mental hospitals, chronic disease hospitals, nursing homes, and other long-term care institutions for the aged.[1]

Members of the dental team are challenged by the need to help the aging population learn about personal care and seek professional care that will provide continuing oral comfort and function. As the percentage of people in the older group has increased, the total number of older patients in a general or adult practice has grown. An increasing number of dental hygienists specialize in the care of the elderly and are employed in long-term care and resident facilities for the aged.

Tooth loss increases with age, but not because of age. Dental caries and periodontal diseases are the major causes of tooth loss. Periodontal diseases in the older population represent the cumulative effects of long-standing, undiagnosed, untreated, or neglected chronic infection.

With application of current knowledge of preventive measures for oral diseases in younger age groups, it is anticipated that future generations of older people will not be subjected to the severe effects of uncontrolled and untreated oral diseases. Key words relating to older patients are defined in table 46–1.

AGING

When aging is defined from a chronologic viewpoint, the aging population may be recognized as the "older population" (age 55 and over), the "elderly" (age 65 and over), the "aged" (75 years and older), and the "very old" (85 years and over).[2] Biologic age is not synonymous with chronologic age, and hence, signs of aging appear at different chronologic ages in different individuals. In other words, some people are old at 45 years, whereas others are not old at 75 years.

The degree of general health and physical activity provides a workable classification not based on age. Relative to the degree of impairment, older persons may be *functionally independent, frail,* or *functionally dependent.* Another term for the functionally independent is the *well elderly,* a more descriptive term for the many healthy, active, productive people who happen to be older than what is considered to be a reasonable retirement age.[3]

Senescence, the process or condition of growing old, has sociocultural, as well as physiologic and chronologic, implications. Normal aging should not be confused with the effects of pathologic influences that accelerate the aging process. Each age period brings changes in body metabolism, activity of the cells, endocrine balance, and mental processes.

An older person's health status is influenced by many factors. Both biologic and environmental factors influence longevity. Genetically, a person may belong to a family of healthy people who have exhibited great

TABLE 46–1
KEY WORDS: GERODONTIC PATIENT

Alzheimer's disease (altz'hī-merz): a presenile dementia of unknown cause beginning at middle age, affecting nerve cells of the frontal and temporal lobes of the cerebrum, and leading to speech defects and progressive loss of mental faculties.

Dysphagia (dĭs-fa'jē-ah): difficulty in swallowing.

Emphysema (em'fĭ-sē'mah): pathologic accumulation of air in tissues or organs; general use refers to **chronic pulmonary emphysema,** in which the terminal bronchioles become plugged with mucus, the lung tissue loses elasticity, and breathing difficulties ensue.

Geriatric dentistry: the branch of dentistry that deals with the special knowledge, attitudes, and technical skills required in the provision of oral health care for older adults.

Geriatrics (jer'ē-at'rĭks): the branch of medicine that deals with the problems of aging and diseases of the elderly.

Gerontology: study of the aging process; includes the biologic, psychologic, and sociologic sciences.

Hemostasis (hē'mō-stā'sĭs): arrest of the escape of blood by either natural (clot formation or vessel spasm) or artificial (compression or ligation) means, or the interruption of blood flow to a part.

Life expectancy: average number of years that a person can be expected to live; expectancy from birth in 1900 averaged 47 years, in 1990 averaged 74 years, and the projected figure for the year 2000 is 76 years; expectancy for the female population is about 7 years longer than that for the male population.

Osteopenia (os'tē-ō-pē'nē-ah): reduced bone mass caused by decrease in rate of osteoid (new young bone) synthesis to a level insufficient to compensate normal bone destruction.

Osteoporosis (os'tē-ō-po-rō'sĭs): abnormal rarefaction of bone related to lifetime calcium deficiency and lack of exercise.

Senility (sĕ-nĭl'ĭ-tē): old age; loss of mental, physical, or emotional control; caused by physical and/or mental deterioration.

resistance to disease factors. Another person may have inherited a specific disease state. Even inherited diseases, for example, diabetes or sickle cell anemia, may be controllable through treatment or genetic counseling.

CHARACTERISTICS OF AGING

Changes with aging vary among individuals and among organs and tissues of the same individual. It may be difficult to separate physiologic manifestations of aging from those of disease or the aftereffects of disease.

I. GENERAL PHYSIOLOGIC CHANGES

During aging, an overall gradual reduction in functional capacities occurs in most organs, with a decrease in cell metabolism and numbers of active cells. The tissues may show signs of dehydration, atrophy, fibrosis, reduced elasticity, and diminished reparative ability. Many of these characteristics cannot be separated from pathologic changes.

A. Skeletal System

1. Skeletal integrity is significantly influenced by an insufficient intake of calcium, phosphorus, and fluoride (page 440).
2. Bone volume (mass) decreases gradually after the age of 40, depending on diet, nutrition, and exercise.
3. Osteoporosis is common in individuals older than age 60, and the incidence increases with age (page 636).

B. Basal Metabolism
Basal metabolism is lowered.

C. Skin

1. The skin may become thin, wrinkled, and dry, with pigmented spots, loss of tone, and atrophy of the sweat glands.
2. Reduced tolerance to temperature extremes and solar exposure is evident.

D. Locomotor System
Older patients may experience loss of muscle mass, development of unsteadiness and tremor, diminishing of muscular strength, and decreased speed of response. Posture may become stooped; joints may stiffen as a result of loss of elasticity in the ligaments.

E. Gastrointestinal System

1. Production of hydrochloric acid and other secretions gradually decreases.
2. Peristalsis is slowed.
3. Evaluation of digestive disorders is complicated by the general indiscriminate use of self-medications.

F. Cardiovascular System (Chapter 58)
Effects of aging on the cardiovascular system include the following:

1. Tendency toward increased blood pressure usually secondary to disease.
2. Arteriosclerosis, with decreased circulation to the tissues.
3. Reduced cardiac output; increased heart size.
4. Postural hypotension; with dizziness or weakness when sitting up from recumbent position.

G. Respiratory System

1. Vital capacity is progressively diminished.
2. Decreased pulmonary efficiency may be related to life-style and lack of exercise.

3. Chronic bronchitis and emphysema are of particular concern.

H. Special Senses (Chapter 53)
1. *Vision.* Decline in accommodation and color and depth perception, and difficulty in adapting from light to dark.
2. *Hearing.* Reduced hearing ability, with a loss of sensitivity to high tones.

II. DISEASES IN THE ELDERLY PERSON
With increasing age, the incidence of chronic mental and physical diseases increases. A patient may have more than one condition. Diseases that are most common among elderly patients are arthritis, heart disease, hypertension, and hearing impairment.

A. Increased Susceptibility to Infection[4]
With aging, an increased susceptibility to infection may be related to one or more of the following:
1. Lowered capacity in cell-mediated and humoral immunity and nonspecific host defenses.
2. Altered skin and mucosal barriers. In the oral cavity, the flora of the mucosa can be changed, especially when systemic conditions or medications lead to xerostomia.
3. Interaction of nutritional factors with underlying chronic conditions.

B. Response to Disease
1. *Course and Severity.* Although the diseases that affect the elderly person also occur in younger persons, the course and effects of the diseases may differ. In the elderly person, disease may occur with greater severity and have a longer course, with slower recovery.
2. *Pain Sensitivity.* May be lessened.
3. *Temperature Response.* May be altered so that a patient may be very ill without the expected increase in body temperature.
4. *Healing*
   a. Decreased healing capacity.
   b. More prone to secondary infection.

C. Osteoporosis
Osteoporosis is a bone disease involving loss of mineral content and bone mass. Although most prominent in postmenopausal women, the condition may also occur at other ages and in men.
1. *Causes*
   a. Endocrine; hormonal disturbances; depletion of estrogen after menopause.
   b. Calcium deficiency; defective absorption of calcium.
   c. Steroid therapy or hypercortisonism.
2. *Risk Factors.* Several risk factors have been identified, some of which usually work together. From this list of risk factors, a list of

methods for long-term prevention can be derived.
   a. Female sex.
   b. Caucasian or Asian ethnicity (worldwide, Blacks are least affected).
   c. Positive family history.
   d. Low calcium intake (lifelong).
   e. Early menopause or early surgical removal of ovaries.
   f. Sedentary lifestyle; lack of exercise.
   g. Alcohol abuse.
   h. High sodium intake.
   i. Cigarette smoking.
   j. High caffeine intake.
3. *Symptoms.* Osteoporosis develops over many years; therefore a long asymptomatic period of bone change occurs with no clinical symptoms.
   a. Backache; stooping of the posture.
   b. Fractures; may have spinal crush fractures with periodic acute pain.
   c. Evidence of bone changes in the mandible; residual ridge resorption.
4. *Treatment.* A patient with osteoporosis may be treated with medications, such as calcium, sodium fluoride, vitamin D, or possibly, estrogens. Activity and exercise require caution and preventive measures to avoid accidental falls.

Severe involvement of the spine may require orthopedic support and medication for pain. Questions regarding the patient's medical history can elicit factors of importance.

D. Alzheimer's Disease[5,6]
Alzheimer's disease is one of the nonreversible types of dementia. Dementia is severe impairment of the intellectual abilities, notably thinking, memory, and personality. At least one half of the patients with dementia have Alzheimer's disease. The causes include cerebrovascular disease and alcoholism (page 778).
1. *Symptoms.* The common impairments of Alzheimer's disease may be divided into three or four overlapping stages that may extend over many years. In table 46–2, characteristics are divided into early, middle, advanced, and terminal stages.
2. *Appointment Considerations.* During the early stages, perhaps even before a diagnosis of Alzheimer's disease has been made, the patient will be attending routine dental and dental hygiene appointments.
   a. An early sign of the disease may be a slow decline of interest in oral hygiene and personal care. Review of the patient's medical and dental history at each maintenance appointment may reveal lapses in memory and other items listed under the "Early Stage" in table 46–2. An op-

TABLE 46-2
COMMON IMPAIRMENTS ASSOCIATED WITH ALZHEIMER'S DISEASE

Early Stage
Forgetfulness
Personality changes
Employment performance difficulty
Social withdrawal
Apathy
Errors in judgment
Inattentiveness
Personal hygiene neglect

Middle Stage
Disorientation
Loss of coordination
Restlessness/anxiety
Language difficulty
Sleep pattern disturbance
Progressive memory loss
Catastrophic reactions
Pacing

Advanced Stage
Profound comprehension difficulty
Gait disturbances
Bladder and bowel incontinence
Hyperoralia
Inability to recognize family members
Seizures
Aggression
Lack of insight into deficits

Terminal Stage
Physical immobility
Contractures
Dysphagia
Emaciation
Mutism
Pathologic reflexes
Unawareness of environment
Total helplessness

(From Fabiszewski, K.J.: Caring for the Alzheimer's Patient, *Gerodontology*, 6, 53, Summer, 1987, © Beech Hill Enterprises, Inc. Used by Permission.)

portunity may be found to help a patient seek professional evaluation and care.

b. Later stages may require that the patient reside in a long-term care facility. Dental hygienists in specialized facilities develop particular techniques for the variety of patients to be served.

ORAL FINDINGS IN AGING

As mentioned earlier in this chapter, changes related to aging must be separated from the long-term effects of chronic diseases.

I. SOFT TISSUES
A. Lips
1. *Tissue Changes.* Dry, purse-string opening results from dehydration and loss of elasticity within the tissues.
2. *Angular Cheilitis.*[7] Angular cheilitis is not specifically an age-related lesion, but is frequently seen among elderly persons. It appears as skin folds with fissuring at the angles of the mouth, and is related to reduced vertical dimension or inadequate support of the lips. Contributing factors are summarized on page 650.

B. Oral Mucosa
Degenerative changes take several forms. The surface texture is affected by changes in lubrication of the tissue with decreased secretion of the salivary and mucous glands. Xerostomia is not a result of aging, but is associated with certain diseases and medications.
1. *Atrophic Changes.* The tissue may become thinner and less vascular, with a loss of elasticity. Clinically, the smooth shiny appearance is related to thinning of the epithelium.
2. *Hyperkeratosis.* White, patchy areas develop as a result of irritation from sharp edges of broken teeth, restorations, or dentures, and from use of tobacco.
3. *Capillary Fragility.* Facial bruises and petechiae of the mucosa are common.

C. Tongue
1. *Atrophic Glossitis (Burning Tongue).* The tongue appears smooth, shiny, and bald, with atrophied papillae. The condition is related to anemia that results from a deficiency of iron or combinations of deficiencies. Elderly people have deficiency anemias more frequently than do those in other age groups because of nutritional factors, but not because of aging specifically.
2. *Taste Sensations.* Taste buds are not reduced in number. Taste may be reduced or abnormal taste reactions may occur, primarily in people with a disease condition, but changes are not routinely observed in the healthy elderly person.[8]
3. *Sublingual Varicosities*
   a. Clinical appearance. Deep, red or bluish nodular dilated vessels on either side of the midline on the ventral surface of the tongue.
   b. Significance. Although frequently occurring, these varicosities do not necessarily have a direct relation to systemic conditions.

D. Xerostomia
Dryness of the mouth is found frequently in older people in conjunction with pathologic

states, drug-induced changes, or radiation-induced degeneration of the salivary glands. Healthy people continue to have normal salivary flow.[9] Xerostomia is described in detail on page 204.

II. TEETH
A. Color
The teeth may show color changes from long use of tobacco or foods with coloring agents, such as tea or coffee. Dark intrinsic stains from dental restorations may be evident.

B. Attrition
The teeth of elderly people frequently show signs of wear, which may be the long-term effects of diet, occupational factors, or bruxism. Figure 14–6, page 238, illustrates incisal wear. Attrition may be accompanied by chipping, and teeth may seem more brittle, particularly when compared with teeth of young people.

C. Abrasion
Abrasion at the neck of a tooth may be the result of extended use of a hard toothbrush in a horizontal direction with an abrasive dentifrice. With current preventive measures, use of soft-textured brushes, and attention to abrasiveness of dentifrices, future generations will be less likely to exhibit such tooth alterations.

D. Dental Caries
1. *Root Caries.* With roots exposed by periodontal infections, an increase in caries of the cementum can result. Root caries is described on page 236. An increase in caries with age is the result of root exposure, not of age.

   Periodontal therapy with continuing maintenance may influence the extent of root caries. In one group of patients with untreated moderate to severe periodontitis, root caries steadily increased with age, until 86% in the over-60 age group were affected. In another group, comparable in age and disease severity but who had received periodontal treatment and regular maintenance, the dental caries incidence tapered off after 60 years, from 51% in the 50- to 59-year-old age group to 42% in those older than 60.[10]
2. *Rampant Caries.* Sometimes called "retirement caries."[11] A noticeable increase in dental caries may occur after age 65. Factors influencing the development of dental caries include the following:
   a. Xerostomia. Tooth-protection factors of the saliva are missing (page 204).
   b. Masticatory abilities. Oral conditions and, possibly, tooth loss make mastication difficult. This leads to changes in food selections.
   c. Life-style. After retirement, without a daily work schedule, snacking and irregular mealtimes may lead to poor food selections and an excessively cariogenic diet.

E. Dental Pulp[12]
Whether pulpal changes can be considered results of aging is questionable. The pulpal changes develop as reactions to dental caries, restorations, bruxism, and other assaults during the elderly person's long life. The changes noted here may be observed at younger ages, but are seen more frequently in older people.
1. Narrowing of pulp chambers and root canals; increased deposition of secondary dentin.
2. Progressive deposition of calcified masses (pulp stones or denticles).

III. PERIODONTIUM
A. Clinical Findings
The periodontal tissues reflect the health and disease of the patient over the years. One of the following may apply to any patient.
1. *The Healthy Periodontium.* Healthy tissues that have been maintained over the years may have had a minimum of disease. The radiographs show little if any bone recession, the gingiva are firm, and the appearance is normal in every way. Probing reveals minimal sulcus depth with no bleeding. The teeth are not mobile.
2. *The Patient with Periodontal Infection.* Neglect or omission of preventive measures and therapy over the years may have resulted in a chronic periodontal infection with extension of tissue destruction into the bone, periodontal ligament, and cementum. Loss of attachment, deep periodontal pockets, tooth mobility, and radiographic signs of periodontitis may be present.
3. *The Treated Patient.* Although the patient was subject to periodontal infection, treatment was completed, and the tissues were maintained in health through personal care and professional supervision. The tissues may show the effects of the treated disease, such as scar tissue. Areas of recession with exposed cementum may also be evident. The teeth are not mobile.

B. Tissue Changes Related to Aging
1. *Bone*
   a. Osteoporosis may be present; related to nutritional and hormonal factors.
   b. Depressed vascularity, a reduction in metabolism, and reduced healing power affect bone.
2. *Cementum.* Increased thickness has been demonstrated. In one series of measurements, the average overall thickness of the cementum at 20 years of age was 0.095 mm,

whereas cementum from 60-year-old persons measured 0.215 mm.[13]

3. *Gingiva.* Most gingival changes can be traced to the effects of infection or to anatomic factors. For example, gingival recession is common in older individuals. Predisposing factors may be a lack of sufficient attached gingiva or malposition of the teeth.

Precipitating factors may be vigorous inappropriate toothbrushing, laceration, inflammation, or dental treatment, such as the placement of a rubber dam on an area with minimum attached gingiva.

PERSONAL FACTORS

The following list should not be considered typical of all elderly patients, because many are well adjusted. These characteristics are suggested to help the dental team members understand an older person's attitudes and actions.

I. INSECURITY
A. Related to reduced economic status, self-respect, and feeling of being needed.
B. Inability to work.
C. Reduced activity.
  a. Physical limitations.
  b. Overprotection by family.
D. Rejection by family.
E. Anxiety over health.

II. DEPRESSION
A. Limited physical power; sensitivity about shortcomings of impaired vision, hearing, and lack of motor control.
B. Changes in physical appearance.
C. Loneliness.
  1. Loss of spouse and friends.
  2. Need for attention and concern from others; companionship.

III. INABILITY TO ADJUST TO CHANGES IN MODE OF LIFE
Tendency to develop fixed habits and ideas.

IV. SLOWING OF VOLUNTARY RESPONSES
Voluntary responses, association of thoughts, and speed of vocalization may all be slowed.

V. TENDENCY TO INTROSPECTION
Narrowing of interests; living in the past.

DENTAL HYGIENE CARE

When planning and conducting appointments for an older patient, many of the procedures included in Chapter 50 (page 679) can be applied. Certain aging patients have physical and sensory limitations, and for those persons, adaptations are needed. It should be appreciated, however, that many members of the elderly population are independent, agile, and healthy people without systemic disease and who are not dependent on medications.

Care for the older patient should be planned in terms of comprehensive, not palliative, treatment. Long-term maintenance for the prevention of oral disease must be the basic objective.

Many elderly people do not seek dental and dental hygiene care except when an emergency arises. A primary reason for the limited attention to professional care may be a lack of perceived need. Other reasons relate to physical and mental disabilities, chronic disease, and physical barriers, such as transportation or accessibility of the dental office. Financial resources have not been a major reason.[14]

I. APPOINTMENT FACTORS
A. Office or Clinic Facilities
Attention to dental office arrangement that eliminates physical barriers is important. An aged person's impaired vision, feebleness, or lack of motor control must be considered.

Hazards, such as small rugs, which can slide on polished floors, loose corners of rugs, which can be tripped over, and irregularities in floor levels, can be eliminated. Other considerations related to architectural barriers and how to assist an elderly person who may be disabled are described on pages 682–684.

B. Patient History
Preparation of a careful and detailed medical and dental history takes on particular significance. Basic procedures for preparation of the history are described in Chapter 6.

Suggestions for good communication include the following:
1. Eliminate distracting background music or sounds.
2. Sit facing the patient, because hearing may be a problem. Other suggestions for the hearing-impaired patient are described on pages 734–740.
3. Do not shout; just increase volume and speak slowly and clearly.
4. Be courteous at all times; show respect for age. Do not call the patient by his/her first name unless the patient suggests doing so.
5. Present one idea at a time; be a good listener; older people do not like to be hurried.
6. Develop trust; reduce anxiety.

C. Medications
Older patients use more drugs and have more prescriptions, as well as more over-the-counter drugs, than does any other age group. Many

have more than one chronic disease or disability requiring medication.

1. *Obtain the Correct List.* Ask the patient to bring in either the bottles that contain the various medications (over-the-counter as well as prescription items) or a written copy of the labels so that a list may be kept in the patient's record. The patient's physician may be the best source for an accurate list.

    The list of medications must be checked at each maintenance appointment. Changes in health status can mean changes in prescriptions.

2. *References for Checking Drugs.* Each practice center or clinic needs current references, such as the *Physician's Desk Reference (PDR),* *Merck Manual,* and pharmacology textbooks.

    Prescriptions reported by patients need to be reviewed for (1) potential adverse side effects, (2) possible drug interactions with products recommended or used during the appointment, and (3) a clear understanding of the patient's state of health to assure the clinician that the recommended procedure is right for the patient.

3. *Effects on Appointment.* Table 46–3 provides a partial list of effects of medications and the general classes of drugs that can produce each effect. Although the drug effects apply to all age groups, the elderly patient not only has more chronic disease and more prescriptions, but also can be more sensitive. Consultation with the patient's physician carries particular significance.

D. Need for Antibiotic Premedication

Many conditions that require prophylactic coverage are found fairly frequently in the elderly person. Those with uncontrolled diabetes or those who receive chemotherapeutic or steroid treatments may have an increased susceptibility to infection. When the patient has a prosthetic joint replacement, heart valve or aortic prosthesis, pacemaker, or a history of other conditions listed on pages 102 and 103, premedication is indicated.

E. Vital Signs

Blood pressure determination is recommended for each visit (pages 113 and 114).

F. Intraoral and Extraoral Examination

The need for careful, periodic examination of the oral mucosa from lips to throat cannot be overstressed at any age, but is especially crucial for the elderly patient because oral cancer occurs with increasing frequency with advancing years. Many, in fact most, oral lesions exist without the patient being aware of them.

**TABLE 46–3
EFFECTS OF MEDICATIONS**

Effect of Medication Adjust Procedure	Drug Classes Involved
Abnormal Hemostasis	Aspirin Warfarin (Coumadin) Dipyridamole
Need to Minimize Vasoconstrictor Use	Antiarrhythmics Cardiac glycosides Sublingual and systemic nitrates Tricyclic antidepressants
Decreased Tolerance for Stress	Beta-blockers Calcium-channel blockers Cardiac glycosides Sublingual and systemic nitrates
Altered Host Resistance	Long-term antibiotics Insulin Oral hypoglycemics Systemic corticosteroids
Xerostomia	Antianxiety agents Anticholinergics Antidepressants Antihistamines/decongestants Antihypertensives Antiparkinsons Antipsychotics Chemotherapy agents Diuretics
Movement Disorders	Antipsychotics Levodopa Lithium
Gingival Overgrowth	Phenytoin Nifedipine Cyclosporine

(Adapted from Levy, S.M., Baker, K.A., Semla, T.P., and Kohout, F.J.: Use of Medications with Dental Significance by a Noninstitutionalized Elderly Population, *Gerodontics, 4,* 119, June, 1988.)

For some early surface lesions, biopsy is definitely indicated. For others, a cytologic smear can be prepared as directed by the dentist (page 126).

II. PREVENTIVE TREATMENT PROGRAM

Older patients need to have frequent appointments to maintain their oral health at a high level through supervision on a regular basis. The content of a treatment plan resembles that for other age groups, and emphasis on plaque control dominates. Appointment suggestions are summarized in table 46–4. The dental hygiene appointments may include the following:

TABLE 46-4
ADAPTATIONS IN TREATMENT PROCEDURES FOR THE GERODONTIC PATIENT

Appointment Factors	Characteristic of the Gerodontic Patient	Dental Hygiene Implication
Medical History Review	Many forms of chronic diseases Variety of medications used	Poor medical prognosis may limit extent of total treatment Need for antibiotic premedication for decreased immune response
Appointment Planning	Low stress tolerance Tires more easily than does a younger patient	Morning appointments Shorter appointments Need for frequent maintenance appointments to provide high-level preventive care Appreciation of the real effort patient has made to get there
	Slower voluntary responses Sensitivity about shortcomings of lack of motor control	Do not rush Do not make the patient feel old by obvious physical assistance
	Lowered tolerance to extremes of heat and cold; less body cooling through perspiration Impaired hearing; difficulty in hearing when there are distractions	Adjust room temperature Speak clearly and slowly; provide written memorandum of date and time of each appointment Eliminate background noises and music
Instrumentation	Loss of elasticity of lips and oral mucosa	Difficulty in retraction may provide patient discomfort
	Slowing of voluntary responses Cannot adjust to sudden muscular demands	Do not demand quick response to request for change of position of head, rinsing
	Pulp recession: variable pain threshold	Ask patient before administering anesthesia; the patient may not need it
	Reduction in growth and repair processes Decreased resistance to infection Healing slowed	Provide as little trauma to gingiva as possible during instrumentation Suggest postoperative care procedures to promote healing
	Inability to recover readily from stresses and strains Unsteadiness; tendency to postural hypotension	At completion of appointment, straighten chair back slowly and let patient sit up for short time before dismissing; assist out of chair.

A. Plaque Control
Plaque control is described in detail in a subsequent section.

B. Periodontal Care
Treatment with complete scaling, root planing, and follow-up to assess need for additional therapy.

C. Dental Caries Control
1. Diet survey covering several days (pages 425–429).
2. Diet adjustment to eliminate cariogenic foods and make appropriate substitutions.
3. Emphasis on prevention of rampant root caries.
4. Fluoride therapy by use of daily self-applied

preparations by dentifrice, rinse, or brush-on gel as needed (pages 449–453).

D. Xerostomia
Use of a saliva substitute (page 205).

III. BACTERIAL PLAQUE CONTROL
A. Objectives
Basic objectives do not differ from those for younger people: infection must be eliminated and controlled.

Older individuals need to be as interested in their health and appearance as do people of any age. Esthetic deterioration may create emotional unhappiness, and when aging persons feel insecure or unwanted, they may lose their interest in personal oral care and diet. Motivation through expression of sincere interest on the part of dental personnel can be an influencing factor in helping the patient to better health.

Certain people fear dentures because they associate them with "old" people. Patients with partial dentures may already have been impressed with the need for preserving the remaining teeth. Here, in the desire to save the teeth, lies the appeal for preventive measures for both the teeth and their supporting structures, and good use should be made of this very real motivating force.

B. Approach to Instruction

In patient instruction, do not try to change all lifelong habits because doing so may create frustration and unhappiness. Self-confidence, which has diminished because of lowering of physical capabilities and emotional satisfaction, must be built up. Major changes required because previous habits were detrimental must be brought about gradually if cooperation is to be expected. A more optimistic attitude is placed about the degree of oral health the elderly patient can be expected to achieve.

C. Dental Plaque Formation

The incidence and severity of periodontal diseases increase with age as an effect of disease accumulation. The amount of periodontal destruction reflects the length of time the tissues have been exposed to disease-producing factors, primarily plaque microorganisms.

Several factors can contribute to a more rapid accumulation of plaque in the older patient. Some of these are listed here.

1. *Anatomic*
   a. Gingival recession with wide embrasures that result from periodontal destruction provides a larger surface area for plaque retention.
   b. Exposed cementum with areas of abrasion or dental caries at the neck of a tooth can create undercut areas where special adaptation of plaque removal devices is needed.

2. *Plaque Retention and Removal*
   a. Exposed untreated cementum may hold plaque more readily than does enamel. Cementum planed smooth is less likely to hold plaque, and plaque removal efforts are more successful.
   b. Decreased saliva production reduces or eliminates the cleansing and lubricating effects of saliva.
   c. Restorations and prostheses provide a more complex dentition for personal care. Plaque removal requires more time, patience, and motivation.
   d. Deficient restorations may have overhanging margins that provide areas of plaque retention.
   e. Lack of dexterity related to disabling conditions resulting from chronic diseases, such as arthritis and Parkinsonism, makes plaque removal more difficult.

D. Specific Recommendations

Toothbrushing and other plaque control procedures, as well as methods for the care of fixed and removable prostheses, are selected as for other adult patients. A power-assisted brush may help certain patients, particularly those with impaired motor function. Adaptations to alter the handle of a manual brush are described on pages 692–694.

Because of increased exposure of root surfaces, attention must be paid to dentifrice selection to prevent effects of abrasion and to prevent root caries. Certain patients may need instruction in desensitizing procedures (page 557). The use of a fluoride dentifrice and a daily fluoride mouthrinse can contribute to both dental caries prevention and desensitization.

When a saliva substitute is recommended for patients with dry mouth, specific instructions must be given. Information about where to obtain available preparations is needed.

Instruction and motivation techniques are best applied gradually and regularly at frequent intervals. Suggestions for adaptations of instruction to the physical and personal characteristics of the patient are listed in table 46–5.

IV. DIET AND NUTRITION
A. Dietary Habits

1. *Nutritional Deficiencies.* Dietary and resulting nutritional deficiencies are common in older people. For example, characteristic changes, such as burning tongue, angular cheilitis, and atrophic glossitis, may be related to vitamin B deficiencies. Unfortunately, many people believe that a diet rich in nutritive elements is important only for children.

2. *Factors Contributing to Dietary and Nutritional Deficiencies*
   a. Limited budget.
   b. Lives alone or eats alone.
   c. Does not eat regular meals; frequently uses nonnutritious snacks and foods for entertaining.
   d. Alcoholism.
   e. Lacks interest in shopping for or preparing food.
   f. Acuteness of senses lowered; may seek highly seasoned or sweetened foods.
   g. Childish likes and dislikes; unusual cravings.

TABLE 46-5
CHARACTERISTICS AFFECTING INSTRUCTION FOR THE GERODONTIC PATIENT

Characteristic of the Gerodontic Patient	Suggested Relation to Patient Instruction
Tendency for introspection; desire for attention	Patience needed in taking time to listen to complaints and accounts of past experiences
Feelings of insecurity Deprivation of physical capabilities Touchy sensitiveness, exaggerated imaginary or real pains, or attitudes of suspicion	Sympathetic understanding needed Build up self-confidence
Resistance to change; tendency to maintain fixed habits	Should not attempt to change all lifelong habits, only detrimental habits
Vision impaired	For the patient who wears prescription eyeglasses, make sure the glasses are worn while instruction is being given Recommend that eyeglasses be worn at home while performing plaque control procedures
Hearing impaired; loss of sensitivity to higher tones	Speak distinctly in normal voice. Look directly at patient while speaking; many are lip readers
Slowing of voluntary responses Slowing of speed of thought associations Difficulty in timing sequential events; skills become separate movements, as by a child Least comfortable when must respond quickly to demanding sequential stimuli Rate of learning changed, ability to learn not changed Changes in speed of vocalization	Make suggestions gradually, over a series of appointments Do not demand learning a completely new procedure; adapt procedure already used Guide patient's demonstration of toothbrushing to prevent embarrassment Do not expect perfection; go slowly, anticipate difficulties, give cues, clues Distinguish between slowness of learning and inability to learn
Memory shortened, mainly the result of lack of attention, lack of interest, or more selection of what patient wants to remember	Use motivating factors carefully. Provide written instructions; spoken instructions may be forgotten or misunderstood
Need for personal achievement	Help patient gain sense of accomplishment; commend for any success, however minor Never compare the patient's condition with that of other patients

h. Tendency to follow food habits of lifetime; ignores newer knowledge of food preparation methods and dietary needs.

i. Inadequate masticatory efficiency because of tooth loss or dentures that no longer fit properly.

j. Adverse food selection may result from social embarrassment over inability to chew.

k. Adaptations in eating habits, made to compensate for deficiency, may interfere with adequate digestion and absorption of nutrients.

l. May follow dietary fads that provide only a limited and unbalanced diet.

m. Loss of appetite, which may have physiologic, social, or economic causes.

n. Lack of self-discipline; feeling that aging brings privilege to eat only preferred foods.

B. Dietary Needs of the Aged

The total nutritional needs of older persons are not different from those of younger persons, but they should cut down the quantity, particularly of calories. Caloric intake must be decreased to control weight. Protein, vitamins, and minerals are particularly important for body function, repair, and resistance to disease.

A necessary objective in geriatric nutrition is to retard the progression of diet-induced chronic diseases. Examples of these are atherosclerosis related to disorders of glucose and lipid metabolism, anemias related to iron and folic acid deficiencies, and osteoporosis resulting from calcium and fluoride deficiency.

In addition to a better intake of calcium in the diet, recent research has shown that fluoride intake over the years is beneficial in the prevention of osteoporosis and fractures of the bones.[15] The relationship between fluoride in the drinking water and the decreased prevalence of osteoporosis was described on page 440.

C. Instruction in Diet and Oral Health

1. *Dietary Analysis.* A 4- or 5-day record of the patient's diet can provide information to guide recommendations to be made. Difficulties in showing the procedure to the patient and obtaining accurate results may seem insurmountable. Inaccuracy of recent memory is a problem with some elderly people, so that even the 24-hour dietary record prepared during the appointment may not be complete.

   The first consideration in making recommendations for aging patients is that a well-balanced diet be used with limited amounts of cariogenic foods for dental caries prevention. Food for an adequate diet is shown in figure 28–1 on page 424.

2. *Motivation.* Appeal to the patient is made through personal concerns for the relationships of dietary deficiencies to appearance, lowered resistance to disease, and premature aging, which may inspire the patient to improve daily habits. Educational materials are available to study with, and to give to, the patient.

TECHNICAL HINTS

SOURCES OF MATERIALS

American Dental Association
  Department of Salable Materials
  211 E. Chicago Avenue
  Chicago, IL 60611

Department of Dental Hygiene
  University of Rhode Island
  Kingston, RI 02881

The Why, When, and How, Preventive Oral Hygiene Care for the Elderly, Homebound or Nursing Home Residents (Revised)

REFERENCES

1. **American Association of Retired Persons and the Administration on Aging,** United States Department of Health and Human Services: *A Profile of Older Americans, 1985.* American Association of Retired Persons, 1909 K Street, N.W., Washington, D.C. 20049.
2. **World Health Organization:** *Planning and Organization of Geriatric Services.* Geneva, World Health Organization, Technical Report Series, No. 548, 1974, p. 11.
3. **Roddy,** J.A.: Dental Needs: The Well Elderly, *Dentalhygienistnews, 3,* 13, Fall, 1990.
4. **Terpenning,** M.S. and Bradley, S.F.: Why Aging Leads to Increased Susceptibility to Infection, *Geriatrics, 46,* 77, February, 1991.
5. **Fabiszewski,** K.J.: Caring for the Alzheimer's Patient, *Gerodontology, 6,* 53, Summer, 1987.
6. **Niessen,** L.C. and Jones, J.A.: Alzheimer's Disease: A Guide for Dental Professionals, *Spec. Care Dentist., 6,* 6, January/February, 1986.
7. **Ibsen,** O.A.C. and Phelan, J.A.: *Oral Pathology for the Dental Hygienist.* Philadelphia, W.B. Saunders Co., 1992, pp. 38–39, 193, 196.
8. **Baum,** B.J.: Current Research on Aging and Oral Health, *Spec. Care Dentist., 1,* 105, May/June, 1981.
9. **Baum,** B.J.: Age Changes in Salivary Glands and Salivary Secretion, in Holm-Pedersen, P. and Löe, H., eds.: *Geriatric Dentistry.* St. Louis, Mosby, 1986, pp. 114–122.
10. **Hix,** J.O. and O'Leary, T.J.: The Relationship Between Cemental Caries, Oral Hygiene Status and Fermentable Carbohydrate Intake, *J. Periodontol., 47,* 398, July, 1976.
11. **Chase,** R.H.: The Management of "Retirement Caries," *J. Mich. Dent. Assoc., 57,* 178, April, 1975.
12. **Seltzer,** S. and Bender, I.B.: *The Dental Pulp. Biologic Considerations in Dental Procedures,* 3rd ed. St. Louis, Ishiyaku EuroAmerica, 1990, pp. 324–348.
13. **Zander,** H.A. and Hurzeler, B.: Continuous Cementum Apposition, *J. Dent. Res., 37,* 1035, November-December, 1958.
14. **Kiyak,** H.A.: Barriers to the Utilization of Dental Services by the Elderly, in Chauncey, H.H., Epstein, S., Rose, C.L., and Hefferren, J.J., eds.: *Clinical Geriatric Dentistry, Biomedical and Psychosocial Aspects.* Chicago, American Dental Association, 1985, pp. 157–168.
15. **Simonen,** O. and Laitinen, O.: Does Fluoridation of Drinking-water Prevent Bone Fragility and Osteoporosis? *Lancet, 2 (8452),* 432, August 24, 1985.

SUGGESTED READINGS

Clark, D.C., Morgan, J., and MacEntee, M.I.: Effects of a 1% Chlorhexidine Gel on the Cariogenic Bacteria in High-risk Elders: A Pilot Study, *Spec. Care Dentist., 11,* 101, May/June, 1991.

Compton, S.: Dental Implantology and the Older Adult. Implications for Oral Hygiene Maintenance, *Can. Dent. Hyg./Probe, 26,* 121, Autumn, 1992.

Drake, C.W., Beck, J.D., and Strauss, R.P.: The Accuracy of Oral Self-perceptions in a Dentate Older Population, *Spec. Care Dentist., 10,* 16, January/February, 1990.

Goodman, H.S., Ickrath, M.C., and Niessen, L.C.: Managing Patients with Alzheimer's: The Primary Care Role of Dentists, *J. Am. Dent. Assoc., 124,* 75, May, 1993.

Hunt, R.J., Drake, C.W., and Beck, J.D.: *Streptococcus mutans,* Lactobacilli, and Caries Experience in Older Adults, *Spec. Care Dentist., 12,* 149, July/August, 1992.

Jorgensen, J.E.: A Dentist's Social Responsibility to Diagnose Elder Abuse, *Spec. Care Dentist., 12,* 112, May/June, 1992.

King, L.J.: The Senior Patient: Emphasizing the Individual, *Access, 6,* 7, March, 1992.

MacEntee, M.I.: Does the Dental Profession Care for Disabled Elders? Some Practical Questions, *Can. Dent. Assoc. J., 56,* 215, March, 1990.

MacEntee, M.: Oral Health in Old Age—Practical Problems and Practical Solutions, *Can. Dent. Hyg./Probe, 26,* 116, Autumn, 1992.

Moody, G.H., Drummond, J.R., and Newton, J.P.: Alzheimer's Disease, *Br. Dent. J., 169,* 45, July 21, 1990.

Morse, D.R., Esposito, J.V., Schoor, R.S., and Gorin, R.: A Cross-sectional Radiographic Study of Aging Changes of Teeth and Supporting Structures, *Compendium, 14,* 241, February, 1993.

Niessen, L.C., Mash, L.K., and Gibson, G.: Practice Management Considerations for an Aging Population, *J. Am. Dent. Assoc., 124,* 55, March, 1993.

Norlen, P., Ostberg, H., and Bjorn, A.-L.: Relationship Between General Health, Social Factors and Oral Health in Women at the Age of Retirement, *Community Dent. Oral Epidemiol., 19,* 296, October, 1991.

Ship, J.A.: Oral Health of Patients with Alzheimer's Disease, *J. Am. Dent. Assoc., 123,* 53, January, 1992.

Sidhu, S.K., Soh, G., and Henderson, L.J.: Effect of Dentin Age on Effectiveness of Dentin Bonding Agents, *Oper. Dent., 16,* 218, November-December, 1991.

Vosburg, F.: The Behavior of the Geriatric Patient, *Can. Dent. Assoc. J., 56,* 211, March, 1990.

Widdop, F.T.: Caring for the Dentate Elderly, *Int. Dent. J., 39,* 85, June, 1989.

Medications (References for Table 46–3)

Levy, S.M., Baker, K.A., Semla, T.P., and Kohout, F.J.: Use of Medications with Dental Significance by a Noninstitutionalized Elderly Population, *Gerodontics, 4,* 119, June, 1988.

Matthews, T.G.: Medication Side Effects of Dental Interest, *J. Prosthet. Dent., 64,* 219, August, 1990.

Mazer, M.S.: Geriatric Pharmacology and Dental Implications, *Gen. Dent., 40,* 215, May-June, 1992.

McDermott, R.E., Hoover, J.N., and Gaucher, C.: Self-reported Medical Conditions and Drug Use Among Elderly Dental Patients, *Can. Dent. Assoc. J., 56,* 219, March, 1990.

Saunders, R.H. and Handelman, S.L.: Effects of Hyposalivatory Medications on Saliva Flow Rates and Dental Caries in Adults Aged 65 and Older, *Spec. Care Dentist., 12,* 116, May/June, 1992.

Soon, J.A.: Effects of Drug Therapy on Oral Health of Older Adults, *Can. Dent. Hyg./Probe, 26,* 118, Autumn, 1992.

Streckfus, C.F., Strahl, R.C., and Welsh, S.: Anti-hypertension Medications: An Epidemiological Factor in the Prevalence of Root Decay among Geriatric Patients Suffering from Hypertension, *Clin. Prev. Dent., 12,* 26, August-September, 1990.

Tomaselli, C.E.: Pharmacotherapy in the Geriatric Population, *Spec. Care Dentist., 12,* 107, May/June, 1992.

Wynn, R.L.: The Top 20 Prescribed Medications in 1991, *Gen. Dent., 40,* 374, September-October, 1992.

Assessment

Applegate, W.B., Blass, J.P., and Williams, T.F.: Instruments for the Functional Assessment of Older Patients, *N. Engl. J. Med., 322,* 1207, April 26, 1990.

Brangan, P.P.: Oral Changes in Older Adults, *Dentalhygienistnews,* 4, 4, Spring, 1991.

Campbell, P.R.: The Extra/Intraoral Exam and the Elderly Patient, *Dentalhygienistnews, 6,* 23, Spring, 1993.

Mohajery, M. and Brooks, S.L.: Oral Radiographs in the Detection of Early Signs of Osteoporosis, *Oral Surg. Oral Med. Oral Pathol., 73,* 112, January, 1992.

Shamburek, R.D. and Farrar, J.T.: Disorders of the Digestive System in the Elderly, *N. Engl. J. Med., 322,* 438, February 15, 1990.

Wolff, A., Ship, J.A., Tylenda, C.A., Fox, P.C., and Baum, B.J.: Oral Mucosal Appearance is Unchanged in Healthy, Different-aged Persons, *Oral Surg. Oral Med. Oral Pathol., 71,* 569, May, 1991.

Periodontics

Holm-Pedersen, P.: Periodontal Treatment and Prophylaxis in the Frail Elderly, *Int. Dent. J., 41,* 225, August, 1991.

Holm-Pedersen, P., Agerbaek, N., and Theilade, E.: Experimental Gingivitis in Young and Elderly Individuals, *J. Clin. Periodontol., 2,* 14, February, 1975.

Holm-Pedersen, P., Folke, L.E.A., and Gawronski, T.H.: Composition and Metabolic Activity of Dental Plaque from Healthy Young and Elderly Individuals, *J. Dent. Res., 59,* 771, May, 1980.

Matheny, J.L., Johnson, D.T., and Roth, G.I.: Aging and Microcirculatory Dynamics in Human Gingiva, *J. Clin. Periodontol., 20,* 471, August, 1993.

Papapanou, P.N. and Linde, J.: Preservation of Probing Attachment and Alveolar Bone Levels in 2 Random Population Samples, *J. Clin. Periodontol., 19,* 583, September, 1992.

Papapanou, P.N., Lindhe, J., Sterrett, J.D., and Eneroth, L.: Considerations on the Contribution of Aging to Loss of Periodontal Tissue Support, *J. Clin. Periodontol., 18,* 611, September, 1991.

Savitt, E.D. and Kent, R.L.: Distribution of *Actinobacillus actinomycetemcomitans* and *Porphyromonas gingivalis* by Subject Age, *J. Periodontol., 62,* 490, August, 1991.

Socransky, S.S. and Manganiello, S.D.: The Oral Microbiota of Man from Birth to Senility, *J. Periodontol., 42,* 485, August, 1971.

van der Velden, U.: Effect of Age on the Periodontium, *J. Clin. Periodontol., 11,* 281, May, 1984.

Diet and Nutrition

Ernest, S.L.: Dietary Intake, Food Preferences, Stimulated Salivary Flow Rate, and Masticatory Ability in Older Adults with Complete Dentitions, *Spec. Care Dentist., 13,* 102, May/June, 1993.

Ham, R.J.: Indicators of Poor Nutritional Status in Older Americans, *Am. Fam. Physician, 45,* 219, January, 1992.

Hardy, D.L. and Miller, J.R.: Nutritional Assessment of the Geriatric Patient. The Role of the Dental Hygienist, *Access, 7,* 34, March, 1993

Lightfoot, C.: Nutrition Concerns of and for Senior Canadians, *Can. Dent. Hyg./Probe, 26,* 124, Autumn, 1992.

The Edentulous Patient

The completely edentulous patient needs an appointment at least annually for careful observation of the oral tissues, as well as for supervision of bacterial plaque control for the dentures and care of the mucosa. Instruction for the patient who receives new dentures is also a concern, because preventive procedures are necessary for the patient's general and oral health. Terminology related to the edentulous patient and dentures is defined in table 47–1.

Of the completely edentulous population, particularly in the older age groups, some individuals have dentures they do not wear, others have full dentures but wear only one of them, and still others have no dentures. When there is a single denture, more frequently the maxillary denture is worn. It is not unusual to find that the same dentures have been worn for many years without having the dentures or the supporting oral tissues examined.

Dentures occasionally must be constructed to replace primary teeth. The teeth may be congenitally missing (anodontia) or may have required extraction because of rampant caries or trauma. Nursing caries, which can result in severe breakdown of the teeth soon after eruption, was described on page 234.

To provide esthetics and function, dentures can be constructed for the accepting child who is able to cooperate. As the permanent teeth begin to erupt, parts of the denture are cut away (figure 47–1). A supervised caries prevention program is initiated for protection of the permanent dentition.

THE EDENTULOUS MOUTH

I. BONE
A. Residual Ridges
After the teeth are removed, the residual ridges enter into a continuing process of remodelling. The alveolar bone, which had supported the teeth, undergoes resorption. The rate and amount of bony resorption vary with each individual. The major bony changes occur during the first year after the teeth are removed, but changes continue throughout life. Mandibular bone loss is generally as much as four times greater than maxillary bone loss.[1] Because of the oral changes, it is usually necessary to have dentures rebased or remade at intervals.

B. Tori
The tori that interfere with dentures are benign bony outgrowths. Because of the size, shape, or location, a torus often must be removed surgically before a denture can be constructed.
1. *Torus Palatinus.* Bony enlargement located over the midline of the palate.
2. *Torus Mandibularis.* Bony mass(es) generally located on the lingual side of the mandibular arch in the premolar area; may appear as a radiopaque area in the region of the premolars.

TABLE 47-1
KEY WORDS: EDENTULOUS PATIENT*

Anodontia (an'o-don'she-ah): congenital absence of all teeth, primary and permanent.

Complete denture prosthodontics: that body of knowledge and skills pertaining to the restoration of the edentulous arch with a removable prosthesis.

Denture: an artificial substitute for missing natural teeth and adjacent tissues.

  Complete denture: a removable dental prosthesis that replaces the entire dentition and associated structures of the maxilla or mandible.

Denture adhesive: a material used to adhere a denture to the oral mucosa; over-the-counter product that can be misused without professional instruction.

Denture characterization: modification of the form and color of the denture base and teeth to produce a more lifelike appearance.

Denture placement: the process of directing a prosthesis to a desired oral location; introduction of a prosthesis into a patient's mouth; other terms used are denture **delivery** or denture **insertion.**

Immediate denture: a complete denture fabricated for placement immediately following the removal of the natural teeth and/or other surgical preparation of the dental arches.

Implant prosthesis: any prosthesis that utilizes dental implants in part or whole for retention, support, and stability; the prosthesis may be a complete denture.

Overdenture: a removable denture that covers and is partially supported by one or more remaining natural teeth, roots, and/or dental implants and the soft tissue of the residual alveolar ridge; also called overlay denture.

* Definitions are taken from or adapted from and in harmony with the Glossary of Prosthodontic Terms, 6th ed., 1993, from the Academy of Prosthodontics Foundation.

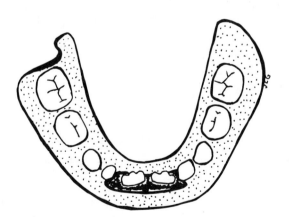

FIG. 47-1. Denture for a Young Child. As permanent teeth erupt, parts of the denture are cut away. Shown are denture alterations for the mandibular right first permanent molar and the mandibular incisors.

II. MUCOUS MEMBRANE

As described on pages 181 and 182, the oral mucosa is composed of masticatory, lining, and specialized mucosa. The edentulous ridges and the hard palate are covered with masticatory mucosa, which is continuous with the lining mucosa that covers the floor of the mouth, vestibules, and cheeks.

The mucous membrane covering the bony ridges is made up of two layers, the lamina propria and the surface stratified squamous epithelium, which is keratinized in the healthy mouth. Underneath the mucous membrane is the submucosa, which is attached to the underlying bone.

The submucosa is composed of connective tissue with vessels, nerves, adipose tissue, and glands. The support or cushioning effect for the denture depends on the makeup of the submucosa, which varies in different parts of the mouth.

When an edentulous mouth is examined clinically and the lips and cheeks are retracted using a tension test technique (page 217), a line of demarcation similar to the mucogingival junction is apparent, separating the attached tissue over the bony ridge and the loose lining mucosa of the vestibule. Frenal attachments can be observed readily.

III. THE PATIENT WITH NEW DENTURES
A. Patient Counseling

The preparation for denture insertion has to begin well in advance of the day the dentures are delivered. The patient needs a clear idea of what to expect and what procedures will be followed. Successful after-care and denture satisfaction depend to a large extent on conditioning the patient to the adjustments to be made and to the period of practice and learning with the new dentures that can be expected.

Many dental teams prepare their own printed educational materials, whereas others use those available from outside sources.

The preliminary counseling is followed through the initial postinsertion appointments, particularly to teach denture hygiene and to arrange for continuing maintenance appointments during the following years.

B. Postinsertion Care

1. *Immediate Denture.* The patient receiving an immediate denture is instructed to leave the denture in place for 24 to 48 hours to aid in the control of bleeding and swelling. When the patient returns and the denture is removed, the mouth is rinsed and appropriate instructions are given. After initial healing, the denture care and other instructions are similar to those presented in table 47-2.

2. *New Dentures over Healed Ridges*
   a. Appointments. Following insertion, adjustment appointments are scheduled

TABLE 47–2
PATIENT INSTRUCTION FOR COMPLETE DENTURES

Item	Factors to Teach

Food Selection	Use foods from the Food Guide Pyramid (page 424)
	Check each day's diet to fulfill needs for a balanced diet
	Older patients: use foods to prevent diet-induced chronic diseases (pages 643 and 644)
	New denture wearer:
	   Avoid foods that need incising
	   Avoid raw vegetables, fibrous meats, and sticky foods until experience has been gained
	   Cut food into small pieces
	Practiced denture wearer:
	   Select a variety of foods, but do not expect the same efficiency as with the natural teeth

Incision or Biting	Use the canine and premolar area. Insert for biting at the angle of the mouth. Push back as the food is incised; do not pull or tear the food in a forward direction
Chewing	Take small portions Try to chew with some food on each side at the same time to stabilize the denture Be patient and practice
Salivary Flow	Anticipate an increased flow of saliva when a new denture is worn
Speaking	Speak slowly and quietly Practice by reading aloud at home, preferably in front of a mirror Repeat and practice words that seem the most difficult
Sneezing, Coughing, Yawning	Anticipate loss of denture retention Cover mouth with hand and handkerchief
Denture Hygiene	Thoroughly clean dentures twice each day Immerse dentures in chemical solution and brush for plaque removal. Rinse thoroughly Complete denture care is described on pages 385–388 Devices to aid a disabled person are shown on page 696
Mucosa	Tissues need to rest each day. Preferable to leave the dentures out while sleeping Brush and massage the mucosa to clean away plaque and debris and stimulate circulation
Storage of Dentures	After careful cleaning to remove all bacterial plaque, store the dentures in water (or cleaning solution) in a covered container Place in a safe place inaccessible to children or house pets Change water or cleaning solution daily and wash the container
Over-the-counter products	Never attempt to alter the denture for relief of discomfort Do not buy and use self-reline materials, adhesives, or other additives without consulting the dentist. They may be harmful to the dentures and/or the oral tissues. Consult the dentist for advice about all denture problems
Maintenance	Understand the importance of the dentist's examination of the denture fit, occlusion, and wear, and the condition of the oral mucosa First year: expect reline, rebase, or remake of dentures because bone remodeling is greatest during the first year. Subsequent appointment: an examination each year for most patients, provided the denture hygiene is ideal. Other patients in the cancer-susceptible category need an examination every 3 months

routinely because adjustments can be expected. The first appointment is made within 48 hours of the time of insertion, and additional appointments are made in accord with individual needs.

b. Instructions.[2] Too many instructions given on the day of insertion may only confuse the patient. Basic denture care and other procedures of immediate concern can be reviewed. Slow repetition over several periods helps the patient to develop adequate denture management and hygiene habits.

Basic information for the new denture

wearer is provided in table 47–2. Denture cleaning methods are described with other plaque control procedures for the care of dental prostheses on pages 385–388.

DENTURE-RELATED ORAL CHANGES

The condition of the mucous membranes, salivary glands, and alveolar bone is influenced by dietary and nutritional deficiencies, age, and various chronic diseases. Tissue alterations for an older patient were described on page 637. Some of the denture-related changes are listed here.

I. BONE CHANGES
A. Alveolar Ridge Remodeling[3]
The continuing reduction in the size of the residual ridge may lead to loss of denture support, loss of facial height and lip support, increased prominence of the chin, possible temporomandibular joint manifestations, and occlusal disharmony.

B. Compensations by the Patient
1. Patients may adapt to the bone changes by making compensating adjustments in the way they wear and manage the dentures.
2. Other patients may resort to drugstore remedies, such as pads, adhesives, or self-reline materials, which may be detrimental and cause further oral damage.[4]

C. Treatment by the Dentist
Dentures need relining, rebasing, or remaking periodically.

II. ORAL MUCOSA
The tissue reaction under a denture varies considerably among individuals. Whereas one mouth may have thinning of the mucosa, submucosa, and particularly, the epithelium with an absence of keratinization, another may have normal keratinization or hyperkeratinization.

Factors that influence the mucosa include systemic conditions that alter host response, aging, denture and tissue hygiene, wearing the denture constantly, xerostomia, and fit and occlusion of the denture itself.

III. XEROSTOMIA
The causes of xerostomia were described on page 204. Diminished salivary flow can influence denture retention and tissue lubrication, as well as reduce the resistance of the oral mucosa to trauma and infection.

A. Lubrication
The oral mucosa needs saliva for protection against frictional irritation by the denture.

B. Retention
The film of saliva between the denture and the mucosa contributes to retention of the denture.

IV. SENSORY CHANGES
A. Tactile Sense
With the dentures in place, sensitivity may be diminished to small objects in the mouth, such as small bones or bits of nut shells.

B. Taste
Occasionally, patients indicate that, since they have been wearing dentures, food has a different taste for them. Although the taste buds that are located in the tongue papillae are not affected by the dentures, the taste buds of the palate are covered by the maxillary denture and therefore are ineffective for taste perception. Denture hygiene must be meticulous to assure that the denture does not develop thick odoriferous plaque, which may alter food flavors.

DENTURE-INDUCED ORAL LESIONS

When the mouth is examined extraorally and intraorally, the dentures are removed and the mucosa is carefully and thoroughly examined. The patient may tell of an area that has been sensitive and thus helpfully call attention to a specific visible lesion. On the other hand, a patient may be unaware of chronic mucosal lesions, which are often asymptomatic. Because tissue changes may be important indicators of serious disease, such as oral cancer, the intraoral examination must be conducted thoroughly with good illumination.

I. PRINCIPAL CAUSES OF LESIONS UNDER DENTURES
The factors that singly or in combination cause most oral lesions under dentures are infection, trauma, ill-fit of the dentures, inadequate oral hygiene, and wearing the dentures all the time, without relief for the tissues.

A. Ill-fitting Dentures
Because tissue changes under dentures occur gradually over a long period, the patient may not be aware of developing disease. The patient may not realize or may not have been informed of the importance of having regular professional examinations of the dentures and the oral mucosa.

B. Lack of Oral Hygiene
The dentures and the oral mucosa need daily care. Neglected dentures can accumulate heavy plaque and calculus that may irritate the mucosa and cause infection.

C. Continuous Wearing of Dentures
Dentures need to be removed for a part of every 24 hours so that the mucosa can have a rest from the pressure of the hard acrylic during occlusion, bruxism, and clenching. The rest period also allows the tissue to recover in its natural

environment, where the tongue and saliva provide a cleansing effect.

II. INFLAMMATORY LESIONS
A. Localized Inflammation (Sore Spots)
1. *Appearance.* Isolated red inflamed area, sometimes ulcerated.
2. *Contributing Factors.* Trauma from an ill-fitting denture, rough spot on a denture surface, tongue bite.

B. Generalized Inflammation
1. *Other Names.* "Denture sore mouth," "denture stomatitis."
2. *Appearance.* Generalized redness over the tissues that support the denture. The patient may have pain and a burning sensation. This occurs more frequently in the maxilla.
3. *Contributing Factors*
   The following may occur singly or in combinations.
   a. Denture trauma from the fit, occlusion, or parafunctional habits.
   b. Inadequate denture hygiene and care of the mucosa.
   c. Chemotoxic effect from residual cleansing paste or solution not thoroughly rinsed from the denture.
   d. Allergy to the denture base (rare).
   e. Continuous denture wearing without relief for the tissues.
   f. Patient self-treatment with over-the-counter products for relining.
   g. Systemic influence on the tolerance of the tissues to trauma and lowered resistance to infection; for example, vitamin and other nutritional deficiencies and immunosuppressant therapy, such as chemotherapy.
   h. *Candida albicans* infection.[5] *C. albicans* is a customary member of the oral flora of people with or without teeth. In denture stomatitis, or in recognizable candidiasis or moniliasis, the numbers of the yeast-like fungus increase. Conditions that promote *C. albicans* overgrowth are depression of defense mechanisms by immunosuppressants, radiation therapy, or prolonged antibiotic therapy.

III. ULCERATIVE LESIONS
Localized ulcer-shaped lesions usually are related to an overextended denture border. The ulcer may resemble a cancerous lesion and should be biopsied if it persists longer than expected of a healing traumatic ulcer.

IV. PAPILLARY HYPERPLASIA
A. Appearance
Papillary hyperplasia is located on the palatal vault, rarely outside the confines of the bony

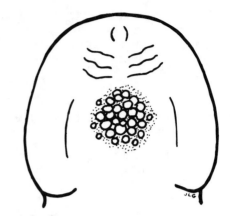

FIG. 47–2. Papillary Hyperplasia. Outline of an edentulous palate shows the characteristic location of papillary hyperplasia within the bony ridges.

ridges (figure 47–2). The overall lesion appears as a group of closely arranged, pebble-shaped, red, edematous projections.

B. Contributing Factors
The cause is unknown but it is associated with poor denture hygiene, ill-fitting dentures, and possible *Candida albicans* infection.

V. DENTURE IRRITATION HYPERPLASIA (EPULIS FISSURATUM)
Long-standing, chronic inflammatory tissue appears in single or multiple elongated folds related to the border of an ill-fitting denture.

VI. ANGULAR CHEILITIS[6]
A. Appearance
Angular cheilitis appears as fissuring at the angles of the mouth, with cracks, ulcerations, and erythema. Sometimes it is dry with a crust; other times, it is moist from saliva.

B. Contributing Factors
Angular cheilitis is usually initiated by lack of support of the commissure because of overclosure and by moistness from drooling. Secondarily, a riboflavin deficiency or an infection by *Candida albicans* or other organisms may be involved.

PREVENTION AND MAINTENANCE

I. DEVELOPMENT OF ATTITUDE AND UNDERSTANDING BY THE PATIENT
For continuing oral health and appropriate denture service, the patient needs to understand the following:
   A. Purposes of regular maintenance appointments for finding early signs of disease, particularly chronic irritations and oral cancer.

B. Reasons why the dentist must supervise the function and fit of the dentures.

C. Damage that can result from wearing ill-fitting dentures for long periods of time (years) without tissue and denture examination.

D. Harmful effects to the oral tissue and damage to the dentures that can result from the unsupervised use of commercial products for denture retention or relief, or of home repair kits.

II. DAILY PREVENTIVE MEASURES
A. Denture Hygiene

Dentures must be cleaned after each meal. Details were explained on pages 385–387. Cleansing solutions must be changed daily.

B. Oral Mucosa

1. Brush to clean and massage.
2. Digital massage (page 389).

C. Rest for the Tissues

For most patients, having the dentures out while sleeping is the best procedure to provide rest for the oral tissues. When this is impossible, the patient should remove the denture for as long a daytime period as possible, such as while bathing. While the dentures are out of the mouth, they can be placed in a container with cleaning solution, and the mucosa can be cleaned and massaged.

D. Diet and Nutrition

The teaching of food selection cannot be overemphasized. For denture wearers, an emphasis on using foods from the basic food groups as shown in the pyramid (figure 28–1, page 424) is necessary. Control of weight and avoidance of foods that are related to specific chronic conditions are important. A dietary analysis can provide a foundation for making specific recommendations.

The diet problems of the elderly patient have been described on pages 643 and 644. Factors that contribute to dietary deficiencies in patients of any age are magnified when dentures are ill-fitting and masticatory efficiency is decreased. The patient tends to overlook food value and to select foods that are within the limits of chewing ability or that can be swallowed without chewing.

E. Relief from Xerostomia

The use of saliva substitute may be recommended (page 204).

F. Dental Caries Control for Overdenture Wearers

Meticulous denture hygiene and bacterial plaque control for the natural teeth is mandatory. Care of the overdenture is described on page 390.

Sodium fluoride dentifrice is used while brushing the teeth. Daily fluoride application is made by placing gel drops inside the overdenture (page 390).

III. PROFESSIONAL SUPERVISION
A. Appointment Frequency

1. *First Year.* After the initial adjustments, the patient can expect the dentures to need reline, rebase, or remake in 6 months to 1 year.
2. *Subsequent Maintenance Period*
   a. For most patients, one appointment each year may be adequate.
   b. For patients who are careless with denture and tissue care, at least two appointments each year are recommended.
   c. For patients who are at high cancer risk because of age, tobacco use, and alcohol-drinking habits or have a previous history of cancer, examination three to four times per year should be scheduled.

B. Maintenance Appointment

Maintenance procedures as described on pages 599 and 600 are followed with necessary adaptations for the edentulous patient.

1. *Procedures*
   a. Review patient history; make necessary additions to the record.
   b. Determine blood pressure.
   c. Perform an extraoral and intraoral examination.
   d. Examine dentures for cleanliness and evidences of patient care
      i. Ask patient to describe the personal hygiene care procedures used routinely.
      ii. Supplement with additional demonstration and instruction when the care is less than adequate.
   e. Clean the dentures to remove calculus and stain. Procedures are described on pages 571 and 572.
2. *Procedures for the Dentist*
   a. Review the complete assessment.
   b. Examine the oral tissues and the fit and occlusion of the dentures.
   c. Treat as needed.
3. *Subsequent Appointment*
   Make necessary appointments for continuing current treatment or for maintenance.

DENTURE MARKING FOR IDENTIFICATION[7]

The need for denture marking is apparent in a variety of situations. A universal system for marking would be ideal. Marking is required by law in some countries and in most states of the United States. In forensic dentistry, or for identification of victims of war, such disasters as flood or fire, or transportation catastrophe, the dentition has been used increasingly as a means of identification.

Dentures provide a method for immediate identification. Prompt identification can be urgent when an individual is found unconscious from illness or injury or suffering from amnesia as a result of psychiatric or traumatic causes, as well as from senility.

The dentures of people in long-term residence or care facilities should be marked. Mislaid dentures can be returned and mix-ups by the direct care staff can be prevented. An important contribution to an oral health program is to introduce a plan for denture marking.

I. CRITERIA FOR AN ADEQUATE MARKING SYSTEM

Information on the denture must be specific so that rapid identification is possible.

A. Relative to the Denture

1. Must have no adverse effects on denture material.
2. Must not change the strength, surface texture, or fit of the denture.
3. Must be cosmetically acceptable; the label must be placed in an inobtrusive position.

B. Relative to the Procedure

1. Readily learned and simple to carry out.
2. Inexpensive.
3. Durable result. When the information is incorporated during denture processing, indefinite durability can be expected. A surface marker for a denture already in use should be able to withstand denture cleaning methods for a reasonable period of time.

C. Characteristics of the Material Used

1. *Fire and Humidity Resistant.* When the label is placed inside the posterior section of a denture, the surrounding tongue and maxillofacial parts offer protection except in the most severe conflagration.
2. *Radiopaque.* A metal marker can be of use as a means of identification by radiographic examination in the event the radiolucent acrylic denture is accidentally swallowed.

II. INCLUSION METHODS FOR MARKING
A. New Dentures

A typewritten or printed enclosure is inserted as a denture is being processed. Labels are positioned on the impression surfaces of the maxillary and mandibular dentures (figure 47-3). They are covered, just before the final closure of the flask, with a clear acrylic material.

A label may be typewritten on onionskin paper or the tissue paper that separates sheets of packaged baseplate wax.[7,8] Another system uses a thin metal strip for the insert. Stainless steel matrix bands, orthodontic bands, and thin metal strips (shim stock) have been used.[9]

B. Existing Dentures[10]

1. Clean the dentures thoroughly.
2. Use a No. 6 or 8 round bur and an inverted cone to cut small, shallow, box-like preparations in the posterior buccal flange of the maxillary denture and the lingual posterior flange of the mandibular denture (figure 47-4). Do not go through to the impression surface.
3. Typewrite two copies of the patient's initials (or other choice of identification) on onionskin paper, and trim the papers to fit the box-like preparations.

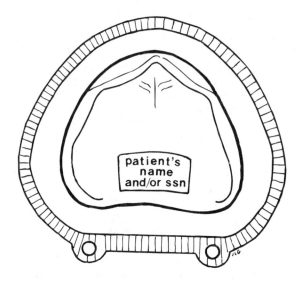

FIG. 47-3. Inclusion Marker for New Denture. The label is inserted on the impression surface as the denture is being processed. On the flasked maxillary denture shown, the marker is positioned near the posterior border.

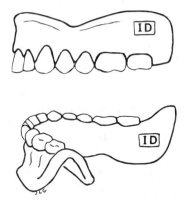

FIG. 47-4. Surface Markers for Dentures. The labels are placed on the external denture surfaces for existing dentures. As shown, the markers are on the maxillary buccal flange and the mandibular lingual flange.

4. Cover the paper with cold-cure clear acrylic and fill to a slight excess; after the acrylic has cured, polish to a smooth finish.

III. SURFACE MARKERS

Surface markers are not as durable, but instruction can be provided for persons not trained in dental laboratory methods. In a skilled nursing facility or other long-term institution that has no resident dentist or dental hygienist, it may be important to teach a nurse or other staff member to mark dentures of residents as they are admitted. The methods described as follows have been used for this purpose.

A. Indelible Pen or Ballpoint

After cleaning and drying the denture, a small area near the posterior of the outer or polished denture surface is rubbed with an emery board until it is rough (figure 47–4). The name, initials, or other identification is printed on the roughened area with an indelible pen and dried. Two or three coats of a fingernail acrylic (heavy nail protector) are painted over the area; each layer is dried before applying the next. Surface markings have been found to last at least 6 months.[11] Light-cured materials may also be used.[12,13]

B. Engraving Tool

An engraving tool is used to enter the name on the denture, and the grooves created are darkened with a special pencil before a sealing liquid is applied. Materials are available in a commercial kit.[14]

IV. INFORMATION TO INCLUDE ON A MARKER

For residents of a home or institution, using only the person's name and initials should suffice for temporary surface marking.

In a community, country, or international situation, the name alone would not provide enough identification, and the social security number, armed services serial number, or the equivalent in other countries should be included.

Other identification, such as blood type and vital drug or disease condition, has been suggested. In certain countries, the dentist's registration or hospital number has been used. In Sweden, the patient's date of birth and national registration number have been marked on the dentures. The markings that can provide *immediate* identification are the most significant.

FACTORS TO TEACH THE PATIENT

I. Dentures are not permanent appliances.
II. Dentures and tissues must be examined at least once a year. Teach frequency of maintenance appointments for the individual, depending in part on that individual's ability to clean the dentures and maintain them free from plaque, stain, and calculus.
III. Dentures may need replacement periodically. Tissues under the denture change.
IV. Avoid use of drugstore remedies, reliners, and other home-applied materials unless the dentist has provided specific instruction.
V. Specific methods of care for dentures.
VI. Leaving the dentures out of the mouth overnight in accord with dentist's directions.
VII. Where to obtain and how to use a saliva substitute.

REFERENCES

1. **Tallgren,** A.: The Continuing Reduction of the Residual Alveolar Ridges in Complete Denture Wearers: A Mixed-longitudinal Study Covering 25 Years, *J. Prosthet. Dent., 27,* 120, February, 1972.
2. **Gallagher,** J.B.: Insertion and Postinsertion Care, in Clark, J.W., ed.: *Clinical Dentistry,* Volume 5, Revised Edition—1984. Philadelphia, J.B. Lippincott Co., Chapter 14, pp. 1–27.
3. **Atwood,** D.A.: Bone Loss of Edentulous Alveolar Ridges, *J. Periodontol., 50,* 11, Special Issue, 1979.
4. **Welker,** W.A.: Prosthodontic Treatment of Abused Oral Tissues, *J. Prosthet. Dent., 37,* 259, March, 1977.
5. **Iacopino,** A.M. and Wathen, W.F.: Oral Candidal Infection and Denture Stomatitis: A Comprehensive Review, *J. Am. Dent. Assoc., 123,* 46, January, 1992.
6. **Shafer,** W.G., Hine, M.K., and Levy, B.M.: *A Textbook of Oral Pathology,* 4th ed. Phialdelphia, W.B. Saunders Co., 1983, pp. 556–557.
7. **American Dental Association,** Council on Prosthetic Services and Dental Laboratory Relations: *Techniques for Denture Identification.* Chicago, American Dental Association, 1984, 12 pp.
8. **Dentsply International, Inc.:** *Method for Placing Permanent Record Data in Denture Base Without Affecting Tissue Adaptation,* Technical Bulletin, Dentsply International, Inc., York, PA 17404.
9. **Turner,** C.H., Fletcher, A.M., and Ritchie, G.M.: Denture Marking and Human Identification, *Br. Dent. J., 141,* 114, August 17, 1976.
10. **Bauer,** T.L.: Technique for Denture Identification, *J. Indiana Dent. Assoc., 58,* 28, No. 6, 1979.
11. **Deb,** A.K. and Heath, M.R.: Marking Dentures in Geriatric Institutions. The Relevance and Appropriate Methods, *Br. Dent. J., 146,* 282, May 1, 1979.
12. **Richards,** E.E., Williams, J.E., and Gauthier, G.: A Modified Light-cured Denture Identification Technique, *Spec. Care Dentist., 12,* 81, March/April, 1992.
13. **Lamb,** D.J.: A Simple Method for Permanent Identification of Dentures, *J. Prosthet. Dent., 67,* 894, June, 1992.
14. **Identure,** Geri, Inc., P.O. Box 9086, North St. Paul, MN 55109.

SUGGESTED READINGS

Burt, B.A. and Eklund, S.A.: *Dentistry, Dental Practice, and the Community,* 4th ed. Philadelphia, W.B. Saunders Co., 1992, pp. 83–89.
Catelli, W.F., Engstrom, H.I.M., Hollender, L.G., and Feller, R.P.: Panoramic Radiographic Examination of Patients Who Are Edentulous, *Spec. Care Dentist., 7,* 114, May-June, 1987.

Granström, G.: Upper Airway Obstruction Caused by a Do-it-yourself Denture Reliner, *J. Prosthet. Dent., 63,* 495, May, 1990.

Hardy, D.L.: Dental Hygiene Care of the Denture Patient, *Dentalhygienistnews, 5,* 22, Fall, 1992.

Keur, J.J., Campbell, J.P.S., McCarthy, J.F., and Ralph, W.J.: Radiological Findings in 1135 Edentulous Patients, *J. Oral Rehabil., 14,* 183, March, 1987.

Marsh, P.D., Percival, R.S., and Challacombe, S.J.: The Influence of Denture-wearing and Age on the Oral Microflora, *J. Dent. Res., 71,* 1374, July, 1992.

Niedermeier, W.H.W. and Krämer, R.: Salivary Secretion and Denture Retention, *J. Prosthet. Dent., 67,* 211, February, 1992.

Smedley, T.C., Friedrichsen, S.W., and Cho, M.H.: A Comparison of Self-assessed Satisfaction Among Wearers of Dentures, Hearing Aids, and Eyeglasses, *J. Prosthet. Dent., 62,* 654, December, 1989.

Witt, S. and Hart, P.: Cross-infection Hazards Associated with the Use of Pumice in Dental Laboratories, *J. Dent., 18,* 281, October, 1990.

Denture Pathology

Allen, C.M.: Diagnosing and Managing Oral Candidiasis, *J. Am. Dent. Assoc., 123,* 77, January, 1992.

Arendorf, T.M. and Walker, D.M.: Denture Stomatitis: A Review, *J. Oral Rehabil., 14,* 217, May, 1987.

Cook, R.J.: Response of the Oral Mucosa to Denture Wearing, *J. Dent., 19,* 135, June, 1991.

Jennings, K.J. and MacDonald, D.G.: Histological, Microbiological, and Haematological Investigations in Denture-induced Stomatitis, *J. Dent., 18,* 102, April, 1990.

Könönen, E., Asikainen, S., Alaluusua, S., Könönen, M., Summanen, P., Kanervo, A., and Jousimies-Somer, H.: Are Certain Oral Pathogens Part of Normal Oral Flora in Denture-wearing Edentulous Subjects?, *Oral Microbiol. Immunol., 6,* 119, April, 1991.

Lai, K., Santarpia, R.P., Pollock, J.J., and Renner, R.P.: Assessment of Antimicrobial Treatment of Denture Stomatitis Using an *In Vivo* Replica Model System: Therapeutic Efficacy of an Oral Rinse, *J. Prosthet. Dent., 67,* 72, January, 1992.

Moskona, D. and Kaplan, I.: Oral Lesions in Elderly Denture Wearers, *Clin. Prev. Dent., 14,* 11, September/October, 1992.

Phelan, J.A. and Levin, S.M.: A Prevalence Study of Denture Stomatitis in Subjects with Diabetes Mellitus or Elevated Plasma Glucose Levels, *Oral Surg. Oral Med. Oral Pathol., 62,* 303, September, 1986.

Radford, D.R. and Radford, J.R.: A SEM Study of Denture Plaque and Oral Mucosa of Denture-related Stomatitis, *J. Dent., 21,* 87, April, 1993.

Denture Sanitation

DePaola, L.G. and Minah, G.E.: Isolation of Pathogenic Microorganisms from Dentures and Denture-soaking Containers of Myelosuppressed Cancer Patients, *J. Prosthet. Dent., 49,* 20, January, 1983.

Mäkilä, E. and Taulio-Korvenmaa, A.: Denture and Oral Brush for Elderly People, *Proc. Finn. Dent. Soc., 84,* 197, No. 3, 1988.

Moore, T.C., Smith, D.E., and Kenny, G.E.: Sanitization of Dentures by Several Denture Hygiene Methods, *J. Prosthet. Dent., 52,* 158, August, 1984.

Stafford, G.D., Arendorf, T., and Huggett, R.: The Effect of Overnight Drying and Water Immersion on Candidal Colonization and Properties of Complete Dentures, *J. Dent., 14,* 52, April, 1986.

Denture Identification

Cunningham, M. and Hoad-Reddick, G.: Attitudes to Identification of Dentures: The Patients' Perspective, *Quintessence Int., 24,* 267, April, 1993.

Fiske, J., Graham, T., and Gelbier, S.: Denture Identification for Elderly People, *Br. Dent. J., 161,* 448, December 20, 1986.

Goshima, T., Gettleman, L., Goshima, Y., and Yamamoto, A.: Evaluation of Radiopaque Denture Liner, *Oral Surg. Oral Med. Oral Pathol., 74,* 379, September, 1992.

Harrison, A.: A Simple Denture Marking System, *Br. Dent. J., 160,* 89, February 8, 1986.

Oliver, B.: A New Inclusion Denture Marking System, *Quintessence Int., 20,* 21, January, 1989.

The Oral and Maxillofacial Surgery Patient

Oral and maxillofacial surgery is the specialty of dentistry that includes the diagnostic, surgical, and adjunctive treatment of diseases, injuries, and defects involving both the functional and the esthetic aspects of the hard and soft tissues of the oral and maxillofacial regions.[1] Table 48–1 lists types of treatment included in this specialty with examples.

The practice of an oral surgeon may be primarily in a group clinical setting, in a hospital, or in a private office with outpatient hospital facilities available. With the oral surgeon is a team of specially trained individuals that might include surgical assistants, anesthetists, registered nurses, and dental hygienists.

The surgeon is involved with various dental practitioners, including general dentists and specialists. Maxillofacial surgery can be programmed, for example, with prosthodontists, orthodontists, implantologists, and specialists caring for any of the patients suggested by the list in table 48–1. Terminology that relates to maxillofacial surgery is defined in table 48–2.

Surgery for treatment of diseases and correction of defects of the periodontal tissues is categorized specifically as *periodontal surgery*. Within the scope of periodontal surgery are procedures for pocket elimination, gingivoplasty, treatment of furcation involvements, correction of mucogingival defects, and treatment for bony defects about the teeth. Preparation for periodontal surgery is not specifically described in this chapter.

PATIENT PREPARATION

I. OBJECTIVES

Dental hygiene care and instruction prior to oral and maxillofacial surgery may contribute to the patient's health and well-being by one or more of the following:

A. Reduce Oral Bacterial Count
1. Aid in the preparation of an aseptic field of operation.
2. Make postoperative infection less likely or less severe.

B. Reduce Inflammation of the Gingiva and Improve Tissue Tone
1. Lessen local bleeding at the time of the surgery.
2. Promote postoperative healing.

C. Remove Calculus Deposits
1. Remove a source of plaque retention and thus improve gingival tissue tone.
2. Prevent interference with placement of surgical instruments.
3. Prevent pieces of calculus from breaking away.
   a. Danger of inhalation, particularly when a general anesthetic is used.
   b. Possibility of calculus falling into a socket or other surgical area and acting as a foreign body to inhibit healing.

D. Instruct in Preoperative Personal Oral Care Procedures
Such instruction contributes to reducing inflammation and thus improves tissue tone and helps to prepare the patient for postoperative care.

E. Instruct in the Use of Foods
The patient should be instructed about foods that provide the elements essential to tissue building and repair during pre- and postoperative periods.

655

TABLE 48–1
CATEGORIES OF ORAL AND MAXILLOFACIAL TREATMENTS

Dentoalveolar Surgery
  Exodontics
  Impacted tooth removal
  Alveolar bone surgery: alveoloplasty
Infections
  Abscesses
  Osteomyelitis
Traumatic Injury
  Fractures of jaws, zygoma
  Fracture of teeth, alveolar bone
Neoplasms
  Cysts
  Tumors
Dental Implant Placement
Preprosthetic Reconstruction
  Maxillofacial prosthetics
Orthognathic Surgery
  Prognathism correction
  Facial esthetics
Cleft Lip/Palate
Temporomandibular Disorders (TMD)
Salivary Gland Obstruction

TABLE 48–2
KEY WORDS: ORAL AND MAXILLOFACIAL SURGERY

Exodontics (ek′sō-don′tiks): branch of dentistry dealing with the surgical removal of teeth.
Exostosis (ek′sos-tō′sis): benign new growth projecting from the surface of bone.
Intermaxillary fixation (in′ter-mak′sǐ-lār′ē): fixation of the maxilla in occlusion with the mandible held in place by means of wires and elastic bands; the healing parts are stabilized following fracture or surgery.
Maxillofacial; ;(mak-sǐl′-ō-fā′shal): pertaining to the jaws and the face.
Maxillofacial prosthetics: the branch of prosthodontics concerned with the restoration of the mouth and jaws and associated facial structures that have been affected by disease, injury, surgery, or a congenital defect.
Miniplate osteosynthesis: a method of internal fixation of mandibular fractures utilizing miniaturized metal plates and screws made of titanium or stainless steel.
Orthognathic surgery: surgery to alter relationships of the dental arches and/or supporting bone; usually coordinated with orthodontic therapy.
Orthognathics (or′thog-na′thiks): science dealing with the causes and treatment of malposition of the bones of the jaws.
Trismus (triz′mus): motor disturbance of the trigeminal nerve with spasm of masticatory muscles and difficulty in opening the mouth (lockjaw).

For the patient who will have teeth removed and complete or partial dentures inserted, the importance of a diet containing all essential food groups should be emphasized.

F. Interpret the Dentist's Directions

Explanation should be given for the immediate preoperative preparation with respect to rest and dietary limitations, particularly when a general anesthetic is to be administered.

G. Motivate the Patient Who Will Have Teeth Remaining

The patient who will have teeth remaining after surgery should be motivated to prevent further tooth loss through routine dental and dental hygiene professional care and personal oral care procedures.

II. PERSONAL FACTORS

The extent of the surgery to be performed and previous experiences affect the patient's attitude. Many patients who are in the greatest need of preoperative dental hygiene care and instruction may be people who have neglected their mouths for many years. They have been indifferent to or unaware of the importance of obtaining adequate care. Their only visits to a dentist may have been to have a toothache relieved by extraction. Their knowledge of preventive measures may be limited. A few of the characteristics are suggested here.

A. Apprehensive and Fearful

1. Apprehensive and indifferent toward need for personal care of teeth that are to be removed.
2. Fearful of all dental procedures, particularly oral surgery and anesthesia.
3. Fearful of cancer or other disease.
4. Fearful of personal appearance after surgery.

B. Impatient

When teeth have caused discomfort and pain, the patient may have difficulty understanding the need for delay while oral hygiene procedures are accomplished.

C. Ashamed

Of appearance or of having neglected the teeth.

D. Resigned

Feeling of inevitableness of the situation; lack of appreciation for natural teeth.

E. Discouraged

Over tooth loss or development of soft tissue lesions.

F. Resentful

1. Toward time lost from work.
2. Toward the financial aspects of dental care.
3. Toward inconvenience and discomfort.

DENTAL HYGIENE CARE

A review of the patient's record shows preliminary procedures that need to be completed. For example, a thorough intraoral and extraoral examination, a recording of vital signs, photographs, and additional radiographs may be required. The patient's medical and dental history reveals essential information relative to the need for prophylactic antibiotics or other precautions.

I. PRESURGERY TREATMENT PLANNING

The pending date for the operation and the patient's attitude may limit the time to be spent.

A. First Appointment

1. Develop rapport; explain purposes of presurgical appointments.
2. Explain and demonstrate bacterial plaque control principles.
3. Present dietary record form for completion before the next appointment (page 426).
4. Perform scaling to prepare for tissue healing.
5. Give postappointment instruction for rinsing with basic saline or with chlorhexidine 0.12% for tissue conditioning.

B. Second Appointment

1. Observe gingival tissue response; apply disclosing agent. Review disease control procedures. Introduce the use of dental floss or other interdental aids when applicable.
2. Receive the dietary record and review it with the patient (pages 427–429). Present diet recommendations.
3. Complete or continue the scaling. More than two appointments may be needed for patients who will have surgery for oral cancer or who have a cardiovascular or other condition for which all periodontal and dental treatment must be completed. When radiation or chemotherapy will be used following surgery for oral cancer, or when a prosthetic heart valve or total joint replacement will be involved, complete oral care is necessary as described on pages 670 and 671.

II. PATIENT INSTRUCTION
A. Bacterial Plaque Control

1. *Brush.* Soft.
2. *Technique.* For a patient who may not have practiced careful brushing on a regular plan, a simple brushing technique is preferred. Time for establishing habits may be limited until postoperative healing is complete. Use of disclosing agent for the patient's own evaluation is important.

B. Auxiliary Procedures

Interdental plaque removal and care of fixed and removable prostheses are included in instruction (Chapters 23 and 24). The patient who is to have multiple extractions for the placement of an immediate denture or other prosthesis, such as an obturator following cleft palate, tumor, or other surgery, needs postoperative instruction for the specific care of the prosthesis.

III. INSTRUMENTATION

Scaling procedures are of primary importance. Stain removal procedures may be contraindicated because of the condition of the gingival tissues.

A. Scaling

1. *Problems*
   a. Teeth with large carious lesions.
   b. Mobile teeth.
   c. Edentulous areas.
   d. Sensitive, enlarged gingival tissue that bleeds readily.
2. *Suggestions for Procedure*
   a. Use topical or local anesthetic.
   b. Maintain a clear field, using evacuation techniques.
   c. Use alternate finger rests to adapt to mobile teeth or edentulous areas: stabilize mobile teeth during scaling strokes.
   d. Ultrasonic scaling may be the technique of choice; high power evacuation is essential. When used, an antimicrobial mouthrinse is used first to lessen the bacterial count of the aerosols produced.

B. Stain Removal

1. *Contraindications*
   a. Enlarged, inflamed, sensitive gingiva.
   b. Deep pockets.
   c. Profuse hemorrhage.
2. *Effects*
   a. Irritation to tissue by polishing abrasive and action of rubber polishing cup.
   b. Abrasive particles forced into the gingival tissues by movement of rubber cup.

C. Rinsing Instruction

1. *Objectives.* To promote tissue healing following scaling and to remove debris; to initiate the habit of rinsing for postoperative care later.
2. *Rinsing Solution.* Warm, mild, hypertonic salt solution (pages 526 and 527).
3. *Frequency.* Recommended for several times each day after the surgical procedure as instruction by oral surgeon.

D. Follow-up Evaluation

Scaling and planing should be planned for a few weeks after oral surgery. Such an appointment should not be scheduled until healing has progressed favorably.

IV. PATIENT INSTRUCTION: DIET SELECTION[2]

The nutritional state can influence the resistance to infection and wound healing, as well as general recovery powers. Nutritional deficiencies can occur because of the inability to ingest adequate nutrients orally.

Specific recommendations of what to include and not to include in the diet should be given to the patient. Postoperative suggestions may differ from preoperative; for example, when difficulty in chewing is a postoperative problem, a liquid or soft diet may be required. When major oral surgery requires hospitalization, tube feeding may be necessary during the initial healing period. Tube feeding is described on page 665.

A. Nutritional and Dietary Needs

Diets outlined are designed to include the essential foods from the Food Guide Pyramid (figure 28–1, page 424).

1. *Essential for Promotion of Healing.* Protein and vitamins, particularly vitamin A, vitamin C, and riboflavin.
2. *Essential for Building Gingival Tissue Resistance.* A varied diet that includes adequate portions of all essential food groups.
3. *Essential for Providing Gingival Stimulation.* Firm, fibrous foods that require mastication, especially fresh fruits and vegetables. Possibilities for making recommendations in this area are limited by the patient's masticatory deficiencies.
4. *Essential for Dental Caries Prevention.* Foods without fermentable carbohydrate. When a patient has not been able to masticate properly, the diet employed frequently may have included many soft and cariogenic foods.

B. Suggestions for Instruction

1. Provide instruction sheets that show specific pre- and postsurgery meal plans. Foods for liquid and soft diets are listed on pages 665 and 666.
2. Express nutritional needs in terms of quantity or servings of foods so that the patient clearly understands.
3. For the patient who will receive dentures, careful instruction must be provided over a period of time. At the preoperative appointment, only an introduction can be given, particularly because the patient is probably more concerned about the operation than about the aftereffects.

   When the patient loses the teeth because of dental caries, the diet has likely been high in fermentable carbohydrates. Emphasis should be placed on helping the patient include nutritious foods for the general health of the body and, more specifically, the health

of the alveolar processes, which will support the dentures.

V. PREOPERATIVE INSTRUCTIONS[3,4]

At the appointment just prior to the oral surgery appointment, instructions relative to the surgical procedure should be discussed with the patient. The objective is to let the patient know what to expect so that full cooperation is possible. The patient may have concerns about the anesthesia, the surgical procedure, and the outcome.

A. Explain the general procedures for anesthesia and surgery.
B. Provide printed preoperative instructions. Information in the printed instructions should include the following:

1. *Food and Liquid Intake.* Specify the number of hours before the time of the operation when the patient should stop further intake of food and fluids.
2. *Alcohol and Medications Restrictions.* Certain proprietary self-medications are not compatible with the anesthetic and drugs to be used during and following the surgical procedure. The patient should be instructed to discontinue use.
3. *Transport to and from the Appointment.* When a general anesthetic or light sedation is used, the patient should not drive. Plans for someone to accompany and assist the patient should be made.
4. *The Night Before the Appointment.* In addition to food and alcohol restrictions, a good night's rest is advocated.
5. *Personal Items*
   a. Clothing. The clothing worn should be loose and comfortable. The sleeves should be easily drawn up over the elbows.
   b. Care of contact lenses and prostheses. The patient will be asked to remove contact lenses and prostheses, and should bring containers for their safe keeping.

VI. POSTOPERATIVE CARE
A. Immediate Instructions

Printed postoperative instructions are provided following all oral operations. The prepared material is reviewed with the patient after surgery. Specific details vary, but basic information for postoperative instruction sheets includes the following:

1. *Control Bleeding.* Keep the sponge in the mouth over the surgical area for ½ hour; then discard it. When bleeding persists at home, place a gauze pad or cold wet teabag over the area and bite firmly for 30 minutes.
2. *Rinsing.* Do not rinse for 24 hours after the surgical appointment. Then use warm salt water (½ teaspoonful salt in ½ cup [4 ounces]

3. Disfigurement, changes in appearance, and pain.
4. Extended hospitalization.
5. Financial stress.

B. During and Following Therapy

1. Preoccupation with details of examinations, treatments, symptoms, or medications.
2. Depression and grief, which may lead to withdrawal and isolation.
3. Major concerns include obvious facial deformity, speech difficulty, swallowing difficulty, drooling, and odors from debris collection and tissue changes.

II. SUGGESTIONS FOR APPROACH TO PATIENT

A. Provide explanations before and after therapy to prevent misconceptions and apprehensions and to attempt to allay fears.
B. Provide paper and pencil for patient with a speech difficulty to write questions and requests.
C. Show acceptance. Acknowledge the appropriateness of the patient's concerns.
D. Express empathy, but avoid oversolicitousness.
E. Help to direct thoughts and efforts toward restoration of functional activity.
F. Instill trust and security by demonstrating genuine interest.
G. Assist the patient who was alcoholic, used tobacco products excessively, or had other habits that have to be eliminated. The patient may need the help of psychiatry, Alcoholics Anonymous, or other type of support organization.

DENTAL HYGIENE CARE[14,15]

In the not too distant past, the patient with oral cancer was doomed to complete tooth removal or at least removal of all teeth in the line of radiation. When the teeth were left in the mouth, severe radiation caries inevitably developed. A high percentage of patients had osteoradionecrosis. Now, many teeth are saved, restored, and preserved by an intensive daily preventive program of bacterial plaque control and self-applied fluoride by gel trays or brush-on.

The dental hygienist's contribution to the preparation of the patient for cancer therapy and the continued supervision of oral health and preventive techniques during treatment and regularly thereafter has special significance. Bacterial plaque control, irrigation, rinsing, fluoride application, dietary factors for general health and dental caries prevention, along with specific instrumentation for the health of the periodontal tissues, are major areas of attention.

I. PATIENT INSTRUCTION
A. Bacterial Plaque Control

A complete instruction series (pages 414–417) should be started before cancer treatment, with careful supervision. The patient must understand the reasons for intensive oral health care. Scaling and root planing can be accomplished within the same series of appointments. Time is usually an important factor when a malignant tumor is involved.

1. *Toothbrushing.* Sulcular brushing with a soft nylon brush is recommended for the following reasons:
   a. "Radiation caries" occurs primarily at the cervical third, about the necks of the teeth. Emphasis must be placed on keeping the cervical areas plaque-free.
   b. Control of gingival health with prevention of gingivitis is necessary. Fewer side effects develop from chemotherapy when optimum oral health is maintained.[16]
   c. Sensitivity of teeth is associated most frequently with the cervical third. Brushing with a desensitizing dentifrice with fluoride can help alleviate sensitivity and prevent dental caries (pages 452 and 557).
2. *Tongue Brushing.* Bacteria and debris collect on a dry tongue.
3. *Dental Floss.* Proximal surface plaque must be removed. Other interdental devices may be helpful.

B. Nutrition and Diet

Every possible attempt to improve the general health must be made. If the patient is malnourished and debilitated, a high protein diet is needed. Reduction of cariogenic foods is essential to the dental caries prevention program.

A hospitalized patient is under the supervision of a physician who gives diet prescription orders to the hospital dietitian. The private or clinic physician may make specific recommendations to the patient. Within the framework of the physician's orders, the dental hygienist may also help the patient and the person who prepares the patient's food at home. Instructions in the preparation of foods in a blender may be needed (page 665).

Because the mouth may be sore and tender, a topical anesthetic in the form of a troche may be needed before eating. During the treatment phase and immediately following radiation therapy, swallowing may be difficult, and because of xerostomia, liquids are needed with meals to moisten the food for swallowing. Because the patient suffers from a loss of appetite and difficulty in eating, weight loss is common. Diet selection can be very important so that proper nutrients are included within the limited diet.

C. Other Instruction

1. *Reduction of Sources of Irritation to the Mucosa.* The patient must not use alcohol or tobacco.
2. *Care of Dental Prostheses.* Frequently, prostheses are not worn during the period of cancer therapy. The use of a saliva substitute can provide relief, and allow the patient to wear dentures with comfort.

    Meticulous denture hygiene must be maintained when the dentures are worn. Instruction and frequent supervision of cleansing procedures can be very important to most patients.

II. INSTRUMENTATION

A. Mouth Preparation for Radiation and Surgery

Although complete periodontal treatment before treatment of oral cancer is ideal, time frequently contraindicates prolonged procedures. Minimum preparation, therefore, includes complete nonsurgical therapy with calculus removal and root planing. Excessive manipulation of tissues and instrumentation within the few days preceding oral surgery should be avoided.

Whenever possible, the following should be completed:

1. Scaling and root planing. These may be accomplished in conjunction with bacterial plaque control instruction in a series of quadrant treatments.
2. Removal of all rough and overhanging margins and finishing all restorations.

B. Continuing Treatment

Repeated scaling and root planing are needed at frequent maintenance appointments to supplement plaque control efforts by the patient.

III. FLUORIDE

A. Dentifrice

Use of a fluoride dentifrice is basic to fluoride therapy. The tissues may not tolerate a highly flavored dentifrice during the period when the mucosa is inflamed. A bland dentifrice with fluoride may be recommended.

B. Gel Tray Applications

The patient must receive daily fluoride applications while receiving radiation therapy. The incidence of postirradiation caries can be reduced by use of a custom tray with a fluoride gel or by brushing with the gel after regular brushing.[15]

1. *Application by Patient.* The patient can be trained to make the application. During radiation therapy, the patient may be preoccupied or too uncomfortable to have interest in carrying out the procedure because it may appear to have no immediate benefit.

    When it seems apparent that the patient

may neglect the fluoride, the topical daily application must be made, if possible, by a family member after instruction.

2. *Procedure.* Prepare custom trays before the radiation therapy starts, one for each dental arch. Fluoride gel is placed in the tray and fitted over the teeth for 5 minutes. The patient does not rinse after removal.
3. *Effect on Sensitivity of the Teeth.* Topical fluoride on a daily basis benefits the patient by lessening tooth sensitivity.

IV. SALIVA SUBSTITUTE

A patient undergoing radiation therapy for cancer of the head and neck may have a drop in saliva flow of as much as 60% during the first week and 95% by the sixth week.[17] Severe discomfort with drying, cracking, and bleeding of the mucosa, difficulty during mastication and swallowing, which can affect nutritional factors, food particles clinging to the teeth and gingiva with increased bacterial plaque, inability to wear prostheses, and increased susceptibility to dental caries are major effects from xerostomia.

The increase in dental caries following irradiation is caused by a lack of saliva and not by the direct radiation to the tooth. Information about xerostomia is in Chapter 12 on pages 204 and 205.

Instructions to the patient are simple, and no limitations are placed on the frequency of use. The only contraindication is if a patient is on a low-sodium diet. The patient is instructed to place a drop or two in the mouth and spread the gel around with the tongue.

V. MAINTENANCE

A. Preventive Self-Care

The importance of prevention and control throughout the patient's life cannot be overemphasized. All the steps for care of the gingiva and teeth should be continued daily.

B. Frequency of Appointments

Examination of the oral mucosa and supervision of gingival and dental health are carried out daily during therapy, weekly following the completion of therapy, and then monthly as indicated by the condition of the oral tissues.

The dental hygiene appointment includes at least the following:

1. Extraoral and intraoral soft tissue examination.
2. Gingival examination with probing measurements and evaluation of bleeding, tooth mobility, and other signs of periodontal infection.
3. Evaluation of bacterial plaque and plaque removal procedures. Review of techniques to motivate and encourage the patient.
4. Instrumentation. Scaling and planing as needed must be completed. Patients receiving immunosuppressive drugs need antibi-

otic premedication prior to instrumentation. Consultation with the patient's physician/oncologist is indicated.

5. Review of fluoride procedures with a check to be certain the patient has refilled the fluoride prescription.

TECHNICAL HINTS

I. PREPARATION OF HISTORY

Preparation of a medical and dental history for all patients should include questions relative to radiation therapy received. Radiation during childhood should be recorded as well as that during adulthood.

II. PATIENT REFERRAL

When a patient is referred to a specialist or specialty clinic, a check must be made to ascertain that the patient arrives for the appointment. Frightened patients may become confused or may postpone the visit if they do not realize the urgency of the condition.

III. SOURCE OF MATERIAL

American Cancer Society
1599 Clifton Road N.E.
Atlanta, GA 30329
Local cancer society addresses can be obtained from the Atlanta office or local telephone book.

FACTORS TO TEACH THE PATIENT

I. The importance of oral soft tissue screening and complete oral examination at regular frequent intervals.

II. Plaque control methods, gel-tray application, use of saliva substitute, and all other details of personal care.

III. Why use of alcohol and tobacco must be stopped.

IV. Instruction for family members in oral health care for the sick and helpless patient.

REFERENCES

1. **Cancer Statistics,** 1993, *CA.*, *43*, 9, January/February, 1993.
2. **Silverman,** S. and Shillitoe, E.J.: Etiology and Predisposing Factors, in Silverman, S., ed.: *Oral Cancer*, 3rd ed. Atlanta, GA, American Cancer Society, 1990, pp. 7–39.
3. **Silverman,** S., Gorsky, M., and Greenspan, D.: Tobacco Usage in Patients with Head and Neck Carcinomas: A Follow-up Study on Habit Changes and Second Primary Oral/Oropharyngeal Cancers, *J. Am. Dent. Assoc., 106*, 33, January, 1983.
4. **Galante,** M., Phillips, T.L., Silverberg, I.J., and Fu, K.: Treatment, in Silverman, S., ed.: *Oral Cancer*, 3rd ed. Atlanta, GA, American Cancer Society, 1990, pp. 65–80.
5. **Harrison,** L.B. and Fass, D.E.: Radiation Therapy for Oral Cavity Cancer, *Dent. Clin. North Am., 34*, 205, April, 1990.
6. **Fleming,** T.J.: Oral Tissue Changes of Radiation-oncology and Their Management, *Dent. Clin. North Am., 34*, 223, April, 1990.
7. **Jansma,** J.: *Oral Sequelae Resulting from Head and Neck Radiotherapy.* Groningen, Drukkerij van Denderen B.V., 1991, pp. 5–50, 117–136.
8. **Smeltzer,** S.C. and Bare, B.G.: *Brunner and Suddarth's Textbook of Medical-Surgical Nursing*, 7th ed. Philadelphia, J.B. Lippincott Co., 1992, pp. 353–358.
9. **Peterson,** D.E. and Sonis, S.T., eds.: *Oral Complications of Cancer Chemotherapy.* The Hague/Boston/London, Martinus Nijhoff Publishers, 1983, pp. 1–12.
10. **Toth,** B.B., Martin, J.W., and Fleming, T.J.: Oral Complications Associated with Cancer Therapy. An M.D. Anderson Cancer Center Experience, *J. Clin. Periodontol., 17*, 508, August, 1990 (Part II).
11. **Rosenberg,** S.W.: Oral Care of Chemotherapy Patients, *Dent. Clin. North Am., 34*, 239, April, 1990.
12. **Sonis,** S.T., Sonis, A.L., and Lieberman, A.: Oral Complications in Patients Receiving Treatment for Malignancies Other than of the Head and Neck, *J. Am. Dent. Assoc., 97*, 468, September, 1978.
13. **Allen,** J.: The Psychosocial Effects of Cancer and Its Treatment in the Elderly, *Spec. Care Dentist., 4*, 13, January/February, 1984.
14. **Joyston-Bechal,** S.: Prevention of Dental Diseases Following Radiotherapy and Chemotherapy, *Int. Dent. J., 42*, 47, February, 1992.
15. **Barker,** G.J., Barker, B.F., and Gier, R.E.: *Oral Management of the Cancer Patient. A Guide for the Health Care Professional*, 4th ed. Kansas City, MO, Biomedical Communications, University of Missouri-Kansas City, School of Dentistry, June, 1992, 24 pp.
16. **Lindquist,** S.F., Hickey, A.J., and Drane, J.B.: Effect of Oral Hygiene on Stomatitis in Patients Receiving Cancer Chemotherapy, *J. Prosthet. Dent., 40*, 312, September, 1978.
17. **Shannon,** I.L., Starcke, E.N., and Wescott, W.B.: Effect of Radiotherapy on Whole Saliva Flow, *J. Dent. Res., 56*, 693, June, 1977.

SUGGESTED READINGS

Al-Joburi, W., Clark, C., and Fisher, R.: A Comparison of the Effectiveness of Two Systems for the Prevention of Radiation Caries, *Clin. Prev. Dent., 13*, 15, September–October, 1991.

Allard, W.F., El-Akkad, S., and Chatmas, J.C.: Obtaining Preradiation Therapy Dental Clearance, *J. Am. Dent. Assoc., 124*, 88, June, 1993.

Bredfeldt, G.W.: Prosthetic Rehabilitation of the Oral Cancer Patient: A Clinical Report, *Spec. Care Dentist., 12*, 211, September/October, 1992.

Karr, R.A., Kramer, D.C., and Toth, B.B.: Dental Implants and Chemotherapy Complications, *J. Prosthet. Dent., 67*, 683, May, 1992.

Kaugars, G.E., Brandt, R.B., Chan, W., and Carcaise-Edinboro, P.: Evaluation of Risk Factors in Smokeless Tobacco-associated Oral Lesions, *Oral Surg. Oral Med. Oral Pathol., 72*, 326, September, 1991.

Liu, R.P., Fleming, T.J., Toth, B.B., and Keene, H.J.: Salivary Flow Rates in Patients with Head and Neck Cancer 0.5 to 25 Years after Radiotherapy, *Oral Surg. Oral Med. Oral Pathol., 70*, 724, December, 1990.

Marciani, R.D. and Ownby, H.E.: Treating Patients Before and After Irradiation, *J. Am. Dent. Assoc., 123*, 108, February, 1992.

Nguyen, A.-M.H.: Dental Management of Patients Who Receive Chemo- and Radiation Therapy, *Gen. Dent., 40*, 305, July–August, 1992.

Piro, J.D., Battle, L.W., Harrison, L.B., and D'Elia, M.J.: Conversion of Complete Dentures to a Radiation Shield Prosthesis, *J. Prosthet. Dent., 65,* 731, June, 1991.

Reed, J.R.: Head and Neck Radiation Patients in a Small Town: Coordinating Dental Treatment with Radiation Therapy, *Gen. Dent., 39,* 258, July–August, 1991.

Salisbury, P.L., Stump, T.E., and Randall, M.E.: Interstitial Radioactive Implants for Oral and Oropharyngeal Cancer: Dentistry's Role, *Spec. Care Dentist., 11,* 63, March/April, 1991.

Thomas, J.E. and Faecher, R.S.: A Physician's Guide to Early Detection of Oral Cancer, *Geriatrics, 47,* 58, January, 1992.

Valdez, I.H.: Radiation-induced Salivary Dysfunction: Clinical Course and Significance, *Spec. Care Dentist., 11,* 252, November/December, 1991.

Zablow, A.I., Eanelli, T.R., and Sanfilippo, L.J.: Electron Beam Therapy for Skin Cancer of the Head and Neck, *Head Neck, 14,* 188 May–June, 1992.

Children

Childers, N.K., Stinnett, E.A., Wheeler, P., Wright, J.T., Castleberry, R.P., and Dasanayake, A.P.: Oral Complications in Children with Cancer, *Oral Surg. Oral Med. Oral Pathol., 75,* 41, January, 1993.

Fayle, S.A. and Curzon, M.E.J.: Oral Complications in Pediatric Oncology Patients, *Pediatr. Dent., 13,* 289, September/October, 1991.

Hsu, E.Y.: Cancer in Children, *Can. Dent. Assoc. J., 58,* 119, February, 1992.

Krywulak, M.L.: Dental Considerations for the Pediatric Oncology Patient, *Can. Dent. Assoc. J., 58,* 125, February, 1992.

Simon, A.R. and Roberts, M.W.: Management of Oral Complications Associated with Cancer Therapy in Pediatric Patients, *ASDC J. Dent. Child., 58,* 384, September–October, 1991.

Soft Tissues

Bergmann, O.J., Ellegaard, B., Dahl, M., and Ellegaard, J.: Gingival Status During Chemical Plaque Control with or Without Prior Mechanical Plaque Removal in Patients with Acute Myeloid Leukaemia, *J. Clin. Periodontol., 19,* 169, March, 1992.

Carl, W.: Local Radiation and Systemic Chemotherapy: Preventing and Managing the Oral Complications, *J. Am. Dent. Assoc., 124,* 119, March, 1993.

Carl, W. and Emrich, L.S.: Management of Oral Mucositis During Local Radiation and Systemic Chemotherapy: A Study of 98 Patients, *J. Prosthet. Dent., 66,* 361, September, 1991.

DeBeule, F., Bercy, P., and Ferrant, A.: The Effectiveness of a Preventive Regimen on the Periodontal Health of Patients Undergoing Chemotherapy for Leukemia and Lymphoma, *J. Clin. Periodontol., 18,* 346, May, 1991.

Epstein, J.B., McBride, B.C., Stevenson-Moore, P., Merilees, H., and Spinelli, J.: The Efficacy of Chlorhexidine Gel in Reduction of *Streptococcus mutans* and *Lactobacillus* Species in Patients Treated with Radiation Therapy, *Oral Surg. Oral Med. Oral Pathol., 71,* 172, February, 1991.

Epstein, J.B., Vickars, L., Spinelli, J., and Reece, D.: Efficacy of Chlorhexidine and Nystatin Rinses in Prevention of Oral Complications in Leukemia and Bone Marrow Transplantation, *Oral Surg. Oral Med. Oral Pathol., 73,* 682, June, 1992.

Reynolds, M.A., Minah, G.E., Peterson, D.E., Weikel, D.S., Williams, L.T., Overholser, C.D., DePaola, L.G., and Suzuki, J.B.: Periodontal Disease and Oral Microbial Successions During Myelosuppresive Cancer Chemotherapy, *J. Clin. Periodontol., 16,* 185, March, 1989.

Care of Patients with Disabilities

Many types of disabilities require special attention and adaptations during dental and dental hygiene appointments. The general term disability refers to any reduction of a person's activity that has resulted from an acute or chronic health condition and affects motor, sensory, or mental functions.

A disability may be permanent or temporary. A temporary impairment may be physical, such as a fracture of a leg, or physiologic with physical limitations, such as during pregnancy. Chronic systemic diseases may result in crippling disabilities. The causes of disabilities may be factors of heredity, systemic disease, trauma, or combinations of these. Table 50–1 supplies key words and definitions pertaining to impairments, disabilities, and handicaps. As defined by the *United States Americans with Disabilities Act (ADA)*, an individual with a disability is a person who *"has a physical or mental impairment that substantially limits a major life activity."*[1]

The *International Classification of the World Health Organization* clarifies the meaning of impairment, disability, and handicap.[2] An *impairment* is an abnormality of structure or function of a limb or body organ, whereas the *disability* is the inability to perform a task or activity as a result of the impairment. The *handicap* is the disadvantage or limitation that an individual has when compared to others of the same age, sex, and background that has resulted from the impairment and the disability. Table 50–2 lists categories and examples of each.

Current trends toward deinstitutionalization have brought alternative living, educational, and work arrangements to many individuals with physical and mental disabilities. Children taken out of institutional life and trained for community living in transitional homes are being integrated or "mainstreamed" into regular school and health programs.

Through a program of rehabilitation, persons with disabilities may receive vocational, educational, placement, medical, and dental services as needed. Specially staffed community housing for group living has been made available.

DENTAL AND DENTAL HYGIENE CARE

Oral health for the individual with a disability takes on more than usual significance and presents a challenge to dental personnel. For the patient, the disability provides enough of a burden without additional oral problems, which can reduce an already lowered potential for normal living. Preventive measures, particularly fluoridation and other means for protecting the teeth with fluoride, must be encouraged and promoted through community effort and personal instruction to minimize oral problems.

Imagination, ingenuity, and flexibility are necessary for those involved in treating people with disabilities. Individualization and modification of usual procedures are necessary in addition to the material described in this chapter. Patience, calmness, and kindness are keys to approaching the special patient.

I. OBJECTIVES

The dental team can make a significant contribution to the well-being, independent mobility, and sense of personal value of a patient with a disability. Whether employed in private practice, working in an institutional or community clinical and educational setting, or contributing on a volunteer basis, the dental team must have as its objectives to

679

TABLE 50-1
KEY WORDS AND ABBREVIATIONS: IMPAIRMENT, DISABILITY, HANDICAP

Accessibility standards: the ADA prohibits discrimination on the basis of a disability and requires places of public accommodation and commercial facilities to meet requirements of accessibility by removing architectural, transportation, and communication barriers.

ADA: Americans with Disabilities Act (U.S.A. 1991).

Barrier-free: area that is freely accessible to all without discrimination on the basis of a disability; obstacles to passage or communication have been removed.

Behavior modification: an approach to correction of undesirable conduct that focuses on changing observable actions; modification of behavior is accomplished through systematic manipulation of the environmental and behavioral variables related to the specific behavior to be changed.

Behavior therapy: an approach in which the focus is on the patient's observable behavior, rather than on conflicts and unconscious processes presumed to underlie the maladaptive behavior; accomplished through systematic manipulation of the environmental and behavioral variables related to the specific behavior to be modified.

Deinstitutionalization: returning patients to home and community as quickly as possible after treatment rather than housing them permanently or for long periods in custodial institutions; the elimination of mental health institutions, for example, has been made possible (1) by the use of new medications that control the symptoms of illness and (2) by community health centers that serve as support.

Desensitization: the treatment of phobias and related disorders by intentionally exposing the patient, in imagination or real life, to emotionally distressing stimuli; desensitization of a fearful patient to accept dental treatment might consist, for example, of short exposures to the dental chair, instruments, air syringe, and the sound of a handpiece along with building trust in the dental team members.

Developmental disability: a substantial handicap of indefinite duration with onset before the age of 18 years, attributable to mental retardation, autism, cerebral palsy, epilepsy, or other incurable neuropathy.

Disability: any restriction or lack of ability (resulting from an impairment) to perform an activity in the manner or within the range considered normal for a human being of the same age, sex, and background.

Handicap: a disadvantage for an individual, resulting from an impairment or a disability, that limits or prevents fulfillment of a role that is within the normal for a human of the same age, sex, and social and cultural factors as the affected individual.

Impairment: any loss or abnormality of psychologic, physiologic, or anatomic structure or function.

Mainstreaming: integration of people with disabilities into their community through programs of rehabilitation; process by which persons with special needs (educational, physical, psychologic) are included within the mainstream of society rather than segregated.

Normalization: making available to all individuals patterns and conditions of everyday life that are as close as possible to the norms and patterns of the mainstream of society.

A. Motivate the patient and the caregiver. Personal oral care practices conducive to maintaining healthy oral tissue with freedom from infection must be developed.

B. Contribute to the patient's general health, of which oral health is an integral part. Prevention of tooth loss increases the ability to masticate food, which, in turn, is essential to prevent malnutrition and to increase resistance to infection.

C. Prevent the need for extensive dental and periodontal treatment that the patient may not be able to undergo because of lowered physical stamina or the inability to cooperate. Dentures or other removable appliances can be hazardous for certain patients or impossible for others.

D. Aid in the improvement of appearance, thereby contributing to social acceptance. An untidy person with unclean teeth and halitosis (from local causes) is much less acceptable socially than is one with a clean mouth.

E. Make appointments pleasant and comfortable experiences.

II. TYPES OF CONDITIONS

A variety of impairments are found among persons with disabilities. An individual may have more than one type of crippling or limiting problem. The lists in table 50–2 are representative. Many of the diseases and syndromes with symptoms of impairments are described in the various chapters throughout Section VI of this book.

III. PRETREATMENT PLANNING

Most patients with disabilities can be treated in the private dental office setting. Only a relatively few need hospitalization because of marked difficulties in management or because of a systemic condition that would require special medical supervision.

A. Preliminary Information

Information about the younger and/or dependent, mentally retarded, or elderly senile patient is obtained from a parent, relative, advocate, or other person responsible for the patient. The essential information can be obtained in advance by telephone or interview.

TABLE 50–2
IMPAIRMENTS, DISABILITIES, AND HANDICAPS

Impairments	Disabilities	Handicaps

Intellectual impairments
  Mental retardation
  Memory, thinking
Psychologic impairments
  Consciousness
  Perception
Language impairments
  Communication
  Voice function
Aural impairments
  Hearing impairment
  Auditory sensitivity
Ocular impairments
  Visual acuity
  Blindness
Visceral impairments
  Internal organs
  Impaired mastication, swallowing
Skeletal impairments
  Mechanical and motor
  Deficiency of parts
  Paralysis
Disfiguring Impairments
  Structural deformity
Generalized, sensory impairment
  Susceptible to trauma
	Behavior disabilities
	  Awareness
	  Motivation
	Communication disabilities
	  Speaking
	  Listening
	Personal care disabilities
	  Personal hygiene
	  Dressing
	Locomotor disabilities
	  Ambulation
	  Transport
	Body disposition disabilities
	  Subsistence
	Dexterity disabilities
	  Daily activity
	  Grasping
	Situational disabilities
	  Environmental temperature
	  Dependence
	  Endurance
	Particular skill disability
	  Task fulfillment
	  Learning ability
	  Dexterity
		Orientation handicap
		  To surroundings
		  Relates to behavior and communication
		    disability
		Physical independence handicap
		  Dependence on others
		Mobility handicap
		  Reduced mobility
		  Dwelling restriction
		Occupation handicap
		  Adjusted occupation
		  Restricted because of disability
		Social integration handicap
		  Restricted participation
		  Socially isolated
		Economic self-sufficiency handicap
		  Fully self-sufficient
		  Impoverished

(From World Health Organization: *International Classification of Impairments, Disabilities and Handicaps*, Geneva, 1980.)

Medical and other record forms can be mailed to the home for completion. Advance information permits the dental team to be prepared for the patient so that valuable appointment time is not wasted and complete attention can be devoted to the patient's needs.

B. Records and Forms

1. *Medical History*. In addition to the usual topics covered by questions (pages 92–95), information relative to the disabling condition is needed. At least the following should be included:
   a. Specific disabling condition. When diagnosed, history of treatments, hospitalizations, current medications and other therapy, names and addresses of specialists involved.
   b. Record of institutionalization.
   c. History of communicable diseases; most recent blood tests; immunizations.
   d. Seizures. History, frequency, treatment.
   e. Muscular coordination. Mobility, dexterity.
   f. Communication. Speech, vision, hearing.
   g. Mental capacities. Schooling, special classes.
   h. Degree of independence. Self-care, ability to dress and feed self and to perform own oral care with brush, floss, other aids.
   i. Dietary restrictions.
2. *Dental History*
   a. Previous dental experiences. Patient's attitude, ability to cooperate.
   b. Difficulties in obtaining appointments in other locations.
   c. Most recent care. Scaling, restorations, extractions, other.
   d. Oral infections and oral habits.
   e. Fluoride history. Fluoridation, dietary supplements, self- or professionally applied topical methods, including years, ages, and frequency.
   f. Current home care methods. Aids and special devices, frequency, degree of self-care.
   g. Patient/parent. Concepts of perceived needs, attitudes, and apparent emphasis on dental care.
3. *Consent Forms*. Consent forms for minor, dependent, and/or incompetent patient must be signed by parent or legal guardian.

C. Consultations with Physicians and Other Specialists

Medical aspects of the patient's care are integrated into treatment planning for oral care. The physician can supply information the dentist can apply in the selection of antibiotic, sedative, or other necessary pharmaceutical agents. Additional pertinent information may be obtained from other medical specialists and the social worker.

D. Discussion with Parent or Other Caregiver

1. Determine familial interrelationships. Many parents devote their lives to the care of their disabled child. Dental personnel must make every effort to learn from the parents or other caregivers the capabilities of the patient and the methods most effective for gaining cooperation. The names, ages, and interrelationships of other family members can prove helpful.

   Families may overindulge the special child. Sweets may be used as rewards or bribes to pacify. Poor behavior may be condoned.

2. Describe to the parent the cooperation and assistance needed. Special help may be needed during the appointment and for supervision of oral care on a daily basis in the total preventive care program.

3. Solicit parental help in preparing the patient for the appointments. Ask that procedures and facilities be described in advance in a pleasant and positive manner to reassure the patient.

4. Invite the patient to the office or clinic before the appointment to see the facility and become familiar with the surroundings and staff.

5. List special aids the patient must bring to the appointment, such as a transfer board for transfer into the dental chair, hearing aid, dental prostheses and bacterial plaque control devices currently in use.

APPOINTMENT SCHEDULING

I. DETERMINE SPECIAL REQUIREMENTS

Determine whether special requirements of the patient's daily schedule influence time selection. The cooperation of the patient may be decreased if basic routines are disturbed. Some examples follow:

A. Appointment for the diabetic patient must not interfere with medication, meal, or between-meal eating schedules.

B. Elderly person who rises early may feel better during a morning appointment.

C. Arthritic patient may have greater mobility late in the morning or in the afternoon.

D. Child's nap schedule should be respected.

E. Early morning appointment may be difficult for a patient who requires a long time for morning preparation, such as a patient with a spinal cord injury or colostomy.

II. EFFECT OF TRANSPORTATION REQUIREMENTS

A. A family member who accompanies the patient should not be expected to lose a day's work if the dental appointment can be accommodated otherwise. Families may have limited financial resources because of expenses related to treatment of the person with the disability.

B. Wheelchair patient may need to reserve a public wheelchair transport vehicle and, thus, may be limited by the schedule.

III. TIME OF APPOINTMENT

A. Arrange a time when the patient will not have to wait a long time after arrival. If daily appointments tend to run increasingly off schedule by late morning or afternoon, the patient with a disability should be scheduled for the appointment at the start of the day or for the first appointment in the afternoon.

B. Schedule a difficult patient when the clinician is at optimum energy or patience.

C. Allow sufficient time so that the patient does not feel rushed; many persons with disabilities cannot hurry.

IV. FOLLOW-UP

The frequency of maintenance appointments must be individualized. The time depends on the patient's oral problems and general disabilities. Frequent appointments are encouraged for the following reasons:

A. To decrease length of single appointment by keeping the oral tissues at an optimum level of health.

B. To assist the patient whose disability limits the ability to perform personal oral hygiene techniques.

C. To provide motivation through monitoring of plaque and review of procedures for the patient and the parent or other caregiver involved.

BARRIER-FREE ENVIRONMENT

A variety of factors can explain the general lack of dental and dental hygiene care of the elderly patient or of individuals of any age who are disabled. One of the more significant reasons is the existence of physical barriers confronting patients who may attempt to keep appointments. Fear of not being able to cope with architectural barriers, fear of falling, or fear of attracting

C. Crutches

1. Dental chair is positioned upright at a level with patient's knees. Some patients need the chair higher so seating does not require knees to be bent.
2. Clinician assists, as directed by patient, while patient lowers into the chair; the legs are lifted onto the dental chair.
3. After the appointment, with patient seated on the side of the dental chair, pass the crutches together to one hand. The patient usually uses the other hand to push up. If assistance in rising is requested, the clinician can hook an arm under the patient's arm as directed.

D. Cane

1. Dental chair is positioned at the level of the patient's knees or higher if the patient may have difficulty in bending the knees.
2. Patient may need assistance in lifting the legs onto the dental chair.
3. After the appointment, when the patient is seated on the side of the dental chair, the clinician passes the cane to the patient and assists patient to rise only as directed.

PATIENT POSITION AND STABILIZATION

The objectives in patient positioning and stabilization are to let the patient feel comfortable and secure while the professional person performs in a position that provides adequate illumination, visibility, and accessibility. A hyperactive patient or a patient with involuntary muscle movements can wear a special stabilizing device to enable the clinician to work and to prevent damage to the oral tissues by accidental movement of instruments.

I. CHAIR POSITION

A. Tip Chair Back Slowly

Immediately after a patient with cerebral palsy or other condition that involves a lack of muscle control is in the dental chair, start to tip the chair back to provide balance so that the patient cannot fall. While tipping back the chair, place one hand on the patient's shoulder to offer assurance and support. Never place the chair back quickly. Advance in steps to allow the patient to adjust.

B. Chair Up

A patient with a respiratory complication must have the chair back up. A patient with a cardiac disease or a patient wearing a pacemaker should be asked "How many pillows do you use at night?" The chair can be adjusted accordingly.

II. BODY ADJUSTMENTS

During the appointment, patients with a spinal cord injury must do a "push up" and patients with quadriplegia must shift their weight every 20 minutes for 10 to 15 seconds. By doing so, the patient can maintain good circulation and healthy tissue of the buttocks, where there is no sensation. The procedure is a preventive measure for decubitus ulcers and should be a consideration during long dental procedures (page 714).

III. BODY STABILIZATION

A restraint can be used to limit body movement and provide support for paralyzed limbs. When a restraint of any type is to be used, it should be explained to the patient. The patient must understand that the devices are used to help the clinician and to make the patient more comfortable, and are by no means a form of punishment.

A. Body Enclosure Restraints

Although a small patient may be held by a parent, such positioning can be tiring and insecure. Better cooperation is usually obtained by the use of positive restraints, such as commercial wraps, which are available, or improvised wraps.

1. *Pediwrap.* The *Pediwrap* is made of nylon mesh and encloses the patient from neck to ankles. It is available in 3 sizes to fit infants and children through 10 years of age.[7] It is frequently used with support straps about the patient's legs and arms.
2. *Papoose Board.* A *Papoose board* is a board with padded wraps to enclose a patient (figure 50-3). It is available in three sizes from a small child size to an adult size.[8]
3. *Bedsheet or Blanket.* The parent can bring from home a blanket or sheet that is familiar to the patient. The sheet or blanket is folded firmly around the patient twice and held securely by a Velcro strap around the body. Support straps about the legs and body provide the patient with additional control.

B. Support Straps

Adhesive tape (2 or 3 inches wide), canvas, or Velcro straps may be used with or without a body enclosure restraint. A soft restraint may be made from a soft material, such as flannel, with a padded section to place over the wrists, ankles, or where needed. Ties 4 to 6 inches wide may be passed around the dental chair or may be tied to the arms of the chair.

C. Head Stabilization

1. *Arm of Clinician.* From a working position at 12 o'clock (top of patient's head), the nondominant arm is placed around the patient's head to hold it in position.
2. *Mouth Prop* (page 702).

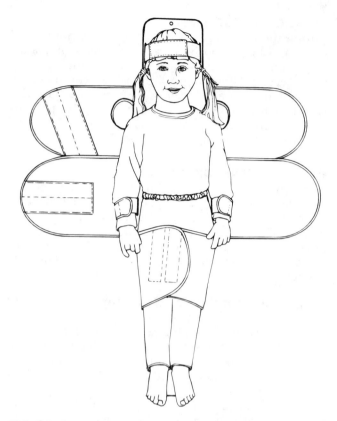

FIG. 50–3. Papoose Board. *Stabilization is accomplished by three body wraps and a head restrainer. The arms are secured at the wrists, as shown, before the large center wrap is closed. (From King, E.M., Wieck, L., and Dyer, M.: Illustrated Manual of Nursing Techniques. Philadelphia, J.B. Lippincott Co., 1977, page 311.)*

CLINIC PROCEDURES FOR ASSESSMENT OF PATIENT

As many as possible of the procedures for assessment are accomplished at the first appointment. The goals should be the same for all patients, namely, to prepare the assessment material to be reviewed and analyzed for treatment planning.

The patient may not be able to complete all the steps in the assessment, and extra time may be needed for orientation. Each clinic procedure is prefaced by an explanation and demonstration. Several trials may be needed.

I. PATIENT HISTORIES

Certain patients require prophylactic antibiotics prior to instrumentation (pages 102 and 103). Suggestions for preparing the medical history are on page 681.

II. VITAL SIGNS: BLOOD PRESSURE DETERMINATION

For the patient who will be examined in a body enclosure restraint, blood pressure determination must be accomplished early in the appointment, before application of the restraint.

III. EXTRAORAL AND INTRAORAL EXAMINATION

When a mouth prop is needed to perform intraoral procedures, the intraoral pathologic examination can be made in conjunction with the gingival and dental examinations. The mouth prop is placed first on one side and then on the other.

IV. PHOTOGRAPHS

Depending on the treatment, photographs may be requested by the dentist. A patient requiring orthodontic therapy, maxillofacial surgery, or other special treatment may need to be photographed.

V. RADIOGRAPHIC SURVEY
A. Periapical Survey

Because the most diagnostic information can be gained from periapical and bitewing surveys, the attempt should be made to obtain as many of the essential exposures as possible.

1. Use a mouth prop, film holder, and much patience. When help is needed, the parent or caregiver can assist.
2. Patient and parent or other caregiver wear lead aprons: person holding the film in mouth can wear a lead glove. Dental personnel never hold film for a patient.

B. Extraoral, Occlusal, Panoramic

The overall views provided by occlusal or extraoral surveys can aid in locating anomalies, retained root tips, impactions, and other abnormalities, but such surveys are not substitutes for the detail provided by periapical radiographs. For example, a periapical film is needed to identify root fracture and apical disorders that may be present in the patient with cerebral palsy who bruxes heavily and may traumatize anterior teeth.

VI. STUDY CASTS[9]

Study casts are needed for orthodontic, prosthetic, and phases of restorative therapy or for documentation and recording purposes. With adequate patient preparation and orientation, cooperation can be obtained. Suggestions for technique are listed here.

A. Use a comfortable tray and bead with a soft wax (page 168). A flexible tray may prove easier to insert.
B. Practice the insertion and removal several times to prepare the patient. Practicing tray insertion may be started at one appointment and the actual impression made at another.
C. Apply a topical anesthetic to the intraoral tissues when the patient has a gag reflex.
D. Use fast-setting alginate and warm water.

VII. GINGIVAL EXAMINATION

Despite difficulties, a thorough assessment must be made. Procedures for examination were described on pages 209–217. Clinical aspects, including the degree of inflammation, pockets, mucogingival involvement, frenal attachments, and tooth mobility, are detected and recorded. Information from the radiographs is used to confirm the presence and degree of periodontal destruction.

Assessment of the amount, extent, and location of calculus is needed so that an appropriate estimate of scaling requirements may be made for the dental hygiene treatment plan. Overall oral cleanliness and the presence of plaque and materia alba provide a prevue to plaque control instruction needs.

VIII. DENTAL EXAMINATION

A. Number, size, color, and occlusion of the teeth.
B. Dental caries.
C. Supernumerary teeth, malformations, and other irregularities that frequently are associated with certain developmental disabilities.

ORAL MANIFESTATIONS

Oral diseases of disabled individuals are not different in kind from those of nondisabled persons. The two principal diseases found are dental caries and periodontal infections. Other oral findings described later include congenital malformations, oral injuries, and malocclusions. In the chapters devoted to describing specific individuals with disabilities, oral characteristics of each are included.

For a majority of patients with disabilities, dental and dental hygiene treatment is not different once the patient is in the dental chair, sedated if needed, and stabilized physically. For a few other patients, an oral manifestation can be caused by, or be a result of, the patient's disabling condition or the treatment for it. Examples are included here.

I. CONGENITAL MALFORMATIONS
A. Cleft Lip or Palate (Page 617)
B. Other Craniofacial Anomalies
C. Tooth Defects

An increased incidence of malformations has been observed with developmental disabilities, for example,
1. Variations in number and structure of teeth.
2. Dentinogenesis imperfecta, amelogenesis imperfecta, enamel hyperplasia, and other abnormalities of tooth structure.

II. ORAL INJURIES
A. Attrition

Attrition caused by bruxism is particularly common among individuals with cerebral palsy and mental retardation.

B. Trauma to Teeth and Soft Tissues

Trauma to teeth and soft tissues may result from accidents (instability, falling), self-abuse, or seizures. The individual with epilepsy is particularly susceptible to accidents. Chipped and fractured teeth, as well as residual scars in the tongue and lips, may be seen frequently.

Because of personal limitations and living a protected life, many patients with disabilities are not exposed to contact sports, traffic accidents, and other accident-prone situations. The incidence of facial trauma may be expected to be less.

III. FACIAL WEAKNESS OR PARALYSIS

When a patient has muscle weakness or paralysis of one side of the face, bilateral mastication is not possible. Plaque usually collects more heavily, and food debris is retained on the involved side. Certain patients may have bilateral weakness.

IV. MALOCCLUSION

Malocclusion is frequently found among persons with developmental disabilities. Factors contributing to problems of occlusion include skeletal and muscular deformities, macroglossia, congenitally missing teeth, and such oral habits as tongue thrust and mouth breathing.

V. DENTAL CARIES

Survey summaries vary, so generalizations cannot be made concerning the prevalence of dental caries in disabled persons. Studies have shown a high incidence of *untreated* dental caries, as well as many missing teeth, which may be a reflection of the type of dental care the patient has or has not received. The dentist may have been unable to cope with the problems presented by the individual with a disability, and therefore, more extractions than restorations were performed.[10]

The more fortunate patients with fewer carious lesions and extractions may have lived in a community with fluoridated water or had the benefit of supplements, such as tablets, rinses, or professional topical fluoride applications. They may also have had knowledgeable parents who were able to control the exposures to carbohydrates in the diet.

VI. GINGIVAL AND PERIODONTAL DISEASES[11]

Gingival and periodontal diseases have been shown to have an increased incidence, especially in individuals with mental retardation and those with physical conditions that prevent daily self-care. Patients with Down's syndrome have a greater incidence of severe periodontal disease with bone loss at an earlier age than that of other individuals with mental retardation (page 754).

Many patients with disabilities have poor oral hygiene and heavy calculus deposits. Factors related to plaque control are described on page 691, and calculus is reviewed on page 702.

VII. THERAPY-RELATED ORAL FINDINGS

A. Phenytoin-induced Gingival Overgrowth

Patients whose treatment for seizures requires phenytoin (Dilantin) may be susceptible to a slight to severe gingival enlargement. The severity of the enlargement usually depends on the maintenance of healthy gingival tissue associated with adequate daily plaque control. A description of phenytoin-induced gingival overgrowth is included in Chapter 54, page 744.

B. Chemotherapy

Oral ulcerations, mucositis, and susceptibility to infection are frequent manifestations following cancer chemotherapy (page 674). Patients with leukemia have a high incidence of oral manifestations, including lymphadenopathy, gingival changes with bleeding, and petechiae, that are more severe following chemotherapy.

C. Radiation Therapy

When radiation therapy of the head and neck area involves the cells of the salivary glands, xerostomia can result and contribute to an increased incidence of dental caries. The symptoms and treatment aspects of radiation therapy are described on pages 673 and 674.

DENTAL HYGIENE TREATMENT PLAN

Parts of the total treatment plan that are to be accomplished by the dental hygienist can be identified under preventive, educational, and therapeutic services. Choice of procedures depends on the findings of the clinical examination and includes some or all of the items listed here.

I. PREVENTIVE THERAPY
A. Bacterial Plaque Control

B. Fluoride Program
1. Supervision of self-applied daily fluoride.
2. Periodic professionally applied topical fluoride.

C. Pit and Fissure Sealants

D. Use of Artificial Saliva for Xerostomia

II. EDUCATIONAL
A. Orientation
Patient orientation to each dental hygiene and dental procedure.

B. Counseling
Parental counseling starting as early as possible after an infant is known to have a disability.

C. Instruction in Disease Control
1. Plaque control for natural teeth and appliances.
2. Daily fluoride, systemic and/or topical.
3. Dietary and nutritional effects.

III. THERAPEUTIC
A. Patient's plaque control for therapeutic purposes until tissue health is attained, followed by planned maintenance.
B. Complete scaling and root planing.
C. Removal of overhanging fillings.
D. Re-evaluation for additional periodontal therapy.
E. Restorative phase; finishing restorations.

DISEASE PREVENTION AND CONTROL

I. PREVENTIVE PROGRAM COMPONENTS[12]
A. Bacterial plaque control.
B. Fluorides.
C. Pit and fissure sealants.
D. Diet counseling.
E. Regular professional examinations and treatment at intervals as recommended by the dentist and dental hygienist.

II. FUNCTIONING LEVELS
For a patient who does not have a mental or physical disability, neglect of personal oral hygiene usually can be explained by either a lack of knowledge and understanding about the need for plaque removal and how it is accomplished or a lack of motivation to carry out the necessary daily routines. For certain patients with disabilities, the problem of disease control becomes greatly magnified because of a lack of the necessary mental and/or physical coordination to carry out even the simplest of oral hygiene measures.

Depending on the severity of the disability, many patients need either complete or partial assistance. Assistance must be provided by parents and other family members when living at home, or by an aide or other caregiver responsible for the patient's care in a residence or institutional setting. There is a twofold responsibility to teach and supervise the patient and the patient's caregivers. Suggestions for in-service education are on pages 699–701.

A *high, moderate,* or *low* functioning level refers to the daily living skills (bathing, toothbrushing, dressing, for example) an individual can do alone, what range or degree of assistance is needed, or whether the person depends on others for complete care. The functioning levels have also been called *self-care, partial care,* or *total care.*[13] In another concept, the terms *supervised,*

4. **Metal Dynamics Corporation,** 9324 State Road, Philadelphia, PA 19114.

5. **Posnick,** W.R. and Martin, H.H.: Wheel Chair Transfer Techniques for the Dental Office, *J. Am. Dent. Assoc., 94,* 719, April, 1977.

6. **Stiefel,** D.J., Schubert, M.M., Hale, J.M., and Friedel, C.A.: *Wheelchair Transfers in the Dental Office.* Disability Dental Instruction, 4919 Northeast 86th Street, Seattle, WA 98115, 42 pp.

7. **Clark Associates,** P.O. Box 517, Charlton, MA 01508.

8. **Olympic Medical Corporation,** 4400 7th Avenue South, Seattle, WA 98108.

9. **Koster,** S.: Orthodontic Treatment of Handicapped Persons, in Wei, S.H.Y. and Casko, J., eds.: *Orthodontic Care for Handicapped Persons.* Proceedings of a Workshop, University of Iowa, Iowa City, IA, 1977, p. 31.

10. **Nowak,** A.J.: Dental Care for the Handicapped Patient—Past, Present, Future, in Nowak, A.J.: *Dentistry for the Handicapped Patient.* St. Louis, Mosby, 1976, p. 11.

11. **Steinberg,** A.D.: Periodontal Evaluation and Treatment Considerations with the Handicapped Patient, in Nowak, A.J.: *Dentistry for the Handicapped Patient.* St. Louis, Mosby, 1976, pp. 302–328.

12. **Nowak,** A.J.: *Dentistry for the Handicapped Patient.* St. Louis, Mosby, 1976, pp. 167–192.

13. **Troutman,** K.C.: Prevention of Dental Disease for the Handicapped, in DePaola, D.P. and Cheney, H.G., eds.: *Preventive Dentistry.* Preventive Dental Handbook Series, Vol. 2. Littleton, MA, PSG Publishing, 1979, pp. 205–224.

14. **Meador,** H.G.: Toothbrushing: A Sensible Approach for the Mentally Retarded, *Dent. Hyg., 53,* 462, October, 1979.

15. **Duncan,** J.L.: Incorporating Oral Hygiene Procedures in Geriatric Nursing Homes, *Dent. Hyg., 53,* 519, November, 1979.

16. **Price,** V.E.: Toothbrush Modifications for the Handicapped, *Dent. Hyg., 54,* 467, October, 1980.

17. **Sroda,** R. and Plezia, R.A.: Oral Hygiene Devices for Special Patients, *Spec. Care Dentist., 4,* 264, November–December, 1984.

18. **Fred Sammons Inc.,** Box 32, Brookfield, IL 60513.

19. **Albertson,** D.: Prevention and the Handicapped Child, *Dent. Clin. North Am., 18,* 595, July, 1974.

20. **Ettinger,** R.L. and Pinkham, J.R.: Oral Hygiene and the Handicapped Child, *J. Int. Assoc. Dent. Child., 9,* 3, July, 1978.

21. **Williams,** N.J. and Schuman, N.J.: The Curved-bristle Toothbrush: An Aid for the Handicapped Population, *ASDC J. Dent. Child., 55,* 291, July–August, 1988.

22. **Mulligan,** R.A.: Design Characteristics of Electric Toothbrushes Important to Physically Compromised Patients, *J. Dent. Res., 59,* 450, Abstract 731, Special Issue A, March 1980.

23. **Ettinger,** R.L. and Pinkham, J.R.: Dental Care for the Homebound—Assessment and Hygiene, *Aust. Dent. J., 22,* 77, April, 1977.

24. **National Foundation of Dentistry for the Handicapped,** National Fluorides Task Force: A Guide to the Use of Fluorides for the Prevention of Dental Caries with Alternative Recommendations for Patients with Handicaps, *J. Am. Dent. Assoc., 113,* 506, September, 1986.

25. **Ripa,** L.W. and Cole, W.W.: Occlusal Sealing and Caries Prevention: Results 12 Months After a Single Application of Adhesive Resin, *J. Dent. Res., 49,* 171, January, 1970.

26. **Richardson,** B.A., Smith, D.C., and Hargreaves, J.A.: A 5-year Clinical Evaluation of the Effectiveness of a Fissure Sealant in Mentally Retarded Canadian Children, *Community Dent. Oral Epidemiol., 9,* 170, August, 1981.

27. **Feigal,** R.J. and Jensen, M.E.: The Cariogenic Potential of Liquid Medications: A Concern for the Handicapped Patient, *Spec. Care Dentist., 2,* 20, January–February, 1982.

28. **Gertenrich,** R.L. and Hart, R.W.: Utilization of the Oral Hygiene Team in a Mental Health Institution, *ASDC J. Dent. Child., 39,* 174, May–June, 1972.

29. **Pattison,** A.M. and Pattison, G.L.: *Periodontal Instrumentation,* 2nd ed. Norwalk, CT, Appleton & Lange, 1992, pp. 355–408.

SUGGESTED READINGS

Belles, M.T.: Long-term Care Facilities: An In-service Education Program, *Dentalhygienistnews, 6,* 14, Spring, 1993.

Bowers, S.A.: Litigation and Legislation Update. The Americans with Disabilities Act., *Am. J. Dent. Orthod. Dentofacial Orthop., 100,* 290, September, 1991.

Ferguson, F.S., Berentsen, B., and Richardson, P.S.: Dentists' Willingness to Provide Care for Patients with Developmental Disabilities, *Spec. Care Dentist., 11,* 234, November/December, 1991.

Finger, S.T. and Jedrychowski, J.R.: Parents' Perception of Access to Dental Care for Children with Handicapping Conditions, *Spec. Care Dentist., 9,* 195, November–December, 1989.

Judd, P.L. and Kenny, D.J.: Feeding Disorders Research and Teams: A New Challenge for Dentistry, *Spec. Care Dentist., 8,* 201, September–October, 1988.

Kaz, M.E. and Schuchman, L.: Oral Oral Health Care Attitudes of Nursing Assistants in Long-term Care Facilities, *Spec. Care Dentist., 8,* 228, September–October, 1988.

Lange, B.M., Entwistle, B.M., and Lipson, L.F.: *Dental Management of the Handicapped: Approaches for Dental Auxiliaries.* Philadelphia, Lea & Febiger, 1983, 169 pp.

Lo, G.L., Soh, G., Vignehsa, H., and Chellappah, N.K.: Dental Service Utilization of Disabled Children, *Spec. Care Dentist., 11,* 194, September/October, 1991.

Mills, S.H.: Deinstitutionalization and Clinical Dental Practice, *Gen. Dent., 37,* 138, March–April, 1989.

Ramsey, W.O.: Valved Feeding Devices: Adjuncts in Rehabilitation of the Oral Phase of Swallowing, *Int. J. Periodontics Restorative Dent., 10,* 321, No. 4, 1990.

Waldman, H.B.: Respite Care: A New Social Program for Children at Risk, *ASDC J. Dent. Child., 58,* 241, May–June, 1991.

Patient Management

Adair, S.M. and Durr, D.P.: Modification of Papoose Board® Restraint to Facilitate Airway Management of the Sedated Pediatric Dental Patient, *Pediatr. Dent., 9,* 163, June, 1987.

Barker, D.T.: A Motorized Surgery Unit for Treatment of the Handicapped Patient, *Br. Dent. J., 162,* 436, June 6, 1987.

Casamassimo, P.S.: A Primer in Management of Movement in the Patient with a Handicapping Condition, *J. Mass. Dent. Soc., 40,* 23, Winter, 1991.

Felder, R.S., Gillette, V.M., and Leseberg, K.: Wheelchair Transfer Techniques for the Dental Office, *Spec. Care Dentist., 8,* 256, November–December, 1988.

Fenton, S.J., Fenton, L.I., Kimmelman, B.B., Shellhart, W.C., Sheff, M.C., Scott, J.P., Staggers, J.A., and Portugal, B.V.: ADH ad hoc Committee Report: The Use of Restraints in the Delivery of Dental Care for the Handicapped—Legal, Ethical, and Medical Considerations, *Spec. Care Dentist., 7,* 253, November–December, 1987.

Frankel, R.I.: The Papoose Board® and Mothers' Attitudes Following Its Use, *Pediatr. Dent., 13,* 284, September/October, 1991.

Jacobs, W., Lipp, M., Daubländer, M., and Jakobs-Hannegrefs, E.: Dental Treatment of Handicapped Patients with Conscious Sedation, *Anesth. Prog., 36,* 144, July–October, 1989.

Kamen, S., Crespi, P., and Ferguson, F.S.: Dental Management of the Physically Handicapped Patient, in Thornton, J.B and Wright, J.T., eds.: *Special and Medically Compromised Patients in Dentistry.* St. Louis, Mosby YearBook, 1989, pp. 24–48.

Kaminsky, S.B., Kaurich, M.J., and Chenderlin, J.: Managing Cooperative Nonambulatory Patients: Transfers to the Dental Chair, *Gerodontics, 4,* 1, February, 1988.

Malamed, S.F., Gottschalk, H.W., Mulligan, R., and Quinn, C.L.: Intravenous Sedation for Conservative Dentistry for Disabled Patients, *Anesth. Prog., 36,* 140, July–October, 1989.

McCord, J.F., Moody, G.H., and Blinkhorn, A.S.: Overview of Dental Treatment of Patients with Microstomia, *Quintessence Int., 21,* 903, November, 1990.

Moulding, M.B. and Koroluk, L.D.: An Intraoral Prosthesis to Control Drooling in a Patient with Amyotrophic Lateral Sclerosis, *Spec. Care Dentist., 11,* 200, September/October, 1991.

Parker, C.B. and White, S.P.: Intra-oral Remote Control. An Access Device for the Severely Disabled, *Br. Dent. J., 169,* 302, November 10, 1990.

Spencer, P.R.: Techniques for Transporting the Handicapped Patient in the Dental Setting, *Dent. Assist., 57,* 16, January/February, 1988.

Williams, E.O. and Seals, R.R.: Treating Patients in Wheelchairs, *J. Prosthet. Dent., 67,* 431, March, 1992.

Bacterial Plaque Control

Brownstone, E.: Handicapped Dental Patients: Mechanical Methods and Modifications for Oral Hygiene Care, *Can. Dent. Hyg./Probe, 24,* 32, Spring, 1990.

Fitchie, J.G., Reeves, G.W., Comer, R.W., Gatewood, R.S., Campbell, E.A., and Rommerdale, E.H.: Oral Hygiene for the Severely Handicapped: Clinical Evaluation of the University of Mississippi Dental Care System, *Spec. Care Dentist., 8,* 260, November–December, 1988.

Kalaga, A., Addy, M., and Hunter, B.: The Use of 0.2% Chlorhexidine Spray as an Adjunct to Oral Hygiene and Gingival Health in Physically and Mentally Handicapped Adults, *J.. Periodontol., 60,* 381, July, 1989.

Soncini, J.A. and Tsamtsouris, A.: Individually Modified Toothbrushes and Improvement in Oral Hygiene and Gingival Health in Cerebral Palsy Children, *J. Pedod., 13,* 331, Summer, 1989.

Stiefel, D.J., Truelove, E.L., Chin, M.M., and Mandel, L.S.: Efficacy of Chlorhexidine Swabbing in Oral Health Care for People with Severe Disabilities, *Spec. Care Dentist., 12,* 57, Marsh/April, 1992.

The Patient Who Is Homebound, Bedridden, or Helpless

HOMEBOUND PATIENTS

Within recent years, efforts have been made through research and organized programming to attend to the oral health needs of people with a chronic illness and a disability. Patients of all age groups who are confined to hospitals, hospices, institutions, nursing homes, skilled nursing facilities, or private homes need special adaptations for oral care. Portable equipment is available, and special training for dental personnel is encouraged.

Dental care for the chronically ill must be completed in a variety of surroundings. For the hospitalized person, dental clinics frequently are available to provide care for in-patients. Those who are not hospitalized may be confined to their homes or may be able to be transported to the dental office or clinic in a wheelchair, depending on the severity and extent of disability.

Private practice clinicians have occasion to attend to patients confined to their homes. Dental hygiene procedures lend themselves to care for the bedridden because nearly the entire treatment can be completed with manual instruments. Instruction in personal oral preventive procedures has particular significance for the comfort, as well as the health, of the patient. Suggestions relative to planning and conducting a home visit are included in this chapter. Key words and definitions are included in table 51–1.

I. OBJECTIVES
A. Aid in preventing dental caries and periodontal infections that require extensive treatment.
B. Assist in preventing further complication of the patient's state of health by lessening oral care problems.
C. Contribute to the patient's comfort, mental ease, and general well-being.
D. Encourage adequate personal care procedures, whether performed by the patient or a caregiver.
E. Contribute to general rehabilitation or habilitation of the patient.
F. Provide palliative care for the individual with a shortened life span.

II. PREPARATION FOR THE HOME VISIT
A. Understanding the Patient
1. Consider the characteristics associated with the particular chronic illness or disease.
2. Consider special problems related to age. (For example, for the gerodontic patient, see Chapter 46.)
3. Review patient's medical history (by telephone, if preliminary visit is not practical) to determine unusual precautions that must be taken. Arrange with physician and dentist when premedication is indicated (pages 102 and 103).

B. Instruments and Equipment
1. *Protective Barriers.* Mask, protective eyewear, gloves.
2. *Instruction Materials.* Toothbrush, interdental aids (several types, until needs of patient are known).
3. *Sterile Equipment.* Sterile instruments and other items are transported in the sealed packages in which they were sterilized.
4. *Disposable Items.* Gauze sponges, cotton rolls and pellets, wood points, fluoride application trays, and other essential disposable items

705

are prepared in packages that are convenient to open and use at the bedside.

5. *Pharmaceuticals.* Such substances as the disclosing agent, postoperative antiseptic, polishing agent, and topical fluoride preparation are carried in small, tightly closed bottles.

6. *Coverall.* A large plastic drape is of particular importance, because in certain types of illness the patient's coordination during rinsing may be limited.

7. *Emesis Basin for Patient Rinsing.* Although a small basin undoubtedly would be available at the home, the kidney-shaped emesis basin facilitates the rinsing process.

8. *Lighting.* Adaptation of available possibilities.
   a. Headlight or reflector. Dentist may have as part of the office equipment; with practice, the dental hygienist can learn to use with ease.
   b. Photography spot light. Might be available either from the dentist or from the patient's home; need a type with a narrow, concentrated beam.
   c. Gooseneck lamp. Might be available in patient's home; need bulb of adequate wattage.

9. *Miscellaneous Items Usually Available at the Home.* Arrangements must be planned (by telephone) in advance of appointment.

a. Large towels. For covering pillows.
b. Pillows. Types of pillows available that may be firm enough to assist in maintaining patient's head in reasonably stationary position.
c. Hospital bed. Can be adjusted most effectively for patient's position.
d. Container for prosthesis.

C. Appointment Time

Arrange during the patient's usual waking hours at as convenient a time as possible in relation to nursing care and mealtime schedule.

III. APPROACH TO PATIENT

Because a majority of patients who come to the dental office are active people with good general health, the adjustment to the relatively helpless, chronically ill person is sometimes difficult. One may tend to be oversolicitous, an attitude that may not contribute to the development of a cooperative patient.

Usually, a direct approach with gentle firmness is most successful. Establishment of rapport with the patient depends in part on whether the patient has requested and anticipated the appointment or whether those caring for the patient have insisted on and arranged for the visit.

A. Personal Factors

Frequently, the well-adjusted chronically ill person may be more appreciative of the care provided than is the healthy patient who comes to the dental office. The ill patient may also be well aware of the difficulties under which the clinician is working. The cooperation obtained frequently depends on the patient's attitude toward the illness or disability.

A prolonged illness that may have been accompanied by suffering is not conducive to a healthy outlook on life. Monotonous confinement contributes to the development of characteristics such as those that follow.

1. Unable to maintain a cheerful attitude.
2. Bored or dissatisfied with sameness of daily routine.
3. Easily depressed.
4. Discouraged about recovery; leads to mental state that may retard recovery.
5. Sensitive and easily offended.
6. Demanding; enjoys being waited on if used to having prompt attention to each request.
7. Indifferent to personal appearance and general rules of personal hygiene.
8. Preoccupied with details of medical examinations, tests, treatment, medications, and symptoms.

B. Suggestions for General Procedure

1. Request the caregiver to be present to assist as needed and to learn method for care of the patient's mouth on a daily basis. Other

visitors should be asked to remain out of the room during the appointment to prevent distraction of patient.

2. Introduce each step slowly to be sure patient knows what is being done.

3. Do not make the patient feel rushed. Listen attentively; socializing is one of the best ways to establish rapport.

4. Regardless of inconvenience of arrangements, plan two or more appointments when extensive scaling is required.
   a. Need to avoid tiring the patient.
   b. Need for observing tissue response.
   c. Need to give encouragement in plaque control procedures.

IV. DENTAL HYGIENE CARE AND INSTRUCTION

A. The Working Situation

Because many patients can sit up in a chair or wheelchair for at least 1 or 2 hours each day, only rarely must procedures be performed while the patient is in bed. For the patient in a chair, a kitchen or large bathroom may be most satisfactory for working. In either situation, ingenuity is needed to arrange patient position, head stabilization, and proper lighting to maintain patient comfort and yet provide access for the clinician.

1. *Patient in Bed*
   a. Hospital bed. Adjust to lift patient's head to desirable height.
   b. Ordinary bed. Use firm pillows to support patient.

2. *Patient in Wheelchair.*
   a. Portable headrest may be attached to back of plain chair or wheelchair.
   b. Although the chair can be backed against a wall and a pillow inserted for the head, the patient preferably should be moved to a davenport or chair where a more stable headrest could be provided.

3. *Small Patient.* Positions for plaque control described on page 697 and shown in figure 50–10 may be applicable during treatment.

4. *Suggestions for Lighting*
   a. Overhead lighting. Turn off to reduce shadows in the mouth.
   b. Headlight. Usually the most convenient and efficient form of lighting because of concentrated beam.
   c. Head reflector. Reflect light from bed lamp attached to bed behind patient's head.
   d. Gooseneck or photographer's light. Care must be taken not to direct the light into patient's eyes.

5. *Instrument Arrangement.* Use instruments directly from a sterile package or cassette.

B. Assessment Treatment Plan
1. Vital signs.
2. Extraoral/intraoral examination.
3. Periodontal assessment.
4. Dental examination.

C. Personal Oral Care
Provide specific instruction for caregiver of helpless or uncoordinated patient. Demonstrate in patient's mouth. A power-assisted toothbrush may prove valuable for certain patients (page 344).

D. Instrumentation
Scaling is complicated by instability of the head. A mouth prop may be needed when patient has difficulty holding the mouth open.

E. Fluoride Application
Selection of method for fluoride application varies with the patient and the home situation. The use of self-care techniques depends on the patient's disability and the cooperation of the caregiver. The greatest benefit is obtained from a daily mouthrinse, chewable tablet, or gel applied in a mouthguard tray or brushed on (pages 449–453).

F. Dietary Suggestions
1. Consultation with physician concerning a prescribed diet is necessary. When significant relationships of diet to oral health are suspected, they should be reported to the physician. The patient's problem then can be discussed with the physician and dietary adjustments made.
2. Cariogenic foods should be avoided as snacks. The patient and those who provide the patient's food need specific suggestions for food substitutes that are noncariogenic.
3. Factors influencing suggestions for diet
   a. Patient's appetite may be poor, particularly if the patient is discouraged about the state of health.
   b. The patient who is finicky in food selection may have affected the general nutritional state or may have used cariogenic foods in excess.
   c. Monotony of meals may have lessened the desire to eat.

G. Appointment Plan for Maintenance

THE HELPLESS OR UNCONSCIOUS PATIENT

Personal oral care procedures for the unconscious patient are accomplished by the caregiver when self-care by the patient is impossible. Planning and conducting an oral health in-service program for a nursing staff and other caregivers are described on pages 699–701.

Understanding the possible procedures for oral care of hospitalized patients is important to all dental hygienists, whether or not they are employed in a hospital, if they are to appreciate ramifications of dental hygiene care for the many types of patients with special needs.

Skill is required to carry out routine methods of toothbrushing, rinsing, and cleaning of removable dentures for the conscious patient who is able to cooperate. Methods must be adapted when the patient's head cannot be elevated. When the patient's illness or injury involves the oral cavity, the advice and recommendations of the attending oral surgeon are followed.

Maintenance of oral cleanliness for the acutely ill or unconscious patient requires special procedures because of the complete helplessness of the patient. Objectives and methods described in the following sections have application for patients with other special needs, for example, the patient with a fractured jaw (pages 660–666) or severe mental retardation (pages 750–751).

I. OBJECTIVES OF CARE

A. Prevent debris in the mouth from being aspirated and clogging air passages.

B. Minimize the possibility of oral infection.

C. Clean the mouth and provide comfort for the patient.

II. CARE OF REMOVABLE DENTURES

A. Remove dentures from the patient's mouth. Usual hospital policy requires removal of dentures when a patient is unconscious.

B. Procedure for removal is described on page 572.

C. Clean the dentures (pages 383–388) and store in water in a covered container by the patient's bedside. Fresh water or denture cleanser must be provided daily to prevent bacterial growth.[2]

III. GENERAL MOUTH CLEANING
A. Edentulous and Dentulous

1. Clean the mouth at least three times each day to prevent dryness and sordes. Sordes is a crust-like material that collects on the lips, teeth, and gingiva of a patient with a fever or dehydration in a chronic debilitating disease.

2. Toothbrushing and flossing are essential for mechanical plaque removal. Other devices, such as swabs or gauze sponges, are much less effective and more time consuming.[3]

B. Brushing and Flossing

1. *Patient Who Can Rinse.* When unable to manipulate brush or floss but able to rinse and expectorate, a patient can be propped upright and an emesis basin used.

2. *Patient Who Cannot Participate.* Suction is a necessity. When suction is used, an assistant is needed, except for the suction toothbrush described in the following section.

3. *Brush.* A power-assisted brush may be more efficient and thorough than a manual brush when a caregiver must brush a helpless patient's teeth. A mouth prop can be placed in one side while the other side is retracted.

IV. TOOTHBRUSH WITH SUCTION ATTACHMENT

The toothbrush with attached suction provides an efficient and safe method for patient care.

A. Description of the Brush[4,5]

1. Soft-textured nylon brush with the hole drilled between the bristles in the middle of the head of the brush.

2. Small plastic tubing inserted into hole; end adjusted slightly below level of brushing plane.

3. Other end of tubing passed across back of brush handle and attached to handle by small rubber bands (figure 51–1).

4. Tubing is connected by an adapter to aspirator or suction outlet.

5. Suction brushes are also manufactured commercially (see *Technical Hints* at the end of chapter).

B. Procedure for Use of Brush

The detailed procedure should be outlined for hospital personnel and included in the nursing procedures manual. An abbreviated outline of the basic steps is included here.

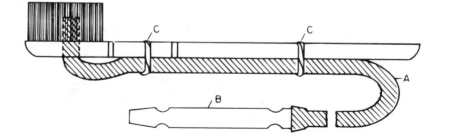

FIG. 51–1. Suction Toothbrush. A. Plastic tubing. **B.** Adapter for attachment of the tubing to an aspirator or suction outlet. **C.** Small rubber bands attach the tubing to the brush handle. The plastic tube is inserted through a hole in the head of the brush and extended to a level slightly below the brushing plane.

1. Prepare patient
   a. Although not able to respond in a usual manner, the patient may be aware of what is going on.
   b. Tell patient that the teeth are going to be brushed, and thereafter maintain a one-way conversation despite patient's inability to respond verbally.
   c. Turn patient on a side and place a pillow at the back for support.
   d. Place a face towel under patient's chin and over bedding.
2. Attach toothbrush to suction outlet and lay brush on towel near patient's mouth.
3. Place a rubber bite block on one side of the patient's mouth between the teeth. String tied to bite block is fastened to the patient's gown with a safety pin.
4. Dip brush in fluoride mouthrinse; turn on suction.
5. Gently retract lip and carefully apply the appropriate toothbrushing procedures; apply suction over each tooth surface with particular care at each interproximal area. Moisten brush frequently.
6. Move bite block to opposite side of mouth and continue brushing procedure.
7. Place brush in cup of clear water to allow water to be sucked through to clear the tubing during the procedure if there is clogging and to clean the tube after brushing.
8. Remove bite block; wipe patient's lips with paper wipe and apply a water-based lubricant, such as plain hydrous lanolin.
9. Wash brush and bite block; prepare materials for next use.

V. RELIEF FOR XEROSTOMIA
A. Use Saliva Substitute
Swab the oral mucosa using a saliva substitute. Lemon and glycerin swabs formerly were used by hospital personnel, but the acidic effect of the lemon led to demineralization of enamel, and the drying effect of the glycerin was contradictory to the intended outcome.[6,7] Swabs prepared with saliva substitute are available to relieve xerostomia and can be used as frequently as needed throughout the day and night.[8]

B. Alcohol and Glycerin
Avoid products that contain alcohol or glycerin, that are drying to the oral tissues.

TECHNICAL HINTS

I. SOURCES FOR SUCTION TOOTHBRUSHES
Ora Genics
5699 S.E. International Way, Unit D.
Milwaukie, OR 97222
Vac-U-Brush

Trademark Corp.
1053 Headquarters Park
Fenton, MO 63026-2033
Plak-Vac

II. INSURANCE
Check practice liability insurance for alternate practice settings, such as a private home or nursing care facility.

REFERENCES

1. **National Hospice Organization (NHO),** 1978, in Zimmerman, J.M.: *Hospice Complete Care for the Terminally Ill,* 2nd ed. Baltimore-Munich, Urban & Schwarzenberg, 1986, p. 17.
2. **DePaola,** L.G. and Minah, G.E.: Isolation of Pathogenic Microorganisms from Dentures and Denture-soaking Containers of Myelosuppressed Cancer Patients. *J. Prosthet. Dent., 49,* 20, January, 1983.
3. **Seto,** B.G., Wolinsky, L.E., Tsutsui, P., and Avera, C.: Comparison of the Plaque-removing Efficacy of Four Nonbrushing Oral Hygiene Devices, *Clin. Prev. Dent., 9,* 9, March–April, 1987.
4. **Capps,** J.S.: New Device for Oral Hygiene, *Am. J. Nurs., 58,* 1532, November, 1958.
5. **Tronquet,** A.A.: Oral Hygiene for Hospital Patients, *J. Am. Dent. Assoc., 63,* 215, August, 1961.
6. **Daeffler,** R.J.: Oral Care, *Hospice J., 2,* 81, Spring, 1986.
7. **Poland,** J.M.: Xerostomia in the Oncologic Patient. Combating Complications of Treatment, *Am. J. Hospice Care, 4,* 31, May/June, 1987.
8. **Moi-stir Oral Swabsticks,** Kingswood Laboratories, Inc., 10375 Hague Road, Indianapolis, IN 46256.

SUGGESTED READINGS

Aldred, M.J., Addy, M., Bagg, J., and Finlay, I.: Oral Health in the Terminally Ill: A Cross-sectional Pilot Survey, *Spec. Care Dentist., 11,* 59, March/April, 1991.

Allman, R.M.: Pressure Ulcers Among the Elderly, *N. Engl. J. Med., 320,* 850, March 30, 1989.

Anderson, J.L.: Dental Treatment for Homebound and Institutionalized Patients, in Nowak, A.J.: *Dentistry for the Handicapped Patient.* St. Louis, Mosby, 1976, pp. 211–224.

Baker, K.A., Levy, S.M., and Chrischilles, E.A.: Medications with Dental Significance: Usage in a Nursing Home Population, *Spec. Care Dentist., 11,* 19, January/February, 1991.

Brown, J.O. and Hoffman, L.A.: The Dental Hygienist as a Hospice Care Provider, *Am. J. Hosp. Palliat. Care, 7,* 31, March–April, 1990.

Casamassimo, P.S., Coffee, L.M., and Leviton, F.J.: A Comparison of Two Mobile Treatment Programs for the Homebound and Nursing Home Patient, *Spec. Care Dentist., 8,* 77, March–April, 1988.

Gordon, S.R. and McLain, D.: Dental Needs Related to Primary Cause for Institutionalization, *Spec. Care Dentist., 11,* 49, March/April, 1991.

Harris, N.O. and Christen, A.G.: Primary Preventive Dentistry in a Hospital Setting, in Harris, N.O. and Christen, A.G.: *Primary Preventive Dentistry,* 3rd ed. Norwalk, CT, Appleton & Lange, 1991, pp. 467–496.

Hartley, M.S.: The Older Patient, *RDH, 11,* 14, June, 1991.

Hoyen-Chung, D.J.: Oral Hygiene Training Programmes in Long-stay Hospitals, *Br. Dent. J., 167,* 178, September 9, 1989.

Jobbins, J., Bagg, J., Finlay, I.G., Addy, M., and Newcombe, R.G.:

Oral and Dental Disease in Terminally Ill Cancer Patients, *Br. Med. J., 304,* 1612, June 20, 1992.

Kambhu, P.P. and Levy, S.M.: An Evaluation of the Effectiveness of Four Mechanical Plaque-removal Devices when Used by a Trained Care-provider, *Spec. Care Dentist., 13,* 9, January/February, 1993.

Kemper, P. and Murtaugh, C.M.: Lifetime Use of Nursing Home Care, *N. Engl. J. Med., 324,* 595, February 28, 1991.

Krust, K.S. and Schuchman, L.: Out-of-office Dentistry: An Alternative Delivery System, *Spec. Care Dentist., 11,* 189, September/October, 1991.

Libow, L.S. and Starer, P.: Care of the Nursing Home Patient, *N. Engl. J. Med., 321,* 93, July 13, 1989.

MacEntee, M.I., Weiss, R.T., Waxler-Morrison, N.E., and Morrison, B.J.: Opinions of Dentists on the Treatment of Elderly Patients in Long-term Care Facilities, *J. Public Health Dent., 52,* 239, Summer, 1992.

Markitziu, A., Leviner, E., and Sela, M.: Overdentures for Patients Who Are Chronically Ill: A 4-year Follow-up, *Spec. Care Dentist., 9,* 42, March–April, 1989.

McFall, D.B.: Choosing a Portable Delivery System, *Dentalhygienistnews, 5,* 14, Spring, 1992.

Rhymes, J.A.: Clinical Management of the Terminally Ill, *Geriatrics, 46,* 57, February, 1991.

Shaver, R.D.: Portable Dentistry Benefits Homebound and Providers, *N.Y. State Dent. J., 57,* 30, October, 1991.

Smith, D.M.: Are We Missing an Important Segment of the Population? *RDH, 12,* 30, March, 1992.

Strayer, M.S. and Ibrahim, M.F.: Dental Treatment Needs of Homebound and Nursing Home Patients, *Community Dent. Oral Epidemiol., 19,* 176, June, 1991.

Williams, J.N. and Butters, J.M.: Sociodemographics of Homebound People in Kentucky, *Spec. Care Dentist., 12,* 74, March/April, 1992.

The Patient with a Physical Impairment

Many diseases of the locomotor system and nervous system have as a symptom or leave as a chronic after-effect loss of function in the form of a physical impairment.

This chapter contains brief descriptions of selected diseases or conditions to illustrate the types of care necessary and the adaptations that must be made by the patient, as well as by the professional person, during treatment appointments. Table 52–1 lists key words and their definitions relating to physical impairments and disabilities.

General suggestions that may be adapted to a variety of patients with disabilities were described in Chapter 50. From those descriptions, methods and materials can be selected as they apply in the situations created by the different disorders included in this chapter and encountered in practice.

SPINAL CORD DYSFUNCTIONS

There are many causes of disruption of spinal cord function. Major causes are listed here with examples provided in parentheses.

  I. Trauma (spinal cord injury).
  II. Neoplasms (within the cord or extradural).
  III. Viral or bacterial infections (poliomyelitis).
  IV. Progressive degenerative disorders (multiple sclerosis).
  V. Vascular accidents (hemorrhage, thrombus, embolus, hematoma).
  VI. Compression from an arthritic spur (spondylitic osteoarthritis).
  VII. Congenital anomalies or deformities (myelomeningocele, meningocele, spina bifida).

SPINAL CORD INJURY

Spinal cord injury is the impairment of spinal cord function resulting from the application of an external traumatic force. The effect is partial or complete paralysis to a degree related to the spinal cord level and the extent of the injury.

I. OCCURRENCE
At least one half of the trauma cases result from motor vehicle accidents; other causes are falls, diving accidents, and violence, such as from gunshot or stabbing wounds. Most patients are teenage or young adult men.

II. THE INITIAL INJURY
Total or partial loss of sensory, motor, and autonomic function occurs below the level of injury. The injury may be diagonal and leave one side with better function than the other at that particular level.

A. Types of Injury
Damage to the spinal cord may result from one or more of the following:
  1. Fracture, dislocation, or both, of one or more vertebrae.
  2. Compression, stretching, bending, or severing of the spinal cord.

B. Emergency Patient Care[1,2]
At the scene of an accident, severe damage can be done by inexpert care. The patient should be placed in a supine position, but when back injury is suspected, the arms and legs should be straightened with caution. Any twisting motion may produce irreversible injury to the spinal cord by bony fragments cutting into or severing

711

TABLE 52–1
KEY WORDS AND ABBREVIATIONS:
PHYSICAL IMPAIRMENTS

Akinesia (ah′-kĭ-nē′zē-ah): abnormal absence of movements.

Ankylosis (ang′kĭ-lō′sĭs): abnormal immobility or consolidation.

   Bony ankylosis: union of bone with bone or bone with tooth resulting in complete immobility; the periodontal ligament of an ankylosed tooth is completely obliterated.

Aphasia (ah-fā′zē-ah): defect in, or loss of power of, expression by speech, writing, or signs, or of comprehension of spoken or written language.

Ataxia (ah-tak′sē-ah): failure of muscular coordination; irregularity of muscle action.

Atrophy (at′rō-fē): wasting; decrease in size; occurs when muscle fibers are not used or are deprived of their blood supply, or when the nerve connection is interrupted.

Bradykinesia (brăd′ē-kĭn-nē′sē-ah): abnormal slowness of movements.

Cerebrovascular accident (CVA): a focal neurologic disorder caused by destruction of brain substance as a result of intracerebral hemorrhage, thrombosis, embolism, or vascular insufficiency; also called stroke.

Decubitus ulcer (dē-ku′bĭ-tus): ulcer that usually occurs over a bony prominence as a result of prolonged, excessive pressure from body weight; also called pressure sore or bed sore.

Demyelinate (dē-mī′ĕ-lin-āt): destruction/removal of the myelin sheath of a nerve.

Dysphagia (dĭs-fa′ze-ah): difficulty in swallowing.

Hypercholesterolemia (hī′per-kō-les′ter-ol-ē′mē-ah): excess of cholesterol in the blood.

Ischemia (is-kē′mē-ah): deficiency of blood caused by functional construction or actual obstruction of a blood vessel.

Kyphosis (kī-fō′sĭs): abnormally increased convexity in the curvature of the thoracic spine (viewed from the side).

Microcephaly (mī′krō-sef′ah-lē): head that is small in relation to rest of the body; contrast with **macrocephaly,** head that is large in relation to rest of the body.

Myopathy (mī-op′ah-thē): any disease of muscle.

Orthosis (or-thō′sĭs): orthopedic appliance or apparatus used to support, align, prevent, or correct deformities or to improve the function of a movable part of the body.

Paralysis (pah-ral′ĭ-sis): a symptom of the loss or impairment of motor function in a body part caused by a lesion of the neural or muscular mechanism.

   Diplegia (dī-ple′jē-ah): paralysis of like parts on either side of the body.

   Hemiplegia (hem′e ple′jē-ah): paralysis of one side of the body; usually caused by CVA or a brain lesion.

   Paraplegia (par′ah-ple′jē-ah): paralysis of the legs and in some cases the lower part of the body.

   Quadriplegia (kwod′rĭ-ple′jē-ah): paralysis of all four limbs from neck down; tetraplegia.

   Triplegia (trī-ple′jē-ah): paralysis of three limbs; hemiplegia with additional paralysis of one limb on the opposite side.

Paresis (pah-rē′sis): slight or incomplete paralysis.

Sclerosis (sklĕ-rō′sĭs): induration or hardening; especially hardening from inflammation and in disease of the interstitial substance.

Shunt: passage between two natural channels; to bypass or drain an area.

   Ventriculoatrial shunt: surgical creation of a communication between a cerebral ventricle and a cardiac atrium by means of a plastic tube; for relief of hydrocephalus.

   Ventriculoperitoneal shunt: communication between a cerebral ventricle and the peritoneum by means of a plastic tube; for relief of hydrocephalus.

TIA: transient ischemic attack; brief episode of cerebral ischemia that results in no permanent neurologic damage; symptoms are warning signals of impending CVA (stroke.).

Visceral (vĭs′er-al): pertaining to internal organs (digestive, respiratory, urogenital, endocrine, spleen, heart, and great vessels).

---

the cord. When transfer is made, the patient must be moved by at least four persons and placed on a board for transport.

C. Spinal Shock

Immediately after the injury, spinal shock causes a complete loss of reflex activity. The result is a flaccid paralysis below the level of injury. The state of spinal shock may last from several hours to 3 months.

III. CHARACTERISTICS OF SPINAL CORD INJURY

The pattern of signs and symptoms depends on the nature and level of injury to the spinal cord. There

are 7 cervical (C), 12 thoracic (T), and 5 lumbar (L) vertebrae, with paired spinal nerves extending from each.

The areas of the body that are controlled at the different levels are illustrated in figure 52–1. The patient's condition is referred to by the letter C, T, or L, followed by the specific vertebra number where the injury occurred. The most severely disabled patients have a lesion level above C6, which refers to the sixth cervical vertebral level.

A. Sensorimotor Effects

   1. *Complete Lesion.* A complete transection or compression of the spinal cord leaves no sen-

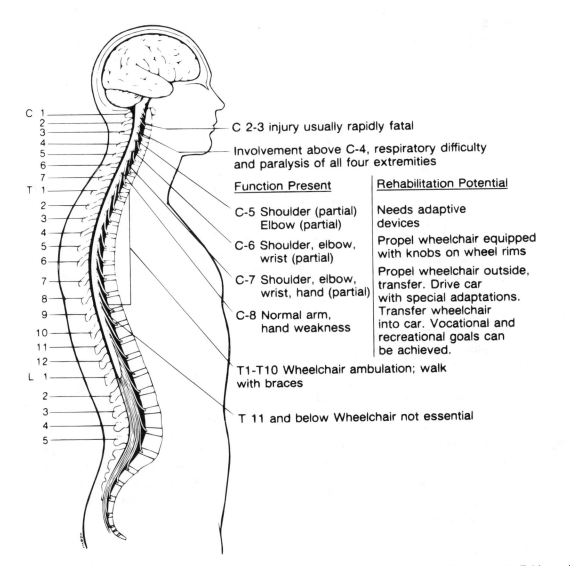

C 2-3 injury usually rapidly fatal

Involvement above C-4, respiratory difficulty and paralysis of all four extremities

Function Present	Rehabilitation Potential
C-5 Shoulder (partial) Elbow (partial)	Needs adaptive devices
C-6 Shoulder, elbow, wrist (partial)	Propel wheelchair equipped with knobs on wheel rims
C-7 Shoulder, elbow, wrist, hand (partial)	Propel wheelchair outside, transfer. Drive car with special adaptations.
C-8 Normal arm, hand weakness	Transfer wheelchair into car. Vocational and recreational goals can be achieved.

T1-T10 Wheelchair ambulation; walk with braces

T 11 and below Wheelchair not essential

FIG. 52–1. Levels of Spinal Cord Injury. On the left, the vertebrae are designated as C (cervical), T (thoracic), and L (lumbar). The effects of spinal cord injury depend on the level of injury, as shown by the information under Function Present at the specific level. The most severely disabled patient has a lesion above level C6. (From Smeltzer, S.C. and Bare, B.G.: *Brunner and Suddarth's Textbook of Medical-Surgical Nursing,* 7th ed. Philadelphia, J.B. Lippincott Co., 1992, page 1739.)

sation or motor function below the level of the lesion.

2. *Incomplete Lesion.* Partial transection or injury of the spinal cord leaves some evidence of sensation or motor function below the level of the lesion. The sensation and motor function may return within a few hours after injury, and maximum return may occur in 6 months to 1 year.

B. Other Possible Effects

1. Impairment of voluntary bladder and bowel control.
2. Impairment of sexual function.
3. Impairment of vasomotor and body temperature regulatory mechanisms.

IV. SECONDARY COMPLICATIONS THAT MAY OCCUR[3,4]

Most of the complications described here do not occur in patients with lesions below the T6 level.

A. Respiratory Function

Respiratory difficulties may occur. During dental hygiene therapy, attention to patient position and continuous suction to keep passageways clear are vital. Some quadriplegic patients are unable to elicit a functional cough and need assistance. By placing manual pressure over the abdomen, below the diaphragm, after the patient has inhaled, the patient may be assisted while an attempt to cough is made.[3]

B. Tendency for Pressure Sores

A pressure sore (decubitus ulcer) is caused by pressure exerted on the skin and subcutaneous tissues by bony prominences and the object on which they rest, such as a mattress. The result is tissue anoxia or ischemia. The cutaneous tissue becomes broken or destroyed, thereby leading to destruction in the subcutaneous tissue. The ulcer that forms may be very slow to heal and may become infected by secondary bacterial invasion. Anemia and poor nutrition may also contribute.

Prevention of pressure can be accomplished by the use of padding and by regular turning of the patient. The dental chair can be positioned to prevent pressure. The patient may be asked to bring special padding to be used during the appointment, and also may be asked to provide instruction for the dental personnel so correct procedures can be followed.

C. Spasticity

As spinal shock subsides, muscle-reflex spasticity develops from a slight to a severe degree. Stimuli, such as pressure sores, infections, and sensory irritation, may bring on a spasm. Before dental hygiene treatment, the patient should be asked about susceptibility to spasms and to describe the procedure to follow should one occur.

D. Body Temperature

High-level quadriplegic patients are unable to regulate body temperature. A blanket may be needed in colder weather and air cooling during summer. When air conditioning is not available, the patient's temperature should be monitored. In the event of a rise in temperature, treatment should be postponed.

E. Vulnerability to Infection

Infections related to elimination, decubitus ulcer, and respiratory problems are the most common.

F. Autonomic Dysreflexia

1. *Definition.* Autonomic dysreflexia, or hyperreflexia, is a life-threatening *emergency* condition in which the blood pressure increases sharply. It may occur in patients with lesions at T6 or above, but not below that level. A variety of stimuli may precipitate dysreflexia, especially an irritation to the bowel or bladder.
2. *Symptoms*
   a. Increased blood pressure with slowed pulse rate. The blood pressure may rise to 300/160 mm Hg.
   b. Pounding headache.
   c. Flushing, chills, perspiration, stuffy nose.
   d. Restlessness; increased spasticity.
3. *Emergency Care*[3]
   a. Position chair upright gradually. Do NOT recline the chair, because increased blood pressure in the brain could result.
   b. Monitor the blood pressure.
   c. Call for medical aid.
   d. Check bladder distention and unclamp catheter.

V. PERSONAL FACTORS

The typical patient is a young man, possibly a former athlete. Depression and discouragement along with the pain and pressure of treatment and rehabilitation make psychiatric therapy necessary for many patients.

Physical and occupational therapists provide self-care training and preparation for discharge from the rehabilitation hospital. As much responsibility as possible is given the patient for personal care. Daily oral care, which at first may have been carried out by the nursing care staff, gradually should become a part of the daily hygiene routine accomplished by the patient, depending on the cord level of injury.

VI. DENTAL HYGIENE CARE

Emergency dental care may be needed during the patient's hospital period of recovery and treatment.

By the time the patient is able to be transported to a dental office or clinic, physical and psychologic preparation for daily living is at a stage where the patient has developed a stable routine.

Most of the information necessary for patient management and instruction is presented in Chapter 50. A few special considerations are described here.

A. Dental Chair Position

1. Wheelchair transfers (page 685).
2. Chair angle[3]
   a. For the patient with a gravity-drained urinary appliance, the chair may be adjusted to accommodate the drainage, or the patient should be uprighted at intervals to allow drainage to take place. The bag may require emptying during the appointment.
   b. The chair angle should not be changed abruptly because of the patient's susceptibility to postural hypotension.
   c. Change the patient's body position in the chair by lifting and turning at intervals to prevent pressure sores and pain in muscles and joints. The use of padding was mentioned earlier in this section.

B Four-handed Dental Hygiene

An assistant is a necessity. Precautions for the patient with spinal cord injury relate to the problems of respiration, pressure sores, spasms, autonomic dysreflexia, temperature control, and other factors that were described earlier. Assistance is definitely needed in many ways, including the following:

1. Assist in wheelchair transfer and in turning the patient at intervals.

tient's limitations must be recorded so that adaptations can be made during the appointment.

B. Child

1. *Learning Ability*
   a. Sensory defects often mask a child's intellectual capacity because responses cannot be the same as in other children.
   b. Blind children may learn to speak later than sighted children and may start school when they are a year or two older.
   c. A blind child takes longer than does the sighted child to cover the same amount of material; therefore, the educational level for the blind child may be different from that for the sighted child of the same chronologic age.
   d. Blind children are deprived of the opportunity to learn by imitation.
2. *Personal Factors.* Environment influences the child's adjustment, and parental attitude affects the blind child as it does the sighted child. When the parent is overindulgent and protective, the child may be self-centered, dependent, and emotionally less stable.

C. Adult

The adult who has always been blind or has been so since childhood has made adjustments and may be employed in a limited but useful occupation. The greater number of those who become blind after adulthood experience an immediate natural reaction of depression and feeling of helplessness.

When loss of vision is incipient, the reactions of shock and upheaval usually are less, but dread, worry, and anxiety may be experienced for years in anticipation. When the patient begins to accept the disability, efforts for rehabilitation are made easier, Independence and self-confidence should be developed, and the patient must be helped to avoid helplessness.

III. DENTAL HYGIENE CARE: TOTALLY BLIND
A. Factors in Patient Care

1. A blind person can perceive a new experience readily if told about it in detail.
2. Because of the visual disability, the patient must rely more on other senses and cultivate them.
3. A blind person must be neat and orderly. If something is put down, it must be located readily again.
4. A blind person does things deliberately and slowly to gain perception and prevent accidents.
5. Effective conversation with a blind person can best be accomplished by speaking as on a telephone.
6. A blind person learns to interpret and rely on tone of voice more than do persons with sight who can watch facial expressions.

B. Patient Reception and Seating

1. Lower dental chair prior to receiving patient; move other dental equipment, such as the bracket tray and clinician's stool, from pathway.
2. Guide to dental chair. Patient holds arm and is led without being pushed or pulled (figure 53–1).
3. Provide forewarnings of potential hazards in the pathway.
4. Instruct patient of step up to conventional dental chair.
5. The patient who has become familiar with office arrangement from previous appointments should be informed of changes to prevent embarrassment.
6. When leaving the treatment room during the appointment, explain absence; prevent embarrassment of patient speaking to someone who is not there; speak when re-entering the room.

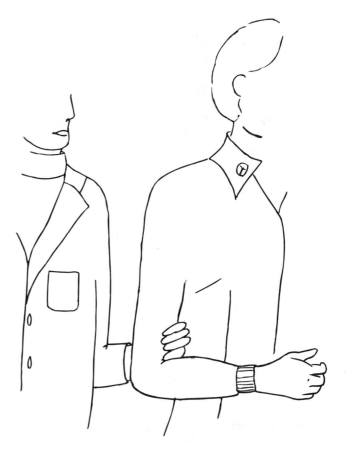

FIG. 53–1. Escorting a Blind Person. *The blind person holds the arm of the guide just above the elbow and walks beside and slightly behind. The guide verbally gives advance notice of approaching changes. The blind person can sense the body motion of the guide and anticipate changes.*

C. The Dog Guide

1. Do not distract a dog guide on duty by speaking to or touching it.
2. Ask the patient where the best place would be for the dog to stay during the appointment. The dogs are gentle, carefully trained animals, and may lie quietly in a corner of the treatment room as directed by the patient.

D. Introduce Clinical Procedures

1. Describe each step in detail before proceeding. Explain instruments, materials, and how each will be applied. Mention flavors.
2. Permit patient to handle instruments, such as a mouth mirror. This applies particularly to a child patient who is not familiar with dental procedures.
3. Use other instruments of a similar size and shape when describing scalers or explorers because handling sharp instruments would be dangerous for the patient.
4. Prepare patient for power-driven instruments.
   a. Avoid surprise applications of compressed air, water from syringe, or power-driven instruments.
   b. Apply moving rubber cup to child's finger. When power-driven instruments disturb the patient, a porte polisher may be used when stain removal is considered necessary.
5. Speak before touching the patient. By maintaining contact of a finger on a tooth or through retraction while changing instruments, repeated orientation can be avoided.
6. Rinsing
   a. Use evacuator when possible.
   b. Without evacuation, explain the water syringe and place rinsing cup in the patient's hand each time. Do not expect the patient to pick it up from unit.
   c. Help the patient avoid embarrassment if water is spilled.

E. Instructions for Patient

1. Give instructions clearly and concisely.
2. Visual aids, such as models, may be used if described in detail and given to the patient to handle.
3. Demonstrate toothbrushing in patient's mouth.

IV. DENTAL HYGIENE CARE: PARTIALLY SIGHTED

Persons with sight often underestimate the degree and fail to realize how useful a little vision can be. Patience in helping a patient to make full use of available vision, without oversolicitousness, is important. Although many of the procedures described for the totally blind person can be applied to the partially sighted person, a few additional hints are suggested here.

Elderly patients with failing sight rarely admit such an impairment. Sight failure in the aged individual or lowered vision in a person of any age may be suspected from the patient's unusual squinting, blinking, or lack of continued attention. Procedures can be adapted without mention of sight to the patient.

A. Patient Position

Adjust for patient comfort. Tilting back a patient with glaucoma may increase pain and pressure in the eyes.

B. Light

Avoid glare of the operating light in the patient's eyes. Sensitivity to light is characteristic of many eye conditions.

C. Patient Instruction

1. Position patient for best vision. For example, a patient with glaucoma has no peripheral vision; thus instruction should be given directly from the front.
2. Do not expect patient to see fine detail, such as that in a radiograph or on a small model.
3. Work patiently and give instruction slowly. Patient may have slow visual accomodation.
4. Present the patient's eyeglasses before beginning instruction.

HEARING IMPAIRMENT

When hearing is impaired to the extent that it has no practical value for the purpose of communication, a person is considered deaf. When hearing is defective but functional with or without a hearing aid, the terms "hard of hearing" or "hearing impaired" are used.

I. CAUSES OF HEARING IMPAIRMENT

The auditory system includes the anatomic parts from the outer ear to the termination of the auditory nerve in the brain. The cause of hearing loss may be associated with the outer, middle, or inner ear mechanisms, singly or in combinations.

Many factors may contribute to deafness. Heredity, prenatal infection in the mother, especially rubella, and birth trauma are significant in the earliest years. Chronic inner ear infections, infectious diseases (meningitis), trauma, and toxic effects of drugs have all been implicated.

II. TYPES OF HEARING LOSS

A. Conductive Hearing Loss

Outer or middle ear involvement of the conduction pathways to the inner ear.

B. Sensorineural Hearing Loss

Damage to the sensory hair cells of the inner ear or the nerves that supply the inner ear.

C. Mixed Hearing Loss

Combination of conductive and sensorineural.

D. Central Hearing Loss

Damage of the nerves or nuclei of the central nervous system in the brain or the pathways to the brain.

III. CHARACTERISTICS SUGGESTING HEARING IMPAIRMENT

Partial deafness may not have been diagnosed, or certain patients, particularly an elderly person, may not admit hearing limitation. Clues to the identification of a hearing problem are listed as follows.

A. Lack of attention; fails to respond to conversational tone.
B. Intentness; strained facial expression; stares at others.
C. Turns head to one side; hearing may be good on one side only.
D. Gives unexpected answer unrelated to question; does one thing when told to do another.
E. Frequently asks others to repeat what was said.
F. Unusual speech tone.

IV. HEARING AIDS

A hearing aid is an electronic device that amplifies and shapes sound waves that enter the external auditory canal. Current hearing aids are more technically advanced, more esthetic in their invisibility, and more commonly used. Standards for the manufacture and distribution of hearing aids are set by the U.S. Food and Drug Administration. A medical evaluation is required along with extensive audiologic testing.

Figure 53–2 shows 5 types of hearing aids that are available. The small units may be difficult to operate

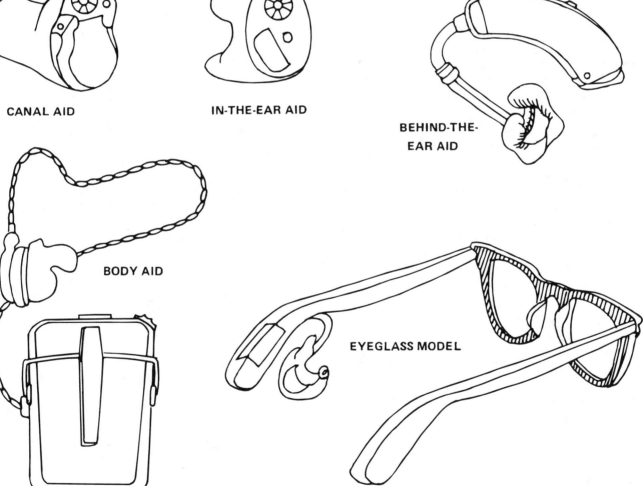

CANAL AID   IN-THE-EAR AID   BEHIND-THE-EAR AID

BODY AID   EYEGLASS MODEL

FIG. 53–2. Types of Hearing Aids. Hearing aids are electronic devices made with tiny controls to amplify sounds. The hearing aids may be able to fit over or inside the ear, connect to eyeglasses, or be fastened to clothing. (From Series 2: *The Ear and Hearing.* Gallaudet University, 1986. Used with permission.)

for people without finger dexterity. The aids are delicate and require special instruction for care.

A. Body Aid Model
The unit is in a case for carrying in a pocket or attaching to clothing.

B. Eyeglass Model
A thickened temple bar of the eyeglasses holds the essential parts, and the earmold is connected by a small tube.

C. Behind-the-Ear Model
The device hooks over the ear and contains tone controls.

D. In-the-Ear Model
Because the unit is practically invisible and lightweight, the in-the-ear model has been a frequent choice.

E. Canal Aid
This model fits entirely within the canal and is the most cosmetically acceptable of all types. It may take extra skill to adjust and remove.

V. MODES OF COMMUNICATION[2]
A person with a hearing loss may learn a particular way of personal communication. Choices include speaking, speechreading, writing, and manual communication. Manual communication includes using sign language or "signing" and fingerspelling.

A. Sign Language
The American manual alphabet is shown in figure 53–3.[3] A few examples of signs are shown in figure 53–4.

Although a universal sign language has not been recognized, many countries have their own. The British Sign Language (BSL), for example, has been in use for more than a century. Schools for the deaf have combined their teaching of spoken and written English with emphasis on use of residual hearing and lip-reading skills.[4]

B. Fingerspelling
Spelling "in the air" is often combined with sign language. Certain words cannot be readily signed, so spelling may be easier than stopping to write.

C. Oral Communication
Oral communication by a deaf person means a combination of some speech, residual hearing, and speechreading. The use of residual hearing is emphasized in the education of young deaf children.

D. Speechreading
Speechreading consists of recognizing spoken words by watching the lips, face, and gestures. Because many of the mouth movements for spoken words have the same appearance as one or more other words, speechreading may need to be combined with another method of communication.

VI. DENTAL HYGIENE CARE
Patients with hearing problems are of all ages; some have been deaf all their lives, and others lost their hearing later in life. Each has special problems. Determination of the mode of communication is an important step at the start.

When the patient's preferred mode of communication is sign language and the clinician does not know sign language, or when the patient lipreads but cannot read the clinician's lips, writing on a pad of paper may be the first choice. If an involved treatment plan must be reviewed or if other need for lengthy communication exists, and no family member is available to help, the services of a sign language interpreter may be necessary.

A. Patient with Hearing Aid
1. Be careful not to touch a hearing aid when it is operating.
2. Ask patient to turn off or remove a hearing aid when a power-driven dental instrument, particularly an ultrasonic scaler, will be used. The noise can be amplified many times, much to the discomfort of the patient.

B. Patient with Partial Hearing Ability
1. Speak clearly and distinctly; direct speaking to side of "good" ear, if hearing is impaired on one side only.
2. Eliminate interfering noises from street outside or from saliva ejector suction.

C. Speech Reader
1. Be sure patient is looking; do not turn to side; speak directly.
2. Speaker's face must be clearly visible so patient can read lips easily; difficult when dental light is directed to patient's face or the clinician has back to window.
3. Speak in normal tone; do not accentuate words; pause more frequently than usual.
4. Do not raise voice; raising voice can distort lip movements and make lipreading more difficult.
5. When patient cannot understand, use alternate words to express the same thought; many letters and combinations of letters look the same on the lips; others are not visible at all.
6. Keep calm; display of irritation or annoyance over difficulties in conversing discourages or upsets the patient.
7. Write proper names or unusual words the patient fails to understand.

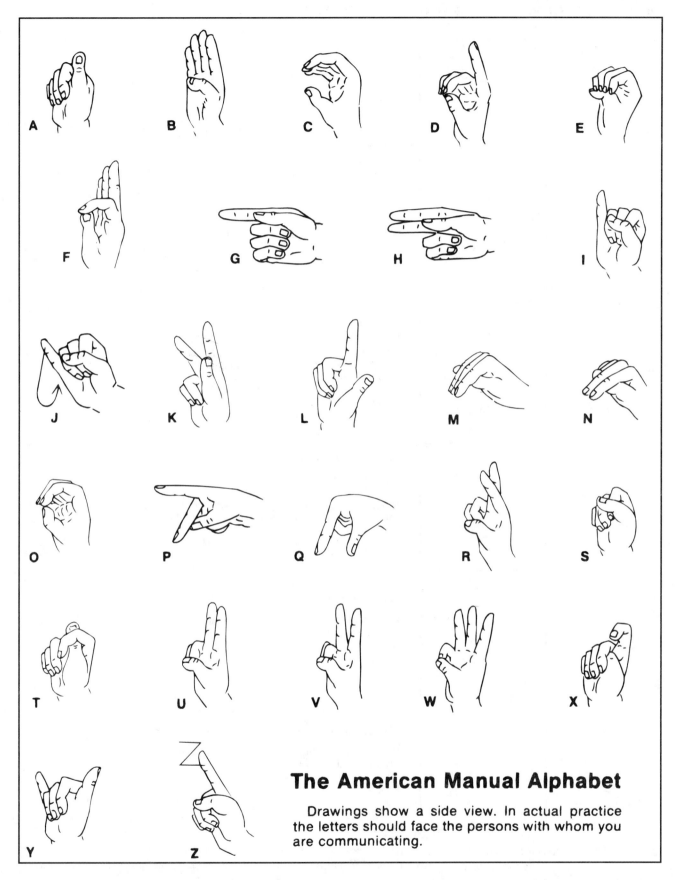

The American Manual Alphabet

Drawings show a side view. In actual practice the letters should face the persons with whom you are communicating.

FIG. 53–3. American Manual Alphabet. Fingerspelling is used in combination with signs and lip reading. (From Riekehof, L.L.: *The Joy of Signing*, Second Edition, Gospel Publishing House, Springfield, Missouri. Copyright 1987. Reproduced by permission.)

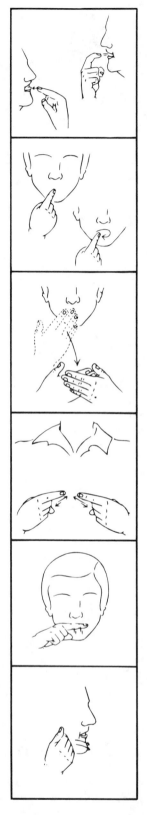

TEETH

Run the tip of the bent index finger across the teeth.
Usage: strong white *teeth*.

TONGUE

Touch the tip of the tongue with the index finger.
Usage: A look at your *tongue* tells the doctor something.

MOUTH

Point to the mouth.
Usage: The dentist looked into my *mouth*.

LIPS

Trace the lips with the index finger.
Usage: Your *lips* are easy to read.

GOOD, WELL

Touch the lips with the fingers of the right hand and then move the right hand forward placing it palm up in the palm of the left hand.
Origin: It has been tasted and smelled and offered as acceptable.
Usage: *good* food; doing *well* at work.

PAIN, ACHE, HURT

The index fingers are jabbed toward each other several times.
Note: This sign is generally made in front of the body but may be placed at the location of the pain, as: headache, toothache, heartache, etc.
Usage: suffered *pain* after the accident; *aching* all over; my knee *hurts*; have an *earache*.

TOOTHBRUSH

Using the index finger as a brush, imitate the motion of brushing the teeth.
Usage: *brushing teeth* twice a day.

DAILY, EVERY DAY

Place the side of the "A" hand on the cheek and rub it toward the chin several times.
Origin: Indicating several tomorrows.
Usage: *daily* bread.
     drive to work *every day*.

FIG. 53–4. Examples of Signing. Selected words that may be used during a patient's dental appointment. (From Riekehof, L.L.: *The Joy of Signing,* Second Edition, Gospel Publishing House, Springfield, Missouri. Copyright 1987. Reproduced by permission.)

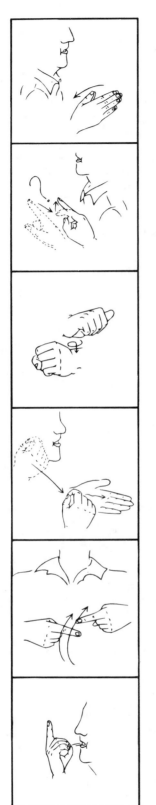

ASK, REQUEST

Place the open hands palm to palm and draw them toward the body.
Origin: Hands held as in prayer.
Usage: *Ask* for help. What is your *request?*

QUESTION

Draw a question mark in the air with the index finger; draw it back and direct it forward as if placing the dot below the question mark.
Usage: That *question* is hard to answer.

ENGAGEMENT, APPOINTMENT, RESERVATION

Make a small circle with the right "A" hand and then place the wrist on the wrist of the left "S" which is facing right.
Origin: Indicating one is bound.
Usage: a dinner *engagement* tonight.
a 4 o'clock *appointment.*
a plane *reservation.*

SECRETARY

Take an imaginary pencil from the ear, write into the left hand and make the "PERSON" ending.
Origin: A person who takes notes.
Usage: Teri is my good *secretary.*

COME

Index fingers rotating once around each other move toward the body. Or, use the open hand in a beckoning motion.
Origin: Using the hands in a natural motion.
Usage: When can you *come* to my home?
Come, I'm waiting for you. (Use second description.)

DENTIST

Place the right "D" at the teeth.
Origin: The initial sign at the teeth.
Usage: Let the *dentist* check your teeth.

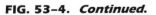

FIG. 53–4. *Continued.*

8. When wearing a mask, communication by writing notes is necessary.

D. Sign Language

All the points previously mentioned for the speech reader apply to patients who use sign language because lips are read along with signs.

E. General Suggestions

1. For written messages, use a clipboard with a marker-type pen attached and large paper, at least $8\frac{1}{2} \times 11$ inches. Write clearly.
2. Do not startle the patient by tapping to gain attention.
3. Plan in advance for a signal the patient can give to show reaction or discomfort.
4. Teach by demonstration
   a. Use mirror and show bacterial plaque removal methods directly on teeth.
   b. Younger child may be taught to rinse by watching and imitating.
   c. Provide reassurance and approval by maintaining eye contact and smiling.
5. Person with hearing loss should always have a written appointment card to assure complete understanding. Use the state TDD relay to call a deaf patient directly with appointment reminders.
6. Use judgment in prolonging conversation with deaf person. Certain patients are under tension and tire easily, whereas others enjoy the opportunity to communicate.

TECHNICAL HINTS

I. BASIC SKILLS
Learning basic sign language and finger spelling can provide health-care workers with an added skill.

II. SOURCES OF MATERIALS AND INFORMATION
American Foundation for the Blind
15 East 16th Street
New York, NY 10011
National Society to Prevent Blindness and Its Affiliates
79 Madison Avenue
New York, NY 10016
National Academy, Gallaudet University
800 Florida Avenue, N.E.
Washington, D.C. 20002
(Professional and Community Training Program)

REFERENCES

1. **Engar,** R.C. and Stiefel, D.J.: *Dental Treatment of the Sensory Impaired Patient.* Disability Dental Instruction, 4919 NE 86th Street, Seattle, WA 98115, 65 pp.
2. **National Information Center on Deafness and National Association of the Deaf:** *Deafness: A Fact Sheet.* Washington, D.C., Gallaudet University, 1989.
3. **Riekehof,** L.L.: *The Joy of Signing,* 2nd ed. Springfield, MO, Gospel Publishing House, 1987.
4. **Manley,** M.C.G., Leith, J., and Lewis, C.: Deafness and Dental Care, *Br. Dent. J., 161,* 219, September 20, 1986.

SUGGESTED READINGS

Brock, A.M.: Communicating with the Elderly Patient, *Spec. Care Dentist., 5,* 157, July–August, 1985.
Dahle, A.J., Wesson, M.D., and Thornton, J.B.: Dentistry and the Patient with Sensory Impairment, in Thornton, J.B. and Wright, J.T., eds.: *Special and Medically Compromised Patients in Dentistry.* Littleton, MA, PSG Publishing Co., 1989, pp. 63–72.
Kanar, H.L.: The Blind and the Deaf, in Nowak, A.J.: *Dentistry for the Handicapped Patient.* St. Louis, Mosby, 1976, pp. 121–133.
Lange, B.M., Entwistle, B.M., and Lipson, L.F.: *Dental Management of the Handicapped: Approaches for Dental Auxiliaries.* Philadelphia, Lea & Febiger, 1983, pp. 11–38.

Hearing Impairment
Graves, C.E. and Portnoy, E.J.: Identifying Hearing Impairment among Older Adults, *J. Dent. Hyg., 65,* 138, March–April, 1991.
Hollingsworth, R.A.: Sign for the Times, *RDH, 12,* 40, June, 1992.
Merrell, H.B. and Claggett, K.: Noise Pollution and Hearing Loss in the Dental Office, *Dent. Assist., 61,* 6, Third Quarter, 1992.
Nadol, J.B.: Hearing Loss, *N. Engl. J. Med., 329,* 1092, October 7, 1993.
O'Brien, S.: A Special Challenge, *RDH, 9,* 18, March, 1989.
Zazove, P. and Kileny, P.R.: Devices for the Hearing Impaired, *Am. Fam. Physician, 46,* 851, September, 1992.

Visual Impairment
Cohen, S., Sarnat, H., and Shalgi, G.: The Role of Instruction and a Brushing Device on the Oral Hygiene of Blind Children, *Clin. Prev. Dent., 13,* 8, July–August, 1991.
Hunter, L.H.: "The Way We See It"—Dental Health for the Visually Handicapped, *Dental Health (London), 27,* 3, June/July, 1988.
O'Donnell, D.: The Prevalence of Nonrepaired Fractured Incisors in Visually Impaired Chinese Children and Young Adults in Hong Kong, *Quintessence Int., 23,* 363, May, 1992.
O'Donnell, D. and Crosswaite, M.A.: Dental Health Education for the Visually Impaired Child, *Dent. Health (London), 30,* 8, February/March, 1991.
Schein, J.: Keeping an Eye on Your Vision, *RDH, 9,* 28, August, 1989.

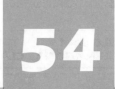

The Patient with Epilepsy

Epilepsy is not a disease entity, but is rather a term used to describe a symptom or group of symptoms of disordered function of the central nervous system. A person with epilepsy may be susceptible to recurrent involuntary loss of consciousness or awareness with or without convulsive movements or spasms. Some patients may have convulsions without loss of consciousness.

The patient's medical history should reveal a susceptibility to seizures, and the physician must be contacted when additional information other than that provided by the patient is required. The well-controlled patient who is under anticonvulsant medication usually presents no specific problems. An uncontrolled patient may require special treatment. A knowledge of symptoms is important in all cases, and dental personnel should know and be able to apply emergency measures in or out of the dental office.

Care of the oral cavity becomes important for its relationship both to general health and to oral accidents that may occur during a severe attack. All patients are advised by their physicians to live a moderate life-style and pay strict attention to general health rules.

Occupation may be limited because the person with epilepsy cannot be permitted to participate in activities that provide hazards in the event of a seizure. Such limitation is particularly depressing to adults who acquire epilepsy after reaching the working age and thus may be required to change their vocation.

DESCRIPTION[1,2,3]

A seizure is a convulsive disorder that results from a transient, uncontrolled alteration in brain function.

The effect is an abrupt onset of symptoms that may be of a motor, sensory, or psychic nature, depending on which brain cells are involved.

I. TYPES OF SEIZURES

The two basic types of seizures are *generalized* and *partial*. The international classification of seizures is outlined in table 54–1.

A seizure that is focal in origin and involves only a part of the brain is called a partial seizure. A generalized seizure, on the other hand, is not specific in area of origin and affects the entire brain at the same time. Terminology used in table 54–1 and in the study of seizures is defined in table 54–2.

II. ETIOLOGY OF SEIZURES[3]

In addition to epilepsy, seizures can be a symptom of many different conditions from birth throughout life. During infancy, seizures can be related to maternal infection (rubella), birth injury, or congenital abnormalities, whereas in older children, additional causes include trauma, infections, toxins, and cerebral degenerative diseases. In middle age and older, vascular disease and tumors are added to the list.

The causes can be divided into primary and secondary.

A. Primary (Idiopathic) Epilepsy

Genetic predisposition to seizures or to other neurologic abnormalities for which seizure may be a symptom.

B. Secondary (Symptomatic) Epilepsy

1. Congenital conditions, such as maternal infection (rubella).
2. Perinatal injuries.
3. Brain tumor.

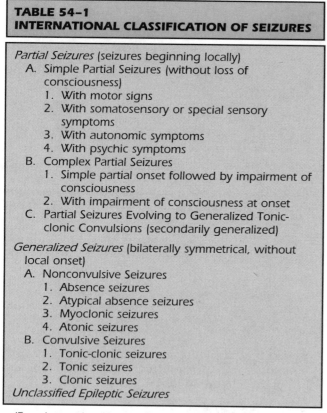

(From International League Against Epilepsy, Commission on Classification and Terminology: Proposal for Revised Clinical and Electroencephalographic Classification of Epileptic Seizures, *Epilepsia, 22,* 489, August, 1981.)

4. Trauma (head injury).
5. Infection (meningitis, encephalitis).
6. Degenerative brain disease.
7. Metabolic and toxic disorders, including alcoholism and drug addiction; seizures are common during drug withdrawal.

C. Potential Causes of Emergency

In dental and dental hygiene practice, seizures that may be most likely to require emergency procedures are caused by:[3]
1. Epilepsy.
2. Hypoglycemia.
3. Anoxia/hypoxia secondary to syncope.
4. Local anesthetic overdose (page 846).

CLINICAL MANIFESTATIONS

I. POSSIBLE PRECIPITATING FACTORS

A. Psychologic stress; apprehension.
B. Fatigue; sleep deprivation.
C. Sensory stimuli, such as flashing lights, noises, peculiar odors.
D. Alcohol use; withdrawal from alcohol or other substances.

TABLE 54–1
INTERNATIONAL CLASSIFICATION OF SEIZURES

Partial Seizures (seizures beginning locally)
A. Simple Partial Seizures (without loss of consciousness)
  1. With motor signs
  2. With somatosensory or special sensory symptoms
  3. With autonomic symptoms
  4. With psychic symptoms
B. Complex Partial Seizures
  1. Simple partial onset followed by impairment of consciousness
  2. With impairment of consciousness at onset
C. Partial Seizures Evolving to Generalized Tonic-clonic Convulsions (secondarily generalized)

Generalized Seizures (bilaterally symmetrical, without local onset)
A. Nonconvulsive Seizures
  1. Absence seizures
  2. Atypical absence seizures
  3. Myoclonic seizures
  4. Atonic seizures
B. Convulsive Seizures
  1. Tonic-clonic seizures
  2. Tonic seizures
  3. Clonic seizures
Unclassified Epileptic Seizures

TABLE 54–2
KEY WORDS: SEIZURES

Absence: a generalized seizure of sudden onset characterized by a brief period of unconsciousness. Formerly called **petit mal.**

Ataxia (ah-tak′sē-ah): failure of muscular coordination; irregularity of muscular action.

Atonic: relaxed; without normal tone or tension.

Aura (aw′rah): warning sensation felt by some people immediately preceding a seizure; may be flashes of light, dizziness, peculiar taste, or a sensation of prickling or tingling.

Automatism (aw-tōm′ah-tizm): involuntary motor activity, such as lip smacking or repeated swallowing.

Autonomic symptoms: pallor, flushing, sweating, pupillary dilation, cardiac arrhythmia, incontinence.

Clonic: alternate contraction and relaxation of muscle; **clonic phase** is the convulsion phase of a seizure.

Consciousness: degree of awareness and/or responsiveness of a person to externally applied stimuli.

Convulsion: violent spasm.

Cryptogenic (krĭp′tō-jen′ik): a disorder for which the cause is hidden or occult.

Electroencephalography (e-lek′trō-en-sef′ah-log′rah-fē): the recording of changes in electric potentials in various areas of the brain by means of electrodes placed on the scalp or on/in the brain itself and connected to a vacuum-tube radio amplifier that amplifies the impulses more than a million times; the impulses move an electromagnetic pen that records the brain waves; a clinical test used for partial diagnosis of epilepsy.

Grand mal (grahn mahl): former name for a generalized or major seizure as contrasted with **petit mal** (pĕ-tē′mahl), a minor or relatively mild seizure.

Ictal (ik′tal): pertaining to or resulting from a stroke or an acute epileptic seizure.

Myoclonus (mi′ŏk-lō′nus): isolated or repetitive shock-like contractions of a muscle or group of muscles; *adj.* myoclonic.

Paresthesia (par′es-thē′zē-ah): an abnormal sensation, such as burning, prickling, or tingling.

Paroxysm (par′ok-sizm): sharp spasm or convulsion; sudden recurrence or intensification of symptoms.

Prodrome (prō′drōm): a premonitory symptom; a symptom indicating the onset of a disease or condition; *adj.* prodromal.

Psychic (sī′kik): pertaining to the mind or psyche.

Seizure (sē′zhur): paroxysmal spell of transitory alteration in consciousness, motor activity, or sensory phenomenon; convulsion.

Spasm (spazm): sudden involuntary contraction of a muscle or group of muscles; may be tonic or clonic; may vary from small twitches to severe convulsions.

Status epilepticus (sta′tus ĕp′ĭ-lĕp′tĭ cus): rapid succession of epileptic spasms without intervals of consciousness; life threatening; emergency care urgent.

Tonic (ton′ik): state of continuous, unremitting action of muscular contraction; patient appears stiff.

Tonic-clonic: in a seizure, a sudden sharp tonic contraction of muscles followed by clonic convulsive movements.

II. AURA

Not all patients have a warning, or aura, before a seizure. A patient with a warning may seek a safe place to sit or lie down in privacy. In the dental environment, the patient can inform the personnel, so that procedures can be terminated and brief preparations made.

The aura may be a special sensory stimulus, a sensation of numbness, tingling, or a twitching or stiffness of certain muscles.

III. PARTIAL SEIZURES

A. Simple

Seizures may include a brief staring spell, a shake of a finger or hand, and/or a jerk of muscles about the mouth. Although dizziness and jumbled speech may occur, loss of consciousness does not result.

B. Complex

1. Trance-like state with confusion lasts usually for a few minutes, sometimes for hours.
2. Consciousness is impaired to varying degrees.
3. Patient may manifest purposeless movements or actions followed by confusion, incoherent speech, ill humor, bad temper; does not remember what happened during the attack.

IV. GENERALIZED ABSENCE

A. Loss of consciousness for 5 to 30 seconds.
B. Patient usually does not fall; posture becomes fixed; may drop whatever is being held.
C. May become pale.
D. May have rhythmic twitching of eyelids, eyebrows, or head.
E. Attack ends as abruptly as it begins. Patient resumes activities; may or may not be aware of attack.

V. GENERALIZED TONIC-CLONIC

A. Loss of consciousness is sudden and complete; the patient falls. A patient may slide out of the dental chair.
B. The entire voluntary musculature experiences continuous contraction, which is the *tonic* (tension with rigidity) phase. The *clonic* movements follow, with intermittent muscular contraction and relaxation.
C. Muscles of the chest and pharynx may contract at the same time, thus forcing air out. The result is a peculiar sound known as the "epileptic cry."
D. Color is pale at first; then the superficial veins become gorged. The chest becomes fixed and aeration of blood ceases, leading to cyanosis of the face.
E. Pupils dilate.
F. Intermittent muscular contractions follow, rapidly at first, then less frequently. If the tongue is between the teeth, it may be bitten.

G. The incident lasts from 1 to 3 minutes; the bladder, and rarely the rectum, may be emptied.
H. Respiration begins to return. Saliva, which previously could not be swallowed, may become mixed with air and appear as foam.
I. Postconvulsive coma is characterized by fixed or sluggish pupils, noisy respiration, profuse perspiration, cyanosed lips, and complete relaxation of body muscles.
J. Patient emerges in a cloudy state.
K. Postconvulsive phase includes headache, muscle aches, and drowsiness. Patient usually falls into a deep sleep.

VI. TREATMENT

Anticonvulsant drugs are used to prevent seizures.[4,5] The most frequently prescribed medications for generalized tonic-clonic seizures are phenytoin, carbamazepine, valproic acid, phenobarbital sodium, and primidone. Each has its own side effects.

Patients whose epilepsy is caused by a brain tumor undergo surgery for tumor removal. Anticonvulsant medication is usually necessary following the surgery.

In addition to medication, patients frequently need psychologic or psychiatric support therapy to aid in coping with problems during rehabilitation. Psychologic stress may increase the frequency of seizures.

ORAL FINDINGS

Epilepsy in itself produces no oral changes. Specific effects relate to anticonvulsant therapy using phenytoin and to the results of oral accidents during seizures.

I. GINGIVAL MANIFESTATION

Phenytoin-induced gingival overgrowth occurs in 25 to 50% of persons using phenytoin for treatment. The condition occurs more frequently in institutionalized than in noninstitutionalized populations. No other anticonvulsant drug produces such an unusual side effect. Other drugs that produce a similar gingival enlargement are described on page 203.

Phenytoin has been used in the treatment of many conditions other than epilepsy. These include behavior problems, stuttering, headaches, neuromuscular disturbances, and cardiac conditions. The presence of gingival enlargement and a history of phenytoin use should not lead to the assumption that the patient has epilepsy.

II. EFFECTS OF ACCIDENTS DURING SEIZURES

A. Scars of Lips and Tongue

During generalized tonic-clonic seizures, the oral tissues, particularly tongue, cheek, or lip, may be bitten. Scars may be observed during the extraoral/intraoral examination, and the cause may be differentiated from other types of healed wounds.

B. Fractured Teeth

During the tonic and clonic movements, the teeth may be clamped and bruxing may be forceful enough to fracture teeth.

PHENYTOIN-INDUCED GINGIVAL ENLARGEMENT (OVERGROWTH)

Gingival enlargement is one of several side effects from treatment with phenytoin. The condition is also called Dilantin hyperplasia, Dilantin-induced hyperplasia, diphenylhydantoin-induced hyperplasia, diphenylhydantoin gingival hyperplasia, Dilantin-induced gingival fibrosis, and phenytoin-induced hyperplasia.

I. SIDE EFFECTS OF PHENYTOIN

In addition to gingival overgrowth, other long-term side effects may influence dental hygiene appointments. During history preparation and the extraoral/intraoral examination, the effects described as follows can aid in understanding the patient and planning treatment.

A. General Effects that May Occur[6]

Drowsiness, gastric distress, skin rash, ataxia, and restlessness are not uncommon. Increased growth of body and facial hair may occur in women.

B. Nutritional Influences

Vitamins K, D, and folic acid are affected by anticonvulsant drugs. A megaloblastic anemia can result from a low folic acid blood level, which is described on page 808. Epithelial changes, such as glossitis, angular cheilitis, and ulcerations of the lips, tongue, and buccal mucosa, may be observed.[7,8]

C. Fetal Hydantoin Syndrome[6,9]

Children of women receiving anticonvulsant therapy during pregnancy are more susceptible to malformations. They may have craniofacial abnormalities, growth retardation, mental deficiency, congenital heart defects, and cleft lip and/or palate.

II. OCCURRENCE[10]

A. Age

Incidence is greater in younger patients than in older patients just beginning therapy.

B. Initial Enlargement

The gingiva may start to enlarge within a few weeks or even after a few years following the initial administration of the drug.

C. Dosage and Length of Treatment

The size of the dose and the length of treatment are not necessarily factors in the incidence or nature of the gingival enlargement.

D. Sites

The anterior gingiva are usually more affected than are the posterior, and the maxillary more than the mandibular. Facial and proximal areas are usually larger than lingual and palatal areas.

E. Edentulous Areas

Although rare, an overgrowth of tissue may occur in an edentulous area. A source of trauma, irritation from a denture, or the presence of a dental implant, retained roots, or unerupted teeth usually have been associated with the overgrowth.[11,12]

III. TISSUE CHARACTERISTICS

A. Early Clinical Features

The overgrowth appears as a painless enlargement of interdental papillae with signs of inflammation. Eventually, the tissue becomes fibrotic, pink, and stippled, with a mulberry- or cauliflower-like appearance (figure 54–1B).

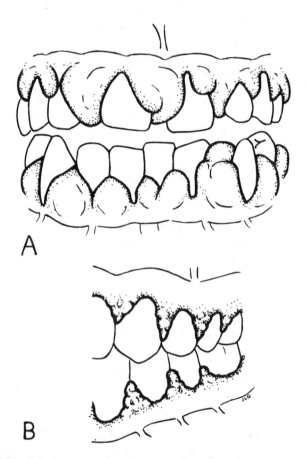

FIG. 54–1. Phenytoin-induced Gingival Enlargement. A. Papillary enlargement with cleft-like grooves. Note the effect of the pressure of the fibrotic tissue on the position of teeth. Maxillary incisors and the mandibular left canine have been wedged away from normal positions. **B.** Mulberry-like shape of interdental papillae.

B. Advanced Lesion

With time, the tissue increases in size, extends to include the marginal gingiva, and covers a large portion of the anatomic crown. Often, cleft-like grooves are between the lobules (figure 54–1A).

C. Severe Lesion

Large, bulbous gingiva may cover the enamel, tend to wedge the teeth apart, and interfere with mastication. Note the severe growth about the mandibular left canine in figure 54–1A.

D. Microscopic Appearance

During therapy, phenytoin is present in the saliva, blood, gingival sulcus fluid, and bacterial plaque. The number of fibroblasts and the amount of collagen in the tissue are increased. The stratified squamous epithelium is thick, with long rete pegs. Inflammatory cells are in greatest abundance near the base of the pockets.

IV. COMPLICATING FACTORS
A. Plaque and Gingivitis

Adequate plaque control, particularly if started before the administration of phenytoin, may decrease the extent of gingival overgrowth.[10,13,14] Application of antiplaque agents (stannous fluoride,[15] chlorhexidine[16]) has been effective in decreasing bacterial plaque formation and gingival overgrowth.

B. Other Contributing Factors

Mouth breathing, overhanging and other defective restorations, large carious lesions, calculus, and other plaque-retaining factors encourage gingival overgrowth. Treatment must include removal of overhangs and calculus and restoration of carious lesions.

V. TREATMENT OF PHENYTOIN-INDUCED GINGIVAL OVERGROWTH
A. Conservative Treatment

Scaling with a concentrated program of bacterial plaque control may help early lesions to regress. Once the tissue has become fibrotic, however, shrinkage cannot be expected.

A program of prevention and control should be started prior to, or simultaneously with, the initial administration of phenytoin.

B. Change in Drug Prescription

Phenytoin alone or with phenobarbital has been a drug of choice for use with patients subject to generalized seizures since the drug was introduced in 1938. Other drugs in current use do not induce gingival enlargement. When the patient has a severe problem and is faced with embarrassment and social problems because of the appearance of the gingiva, the physician could be approached concerning the possibility of changing the prescription to a different drug. If possible, such a change should be made just prior to gingivectomy or other surgical removal procedure that may be planned.

C. Surgical Removal

Assuming a sufficient band of attached gingiva exists, one surgical procedure that has been used for tissue removal has been gingivectomy. Prior to surgery, a regulated program of plaque control should be introduced and continued as soon as surgical dressings have been removed.[13]

DENTAL HYGIENE CARE

For the patient with epilepsy, general health has special significance, and oral health contributes to general health. For the patient with phenytoin-induced gingival enlargement, emphasis in appointments is on a rigid oral hygiene program if the gingival enlargement is to be kept to a minimum.

I. PATIENT HISTORY

Except in an unusual situation, most patients with epilepsy have had a thorough medical examination prior to the dental appointment. In preparing the patient history, however, all patients should be asked whether they ever had a seizure or currently have recurrent or occasional seizures. When the answer is positive, additional questioning is indicated.

A. History of Seizures

Questioning includes type, frequency, severity, and duration of episodes. The precipitating factors, need for any special premedication, and all information that may have application during the dental and dental hygiene appointments must be carefully documented.

B. Medications

The type, dosage, effectiveness in seizure control, and known side effects of medication are recorded. Patients using valproic acid may be subject to blood coagulation defects and should be questioned concerning bleeding and ease of bruising.[17] Prior to deep scaling or surgical procedures, when bleeding can be expected, blood testing for platelet count and bleeding time provides important information for the prevention of an emergency situation.

II. PATIENT APPROACH
A. Provide a calm, reassuring atmosphere.
B. Treat with patience and empathy; avoid oversolicitousness.
C. Encourage self-expression, particularly if the patient tends to be quiet and withdrawn and has narrowed interests.
D. Recognize possible impairment of memory when reviewing personal oral care procedures.
E. Help patient to develop interest in caring for the mouth; commend all little successes.

F. Drugs used in treatment tend to make patient drowsy.
   1. Be understanding when patient is late or misses an appointment.
   2. Plan telephone reminder at opportune time if patient is chronically late.
   3. Do not mistake drowsiness (effect of drugs) for inattentiveness.

III. TREATMENT PLAN: INSTRUMENTATION

The treatment needs of a patient with phenytoin-induced gingival enlargement were described earlier. The dental hygiene treatment, planned within the total treatment plan, is determined by whether the patient is just starting phenytoin therapy or, if already receiving phenytoin, by the severity of the gingival enlargement.

A. Prior to and at the Start of Phenytoin Therapy

A rigorous plaque control program and complete scaling are introduced in preparation for phenytoin therapy. The patient (and parents) must understand that, with controlled oral hygiene and emphasis on all phases of prevention, gingival enlargement can be prevented to a large degree.[13,14,15]

B. Initial Appointment Series for Patient Treated with Phenytoin

Weekly appointments for complete plaque control instruction and scaling are planned with the following objectives:

1. *Slight or Mild Gingival Overgrowth.* Conservative treatment, including frequent thorough scalings, can be expected to lead to tissue reduction, provided the patient cooperates in daily plaque control. Frequent maintenance appointments can contribute to function and comfort with minimum periodontal involvement.

2. *Moderate Gingival Overgrowth.* After the initial series of weekly plaque instruction and scalings, re-evaluation of the tissue can determine whether further procedures are needed. An optimum level of oral health may be attained by changing the medication to another anticonvulsant drug, using surgical pocket removal, and continuing frequent maintenance appointments.

3. *Severe Fibrotic Overgrowth.* Initial scaling and plaque control are carried out to prepare the mouth for surgical pocket removal. Plans for changing the drug or altering the dose should be discussed with the patient's physician.

C. Maintenance Appointment Intervals

Frequent appointments on a 1-, 2- or 3-month plan are indicated, depending on the severity of the gingival enlargement and the ability and motivation of the patient to maintain the oral health. Most patients need continuing assistance and supervision, and their response is influenced by the instruction and devotion of the dental personnel.

IV. TREATMENT PLAN: PREVENTION

Daily plaque removal and fluoride therapy, the use of pit and fissure sealants, and dietary control all have a vital part in the care of the patient with a convulsive disorder. Initiation of preventive measures as soon as possible after the disorder has been diagnosed can contribute to the total health and well-being of the patient.

EMERGENCY CARE[3]

When a seizure occurs, no attempt should be made to stop the convulsion or to restrain the patient. An outline for procedure appears in table 61–3 on page 846. Some additional suggestions regarding patient care during a generalized seizure that are applicable in a dental office are included here.

I. OBJECTIVES

A. To prevent body injury.
B. To prevent accidents related to the oral structures, such as:
   1. Tongue bite.
   2. Broken or dislocated teeth.
   3. Dislocated or fractured jaw.
   4. Broken fixed or removable dentures.
C. To assure adequate ventilation.

II. PREPARATION FOR APPOINTMENT

When the patient's medical history indicates epilepsy, precautions may prevent complications should a seizure occur.

A. Put emergency materials in a convenient place.
B. Have patient remove dentures for duration of appointment.
C. Provide a calm and reassuring atmosphere.
D. Have other dental personnel available in case of an emergency.

III. EMERGENCY PROCEDURE (Figure 54–2)

The dental clinic or office team has assigned responsibilities during any emergency as described in Chapter 61 and outlined in Figures 61–2 and 61–3 on pages 833–834. Initiation of procedure for seizure emergency follows the usual practice.

A. Terminate procedure; call for assistance; place medical emergency call.
B. Position patient; lower chair and tilt to supine; raise feet.
C. Push aside movable equipment and instrument trays.
D. Loosen tight belt, collar, necktie.

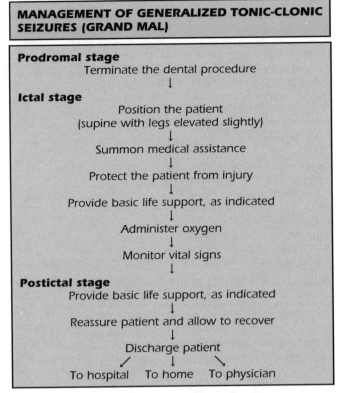

FIG. 54–2. Emergency Procedure During a Seizure. (From Malamed, S.F.: *Medical Emergencies in the Dental Office*, 4th ed. St. Louis, Mosby, 1993, page 295.)

E. DO NOT place (or force) anything between the teeth.

F. Establish airway; check for breathing obstruction; provide basic life support when indicated.

G. Monitor vital signs.

H. Stay beside patient to prevent personal injury.

IV. POSTICTAL PHASE

A. Complete the *Record of Emergency* (figure 61–1, page 831).

B. Allow patient to rest.

C. Talk to patient in a low, reassuring tone. Ask onlookers to leave the patient in privacy.

D. Check oral cavity for trauma to teeth or tissues. Palliative care can be administered. When a tooth is broken, the piece must be located so that aspiration can be prevented.

TECHNICAL HINTS

I. Never use a glass syringe or other breakable instrument when a seizure could occur.

II. When a patient vomits during a seizure, use high-power evacuator with wide tip to remove material from the mouth as a first aid measure against aspiration of vomitus into the airway.

REFERENCES

1. **International League Against Epilepsy,** Commission on Classification and Terminology: Proposal for Revised Clinical and Electroencephalographic Classification of Epileptic Seizures, *Epilepsia, 22,* 489, August, 1981.

2. **International League Against Epilepsy,** Commission on Classification and Terminology: Proposal for Revised Classification of Epilepsies and Epileptic Syndromes, *Epilepsia, 30,* 389, July/August, 1989.

3. **Malamed,** S.F.: *Handbook of Medical Emergencies in the Dental Office,* 4th ed. St. Louis, Mosby, 1993, p. 279–298.

4. **Scheuer,** M.L. and Pedley, T.A.: The Evaluation and Treatment of Seizures, *N. Engl. J. Med., 323,* 1468, November 22, 1990.

5. **Bruni,** J.: Epilepsy in Adolescents and Adults, in Rakel, R.E., ed.: *Conn's Current Therapy.* Philadelphia, W.B. Saunders Co., 1993, pp. 851–860.

6. **Felpel,** L.P.: Anticonvulsants, in Neidle, E.A. and Yagiela, J.A.: *Pharmacology and Therapeutics for Dentistry,* 3rd ed. St. Louis, Mosby, 1989, pp. 208–218.

7. **Mallek,** H.M. and Nakamoto, T.: Dilantin and Folic Acid Status. Clinical Implications for the Periodontist, *J. Periodontol., 52,* 255, May, 1981.

8. **Poppell,** T.D., Keeling, S.D., Collins, J.F., and Hassell, T.M.: Effect of Folic Acid on Recurrence of Phenytoin-induced Gingival Overgrowth Following Gingivectomy, *J. Clin. Periodontol., 18,* 134, February, 1991.

9. **Delgado-Escueta,** A.V. and Janz, D.: Consensus Guidelines: Preconception Counseling, Management, and Care of the Pregnant Woman with Epilepsy, *Neurology, 42,* 149, Supplement 5, April, 1992.

10. **Hassell,** T.M.: *Epilepsy and the Oral Manifestations of Phenytoin Therapy.* Monographs in Oral Science, Volume 9. London, S. Karger, 1981, pp. 116–127.

11. **Bredfeldt,** G.W.: Phenytoin-induced Hyperplasia Found in Edentulous Patients, *J. Am. Dent. Assoc., 123,* 61, June, 1992.

12. **McCord,** J.F., Sloan, P., and Hussey, D.J.: Phenytoin Hyperplasia Occurring under Complete Dentures: A Clinical Report, *J. Prosthet. Dent., 68,* 569, October, 1992.

13. **Pihlstrom,** B.L.: Prevention and Treatment of Dilantin-associated Gingival Enlargement, *Compendium, 11,* S506, Supplement 14, 1990.

14. **Allen,** S.: The Role of the Dental Hygienist in the Prevention, Control and Treatment of Dilantin Hyperplasia, *Can. Dent. Hyg./ Probe, 20,* 139, December, 1986.

15. **Steinberg,** S.C and Steinberg, A.D.: Phenytoin-induced Gingival Overgrowth Control in Severely Retarded Children, *J. Periodontol., 53,* 429, July, 1982.

16. **O'Neil,** T.C.A. and Figures, K.H.: The Effects of Chlorhexidine and Mechanical Methods of Plaque Control on the Recurrence of Gingival Hyperplasia in Young Patients Taking Phenytoin, *Br. Dent. J., 152,* 130, February 16, 1982.

17. **Hassell,** T.M., White, G.C., Jewson, L.G., and Peele, L.C.: Valproic Acid: A New Antiepileptic Drug with Potential Side Effects of Dental Concern, *J. Am. Dent. Assoc., 99,* 983, December, 1979.

SUGGESTED READINGS

Buehler, B.A., Delimont, D., van Waes, M., and Finnell, R.H.: Prenatal Prediction of Risk of the Fetal Hydantoin Syndrome, *N. Engl. J. Med., 322,* 1567, May 31, 1990.

Hansotia, P. and Broste, S.K.: The Effect of Epilepsy or Diabetes Mellitus on the Risk of Automobile Accidents, *N. Engl. J. Med., 324,* 22, January 3, 1991.

Hecht, J.T. and Annegers, J.F.: Familial Aggregation of Epilepsy and Clefting Disorders: A Review of the Literature, *Epilepsia, 31,* 574, September–October, 1990.

Leppik, I.E.: Antiepileptic Medications, *Compendium, 11,* S490, Supplement 14, 1990.

Pellock, J.M., ed.: Seizure Disorders, *Pediatr. Clin. North Am., 36,* 265–460, April, 1989.

Rosa, F.W.: Spina Bifida in Infants of Women Treated with Carbamazepine During Pregnancy, *N. Engl. J. Med., 324,* 674, March 7, 1991.

Schraeder, P.L.: The Risks of Having Epilepsy, *Compendium, 11,* S497, Supplement 14, 1990.

Yerby, M.S., Leavitt, A., Erickson, D.M., McCormick, K.B., Loewenson, R.B., Sells, C.J., and Benedetti, T.J.: Antiepileptics and the Development of Congenital Anomalies, *Neurology, 42,* 132, Supplement 5, April, 1992.

Phenytoin-induced Gingival Enlargement

Brown, R.S., Beaver, W.T., and Bottomley, W.K.: On the Mechanism of Drug-induced Gingival Hyperplasia, *J. Oral Pathol. Med., 20,* 201, May, 1991.

Brown, R.S., DiStanislao, P.T., Beaver, W.T., and Bottomley, W.K.: The Administration of Folic Acid to Institutionalized Epileptic Adults with Phenytoin-induced Gingival Hyperplasia. A Double-blind, Randomized, Placebo-controlled, Parallel Study, *Oral Surg. Oral Med. Oral Pathol., 71,* 565, May, 1991.

Dahllöf, G., Axiö, E., and Modéer, T.: Regression of Phenytoin-induced Gingival Overgrowth after Withdrawal of Medication, *Swed. Dent. J., 15,* 139, No. 3, 1991.

Fitchie, J.G., Comer, R.W., Hanes, P.J., and Reeves, G.W.: The Reduction of Phenytoin-induced Gingival Overgrowth in a Severely Disabled Patient: A Case Report, *Compendium, 10,* 314, June, 1989.

Hall, W.B.: Dilantin Hyperplasia: A Preventable Lesion? *Compendium, 11,* S502, Supplement 14, 1990.

Hassell, T.M., Harris, E.L., Boughman, J.A., and Cockey, G.C.: Gingival Overgrowth: Hereditary Considerations, *Compendium, 11,* S511, Supplement 14, 1990.

Jones, J.E., Weddell, J.A., and McKown, C.G.: Incidence and Indcations for Surgical Management of Phenytoin-induced Gingival Overgrowth in a Cerebral Palsy Population, *J. Oral Maxillofac. Surg., 46,* 385, May, 1988.

Natelli, A.A.: Phenytoin-induced Gingival Overgrowth: A Case Report, *Compendium, 13,* 786, September, 1992.

Penarrocha-Diago, M., Bagán-Sebastián, J.V., and Vera-Sempere, F.: Diphenylhydantoin-induced Gingival Overgrowth in Man: A Clinico-pathological Study. *J. Periodontol., 61,* 571, September, 1990.

Thomason, J.M., Seymour, R.A., and Rawlins, M.D.: Incidence and Severity of Phenytoin-induced Gingival Overgrowth in Epileptic Patients in General Medical Practice, *Community Dent. Oral Epidemiol., 20,* 288, October, 1992.

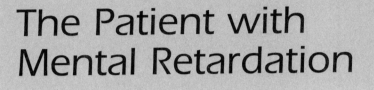

The Patient with Mental Retardation

With trends toward deinstitutionalization and emphasis on special training and education in local agencies and schools, more people with mild and moderate mental retardation have appeared in private dental offices and clinics, as well as in school and community dental facilities. Opportunities are available in all settings to contribute to the health and well-being of this special group.

MENTAL RETARDATION

Mental retardation refers to significantly subaverage general intellectual functioning that exists concurrently with deficits in adaptive behavior. Mental retardation is one of several developmental disorders that usually are first diagnosed in infancy, childhood, or adolescence. Table 55–1 lists the major categories of developmental disorders, and table 55–2 provides descriptive terminology and other key words.

The levels of intellectual functioning are designated *mild, moderate, severe,* and *profound.* Standardized intelligence tests are used to determine individual levels. The Intelligence Quotient (IQ) expresses the test results. A category of *Unspecified Mental Retardation* is used when standard tests cannot be performed because of lack of cooperation, severe impairment, or infancy.

Adaptive functioning refers to the person's effectiveness in social skills, communication, and daily living skills, as well as to how standards of personal independence and social responsibility characteristic of the age and cultural group are met. Adaptive functioning is influenced by such factors as motivation, education, and social and vocational opportunities and has more

chance for improvement by remedial efforts than does IQ, which tends to be more fixed.[1]

Adaptive functioning is described briefly for each of the categories listed in the following sections. An understanding of expected capabilities can help to provide necessary background information for teaching basic oral care procedures.

I. MILD RETARDATION
A. IQ
50–55 to approximately 70.

B. Adaptive Functioning
1. *Child.* In special classes for the educable, the child advances to a level of third to sixth grade. Practical skills can be learned.
2. *Adult.* At adult level, the individual cares for personal hygiene and other necessities, with reminders. Communication is good, although the attention span and memory are less than average. Activities that do not require involved planning or rapid implementation can be carried out satisfactorily. Most educable individuals can engage in semi-skilled or simple skilled work with guidance, and so maintain themselves.

II. MODERATE RETARDATION
A. IQ
35–40 to 50–55.

B. Adaptive Functioning
1. *Child.* A marked developmental lag occurs in the early years, but the child can be trained in personal care and hygiene with help. These children attend classes and learn simple habits and skills, but they do not learn to read

749

TABLE 55–1 DEVELOPMENTAL DISORDERS*
Mental Retardation
Mild, moderate, severe, profound
Learning Disorders
Reading
Mathematics
Written expression
Motor Skills Disorders
Coordination
Pervasive Developmental Disorder
Autistic disorder
Disruptive Behavior Disorders
Overaggressiveness, hostility, hyperactivity, inattention, impulsiveness
Poor attention span
Conduct disorder; delinquency
Use of alcohol; stealing; destructive acts
Anxiety Disorders
Chronic anxiety, timid, inhibited
Unrealistic fears of the unfamiliar
Fear of separation
Overanxious
Feeding Disorders
Failure to eat adequately
Pica
Rumination disorder
Tic Disorders
Tourette's syndrome
Chronic motor or vocal tic disorder
Speech and Language Disorders
Expressive language
Voice disorder (pitch, tone)
Stuttering
Elective mutism

* Disorders usually first diagnosed during infancy, childhood, or adolescence.

TABLE 55–2 KEY WORDS: MENTAL RETARDATION
Autism (aw'tizm): a syndrome beginning in infancy characterized by extreme withdrawal and an obsessive desire to maintain the status quo.
Hyperactivity (hi'per-ak-tiv'ĭ-tē): abnormally increased activity.
Developmental hyperactivity (hyperkinesia): characterized by constant motion, fidgetiness, excitability, impulsiveness, and a short attention span.
Intelligence quotient (IQ): numeric rating determined through psychologic testing that indicates the approximate relationship of a person's mental age (MA) to chronologic age (CA).
Mutism (mu'tizm): inability or refusal to speak; deafness may prevent learning to speak.
Elective mutism: persistent refusal to talk in children with demonstrated ability to speak.
Pervasive: throughout entire individual; entire development is severely and markedly impaired, as in autism.
Pica (pi'kah): persistent craving/eating of nonnutritive substances or unnatural articles of food.
Rumination (roo'mĭ-na'shun): repeated regurgitation of food in the absence of any associated gastrointestinal illness.
Tic: an involuntary, sudden, rapid, recurrent, nonrhythmic, stereotyped motor movement or vocal sound.
Tourette's syndrome: multiple motor and one or more vocal tics; may involve squatting, twirling, grunts, barks, sniffs, and coprolalia.
Coprolalia (kop'rō-lā'lē-ah): involuntary utterance of vulgar or obscene words.

and write. They speak in short sentences, and understand best when single-thought, short sentences are used. They participate well in group activities.

2. *Adult.* As adults, these individuals attend to personal care, with reminders, and have a relatively short attention span and memory. Although they may have problems of coordination, they perform simple tasks and are conscientious about taking responsibility for errands and helpful duties. Although not completely capable of self-maintenance, many do unskilled work with direct supervision.

III. SEVERE RETARDATION
A. IQ
20–25 to 35–40.

B. Adaptive Functioning
1. *Child.* Children at this level can benefit from systematic habit training and may make at-

tempts at personal care and dressing with assistance. They usually walk, use some speech, and respond to directions.

2. *Adult.* Adults conform to a daily routine and may help with household and other small tasks, in spite of a limited attention span. Some personal care with supervision is possible.

IV. PROFOUND RETARDATION
A. IQ
Below 20 or 25.

B. Adaptive Functioning
1. *Child.* Delays occur in all phases of development, and close supervision and care are necessary.

2. *Adult.* Many remain inert and placid throughout the early years and never learn to sit up. A few may learn a few words, but as a group, their ability to interact is lacking. Nursing care is needed, and many cannot feed themselves.

ETIOLOGY OF MENTAL RETARDATION[1]

Mental retardation represents a more or less important symptom in well over 200 different conditions. Many of these are rare. A variety of means of classification is found in the literature. It has been convenient to divide the causes into factors operating before birth, at birth, and after birth.

A majority of cases of mental retardation results from prenatal influences; a small number is effected as injuries at birth. Diagnosis may be complicated and difficult, and many cases can only be classified as of unknown origin.

I. MAJOR CAUSATIVE FACTORS[1]
   A. Genetic; chromosomal.
   B. Early alterations of embryonic development.
   C. Pregnancy and perinatal problems.
   D. Physical disorders acquired in childhood.
   E. Environmental influences.
   F. Unknown.

II. EXAMPLES DURING PRENATAL PERIOD
A. Infections
   Brain damage can result from maternal infection during pregnancy. Serious infections during the first trimester are most likely to cause physical malformations.
   1. *Congenital Rubella Syndrome.* German measles virus infection during the first trimester may result in abnormalities, and mental retardation may occur. The rubella syndrome also may include cataracts, cardiac anomalies, deafness, and microcephaly.
      Immunization with rubella vaccine has reduced the incidence of the disease in the general population. Because more prospective mothers now are immune than were in the past, retardation related to the virus infection has been reduced.
   2. *Congenital Syphilis.* Transfer of syphilis from the mother leads to numerous symptoms, and when the central nervous system is involved, hydrocephalus, convulsions, and mental retardation can result. Hutchinson's triad, which is associated with the late stage of congenital syphilis, includes deafness, interstitial keratitis, and dental defects. Hutchinsonian incisors, which are notched and tapered, mulberry molars, and microdontia are typical (figure 14–5, page 237).
   3. *Neonatal Congenital Toxoplasmosis.* Infection of the fetus transplacentally may lead to miscarriage, stillbirth, or a living baby with severe clinical disease. The effects may include hydrocephalus or microcephalus, blindness, and mental retardation.

B. Drugs Used During Pregnancy
   1. *Contraindicated Drugs.* Table 43–2 (page 607) lists drugs contraindicated during pregnancy and the possible adverse effects the drugs can have on the fetus. Birth malformations and syndromes that include mental retardation are identified.
   2. *Fetal Alcohol Syndrome (FAS).* The signs and symptoms of FAS are described on page 778, and the facial features are shown in figure 57–1.

C. Metabolic Disorders
   1. *Phenylketonuria (PKU).* Phenylketonuria results from an error of metabolism in which the enzyme necessary for digestion of the amino acid phenylalanine is missing. Severe mental retardation is a consequence. Early recognition of the missing enzyme with early dietary control lessens the severity of retardation. Many states require blood and urine screening tests soon after an infant is born. A diet free from animal and vegetable protein is necessary.
   2. *Congenital Hypothyroidism.* Cretinism is usually the result of partial or complete absence of the thyroid gland at birth. Mental retardation accompanies a variety of physical symptoms related to defective development.

D. Chromosomal Abnormality
   Down's syndrome is described in a separate section on pages 752–754.

III. EXAMPLES DURING BIRTH
A. Mechanical Injury at Birth
   Damage leading to mental retardation may have a variety of causes, including difficulties of labor and delivery.

B. Hypoxia
   Asphyxiation from prolonged oxygen deficiency may result from labor complications.

IV. EXAMPLES DURING POSTNATAL PERIOD
A. Infections
   Cerebral infection may be caused by a wide variety of organisms. Examples of diseases that may have this effect are encephalitis and meningitis.

B. Postnatal Trauma
   Accidents may result in a fractured skull or prolonged unconsciousness.

C. Nutritional Disorder
   Dietary imbalances and inadequacies, debilitating diseases, or parasitic diseases can lead to slow development and retardation.

GENERAL CHARACTERISTICS

I. PHYSICAL FEATURES

Because most individuals with mental retardation are in the borderline and mild categories, no unusual physical characteristics should be expected at initial patient evaluation, other than those present in the usual population of normal intelligence.

Within the low-moderate, severe, and profound groups, certain physical variations appear more frequently. Facial or other characteristics may be pathognomonic for a particular condition or syndrome; that is, there may be an identifying characteristic that is specific for that condition and rarely occurs in other syndromes.

Skull anomalies include microcephaly (smaller), hydrocephalus (larger, contains fluid), spherical, conical, or otherwise asymmetrical shapes. Other features, such as asymmetries of the face, malformations of the outer ear, anomalies of the eyes, or unusual shape of the nose, may be present. Growth and physiologic development are generally delayed.

II. ORAL FINDINGS

A higher incidence of oral developmental malformations has been observed, some specifically associated with particular syndromes or conditions. Oral findings that have been observed to occur more frequently in individuals with mental retardation than in those with normal intelligence include the following:

A. Lips

Thickness of the lips is common.

B. Tooth Anomalies

Teeth may be imperfectly formed; eruption patterns may be delayed or irregular.

C. Periodontal Conditions[2,3]

Gingivitis and periodontitis are common in individuals with mental retardation. Patients with Down's syndrome have more severe disease than do those from other groups with mental retardation. The incidence is greater among the institutionalized patients when compared with those living in the community.[4]

D. Habits

Incidence of clenching, bruxing, mouthbreathing, and tongue thrusting is increased.

E. Dental Caries[2,3]

The factors that are effective in the prevention of dental caries in the special group are the same as those in a population of normal intelligence. These factors include exposure to fluoridation and other forms of fluoride, form and frequency of cariogenic foods in the diet, and the control of bacterial plaque.

Studies have shown that, when all degrees of retardation are grouped together, dental caries incidence is generally higher for noninstitutionalized than for institutionalized patients, particularly among the profoundly retarded group.[2] Institutionalized individuals have a controlled diet with less food available between meals. They also may have less accessibility to snacks containing refined carbohydrates, except those brought by visitors.

The private water supply for many institutions has been fluoridated. This may be equally true of the community water supply where the noninstitutionalized individuals reside.

When the figures for dental caries incidence are separated according to degree of retardation, the severely and profoundly retarded patients have been shown to have significantly more dental caries.[2]

DENTAL AND DENTAL HYGIENE CARE AND INSTRUCTION

Procedures for management and care of the patient with a disability were described in Chapter 50 with suggestions for various types of adaptations. The patient with mental retardation may have physical and sensory disabilities or systemic disease problems; therefore, information from various chapters can be applied during treatment. Patients with any type of mental retardation need basic periodontal therapy consisting of intensive daily plaque control, scaling, and frequent maintenance supervision.

In the following pages, the special characteristics and problems of patients with Down's syndrome and the syndrome of autism are described.

DOWN'S SYNDROME

A special and unique group of individuals with mental retardation has a chromosomal abnormality manifested in Down's syndrome or trisomy 21 syndrome. The incidence of Down's syndrome in the United States is approximately 1 in 800 live births and stillbirths.[5]

Formerly, the incidence of births of babies with Down's syndrome increased with advancing maternal age. In recent years, however, the average age of mothers of infants with Down's syndrome has decreased.[6] Also, statistical evidence shows that the father can be the source of the chromosomal abnormality.[7]

Patients with Down's syndrome have a combination of characteristic abnormalities that is relatively constant. They tend to resemble one another.

I. PHYSICAL CHARACTERISTICS[5]
A. Stature

Small, with a short neck; awkward, waddling gait; general growth retardation.

21. **Snow,** M.K. and Stiefel, D.J.: *Dental Treatment of the Mentally Retarded.* Disability Dental Instruction, 4919 NE 86th Street, Seattle, WA 98115, 15 pp.

SUGGESTED READINGS

Becking, A.G. and Tuinzing, D.B.: Orthognathic Surgery for Mentally Retarded Patients, *Oral Surg. Oral Med. Oral Pathol., 72,* 162, August, 1991.

Belanger, G. and Casamassimo, P.S.: Dental Management of the Mentally Retarded Adult, in Thornton, J.B. and Wright, J.T., eds.: *Special and Medically Compromised Patients in Dentistry.* St. Louis, Mosby, 1989, pp. 10–23.

Bickley, S.R.: Dental Care for the Mentally Handicapped—A Duty or a Pleasure? *Dent. Health (London), 27,* 3, February–March, 1988.

Davila, J.M. and Menendez, J.: Relaxing Effects of Music in Dentistry for Mentally Handicapped Patients, *Spec. Care Dentist., 6,* 18, January–February, 1986.

Dicks, J.L. and Banning, J.S.: Evaluation of Calculus Accumulation in Tube-fed, Mentally Handicapped Patients: The Effects of Oral Hygiene Status, *Spec. Care Dentist., 11,* 104, May/June, 1991.

Dura, J.R., Torsell, A.E., Heinzerling, R.A., and Mulick, J.A.: Special Oral Concerns in People with Severe and Profound Mental Retardation, *Spec. Care Dentist., 8,* 265, November–December, 1988.

Eyman, R.K., Grossman, H.J., Chaney, R.H., and Call, T.L.: The Life Expectancy of Profoundly Handicapped People with Mental Retardation, *N. Engl. J. Med., 323,* 584, August 30, 1990.

Hunt, N.: *The World of Nigel Hunt; the Diary of a Mongoloid Youth.* New York, Garrett, 1967, 126 pp.

Kendall, N.P.: Oral Health of a Group of Non-institutionalized Mentally Handicapped Adults in the UK, *Community Dent. Oral Epidemiol., 19,* 357, December, 1991.

Minihan, P.M. and Dean, D.H.: Meeting the Needs for Health Services of Persons with Mental Retardation Living in the Community, *Am. J. Public Health, 80,* 1043, September, 1989.

Øilo, G., Hatle, G., Gad, A.-L., and Dahl, B.L.: Wear of Teeth in a Mentally Retarded Population, *J. Oral Rehabil., 17,* 173, March, 1990.

Platt, L.D. and Carlson, D.E.: Prenatal Diagnosis—When and How? *N. Engl. J. Med., 327,* 636, August 27, 1992.

Taylor, R.: Finding Rewards Treating Special Patients, *RDH, 9,* 28, October, 1989.

Wakham, M.D., Burtner, A.P., McNeal, D.R., Garvey, T.P., and Bedinger, S.: Pica: A Peculiar Behavior with Oral Involvement, *Spec. Care Dentist., 12,* 207, September/October, 1992.

Willette, J.C.: Lip-chewing: Another Treatment Option, *Spec. Care Dentist., 12,* 174, July/August, 1992.

Williams, C.A., Weber, F.T., McKim, M., Steadman, C.I., and Kane, M.A.: Hepatitis B Virus Transmission in a Public School: Effects of Mentally Retarded HBsAG Carrier Students, *Am. J. Public Health, 77,* 476, April, 1987.

Down's Syndrome

Barnett, M.L.: The Prevalence of Mitral Valve Prolapse in Patients with Down's Syndrome: Implications for Dental Management, *Oral Surg. Oral Med. Oral Pathol., 66,* 445, October, 1988.

Klaiman, P. and Arndt, E.: Facial Reconstruction in Down Syndrome: Perceptions of the Results by Parents and Normal Adolescents, *Cleft Palate J., 26,* 186, July, 1989.

Klaiman, P., Witzel, M.A., Margar-Bacal, F., and Munro, I.R.: Changes in Aesthetic Appearance and Intelligibility of Speech after Partial Glossectomy in Patients with Down Syndrome, *Plast. Reconstr. Surg., 82,* 403, September, 1988.

Randall, D.M., Harth, S., and Seow, W.K.: Preventive Dental Health Practices of Non-institutionalized Down Syndrome Children: A Controlled Study, *J. Clin. Pediatr. Dent., 16,* 225, Spring, 1992.

Down's Syndrome: Periodontal

Barnett, M.L., Press, K.P., Friedman, D., and Sonnenberg, E.M.: The Prevalence of Periodontitis and Dental Caries in a Down's Syndrome Population, *J. Periodontol., 57,* 288, May, 1986.

Barr-Agholme, M., Dahllof, G., Linder, L., and Modéer, T.: *Actinobacillus actinomycetemcomitans, Capnocytophaga* and *Porphyromonas gingivalis* in Subgingival Plaque of Adolescents with Down's Syndrome, *Oral Microbiol. Immunol., 7,* 244, August, 1992.

Modéer, T., Barr, M., and Dahllöf, G.: Periodontal Disease in Children with Down's Syndrome, *Scand. J. Dent. Res., 98,* 228, June, 1990.

Reuland-Bosma, W. and van Dijk, J.: Periodontal Disease in Down's Syndrome: A Review, *J. Clin Periodontol., 13,* 64, January, 1986.

Reuland-Bosma, W., van Dijk, L.J., and van der Weele, L.: Experimental Gingivitis Around Deciduous Teeth in Children with Down's Syndrome, *J. Clin Periodontol., 13,* 294, April, 1986.

Reuland-Bosma, W., van den Barselaar, M.Th., van de Gevel, J.S., Leijh, P.C.J., deVries-Huiges, H., and The, H.T.: Nonspecific and Specific Immune Responses in a Child with Down's Syndrome and Her Sibling. A Care Report, *J. Periodontol., 59,* 249, April, 1988.

Reuland-Bosma, W., Liem, R.S.B., Jansen, H.W.B., van Dijk, L.J., and van der Weele, L.T.: Cellular Aspects of and Effects on the Gingiva in Children with Down's Syndrome During Experimental Gingivitis, *J. Clin Periodontol., 15,* 303, May, 1988.

Reuland-Bosma, W., Liem, R.S.B., Jansen, H.W.B., van Dijk, L.J., and van der Weele, L.T.: Morphological Aspects of the Gingiva in Children with Down's Syndrome During Experimental Gingivitis, *J. Clin Periodontol., 15,* 293, May, 1988.

Shapira, J., Stabholz, A., Schurr, D., Sela, M.N., and Mann, J.: Caries Levels, *Streptococcus mutans* Counts, Salivary pH, and Periodontal Treatment Needs of Adult Down Syndrome Patients, *Spec. Care Dentist., 11,* 248, November/December, 1991.

Stabholz, A., Mann, J., Sela, M., Schurr, D., Steinberg, D., Dori, S., and Shapira, J.: Caries Experience, Periodontal Treatment Needs, Salivary pH, and *Streptococcus mutans* Counts in a Preadolescent Down Syndrome Population, *Spec. Care Dentist., 11,* 203, September/October, 1991.

Ulseth, J.O., Hestnes, A., Stovner, L.J., and Storhaug, K.: Dental Caries and Periodontitis in Persons with Down Syndrome, *Spec. Care Dentist., 11,* 71, March/April, 1991.

Autism

Davila, J.M. and Jensen, O.E.: Behavioral and Pharmacological Dental Management of a Patient with Autism, *Spec. Care Dentist., 8,* 58, March–April, 1988.

Lowe, O. and Lindemann, R.: Assessment of the Autistic Patient's Dental Needs and Ability to Undergo Dental Examination, *ASDC J. Dent. Child., 52,* 29, January–February, 1985.

Shapira, J., Mann, J., Tamari, I., Mester, R., Knobler, H., Yoeli, Y., and Newbrun, E.: Oral Health Status and Dental Needs of an Autistic Population of Children and Young Adults, *Spec. Care Dentist., 9,* 38, March–April, 1989.

Bacterial Plaque Control and Chlorhexidine

Bratel, J. and Berggren, U.: Long-term Oral Effects of Manual or Electric Toothbrushes Used by Mentally Handicapped Adults, *Clin. Prev. Dent., 13,* 5, July/August, 1991.

Bratel, J., Berggren, U., and Hirsch, J.M.: Electric or Manual Toothbrush? A Comparison of the Effects on the Oral Health of Mentally Handicapped Adults, *Clin. Prev. Dent., 10,* 23, May–June, 1988.

Burtner, A.P., Low, D.W., McNeal, D.R., Hassell, T.M., and Smith, R.G.: Effects of Chlorhexidine Spray on Plaque and Gingival Health in Institutionalized Persons with Mental Retardation, *Spec. Care Dentist., 11,* 97, May/June, 1991.

Chikte, U.M., Pochee, E., Rudolph, M.J., and Reinach, S.G.: Evaluation of Stannous Fluoride and Chlorhexidine Sprays on Plaque and Gingivitis in Handicapped Children, *J. Clin Periodontol., 18,* 281, May, 1991.

Kalaga, A., Addy, M., and Hunter, B.: The Use of 0.2% Chlorhexidine Spray as an Adjunct to Oral Hygiene and Gingival Health in Physically and Mentally Handicapped Adults, *J. Periodontol., 60,* 381, July, 1989.

Marchesani, J., Carrel, R., Chialastri, A.J., and Binns, W.H.: The Vehicle of Toothpaste in the Control of Plaque and Calculus, *J. Pedod., 12,* 327, Summer, 1988.

Ozeki, M., Zinda, K., Matsumoto, S., Ohkouchi, K., Kobayashi, Y., and Moriyama, T.: Bacteriological Examination of Fissure Plaques from Seriously Mentally Retarded Adults, *Caries Res., 24,* 318, No. 5, 1990.

Shaw, L., Shaw, M.J., and Foster, T.D.: Correlation of Manual Dexterity and Comprehension with Oral Hygiene and Periodontal Status in Mentally Handicapped Adults, *Community Dent. Oral Epidemiol., 17,* 187, August, 1989.

Stabholz, A., Shapira, J., Shur, D., Friedman, M., Guberman, R., and Sela, M.N.: Local Application of Sustained-release Delivery System of Chlorhexidine in Down's Syndrome Population, *Clin. Prev. Dent., 13,* 9, September/October, 1991.

Stiefel, D.J., Truelove, E.L., Chin, M.M., and Mandel, L.S.: Efficacy of Chlorhexidine Swabbing in Oral Health Care for People with Severe Disabilities, *Spec. Care Dentist., 12,* 57, March/April, 1992.

The Patient with a Mental Disorder

A mental disorder is an illness with behavioral and psychologic manifestations associated with impairment in functioning. The causes may be related to biologic, psychologic, genetic, physical, or chemical disturbances.[1]

With the discovery and approval of new psychotropic drugs for more effective therapy, and with the current policy of deinstitutionalization, more individuals with mental disorders are seeking dental and dental hygiene care in dental offices and clinics. Dental hygiene care for a person with a psychiatric illness, or for one who may be undergoing an emotional crisis, poses an increased challenge.[2,3]

The American Psychiatric Association has classified the more than 200 types of mental disorders in the document *Diagnostic and Statistical Manual (DSM)*.[4] The DSM is in accord with the International Classification of Diseases (ICD) published by the World Health Organization.[5]

The classification of primary mental disorders is shown in table 56–1. Each major category can be divided into four divisions, namely, *Primary Disorders, Substance-induced Disorders, Secondary to a Nonpsychiatric Disorder*, and *Not Otherwise Specified (NOS)*.[6] Each disorder has characteristic signs and symptoms. Terminology related to the disorders is listed and defined in table 56–2.

This chapter includes descriptions of the most frequently encountered psychiatric disorders, namely, schizophrenia, mood disorders, anxiety disorders, and eating disorders. Other disorders are described elsewhere in the text, for example, alcoholism (Chapter 57), other substance abuse (Chapter 8), and Alzheimer's disease (Chapter 46).

Knowledge of the types of mental disorders and their signs and symptoms can help the clinician to recognize a patient's needs and understand the patient's behaviors. Confidence and trust by the patient are essential for communication and the patient's acceptance of clinical care.

SCHIZOPHRENIA

Schizophrenia is a complex, chronic mental disorder. Disturbances in feeling, thinking, and behavior significantly impair function to a level below normal for the individual. Schizophrenia is a major psychotic illness in which the individual may be out of touch with reality. Symptoms include delusions, hallucinations, disorganized thinking, and incoherence.

The onset is usually between the ages of 15 and 35 years. The incidence in both men and women is similar.

Although the cause is not fully understood, genetic factors can make an individual more vulnerable. Periods of remission and recurrence may occur. Symptoms may be triggered by various social, psychologic, or environmental stresses.

I. SUBTYPES OF SCHIZOPHRENIA[7]
Once diagnosed, schizophrenia then can be classified into one of several subtypes depending on the patterns of behavior shown by the symptoms in table 56–3.
  A. Positive (paranoid) type with delusions or hallucinations.
  B. Disorganized type with disorganized speech and behavior.
  C. Catatonic type with stupor, agitation, stereotyped movements, and extreme negativism.
  D. Deficit type with negative symptoms.

759

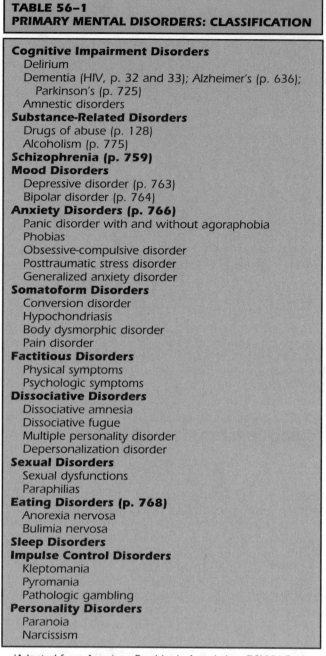

TABLE 56–1
PRIMARY MENTAL DISORDERS: CLASSIFICATION

Cognitive Impairment Disorders
 Delirium
 Dementia (HIV, p. 32 and 33); Alzheimer's (p. 636);
  Parkinson's (p. 725)
 Amnestic disorders
Substance-Related Disorders
 Drugs of abuse (p. 128)
 Alcoholism (p. 775)
Schizophrenia (p. 759)
Mood Disorders
 Depressive disorder (p. 763)
 Bipolar disorder (p. 764)
Anxiety Disorders (p. 766)
 Panic disorder with and without agoraphobia
 Phobias
 Obsessive-compulsive disorder
 Posttraumatic stress disorder
 Generalized anxiety disorder
Somatoform Disorders
 Conversion disorder
 Hypochondriasis
 Body dysmorphic disorder
 Pain disorder
Factitious Disorders
 Physical symptoms
 Psychologic symptoms
Dissociative Disorders
 Dissociative amnesia
 Dissociative fugue
 Multiple personality disorder
 Depersonalization disorder
Sexual Disorders
 Sexual dysfunctions
 Paraphilias
Eating Disorders (p. 768)
 Anorexia nervosa
 Bulimia nervosa
Sleep Disorders
Impulse Control Disorders
 Kleptomania
 Pyromania
 Pathologic gambling
Personality Disorders
 Paranoia
 Narcissism

(Adapted from American Psychiatric Association, DSM-IV Options Book, 1991, pp. B:2–B:10.)

E. Residual type with symptoms from the residual list (table 56–3).

II. SYMPTOMS OF SCHIZOPHRENIA

The disturbance progresses from subchronic to remission with acute exacerbations of varying frequencies. The three phases are described as *prodromal, active,* and *residual.* Prodromal symptoms may appear as signs of deterioration for as long as 1 year before the active phase.

Table 56–3 shows the symptoms of each phase. Ac-tive-phase symptoms are *positive,* those that reflect un-usual, profound behavior, or *negative,* those that show the absence of behavior that might be expected normally.

Rates of alcohol and drug abuse are high among patients with schizophrenia. Many patients diagnosed with schizophrenia also qualify for a diagnosis of alcoholism. Drug and alcohol abuse can increase psychiatric symptoms and lead to poor treatment compliance, increased hospitalization, homelessness, and suicide.[8]

III. TREATMENT OF SCHIZOPHRENIA

The response to initial treatment is a critical predictor of the long-term prognosis. The prognosis has generally been considered guarded to poor. Evidence shows that, although deterioration may occur during the early years, the condition may stabilize with treatment during middle age.[9]

A. Pharmacotherapy

The objectives of treatment are to reduce or alleviate the delusions, hallucinations, and other positive symptoms (table 56–3) and to enable the patient to function in daily living. The use of antipsychotic medications has improved the outcomes of treatment and led to the process of deinstitutionalization.

Schizophrenia is associated with an excess of dopamine at specific synapses in the brain. Medications are used to block dopamine receptors.[10]

1. *Antipsychotic Medications*[10,11,12]
    a. Phenothiazines (for example, chlorpromazine [Thorazine])
    b. Butyrophenones (for example, haloperidol [Haldol])
    c. Thioxanthenes (for example, thiothixene [Navane])
    d. Atypical (for example, clozapine)[13]
2. *Adverse Effects of Medications.* Careful monitoring is essential because side effects can be severe.[14] For example, weekly white blood cell counts are needed during clozapine therapy because of the high risk of agranulocytosis.[13] Table 56–4 lists a few of the many side effects of antipsychotic medication with suggestions for appointment adaptations.
3. *Maintenance.* After an acute episode, the dosage is adjusted for the remission period. A minimal effective dose is important because of the risk of tardive dyskinesia. Noncompliance in continuing medication is a common cause of psychotic relapse and rehospitalization.[15]

B. Psychosocial Therapy[15]

Long-term treatment for psychosocial and vocational recovery after an acute psychotic episode must include family and all those close to the patient. Psychotherapy may include a variety of vocational rehabilitation efforts and training in social skills.

I. PHASES AND SYMPTOMS

A. Depressive Phase

The characteristics for major depression (table 56–5) and for a depressed episode of bipolar disorder are identical except that the patient with bipolar depression must have had a manic episode.

B. Manic Phase

Mania is characterized by excessive elation, hyperactivity, and accelerated thinking and speaking. A severe manic episode causes marked impairment in occupational and social functioning. Characteristics of a manic episode are listed in table 56–6.

C. Mixed

The "mixed" category is used when symptoms of depression and mania are concurrent or when rapid changes between the two states occur within days or weeks.

II. TREATMENT OF BIPOLAR DEPRESSION

Three distinct treatment strategies apply, one for the manic phase, one for the depressive phase, and one for the normal phase, which requires maintenance therapy. Treatment for the depressive phase was described under major depression on page 763.

Both pharmacotherapy and psychotherapy are used for the manic phase. Initially, hospitalization may be needed to protect the individual from harm to self or others.[29]

A. Pharmacotherapy[22,29]

1. Sedation may be needed for the acute stage of mania when the patient is severely agitated.
2. Antimanic medication: lithium carbonate.
   a. Medication of choice for mood stabilization in the manic phase.
   b. Prevents recurrence of bipolar disorder when given on a maintenance drug level.[27]
   c. Possible side effects include gastrointestinal irritation, fine hand tremor, thirst, polyuria, and muscular weakness. Prolonged use may lead to renal tube damage and hypothyroidism.
   d. Frequent monitoring is important to guard against lithium toxicity, which can occur with long-term drug use.[22,27]
3. Antidepressant therapy may be needed for the patient with moderate to severe bipolar depression to protect against a drug-induced switch to mania.

B. Psychotherapy

Psychotherapy can help to lower stress factors and uncover early warning signs of an approaching high or low mood. Psychosocial support is important to help the patient to prevent relapse.

III. DENTAL HYGIENE CARE

A. Personal Factors

Characteristics of an individual during a manic episode can be studied in table 56–6. During the manic phase, the patient is overactive, restless, and in constant motion, and behaves in an aggressive, fearless manner. Many patients talk quickly, jump from thought to thought, and have a short attention span. A tendency to argue and become irritable may be apparent if pressured in any way.

B. Oral Health Implications[30]

1. Oral hygiene needs are often unmet.
2. Patient unlikely to report injury or illness; complete oral assessment can be especially significant.
3. Gingival tissues may appear abraded and lacerated because of over-eager grandiose brushing motions.
4. Xerostomia from long-term use of medications may require use of a saliva substitute. A complete preventive program with daily fluoride therapy and an anticariogenic diet against rampant dental caries is important.
5. Lithium may impart a metallic taste in the mouth.

C. Appointment Suggestions[30,31]

Lithium medication and other treatment usually provide control for the nonhospitalized patient. The need for protecting the patient and others from overactive behavior may not be experienced in the private clinical setting because elective dental and dental hygiene appointments usually are postponed until the patient is under medical control.

1. Simplify the surroundings; provide a comfortable uncluttered environment.

TABLE 56–6
CHARACTERISTICS OF MANIC EPISODE

- Inflated self-esteem or grandiosity
- Decreased need for sleep
- More talkative than usual or pressure to keep talking
- Flight of ideas or subjective experience that thoughts are racing
- Distractibility (that is, attention easily drawn to unimportant or irrelevant external stimuli)
- Increase in goal-directed activity (socially, at work or school, or sexually) or psychomotor agitation
- Excessive involvement in pleasurable activities that have a high potential for painful consequences (for example, engages in unrestrained buying sprees, sexual indiscretions, or foolish business investments)

(Adapted from American Psychiatric Association: DSM-IV Options Book, 1991.)

2. Do not rush the patient, as doing so can lead to anger and hostility.
3. Use quiet persuasion; keep the voice firm and low-pitched with a coaxing quality.
4. When applicable, help the patient's caregiver to learn procedures for dental caries prevention and periodontal health.
5. Patient instruction is difficult because the patient has a short attention span and may not like fine detail. Avoid long descriptions.

POSTPARTUM MOOD DISTURBANCES

The puerperium is the 6-week period after childbirth when the body undergoes physical and physiologic changes. During the entire postpartum period, many physiologic and psychologic stresses are related to the changes taking place in the mother's life. Degrees of emotional reactions are evident and range from postpartum blues to psychosis. Postpartum psychosis is considered a major psychiatric emergency.[32]

I. POSTPARTUM BLUES
A period of postpartum blues is considered a normal state after giving birth. It may last a few days and clear spontaneously.

II. POSTPARTUM PSYCHOSIS
Postpartum or puerperal psychosis is characterized by severe depression. The condition is more typical following the birth of a first baby.

A. Underlying Causes
1. Secondary to pre-existing mental illness, such as bipolar disorder or schizophrenia.
2. Conflicts about motherhood, such as unwanted pregnancy, fears about mothering, and marital problems.

B. Symptoms
1. *Early.* Complaints of insomnia, restlessness, tearfulness, fatigue, and emotional unsteadiness.
2. *Progressive.* Confusion, irrationality, and obsessive concerns about the baby. Thoughts of bringing harm to the baby or oneself are not unusual.

C. Treatment
Without treatment, risk of suicide, infanticide, or both exists. A favorable outcome can be expected with appropriate treatment, family support, and no pre-existing illness.
1. *Suicidal Precautions.* Baby should not be left alone with mother.
2. *Pharmacotherapy.* In accord with symptoms of depression.
3. *Psychotherapy.* Individual and marital. Arrangements for assistance at home must be made before hospital release.

4. *Extended Treatment.* Counseling in infant care with observation for emergence of major mood disorder.[32]

ANXIETY DISORDERS

Anxiety is experienced as apprehension, tension, or dread that results from the anticipation of danger, the source of which is unknown or unrecognized. Anxiety is the result of feeling a threat to the person's being, self-esteem, or identity. Fear, on the other hand, is an emotional or physiologic response to a recognized source of danger.

In normal life, some mild anxiety provides an effective stimulus to improved performance. As a psychiatric symptom, anxiety can be excessive, irrational, and beyond the control of the individual.

I. TYPES AND SYMPTOMS OF ANXIETY DISORDERS
The several types of anxiety disorders are listed in table 56–7. The disorders have symptoms of fear, excess worry, and avoidance behavior that are revealed in a variety of ways and degrees of severity. The symptoms also vary in the degree of occupational and social dysfunction that can be produced. Certain patients may have secondary problems of alcohol and other substance abuse. The abuse may be the result of an attempt at self-medication.

A. Panic Attack[33]
The symptoms that may occur in a panic attack are listed in table 56–8. The panic attack itself is a symptom in several of the anxiety disorders. An overwhelming sense of impending doom is the cardinal symptom of the attack.

A panic attack may be unexpected (uncued) or "situationally bound" (cued). A situationally bound panic attack invariably results from ex-

**TABLE 56–7
ANXIETY DISORDERS**

- Panic disorder without agoraphobia
- Panic disorder with agoraphobia
- Agoraphobia without history of panic disorder
- Specific phobia
- Social phobia
- Obsessive-compulsive disorder
- Posttraumatic stress disorder
- Generalized anxiety disorder
- Secondary anxiety disorder caused by a nonpsychiatric medical condition
- Substance-induced (intoxication/withdrawal) anxiety disorder

(Adapted from American Psychiatric Association: DSM-IV Options Book, 1991, p. B:7.)

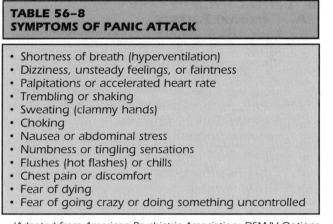

**TABLE 56–8
SYMPTOMS OF PANIC ATTACK**

- Shortness of breath (hyperventilation)
- Dizziness, unsteady feelings, or faintness
- Palpitations or accelerated heart rate
- Trembling or shaking
- Sweating (clammy hands)
- Choking
- Nausea or abdominal stress
- Numbness or tingling sensations
- Flushes (hot flashes) or chills
- Chest pain or discomfort
- Fear of dying
- Fear of going crazy or doing something uncontrolled

(Adapted from American Psychiatric Association: DSM-IV Options Book, 1991, pp. H:1–H:2.)

posure to a specific trigger. Such triggers are most characteristic of social and specific phobias that are described in this section.

B. Panic Disorder[34]

Panic disorder is characterized by recurrent panic attacks that are usually unexpected. Panic disorder may occur alone or with agoraphobia.

Agoraphobia is the fear of being in places or situations from which escape might be difficult or embarrassing or in which help might not be available in the event of a panic attack. The fear is of open spaces, of crowds, or of going outside the home alone and away from a safe place.

C. Agoraphobia Without History of Panic Disorder

Agoraphobic fear may be related to a genuine medical concern. An example is a nonpsychiatric medical condition, such as a heart attack after which the patient avoids leaving home, especially alone.

D. Phobic Disorder[35]

A phobia is a persistent, unrealistic pathologic fear out of proportion to the stimulus from a particular object or situation. The patient must avoid the phobic stimulus, endure it with marked stress, or have an anxiety reaction, perhaps in the form of a panic attack (table 56–8).

1. *Specific Phobia.* Examples include fear of heights, such as riding in an elevator or airplane, certain animals, fire, or the sight of blood.
2. *Social Phobia.* Examples include the inability to speak in public or to be in a situation in which the individual can be exposed to possible scrutiny and thus fears that he or she may show humiliating anxiety symptoms.

E. Obsessive-Compulsive Disorder[36]

Obsessive thoughts and compulsive actions characterize this disorder. The individual may recognize the self-generated thoughts or actions as excessive and unreasonable. The disorder may begin in early childhood or early adulthood, and unless specific treatment is introduced, the condition may last throughout life.

1. *Obsessions.* An obsession is a repetitive intrusive thought or impulse. Preoccupation with a single idea can result in neglect of daily work and other responsibilities.
2. *Compulsions.* Compulsions are repetitive, ritualistic behaviors or mental acts that the individual is compelled to perform against the person's conscious wishes or standards. Examples are counting, frequent handwashing, and checking and rechecking.

F. Post-traumatic Stress Disorder

In this disorder, an initiating traumatic event has occurred outside the range of usual human experience. It may be destruction to the home or family, or may result from a manmade disaster, such as war, imprisonment, torture, rape, or other exposure associated with intense horror, fear, or serious threat to life. A child may have stress disorder brought on by physical or sexual abuse.

Flashbacks of the traumatic experience and the attendant terror may be precipitated by a stimulus that can be readily associated with the original event. Through dreams or recollections, the patient may have the feeling of reliving the event. Symptoms of depression or panic attacks may be evident in an acute episode.

G. Generalized Anxiety Disorder[33]

The person with generalized anxiety disorder shows persistent, pervasive anxiety and worry. This disorder is not associated with life-threatening fears or "attacks." The anxiety is usually not associated with a specific event, as is a phobia. It may be complicated by depression or alcohol abuse.

Symptoms include motor tension (trembling, restlessness, easy fatigability); autonomic hyperactivity (sweating, dry mouth, difficulty in swallowing, shortness of breath); tachycardia; and hyperarousal (edginess, irritability, difficulty in concentrating, insomnia). Gastrointestinal disturbances are common. The worry and the symptoms impair social and occupational functioning.

II. TREATMENT OF ANXIETY DISORDERS[34,35]
A. Basic Therapeutic Approach

1. Eliminate the intake of caffeine, alcohol, and drugs of abuse. Anxiety disorders are frequently complicated by alcohol abuse.
2. Diagnose and treat other medical and psychiatric problems. Anxiety disorders may emerge with depression, which should be

treated first or at least simultaneously (Depression, page 763).

3. Exercise. Participation in vigorous aerobics or an active sport helps to eliminate physical and psychologic symptoms and enhances the patient's sense of control. Working and keeping busy are important.

B. Cognitive-behavioral Therapy

For phobic disorders, compulsive actions, and the event associated with a posttraumatic stress disorder, repeated exposure to a feared object, act, or situation may help to overcome the problem. The support of family and friends can be significant.

A skilled behavioral therapist is usually needed. Relaxation, biofeedback, and other behavioral therapies have shown selective successes. Treatment can help in many ways; for example, acceptance of dental and dental hygiene therapy may be facilitated in a resistant patient.[36]

C. Psychotherapy

Although not specifically related to the treatment of anxieties, psychotherapy can be valuable as an adjunct when significant interpersonal problems exist.

D. Pharmacotherapy

As few medications as possible should be used. Treatment can best be focused on the patient's sleeping habits, physical activity, and attainment of personal control in general. Determination of a patient's specific problem is essential because treatment for each disorder is different. When treatment is indicated, antianxiety and antidepressant medications are the drugs of choice.

1. *Antianxiety Medications.*[34,37,38] Benzodiazepines are most frequently used. They are available as very fast, fast, intermediate, and slow preparations.
   a. Objectives. Reduce tension and relieve anxiety; induce sleep.
   b. Prescription. Short-term basis for immediate need only; gradual discontinuance to prevent withdrawal symptoms.
   c. Complications. Existing addictions to nicotine, caffeine, alcohol.
   d. Possible side effects. Confusion, dizziness, muscle weakness, difficulty in speaking, skin rash.
   e. Adverse effects. Potential for addiction, withdrawal symptoms, diminished alertness (drowsiness), impaired eye-hand coordination, xerostomia.
2. *Antidepressant Medication.*[34] Antidepressants may be used in the treatment of panic attack. The side effects were described on page 763.

III. DENTAL HYGIENE CARE

A. Personal Factors

Each anxiety disorder has its own specific characteristics. Individuals suffering from an anxiety disorder maintain contact with reality and may be aware of the type of their disorder. Relationships with other people are often strained.

Physical complaints, such as rapid heart beat, hyperventilation, tightness in the throat, and constant fatigue, are common. Such symptoms may lead to an anxiety about the anxiety.

B. Oral Implications

1. Hypersensitivity of the teeth, related to patient's general tenseness and irritability, may be present.
2. Xerostomia related to medications can cause severe problems for periodontal infections and dental caries. Candy or cariogenic beverages used to allay dry mouth lead to enamel and root caries.
3. Oral cleanliness may not be present, even in a patient with an obsession for cleanliness. The opposite may be true, however, and a patient may perform such excessive, vigorous brushing that gingival and dental abrasion result.

C. Appointment Suggestions[36,39]

1. Help the patient to feel in control. Patient may appear very nervous, jumpy, and tense. Accept the patient without judgment or criticism. Attempting to change behavior could cause symptoms of panic attack.
2. Explain each step to the patient and keep communication as open as possible. When the patient must remain still, such as during sealant placement, explain and then distract with trivial encouragement.
3. Effective pain control is needed for these highly nervous, anxious patients. Use local anesthesia for scaling and root planing. Provide gentle, painless injections.
4. Appointments are best scheduled in the morning; patient should not have to wait in the reception area unnecessarily; length of appointment can be minimized and planned to prevent stress.
5. Watch for symptoms of panic attack (table 56–8), such as sweating or hyperventilation. Allow the patient to sit up and enjoy short breaks.

EATING DISORDERS

Anorexia nervosa, bulimia nervosa, and bulimarexia (a combination of the two) are examples of serious eating disorders. They occur primarily in adolescent girls and young adult women, but men and people of other age groups may be involved. The incidence and awareness of the conditions have increased possibly because of better recognition and diagnosis.

Identification by dental professionals of the oral manifestations can lead to detection of the patient's problem. Referral and medical evaluation may be life saving because serious medical problems may exist and psychiatric therapy may be indicated. Because of patient resistance and denial, however, referral for help may be difficult or impossible.

An interdisciplinary team approach for successful rehabilitation of an individual with an eating disorder involves, at the least, the medical, psychiatric, nutritional, dental, and dental hygiene professions. Sometimes dental and dental hygiene care must be postponed until the eating disorder is under control. For other patients, definitive dental care can provide the patient with confidence and encouragement through improved esthetics and relief from tooth sensitivity.[40]

ANOREXIA NERVOSA

The syndrome anorexia nervosa is characterized by a refusal of the individual to maintain body weight over the minimal normal weight for age and height. The aversion to eating results in life-threatening weight loss.

Anorexia involves self-imposed starvation that results from an obsessive desire to be thin and a marked fear of gaining weight. Perceptual disturbances relative to body image are present (figure 56–1). The course of the disease may continue until hospitalization is necessary to prevent death.

I. SIGNS AND SYMPTOMS[41]

The characteristics of anorexia nervosa are listed in table 56–9. The two types are the bulimic and the nonbulimic, as defined in the table. Many anorectic persons have major depression or a family history of major depression or bipolar disorder.

A. General Characteristics[42,43,44]

1. Severe weight loss with emaciation; "waif-like" appearance.
2. Refusal to eat, yet a preoccupation with food; strange habits, such as hoarding but not eating food (except in the bulimic type, when recurrent episodes of binge eating do occur).
3. Hyperactivity and excessive exercising.
4. Abuse of diuretics and laxatives.
5. Dry, flaky skin, brittle fingernails; hair growth on the arms and face.

B. Medical Complications

1. *Malnutrition and Dehydration.*
2. *Vital Signs.* Low pulse rate, hypotension, decreased respiratory rate, and low body temperature.

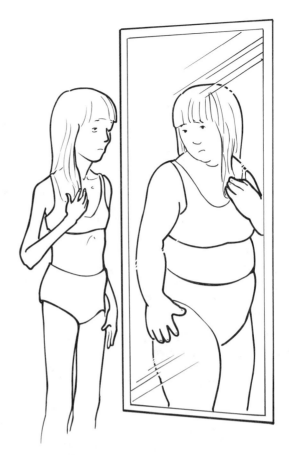

FIG. 56–1. Anorexia Nervosa. The person with anorexia typically has a distorted body self-image. Although small and waif-like in real life, the mirror image appears as an overweight individual.

TABLE 56–9
CHARACTERISTICS OF ANOREXIA NERVOSA

- Refusal to maintain body weight over a minimally normal weight for age and height.
- Intense fear of gaining weight or becoming fat, even though underweight.
- Disturbance in the way in which one's body weight or shape is experienced.
  Places undue importance on body weight or shape in self-evaluation.
  Denies the seriousness of the current low body weight.
- In females, absence of menstrual cycles when otherwise expected to occur.
- Types
  Bulimic type: during the episode of anorexia nervosa, the person engages in recurrent episodes of binge eating.
  Nonbulimic type: during the episode of anorexia nervosa, the person does not engage in recurrent episodes of binge eating.

(Adapted from American Psychiatric Association: DSM-IV Options Book, 1991, p. N:1.)

3. *Metabolic Changes.* Gastrointestinal, cardio-vascular, hematologic, and renal system disturbances.
4. *Amenorrhea.*

II. TREATMENT OF ANOREXIA[45]

Medical and psychiatric therapies are necessary, with hospitalization for the severely ill patient. The primary objectives are to promote weight gain and restore the nutritional status. Treatment may require months or even years.

Pharmacotherapeutic agents are not usually involved, although the patient may be taking antidepressants, tranquilizers, antipsychotics, or antianxiety medication. Vitamin supplements may have been prescribed.

Psychotherapy varies and involves individual behavior modification, as well as group and family therapies. Professional therapists can help the individual to discover the underlying causes of the problems and the sources of the anorectic and bulimic behaviors.

III. DENTAL HYGIENE CARE
A. Personal Factors

The individual with anorexia is usually engaged in excessive exercise and preoccupied with food and weight loss. Depression may be apparent and shown by crying spells, sleep disturbances, and even thoughts of suicide. The person frequently is a high achiever and highly motivated scholastically, but is socially isolated, withdrawn, and shy.

B. Oral Implications
1. Xerostomia leading to enamel and cervical cemental dental caries.
2. Perimylolysis and other findings of bulimia can be noted in the bulimic-type anorexia (see next section).

C. Appointment Suggestions
1. Respect the patient's shy, anxious manner. Gently encourage the patient to talk to develop rapport.
2. Be aware that answers to medical and personal history questions concerning diet, medications, use of laxatives and diuretics, and weight and weight loss may bring strong suspicions of anorexia or bulimarexia.
3. Assess the nutritional status through use of a dietary analysis.
4. Record vital signs.
5. Introduce a concentrated preventive program. Apply significant points itemized for bulimia (next section).

BULIMIA NERVOSA

Bulimia nervosa is a psychiatric compulsive disorder marked by recurrent episodes of uncontrollable binge eating. The two types of bulimic individuals are known

---

TABLE 56–10
CHARACTERISTICS OF BULIMIA NERVOSA

- Recurrent episodes of binge eating. An episode of binge eating is characterized by both of the following:
  Eating, within any 2-hour period, an amount of food that is definitely larger than most people would eat in a similar period of time.
  A sense of lack of control over eating during the episode, for example, a feeling that one cannot stop eating or control what or how much one is eating.
- Regularly engages in either self-induced vomiting, use of laxatives or diuretics, strict dieting or fasting, or vigorous exercise to prevent weight gain.
  Purging type: regularly engages in self-induced vomiting or the use of laxatives or diuretics.
  Nonpurging type: use of strict dieting, fasting, or vigorous exercise, but does not regularly engage in purging.
- A minimum average of 2 binge-eating episodes a week for at least 3 months.
- Self-evaluation is unduly influenced by body shape and weight.
- The disturbance does not occur exclusively during episodes of anorexia nervosa.

(Adapted from American Psychiatric Association: DSM-IV Options Book, 1991, p. N:2.)

---

as the purging type and the nonpurging type (table 56–10). Because of the fear of becoming overweight, self-induced vomiting after eating or the use of laxatives or diuretics is characteristic of the purging type, whereas the nonpurging type uses strict dieting, fasting, and/or vigorous exercise.

The individual with bulimarexia has bulimic-type anorexia and shows symptoms of both anorexia and bulimia. All these individuals are concerned with body weight and shape.

I. SIGNS AND SYMPTOMS
The characteristics of a person with bulimia nervosa are listed in table 56–10. The illness may last over many years, and may alternate with periods of normal eating or periods of fasting.

A. General Characteristics
1. Normal body weight or slightly overweight is typical in contrast to the thin anorectic person.
2. Food consumed during a binge may include cariogenic items with a high caloric content, sweet taste, and a texture that allows rapid eating. Often, favorite foods are selected.
3. Drug and/or alcohol abuse by the patient or in the family history is not uncommon.

B. Medical Complications
1. Problems include dehydration, electrolyte imbalance, protein malnutrition, and cardiac arrhythmia.

2. Self-medications include abuse of laxatives and diuretics, which contribute to gastrointestinal disturbances.
3. Amenorrhea when the person also has a history of anorexia nervosa.
4. Complications of drug and alcohol abuse.

II. TREATMENT OF BULIMIA[45]

Electrolyte imbalance and metabolic disturbances may necessitate hospitalization. Antidepressants may be prescribed because anxiety and depressive symptoms are common.

Treatment is focused on the psychologic aspects with individual psychotherapy and family group therapy. Behavior modification is particularly important in the attempt to help the patient to practice a normal eating pattern.

III. DENTAL HYGIENE CARE
A. Personal Factors[42,43,46]

The individual with bulimia nervosa tends to be socially extroverted and outgoing in contrast to the shy, introverted person with anorexia. Like the anorectic person, perfectionism in life is sought, especially physical perfection through body shape and weight. The patient is well aware that the eating habits are abnormal, and may suffer low self-esteem and guilt feelings.

B. Oral Findings[44,47]

1. *Perimylolysis.* Perimylolysis is the chemical erosion of the tooth surfaces by acid from the regurgitation of stomach contents. After vomiting, acid is retained by the tongue papillae and provides longer contact with the palatal surfaces of maxillary teeth.

   The earliest evidence of bulimia may be on the smooth palatal surfaces of the teeth. With time, the erosion extends over the occlusal and incisal surfaces. The mandibular teeth are protected in part by the tongue, lips, and cheeks.
2. *Restorations.* Restorations may appear raised because of erosion of the enamel around the margins.
3. *Dental Caries.* An increase in caries incidence is found, particularly in cervical caries. Demineralization results from the pH changes in the saliva, from xerostomia, and from the large quantities of cariogenic foods ingested during binges.
4. *Saliva.* The decrease in quantity, quality, and pH of the saliva limits its buffering and lubricating properties. Dehydration of the oral soft tissues occurs.
5. *Xerostomia.* Body fluid is lost from vomiting and the use of diuretics. Xerostomia is also a side effect of antidepressant medication prescribed for certain patients with bulimia and anorexia.
6. *Hypersensitive Teeth.* The loss of enamel and the exposure of dentin results in thermal sensitivity, which can be especially noticeable for the maxillary anterior teeth.
7. *Oral Trauma*
   a. The soft palate can be traumatized by fingers, comb, pencils, or toothbrush used to induce vomiting. The same implement may injure the mouth at the commissures.
   b. Pharyngeal trauma is caused by a large food bolus that is swallowed or regurgitated.
   c. Callous formation or scars on fingers or knuckles used for self-induced vomiting may be seen.
8. *Parotid Gland.* Enlargement may occur for 2 to 6 days after a binge. A cause for the enlargement is not known, but it has been related to malnutrition.
9. *Bruxism.* Tooth wear related to stress and tension.
10. *Taste.* Impairment of taste perception.

C. Appointment Suggestions[43,44]

1. Patient instruction in cause and prevention of perimylolysis and dental caries.
   a. Reduce use of cariogenic foods; provide list of suggestions for substituting sugarless products.
   b. Improve personal oral care. Show use of appropriate brushing and flossing with additional interdental aids if required for plaque removal.
   c. Do not brush after vomiting. Demineralization of the tooth surface by the acid from the stomach starts immediately on contact. Brushing may abrade the demineralized areas. Remineralization can be helped by an alkaline rinse of sodium bicarbonate or magnesium hydroxide solution to neutralize the acid. A .05% neutral sodium fluoride rinse should also be used.
2. Fluoride therapy to reduce dental hypersensitivity and build resistance of teeth to acid demineralization.
   a. Use fluoride dentifrice with several brushings daily.
   b. Use neutral pH sodium fluoride mouthrinse (.05%) daily.
   c. Custom-fitted tray for daily home application (1.1 neutral sodium fluoride gel) (page 450).
3. Reduction in problems caused by xerostomia.
   a. Advise sugarless mints or chewing gum if patient uses them to stimulate saliva flow.
   b. Recommend saliva substitutes containing fluoride (pages 204 and 205).
4. Reduction in problems caused by hypersensitive teeth. Use sugarless foods and other products, and use fluoride dentifrice,

mouthrinse, and gel tray, to ease the sensitivity. (Additional suggestions can be found in Chapter 37, pages 557 and 558).

PSYCHIATRIC EMERGENCIES

I. PSYCHIATRIC EMERGENCY

A psychiatric emergency in a dental clinic or private dental practice would be rare. The most common causes of emergency include panic attack, atypical drug reaction, and schizophrenic or manic decompensation.[48]

II. RISK PATIENTS FOR EMERGENCIES

A. Patient with a significant psychiatric history.
B. Patient with a known substance abuse history.
C. Patient new to the clinic or office; not known by the practitioners.

III. PREVENTION OF EMERGENCIES

A. Prepare a complete history: collect as much information as possible.
B. Be alert to risks and characteristic symptoms of each disorder.
C. Learn and apply all the principles of stress management.
D. Know the patient's medications and when they are taken. Request that patient (or caregiver if accompanied) have readily available any necessary medication that may be effective in an emergency.
E. Develop rapport with each patient; do not confront or threaten a patient who may react.

IV. PREPARATION FOR AN EMERGENCY

A. Attend to surroundings, such as door access, objects in the room.
B. Arrange for colleagues to be aware of the possible needs of a special patient appointment; plan for an assistant to participate in clinical procedures.
C. Review characteristics of specific emergencies; have necessary equipment ready.
D. Keep names of the patient's case worker, psychiatrist, and responsible family member in the record in a prominent position for ready reference.

V. INTERVENTION

A. Panicked Patient

1. Stay with the patient; request colleague to contact patient's case worker, psychiatrist, or other responsible person.
2. Maintain a calm, serene manner; talk briefly but firmly.
3. Move the patient to a quiet, less stimulating environment. The dental equipment and environment may have contributed to the patient's disturbance.
4. Assist with medication when indicated.

B. Other General Emergencies

See Chapter 61, table 61–3, page 842.

REFERENCES

1. **Kaplan,** H.I. and Sadock, B.J.: *Pocket Handbook of Clinical Psychiatry.* Baltimore, Williams & Wilkins, 1990, p. 1.
2. **Lemon,** S. and Reveal, M.: Dental Hygiene Students' Preparation for Treatment of Patients with Mental Illness, *J. Dent. Educ., 55,* 724, November, 1991.
3. **Reveal,** M. and Lemon, S.: Survey of Dental Hygienists' Perceptions of Their Educational Preparation Regarding Oral Care for the Mentally Ill, *J.D.H., 65,* 20, January, 1991.
4. **American Psychiatric Association:** *Diagnostic and Statistical Manual of Mental Disorders,* 3rd ed.—Revised (DSM–III R). Washington, D.C., American Psychiatric Association, 1987.
5. **World Health Organization:** International Classification of Diseases (ICD-10). Geneva, World Health Organization, 1993.
6. **American Psychiatric Association,** Task Force on DSM-IV: *DSM-IV Options Book: Work in Progress.* Washington, D.C., American Psychiatric Association, 1991, pp. B-14 to B-16.
7. **Ibid.,** F-8 to F-11.
8. **Drake,** R.E., Osher, F.C., and Wallach, M.A.: Alcohol Use and Abuse in Schizophrenia: A Prospective Community Study, *J. Nerv. Ment. Dis., 177,* 408, July, 1989.
9. **Breier,** A., Schreiber, J.L., Dyer, J., and Pickar, D.: National Institute of Mental Health Longitudinal Study of Chronic Schizophrenia: Prognosis and Predictors of Outcome, *Arch. Gen. Psychiatry, 48,* 239, March, 1991.
10. **Felpel,** L.P.: Psychopharmacology, Antipsychotics and Antidepressants, in Neidle, E.A. and Yagiela, J.A.: *Pharmacology and Therapeutics for Dentistry,* 3rd ed. St. Louis, Mosby, 1989, pp. 162–168.
11. **Cowan,** F.F.: *Dental Pharmacology,* 2nd ed. Philadelphia, Lea & Febiger, 1992, pp. 354–360.
12. **Snyder,** N.C.: *Dental Hygiene Clinical Applications in Pharmacology.* Philadelphia, Lea & Febiger, 1987, pp. 189–194.
13. **Baldessarini,** R.J. and Frankenburg, F.R.: Clozapine. A Novel Antipsychotic Agent, *N. Engl. J. Med., 324,* 746, March 14, 1991.
14. **Quock,** R.M.: Clinical Complications in the Psychiatric Dental Patient, *Compendium, 6,* 333, May, 1985.
15. **Kane,** J.M.: Schizophrenic Disorders, in Rakel, R.E., ed.: *Conn's Current Therapy.* Philadelphia, W.B. Saunders Co., 1992, pp. 1071–1074.
16. **Barnes,** G.P., Allen, E.H., Parker, W.A., Lyon, T.C., Armentrout, W., and Cole, J.S.: Dental Treatment Needs among Hospitalized Adult Mental Patients, *Spec. Care Dentist., 8,* 173, July–August, 1988.
17. **Friedlander,** A.H. and Liberman, R.P.: Oral Health Care for the Patient with Schizophrenia, *Spec. Care Dentist., 11,* 179, September/October, 1991.
18. **Steifel,** D.J., Truelove, E.L., Menard, T.W., Anderson, V.K., Doyle, P.E., and Mandel, L.S.: A Comparison of the Oral Health of Persons with and Without Chronic Mental Illness in Community Settings, *Spec. Care Dentist., 10,* 6, January–February, 1990.
19. **Gold,** P.W., Goodwin, F.K., and Chrousos, G.P.: Clinical and Biochemical Manifestations of Depression. Relation to the Neurobiology of Stress (First of Two Parts), *N. Engl. J. Med., 319,* 348, August 11, 1988.

20. **Kaplan** and Sadock: op. cit., pp. 82–85.
21. **Abraham,** I.L., Neese, J.B., and Westerman, P.S.: Depression. Nursing Implications of a Clinical and Social Problem, *Nurs. Clin. North Am., 26,* 527, September, 1991.
22. **Felpel:** op. cit., pp. 168–175.
23. **Potter,** W.Z., Rudorfer, M.V., and Manji, H.: The Pharmacologic Treatment of Depression, *N. Engl. J. Med., 325,* 633, August 29, 1991.
24. **Wynn,** R.L.: Pharmacology Today. Antidepressant Medications, *Gen. Dent., 40,* 192, May–June, 1992.
25. **Kaplan** and Sadock: op. cit., pp. 251–261.
26. **Friedlander,** A.H. and West, L.J.: Dental Management of the Patient With Major Depression, *Oral Surg. Oral Med. Oral Pathol., 71,* 573, May, 1991.
27. **Taylor,** C.M.: *Mereness' Essentials of Psychiatric Nursing,* 13th ed. St. Louis, Mosby, 1990, pp. 235–243.
28. **Yagiella,** J.A., Duffin, S.R., and Hunt, L.M.: Drug Interactions and Vasoconstrictors Used in Local Anesthetic Solutions, *Oral Surg. Oral Med. Oral Pathol., 59,* 565, June, 1985.
29. **Tucker,** G.J.: Psychiatric Disorders in Medical Practice, in Wyngaarden, J.B., Smith, L.H., and Bennett, J.C., eds.: *Cecil Textbook of Medicine,* 19th ed. Philadelphia: W.B. Saunders Co., 1992, p. 2079.
30. **Friedlander,** A.A. and Brill, N.Q.: The Dental Management of Patients with Bipolar Disorder, *Oral Surg. Oral Med. Oral Pathol., 61,* 579, June, 1986.
31. **Taylor:** op. cit., pp. 249–256.
32. **Inwood,** D.G.: Postpartum Psychotic Disorders, in Kaplan, H.I. and Sadock, B.I., eds.: *Comprehensive Textbook of Psychiatry,* 5th ed. Baltimore, Williams & Wilkins, 1989, pp. 852–856.
33. **American Psychiatric Association,** Task Force on DSM-IV: op. cit., pp. H-1 to H-21.
34. **Nagy,** L.M. and Charney, D.S.: Panic Disorder With or Without Agoraphobia, in Rakel, R.E., ed.: *Conn's Current Therapy.* Philadelphia: W.B. Saunders Co., 1992, pp. 1075–1079.
35. **Teicher,** M.H.: Anxiety Disorders, in Rakel, R.E., ed.: *Conn's Current Therapy.* Philadelphia: W.B. Saunders Co., 1992, p. 1056.
36. **Friedlander,** A.H. and Serafetinides, E.A.: Dental Management of the Patient with Obsessive-Compulsive Disorder, *Spec. Care Dentist., 11,* 238, November–December, 1991.
37. **Felpel:** op. cit., pp. 178–188.
38. **Snyder:** op. cit., pp. 57–61.
39. **King,** L.J.: Treating the Anxious Patient, *Access, 5,* 10, September–October, 1991.
40. **Cowan,** R.D., Sabates, C.R., Gross, K.B.W., and Elledge, D.A.: Integrating Dental and Medical Care for the Chronic Bulimia Nervosa Patient: A Case Report, *Quintessence Int., 22,* 553, July, 1991.
41. **American Psychiatric Association:** op. cit., pp. 65–66.
42. **Nadler-Moodie,** M.: *Psychiatric Aspects of General Patient Care.* San Diego, Western Schools, 1991, pp. 9-3, 9-5.
43. **Gross,** K.B.W., Brough, K.M., and Randolph, P.M.: Eating Disorders. Anorexia and Bulimia Nervosa, *ASDC J. Dent. Child., 53,* 378, September–October, 1986.
44. **Montgomery,** M.T., Ritvo, J., Ritvo, J., and Weiner, K.: Eating Disorders: Phenomenology, Identification, and Dental Intervention, *Gen. Dent., 36,* 485, November–December, 1988.
45. **Kaplan** and Sadock: op. cit., pp. 198–200.
46. **Taylor:** op. cit., pp. 380–381.
47. **Knewitz,** J.L. and Drisko, C.L.: Anorexia Nervosa and Bulimia: A Review, *Compendium, 9,* 244, March, 1988.
48. **Storrie-Lombardi,** M.C., Storrie-Lombardi, I.J., Margon, C., and Stiefel, D.J., eds.: *Dental Treatment of the Patient with a Major Psychiatric Disorder.* A Self-instructional Series in Rehabilitation Dentistry. Seattle, University of Washington School of Dentistry, 1987, p. 36.

SUGGESTED READINGS

Avorn, J., Soumerai, S.B., Everitt, D.E., Ross-Degnan, D., Beers, M.H., Sherman, D., Salem-Schatz, S.R., and Fields, D.: A Randomized Trial of a Program to Reduce the Use of Psychoactive Drugs in Nursing Homes, *N. Engl. J. Med., 327,* 168, July 16, 1992.

Eisenberg, L.: Treating Depression and Anxiety in Primary Care. Closing the Gap Between Knowledge and Practice, *N. Engl. J. Med., 326,* 1080, April 16, 1992.

Friedlander, A.H.: The Dental Management of Patients with Schizophrenia, *Spec. Care Dentist., 6,* 217, September–October, 1986.

Friedlander, A.H.: The Dental Management of Depressed Patients, *Spec. Care Dentist., 7,* 65, March–April, 1987.

Friedlander, A.H. and Jarvik, L.F.: The Dental Management of the Patient with Dementia, *Oral Surg. Oral Med. Oral Pathol., 64,* 549, November, 1987.

Friedlander, A.H., Mills, M.J., and Cummings, J.L.: Consent for Dental Therapy in Severely Ill Patients, *Oral Surg. Oral Med. Oral Pathol., 65,* 179, February, 1988.

Haddad, L.M.: Managing Tricyclic Antidepressant Overdose, *Am. Fam. Physician, 46,* 153, July, 1992.

Hede, B. and Petersen, P.E.: Self-assessment of Dental Health among Danish Noninstitutionalized Psychiatric Patients, *Spec. Care Dentist., 12,* 33, January/February, 1992.

Jeste, D.V. and Krull, A.J.: Behavioral Problems Associated with Dementia: Diagnosis and Treatment, *Geriatrics, 46,* 28, November, 1991.

Kinney, R.K., Gatchel, R.J., Ellis, E, and Holt, C.: Major Psychological Disorders in Chronic TMD Patients: Implications for Successful Management, *J. Am. Dent. Assoc., 123,* 49, October, 1992.

Lassen, M.K.: Schizophrenia, *RDH, 6,* 8, March–April, 1986.

Michels, R. and Marzuk, P.M.: Progress in Psychiatry (First of Two Parts), *N. Engl. J. Med., 329,* 552, August 19, 1993.

Mills, S.H.: Deinstitutionalization and Clinical Dental Practice, *Gen. Dent., 37,* 138, March–April, 1989.

Schein, J.: Depression Is Treatable, *RDH, 11,* 20, December, 1991.

Shuman, S.K.: Ethics and the Patient with Dementia, *J. Am. Dent. Assoc., 119,* 747, December, 1989.

Sudram, C.J.: Informed Consent for Major Medical Treatment of Mentally Disabled People. A New Approach, *N. Engl. J. Med., 318,* 1368, May 26, 1988.

ter Horst, G.: Dental Care in Psychiatric Hospitals in the Netherlands, *Spec. Care Dentist., 12,* 63, March/April, 1992.

Anxiety

Enneking, B.A., Milgrom, P., Weinstein, P., and Getz, T.: Treatment Outcomes for Specific Subtypes of Dental Fear: Preliminary Clinical Findings, *Spec. Care Dentist., 12,* 214, September/October, 1992.

Filewich, R.J.: Treatment of the Agoraphobic Dental Patient, *Dent. Clin. North Am., 32,* 723, October, 1988.

Friedlander, A.H. and Eth, S.: Dental Management Considerations in Children with Obsessive-Compulsive Disorder, *ASDC J. Dent. Child., 58,* 217, May–June, 1991.

Jenike, M.A.: Obsessive-Compulsive and Related Disorders (Editorial), *N. Engl. J. Med., 321,* 539, August 24, 1989.

Sandlin, P.D.: Anatomy of Anxiety. A Physician's Overview, *Dent. Clin. North Am., 31,* 1, January, 1987.

Sokol, S.M. and Sokol, C.K.: A Biopsychosocial Approach to the Management of Anxious and Phobic Patients, *Dent. Clin. North Am., 32,* 73, January, 1988.

Weiner, A.A.: Differentiating Endogenous Panic/Anxiety Disorders from Dental Anxiety, *Anesth. Prog., 36,* 127, July–October, 1989.

Weiner, A.A. and Sheehan, D.V.: Differentiating Anxiety-Panic Disorders from Psychologic Dental Anxiety, *Dent. Clin. North Am., 32,* 823, October, 1988.

Eating Disorders

Altshuler, B.D.: Eating Disorder Patients. Recognition and Intervention, *J.D.H., 64,* 119, March–April, 1990.

Bretz, W.A., Krahn, D.D., Drewnowski, A., and Loesche, W.J.: Salivary Levels of Putative Cariogenic Organisms in Patients With Eating Disorders, *Oral Microbiol. Immunol., 4,* 230, December, 1989.

Jensen, Ø.E., Featherstone, J.D.B., and Stege, P.: Chemical and Physical Oral Findings in a Case of Anorexia Nervosa and Bulimia, *J. Oral Pathol., 16,* 399, September, 1987.

Kneisl, C.R., ed.: Eating Disorders (12 articles), *Nurs. Clin. North Am., 26,* 665, September, 1991.

Kopeski, L.M.: Diabetes and Bulimia. A Deadly Duo, *Am. J. Nurs., 89,* 483, April, 1989.

Milosevic, A. and Slade, P.D.: The Orodental Status of Anorexics and Bulimics, *Br. Dent. J., 167,* 66, July 22, 1989.

Monhehen, R.: Anorexia Nervosa, Bulimia, and the Dental Assistant, *Dent. Assist., 58,* 19, July–August, 1989.

O'Reilly, R.L., O'Riordan, J.W., and Greenwood, A.M.: Orthodontic Abnormalities in Patients with Eating Disorders, *Int. Dent. J., 41,* 212, August, 1991.

Riddlesberger, M.M., Cohen, H.L., and Glick, P.L.: The Swallowed Toothbrush: A Radiographic Clue of Bulimia, *Pediatr. Radiol., 21,* 262, No. 4, 1991.

Ruff, J.C., Koch, M.O., and Perkins, S.: Bulimia: Dentomedical Complications, *Gen. Dent., 40,* 22, January–February, 1992.

Schlipf, A.: Health Link, Secret Disorder, *RDH, 11,* 14, April, 1991.

Spigset, O.: Oral Symptoms in Bulimia Nervosa, *Acta Odontol. Scand., 49,* 335, December, 1991.

Tylenda, C.A., Roberts, M.W., Elin, R.J., Li, S.-H., and Altemus, M.: Bulimia Nervosa. Its Effect on Salivary Chemistry, *J. Am. Dent. Assoc., 122,* 37, June, 1991.

3. Less than 10% is excreted directly through the breath, sweat, and urine. The rest is metabolized in the liver.

B. Blood Alcohol Concentration (BAC)[4,5]

1. Within 5 minutes after ingestion, alcohol can be detected in the blood. BAC is measured in milligrams per deciliter (mg/dl).
2. BAC is used in the legal testing of automobile drivers. In most states in the United States, 100 mg/dl (0.1%) or less is the maximum legal driving level. The blood level usually is not measured; it is estimated from the amount present in the expired air and is expressed in percent.

C. Effects of BAC at Various Levels

1. The tolerance level varies among individuals. Whereas the inexperienced drinker may lose self-control and become nauseated with low levels of alcohol, the experienced drinker tolerates a higher level of alcohol without nausea.
2. Ethanol is a powerful depressant of the central nervous system. In low doses, alcohol can act as a disinhibitor and as a relaxant. Euphoria may be produced. In high doses, alcohol can produce analgesic effects, with reduction of anxiety generally accompanied by reduced alertness and reduced judgment.
3. BACs at various levels produce the following characteristic effects.[4,5]

50 mg/dl	sedation, tranquility fine motor coordination reduced unsteadiness on standing
50–100 mg/dl	reduced anxiety enhanced self-esteem reduced critical judgment reduced alertness; slowed reaction time impulsive risk-taking behavior
100–200 mg/dl	intoxication memory deficits possible blackouts increased aggressive behavior
300–400 mg/dl	dilated pupils lowered blood pressure lowered body temperature loss of consciousness
400–500 mg/dl	possibly fatal

D. Liver Metabolism

More than 90% of ingested alcohol is converted into acetaldehyde, then into acetone, and finally into carbon dioxide and water, by action of various liver enzymes. High acetaldehyde levels and chronic alcohol consumption impair liver function and lead to liver damage.

II. HEALTH HAZARDS[6]

Prolonged alcohol use causes many serious medical disorders. The alcohol-dependent person is most seriously afflicted, but even less heavy drinkers may have complications. Alcohol-related illnesses may involve any body system. A few are mentioned here.

A. Immunity and Infection

1. Alcoholic persons have diminished immune response; suppression of immune system defense and disturbed function of neutrophils.
2. Risk for many infections is increased, particularly pulmonary diseases (pneumonia, tuberculosis) and viral infections (hepatitis B).
3. Alcoholic liver disease leads to a depressed responsiveness to vaccines, notably hepatitis B vaccine.[7]

B. Digestive System

1. Alcohol ingestion alters the stomach mucosa, stimulates gastric acid secretion, and affects gastric function.
2. Bleeding lesions may develop with desquamation of the stomach lining (acute gastritis).

C. Nutritional Deficiencies

1. The diet of a person who consumes large quantities of alcohol regularly may be limited because the person loses interest in food and because the alcohol provides an excess of caloric intake.
2. Marked deficiencies can result from the lack of vitamins, minerals, and other essential nutrients.
3. Secondary malnutrition develops because of the direct effects of alcohol on the gastrointestinal tract. Malabsorption and maldigestion occur following cellular changes in the intestinal wall.

D. Liver Disease

1. Alcohol ingestion causes serious damage to the liver, which influences the health of the entire body.
2. Alcoholic hepatitis and cirrhosis are the most common liver complications. Alcohol abuse is the leading cause of cirrhosis, and cirrhosis is a leading cause of death.

E. Cardiovascular Diseases

1. Cardiomyopathy, heart failure, and enlarged heart occur in greater frequency in long-time alcohol consumers.
2. Significant increases in blood pressure are not unusual.
3. Heavy alcohol consumption increases the death rate from cardiovascular disease.

F. Blood Disorders

1. Reduced formation of new blood cells, megaloblastic anemia (page 807), and abnormal

iron storage are related to damaged liver function and nutritional deficiencies.

2. Leukopenia is relatively common in alcohol-dependent people.

G. Neoplasms

1. Alcohol use increases the risk of many types of cancers, including those of the esophagus, stomach, liver, lung, pancreas, colon, and rectum.[6]

2. Alcohol combined with tobacco use has long been associated with increased neoplasms of the oral cavity, pharynx, and larynx (page 670).

H. Brain Damage[8]

Long-term alcohol abuse combined with malnutrition leads to severe damage to both central and peripheral nervous systems. Early changes affect intellectual actions, such as judgment and learning ability. With prolonged and heavy alcohol consumption, chronic brain damage results. The two major disturbances are the following:

1. *Dementia Associated with Alcoholism.* Dementia is a severe impairment second only to Alzheimer's disease as a major cause of mental deterioration. It has many symptoms similar to those of Alzheimer's disease (page 636).

2. *Alcohol Amnestic Disorder (Korsakoff's Syndrome).* This disorder involves severe and persistent memory impairment with other intellectual functions staying relatively intact. It is a result of nutritional deficiency, specifically thiamine deficiency, in conjunction with chronic alcoholism.

I. Reproductive System[6]

Alcohol affects every branch of the endocrine system, directly and indirectly, through the body's organization of the endocrine hormones. Possible effects are listed here.

1. *Female.* Menstrual disturbances, loss of secondary sex characteristics, infertility, and early menopause. Fetal alcohol syndrome is described in the next section.

2. *Male.* Atrophy of testicular tubules, suppression of testosterone, loss of mature sperm cells, feminization, and failure of gonadal function.

III. FETAL ALCOHOL SYNDROME[9,10]

A. Alcohol Use During Pregnancy

The use of alcohol during the prenatal period can be seriously threatening to the health of the baby. Even children born to mothers who have been occasional drinkers, but not alcoholics, may have alcohol-related developmental or behavioral problems. The amount of alcohol, if any, that might be considered "safe" to consume during pregnancy has not been established.

Many women who abuse alcohol have poor health habits and inadequate nutritional intake, use tobacco regularly, and abuse other substances. These other factors may also influence the health of the baby.

Alcohol passes freely across the placenta. Increased incidence of spontaneous abortions and stillbirths has been related to alcohol intake. The most severe effects result in the fetal alcohol syndrome (FAS).

B. Signs and Symptoms

A characteristically abnormal pattern of growth and development can be found in children with fetal alcohol syndrome. The signs and symptoms may be grouped under central nervous system dysfunctions, growth deficiency, facial abnormalities, and other disturbances.

Individually, the signs or symptoms of alcohol-related birth defects cannot be considered specific for alcohol because they appear in other conditions; but grouped together, they form this syndrome.

1. *Central Nervous System*
   a. Mental retardation; learning disabilities.
   b. Poor motor coordination.
   c. Irritability; hyperactivity.

2. *Growth Deficiency*
   a. Prenatal and postnatal growth abnormalities in both length and weight.
   b. Microcephaly.
   c. Reduced adipose tissue; underweight.

3. *Facial Characteristics* (figure 57–1)
   a. Eyes. Short palpebral fissures, epicanthal folds, ptosis.

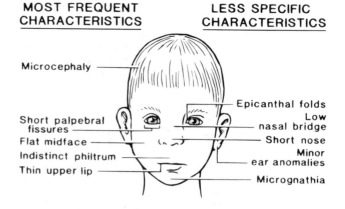

FIG. 57–1. Fetal Alcohol Syndrome. The characteristic abnormal facial features of a child born to a mother who is alcohol-dependent. Growth deficiency is also a recognized feature, as are many other signs of development and behavioral problems. (Adapted from Little, R.E. and Streissguth, A.P.: Alcohol, Pregnancy and the Fetal Alcohol Syndrome Unit in Alcohol Use and Its Medical Consequences: A Comprehensive Teaching Program for Biomedical Education. Project Cork of Dartmouth Medical School. Milner-Fenwick, Inc., 2125 Greenspring Drive, Timonium, MD 21093.)

b. Nose. Short, upturned, with sunken nasal bridge.
c. Mouth. Thin upper lip, smooth philtrum.
d. Midface. Depressed, underdeveloped maxilla.
e. Micrognathia.
f. Ear. Anomalies of shape and position.

4. *Other Disturbances.* Major organ system malformations include cardiac, hepatic, muscular, skeletal, and renal.[9]

WITHDRAWAL SYNDROME[1,2]

Withdrawal consists of the disturbances that occur after abrupt cessation of alcohol intake in the alcohol-dependent person. Withdrawal signs appear within a few hours after drinking has stopped. Even a relative decline in blood concentration can precipitate the syndrome.

I. PREDISPOSING FACTORS
Malnutrition, fatigue, depression, and physical illnesses aggravate withdrawal symptoms.

II. FEATURES
A. Tremor of hands, tongue, eyelids.
B. Nervousness and irritation.
C. Malaise, weakness, headache.
D. Dry mouth.
E. Autonomic hyperactivity; sweating, rapid heart beat, elevated blood pressure.
F. Transient visual, tactile, or auditory hallucinations.
G. Insomnia.
H. Grand mal seizures.
I. Nausea or vomiting.

III. COMPLICATIONS

A. Alcohol Withdrawal Delirium (Delirium Tremens, "DTs")
1. May occur within 1 week of cessation of heavy alcohol intake.
2. Features
   a. Marked autonomic hyperactivity: rapid heart beat, sweating.
   b. Vivid hallucinations (visual, auditory, tactile).
   c. Delusions and agitated behavior; tremor.
   d. Confusion and disorientation.

B. Alcohol Hallucinosis
1. Auditory and visual hallucinations develop within 48 hours after abruptly stopping or reducing heavy alcohol intake of long-standing dependency.

2. Features
   a. May last weeks or months.
   b. Impairment is severe, with schizophrenic symptoms, although schizophrenia is not a predisposing factor.
   c. Delirium is not present.

TREATMENT[11]

The overall objective of treatment is to help the person achieve and maintain total abstinence. An alcohol-dependent person probably can never drink even small amounts of alcohol without eventually resuming dependency.

Treatment includes a combination of medical and psychiatric therapy with self-help. Patients are encouraged not to take other psychoactive drugs, including minor tranquilizers and caffeine.

I. EARLY INTERVENTION
When problem drinkers who are not yet dependent can be identified, counseling may help to reduce and perhaps eliminate the use of alcohol.

II. DETOXIFICATION
The term detoxification applies to the management of acute intoxication and the withdrawal syndrome. A variety of treatments may be involved.

A. Treatment for Immediate Emergencies
An alcoholic may have been in an accident or have a medical emergency other than that of the alcohol withdrawal syndrome. Fractures, head injury, internal bleeding, or other problems may require initial attention. In fact, alcohol dependency may be revealed after a patient is admitted for other reasons and withdrawal symptoms appear within a few hours or days.

B. Removal from Source of Alcohol: Abstinence
One of the advantages of hospitalization is that supervision is available. The patient does not have access to usual sources of alcohol.

C. Rest, Sleep, and Proper Diet
One goal of therapy is to restore general physical health by treating nutritional deficiencies and encouraging a normal daily pattern of sleep and meals.

D. Treatment for Medical Complications
Possible medical complications were described with their systemic effects earlier in this chapter. Most alcoholics have additional illnesses.

E. Relief from Acute Withdrawal Signs
Tranquilizers may be prescribed for short-term use. Vitamins, particularly thiamine, are usually administered.

III. REHABILITATION

A. Counseling and Education

The patient must recognize that alcoholism is a serious disease and must be willing to be helped. Family and work associates may be recruited to cooperate with the program. Behavior therapy and psychotherapy have been used.

B. Disulfiram (Antabuse)[4,11]

The drug disulfiram interferes with the metabolism of alcohol by acting on the enzyme that converts acetaldehyde to acetone in the liver. As a result, acetaldehyde accumulates in the tissues. When both alcohol and disulfiram are taken at the same time, nausea and vomiting with hypotension result, and the patient becomes very ill. The drug acts as a deterrent to provide an adjunct to comprehensive therapy in selected patients.

C. Group Therapy

Alcoholics Anonymous (AA) is one source of possible help for motivated individuals. Other people prefer special clinics and centers for treatment.

AA is a fellowship of men and women who help themselves and others to recover from alcoholism. Al-Anon is a separate program for parents, adult children, siblings, and spouses, as well as other persons concerned with the recovering alcoholic. Alateen is a program for the teenage children.

D. Psychiatry

Treatment is needed for patients with psychiatric disorders. An increased frequency of schizophrenia, psychoneurosis, sociopathy, and manic-depressive diseases is being recognized among alcohol-dependent people.

E. Aftercare Services

Because recovery takes a long time, an extended period of aftercare is needed. Early relapse is more likely when a recovering alcoholic leaves a treatment system too early. A typical follow-up includes weekly aftercare group meetings for 9 to 12 months.

DENTAL HYGIENE CARE

Only a small percentage of individuals with an alcohol-consumption problem are incapacitated, homeless, shabbily dressed, or socially disoriented. Most alcohol-dependent people continue to maintain home, work, and social relationships, at least initially, and many for a span of years.

In dental and dental hygiene practice, patients who consume alcohol include the occasional social drinker, the light to moderate drinker, the problem drinker, the alcohol abuser, and the alcohol-dependent person. The abstainer or "teetotaler" is particularly important to identify because that patient may be a recovering alcoholic.

Many alcoholic patients are polysubstance abusers. They may use other psychoactive drugs, such as cocaine, heroin, amphetamines, marijuana, or assorted sedatives or hypnotics.

I. PATIENT HISTORY

The quality of the content and the frequent updating of the medical history are essential to patient care because of the many general health-related problems of alcohol ingestion that can influence oral health and treatment procedures.

A. Obtain Patient Confidence

Information about substance use and abuse must be obtained from patients of all age levels. Adolescents of all socioeconomic groups may be involved.[12] The number of elderly alcohol consumers is ever increasing; some of these are alcoholics.[13]

Unfortunately, people are hesitant to reveal personal information about alcohol use because of the social stigma attached to alcoholism. A patient first needs to understand the reasons for obtaining the information as a health-safety measure. More than that, the patient must know that personal information will remain confidential.

B. Present Questions Carefully

Questions must be asked privately and without sign of disapproval or judgment. A patient's family members may provide an alert to the patient's problem.

The basic questionnaire or interview format must have a few leading questions to provide basic facts. Care must be taken not to place the patient on the defensive.

1. *Suggested Content for Routine Questions*
   a. Pattern of alcohol consumption, frequency, amount on an average day.
   b. Systemic conditions, suggestions of alcohol-related diseases.
   c. Hospitalizations suggestive of alcohol-related accidents or detoxification program.
   d. Information about medications; self-prescribed, over-the-counter, and prescribed drugs. A relationship to polydrug abuse, alcoholism, or treatment for alcoholism may be evident.
   e. History of drinking problem.
2. *Screening for Alcohol Abuse or Dependency.* Various questionnaires have been used in the attempt to detect alcoholism. One of these, the **CAGE**, has four selected questions. Although these questions may not provide a positive diagnosis, research has shown that they can alert the interviewer and provide a high index of suspicion. One positive reply

can lead to further inquiry. The four questions are as follows[14]:

a. Have you ever felt you ought to **C**ut down on your drinking?

b. Have people **A**nnoyed you by criticizing your drinking?

c. Have you ever felt bad or **G**uilty about your drinking?

d. Have you ever had a drink first thing in the morning to steady your nerves or to get rid of a hangover (**E**yeopener)?

II. PATIENT EXAMINATION[15]

Except for the increased risk of oral cancer in persons who use alcohol heavily, no specific oral finding can be attributed directly to alcohol as the etiologic agent. The characteristics listed here have been observed frequently. When present, they assist in patient evaluation and treatment planning.

A. Extraoral Examination

1. *Breath and Body Odor of Alcohol and of Tobacco.* Many alcohol users are also heavy tobacco users.

2. *Tremor of Hands, Tongue, Eyelids.* Signs of withdrawal.

3. *Skin.* Redness of forehead, cheeks, nose; acne rosacea; dilated blood vessels that produce spider petechiae on the nose.

4. *Face Color.* Light yellowish brown may indicate jaundice from liver disease.

5. *Eyes.* Red, baggy eyes or puffy facial features; bloated appearance.

6. *Evidences of Trauma.* Facial injuries related to falls when intoxicated. Alcohol abusers are especially prone to traumatic accidents.

7. *Lips.* Angular cheilitis related to poor nutrition.

B. Intraoral Examination

1. *Mucosa, Lips, Tongue.* Dry; xerostomia.

2. *Tongue.* Coated; glossitis related to nutritional deficiencies.

3. *Periodontal Infection*

a. Generalized poor oral hygiene; heavy plaque not unusual.

b. Calculus deposits may be generalized, depending on patient neglect.

c. Gingiva that bleeds spontaneously or on probing.

4. *Teeth*

a. Chipped and fractured from falls and injuries; stained from tobacco use.

b. Attrition secondary to bruxism.

c. Erosion secondary to frequent vomiting.

d. Dental caries. Except for neglect of dental care, dental caries incidence may be no different from that for the usual population of the age level. An alcoholic who uses primarily wine or sweetened cocktails and frequently snacks on cariogenic foods is likely to have more carious lesions, particularly if gingival recession and root exposures have occurred. Lack of bacterial plaque removal also favors increased incidence of dental caries.

5. *Evidence of Minimal Dental Care.* Although subject to great variation, the overall tendency is for the alcoholic patient to put off dental and dental hygiene care, sometimes in the interest of money needed to purchase alcohol or, for the polysubstance abuser, additional drugs.

The alcohol-dependent person also may tend to use dental care primarily for emergency purposes for pain relief. The evidence may be noted in a patient who has more missing teeth than treated teeth. The indication can be that dental caries was neglected to the point where extraction was requested.

6. *Dentures.* Chipped, missing; may require frequent repairs.

III. CONSULTATION

Information in the patient history may not reveal accurately the extent of a patient's alcohol use, but clinical observations along with the medical history may provide a high degree of suspicion. From that, further inquiry and consultation with the patient's physician may help to confirm precautions needed during clinical procedures.

When a patient does not have a regular physician and has not had a recent medical evaluation, referral to a physician should be made.

IV. VITAL SIGNS

Routine recording of vital signs is indicated. Blood pressure is frequently increased in the alcoholic. Fluctuations can be particularly significant.

V. CLINICAL TREATMENT PROCEDURES

The clinical procedures for dental hygiene care are greatly influenced by the many health problems that can result from chronic ingestion of alcohol. Some of the effects were described earlier in this chapter.

A. Nonalcoholic Rinses

Preprocedural rinse, antibacterial agents, or any oral hygiene product that contains alcohol must be avoided for all patients suffering from alcoholism. This is absolutely necessary for the recovering alcoholic because recovery depends on a medication-free life-style. The most minute amount of alcohol ingested by a patient being treated with disulfiram can cause an emergency.

B. Scaling and Root Planing

The usual oral tissue response expected following periodontal scaling and root planing may be limited by the changes in the patient's tissues. These can be summarized as follows:

1. Decreased overall reserve that has resulted from degeneration of multiple organ systems.
2. Impaired healing
   a. Prolonged bleeding time; impaired clotting mechanism from chronic liver disease.
   b. Interference with collagen formation and deposition.
   c. Decreased immune system function.
3. Increased susceptibility to infection.

C. Power-driven Instruments

The patient with chronic alcohol abuse or dependency, particularly one who also inhales tobacco smoke, most likely has pulmonary complications. Lung infections are common. Lung abscesses can be caused by bacteria taken into the lungs from the oral cavity or by abnormal breathing during intoxication. Power-driven instruments, particularly ultrasonic scalers and airbrasive stain-removal devices, must be used with caution to prevent inhalation of oral microorganisms by the patient. High-powered suction applied by an assistant is essential.

PATIENT INSTRUCTION

I. BACTERIAL PLAQUE CONTROL

Oral health and cleanliness can be especially important for the patient because of the susceptibility to infection and the high incidence of oral cancer. Motivation may be difficult because many patients with alcohol or polysubstance dependency are preoccupied with alcohol or drugs and place less priority on personal hygiene.

A preventive care program for a recovering alcoholic should become part of the total rehabilitation process.

II. DIET AND NUTRITION
A. Relation of Diet to Alcoholism

1. Alcoholic beverages contain calories; a day's allotment of calories may be ingested when alcohol is used in excess.
2. The calories of alcohol are "empty" calories without nutritional elements, and the balance of the diet can be very limited.
3. Alcohol unfavorably affects the absorption and digestion of many nutrients by the changes it produces in the mucosa of the gastrointestinal tract.
4. Liver damage has a major detrimental influence on the metabolism of nutrients.

B. Dietary Deficiencies

Malnutrition has been associated for many years with alcoholism. The severe malnutrition that has been described applies primarily to the derelict or "skid row" alcoholic who has limited resources for proper food.

Many middle and upper class alcoholics do not consume an acceptable "balanced" diet, but they cannot be considered with the severely malnourished group.

C. Instruction

After a dietary analysis is reviewed with the patient, help can be provided by reviewing the basic dietary needs and encouraging the use of foods from the food guide pyramid (figure 28–1, page 424).

FACTORS TO TEACH THE PATIENT

I. Alcohol abuse is a great risk to overall health.
II. Incidence of oral cancer is increased by the use of alcohol and tobacco.
III. Mixing alcohol with other drugs (prescription or over-the-counter) can lead to medical emergencies. Always check each drug and its actions before using it in combination with alcohol.
IV. Alcoholism is a disease with serious implications. Advise young people of the dangers involved and discourage them from drinking alcohol.
V. Commercial antibacterial and fluoride mouthrinses may contain up to 30% alcohol. Labels must be read carefully. Keep mouthrinse bottles out of reach of children.
VI. Use of alcohol during pregnancy should be avoided because of possible devastating effects on the baby. Be alert to the alcohol content of certain foods and drugs.
VII. Alcohol readily enters breast milk and is transmitted to the infant during nursing.

REFERENCES

1. **American Psychiatric Association:** *Diagnostic and Statistical Manual of Mental Disorders,* 3rd ed.—Revised (DSM-III-R). Washington, D.C., American Psychiatric Association, 1987, pp. 127–134, 173–175.
2. **American Psychiatric Association,** Task Force on DSM-IV: *DSM-IV Options Book: Work in Progress.* Washington, D.C., American Psychiatric Association, 1991, pp. E:10–E:12.
3. **United States Department of Health and Human Services,** Secretary of Health and Human Services: *Seventh Special Report to the U.S. Congress on Alcohol and Health.* Rockville, MD, National Institute on Alcohol Abuse and Alcoholism, January, 1990, pp. 1–8.
4. **Aston,** R.: Aliphatic Alcohols, in Neidle, E.A. and Yagiela, J.A.: *Pharmacology and Therapeutics for Dentistry,* 3rd ed. St. Louis, Mosby, 1989, pp. 594–597.
5. **Theoharides,** T.C., ed.: *Pharmacology.* Boston, Little, Brown and Company, 1992, pp. 323–328.
6. **United States Department of Health and Human Services:** op. cit., 107–138.
7. **Lybecker,** L.A., Mendenhall, C.L., Marshall, L.E., Weesner,

R.E., and Myre, S.A.: Response to Hepatitis B Vaccine (HBVac) in the Alcoholic, *Hepatology, 3,* 807, Abstract 36, May, 1983.

8. **United States Department of Health and Human Services:** op. cit., pp. 87–92.

9. **United States Department of Health and Human Services:** op. cit., pp. 139–161.

10. **Gordis,** E. and Alexander, D.: Progress Toward Preventing and Understanding Alcohol-induced Fetal Injury, *JAMA, 268, 3183,* December 9, 1992.

11. **United States Department of Health and Human Services:** op. cit., pp. 261–280.

12. **Macdonald,** D.I.: Drugs, Drinking, and Adolescence, *Am. J. Dis. Child., 138,* 117, February, 1984.

13. **Friedlander,** A.H. and Solomon, D.H.: Dental Management of the Geriatric Alcoholic Patient, *Gerodontics, 4,* 23, February, 1988.

14. **Ewing,** J.A.: Detecting Alcoholism. The CAGE Questionnaire, *JAMA, 252,* 1905, October 12, 1984.

15. **Friedlander,** A.H., Mills, M.J., and Gorelick, D.A.: Alcoholism and Dental Management, *Oral Surg. Oral Med. Oral Pathol., 63,* 42, January, 1987.

SUGGESTED READINGS

Boffetta, P., Mashberg, A., Winkelmann, R., and Garfinkel, L.: Carcinogenic Effect of Tobacco Smoking and Alcohol Drinking on Anatomic Sites of the Oral Cavity and Oropharynx, *Int. J. Cancer, 52,* 530, Octoer 21, 1992.

Brickley, M.R. and Shepherd, J.P.: Alcohol Abuse in Dental Patients, *Br. Dent. J., 169,* 329, November 24, 1990.

Charness, M.E., Simon, R.P., and Greenberg, D.A.: Ethanol and the Nervous System, *N. Engl. J. Med., 321,* 442, August 17, 1989.

Diamond, I.: Alcohol Myopathy and Cardiomyopathy, *N. Engl. J. Med., 320,* 458, February 16, 1989.

Leonard, R.H.: Alcohol, Alcoholism, and Dental Treatment, *Compendium, 12,* 274, April, 1991.

Lieber, C.S.: Biochemical and Molecular Basis of Alcohol-induced Injury to Liver and Other Tissues, *N. Engl. J. Med., 319,* 1639, December 22, 1988.

Michels, R. and Marzuk, P.-M.: Progress in Psychiatry (Second of Two Parts), *N. Engl. J. Med., 329,* 628, August 26, 1993.

Modell, J.G. and Mountz, J.M.: Drinking and Flying—The Problem of Alcohol Used by Pilots, *N. Engl. J. Med., 323,* 455, August 16, 1990.

Powell, A.H. and Minick, M.P.: Alcohol Withdrawal Syndrome, *Am. J. Nurs., 88,* 312, March, 1988.

Ratcliff, J.S. and Collins, G.B.: Dental Management of the Recovered Chemically Dependent Patient, *J. Am. Dent. Assoc., 114,* 601, May, 1987.

Talamini, R., Franceschi, S., Barra, S., and La Vecchia, C.: The Role of Alcohol in Oral and Pharyngeal Cancer in Non-smokers, and of Tobacco in Non-drinkers, *Int. J. Cancer, 46,* 391, September 15, 1990.

Weisner, C. and Schmidt, L.: Gender Disparities in Treatment for Alcohol Problems, *JAMA, 268,* 1872, October 14, 1992.

Screening/Assessment

Bush, B., Shaw, S., Cleary, P., Delbanco, T.L., and Aronson, M.D.: Screening for Alcohol Abuse Using the CAGE Questionnaire, *Am. J. Med., 82,* 231, February, 1987.

Cyr, M.G. and Wartman, S.A.: The Effectiveness of Routine Screening Questions in the Detection of Alcoholism, *JAMA, 259,* 51, January 1, 1988.

Egbert, A.M.: The Older Alcoholic: Recognizing the Subtle Clinical Clues, *Geriatrics, 48,* 63, July, 1983.

Hennessey, MB.: Identifying the Woman with Alcohol Problems. The Nurse's Role as Gatekeeper, *Nurs. Clin. North Am., 27,* 917, December, 1992.

Robb, N.D. and Smith, B.G.N.: Prevalence of Pathological Tooth Wear in Patients with Chronic Alcoholism, *Br. Dent. J., 169,* 367, December 8/22, 1990.

Fetal Alcohol Syndrome

Gir, A.V., Aksharanugraha, K., and Harris, E.F.: A Cephalometric Assessment of Children with Fetal Alcohol Syndrome, *Am. J. Orthod. Dentofac, Orthop., 95,* 319, April, 1989.

United States Centers for Disease Control and Prevention: Fetal Alcohol Syndrome—United States, 1979–1992, *MMWR, 42,* 339, May 7, 1993.

Waldman, H.B.: Fetal Alcohol Syndrome and the Realities of Our Time, *ASDC J. Dent. Child., 56,* 435, November–December, 1989.

Werler, M.M., Lammer, E.J., Rosenberg, L., and Mitchell, A.A.: Maternal Alcohol Use in Relation to Selected Birth Defects, *Am. J. Epidemiol., 134,* 691, October 1, 1991.

Alcohol in Mouthrinse

Goepferd, S.J.: Mouthwash—A Potential Source of Acute Alcohol Poisoning in Young Children, *Clin. Prev. Dent., 5,* 14, May–June, 1983.

Hornfeldt, C.S.: A Report of Acute Ethanol Poisoning in a Child: Mouthwash Versus Cologne, Perfume and Aftershave, *Clin. Toxicol., 30,* 115, March, 1992.

Leung, A.K.: Acute Alcohol Toxicity Following Mouthwash Ingestion [letter], *Clin. Pediatr., 24,* 470, August, 1985.

Selbst, S.M., DeMaio, J.G., and Boenning, D.: Mouthwash Poisoning, *Clin. Pediatr., 24,* 162, March, 1985.

Tipton, G.A. and Scottino, M.A.: Acute Alcohol Toxicity Following Mouthwash Ingestion in a Child, *Clin. Pediatr., 24,* 164, March, 1985.

Weller-Fahy, E.R., Berger, L.R., and Troutman, W.G.: Mouthwash: A Source of Acute Ethanol Intoxication, *Pediatrics, 66,* 302,

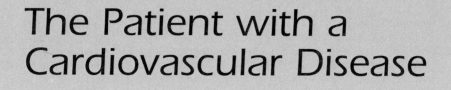

The Patient with a Cardiovascular Disease

Cardiovascular, as the names implies, includes diseases of the heart and blood vessels. Diseases of the heart are the leading causes of death in the United States. Key words and terminology describing the cardiovascular diseases are defined in table 58–1. Prefixes and suffixes to clarify the terminology are listed on pages 851–853.

Patients with cardiovascular conditions are encountered frequently in a dental office or clinic and may be from any age group, although the highest incidence is among older people. A heart disease may be present for many years before the symptoms are recognized. The patients seen in the dental office range from those with no obvious symptoms to the nearly disabled. In severe cases, the nonambulatory patient may require care in the home.

I. CLASSIFICATION
Classification of the diseases is made on either an anatomic or an etiologic basis. In an anatomic system, diseases of the pericardium, myocardium, endocardium, heart valves, and blood vessels are defined. In an etiologic system, the diseases are named by the cause. The principal causes of heart diseases are infectious agents, atherosclerosis, hypertension, immunologic mechanisms, and congenital anomalies.

II. MAJOR CARDIOVASCULAR DISEASES
The five major cardiovascular diseases are congenital heart disease, rheumatic heart disease, infective endocarditis, ischemic heart disease, and hypertensive heart disease. Characteristics and symptoms are complex and overlapping. In this chapter, each of the major diseases is described by its principal symptoms and treatments as well as the applications in dental hygiene care.

CONGENITAL HEART DISEASES

Anomalies of the anatomic structure of the heart or major blood vessels result following irregularities of development during the first 9 weeks *in utero*. The fetal heart is completely developed by the ninth week.

Early diagnosis is important because between one fourth and one half of the infants born with cardiovascular anomalies require treatment during the first year. Treatment usually involves surgical correction.

I. TYPES
Many types of heart defects exist. Those that occur most frequently are the ventricular septal defect, patent ductus arteriosus, atrial septal defect, and transposition of the great vessels.

A diagram of the normal heart is shown in figure 58–1 to provide a comparison with the anatomic changes that may appear in a defective heart. Congenital anomalies either produce abnormal pathways in the blood flow or interfere with the flow itself. The two most common anomalies are described here.

A. Ventricular Septal Defect
In this type of defect, the left and right ventricles are connected through an opening in their dividing wall (septum). The oxygenated blood from the lung, which is normally pumped by the left ventricle to the aorta and then to the entire body, can pass across to the right ventricle as shown in figure 58–2.

When the opening is very small, only a heart murmur and little disability result. If the open-

TABLE 58-1
KEY WORDS: CARDIOVASCULAR DISEASE

Aneurysm (an'ū-rĭzm): sac formed by the localized dilatation of the wall of an artery, a vein, or the heart.

Angina (an-jī'nah): a disease marked by spasmodic suffocative attacks.

　Angina pectoris: acute pain in the chest from decreased blood supply to the heart muscle.

Anoxia (ah-nok'sē-ah): absence of oxygen in the tissues; may be accompanied by deep respirations, cyanosis, increased pulse rate, and impairment of coordination.

Anticoagulant (an'tĭ-kō-ag'ū-lant): a substance that suppresses, delays, or nullifies coagulation of the blood.

Apnea (ap'nē-ah): temporary cessation of breathing.

Arrhythmia (ah-rith'mē-ah): variation from the normal rhythm, especially with reference to the heart.

Arterial blood: oxygenated blood carried by an artery away from the heart to nourish the body tissues.

Asphyxia (as-fik'sē-ah): a condition in which there is a deficiency of oxygen in the blood and an increase in carbon dioxide.

Atheroma (ath'er-ō'mah): lipid (cholesterol) deposit on the intima (lining) of an artery; also called atheromatous plaque.

Bradycardia (brād'e-kar'dē-ah) slowness of heartbeat with slowing of pulse rate to less than 60 per minute.

Cyanosis (sī'ah-nō'sis): bluish discoloration of the skin and mucous membranes caused by excess concentration of reduced hemoglobin in the blood.

Dyspnea (disp'ne-ah) labored or difficult breathing.

Echocardiography (ek'ō-kar'dē-og'rah-fē): recording of the position and motion of the heart walls and internal structures of the heart and neighboring tissue by the echo obtained from beams of ultrasonic waves directed through the chest wall; used to show valvular and other structural deformities; the record produced is called an **echocardiogram.**

Edema (ě-dē'mah): abnormal accumulation of fluid in the intercellular spaces of the body.

Electrocardiography (ē-lek'trō-kar'dē-og'rah-fē): the graphic recording from the body surface of the potential of electric currents generated by the heart as a means of studying the action of the heart muscle; the record produced is called an **electrocardiogram (EKG).**

Embolism (em'bō-lizm): the sudden blocking of an artery by a clot of foreign material, an **embolus,** that has been brought to its site of lodgment by the blood stream; the embolus may be a blood clot (most frequently), or an air bubble, a clump of bacteria, or a fat globule.

Heparin (hep'ah-rin): anticoagulant; prevents platelet agglutination and thrombus formation.

Hypoxia (hi-pok'sē-ah); diminished availability of oxygen to body tissues.

Infarct (in'farkt): localized area of ischemic necrosis produced by occlusion of the arterial supply or venous drainage of the part.

Ischemia (is kē'mē-ah): deficiency of blood to supply oxygen in a part resulting from functional constriction or actual obstruction of a blood vessel.

Lumen (loo'men): the cavity or channel within a tube or tubular organ, as a blood vessel or the intestine.

Murmur (mur'mur): irregularity of heartbeat sound caused by a turbulent flow of blood through a valve that has failed to close.

Myocardium (mī'ō-kar'dē-um): the middle and thickest layer of the heart wall, composed of cardiac muscle.

Occlusion (ŏ-kloo'zhun): blockage; state of being closed.

Sclerosis (skle-rō'sis): induration, hardening.

　Arteriosclerosis: group of diseases characterized by thickening and loss of elasticity of the arterial walls.

Stenosis (stě-nō'sis): narrowing or contraction of a body passage or opening.

Tachycardia (tak'ē-kar'dē-ah): abnormally rapid heart rate, usually taken to be over 100 beats per minute.

Tetralogy (tě-tral'ō-je): a group or series of four.

　Tetralogy of Fallot: congenital, cyanotic malformation of the heart that includes pulmonary stenosis, ventricular septal defect, hypertrophy of the right ventricle, and dextroposition of the aorta.

Thrombus (throm'bus): blood clot attached to the intima of a blood vessel; may occlude the lumen; contrast with embolus, which is detached and carried by the blood steam.

Venous blood: nonoxygenated blood from the tissues; blood pumped from the heart to the lungs for oxygenation.

---

ing is large, the heart enlarges to compensate for overwork.

B. Patent Ductus Arteriosus

A patent ductus arteriosus means the passageway (shunt) is open between the two great arteries that arise from the heart, namely the aorta and the pulmonary artery. Normally, the opening is closed during the first few weeks after birth. When the opening does not close, blood from the aorta can pass back to the lungs, as shown in figure 58–3. The heart compensates

in the attempt to provide the body with oxygenated blood and becomes overburdened.

II. ETIOLOGY

Causes are genetic, environmental, or a combination. Many are unknown.

A. Genetic

Heredity is apparent in some types of defects. An example of a chromosomal defect is Down's syndrome, in which congenital heart anomalies occur frequently (page 754).

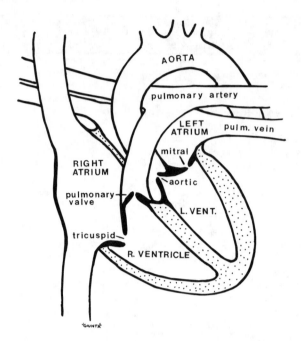

FIG. 58–1. The Normal Heart. The major vessels and the location of the tricuspid, pulmonary, aortic, and mitral valves are shown.

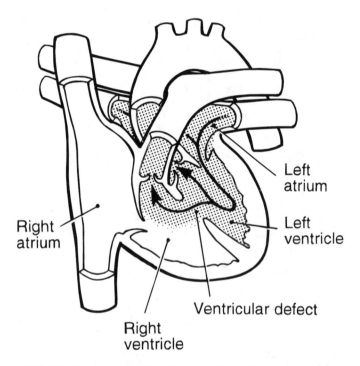

FIG. 58–2. Ventricular Septal Defect. The right and left ventricles are connected by an opening that permits oxygenated blood from the left ventricle to shunt across to the right ventricle and then recirculate to the lungs. Compare with figure 58–1 in which the septum separates the ventricles. (Adapted from Bleck, E.E. and Nagel, D.A.: *Physically Handicapped Children. A Medical Atlas for Teachers.* New York, Grune & Stratton, 1975.)

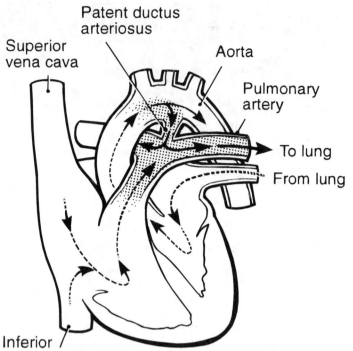

FIG. 58–3. Patent Ductus Arteriosus. An open passageway between the aorta and the pulmonary artery permits oxygenated blood from the aorta to pass back into the lungs. Arrows show directions of flow through the patent ductus. Compare with normal anatomy in figure 58–1. (Adapted from Bleck, E.E. and Nagel, D.A.: *Physically Handicapped Children. A Medical Atlas for Teachers.* New York, Grune & Stratton, 1975.)

B. Environmental

Most congenital anomalies originate between the fifth and eighth weeks of fetal life, when the heart is developing.
1. Rubella (German measles).
2. Drugs.
   a. Chronic maternal alcohol abuse. The fetal alcohol syndrome is described on page 778.
   b. Thalidomide.

III. PREVENTION

A. Use of rubella vaccine for childhood immunization. Vaccination confers indefinite immunity. Vaccination for women of childbearing age is highly advised. The vaccine should not be given during pregnancy, and not within 3 months of becoming pregnant, because of potential risks to the fetus.
B. No medications used during pregnancy without prior consultation with the physician.
C. Appropriate use of radiologic equipment. A lead apron should be used when oral radiographs are made.

**TABLE 58-3
LIFE-STYLE MODIFICATIONS FOR
HYPERTENSION CONTROL AND/OR OVERALL
CARDIOVASCULAR RISK**

- Lose weight if overweight.
- Limit alcohol intake to no more than 1 ounce of ethanol per day (24 ounces of beer, 8 ounces of wine, or 2 ounces of 100 proof whiskey).
- Exercise (aerobic) regularly.
- Reduce sodium intake to less than 100 mmol per day (< 2.3 g of sodium or < 6 g of sodium chloride).
- Maintain adequate dietary potassium, calcium, and magnesium intake.
- Stop smoking and reduce dietary saturated fat and cholesterol intake for overall cardiovascular health. Reducing fat intake also helps to reduce caloric intake—important for control of weight and Type II diabetes.

(From *The Fifth Report of the Joint National Committee on Detection, Evaluation, and Treatment of High Blood Pressure.* National High Blood Pressure Education Program, NIH National Heart, Lung, and Blood Institute, NIH Publication No. 93-1088, January, 1993.)

2. *Cigarette Smoking.* All forms of tobacco must be eliminated.
3. *Other Risk Factors.* Factors that contribute to stress and tension must be decreased or minimized. Risk factors were listed on page 789.

C. Antihypertensive Drug Therapy[5]

1. *Selection of Therapy.* The decision by the physician to prescribe drug therapy at the various levels depends on the severity of the hypertension, as well as on all factors related to the patient's health.
2. *Categories of Drugs Used in Therapy*
   a. Diuretics to promote renal excretion of water and sodium ions.
   b. Sympatholytic agents to modify the sympathetic nerve activity.
   c. Vasodilators to act directly on the blood vessels.
3. *Duration.* Management of hypertension must be considered a lifelong endeavor. Periodic monitoring is essential every 3 to 6 months. Dental personnel can encourage their patients to continue treatment even when a normal reading is maintained. Because many antihypertensive drugs have undesirable side effects, the patient may become discouraged and discontinue treatment.
4. *Side Effects.* The effects of the different drugs prescribed vary, but some of the problems confronted by patients may actually influence the behavior at dental and dental hygiene appointments. Cancellation of an appointment could be anticipated. Side effects may include some or all of the following:
   a. Fatigue.
   b. Gastrointestinal disturbances, including nausea, diarrhea, or cramps.
   c. Xerostomia (potential for dental caries).
   d. Postural hypotension with dizziness and fainting.
   e. Impotence.
   f. Depression.

V. HYPERTENSION IN CHILDREN

Children 3 years of age and older should have blood pressure determinations made at least annually. A variety of cuff sizes are available, and other procedural suggestions are described on pages 112 and 113.

When a child between ages 3 and 12 has a diastolic pressure greater than 90 mm Hg, or if over age 12, greater than 100 mm Hg, further investigation is indicated.[5] Because hypertension has a familial tendency, determining the pressure levels for children of parents known to have hypertension may reveal important information about the health of the child.

HYPERTENSIVE HEART DISEASE[7]

Hypertensive heart disease results from the increased load on the heart because of elevated blood pressure. When the peripheral arterial resistance to the flow of blood pumped from the heart is increased, the blood pressure rises. The heart attempts to maintain its normal output. To cope with the increased workload resulting from the peripheral resistance, muscle fibers are stretched and the heart enlarges.

The effect of hypertension on the heart is at first a thickening of the left ventricle. In later stages, the entire heart is enlarged. This may be discerned by radiographic and medical examination.

Cardiac enlargement has no specific symptoms, but the patient may have symptoms of hypertension, such as headaches, weakness, and others listed on page 790. When undiagnosed and untreated, the severity increases and left ventricular congestive failure occurs, resulting from the disturbance of cardiac function.

ISCHEMIC HEART DISEASE

Ischemic heart disease is the cardiac disability, acute and chronic, that arises from reduction or arrest of blood supply to the myocardium.

The heart muscles (myocardium) are supplied through the coronary arteries, which are branches of the descending aorta. Because of the relationship to the coronary arteries, the disease is often referred to as *coronary heart disease* or *coronary artery disease.*

Ischemia means oxygen deprivation in a local area from a reduced passage of fluid into the area. Ischemic heart disease is the result of an imbalance of the oxygen supply and demand of the myocardium, which in turn, results from a narrowing or blocking of the lumen of the coronary arteries.

I. ETIOLOGY[8]

Other factors may be involved, but the principal cause of the reduction of blood flow to the heart muscle is *atherosclerosis* of the vessel walls, which narrows the lumen, thus obstructing the flow of blood.

A. Definition of Atherosclerosis

Atherosclerosis is a disease of medium and large arteries in which atheromas deposit on and thicken the intimal layer of the involved blood vessel. An atheroma is a fibro-fatty deposit or plaque, containing several lipids, especially cholesterol. With time, the plaques continue to thicken and, eventually, close the vessel (figure 58–4). Some plaques calcify, whereas others may develop an overlying thrombus.

B. Predisposing Factors for Atherosclerosis

Each of the risk factors listed here is significant alone. When these factors occur in combinations, the risk of atherosclerosis, and therefore of ischemic heart disease, is increased. Prevention depends on educational programs along with early identification of persons at risk.

1. Elevated levels of blood lipids; the result of an increased dietary intake of cholesterol, saturated fat, carbohydrate, especially sucrose, alcohol, and calories.
2. Elevated blood pressure.
3. Cigarette smoking.
4. Diabetes.
5. Obesity.
6. Insufficient physical activity.
7. Increased tensions; emotional stress.
8. Family history. Genetic inheritance may not be the fact so much as the perpetuation of familial life-style habits. Diet, smoking habits, tensions, and tendencies toward lack of exercise are typical examples.

II. MANIFESTATIONS OF ISCHEMIC HEART DISEASE

A. Components
1. Angina pectoris.
2. Myocardial infarction.
3. Congestive heart failure.
4. Sudden death.

B. Treatment
1. *Counseling.* With a brief history of angina pain, the patient is counseled to explain the disease, and to reassure the patient that life-style changes are necessary but that a productive life can be led.
2. *Life-style Changes.* Necessary changes in life-style (table 58–3) are encouraged, notably diet, exercise, and no smoking.

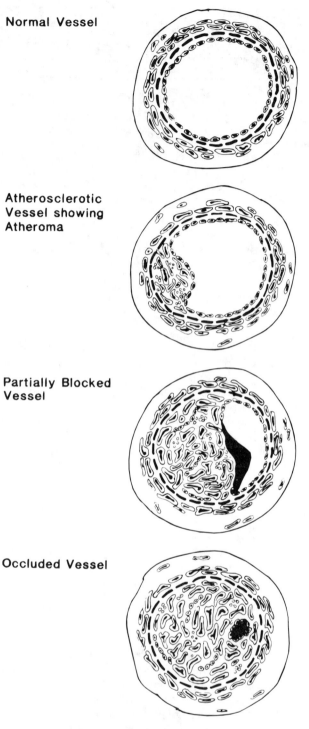

Normal Vessel

Atherosclerotic Vessel showing Atheroma

Partially Blocked Vessel

Occluded Vessel

FIG. 58–4. Atherosclerosis. An atheroma develops within the lining of the normal blood vessel. The atheroma is made of a fatty deposit containing cholesterol. At first, the atheroma is small and no symptoms are apparent; but eventually, it enlarges and completely blocks the vessel, thus depriving the area served by the vessel of oxygen. (From *Arteriosclerosis 1981.* Report of the Working Group on Arteriosclerosis of the National Heart, Lung, and Blood Institute, National Institutes of Health, United States Department of Health and Human Services, NIH Publication No. 81–2034, June, 1981.)

3. *Medications.* A variety of medications may be required depending on individual needs, including

   a. Antianginal (vasodilators). Prevent anginal pain by decreasing systolic blood pressure.
   b. Antihypertensives (diuretics). Blood pressure control.
   c. Antidysrhythmics. Fibrillation; ventricular dysrhythmias.
   d. Beta-adrenergic blocking agents. Decreased heart rate and blood pressure.
   e. Calcium channel blockers. Decreased cardiac workload and act as vasodilators.

4. *Surgery*

   a. Percutaneous transluminal coronary angioplasty (coronary dilation).
   b. Coronary bypass for patients with significant obstruction. The purpose is to "jump-pass" over arteries that have been narrowed with atherosclerosis. The beneficial effects are relief from anginal pains, less workload for the heart, and an in-

crease of oxygen and blood supply to the myocardium. Figure 58–5 shows the use of a vein graft and the internal mammary artery for bypasses.

ANGINA PECTORIS

Angina pectoris is a symptom complex or syndrome of discomfort in the chest and adjacent areas that results from transient and reversible myocardial oxygen deficiency. Although other forms of coronary disease may cause similar pain symptoms, approximately 90% of angina attacks are related to coronary artery atherosclerosis.

I. PREDISPOSING FACTORS
An attack of angina pectoris may be precipitated by exertion or exercise, emotion, or a heavy meal. In the dental office or clinic, a preventive atmosphere of calmness and quiet can do much to alleviate stress.

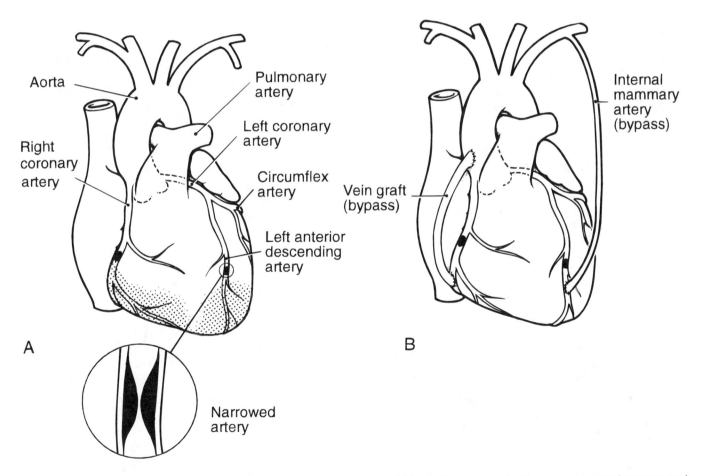

FIG. 58–5. Coronary Bypass Surgery. A. Heart showing infarcted (shaded) areas created by coronary arteries narrowed by atherosclerosis. **B.** Vein graft from saphenous vein connected with aorta to bypass narrowed area of right coronary artery, and internal mammary artery used to bypass narrowed left anterior descending artery.

II. SYMPTOMS

A. Chest Pain

Each person who suffers from angina has a characteristic pattern of pain symptoms. When changes in the usual pain occur, the physician must be notified.

Commonly, the patient has thoracic pain, which is substernal and radiates down the left arm and up to the mandible. It may last for seconds or minutes.

The pain is squeezing or crushing, paroxysmal, or pressing, with a feeling of weight on the chest. The patient stops and tends to stiffen.

B. Other Symptoms

The patient may be pale and also experience faintness, sweating, difficulty in breathing, anxiety, or fear.

III. TREATMENT

A vasodilator, usually nitroglycerin, is administered sublingually.

IV. PROCEDURE DURING AN ATTACK IN THE DENTAL OFFICE

A. Terminate Treatment

Stop the dental or dental hygiene procedure. Call for assistance and the emergency kit or cart.

B. Position Patient

Seat the patient up to a comfortable position; reassure the patient.

C. Administer Vasodilator

Administer nitroglycerin sublingually. Use of the patient's own supply is preferable. Prior to starting procedures of the appointment, the patient's supply should be placed within reach. The patient can be asked when the nitroglycerin was purchased, because the potency is lost after 6 months out of a sealed storage container.

Patient with xerostomia may not have sufficient saliva to moisten the nitroglycerin. A few drops of water from the unit syringe can be placed on the tablet under the tongue.

D. Check Patient Response

Give additional vasodilator. Usually, the first tablet relieves the condition within minutes. When it is suspected that the patient's supply may not be fresh and the first tablet has been ineffective, use of a second tablet from the dental office emergency kit may be advisable.

E. Call for Medical Assistance

When the patient does not respond to the second dose of vasodilator, assume the attack to be a myocardial infarction. Oxygen administration may be indicated.

F. Record Vital Signs

1. Use *Record of Emergency,* figure 61–1, page 831.

2. Measure blood pressure, take pulse rate, and count respirations.

G. Observe Recovery

For the patient who recovers without additional medical assistance, allow a rest period before dismissal. Record vital signs again.

V. SUBSEQUENT DENTAL AND DENTAL HYGIENE APPOINTMENTS

Keep a copy of the *Record of Emergency* in the patient's permanent file for reference when planning future appointments.

MYOCARDIAL INFARCTION

Myocardial infarction is the most extreme manifestation of ischemic heart disease. It is also called *heart attack, coronary occlusion,* or *coronary thrombosis.* It results from a sudden reduction or arrest of coronary blood flow.

The most common artery associated with a myocardial infarction is the anterior descending branch of the left coronary artery. That is also the most common site of advanced atherosclerosis.

I. ETIOLOGY

The immediate cause often is a thrombosis that blocks an artery already narrowed by atherosclerosis. In turn, the blockage creates an area of infarction, which leads to myocardial necrosis of the area. Necrosis of the area can occur within a few hours.

A few patients die immediately or within a few hours. Sudden death may be caused by ventricular fibrillation.

II. SYMPTOMS

A. Pain

1. *Location.* Pain symptoms may start under the sternum, with feelings of indigestion, or in the middle to upper sternum.. Pain may last for extended periods, even hours. When the pain is severe, it gives a pressing or crushing heavy sensation and is not relieved by rest or nitroglycerin.

2. *Onset.* The pain may have a sudden onset, sometimes during sleep or following exercise. The pain may be radial, similar to angina pectoris, which extends to the left arm and mandible.

B. Other Symptoms

Cold sweat, weakness and faintness, shortness of breath, nausea, and vomiting may occur. Blood pressure is lowered.

III. MANAGEMENT DURING AN ATTACK

A. Terminate Treatment

Sit the patient up for comfortable breathing, give nitroglycerin, and reassure the patient.

cautions are needed to prevent hemorrhage, discontinuing the drug can be much more hazardous for the patient than performing dental and dental hygiene therapy with precautions. When extensive surgical procedures are required, the patient may be hospitalized.

I. CLINICAL PROCEDURES
A. Consultation
Information about the patient's prothrombin time is obtained from the physician during an initial consultation. The prothrombin time is a test of the coagulation phase of blood clotting used to monitor therapy with anticoagulants. A therapeutic range of $1\frac{1}{2}$ to $2\frac{1}{2}$ times the normal level is preferred.

B. Treatment Planning
1. *Pretest for Prothrombin Time*
   a. Determine the prothrombin time within 24 hours before an appointment. The patient can have the test made on the day of a dental appointment by preplanning with the physician and the laboratory. Most patients have a routine appointment for monitoring of the blood, and dental appointment dates can be planned to coincide.
   b. Safe level for dental and dental hygiene procedures is considered to be $1\frac{1}{2}$ times the normal, provided precautions are taken during instrumentation and postoperative care.
2. *Quadrant Scaling and Root Planing*
   a. Treat the most healthy quadrant first. The least bleeding will occur.
   b. Teach and emphasize daily bacterial plaque control procedures in a series of appointments to prepare the gingival tissue for instrumentation. Healthy, healed tissue does not bleed as readily or as profusely.
   c. Complete treatment, including removal of all calculus and subgingival plaque and other irritants, is necessary to contribute to the goal of healthy tissue that does not bleed.

C. Local Hemostatic Measures
Instrumentation can be performed for most patients without complication, provided precautions are taken to minimize tissue trauma and control bleeding, and not to dismiss the patient until bleeding has stopped.
1. *Pressure.* Pressure with sponges or cotton pellets packed interdentally can aid in control.
2. *Suture.* Sutures may be used to close and adapt the tissue interdentally following deep scaling and root planing.
3. *Periodontal Dressing.* Placement of a dressing is sometimes advisable to provide pressure and protection from trauma that may initiate postoperative bleeding. Dressing placement is described on page 547

II. POSTOPERATIVE INSTRUCTIONS
The practice by oral surgeons of closely observing patients for 6 to 8 hours following a surgical procedure has application following certain dental and dental hygiene procedures for selected patients. At least, a check that postoperative instructions are being followed is advisable.

Postoperatively, the patient is advised to avoid vigorous toothbrushing and rinsing for several hours or until the next day. The use of extraoral icepacks may be helpful. General postoperative instructions may be found on pages 658 and 659; for the care of an area with a dressing, see table 36–2, page 548.

The use of a soft diet, cool rather than hot foods, and general moderation in activity may be important.

Long-term instruction must emphasize the maintenance of gingival health to prevent future bleeding problems.

CARDIOVASCULAR SURGERY

Cardiac surgery has become widely used. Patients in dental offices and clinics who have had or will have surgery should be identified and need special procedures. Because the patient with a cardiac prosthesis is at risk for infective endocarditis, all possible dental treatment must be completed before the date of cardiac surgery and preventive measures must be emphasized.

I. PRESURGICAL
Before elective cardiac surgery, the patient should be brought to a state of optimum oral health, with all sources of infection removed. All restorations and other dental procedures must be completed.

Patients requiring cardiac surgery need information and motivation relative to the importance of oral health in eliminating a potential source of infective endocarditis. Vigilance in a preventive program including plaque control and self-applied fluorides is essential.

II. POSTSURGICAL
A. Maintenance Appointments
Frequent appointments are necessary for supervision and maintenance.

B. Prophylactic Antibiotics
1. Antibiotic coverage for all dental and dental hygiene procedures for patients with synthetic prostheses is essential. Because of the high susceptibility to infective endocarditis, a special regimen for high-risk patients may be indicated.

2. Patients with implanted vascular autographs generally do not need antibiotic premedication before dental and dental hygiene appointments.[13] An example of an implanted vascular autograph is the use of a patient's own blood vessel to provide a coronary bypass (figure 58–5). The saphenous vein and the internal mammary artery are most commonly used.

TECHNICAL HINTS

I. RECORD PRESCRIPTIONS
Record all prescriptions by date, drug, dose, and directions in the patient's permanent record.

II. DETERMINE STATUS OF PRESCRIPTION
Check that the patient has filled the prescriptions.

III. PREPARE FOR APPOINTMENT
Before each appointment for a patient with a cardiovascular disease.
   A. Determine and record blood pressure.
   B. Review patient history and notes relative to previous appointments to prepare adequately for the current appointment.
   C. Check with the patient to be sure that prescribed medications have been taken and at the proper time.
      1. Antibiotic premedication must be taken 1 hour before the appointment.
      2. Question the patient concerning drugs that may have been taken on the same day as the appointment, such as a sedative, alcoholic beverage, or other that may influence the premedication or the effect of an anesthetic to be given.

IV. SOURCE OF MATERIALS
Local Heart Association
   and
American Heart Association
7320 Greenville Avenue
Dallas, TX 75231

FACTORS TO TEACH THE PATIENT

I. HYPERTENSION THERAPY
Encourage patients who have been diagnosed as hypertensive to continue their prescribed therapy.

II. STRESS REDUCTION PROCEDURES[14]
   A. Select an appointment time that is optimum with respect to time of day when the patient is feeling best and may be less fatigued. Most anxious patients prefer a morning appointment.
   B. Get adequate sleep and rest, and engage in non-fatiguing activities during the 24 hours before the appointment.
   C. Use premedication as prescribed for sleeping the night before. A sedative may be prescribed to be taken 60 minutes before an appointment; at the dental office, if possible. When taken at home 1 hour before, the patient should not drive a car.
   D. Allow time to get to the dental office or clinic; bring own reading material, knitting or sewing, or other relaxing activity in the event waiting is unavoidable.
   E. Eat breakfast, lunch, or other usual between-meal food and take usual medications on schedule.
   F. When other family members, especially children, have dental or dental hygiene appointments, do not add to their stress by relaying personal negative feelings.

REFERENCES

1. **Cotran,** R.S., Kumar, V., and Robbins, S.L.: *Robbins Pathologic Basis of Disease,* 4th ed. Philadelphia, W.B. Saunders Co., 1989, pp. 629–638.
2. **Little,** J.W. and Falace, D.A.: *Dental Management of the Medically Compromised Patient,* 4th ed. St. Louis, Mosby, 1993, pp. 128–135.
3. **Little** and Falace: op. cit., pp. 98–122.
4. **Dajani,** A.S., Bisno, A.L., Chung, K.J., Durack, D.T., Freed, M., Gerber, M.A., Karchmer, A.W., Millard, H.D., Rahimtoola, S., Shulman, S.T., Watanakunakorn, C., and Taubert, K.A.: Prevention of Bacterial Endocarditis. Recommendations by the American Heart Association, *JAMA, 264,* 2919, December 12, 1990.
5. **United States National Institutes of Health,** National Heart, Lung, and Blood Institute: *The Fifth Report of the Joint National Committee on Detection, Evaluation, and Treatment of High Blood Pressure.* Washington, D.C., National Heart, Lung, and Blood Institute, NIH Publication No. 93–1088, January, 1993.
6. **Malamed,** S.F.: *Handbook of Medical Emergencies in the Dental Office,* 4th ed. St. Louis, Mosby, 1993, pp. 128–135.
7. **Cotran,** Kumar, and Robbins: op. cit., pp. 615–617.
8. **Little** and Falace: op. cit., pp. 175–195.
9. **Malamed:** op. cit., pp. 424–449.
10. **Escher,** D.J., Parker, B., and Furman, S.: Pacemaker Triggering (Inhibition) by Electric Toothbrush, *Am. J. Cardiol., 38,* 126, July, 1976.
11. **Martinis,** A.J., Jankelson, B., Radke, J., and Adib, F.: Effects of the Myo-monitor on Cardiac Pacemakers, *J. Am. Dent. Assoc., 100,* 203, February, 1980.
12. **Dreifus,** L.S. and Cohen, D.: Implanted Pacemakers: Medicolegal Implications, *Am. J. Cardiol., 36,* 266, August, 1975.
13. **Lindemann,** R.A. and Henson, J.L.: The Dental Management of Patients with Vascular Grafts Placed in the Treatment of Arterial Occlusive Disease, *J. Am. Dent. Assoc., 104,* 625, May, 1982.
14. **Malamed:** op. cit., pp. 44–48.

SUGGESTED READINGS

Ayoub, E.M: Resurgence of Rheumatic Fever in the United States. The Changing Picture of a Preventable Illness, *Postgrad. Med., 92,* 133, September 1, 1992.

Caplan, L.R.: Diagnosis and Treatment of Ischemic Stroke, *JAMA, 266,* 2413, November 6, 1991.

Carr, M.M. and Mason, R.B.: Dental Management of Anticoagulated Patients, *Can. Dent. Assoc. J., 58,* 838, October, 1992.

Devereux, R.B.: Diagnosis and Prognosis of Mitral-valve Prolapse, *N. Engl. J. Med., 320,* 1077, April 20, 1989.

Gortzak, R.A.Th., Abraham-Inpijn, L., and Oosting, J.: Blood Pressure Response to Dental Check-up: A Continuous Noninvasive Registration, *Gen. Dent., 39,* 339, September–October, 1991.

Hays, G.L., McMahon, J.C., Zimmerman, S.J., Lusk, S.S., and DeVoll, R.E.: Screening for Cardiovascular Disease, *Gen. Dent., 40,* 26, January–February, 1992.

Martinowitz, U., Mazar, A.L., Taicher, S., Varon, D., Gitel, S.N., Ramot, B., and Rakocz, M.: Dental Extraction for Patients on Oral Anticoagulant Therapy, *Oral Surg. Oral Med. Oral Pathol., 70,* 274, September, 1990.

McCarthy, F.M.: Safe Treatment of the Post-heart-attack Patient, *Compendium, 10,* 598, November, 1989.

Sandor, G.K.B., Vasilakos, S.S., and Vasilakos, J.S.: Mitral Valve Prolapse: A Review of the Syndrome with Emphasis on Current Antibiotic Prophylaxis, *Can. Dent. Assoc. J., 57,* 321, April, 1991.

Schein, J.: Correct Medication Can Control Hypertension, *RDH, 9,* 41, October, 1989.

Streckfus, C.F., Strahl, R.C., and Welsh, S.: Anti-hypertension Medications: An Epidemiological Factor in the Prevalence of Root Decay among Geriatric Patients Suffering from Hypertension, *Clin. Prev. Dent., 12,* 26, August–September, 1990.

Syrjänen, J.: Vascular Diseases and Oral Infections, *J. Clin. Periodontol., 17,* 497, Part II, August, 1990.

Wei, J.Y.: Age and the Cardiovascular System, *N. Engl. J. Med., 327,* 1735, December 10, 1992.

Wenger, N.K., Speroff, L., and Packard, B.: Cardiovascular Health and Disease in Women, *N. Engl. J. Med., 329,* 247, July 22, 1993.

Willard, J.E., Lange, R.A., and Hillis, L.D.: The Use of Aspirin in Ischemic Heart Disease, *N. Engl. J. Med., 327,* 175, July 16, 1992.

Infective Endocarditis

Biancaniello, T.M. and Romero, J.R.: Bacterial Endocarditis After Adjustment of Orthodontic Appliances, *J. Pediatr., 118,* 248, February, 1991.

De Geest, A.F.E., Schoolmeesters, I., Willems, J.L., De Geest, H.: Dental Health, Prophylactic Antibiotic Measures and Infective Endocarditis: An Analysis of the Knowledge of Susceptible Patients, *Acta Cardiol., 45,* 441, December, 1990.

Duffin, P.R., McGimpsey, J.G., Pallister, M.L., and McGowan, D.A.: Dental Care of Patients Susceptible to Infective Endocarditis, *Br. Dent. J., 173,* 169, September 19, 1992.

Felder, R.S., Nardone, D., and Palac, R.: Prevalence of Predisposing Factors for Endocarditis among an Elderly Institutionalized Population, *Oral Surg. Oral Med. Oral Pathol., 73,* 30, January, 1992.

Franklin, C.D.: The Aetiology, Epidemiology, Pathogenesis and Changing Pattern of Infective Endocarditis, with a Note on Prophylaxis, *Br. Dent. J., 172,* 369, May 23, 1992.

Knox, K.W. and Hunter, N.: The Role of Oral Bacteria in the Pathogenesis of Infective Endocarditis, *Aust. Dent. J., 36,* 286, August, 1991.

Children

Creighton, J.M.: Dental Care for the Pediatric Cardiac Patient, *Can. Dent. Assoc. J., 58,* 201, March, 1992.

Hallett, K.B., Radford, D.J., and Seow, W.K.: Oral Health of Children with Congenital Cardiac Diseases: A Controlled Study, *Pediatr. Dent., 14,* 224, July/August, 1992.

Spuller, R.L.: The Central Indwelling Venous Catheter in the Pediatric Patient—Dental Treatment Considerations, *Spec. Care Dentist., 8,* 74, March–April, 1988.

Invasive Procedures

Boraz, R.A. and Myers, R.: A National Survey of Dental Protocols for the Patient with a Cardiac Transplant, *Spec. Care Dentist., 10,* 26, January–February, 1990.

Carpendale, J.J., Dykema, R.W., Andres, C.J., and Goodacre, C.J.: Principles Governing the Prosthodontic Treatment of Patients with Cardiac Transplants, *J. Am. Dent. Assoc., 119,* 517, October, 1989.

Harms, K.A. and Bronny, A.T.: Cardiac Transplantation: Dental Considerations, *J. Am. Dent. Assoc., 112,* 677, May, 1986.

Little, J.W. and Rhodus, N.L.: Dental Management of the Heart Transplant Patient, *Gen. Dent., 40,* 126, March–April, 1992.

Shinn, J.A.: Management of a Patient Undergoing Myocardial Revascularization: Coronary Artery Bypass Graft Surgery, *Nurs. Clin. North Am., 27,* 243, March, 1992.

Whittle, J., Conigliaro, J., Good, C.B., and Lofgren, R.P.: Racial Differences in the Use of Invasive Cardiovascular Procedures in the Department of Veterans Affairs Medical System, *N. Engl. J. Med., 329,* 621, August 26, 1993.

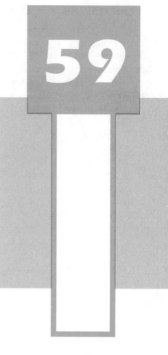

59

The Patient with a Blood Disorder

Oral soft tissue changes, lowered resistance to infection, and bleeding tendencies are major factors to be considered for a patient with a blood disorder. Oral manifestations of blood disorders are generally exaggerated in the presence of bacterial plaque and local predisposing factors.

In this chapter, anemias, leukemias, and hemorrhagic disorders are described. Table 59–1 lists and defines terminology used to describe hematologic conditions. Prefixes, suffixes, and other word derivatives to clarify the terminology are listed on pages 851–853.

ORAL FINDINGS SUGGESTIVE OF BLOOD DISORDERS

Early signs of systemic conditions frequently appear in the oral soft tissues. The patient's medical history may not reveal the existence of a blood disorder, but clinical examination may reveal tissue characteristics suggestive of disease. An important referral for medical examination may lead to diagnosis and treatment of a serious disease. In addition, the findings of a laboratory blood examination may provide essential information for safe and effective treatment.

Oral soft tissue changes that may occur in patients with blood diseases are not necessarily exclusive to systemic blood disorders. The important thing is to recognize change in a previously healthy patient, or an apparently exaggerated response in a patient being examined at an initial appointment.

Findings that may suggest a blood disorder include the following:

A. Gingival bleeding, spontaneously or upon gentle probing.

B. History of difficulty in controlling bleeding by usual procedures.

C. History of bruising easily, with large ecchymoses.

D. Numerous petechiae.

E. Marked pallor of the mucous membranes.

F. Atrophy of the papillae of the tongue.

G. Persistent sore or painful tongue (glossodynia).

H. Acute or chronic infections, such as candidiasis, that do not respond to usual treatment.

I. Severe ulcerations associated with a lack of response to treatment.

J. Exaggerated gingival response to local irritants, sometimes with characteristics of necrotizing ulcerative gingivitis (ulceration, necrosis, bleeding, pseudomembrane).

NORMAL BLOOD[1]

I. COMPOSITION

The blood is composed of 55% plasma fluid and 45% formed elements. The formed elements are categorized by type into *erythrocytes* (red blood cells or corpuscles), *leukocytes* (white blood cells), and *thrombocytes* (platelets). The cell forms and nuclei are shown in figure 59–1.

The red blood cells comprise about 44% and the white blood cells 1% of the 45% total formed elements.

The *hematocrit* is the percentage of packed volume of blood cells, the normal value for which approximates 45%, as shown in table 59–2. The test for the hematocrit is commonly used in general health evaluations.

II. ORIGIN

In adults, all blood cells originate in the bone marrow. The erythrocytes and granulocytes pass through a se-

TABLE 59–1
KEY WORDS: BLOOD DISORDERS

Anaplasia (an' ah-plā'zē-ah): loss of structural differentiation with reversion to a more primitive type of cell.

Aplasia (ah-plā'zē-ah): defective development or congenital absence of an organ or tissue.

Coagulation factor: factor essential to normal blood clotting contained within the blood plasma; designated by Roman numerals I to V and VII to XIII; their absence, diminution, or excess may lead to abnormality of clotting.

Differential cell count: record of the number of white blood cells, including the determination of the percent of each type of cell present; the "differential" is used in the diagnosis of various blood disorders, infections, or other abnormal conditions of the body.

Ecchymosis (ek'ĭ-mō'sis): hemorrhagic spot larger than a petechia in the skin or mucous membrane; nonelevated, blue or purplish.

Epistaxis (ep'ĭ-stak'sis): hemorrhage from the nose.

Erythropoiesis (ĕ-rĭth'rō-poi-ē'sis): formation of red blood cells.

Glossitis (glaw sī'tis): inflammation of the tongue.

Glossodynia (glos'ō-dĭn'e-ah): pain in the tongue.

Hemarthrosis (hem'ar-thro'sis): blood in a joint cavity.

Hematocrit (hē-mat'ō-krit): volume percentage of erythrocytes (red blood cells) in whole blood.

Hematopoiesis (hem'ah-tō-poi-ē'sis): the formation and development of blood cells, usually in bone marrow.

Hemoglobin (he'mo-glo'bin): protein in the erythrocyte that transports molecular oxygen to body cells.

Oxyhemoglobin: oxygenated arterial blood; bright red and about 97% saturated with oxygen; venous blood is a darker color and contains only 20 to 70% oxygen.

Hemolysis (he-mol'ĭ-sis): rupture of erythrocytes with the release of hemoglobin into the plasma.

Leukocytosis (loo'kō-sī-tō'sis): increase in the total number of leukocytes.

Leukopenia (loo'kō-pē'nē-ah): reduction in total number of leukocytes in the blood; count under 5000 per ml.

Lysis (lī'sis): destruction or decomposition, as of a cell, bacterium, or other substance.

Macrocyte (mak'rō-sīt): abnormally large red blood cell; contrast with **microcyte**, abnormally small erythrocyte.

Myelocyte (mī'ĕ-lō-sit): young cell of the granulocyte series; occurs normally in bone marrow; found in circulating blood in certain diseases.

Neutropenia (nu'trō-pē'nē-ah): diminished number of neutrophils (polymorphonuclear leukocytes or PMNs).

Petechia (pĕ-tē'kē-ah): minute, pinpoint, round, nonraised, purplish-red spot in the skin or mucous membrane; caused by hemorrhage.

Phagocytosis (fag'ō-sī-tō'sis): engulfing of microorganisms and foreign particles by phagocytes, such as macrophages.

Purpura (pur'pu-rah): hemorrhage into the tissues, under the skin, and through the mucous membranes; produces petechiae and ecchymoses.

Thrombocytic purpura: when circulating platelets are decreased.

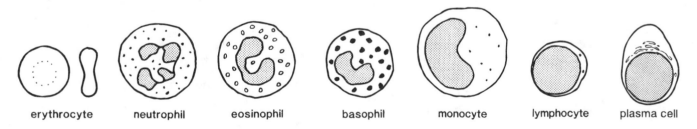

erythrocyte   neutrophil   eosinophil   basophil   monocyte   lymphocyte   plasma cell

FIG. 59–1. Red and White Blood Cells. Diagram shows normal cell forms drawn to scale for comparison of cell size. Note the shape of nuclei in each of the white blood cells. The erythrocyte or red blood cell does not have a nucleus; its biconcave disc shape is shown in the lateral view second from the left.

ries of transformations from the stem cell (cell of origin), the *hemocytoblast,* and leave the bone marrow as mature cells to enter the circulating blood.

The bone marrow also produces the stem cells for the agranulocytes. The lymphocytes and monocytes leave the bone marrow in immature forms and go to the lymphoid tissues for later maturing. In certain blood diseases and cancers, the immature cell forms predominate.

III. PLASMA

The constituents of the fluid portion of the blood are similar to the fluid constituents of the connective tissue. The plasma is comprised 90% of water and 10% of the following:

A. Plasma Proteins
1. Albumin (functions to maintain tissue fluid pressure).

TABLE 59–2
TESTS USED FOR BLOOD EVALUATION

Test	Normal Range*	Causes of Deviations

Hemoglobin	Males: 14–18 g/100 ml
	Females: 12–16 g/100 ml
		Increased in
		    Polycythemia
		    Dehydration
		Decreased in
		    Anemias
		    Hemorrhage
		    Leukemias

Hematocrit (volume of packed red cells)	Males: 40–54%
	Females: 37–47%
		Increased in
		    Polycythemia
		    Dehydration
		Decreased in
		    Anemias
		    Hemorrhage
		    Leukemias

Bleeding Time	Duke: 1–3½ minutes
	Ivy: less than 5 minutes
	Modified Ivy: 2½–10 minutes (Mielke template)
		Prolonged in
		    Disorders of platelet function
		    Thrombocytopenia
		    von Willebrand's disease
		    Leukemias
		    Aspirin and certain other drug use

Clotting Time	Glass tube: 4–8 minutes	Prolonged in
		    Vitamin K deficiency
		    Severe hemophilia
		    Anticoagulant therapy
		    Liver diseases

Prothrombin Time (P.T.)	11–15 seconds	Prolonged in
		    Polycythemia vera
		    Prothrombin deficiency
		    Anticoagulant therapy
		    Vitamin K deficiency
		    Liver diseases
		    Aspirin use

Partial Thromboplastin Time (P.T.T.)	68–82 seconds	Prolonged in
		    Hemophilia A and B
		    von Willebrand's disease
		    Anticoagulant therapy

* The normal range varies with the specificity of the technique used. There is also a range variation, depending on the health facility and the laboratory.

2. Gamma globulins (circulating antibodies essential in the immune system).
3. Beta globulins (transport of hormones, metallic ions, and lipids).
4. Fibrinogen and prothrombin (blood clotting).

B. Inorganic Salts
Sodium, potassium, calcium, bicarbonate, chloride.

C. Gases
Dissolved oxygen, carbon dioxide, and nitrogen.

D. Substances Being Transported
Hormones, nutrients, waste products, enzymes.

IV. RED BLOOD CELLS (ERYTHROCYTES)
A. Description
Although usually called red blood cells, they are more properly termed corpuscles because they have no nuclei (figure 59–1). They are biconcave discs that contain hemoglobin. The cells are sensitive and flexible and change shape readily as they pass through small capillaries.

Table 59–3 contains reference values for blood cells and the names of conditions in which increases or decreases in the normal values occur.

B. Functions
Hemoglobin carries oxygen to the body cells in the form of oxyhemoglobin. Carbon dioxide is transported from the cells.

TABLE 59–3
BLOOD CELLS REFERENCE VALUES

Cell Type	Normal Value	Causes of Increase	Causes of Decrease
Red Blood Cells	Male 4.5–6.0 Female 4.3–5.5 million per mm^3	Polycythemia Dehydration	Anemias Leukemias Hemorrhage
Platelets	150,000–400,000 per mm^3 Wintrobe method: 140,000–440,000 per mm^3	Polycythemia vera Chronic myelocytic leukemia Sickle cell anemia Rheumatic fever Hemolytic anemias Bone fractures	Acute severe infections Cirrhosis of the liver Thrombocytopenic purpura Acute leukemias Aplastic anemias Pernicious anemia
White Blood Cells	5,000–10,000 per mm^3	Inflammation Overexertion Polycythemia vera	Aplastic anemia Granulocytopenia Drug poisoning Thrombocytopenia Radiation Severe infections
DIFFERENTIAL White Cell Count Granulocytes 1. Neutrophils (PMNs)	60–70%	Acute infections Myelogenous leukemia Poisoning Erythroblastosis	Aplastic anemia Granulocytopenia
2. Eosinophils	1–3%	Allergic diseases Dermatitis Hodgkin's disease Scarlet fever	Aplastic anemia Typhoid fever
3. Basophils	1%	Certain chronic infections	Aplastic anemia
Agranulocytes 1. Lymphocytes	20–35%	Lymphocytic leukemia Chronic infections Viral diseases	Aplastic anemia Myelogenous leukemia Radiation
2. Monocytes	2–6%	Monocytic leukemias Tuberculosis Infective endocarditis Hodgkin's disease	Aplastic anemia

The hemoglobin is measured in grams (g) per 100 milliliters (ml). Normal values are shown in table 59–2 and range from 12 to 18 g per 100 ml. The values reflect the anemic state when the hemoglobin is lowered. They also reflect pathologic conditions in which the hemoglobin is increased to a level higher than normal.

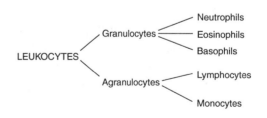

V. WHITE BLOOD CELLS (LEUKOCYTES)
A. Types
White blood cells are divided into two general groups, the granulocytes and the agranulocytes. Granulocytes have granules in their cytoplasm, whereas the agranulocytes do not. They are further subdivided as shown here:

B. Functions
All white cells are amoeboid or motile, thus permitting them to pass through the walls at the terminal ends of capillaries and into the connective tissue. Their work is done within the connective tissue, where they have phagocytic, im-

munologic, and other functions related to the inflammatory process.

The cells respond to an injury or invasion of microorganisms and migrate into the area in large numbers. Neutrophils arrive first and are active in the phagocytosis of foreign material and microorganisms.

The blood functions as a transport medium for the white cells as they pass to areas in the connective tissue where they are needed. Their numbers and proportions in the blood maintain a constant level in health, as shown in table 59–3.

A *differential cell count* of the white blood cells is used in the detection and monitoring of diseased states. Increases and decreases of each cell type can be associated with certain conditions.

C. Agranulocytes

1. *Lymphocytes.* A mature lymphocyte is a small round cell with a round nucleus that nearly fills the cell, leaving only a narrow rim of cytoplasm (figure 59–1). Less mature forms are larger, with more cytoplasm.

   In the connective tissue, certain lymphocytes may differentiate into plasma cells, which produce and secrete antibody. The *plasma cell* is a relatively large oval cell with an eccentric nucleus. Lymphocytes and plasma cells are common in areas of chronic inflammation.

2. *Monocytes.* A monocyte is a large cell with a bean-shaped or indented nucleus. It is actively phagocytic. In the connective tissue, monocytes differentiate into macrophages, which are important in immunologic processes.

D. Granulocytes

1. *Neutrophils.* Neutrophils are the most numerous of all the white blood cells. They are also named polymorphonuclear leukocytes and referred to as "PMNs" or "polys." The nucleus of a neutrophil has three to five lobes connected by thin chromatin threads.

   In circulation, the cells are round, but in the tissues they are more or less amoeboid as they function in phagocytosis. Neutrophils are part of the first line of defense of the body.

2. *Eosinophils.* An eosinophil usually has a two-lobed nucleus and larger, coarser granules than those of a neutrophil. The granules stain a distinct bright pink, so that microscopically the cells can be readily recognized, even though they are few in number. The numbers increase markedly during allergic conditions.

3. *Basophils.* In contrast to the eosinophil or neutrophil, the nucleus of a basophil is usually in "U" or "S" form. The functions of the basophil are related to increasing vascular permeability during inflammation, thus permitting phagocytic cells to pass into the area.

VI. PLATELETS

A platelet is a small round or oval formed element without a nucleus. It is approximately one fourth the size of a red blood cell. Platelets are active in the blood clotting mechanism and essential in the maintenance of the integrity of blood capillaries by closing them at a time of injury. After healing, the platelets participate in clot dissolution.

ANEMIAS

Anemia means a reduction of the hemoglobin concentration, the hematocrit, or the number of red blood cells to a level below that which is normal for the individual. As a result of anemia, oxygen-carrying capacity to the cells is diminished. Oxygen is essential in all body tissues for normal maintenance.

I. CLASSIFICATION BY CAUSE

Anemias are usually classified into three groups by general causes. The categories and an example of each are listed here. Later in the chapter, selected specific anemias with their oral implications are described.

A. Caused by Blood Loss

1. *Acute.* Blood loss from trauma or disease.
2. *Chronic.* An internal lesion with constant slow bleeding, usually of gastrointestinal or gynecologic origin can lead to a chronic loss of blood. An *iron deficiency anemia* can result.

B. Caused by Increased Hemolysis

Hemolysis means the destruction of red blood cells. These types of anemias are called "hemolytic anemias" because of the cell destruction.

1. *Hereditary Hemolytic Disorders*

   Example: *Sickle cell anemia,* which belongs to the group of hereditary disorders called the hemoglobinopathies.

2. *Acquired Hemolytic Disorders*

   Examples: drugs, infections, and certain physical and chemical agents that may cause red cell destruction. In the category of antibody-mediated anemia, *erythroblastosis fetalis* occurs when a mother is Rh negative and develops antibodies against a fetus that is Rh positive. It is sometimes called hemolytic disease of the newborn.

C. Caused by Diminished Production of Red Blood Cells

A nutritional deficiency or bone marrow failure may be the reason for diminished production.

1. *Nutritional Deficiency*
   a. Inadequate dietary choices or inadequate intake.

b. Defective absorption from the gastrointestinal tract.

Example: *pernicious anemia*, which results from a B_{12} vitamin absorption deficiency.

c. Increased demand for nutrients.

Example: *iron deficiency anemia*, which may occur during pregnancy or during a growth spurt.

2. *Bone Marrow Failure*

Example: *aplastic anemia*, which may result from bone marrow failure because of drug use, irradiation, or chemicals. In aplastic anemia, a combination occurs of anemia, neutropenia, and thrombocytopenia, which means a quantitative decrease in all cells formed in the bone marrow.

II. CLINICAL CHARACTERISTICS OF ANEMIA

When a patient's medical history shows the presence of anemia, certain general characteristics may be anticipated for which clinical adaptations may be needed. The general signs and symptoms are

A. Pale and thin skin.
B. Weakness, malaise, easy fatigability.
C. Dyspnea on slight exertion, faintness.
D. Headache, vertigo, tinnitus.
E. Dimness of vision, spots before the eyes.
F. Brittle nails with loss of convexity.

IRON DEFICIENCY ANEMIA

Iron deficiency anemia is a hypochromic microcytic anemia, which means that the hemoglobin is deficient (hypochromic) and the red blood corpuscles are smaller than normal and deficient in hemoglobin (microcytic). In general, it is found more in younger than in older people, and more in females than in males.

I. CAUSES

A. Malnutrition or malabsorption.
B. Chronic infection.
C. Increased body demand for iron over and above the daily intake. Example: during pregnancy.
D. Chronic blood loss. When iron deficiency anemia occurs in men or in postmenopausal women, it usually indicates internal bleeding, and tests are needed to find the source.
1. Causes of internal bleeding
a. Gastrointestinal diseases, such as ulcer, cancer.
b. Drugs, notably aspirin.
c. Hemorrhoids.
2. Excessive menstrual flow.
3. Frequent blood donations.

II. SIGNS AND SYMPTOMS
A. General

Clinical manifestations of iron deficiency anemia include general weakness, headache, pallor, and fatigue on slight exertion.

B. Oral

1. Pallor of the mucosa and gingiva.
2. Tongue changes
a. Atrophic glossitis with loss of filiform papillae. In moderate and severe anemia, when the hemoglobin is at 10 or below, the tongue is smooth and shiny. The patient may have burning, painful sensations (glossodynia).
b. Secondary irritations to the thinned, atrophic mucosa may result from smoking, mechanical trauma, or hot, spicy foods.

III. THERAPY

Iron deficiency anemia is treated with oral ferrous iron tablets. Liquid preparations, which are sometimes used for children, may stain the teeth. Administering the medicine by way of a straw is advised.

MEGALOBLASTIC ANEMIAS

Megaloblastic anemias are characterized by abnormally large (megalo-) red blood cells, many of which are oval shaped. The two principal types of megaloblastic anemias are *pernicious anemia* and *folate deficiency anemia*.

Pernicious anemia is caused by a deficiency of vitamin B_{12}, and folate deficiency anemia is from a deficiency of folate, or folic acid. These two vitamins are essential in red blood cell production in the bone marrow. When one or the other is deficient, the basic precursor cell ("-blast") is altered, thus leading to a derangement in the formation of red blood cells and resultant abnormal, megaloblastic cells.[2] A megaloblastic anemia can result from a deficiency of either vitamin B_{12} or folate, or both together.

I. PERNICIOUS ANEMIA

The implication of "fatality" when the word "pernicious" is used can be misleading, because synthetic vitamin B_{12} is now available for treatment and disease control. The traditional name is still in use, however.

A. Etiologic Factors

Vitamin B_{12} deficiency can be caused by decreased intake (inadequate diet or impaired absorption) or increased requirement (pregnancy, hyperparathyroidism, disseminated cancer). Pernicious anemia is caused by *impaired absorption* of B_{12} because of failure of production of *intrinsic factor (IF)* by the gastric mucosa.

Pernicious anemia is primarily a disease of people over 40 years of age. Frequently, the reason for lack of production of *intrinsic factor* is either chronic atrophic gastritis or surgical removal or partial removal of the stomach.

In the childhood form of the disease, other causes are in effect; no gastric abnormality exists. Although more research is needed, the cause may be either a hereditary inability to produce intrinsic factor, or the intrinsic factor produced may be ineffective.

B. Clinical Findings

1. *General.* Weakness, tingling or numbness of fingers and toes, and weight loss are usually found. Symptoms of central nervous system involvement may include difficulty in walking, some lack of coordination, loss of position sense, and mental confusion.

2. *Oral*
   a. Tongue (atrophic glossitis, burning tongue). The tongue may be painful and inflamed, flabby, red, smooth, and shiny, with loss of filiform papillae. Secondarily, sensitivity to hot or spicy foods and other irritants and painful swallowing may be expected.
   b. Gingiva and mucosa. Soft tissues may be pale and atrophic and appear similar to those in general vitamin B deficiency.

C. Treatment

Vitamin B$_{12}$ is administered by injection twice weekly until the condition is controlled, and then monthly, indefinitely.

The main sources of vitamin B$_{12}$ are meat and dairy products, that is, all foods containing animal protein. Liver is a rich source and was originally used in therapy before the development of synthetic B$_{12}$.

II. FOLATE DEFICIENCY ANEMIA

Folate deficiency anemia has the same characteristics as pernicious anemia, except clinically, no neurologic changes are evident.

A. Etiologic Factors[2]

Folate deficiency can be caused by decreased intake (inadequate diet, impaired absorption), increased requirement (pregnancy, disseminated cancer), or blocked activation (certain drugs impair the utilization of folate).

B. Dietary Factors

Folates are abundant in green vegetables (spinach, lettuce, cabbage, asparagus), yeast, and liver. Only minimal subsistence diets or special diets influenced by such factors as poverty, food fadism, or alcoholism, when the use of alcohol takes precedence over food, are likely to be defi-

cient in folates. Folate deficiency anemia is not uncommon, but it may be more frequently related to malabsorption than to inadequate intake.

SICKLE CELL ANEMIA[3]

Sickle cell anemia is a hereditary form of hemolytic anemia, resulting from a defective hemoglobin molecule. The name is derived from the crescent or "sickle" shape the red corpuscles assume when they become deoxygenated.

The disease occurs primarily in the black population and in white populations of Mediterranean origin. Tests are available for screening and diagnosis of those with sickle cell trait. Genetic counseling can play an important role in prevention. Detection of the presence of sickle cell anemia is possible before birth, so that proper observation and supervision of the infant and young child can be provided.

I. DISEASE PROCESS

Signs and symptoms do not appear until after approximately the sixth month, when hemoglobin has matured. Growth and development may be impaired during the early years. Young children are markedly susceptible to communicable diseases and especially to pneumococcal infections.

The disease abnormality is in the type and solubility of hemoglobin. The defective hemoglobin loses oxygen, and the red blood cells become distorted into sickled shapes (figure 59–2). Increases in blood fluid viscosity result, and blood stasis occurs, which can lead to thrombosis formation and infarction. The sickled cells may collect in the vital organs and lead to serious involvement and organ enlargement, particularly of the liver and spleen. Chronic changes may occur in any organ system of the body.

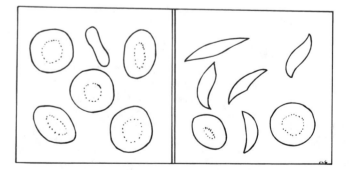

FIG. 59–2. Sickle Cell Anemia. Left, diagrammatic drawing of normal red blood cells. **Right,** sickle shapes of red blood cells of a patient with sickle cell disease.

II. CLINICAL COURSE

A. Severe Hemolytic Anemia

In adults, chronic hemolytic sickle cell disease can be severe. The hematocrit may range between 18 and 30%. The life span of red blood cells normally is from 90 to 120 days, whereas in hemolytic anemia, such as sickle cell anemia, the red blood cell survival rate is about 10 to 15 days.

B. Sickle Cell Crisis

Periodic recurrences of clinical exacerbations of the disease with periods of remission characterize childhood and adolescence. The acute form of the disease is called the sickle cell crisis.

1. *Precipitating Factors.* Crises may appear at any time with or without stimuli. Viral or bacterial infections, other systemic diseases, exertion, trauma, and temperature changes (dehydration in summer, reflex vasospasm in cold weather) may be specific precipitating factors, however.
2. *Clinical Signs and Symptoms.* A crisis is characterized by severe pain. Infarctions occur in various tissues and organs. When the central nervous system becomes involved, symptoms of seizure, stroke, or coma may develop.

   The effects of a crisis may be reversible to some degree, severe physical conditions can result, or a crisis can be fatal. The high mortality rate in young children may be the result of the effects of crisis or of severe infections.

C. Systemic Changes that May Occur

Chronic changes may occur in any organ system at any age. The kidney is a major organ affected; changes in the cardiopulmonary system can result in enlargement of the heart, heart murmurs, and coronary insufficiency. Ocular disturbances even leading to blindness, are not uncommon in adults. Certain patients may be susceptible to cerebrovascular accidents with hemiplegia.

Changes that occur in all bones, including the mandible, result from thrombosis and infarction and from infection.

D. Treatment

1. *Preventive Procedures*
   a. Use folate supplements daily to cope with increased need by the bone marrow.
   b. Avoid and/or promptly treat infections; administer pneumococcal polyvalent vaccine to children.
   c. Obtain genetic counseling for those with sickle cell trait.
2. *Treatment for Disease State*
   Supportive and palliative treatments include those for specific symptoms during crises, such as pain relief and the use of antibiotics for infectious diseases. Oxygen therapy and blood transfusions have limited selective use.

III. ORAL IMPLICATIONS

A. Radiographic Findings[4,5]

Although radiographic findings of bone changes cannot be considered exclusive to sickle cell anemia, the high incidence of characteristics listed here provides a relationship that may, in time, contribute to diagnosis. The bone changes can be observed in patients with sickle cell trait, as well as in those with sickle cell anemia.

1. Decreased radiodensity; increased osteoporosis.
2. Coarse trabecular pattern with large marrow spaces.
3. Significant bone loss in children, indicating the presence of periodontitis.

B. Oral Soft Tissues

The tissues may show the pallor typical of anemias, and because of the specific destruction of tissues in the liver of the patient with sickle cell anemia, the gingiva may have a jaundiced color.

Periodontal evaluation for all ages is likely to reveal pockets, infection, bleeding, and the need for a strict preventive and treatment program.

C. General Suggestions for Appointment Management[6,7]

The objective during therapy is to provide care without precipitating a sickle cell crisis. In general, during a sickle cell crisis, treatment should be limited to emergency relief.

1. Prepare or review the comprehensive medical history.
2. Use prophylactic antibiotics. For a patient so highly susceptible to infection, antibiotics should be considered routine, because any form of tissue manipulation can create a bacteremia.
3. Obtain a hematocrit and a hemoglobin determination immediately prior to each treatment appointment. The patient's physician can provide the interpretation and advise whether the patient is able to have a dental or dental hygiene appointment that day.
4. Teach and supervise a comprehensive preventive program to minimize oral infection and control etiologic factors.

POLYCYTHEMIAS

Polycythemia means an increase in the number and concentration of red blood cells above the normal level. Hemoglobin and hematocrit values are raised. The three general categories are described in the following sections.

I. RELATIVE POLYCYTHEMIA

When a loss of plasma occurs without a corresponding loss of red blood cells, the concentration of cells increases and a relative polycythemia results. The causes of fluid loss may be such conditions as dehydration, diarrhea, repeated vomiting, sweating, or loss of fluid from burns.

Other contributing factors may be smoking, hypertension, obesity, and stress, particularly in middle-aged men.

II. POLYCYTHEMIA VERA (PRIMARY POLYCYTHEMIA)[8]

In contrast to "relative" polycythemia, which results from fluid loss, primary, "absolute," or "true" polycythemia results from an actual increase in the number of circulating red blood cells. In addition to an increased red blood cell count and hemoglobin value, the white cell and platelet counts are also elevated. The viscosity of the blood is increased, thereby affecting the oxygen transport to the tissues.

A. Cause

Polycythemia vera is a neoplastic condition resulting from a bone disorder in which the primitive red cells or stem cells proliferate. It occurs more frequently after age 40 and more often in men.

B. Clinical Signs and Symptoms

Clinical manifestations relate to increased blood volume and viscosity and the tendencies to thrombosis and hemorrhage.

1. *General.* Hemorrhagic spots, such as petechiae or ecchymoses, appear on the skin. The patient suffers from headaches, dizziness, nasal and gastric bleeding, and abdominal pain. Elevated blood pressure and enlarged spleen are found along with high blood test values. A few cases transform into leukemia.
2. *Oral*
   a. The tongue, mucous membranes, and gingiva are deep purplish-red.
   b. The gingiva are enlarged, with bleeding on slight provocation.

C. Treatment

1. Chemotherapy or radiation.
2. Phlebotomy, to reduce the total volume, and particularly the red cell volume, of the blood.

D. Dental Hygiene Treatment Considerations

Increased health of the gingival tissues can result from frequent maintenance appointments for the supervision of personal daily plaque removal procedures. When supplemented by professional treatment, especially calculus removal, bleeding tendencies can be lessened.

III. SECONDARY POLYCYTHEMIA[8]

Secondary polycythemia is also called erythrocytosis, which simply means an increase in numbers of red blood cells. The increased red cell production can result from hypoxia, such as occurs in residents of high altitudes.

Another cause for increased numbers of red blood cells is an increase in the body's production of erythropoietin, a hormone essential to stimulate the development of the red blood cells in bone marrow. A variety of diseases and tumors can cause excess erythropoietin production. Treatment of the underlying condition is necessary to correct the secondary polycythemia.

WHITE BLOOD CELLS

Disorders of the white blood cells may occur because of a decrease (leukopenia) or an increase (leukocytosis) in cell numbers. The types of white blood cells were described in table 59–3 and illustrated in figure 59–1.

I. LEUKOPENIA

A decrease in the total number of white blood cells results when cell production cannot keep pace with the turnover rate or when an accelerated rate of removal of cells occurs, as in certain disease states.

A. Conditions in which Leukopenia Occurs

1. *Specific Infections.* Typhoid fever, influenza, malaria, measles (rubeola), and German measles (rubella) are examples.
2. *Disease or Intoxification of the Bone Marrow.* Chronic drug poisoning, radiation, and autoimmune or drug-induced immune reactions may be implicated.

B. Agranulocytosis[9]

Agranulocytosis, or malignant neutropenia as it is sometimes called, is a rare, serious disease involving the destruction of bone marrow. Drugs or an autoimmune process are the usual causes.

1. *Clinical Course.* With a sharp drop in white blood cells, bacterial invasion may be rapid, and acute illness may develop. Malaise, chills, and fever are followed by extreme weakness. With complete depression of the bone marrow, blood cells cannot be produced, and death can occur within a few days.

   Initial therapy involves terminating the use of a toxic drug that may have caused the condition and using antibiotics and other symptom-relieving measures. Bone marrow transplants may be the only possible, definitive treatment, assuming that a compatible donor is available.
2. *Oral Lesions.* Ulceration in the mouth and pharynx is common in agranulocytosis. Symptoms also include gingival bleeding, increased salivation, and a fetid odor. During the severe illness, only palliative relief is pos-

sible by using a soft diet and attempts at cleaning the mouth with a soft toothbrush, possibly a suction brush (page 344).

II. LEUKOCYTOSIS

An increase in the numbers of circulating white blood cells may be caused by inflammatory and infectious states, trauma, exertion, and other conditions listed in table 59–3. The most extreme abnormal cause of leukocytosis is leukemia.

LEUKEMIAS

Leukemias are malignant neoplasias of immature white blood cells. They are characterized by abnormally large numbers of specific types of leukocytes and their precursors located within the circulating blood and bone marrow and infiltrated into other body tissues and organs.

I. CLASSIFICATION[10]

Leukemias are first named by whether they are acute or chronic and then are subdivided by the maturity and type of white cell predominating, whether lymphocytic, myelocytic, or myelogenous.

A basic classification of leukemias includes the following types:
- A. Acute lymphocytic (lymphoblastic) leukemia (ALL).
- B. Chronic lymphocytic leukemia (CLL).
- C. Acute myelocytic (myeloblastic) leukemia (AML).
- D. Chronic myelocytic leukemia (CML).

II. ETIOLOGY

Specific causes are not known, and extensive research continues. Viral causes have been demonstrated in laboratory research with animals.

Predisposing factors, or leukemogenic agents, which have been shown to influence the development of certain types of leukemias, are ionizing radiation, environmental chemical agents, and genetic factors.

III. DISEASE PROCESS AND EFFECTS

Leukemias are characterized by (1) generalized replacement of bone marrow with proliferating leukemic cells, (2) large numbers of immature white cells in the circulating blood, and (3) widespread infiltrates of white cells throughout the body. The changes that result may be divided into primary and secondary. Tertiary effects also are associated with the treatment given.

A. Primary Changes
The primary changes are those directly related to the increase in numbers of white blood cells.
1. *Bone Marrow.* All the active red marrow is affected; the marrow is replaced by the neoplastic cells.
2. *Lymph Nodes.* Nodes throughout the body are usually enlarged in all forms of leukemia, because of the accumulation of increased numbers of leukemic cells.
3. *Spleen and Liver.* Both liver and spleen are enlarged, the spleen to the greater degree.
4. *Other Leukemic Infiltrates.* Many organs and tissues become involved, for example, the kidneys, adrenals, thyroid, and myocardium. Infiltrates in the gingiva are described in the section, "Oral Manifestations."

B. Secondary Changes
Secondary changes are the result of complications that arise from the destructive effects of the leukemic infiltrates.
1. *Anemia.* Red cells cannot develop because of the infiltrated bone marrow. Severe anemia can result.
2. *Thrombocytopenia.* Abnormal bleeding tendency is a significant characteristic of all forms of leukemia. The platelet count is very low.
3. *Susceptibility to Bacterial Infection.* Circulating white cells do not have their usual defense capacities.
4. *Osteoporosis.* Expansion of the marrow spaces and changes in the bone by the leukemic infiltrate lead to osteoporosis and radiographic radiolucency. Osseous changes in the maxilla and mandible are not uncommon.

IV. CLINICAL SIGNS AND SYMPTOMS
A. Onset
Marked differences exist between the clinical findings of acute and chronic forms of leukemia. The acute diseases appear suddenly and severely, whereas the chronic types are insidious.

B. Physical Symptoms: Acute
1. Fatigue, pallor, weakness (from anemia).
2. Purpura and ecchymoses of the skin, bleeding from the nose and gingiva (from thrombocytopenia).
3. Lymphadenopathy, splenomegaly, hepatomegaly.
4. Fever, indicating an infection (from lowered resistance).
5. Headache, nausea, vomiting, and sometimes seizures and coma (from leukemic infiltration of the meninges).

C. Physical Symptoms: Chronic
1. Low-grade fever, night sweats.
2. Weight loss, weakness, easy fatigability.
3. Anemia with exertional dyspnea.
4. Lymphadenopathy, splenomegaly, hepatomegaly.

V. TREATMENT FOR LEUKEMIA[11]

A. Induction of Remission

The objective at the outset is to return the blood and bone marrow at least to minimally normal blood test levels.

1. Chemotherapy.
2. Irradiation.

B. Preventive Central Nervous System Therapy

Cranial radiation supplemented by chemotherapy is administered for central nervous system infiltration.

C. Stabilization Therapy

Treatment for anemia, bleeding, infections, and other complications is needed.

D. Continuation Therapy

During remission, therapy must be continued to prevent bone marrow relapse. Therapy may be stopped after 2 to 4 years of remission.

Children in remission go to school and participate in normal activities. Physically, the only difference is the loss of hair, a side effect of chemotherapy, which is often reversible if chemotherapy is completed. Remission periods are used for routine dental and dental hygiene therapy.

E. Bone Marrow Transplant

When indicated, transplants may be performed during remission, while the patient is stronger and the numbers of cancer cells may be fewer. Chemotherapy and total body radiation precede the marrow transplant to eradicate leukemic cells and suppress immunoreactivity.

Marrow from an identical twin or matched sibling to prevent graft-versus-host complications is administered intravenously. Autologous bone marrow, which is obtained from the patient during a remission period, has been used.

VI. ORAL MANIFESTATIONS

A high percentage of patients with leukemia have oral complications. Patients with acute leukemias have more oral problems than do those with chronic disease.

The oral lesions may be described as those that result from the effects of the infiltration, of treatment, and of the depression of bone marrow and lymphoid tissue.[11]

A. Leukemic Infiltrate of the Gingiva

Patients with monocytic leukemia tend to have more pronounced gingival lesions than do patients with other forms of leukemia.

The gingiva is grossly enlarged and bluish red, has blunted papillae, and has a soft, spongy consistency. The enlargement may be great enough to cover a large portion of the anatomic crowns of the teeth.

B. Effects of Treatment: Direct Drug Toxicity

Oral complications that result from the use of chemotherapeutic agents include painful ulcerations, spontaneous gingival bleeding, tongue desquamation, xerostomia, and secondary infections. Chemotherapy and its effects are described on page 674.

C. Depression of Bone Marrow and Lymphoid Tissue

1. *Hemorrhagic Manifestations*
   a. Petechiae and ecchymoses may be observed on the lips, soft palate, floor of the mouth, and facial mucosa.
   b. Gingival bleeding appears spontaneously or on gentle provocation.
2. *Increased Susceptibility to Infection.* Bacterial, fungal, viral. Many types of organisms may be found in the local areas of infection, which are often associated with severe ulceration. Candidiasis is a common finding, with white plaques covering varying degrees of the mucosal surfaces.

VII. DENTAL HYGIENE CARE

Selection of procedures centers around the patient's problem of susceptibility to infection and bleeding. During acute exacerbations, the patient is usually very ill, and certain suggestions described here may apply to hospital care. Consultation with the patient's physician, hematologist, or oncologist is mandatory to explain the oral treatment needed and to obtain information about the hematologic status.

A. Preparation for Appointments

1. *Prophylactic Antibiotic Premedication* (page 102). The patient with leukemia is susceptible to infection, and drugs used in therapy are immunosuppressive.
2. *Blood Evaluation.* Complete blood evaluation tests, including a minimum of those listed in table 59–2, are essential shortly before dental and dental hygiene treatment.
3. *Aseptic Techniques.* Patients with leukemia who have had multiple blood transfusions may be carriers of hepatitis and other communicable diseases (pages 22 and 32). Because the patient is also very susceptible to infection, a two-way emphasis on high-level aseptic technique exists.

B. Oral Examination

A careful, thorough examination is needed. Dental and periodontal conditions without symptoms may become acute problems during chemotherapy.

C. Acute Problems During Exacerbation Periods

1. *Gingival Inflammation.* Palliative treatment for grossly enlarged, bleeding, ulcerated gingiva includes frequent warm saline rinses, a nutritious liquid diet with dietary supplements, and plaque removal procedures using a soft toothbrush. A suction toothbrush may be of value in the hospital setting (page 708).

2. *Scaling.* When the platelet and white blood cell counts permit, scaling can be started.

3. *Post-treatment Instructions.* The objective is to control bleeding. The diet should consist of cold, clear liquids for the first 24 hours, and then cool, soft foods. Because suction can disturb clotting, the use of straws should be avoided. Smoking or other use of tobacco is prohibited, and medications that suppress platelet function, such as aspirin, should be avoided. A close follow-up is indicated; the patient should be seen as frequently as possible. A healing time two or three times longer than normal may be expected.

4. *Candidiasis and Other Oral Infections.* Rinsing with nystatin is usually indicated for Candida infection. Treatment for oral lesions associated with chemotherapy is limited and non-specific. A mouthrinse containing a topical anesthetic may be necessary to relieve the pain and discomfort from oral mucosal ulcerations while eating.

D. Oral Care During Remission

Complete preventive care with a supervised plaque removal program, daily self-applied fluoride, sealants, dietary control, and any other measure deemed necessary to obtain and maintain optimum oral health for the individual should be instituted during the remission period. Complete scaling, planing, and all periodontal therapy must be completed along with dental treatments. Although all severe tissue reactions during periods of chemotherapy probably cannot be alleviated, much suffering can be prevented if the oral cavity is in a state of health at the outset.

HEMORRHAGIC DISORDERS

Hemorrhagic disorders have in common tendencies to spontaneous bleeding and moderate to excessive bleeding following trauma or a surgical procedure. Spontaneous bleeding occurs as small hemorrhages into the skin or mucous membranes and other tissues, and appears as petechiae or purpura. Moderate to excessive bleeding or prolonged bleeding may follow dental hygiene therapy, including scaling and root planing. A history or suspicion of a bleeding problem should be fully evaluated before treatment is started.

I. DETECTION
A. Patient's Medical and Dental Histories

A carefully prepared medical history can provide specific information about bleeding disorders and the treatment received by the patient. When no specific disease is mentioned, clues to possible hemorrhagic tendencies must be sought out through interview.

A basic health questionnaire (pages 88 and 97) should include items related to bleeding, bruising, blood transfusions (and for what reasons they were needed), blood disorders, familial blood disorders, and previous abnormal bleeding that may have followed past dental or dental hygiene appointments. Follow-up conversational questioning after "yes-no" answers on a written questionnaire can delve into sufficient detail to determine the need for blood tests before treatment is started.

Additional information is also obtained by consultation with the patient's physician. When blood tests have been made in the past, but are not recent, new reports can be requested.

B. Laboratory Blood Tests

Selected basic tests are listed in table 59–2 with their normal values. Additional tests are frequently needed for a thorough evaluation of specific conditions.

Certain tests may be needed on the same day as treatment, because blood values may fluctuate. For example, the patient using anticoagulants is required to have a prothrombin time determination within 24 hours of appointment time (page 799). A patient with leukemia also needs immediate pre-evaluation, as described on page 812.

The types and numbers of tests vary. For example, the information required prior to subgingival instrumentation and periodontal surgery depends on the severity of the patient's condition. The opinions of dentists and physicians may differ, depending on their previous experiences. For a patient with leukemia, the test recommended may include a prothrombin time, partial thromboplastin time, thrombin time, fibrinogen level, and platelet count, in addition to routine blood counts and a differential white count.[12]

II. TYPES OF HEMORRHAGIC DISORDERS
A. Abnormalities of the Blood Capillaries

In this type of disorder, vascular fragility is increased. Petechial and purpuric hemorrhages in the skin or mucous membranes, including the gingiva can result. A variety of conditions may cause bleeding as a result of an abnormality of the blood vessel walls, including the following:

1. Severe infections (septicemias, severe measles, typhoid fever).
2. Drug reactions (sulfonamides, phenacetin).
3. Scurvy or vitamin C deficiency (impaired collagen of vessel wall).

B. Platelet Deficiency or Dysfunction

1. *Thrombocytopenia.* A lowered number of platelets may be caused by decreased production in the bone marrow. The cause of bone marrow depression may be invasive

disease, such as leukemia, or deficiencies, such as folate or vitamin B_{12} deficiency anemias.

2. *Platelet Dysfunction.* A defect in platelet function interferes with the blood clotting mechanism and leads to a prolonged bleeding time. Defects occur as a result of certain hereditary states, uremia, certain drugs, and von Willebrand's disease. An example of drugs that affect blood clotting is the salicylates (aspirin).[13]

C. Blood Clotting Defects

A possible irregularity or disorder is associated with each of the many clotting factors.

1. *Acquired Disorders.*
   a. Vitamin K deficiency. Vitamin K is essential for prothrombin synthesis and factors VII, IX, X.
   b. Liver disease. Nearly all the clotting factors are produced in the liver. When the liver is not functioning properly, the clotting factors may be altered.

2. *Hereditary Disorders.* At least 30 hereditary coagulation disorders exist, each resulting from a deficiency or abnormality of a plasma protein. Clinically, their signs and symptoms are similar. The following three are described in detail in the next section:
   a. Hemophilia A (factor VIII abnormality).
   b. Hemophilia B (factor IX abnormality).
   c. von Willebrand's disease (von Willebrand factor, which chemically forms a large part of the factor VIII complex; one component affects platelet function).

HEMOPHILIAS[14]

The hemophilias are a group of congenital disorders of the blood clotting mechanism. The three most common types are classic hemophilia A, hemophilia B or Christmas disease, and von Willebrand's disease.

Hemophilias A and B are inherited by males through an X-linked recessive trait carried by females, and von Willebrand's disease is transmitted by an autosomal codominant trait. Rarely is a female affected by hemophilias A or B, but von Willebrand's disease occurs in males and females.

I. LEVEL OF CLOTTING FACTOR

The severity of the disease can be related directly to the level of the clotting factor in the circulating blood. Normal concentrations of the clotting factors are between 50 and 100%.

Patients with severe hemophilia have a clotting factor VIII or IX of less than 1%. They have spontaneous bleeding into muscles, joints, and soft tissues, and severe, prolonged bleeding after minor trauma.

When the hemophilia is less severe, the clotting factor is in the 2 to 5% range. Spontaneous bleeding may be only occasional; gross bleeding occurs after light but definite trauma.

II. EFFECTS AND LONG-TERM COMPLICATIONS

A. Effects of Minor Trauma

Bleeding and bruising from minor trauma vary, depending on the severity of the disease.

B. Hemarthroses

Bleeding into the soft tissue of joints (knees, ankles, elbows) begins in the very young with severe hemophilia. Much swelling, pain, and incapacitation are created.

C. Joint Deformity and Crippling

Permanent joint damage can result, and the patient may need splints, braces, or orthopedic surgery.

D. Intramuscular Hemorrhage

Hemorrhage into the muscles is accompanied by pain and limitation of motion.

E. Oral Bleeding

Bleeding from the gingiva is common and more extensive when periodontal infection is more severe. Because the fear of bleeding, patients may neglect toothbrushing and flossing; doing so can lead to increased plaque accumulation and inflammation. Small children may injure the oral area when they tumble, and severe bleeding can result.

III. HOME INFUSION PROGRAM

Hemophilia care-center teams work with health personnel in the patient's home community to plan and carry out an individual program of instruction for the parents of a young patient and self-care by the patient by age 10, or as soon as the child is capable. The prescribed concentrates of clotting factor can be stored in the home refrigerator and reconstituted as needed for infusion.

The parents and child are taught to recognize the symptoms of the beginning of a bleeding episode or bleeding from injury, and how to administer the treatment. For patients who have bleeding episodes often, such as more than once each week, a prophylactic schedule may be appropriate. Many patients do not require more than one infusion each month, so that routine prophylaxis is not needed.

A sense of security for a patient is provided through contacts with a social worker and local health personnel. Telephone consultations are available on a 24-hour basis with the hemophilia care center, which may be located at a distance. Precautions are taken to arrange for infusion if necessary during school or working hours.

IV. DENTAL HYGIENE CARE

Although prevention and control of bleeding are the central issues when planning appointments for a patient with hemophilia, other factors also require adaptations and attention. A few of these patients are multi-handicapped as a result of internal hemorrhages, which have led to mental and physical problems. Suggestions for appointments from Chapter 50 may prove useful for the patient who has had hemarthroses and orthopedic treatment.

A few patients have suffered brain damage as a result of cerebral hemorrhage and may be limited intellectually. Others have emotional stresses related to the disease and its treatment. New channels for adjustment have opened since patients have been able to develop the responsibility for self-care. This is in contrast to previous requirements of long hospitalizations, childhood separations from family and school, and dependency on others.

A. Preparation for Appointments

1. *Preliminary Evaluation.* The patient's medical and dental histories must include the pertinent hemophilic history with information about the type, severity, treatment, medications used for pain and other symptoms, and family history. Additional information from the hematologist contributes to planning safe and effective appointments.

2. *Factor Replacement.*[12] In preparation for local anesthetic administration, subgingival instrumentation, surgical procedures, or any procedure likely to cause bleeding, replacement therapy is given just prior to the appointment in accord with medical consultation.

   a. **Without inhibitors of Factor VIII** (antihemophilic factor, AHF).

      (1) Factor VIII stimulant (1-desamino-8-D-arginine vasopressin [DDAVP])
      (2) Antifibrinolytic agents
          Epsilon-aminocaproic acid (EACA)
          Tranexamic acid
      (3) Replacement factors
          Cryoprecipitate
          Frozen fresh plasma
          Purified heat-treated AHF
          New ultrapure preparations of AHF
            Monoclonal antibody technique
            Recombinant DNA-produced AHF

   b. **With mild or moderately stable levels of AHF inhibitors.**

      High doses of purified AHF
      Porcine Factor VIII concentrate
      Steroids

   c. **With inducible or high levels of AHF inhibitors.**

      Porcine Factor VIII concentrate
      Prothrombin complex concentrate
      Activated Factor IX
      Plasmapheresis
      Steroids

3. *Premedication.* Prophylactic antibiotic premedication is usually indicated because of the susceptibility to infection. Patients with joint prostheses definitely require antibiotic premedication.[15]

B. Preventive Program

The prevention and control of gingival and dental diseases constitute important aspects of care for patients with hemophilia. Not only are dental and periodontal treatments complicated by necessary special precautions, but spontaneous oral bleeding problems can be at least partially controlled by the elimination of oral infections.

1. *Parental Instruction.* All possible preventive measures should be started while the child is very young, including fluorides, sealants, bacterial plaque control, diet for caries control, and early professional supervision.

2. *Bacterial Plaque Removal.* Complete instruction is given as for any patient. A soft brush is indicated.

   a. Flossing. Teach flossing carefully and correctly to prevent cutting the gingiva and inducing proximal bleeding.

   b. Aids for disabilities. Patients with limited range of motion may benefit from the special adaptations described on pages 692–694.

C. Instrumentation

All instrumentation is performed carefully but thoroughly to minimize tissue trauma and prevent bleeding. Treatment planning for a series of appointments as described on pages 323–326 is appropriate.

1. *Tissue Conditioning.* When oral care has been neglected and the gingiva are soft and spongy, and bacterial plaque is abundant, a tissue conditioning program is advised. Patient instruction in plaque control procedures is given, practiced, and repeated as necessary over a series of appointments. All possible motivational devices can be employed (pages 331 and 413).

   Scaling can be accomplished in small segments. As the tissue begins to shrink, heal, and become more firm, subgingival scaling and root planing can be completed.

2. *Probing and Periodontal Treatment Planning.* Depending on the bleeding tendencies of the gingival tissues, probing and charting for complete periodontal treatment planning may need to be postponed for a few appoint-

ments while tissue conditioning is carried out.

Many patients can be brought to a state of periodontal health through conservative measures of subgingival scaling and root planing. Complete treatment should be accomplished, including periodontal surgery. As with all oral surgery for a patient with hemophilia, coordination with the medical team and hospitalization when indicated can provide the patient with safe and effective treatment.

D. Miscellaneous Treatment Suggestions

Techniques and procedures should be analyzed to make sure that all excess trauma to the patient is prevented. The same procedures should be applied to all patients, but they are more significant with a patient who has a bleeding problem.

1. *Rubber Dam.* A thin rubber dam may be more gentle to the oral tissues than a heavy one. The use of a Young's frame may eliminate pressure, especially at the corners of the mouth. Rubber dam clamps can be checked for sharp corners and placed carefully without damage to the gingival tissues.
2. *Film Placement.* Films can cut and press on the mucous membranes. Care in placement must be exercised.
3. *Impressions.* Beading the rims of the trays protects the mucosa from pressure and damage from a hard, possibly rough surface (page 168).
4. *Evacuation.* High-vacuum suction tips may be sharp. Caution in the use of suction is necessary to prevent pulling the sublingual or other mucosal tissues into the suction tip and causing hematomas.
5. *Periodontal Dressing.* After subgingival scaling and planing, a periodontal dressing can provide pressure and adapt the tissue against the teeth as an aid for the prevention of postappointment bleeding.
6. *Treatment for Hematoma.* Ice pack application may limit the spread of a hematoma as a temporary measure. Prompt replacement therapy may be needed.
7. *Aspirin.* Never suggest the use of aspirin for pain relief of a patient with a bleeding disorder. The bleeding tendency is greatly increased by drug-induced platelet dysfunction.
8. *Frequency of Maintenance Care.* Frequent appointments can aid in keeping the oral tissues in an optimum state of health and help to prevent the need for complex dental treatments.

REFERENCES

1. **Borysenko,** M. and Beringer, T.: *Functional Histology,* 3rd ed. Boston, Little, Brown and Company, 1989, pp. 87–102.
2. **Cotran,** R.S., Kumar, V., and Robbins, S.L.: *Robbins Pathologic Basis of Disease,* 4th ed. Philadelphia, W.B. Saunders Co., 1989, pp. 679–685.
3. **Cotran,** Kumar, and Robbins: op. cit., pp. 666–670.
4. **Sanger,** R.G. and Bystrom, E.B.: Radiographic Bone Changes in Sickle Cell Anemia, *J. Oral Med., 32,* 32, April–June, 1977.
5. **Ibsen,** O.A.C., Phelan, J.A., and Vernillo, A.T.: Oral Manifestations of Systemic Diseases, in Ibsen, O.A.C. and Phelan, J.A.: *Oral Pathology for the Dental Hygienist.* Philadelphia, W.B. Saunders Co., 1992, p. 429.
6. **Smith,** H.B., McDonald, D.K., and Miller, R.I.: Dental Management of Patients with Sickle Cell Disorders, *J. Am. Dent. Assoc., 114,* 85, January, 1987.
7. **May,** O.A.: Dental Management of Sickle Cell Anemia Patients, *Gen. Dent., 39,* 182, May–June, 1991.
8. **Cotran,** Kumar, and Robbins: op. cit., pp. 691, 735–736.
9. **Shafer,** W.G., Hine, M.K., and Levy, B.M.: *A Textbook of Oral Pathology,* 4th ed. Philadelphia, W.B. Saunders Co., 1983, pp. 732–734.
10. **Cotran,** Kumar, and Robbins: op. cit., pp. 722–734.
11. **Little,** J.W. and Falace, D.A.: *Dental Management of the Medically Compromised Patient,* 4th ed. St. Louis, Mosby, 1993, pp. 445–453.
12. **Little** and Falace: op. cit., pp. 423–428.
13. **Snyder,** N.C.: *Dental Hygiene Clinical Applications in Pharmacology.* Philadelphia, Lea & Febiger, 1987, pp. 84–85.
14. **Mosher,** D.F.: Disorders of Blood Coagulation, in Wyngaarden, J.B., Smith, L.H., and Bennett, J.C., eds.: *Cecil Textbook of Medicine,* 19th ed. Philadelphia, W.B. Saunders Co., 1992, pp. 999–1007.
15. **Mulligan,** R.: Late Infections in Patients with Prostheses for Total Replacement of Joints: Implications for the Dental Practitioner, *J. Am. Dent. Assoc., 101,* 44, July, 1980.

SUGGESTED READINGS

Badner, V.M., Lawrence, C., and Mehier, S.: Polycythemia Vera: Dental Management Considerations, *Spec. Care Dentist., 11,* 227, November/December, 1991.

Bergmann, O.J.: Alterations in Oral Microflora and Pathogenesis of Acute Oral Infections During Remission-induction Therapy in Patients with Acute Myeloid Leukaemia, *Scand. J. Infect. Dis., 23,* 355, No. 3, 1991.

Bergmann, O.J., Ellegaard, B., Dahl, M., and Ellegaard, J.: Gingival Status During Chemical Plaque Control with or Without Prior Mechanical Plaque Removal in Patients with Acute Myeloid Leukaemia, *J. Clin. Periodontol., 19,* 169, March, 1992.

Brenneise, C.V., Mattson, J.S., and Commers, J.R.: Acute Myelomonocytic Leukemia with Oral Manifestations: Report of Case, *J. Am. Dent. Assoc., 117,* 835, December, 1988.

Declerck, D. and Vinckier, F.: Oral Complications of Leukemia, *Quintessence Int., 19,* 575, August, 1988.

Dreizen, S.: The Many Faces of Adult Leukemia, *Compendium, 12,* 46, January, 1991.

Epstein, J.B., Vickars, L., Spinelli, J., and Reece, D.: Efficacy of Chlorhexidine and Nystatin Rinses in Prevention of Oral Complications in Leukemia and Bone Marrow Transplantation, *Oral Surg. Oral Med. Oral Pathol.*, *73*, 682, June, 1992.

George, J.N. and Shattil, S.J.: The Clinical Importance of Acquired Abnormalities of Platelet Function, *N. Engl. J. Med.*, *324*, 27, January 3, 1991.

Hou, G.-L. and Tsai, C.-C.: Primary Gingival Enlargement as a Diagnostic Indicator in Acute Myelomonocytic Leukemia. A Case Report, *J. Periodontol.*, *59*, 852, December, 1988.

Imbery, T.A., Camm, J.H., and Anderson, L.D.: Dental Management of a Patient with Aplastic Anemia, *Gen. Dent.*, *40*, 316, July–August, 1992.

Luker, J., Scully, C., and Oakhill, A.: Gingival Swelling as a Manifestation of Aplastic Anemia, *Oral Surg. Oral Med. Oral Pathol.*, *71*, 55, January, 1991.

Miyasaki, K.T.: The Neutrophil: Mechanisms of Controlling Periodontal Bacteria, *J. Periodontol.*, *62*, 761, December, 1991.

Schmitt, R.J., Sheridan, P.J., and Rogers, R.S.: Pernicious Anemia with Associated Glossodynia, *J. Am. Dent. Assoc.*, *117*, 838, December, 1988.

Sickle Cell Anemia

Cherry-Peppers, G., Davis, V., and Atkinson, J.C.: Sickle Cell Anemia: A Case Report and Literature Review, *Clin. Prev. Dent.*, *14*, 5, July/August, 1992.

Crawford, J.M.: Periodontal Disease in Sickle Cell Disease Subjects, *J. Periodontol.*, *59*, 164, March, 1988.

Demas, D.C., Cantin, R.Y., Poole, A., and Thomas, H.F.: Use of General Anesthesia in Dental Care of the Child with Sickle Cell Anemia, *Oral Surg. Oral Med. Oral Pathol.*, *66*, 190, August, 1988.

Patton, L.L., Brahim, J.S., and Travis, W.D.: Mandibular Osteomyelitis in a Patient with Sickle Cell Anemia: Report of Case, *J. Am. Dent. Assoc.*, *121*, 602, November, 1990.

Rada, R.E., Bronny, A.T., and Hasiakos, P.S.: Sickle Cell Crisis Precipitated by Periodontal Infection: Report of Two Cases, *J. Am. Dent. Assoc.*, *114*, 799, June, 1987.

Shroyer, J.V., Lew, D., Abreo, F., and Unhold, G.P.: Osteomyelitis of the Mandible as a Result of Sickle Cell Disease. Report and Literature Review, *Oral Surg. Oral Med. Oral Pathol.*, *72*, 25, July, 1991.

Hemophilia/Bleeding Disorder

Cale, A.E., Freedman, P.D., and Lumerman, H.: Acute Promyelocytic Leukemia Appearing as Spontaneous Oral Hemorrhage: Report of Case, *J. Am. Dent. Assoc.*, *116*, 671, May, 1988.

Kelly, M.A.: Common Laboratory Tests—Their Use in the Detection and Management of Patients with Bleeding Disorders, *Gen. Dent.*, *38*, 282, July–August, 1990.

Luke, K.H.: Comprehensive Care for Children with Bleeding Disorders. A Physician's Perspective. *Can. Dent. Assoc. J.*, *58*, 115, February, 1992.

Mulherin, J.: Of Special Concern, *RDH*, *12*, 22, February, 1992.

Mulherin, J.: Hospital Offers Perfect Setting for RDH to Help Special Patients, *RDH*, *13*, 26, August, 1993.

O'Neil, D.W., Lowe, J.W., and Mariscal, R.: Dentistry and the Hemophiliac: A Review of Current Literature, Part I, *Compendium*, *10*, 86, February, 1989.

O'Neil, D.W., Lowe, J.W., and Mariscal, R.: Dentistry and the Hemophiliac: A Review of Current Literature, Part II, *Compendium*, *10*, 156, March, 1989.

Orlian, A.I. and Karmel, R.: Postoperative Bleeding in an Undiagnosed Hemophilia A Patient: Report of Case, *J. Am. Dent. Assoc.*, *118*, 583, May, 1989.

Sindet-Pedersen, S., Stenbjerg, S., Ingerslev, J., and Karring, T.: Surgical Treatment of Severe Periodontitis in a Haemophilic Patient with Inhibitors to Factor VIII. Report of a Case, *J. Clin. Periodontol.*, *15*, 636, November, 1988.

Tvrdy, J.L. and Muzzin, K.B.: Dental Hygiene Care for the Hemophilia A Patient, *J.D.H.*, *64*, 126, March–April, 1990.

Ublansky, J.H.: Comprehensive Dental Care for Children with Bleeding Disorders—A Dentist's Perspective, *Can. Dent. Assoc. J.*, *58*, 111, January, 1992.

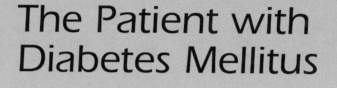

The Patient with Diabetes Mellitus

A preventive dental hygiene program is vital for the patient with diabetes mellitus. The patient with diabetes, particularly one whose condition is unstable or uncontrolled, has a lowered resistance to infection and a delayed healing process. Gingival reactions to bacterial plaque are frequently exaggerated. Periodontal diseases tend to develop with increased severity at an earlier age than in the nondiabetic patient.

The presence of infection, including infection in the oral cavity, may intensify the diabetic symptoms and contribute to difficulty in insulin regulation. The dental team, therefore, has a significant responsibility to provide the patient with oral care and instruction for self-care aimed at maintaining health and preventing gingival and periodontal infections.

Modifications of dental and dental hygiene procedures for the patient may be indicated, depending on the severity and degree of control of the diabetes. No treatment involving tissue manipulation, including subgingival probing and scaling, should be attempted until the diabetic state has been confirmed with the patients physician.

THE DIABETIC SYNDROME: CLASSIFICATION[1,2]

Diabetes mellitus is defined as a genetically heterogeneous group of disorders that is characterized by glucose intolerance. Terminology related to the disorders is listed in table 60–1 with definitions. Prefixes, suffixes, and other word derivations to clarify the terminology are listed on page 851.

I. DIABETES MELLITUS (DM)
  A. Type I. Insulin-dependent diabetes mellitus (IDDM).

  B. Type II. Noninsulin-dependent diabetes mellitus (NIDDM)
    1. Nonobese NIDDM.
    2. Obese NIDDM.
  C. Type III. Associated with other conditions and syndromes, pancreatic disease, hormonal disease, drug- or chemically induced.

II. IMPAIRED GLUCOSE TOLERANCE (IGT)
  A. Nonobese.
  B. Obese.
  C. Associated with other conditions and syndromes, pancreatic disease, hormonal disease, drug- or chemically induced.

III. GESTATIONAL DIABETES (GDM)
IV. PREVIOUS ABNORMALITY OF GLUCOSE TOLERANCE (PREVAGT)
Return to normal glucose tolerance; gestational diabetes, after parturition and obese diabetes, after weight loss.

V. POTENTIAL ABNORMALITY OF GLUCOSE TOLERANCE (POTAGT)
Increased risk in persons with family history or obesity, in mother of neonate weighing more than 9 pounds, in identical twin of diabetic person.

DESCRIPTION

I. TYPE I. INSULIN-DEPENDENT DIABETES MELLITUS (IDDM)
  A. Characteristics
    1. Insulin deficiency.
    2. Dependence on injected insulin to sustain life and prevent ketosis.

818

TABLE 60-1
KEY WORDS AND ABBREVIATIONS: DIABETES MELLITUS

Brittle diabetes: term formerly used to describe very unstable juvenile diabetes; characterized by unexplained oscillation between hypoglycemia and diabetic ketoacidosis.

Gestational diabetes (jes-tā′shun-al): diabetes that occurs during pregnancy.

Gluconeogenesis (gloo′kō-nēō-jenĕ-sis): synthesis of glucose from noncarbohydrate sources, such as amino acids and glycerol; can occur in the liver and kidneys when the carbohydrate intake is insufficient to meet the body's needs.

Hyperpnea (hī′perp-nē′ah): abnormal increase in depth and rate of respiration.

Hypoglycemia (hī′pō-glī-sē′mē-ah): an abnormally low level of glucose in the blood; opposite of **hyperglycemia,** very high blood glucose.

IDDM: insulin-dependent diabetes mellitus.

Insulin (in′su-lin): a powerful hormone secreted by the beta cells in the islets of Langerhans of the pancreas; the major fuel-regulating hormone; enters the blood in response to a rise in concentration of blood glucose and transported immediately to bind with cell surface receptors throughout the body.

Ketoacidosis (kē′tō-ah′si-dō′sis): diabetic coma; too little insulin; accumulation of ketone bodies in the blood.

Ketone bodies: normal metabolic products of lipid (fat) within the liver; excess production leads to urinary excretion of these bodies.

Ketonuria (kē′tō-nu′rē-ah): excess of ketone bodies in the urine.

NIDDM: noninsulin-dependent diabetes mellitus.

Oral glucose tolerance test (OGTT): a test of the body's ability to utilize carbohydrates; aid to the diagnosis of diabetes mellitus. After ingestion of a specific amount of glucose solution, the fasting blood glucose rises promptly in a nondiabetic person, then falls to normal within an hour. In diabetes mellitus, the blood glucose rise is greater and the return to normal is prolonged.

Oral hypoglycemic agent: synthetic drug that lowers the blood sugar level; stimulates the synthesis and release of insulin from the beta cells of the islets of Langerhans in the pancreas; used to treat patients with noninsulin-dependent diabetes mellitus.

Polydipsia (pol′ē-dip′sē-ah): excessive thirst.

Polyphagia (pol′ē-fa′jē-ah): excessive ingestion of food.

Polyuria (pol′e-ū′rē-ah): excessive excretion of urine.

Pruritus (proo-rī′tus): itching.

Retinopathy (ret′ĭ-nop′ah-thē): noninflammatory degenerative disease of the retina; called **diabetic retinopathy** when it occurs with diabetes of long standing.

3. Usually arises in childhood or puberty, but may occur at any age.
4. Abrupt onset of symptoms.
   a. Weight loss, weakness.
   b. Polyuria, polydipsia, polyphagia.
   c. Hyperglycemia from body's inability to utilize glucose.

   B. Former Names
   IDDM has been known as juvenile diabetes, juvenile-onset diabetes, ketosis-prone diabetes, and brittle diabetes.

II. TYPE II. NONINSULIN-DEPENDENT DIABETES MELLITUS (NIDDM)
Types I and II are compared in table 60-2.

   A. Characteristics
   1. Not dependent on insulin for prevention of ketonuria and not prone to ketosis.
   2. Minimal or no symptoms; asymptomatic for years, with slow disease progression.
   3. Onset typical after 35 to 40 years of age, but may occur in younger individuals.
   4. Obese type respresents 60–80% of the diabetic population; condition improves with weight reduction and diet control.
   5. NIDDM incidence has increased in the United States.

   B. Former Names
   NIDDM has been called adult-onset diabetes, maturity-onset diabetes, ketosis-resistant diabetes, and maturity-onset type diabetes of the young.

III. TYPE III. GESTATIONAL DIABETES (GDM)
   A. Characteristics
   1. Begins or is recognized during pregnancy; diabetic women who become pregnant are not included in this category.
   2. Above-normal risk of perinatal complications; increased frequency of fetal loss.
   3. Glucose intolerance may be transitory; patient motivation to maintain normal glucose and body weight influences health of baby.

   B. Postpartum
   1. In the majority of patients, glucose tolerance returns to normal and is reclassified into Class IV—previous abnormality of glucose tolerance.
   2. Others go on to develop overt diabetes in 15 to 20 years, particularly postmenopausally.

ACTION OF INSULIN

Normally, insulin is released from the pancreas in proportion to the amount of glucose in the blood. The beta cells of the pancreas stimulate or inhibit insulin secretion directly in accord with the blood glucose level.

TABLE 60–2
COMPARISON OF CHARACTERISTICS OF INSULIN-DEPENDENT AND NONINSULIN-DEPENDENT DIABETES MELLITUS

Characteristic	Insulin-dependent Diabetes Mellitus	Noninsulin-dependent Diabetes Mellitus
Age of Onset	Usually under 25 years; may appear later	Adulthood, particularly over 40 years; may appear at younger ages
Body Weight	Normal or thin	High percent obese at the time of diagnosis
Onset of Clinical Symptoms	Rapid/abrupt	Slow/insidious
Severity	Severe	Mild
Diabetic Emergency (Ketoacidosis)	Common	Rare
Stability	Unstable	Stable
Insulin Treatment Required	Almost all	Less than 25%
Chronic Manifestations	Uncommon before 20 years; prevalent and severe by age 30	Develop slowly with age

I. FUNCTIONS OF INSULIN

As a powerful hormone, insulin directly or indirectly affects every organ in the body.

    A. Facilitates conversion of glucose to fat in adipose tissue.

    B. Speeds the conversion of glucose to glycogen in the liver and muscles.

    C. Facilitates the transmission of glucose into cells.

    D. Speeds the oxidation of glucose within the cells for energy.

II. EFFECTS OF DECREASED INSULIN

In diabetes, insulin is decreased in amount or function.

    A. With decreased insulin, less glucose is transmitted through cell walls into the cells.

    B. Glucose increases in the circulating blood until a threshold is reached when glucose spills over into the urine.

    C. Without glucose in the cells to use for energy, the cells utilize fat.

       1. End products of fat metabolism (ketones) accumulate in the blood.

       2. Ketones are acid. Usually, when they accumulate, they are neutralized in the blood. When the quantity is large, the neutralizing effect is depleted rapidly and an acid condition (acidosis) results.

       3. In severe, untreated, or inadequately controlled diabetes, acidosis leads to diabetic coma (ketoacidosis).

III. INSULIN COMPLICATIONS

With earlier diagnosis, improved treatment procedures, and better informed patients and their families, emergencies have decreased. Recognizing the earliest symptoms to arrest the development of a crisis stage is increasingly important.

    A. Insulin Reaction

    Too much insulin (hyperinsulinism), with lower levels of blood glucose.

    B. Diabetic Coma (Ketoacidosis)

    Too little insulin (hypoinsulinism). See table 60–3 for a comparison of the characteristics of insulin reaction and diabetic coma, and the respective treatment procedures.

EFFECTS OF DIABETES

I. INFECTION AND DIABETES

    A. Patients with diabetes, particularly those whose disease is inadequately controlled, are more susceptible to infections.

    B. Failure to treat an infection increases the severity of the diabetic state and intensifies the symptoms; it can precipitate diabetic coma.

    C. With infection present, insulin requirements may increase; with elimination of the infection, it may be possible to decrease the prescribed insulin.

    D. Frequently encountered infections involve the urinary tract, skin, lungs (pneumonia or tuberculosis), and the oral cavity, particularly the periodontium.

    E. Factors involved are impaired circulation, alterations in carbohydrate and protein metabolisms, altered nutritional state, or abnormal immunologic response.

TABLE 60-3
COMPARISON OF INSULIN REACTION AND DIABETIC COMA

	Insulin Reaction (Hypoglycemia)	Diabetic Coma (Ketoacidosis)
History (Predisposing Factors)	Too much insulin Too little food: delayed or omitted Loss of food by vomiting or diarrhea Excessive Exercise	Too little insulin: omission of medication or failure to increase dose when requirements increased Too much food Infection Stress Illness of any sort
Cause	Lowered blood glucose with excess insulin in proportion	Decreased glucose utilization when insufficient insulin leads to prolonged increasing acidosis
Occurrence	In insulin-dependent diabetics, particularly the unstable, severe type	Insulin-dependent person who is poorly controlled, unstable, who omits or reduces insulin for emotional or other reasons
Onset	Sudden Slower when long-acting insulin is used	Gradual, over many hours, even days
Physical Findings	Skin: moist, increased perspiration Hunger Headache Tremor Pallor Dilated pupils Dizziness, staggering gait Weakness	Skin: flushed and dry Nausea, vomiting Lack of appetite Dry mouth, thirst Soft, sunken eyeballs Increased urination Abdominal pain
Vital Signs Temperature Respirations Pulse Blood Pressure	Normal or below Normal Fast; irregular Normal or slightly elevated	Elevated when infection Hyperpnea; acetone breath odor Weak; rapid Lowered; person may be in shock
Behavior	Drowsiness Restlessness, anxiety, irritability Incoordination Stupor, confusion Eventual coma, with or without convulsion	Progressive drowsiness Confusion Lethargy Weakness Eventual coma
Treatment	Give sugar to raise the blood glucose level (orange juice, candy, sugar cubes) Revival: prompt Unconscious or unresponsive: treated by injection of glucagon* or may require intravenous glucose	Immediate professional care, hospitalization Keep patient warm Fluids for the conscious patient Insulin injection
Prevention	Smooth regulation of diabetes with steady diet, insulin, exercise	Early diagnosis of diabetes Well-indoctrinated, regulated patient

* *Glucagon*, a hormone produced by the alpha cells of the pancreas, increases blood glucose.

II. DIABETES IN PREGNANCY
A. Effects on Mother
Insulin adjustment, carefully supervised prenatal care, and improved obstetric practices have lessened much of the potential danger for the mother.

B. Effects on Offspring
1. Infants are larger; premature births more frequent; incidence of congenital malformations is high.

2. High perinatal death rate; lower rate with improved prenatal care.

III. LONG-TERM COMPLICATIONS
Patients with controlled diabetes may develop complications later than those whose diabetes is less well controlled. The principal involvements are in the nervous system (neuropathy), kidney (nephropathy), retina (retinopathy), and blood vessels (arteriosclerosis and atherosclerosis).

Kidney disease is most severe in insulin-dependent diabetes, whereas atherosclerotic coronary disease is common in older persons with diabetes. Retinopathy occurs frequently, and diabetes is a leading cause of blindness in the United States.

IV. PERSONAL FACTORS
A. Impact of Personality on Diabetes
1. Problems during treatment may be related to an imbalance between diet and insulin, but often can be influenced by the patient's conscious or subconscious attempt to resist the treatment.
2. Periods of emotional distress bring on alterations in the blood glucose.
3. Changes that lead to acidosis and coma may start during periods of depression, hostility, or anxiety, particularly when such symptoms lead to neglect of diet or insulin.

B. Impact of Diabetes on Personality
1. Reaction to an initial diagnosis may be extremely traumatic, with long-term effects, particularly in a child. An adult patient may suffer fear, frustration, and confusion. Less mature adults show less acceptance, and may reject the diagnosis and try to control their treatment.
2. Adult behavior during the course of treatment can vary from reckless neglect of treatment to the opposite extreme of obsession with details and preoccupation with weighing of foods and extreme attention to personal hygiene.
3. Adolescents may find the restrictions nearly intolerable and their hopes for the future seemingly destroyed. Growing independence and rejection of authority figures (parents and physician) make diabetes control difficult.
4. Younger children may exhibit feelings of oppression, restriction, or suppressed emotions because of subordination and control by the diabetic regimen.
5. Parents' attitudes influence the diabetic child's adjustment.
   a. Overanxious, overprotective parent may precipitate anxiety states or complete dependence of the child.
   b. Overindulgent parent may indirectly lead the child to exploitation or even complete control.
   c. Indifferent or nonchalant parent may give the child feelings of desertion, neglect, or depression.

TREATMENT FOR DIABETES CONTROL

Objectives in patient care are to correct metabolic disturbances, attain the best possible state of general health, and prevent or postpone complications or chronic effects of diabetes. Treatment methods depend on the severity of the disease and on the age, activity, vocation, and psychologic needs, as well as the nutritional and weight problems, of the patient.

I. GENERAL PROCEDURES
A. Methods
1. Immediate treatment to manage the acute symptoms.
2. Elimination of sources of infection, including oral diseases.
3. Patient education for self-care.
4. Diet and exercise.
5. Medication, including insulin for the insulin-dependent patient and oral antidiabetic agents for selected patients.
6. Personal physical and mental hygiene.

B. Self-care
No known cure exists for diabetes. The success of treatment depends on the knowledge, understanding, and attitude of the patient, and on how well the condition is managed on a day-to-day basis throughout life.
1. *Instruction.* Continuing instruction must be provided the patient by the health team, including the physician, registered nurse, dietitian, and other specialists. The dentist and dental hygienist participate to instruct and supervise the patient's oral health practices for the prevention and control of oral diseases.
2. *Components of Self-care*
   a. Objectives. To prevent infections and injuries; prevent glycosuria; and maintain the best possible general health.
   b. Specific instruction. The elements of treatment learned and carried out by the individual include diet management; urine testing; technique of and sites for insulin injection; care of syringe and of insulin; care of the feet to prevent lesions and infections; and what to do in case of acute complications.
   c. Instruction materials. A number of excellent books and other printed materials have been prepared specifically for the patient with diabetes. Review of some of these materials can provide the dental team members with greater insight into the background and knowledge of the patient in preparation for oral health instruction.

II. DIET AND EXERCISE

Diet planning is basic to all diabetic therapy. Exercise is an essential part of the treatment program and contributes to lowering insulin requirements.

A. Fundamentals of the Diabetic Diet

1. *Carbohydrates.* Elimination of concentrated carbohydrates (sugar, frostings, pastries, candy, syrup, and others).
2. *Total Food Intake.* The daily intake may be identical with normal for the patient's age and stature, with appropriate adjustments for growth in the young patient, degree of activity, and occupation. The obese patient needs a weight-reduction diet.
3. *Diet Selection*
   a. Individual quantitative need. As the treatment schedule is planned by the physician and dietitian, the individual needs are determined within the framework of the patient's customary diet. The adequate diabetic diet is calculated so that ideal body weight can be obtained and maintained.
   b. Food exchange system. This widely used system groups foods into six categories, namely, bread, meat, vegetable, milk, fruit, and fat. Each patient is instructed in specific selections from each list. Only the specific amounts are to be eaten and other additions cannot be made. Food exchange means that a certain serving from one group can be exchanged only with an equivalent from the same group.

   At first, all patients are expected to measure and weigh their food so that the size of proper servings can be learned. Patients with severe diabetes may need to weigh and measure for a longer period or indefinitely.

B. Eating Habits

1. *Distribution of Food.* Daily regimen of eating a prescribed caloric intake is essential to balance insulin and blood glucose.
2. *Meals.* Three spaced, on-time meals and three interval feedings are usually indicated. All food, including that used between meals, is counted into the day's total intake.
3. *Intake of Food.* Patient must eat all the food prescribed at the prescribed times. Rejected foods or foods lost through vomiting must be reported because these may explain changes in glucose balance.

III. MEDICATION

A. Insulin Therapy

1. *Types of Insulin.* Insulin is classified as short-acting, intermediate-acting, or long-acting.
2. *Dosage.* Depends on the individual.

   a. Objective is to attain optimum utilization of glucose throughout each 24 hours.
   b. Factors affecting the need for insulin are food intake, illness, stressful events, variations in exercise, or infections.

B. Oral Antidiabetic Agents

Oral antidiabetic (hypoglycemic) agents are used less than in past years because research has revealed significant detrimental side effects. They may still be used when diet control has proved unsuccessful or insulin cannot be used for such reasons as allergy or immune reaction. One group of antidiabetic agents, the sulfonylureas, acts by stimulating insulin release from the beta cells.

ORAL RELATIONSHIPS

The oral mucosa, tongue, and periodontal tissues of a patient with diabetes mellitus may show unusual susceptibility and a tendency toward more marked reactions to injury, infections, and all local irritants than do tissues of nondiabetic persons. Such a response is related to generally lowered resistance and delayed healing processes.

I. PERIODONTAL INVOLVEMENT[3,4,5]

Diabetes is considered a significant risk factor for periodontal infections.

A. Clinical Findings

Marked periodontal disease may be observed at early ages, particularly in patients with insulin-dependent diabetes. Oral findings may include alveolar bone resorption, loss of attachment, increased probing depth, and increased tooth mobility, sometimes accompanied by pathologic tooth migration and other signs of trauma from occlusion. Patients with diabetes are more susceptible to periodontal abscess formation.

B. Contributing Factors

1. Diabetes acts as a conditioning, modifying, and accelerating factor, with local irritants having an important role in the development of periodontal symptoms.
2. Inadequate bacterial plaque control contributes to more severe tissue response because of decreased resistance.

II. DENTAL CARIES
A. Uncontrolled Diabetes

The dental caries rate is generally consistent with the patient's own age group or may be slightly higher related to diminished saliva and dry mouth or to a high carbohydrate diet in the obese.

B. Controlled

With a well-regulated diet, necessarily low in or free of sugar-containing foods, and with a regular eating pattern that excludes permissive and unaccounted-for between-meal snacks, a reduced dental caries rate is frequently observed.

III. OTHER ORAL FINDINGS

In addition to the signs and symptoms of periodontal infections, certain other oral findings may be noted. These occur primarily when diabetes is uncontrolled or poorly controlled. These signs can be important for identifying a previously undiagnosed case of diabetes.

Diabetes does not cause oral disease. The conditions listed here relate to or secondarily result from the lowered resistance and susceptibility to infection that are characteristics of the tissues of patients with diabetes.

A. Lips

Drying, cracking, angular cheilitis.

B. Xerostomia

Alteration in microflora, increased plaque formation.

A dry, sore mouth can lead to diet alterations incompatible with diabetic diet requirements.

C. Mucosa

Edematous, red, possibly ulcerated; burning sensations; poor tolerance for removable prostheses.

DENTAL HYGIENE CARE

Because infection in the oral cavity can alter the course of diabetes and its treatment, the control of oral diseases has a vital role in the maintenance of the patient's health. Frequent and thorough care, with regular supervision of the patient's self-care, is needed. This, in turn, requires gaining the patient's utmost cooperation and confidence.

I. PATIENT HISTORY

The basic medical history obtained from a patient with diabetes is supplemented by additional questioning to provide essential information, such as the type and schedule of medication, dietary requirements, meal schedule, and frequency of medical appointments. A history update at each maintenance appointment can provide significant new information.

Pertinent questions for an undetected diabetic condition apply to weight loss, excess thirst, hunger, and family history of diabetes.

II. CONSULTATION WITH PHYSICIAN

Consultation between the dentist and the physician is necessary before any instrumentation involving tissue manipulation is performed.

A. Information Obtained

1. Degree of control, stability, and severity of the diabetes; susceptibility of the patient to emergency reactions.
2. Other health problems that may influence oral care.
3. Advice relative to a prescription for prophylactic antibiotic therapy.
4. Instructions that have been given the patient about diet, personal care, medication adjustment, or other.

B. Use of Information

The dental hygienist should study and apply information from the patient history and the physician-dentist consultation so that dental hygiene phases of care and instruction are conducted in accord with the health requirements of the patient.

III. APPOINTMENT PLANNING

Stress, including that created during a dental or dental hygiene appointment, increases glycemia and a tendency toward diabetic acidosis and coma. Appointment planning centers around stress prevention.

A. Antibiotic Premedication

Consultation with the patient's physician or specialist in diabetes is necessary.

In general, the patient with well-controlled diabetes can be treated the same as a patient without diabetes. when the patient is first examined and periodontal infection is evident, however, antibiotic premedication may be advisable.

Uncontrolled, unstable diabetes mellitus requires prophylactic antibiotic premedication because of the reduced ability to resist infection.

B. Time

1. *Choice.* Morning, 1½ to 3 hours after the patient's normal breakfast and medication, during the descending portion of the blood glucose level curve.
2. *Long-acting Medication.* Adjust time accordingly.

C. Precautions

1. The patient should not be kept waiting unduly.
2. Do not interfere with the patient's regular meal and between-meal eating schedule.
3. Avoid long periods of stressful procedures; dental and dental hygiene care should be divided into units for short appointments appropriate to the individual's needs.
4. Additional precautions are indicated for the patient with long-term diabetes with complications related to atherosclerosis and other cardiovascular diseases (Chapter 58). The needs of the gerodontic patient may be applied (Chapter 46).

5. Prepare for diabetic emergency when the patient's history reveals diabetic instability or susceptibility to emergencies. Keep sugar cubes or canned orange juice available for the conscious patient as part of the office emergency supplies (page 830, and table 61–3, page 845).

IV. CLINICAL PROCEDURES
A. Instrumentation

1. *Quadrant or Area Scaling.* When a patient is known to have a healing problem, limiting the number of teeth to be completed at each appointment is recommended. For each area, scaling should be completed insofar as possible. A plaque check and review of personal oral hygiene procedures prior to each scaling can improve the health of the tissues and condition them for succeeding scalings.

   With complete scaling and root planing in deep pockets, particularly in areas of furcation involvement, the possibility for periodontal abscess formation may be kept to a minimum.

2. *Postoperative Healing.* Undue trauma to tissues must be avoided to encourage postoperative healing without complications.

B. Fluoride Application

When the gingival tissue has been inflamed or scaling has been extensive, a topical fluoride application can be postponed until the gingival tissue shows improvement following healing and personal oral care by the patient. Home use of fluoride is always encouraged.

V. PATIENT INSTRUCTION
A. Influence of Diabetes Instruction

Many patients with diabetes are already education-oriented because instruction relative to diabetes and self-care procedures by the physician, nurse, and dietitian is an integral part of therapy. Some emphasis on the care of the mouth may have been made. The interrelation of oral tissue infection and the control of diabetes can be reinforced as personal instruction is given.

B. Bacterial Plaque Control

Self-care measures for plaque control are selected on the basis of individual needs (pages 413–414). Continuing supervision with review of recommended procedures is critical to the patient with diabetes because of increased susceptibility to periodontal tissue involvement.

C. Diet

1. Correlate information about dental caries prevention with the elimination of cariogenic foods. Because a diabetic diet limits concentrated sweets, cooperation in caries control measures can be expected.

2. Reinforce principles of a nutritious diet in accord with the instruction provided by the physician.

VI. MAINTENANCE PHASE

A. Appointment for supervision and examination on a regular 2- to 3-month basis.
B. Probe carefully to detect early gingival bleeding and evidence of pocket formation.
C. Soft tissue assessment with attention to areas of irritation related to fixed and removable prosthesis must be carried out at each appointment.
D. Calculus cannot be permitted to accumulate; therefore, routine scaling and planing are required.

PREVENTION OF DIABETES

When diabetes is detected and treated early, complications may be minimized, postponed, or possibly prevented. Mass screening has been used for many years to locate those persons who may have diabetes. Both blood and urine tests have been used for screening, but blood tests have been shown to be the most reliable.

In the universal effort of the health professions and community groups to find early diabetes, dental offices and clinics may become important screening centers. The history-taking and oral examination procedures for dental patients can be extremely useful for singling out diabetic suspects. Suspects can then be referred for a blood test, or an initial screening test can be performed in the dental office.

In addition to the objectives related to the health and well-being of individuals and the community health aspects of case finding, the dentist and dental hygienist have a responsibility to seek out diabetic patients in order that safe and successful dental and periodontal treatment, including the phases of care assigned the dental hygienist, may be carried out. Before proceeding with traumatic, stress-creating treatment in an infection-prone patient, every effort should be made to discover the true systemic condition of each patient.

I. DIABETIC SUSPECTS AMONG DENTAL PATIENTS
A. Patients in a Diabetes-risk Group

From observation and through questions in the patient history, the following may be identified:
1. Individuals with close relatives who have diabetes.
2. Women with abnormal obstetric history, such as multiple spontaneous abortions or stillbirths, or babies over 9 pounds at birth.
3. Obese persons, particularly in the over-40 age group.
4. Those with eye, kidney, or coronary artery disease.

5. Persons with early-onset arteriosclerosis
   a. Premenopausal women with myocardial infarction.
   b. Men having myocardial infarctions before the age of 40.
6. Persons with frequent or chronic infections.

B. Patients with Symptoms Suggestive of Diabetes

Questions in the patient history can be directed to obtain such information as the following:
1. Weight changes; weight loss with increased appetite.
2. Thirst; frequent urination.
3. Slow-healing cuts, bruises, or skin infections, such as boils.
4. Pain in extremities—fingers and toes.
5. Fatigue and drowsiness.
6. Most recent blood tests; whether test was made for blood glucose.

C. Repeat of Patient History

With long-standing patients, it is not unusual for the history to have been completed at an initial visit without follow-up reviews being made periodically. Illnesses, hospitalizations, or other involvements, including a diagnosis of diabetes, may have occurred subsequent to the original history record. At each maintenance appointment, a review history is indicated (pages 95 and 600).

REFERENCES

1. **National Diabetes Data Group,** Harris, M. and Cahill, G., Chairmen: Classification and Diagnosis of Diabetes Mellitus and Other Categories of Glucose Intolerance, *Diabetes, 28,* 1039, December, 1979.
2. **Little,** J.W. and Falace, D.A.: *Dental Management of the Medically Compromised Patient,* 4th ed. St. Louis, Mosby, 1993, pp. 341–360.
3. **Zachariasen,** R.D.: Periodontal Disease and Diabetes Mellitus, *J. Dent. Hyg., 66,* 259, July–August, 1992.
4. **Seymour,** R.A., Heasman, P.A., and Macgregor, I.D.M.: *Drugs, Diseases, and the Periodontium.* Oxford, Oxford University Press, 1992, pp. 20–22, 55–58.
5. **Gottsegen,** R.: Diabetes Mellitus, Cardiovascular Diseases, and Alcoholism, in Schluger, S., Yuodelis, R., Page, R.C., and Johnson, R.H.: *Periodontal Diseases,* 2nd ed. Phialdelphia, Lea & Febiger, 1990, pp. 273–279.

SUGGESTED READINGS

American Diabetes Association: Clinical Practice Recommendations, 1989–1990, *Diabetes Care, 13,* Supplement 1, January, 1990.

Bačić, M., Ciglar, I., Granić, M., Plančak, D., and Sutalo, J.: Dental Status in a Group of Adult Diabetic Patients, *Community Dent. Oral Epidemiol., 17,* 313, December, 1989.

Bauman, D.B.: Controlling Complications for the Diabetic Patient, *Dentalhygienistnews, 2,* 1, Fall, 1989.

Cutler, C.W., Eke, P., Arnold, R.R., and van Dyke, T.E.: Defective Neutrophil Function in an Insulin-dependent Diabetes Mellitus Patient. A Case Report, *J. Periodontol., 62,* 394, June, 1991.

Dahms, W.T.: An Update in Diabetes Mellitus, *Pediatr. Dent., 13,* 79, March–April, 1991.

Gerich, J.E.: Oral Hypoglycemic Agents, *N. Engl. J. Med., 321,* 1231, November 2, 1989.

Gibson, J., Lamey, P.-J., Lewis, M., and Frier, B.: Oral Manifestations of Previously Undiagnosed Non-insulin Dependent Diabetes Mellitus, *J. Oral Pathol. Med., 19,* 284, July, 1990.

Helmrich, S.P., and Ragland, D.R., Leung, R.W., and Paffenbarger, R.S.: Physical Activity and Reduced Occurrence of Non-insulin-dependent Diabetes Mellitus, *N. Engl. J. Med., 325,* 147, July 18, 1991.

Jones, R.B., McCallum, R.M., Kay, E.J., Kirkin, V., and McDonald, P.: Oral Health and Oral Health Behaviour in a Population of Diabetic Outpatient Clinic Attenders, *Community Dent. Oral Epidemiol., 20,* 204, August, 1992.

Malamed, S.F.: *Handbook of Medical Emergencies in the Dental Office,* 4th ed. St. Louis, Mosby, 1993, pp. 230–250.

Parker, R.C., Rapley, J.W., Isley, W., Spencer, P., and Killoy, W.J.: Gingival Crevicular Blood for Assessment of Blood Glucose in Diabetic Patients, *J. Periodontol., 64,* 666, July, 1993.

Pérusse, R., Goulet, J.-P., and Turcotte, J.-Y.: Contraindications to Vasoconstrictors in Dentistry: Part II. Hyperthyroidism, Diabetes, Sulfite Sensitivity, *Oral Surg. Oral Med. Oral Pathol., 74,* 687, November, 1992.

Reichard, P., Nilsson, B.-Y., and Rosenquist, U.: The Effect of Long-term Intensified Insulin Treatment on the Development of Microvascular Complications of Diabetes Mellitus, *N. Engl. J. Med., 329,* 304, July 29, 1993.

Scruggs, R.R., Warren, D.P., and Levine, P.: Juvenile Diabetics' Oral Health and Locus of Control. A Pilot Study, *J. Dent. Hyg., 63,* 376, October, 1989.

Selam, J.-L. and Charles, M.A.: Devices for Insulin Administration, *Diabetes Care, 13,* 955, September, 1990.

Skoczylas, L.J., Terezhalmy, G.T., Langlais, R.P., and Glass, B.J.: Dental Management of the Diabetic Patient, *Compendium, 9,* 390, May, 1988.

Sreebny, L.J., Yu, A., Green, A., and Valdini, A.: Xerostomia in Diabetes Mellitus, *Diabetes Care, 15,* 900, July, 1992.

Tavares, M., DePaola, P., Soparkar, P., and Joshipura, K.: The Prevalence of Root Caries in a Diabetic Population, *J. Dent. Res., 70,* 979, June, 1991.

Thorstensson, H., Falk, H., Hugoson, A., and Kuylenstierna, J.: Dental Care Habits and Knowledge of Oral Health in Insulin-dependent Diabetics, *Scand. J. Dent. Res., 97,* 207, June, 1989.

Thorstensson, H., Falk, H., Hugoson, A., and Olsson, J.: Some Salivary Factors in Insulin-dependent Diabetics, *Acta Odontol. Scand., 47,* 175, June, 1989.

Tracey, M.B. and Rossmann, J.A.: Management of the Diabetic Patient. A Review and Case Report, *J.D.H., 65,* 70, February, 1991.

Twetman, S., Nederfors, T., Stahl, B., and Aronson, S.: Two-year Longitudinal Observations of Salivary Status and Dental Caries in Children with Insulin-dependent Diabetes Mellitus, *Pediatr. Dent., 14,* 184, May–June, 1992.

Zinman, B.: The Physiologic Replacement of Insulin, an Elusive Goal, *N. Engl. J. Med., 321,* 363, August 10, 1989.

Periodontal Infection

Ainamo, J., Lahtinen, A., and Uitto, V.-J.: Rapid Periodontal Destruction in Adult Humans with Poorly Controlled Diabetes. A Report of 2 Cases, *J. Clin. Periodontol., 17,* 22, January, 1990.

Anil, S., Remani, P., Vijayakumar, T., and Hari, S.: Cell-mediated and Humoral Immune Response in Diabetic Patients with Periodontitis, *Oral Surg. Oral Med. Oral Pathol., 70,* 44, July, 1990.

de Pommereau, V., Dargent-Paré, C., Robert, J.J., and Brion, M.: Periodontal Status in Insulin-dependent Diabetic Adolescents, *J. Clin. Periodontol., 19,* 628, October, 1992.

Emrich, L.J., Shlossman, M., and Genco, R.J.: Periodontal Disease in Non-insulin-dependent Diabetes Mellitus, *J. Periodontol., 62,* 123, February, 1991.

Hugoson, A., Thorstensson, H., Falk, H., and Kuylenstierna, J.: Periodontal Conditions in Insulin-dependent Diabetics, *J. Clin. Periodontol., 16,* 215, April, 1989.

Miller, L.S., Manwell, M.A., Newbold, D., Reding, M.E., Rasheed, A., Blodgett, J., and Kornman, K.S.: The Relationship Between Reduction in Periodontal Inflammation and Diabetes Control: A Report of 9 Cases, *J. Periodontol., 63,* 843, October, 1992.

Sandholm, L., Swanljung, O., Rytömaa, I., Kaprio, E.A., and Mäenpää, J.: Periodontal Status of Finnish Adolescents with Insulin-dependent Diabetes Mellitus, *J. Clin. Periodontol., 16,* 617, November, 1989.

Sepälä, B., Sepälä, M., and Ainamo, J.: A Longitudinal Study on Insulin-dependent Diabetes Mellitus and Periodontal Disease, *J. Clin. Periodontol., 20,* 161, March, 1993.

Shlossman, M., Knowler, W.C., Pettitt, D.J., and Genco, R.J.: Type 2 Diabetes Mellitus and Periodontal Disease, *J. Am. Dent. Assoc., 121,* 532, October, 1990.

Tervonen, T., Knuuttila, M., Pohjamo, L., and Nurkkala, H.: Immediate Response to Nonsurgical Periodontal Treatment in Subjects with Diabetes Mellitus, *J. Clin. Periodontol., 18,* 65, January, 1991.

Tervonen, T. and Oliver, R.C.: Long-term Control of Diabetes Mellitus and Periodontitis, *J. Clin. Periodontol., 20,* 431, July, 1993.

Thorstensson, H. and Hugoson, A.: Periodontal Disease Experience in Adult Long-duration Insulin-dependent Diabetics, *J. Clin. Periodontol., 20,* 352, May, 1993.

Microflora

Mandell, R.L., Dirienzo, J., Kent, R., Joshipura, K., and Haber, J.: Microbiology of Healthy and Diseased Periodontal Sites in Poorly Controlled Insulin Dependent Diabetes, *J. Periodontol., 63,* 274, April, 1992.

Morinushi, T. Lopatin, D.E., Syed, S.A., Bacon, G., Kowalski, C.J., and Loesche, W.J.: Humoral Immune Response to Selected Subgingival Plaque Microorganisms in Insulin-dependent Diabetic Children, *J. Periodontol., 60,* 199, April, 1989.

Sandholm, L., Swanljung, O., Rytömaa, I., Kaprio, E.A., and Maenpää, J.: Morphotypes of the Subgingival Microflora in Diabetic Adolescents in Finland, *J. Periodontol., 60,* 526, September, 1989.

Sastrowijoto, S.H., Hillemans, P., van Steenbergen, T.J.M., Abraham-Inpijn, L., and de Graaff, J.: Periodontal Condition and Microbiology of Healthy and Diseased Pockets in Type 1 Diabetes Mellitus Patients, *J. Clin. Periodontol., 16,* 316, May, 1989.

Sastrowijoto, S.H., van der Velden, U., van Steenbergen, T.J.M., Hillemans, P., Hart, A.A.M., de Graaff, J., and Abraham-Inpijn, L.: Improved Metabolic Control, Clinical Periodontal Status and Subgingival Microbiology in Insulin-dependent Diabetes Mellitus. A Prospective Study, *J. Clin. Periodontol., 17,* 233, April, 1990.

61

Emergency Care

It is relatively easy to be skillful in techniques that are repeated frequently. Emergency care is performed only occasionally and, in instances that involve life-saving measures, may be performed once in many years. To be prepared for that rare moment is difficult, but the public expects an individual trained in a health profession to be able to act in an emergency. Periodic review of procedures is necessary if application is to be effective.

Emergencies may occur within or in the vicinity of a dental office or clinic. Readiness involves having not only knowledge of proper procedures, but equipment kept in a convenient place. A quick, handy reference of emergency measures, which may be in the form of a posted chart with characteristic symptoms and related treatment, is important.

The information included in this chapter is basic and is presented with no attempt to mention all types of emergencies that may arise, particularly those of complex traumatic injuries. The principal objectives are to list the symptoms and treatment of the more common emergencies that can occur and to provide a list of the equipment that should be readily available. Other up-to-date references should be kept in the dental office and all dental personnel should familiarize themselves with such sources of information.

Key words and definitions are provided in table 61–1.

PREVENTION OF EMERGENCIES

The permanent records of all patients are handled in a confidential manner. Any identification of a health problem should be within the folder. Prior to each appointment, the record should be reviewed so that preparatory steps can be taken.

Prevention of emergencies requires preparedness, alertness, and anticipation. Some of the procedures that contribute to meeting the requirements are described here.

I. THE PATIENT HISTORY

The carefully prepared and regularly updated medical and personal history, with adequate follow-up consultation with the patient's physician for integration of dental and medical care, can prevent many emergencies by alerting dental personnel to the individual patient's needs and idiosyncrasies. Factors that should be included in the patient's history have been listed on pages 92–95 and include information concerning:
  A. Specific physical conditions that may lead to an emergency.
  B. Diseases for which the patient is (or has been) under the care of a physician and the type of treatment, including medications.
  C. Allergies or drug reactions.

II. RAPPORT AND STRESS MINIMIZATION

Stress and anxiety are the basis for many of the common emergencies that occur in a dental office or clinic. The office atmosphere and the warmth and sincerity of the personnel can help a patient feel accepted and secure.

Reduction of stress includes the following:[1]

  A. Appointment Scheduling
    1. Time of appointment planned in accord with personal health requirements.
    2. Waiting time minimized.
    3. Usual meal time and previous meal checked to prevent hunger anxiety or hypoglycemia.

828

TABLE 61-1
KEY WORDS: EMERGENCIES

Angioneurotic edema (an'jē-ō-nu-rot'ik ĕ-dē'mah): sudden and temporary appearance of large areas of painless swelling in the subcutaneous tissue or submucosa; a symptom related to allergy; also called angioedema.

Arrhythmia (ah-rĭth'mē-ah): variation from normal rhythm, especially the heartbeat.

Basic life support: the phase of emergency cardiac care that supports the ventilation of a victim of respiratory arrest with rescue breathing and supports the ventilation and circulation of a victim of cardiac arrest with cardiopulmonary resuscitation.

Cardiac arrest (kar'dē-ak): sudden and often unexpected stoppage of heart action; circulation ceases and vital organs are deprived of oxygen.

Crepitation (krep'ĭ-tā'shun): dry crackling sound, such as that produced by the grating of the ends of a fractured bone.

Cricothyrotomy (kri'kō-thi-rot'ō-mē): incision through the skin and the cricothyroid membrane to secure a patent airway for emergency relief of upper airway obstruction.

Defibrillation (dē-fib'rĭ-lā'shun): termination of atrial or ventricular fibrillation usually accomplished by electric shock.

Defibrillator (dē-fib'rĭ-lā tor): an apparatus used to produce defibrillation by application of brief electric shock to the heart directly or through electrodes placed on the chest wall.

Fibrillation (fi-brĭ-lā'shun): involuntary muscular contraction caused by spontaneous activation of single muscle cells or fibers.

    Ventricular fibrillation: a cardiac arrhythmia marked by fibrillary contractions of the ventricular muscle caused by rapid repetitive excitation of myocardial fibers without coordinated ventricular contraction; a frequent cause of cardiac arrest.

Hypoxemia (hī'pok-sē'mē-ah): deficient oxygenation of the blood; insufficient oxygenation of the blood eventually leads to **hypoxia,** which is diminished oxygen to body tissues.

Parenteral (pah-ren'ter-al): not through the alimentary canal; administered by subcutaneous, intramuscular, or intravenous injection.

Rescue breathing: a rescuer delivers a volume of 800 to 1200 ml with each ventilation; the exhaled air contains 16 to 17% oxygen, sufficient for the needs of the victim.

Syncope (sin'kō-pē): temporary loss of consciousness caused by a sudden fall in blood pressure resulting in generalized cerebral ischemia; can have serious consequences, particularly in patients with a cardiovascular disease; commonly referred to as **fainting.**

Trendelenburg's position (tren-del'en-bergz): the patient is supine with the heart higher than the head on a surface inclined downward about 45°.

Urticaria (ur'tĭ-ka'rē-ah): vascular reaction of the skin with transient appearance of slightly elevated patches (wheals) that are redder or paler than the surrounding skin; may be accompanied by severe itching; also called hives.

    4. Length of appointment limited to the patient's durability.

B. Medication
1. Premedication when indicated and recommended by the physician and dentist.
2. Pain control during treatment.
3. Patient's own prescriptions. Patients who are subject to emergencies should be instructed to bring their own prescribed medicines; for example, the patient with asthma or one who is subject to attacks of angina pectoris.

C. Post-treatment Care
1. Postcare instructions for prevention and/or relief of discomfort.
2. Follow-up telephone call for anxious patient.

III. OBSERVATION AND VITAL SIGNS
A. Extraoral Examination
The general appearance of the patient on the day of the appointment may suggest indicators that encourage preparation for emergencies.

B. Vital Signs Monitored and Recorded in the Patient's Record (pages 106–114)

IV. PREVENTION OF ACCIDENTS TO FACE AND EYES[2,3,4]
Protective eyewear is indicated for every patient and for the clinician and assistants at all appointments (page 44). Face and eye accidents can result in serious disability and loss of working time; an injured patient may justifiably take legal action. The effects of the preventive measures listed here apply to either a patient or a member of the dental staff.

A. Protective eyewear must be worn by all dental personnel and patients at each appointment.

B. Instruments, medications, and materials being transferred must be carried around the periphery, never over a patient's face.

C. Attention and care must be paid during the use of handpieces, ultrasonic scalers, and other power-driven instruments or implements that create aerosols, spatter, and ejected debris. Handpieces and ultrasonic scalers should be turned on and off only inside the oral cavity. Power-driven instruments should not be in operation while they are being inserted or removed from the patient's mouth. Aerosol production was described on pages 14 and 15.

D. Appropriate working distance from the patient's mouth to the faces of clinicians should be maintained. A distance of 14 to 16 inches from the patient's mouth to the clinician's eyes is recommended (page 72). The faces and eyes of clinician and assistant should not be positioned within the danger zone close to the patient's mouth.

E. Rubber dam should be used for all appropriate procedures to protect the patient's tissues, prevent aspiration, and provide the clinician with improved access and visibility.

EMERGENCY MATERIALS AND PREPARATION

Organization is a key concept in being prepared for an emergency. Group planning and individual acceptance of responsibility can provide the team with efficiency, composure, and freedom from fear at the time of crisis.

I. COMMUNICATION: TELEPHONE NUMBERS FOR MEDICAL AID

Telephone numbers should be posted near each extension from which outside calls can be made.

A. Rescue squads with paramedics (fire, police, flying squad, or 911 in many cities in the United States).

B. Ambulance service.

C. Nearest hospital emergency room.

D. Poison information center.

E. Physicians
1. Patient's physician should be listed in the permanent record in a standard, convenient place.
2. Physicians available for emergency calls.

II. EQUIPMENT FOR USE IN AN EMERGENCY

Every dental office or clinic should have an emergency kit or cart,[5,6] and everyone in the office must be familiar with its contents. The kit should be in order, its contents replenished, and outdated materials replaced as needed.

The emergency equipment should be portable and kept in a place readily accessible to all treatment rooms. Materials are plainly marked and kept separate from other office supplies. Materials included are selected to accomplish emergency treatment by current methods.

The items included in the kit imply proper training in their use. A team should work out additions to the list in keeping with their training and abilities.

A. Essential Equipment

1. *Series E portable oxygen tank*
   a. Low-flow regulator to allow administration at different concentrations.
   b. Delivery systems include nasal cannula, simple face mask, nonrebreather bag, bag-valve mask (Ambu Bag), demand valve.

2. *Airways.* Various sizes for oropharyngeal and nasopharyngeal—child and adults; water-soluble lubricant for insertion of nasopharyngeal airways (petroleum jelly is combustible, hence contraindicated).

3. *Suction Tips.* Wide diameter with smooth edges to prevent damage to mucous membranes.

4. *Blood Pressure Equipment.* Sphygmomanometer, stethoscope; child, regular, and large blood pressure cuffs.

5. *Magill Forceps.* Blunt-ended instrument designed to grasp objects from the mouth or throat.

6. *Cricothyrotomy Equipment.* Included only with advanced training.

B. Injectable Drugs

1. *Essential (critical)*
   a. Antiallergy. Epinephrine 1:1000 in preloaded syringe.
   b. Antihistamine. Chlorpheniramine; diphenhydramine.

2. *Secondary (noncritical)*
   In a clinical setting where trained individuals are available, an emergency kit may contain a variety of drugs for specific emergencies. Included may be an anticonvulsant, analgesic, vasopressor, antihypoglycemic, corticosteroid, antihypertensive, and an anticholinergic.[5]

3. *Equipment*
   a. Syringes. Disposable sterile 2- to 3-ml-capacity syringes (Luer-Lok-Tip) with 18- or 21-gauge disposable needles. Syringes and tourniquet are only included for parenteral drug administration.
   b. Tourniquet. Rubber or Velcro; rubber tubing or the blood pressure cuff can be used.

C. Noninjectable Treatment Items

1. *Essential (critical)*
   a. Oxygen
   b. Vasodilator. Nitrostat tablets (nitroglycerin); nitrolingual spray.

2. *Secondary (noncritical)*
   a. Respiratory stimulant. Aromatic ammonia in gray vaporoles.
   b. Bronchodilator. Albuterol inhaler.
   c. Antihypoglycemic (for conscious person). Frosting mix (tube), sugar cubes.
   d. Antihypertensive. Nifedipine or nitroglycerin capsule form.
   e. Sterile irrigating solution for eyes.
   f. Brown paper bags (for hyperventilation).

D. Supplementary Equipment

1. Pen flashlight.
2. Stopwatch.
3. Scissors.
4. Emesis basin.
5. Blanket (nonallergenic).
6. Board, 12 × 24 inches, to place under patient in a soft dental chair for CPR when patient cannot be moved to floor.
7. Commercial cold pack (nonrefrigerated quick-forming cold bag).
8. Blank pad of *Record of Emergency* (figure 61–1) with pen.

RECORD OF EMERGENCY

NAME _____

ADDRESS _____

Pertinent Medical History _____

Description of Emergency _____

DATE _____ TIME _____

Onset of Emergency _____
CPR Started _____
Ambulance Called _____
Ambulance Arrived _____
Hospital Called _____
Physician Called _____
Patient Left Office _____
Attended by: Self _____
Relative _____
Other _____

Time								
Blood Pressure								
Pulse								
Respiration								
Pupils								
Skin—color —temperature								
Level of Consciousness								
Medication (specify)								
Other Treatment (specify)								

Comments and Summary

Personnel Attending

Signature of Team Director:

FIG. 61–1. Record of Emergency. The form is prepared in duplicate. One copy accompanies the patient to the emergency department, and the second copy is retained in the patient's dental record file.

9. Bandages and dressings are purchased in individual packages and maintained in the sealed sterile state.
   a. Adhesive bandages.
   b. Sterile dressings in sealed envelopes: 2 × 2 inches, and 4 × 4 inches.
   c. Rolled bandage: 1-inch (5 yards); 2-inch (5 yards).
   d. Adhesive tape.
   e. Gauze sponges: 4 × 4 inches.
   f. Inflatable splints (assorted sizes).

III. CARE OF DRUGS

All dental personnel must be familiar with the emergency drugs maintained in the particular office or clinic. Only specially trained, experienced persons should administer injectable medications. If no one on the team has the proper background and experience, the drugs should not be kept in the office with the emergency supplies.[6]

A. Identification

The purpose and method of administration of each drug should be clearly identified with the container. A compartmentalized clear plastic cabinet or box can be particularly useful for this purpose, because the labels and instructions can be seen from the outside and efficient selection can be made.

The replacement date must appear clearly on each item with a limited shelf life. When narcotics are included in the list of drugs available for emergencies, storage in a less accessible place than an emergency kit and purchase in small amounts are indicated to prevent them from being stolen easily.

B. Record of Drugs

A complete record of each available drug is kept. Recorded are the name, dosage, date purchased, address of source if different from the usual local pharmacy, with each itemized record signed by the staff member responsible.

As each drug is used, a specific entry is made. Expiration dates can be checked at routine intervals.

IV. RECORD OF EMERGENCY

Figure 61–1 shows an example of a form that can be used to record the essential information during an emergency. Such a form can be printed into pads for the convenience of having a carbon copy to place in the patient's permanent record when the original accompanies the patient to a hospital or other medical facility.

A. Purposes

1. Organize data collected during the emergency.
2. Serve as a time reference during the monitoring of vital signs.
3. Prepare a record from which the medical personnel can interpret the patient's condition at the time of transfer from the dental facility.

B. Uses

1. Evaluation for planning dental and dental hygiene appointments so that future emergencies for the patient can be avoided.
2. Provide a reference in the event legal questions arise. A well-kept record can be vital, and each emergency, however insignificant the incident may seem, should be recorded.[7]

V. PRACTICE AND DRILL

A. Staff Instruction

Each member of the clinic or office staff must be thoroughly familiar with the location, purpose, effect, and application of each item of equipment and its source.

B. Assignments

Specific responsibilities must be assigned to each staff member to prevent confusion. Each must know the order of procedures in all types of emergencies, however, and be able to assume any role when needed. Moments count, and there is no time for fumbling or discussion.

C. Flowchart

Figure 61–2 shows an example of possible distribution of duties when four people are available to attend the patient, and figure 61–3 shows the distribution when three people are available. Although the chart can be posted for study, it must be memorized by the persons concerned. In a real emergency, no one would have time to consult a flowchart.

1. *Advantages*
   a. Organization efficiently uses personnel.
   b. Sharing responsibility relieves pressure.
   c. Duties can be carried out quietly, without excess discussion.
   d. Necessary work gets done without duplication and without omissions.
2. *Preparation.* The preparation of a flowchart and the assignment of all duties related to emergencies should be a result of planning by the whole team.
3. *Substitutions.* Because a staff member may be absent from the scene at the time of an emergency, each person should know the duties for all positions so that substitutions can be made and duties doubled with a minimum of discussion and no confusion.

D. Drills

1. Regular reviews and rehearsals for each type of emergency should be conducted, preferably on a "surprise" basis, at least once a month. The dentist can use a specific code

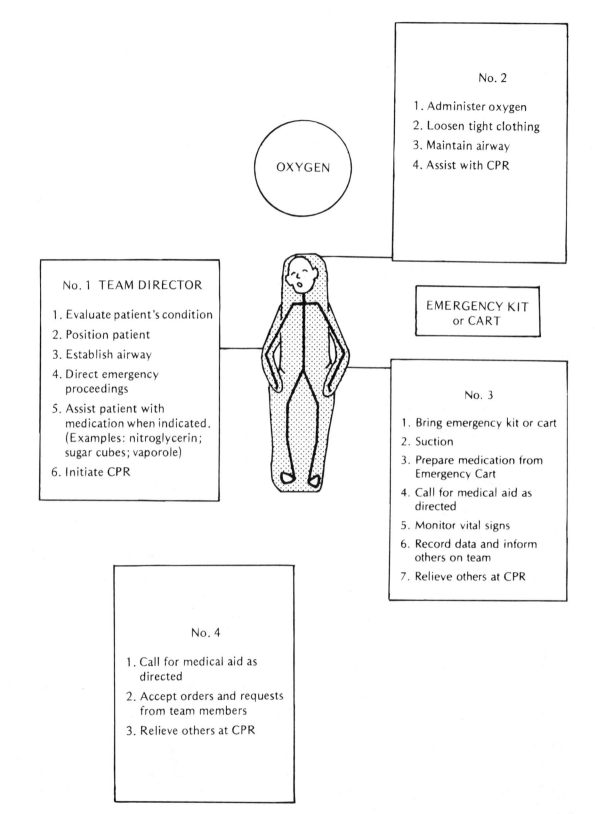

FIG. 61-2. Emergency Team Flowchart: Four People. Suggested distribution of responsibilities to be memorized and practiced by the dental personnel who form the emergency team. Compare with figure 61-3, flowchart for three people.

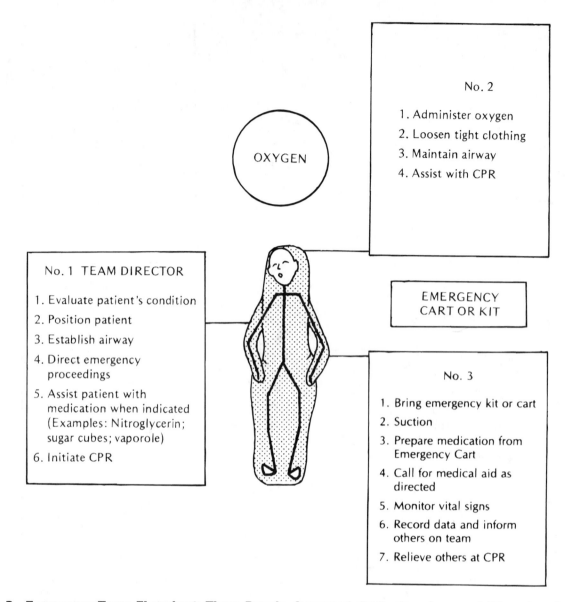

No. 2

1. Administer oxygen
2. Loosen tight clothing
3. Maintain airway
4. Assist with CPR

OXYGEN

No. 1 TEAM DIRECTOR

1. Evaluate patient's condition
2. Position patient
3. Establish airway
4. Direct emergency proceedings
5. Assist patient with medication when indicated (Examples: Nitroglycerin; sugar cubes; vaporole)
6. Initiate CPR

EMERGENCY CART OR KIT

No. 3

1. Bring emergency kit or cart
2. Suction
3. Prepare medication from Emergency Cart
4. Call for medical aid as directed
5. Monitor vital signs
6. Record data and inform others on team
7. Relieve others at CPR

FIG. 61–3. Emergency Team Flowchart: Three People. Suggested distribution of responsibilities when three people are available during an emergency. Compare with figure 61–2, flow chart for four people.

call when an intercom or other message system is available.

2. Practice in the use of all procedures, including oxygen administration, resuscitation, and airway maneuvers, as well as of specific positioning of a patient for all emergencies, is indicated.

3. Equipment and materials can be checked at the time of the drill to assure their availability and that each is in working order. Outdated supplies can be replaced. One staff member should be in charge of the emergency supplies.

4. Keep a record of drills by making a diary of dates and names of those present.

E. New Staff Member

1. Assignment of duties and practice for the new member should be a part of the first working day's orientation.

2. New members must be expected to renew CPR certificates by taking necessary refresher courses within a specified time. Such a procedure is not necessary in a state where a renewal certificate is required for annual licensure.

F. Procedures Manual

A looseleaf manual, reviewed and updated three or four times each year, can provide a valuable study and work reference. It is particularly useful during the orientation of a new member.

The notebook can contain work assignments and check lists for equipment and resources. Direct reference information concerning specific emergencies with their symptoms and initial treatment may be placed in alphabetic order in a specially color-coded section. Members of the team can keep the manual current by bringing references and notes from readings and courses.

BASIC LIFE SUPPORT[8]

Sudden cessation of effective respiration and circulation must be treated immediately. Without breathing and heart action, oxygen cannot be carried to the cells and a deficiency occurs quickly. *Irreversible brain tissue damage may occur within 4 to 6 minutes in the absence of oxygenated blood. After 6 minutes, brain damage nearly always occurs.*

The cause of collapse, respiratory arrest, or cardiac arrest cannot always be determined at the outset. Survival rates depend on prompt entry into emergency medical service (EMS) for state-of-the-art medical attention. Preliminary assessment of the state of consciousness (response, breathing, and pulse rate) must be made quickly, and the EMS activated promptly.

Basic patient care in an emergency is defined by the letters A-B-C.

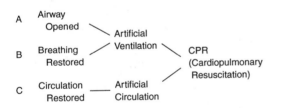

A "D" is sometimes included in the alphabet run to designate definitive care that is required. Examples of definitive care are defibrillation or drug administration by the emergency medical care team or the physicians at a hospital.

It is necessary to keep calm and act promptly, but not hastily. The incorrect procedure may be more harmful than none at all. Each member of the dental team should have participated in courses in emergency procedures and resuscitation techniques while in school and periodically since graduation for refresher, renewal, and updating. This section is intended to provide an outline for reference and review. Abbreviations pertaining to emergency care are listed in table 61-2. The steps described are carried out in rapid succession.

I. QUICKLY LOWER DENTAL CHAIR (IN DENTAL SETTING)
A. Adjust patient for supine position.
B. Remove a round or wedge-shaped accessory

TABLE 61-2
EMERGENCY CARE: ABBREVIATIONS

ACLS:	Advanced Cardiac Life Support
AED:	Automated External Defibrillator
AHA:	American Heart Association
ALS:	Advanced Life Support
BLS:	Basic Life Support
BCLS:	Basic Cardiac Life Support
CAD:	Coronary Artery Disease
CPR:	Cardiopulmonary Resuscitation
ECC:	Emergency Cardiac Care
ECG:	Electrocardiogram
EMD:	Emergency Medical Dispatcher
EMS:	Emergency Medical Service
EMT:	Emergency Medical Technician
EMT-D:	Emergency Medical Technician-Defibrillation

head or shoulder support to permit the head to lie flat and the chin to be raised without resistance.

II. DETERMINE STATE OF CONSCIOUSNESS
A. Tap or gently shake the shoulder and shout "Are you O.K?" If fractures are suspected, the shake must be light.
B. Unconscious patient does not respond.
C. Call for help. When available, use an alert (buzzer) system of an office or clinic.

III. OPEN AIRWAY

A. Head Tilt
Place palm of hand on patient's forehead to apply backward pressure.

B. Head Tilt with Chin Lift
Place palm of hand on the forehead to apply a backward pressure; place fingertips (not thumb) of other hand under the chin with light pressure on the mandible to bring the chin up (figure 61-4).

C. Modified Jaw Thrust
1. Indication. When a neck or spinal injury is suspected, the airway can be opened without extending the neck. DO NOT use head tilt/chin lift maneuver when spinal injury is suspected.
2. Procedure
   a. From over the top of the head, place thumbs on zygoma and grasp angles of the mandible with fingertips.
   b. Lift fingers upward to open airway.
   c. Never tilt the head when spinal injury is suspected.

IV. CHECK BREATHING (3 TO 5 SECONDS)
A. From beside the patient at the shoulder (kneeling if patient is on the floor), place ear

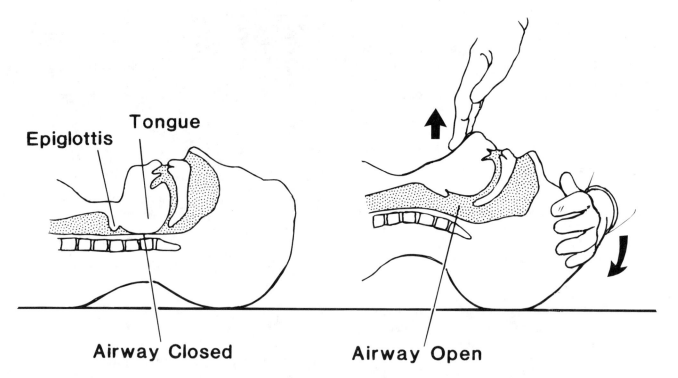

Epiglottis **Tongue**

Airway Closed **Airway Open**

FIG. 61–4. Chin Lift to Open Airway. Left, Unconscious person with tongue falling back against posterior wall of pharynx and obstructing the air passage. **Right,** Head is tilted back and chin is lifted by light pressure under the mandible. When neck injury is suspected, a jaw thrust is used. See text for instructions. (After Malamed, S.F.: *Handbook of Medical Emergencies in the Dental Office,* 3rd ed. St. Louis, Mosby, 1987, page 87).

over the patient's mouth and nose while looking at the chest.

B. LOOK for chest movement.

C. LISTEN for and FEEL air from the nose and mouth.

    1. If patient is unconscious and breathing, check pulse.

    2. If patient is unconscious with no breathing, say, "No breathing," when signalling second rescuer.

D. When NO breathing, immediately administer two full breaths.

    1. Place resuscitation mask on patient.

    2. Place thumbs on each side of mask (to obtain seal).

    3. Place fingers on border of ramus.

    4. Utilize a modified jaw thrust to open airway.

    5. Holding the tight seal around mask, force air in until the chest is seen to rise, then release.

    6. When patient cannot be ventilated, obstruction is apparent. Proceed to airway obstruction management.

V. CHECK PULSE

A. Location

    1. *Adult.* Carotid pulse in neck (figure 61–5).

    2. *Child* (ages 1 to 8 years). Carotid pulse in neck.

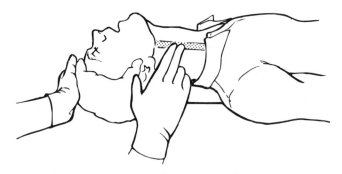

FIG. 61–5. Carotid Pulse. To locate the pulse, two or three fingers are placed on the patient's pharynx. The fingers are then slid down into the groove between the trachea and the neck muscles. With gentle pressure, the pulse can be detected.

    3. *Infant* (younger than 1 year). Brachial pulse of the inner upper arm (figure 7–3, page 110).

B. Determine Need for Cardiopulmonary Resuscitation (CPR)

    1. If pulse present and patient not breathing, *proceed with rescue breathing.*

    2. If NO pulse, but patient breathing, *proceed with CPR.*

VI. ACTIVATE EMERGENCY MEDICAL SERVICES

Telephone 911 or appropriate number for the given community.

RESCUE BREATHING

I. CLEAR THE MOUTH

Turn the patient's head to the side to clear the mouth of mucus, vomitus, and other foreign material. Use suction, gauze, and finger. Dentures should be left in place to provide support unless the dentures are very loose and could cause throat obstruction if displaced.

II. RESCUE BREATHING
A. Place resuscitation mask on patient.
B. Hold with thumbs (on sides of mask) and place fingers on the border of the ramus to obtain a seal.
C. Apply modified jaw thrust to open airway.
D. Deliver 2 breaths (1½ to 2 seconds each breath).
E. Remove mouth and take in fresh air between each breath. The rescuer must take care not to become hyperventilated by taking too many deep breaths.
F. For child or infant, use only enough breath volume for chest to rise and fall.

III. REPEAT THE VENTILATIONS
A. For adult, repeat 1 ventilation every 5 seconds (12 per minute).
B. For child, repeat 1 ventilation every 3 seconds (20 per minute).
C. For infant, repeat 1 ventilation every 3 seconds (20 per minute).
D. Rescue breathing is considered effective when the patient's chest rises with each ventilation.

IV. MAKE A PULSE CHECK EACH MINUTE
A. If no pulse, start CPR.
B. With pulse present, continue rescue breathing.

EXTERNAL CHEST COMPRESSION

There are two mechanisms for blood flow during CPR. One is the principle that rhythmic pressure applied over the lower half of the sternum compresses the heart to produce artificial circulation. The procedure is also called *external cardiac compression.*

The second mechanism involves the intrathoracic pressure, which rises during chest compression. The rise in intrathoracic pressure provides a significant mechanism for movement of blood to the brain. Both cardiac and intrathoracic pressures may be in effect during resuscitation efforts.

Chest compressions are always accompanied by rescue breathing.

I. POSITION
The patient is in a supine position. When working in a dental chair, lower the chair to its lowest position and place a cardiac arrest board or other firm flat object under the patient's back to provide a solid surface for compression.

II. ADULT
A. Locate Point for Compression
1. Run the middle finger of hand 1 along the lower edge of the rib cage to the notch in the midline.
2. With the middle finger in the notch and the index finger beside it, place the heel of hand 2 next to the index finger on the midline of the sternum.
3. Place the heel of hand 1 on top of hand 2 with the fingers in the same direction. Link and close the fingers.
4. Hold the fingers up so that only the heel of hand 2 is on the sternum (figure 61–6).

B. Compression
1. Lean forward over the positioned hands, arms straight, until shoulders are directly over the sternum.
2. Use a firm, steady, vertical pressure (not a blow). The sternum moves down 1½ to 2 inches (figure 61–6).
3. Release pressure but maintain contact and position of the hands with sternum.
4. Compress at a rate of 80 to 100 times per minute.
5. Make the compressions smooth and uninterrupted, with compression and relaxation of equal duration.
6. Use the natural weight of the upper body to prevent pushing from the shoulders or depending on arm strength.
7. As the heart is compressed between the sternum and the spine, blood is forced out of the heart into the circulation.
8. Release of pressure allows blood to flow into the heart.
9. An interruption in compression results in a return of blood flow to zero.

III. CHILD
A. Locate Point for Compression
1. Follow the lower edge of the rib cage to the notch where sternum and ribs meet.
2. Place the middle finger in the notch with the index finger beside it.
3. Place the heel of the other hand next to the index finger.

B. Compression
1. Use the heel of one hand only; compress to a depth of 1 to 1½ inches.

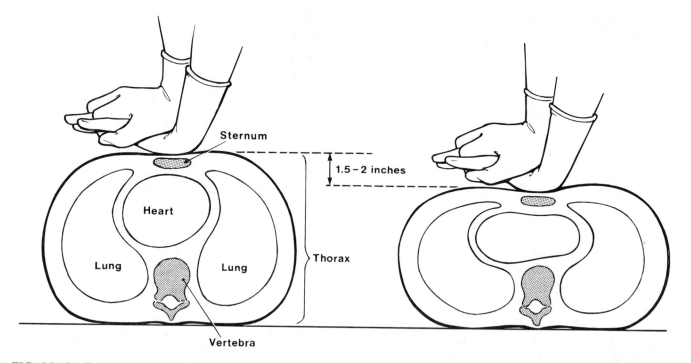

FIG. 61–6. External Chest Compression. Left, Hands in position on the sternum with fingers turned up. **Right,** Application of firm vertical pressure compresses the heart. The sternum should be compressed 1½ to 2 inches and then released. Hands are held in position for the next compression. For an adult, compressions are repeated at a rate of 80 to 100 per minute.

2. Release to allow chest to return to normal level.
3. Compress at a rate of 80 to 100 per minute, using a smooth, even rhythm.
4. Keep fingers up, off the chest.

IV. INFANT
A. Locate Point for Compression
1. Place fingers along the sternum with the index finger just below an imaginary line between the nipples. Lift the index finger. If the fingers are on the xiphoid process, move the fingers closer to the nipples.
2. Use the area under the middle and ring fingers.

B. Compression
1. Compress with 2 fingers to a depth of ½ to 1 inch; release to allow chest to return to normal after each compression.
2. Compress at a rate of at least 100 per minute, using a smooth rhythm.

V. COORDINATED ACTIVITY FOR CPR
A. Lone Rescuer
1. Provide ventilation and compressions.
2. *Adult Patient*
   a. Use ratio 15 compressions followed by 2 lung inflations.
   b. Compress at the rate of 80 to 100 per minute (count "1, and 2 and, 3 and . . .").

c. Check carotid pulse after 4 cycles of compressions and ventilations; continue if no pulse; check pulse regularly.
3. *Child and Infant*
   a. Use a ratio of 5 compressions with a slight pause for 1 ventilation.
   b. Compress at the rate of 80 to 100 per minute for a child; minimum of 100 for an infant.
   c. Reassess pulse after 10 cycles, and every few minutes.

B. Two Rescuers
1. First person begins airway, breathing, and circulation treatment as has been described.
2. Second person calls for medical assistance and ambulance, then promptly takes over compression.
3. Use coordinated rhythm of 1 lung inflation after 5 compressions.
4. The rescuer at the patient's head maintains the open airway, monitors the carotid pulse, and provides rescue breathing.
5. The compressor calls the time for a switch of positions between ventilation and compression.
6. Always finish the cycle with a ventilation and after a pulse check.
7. Start the cycle with a ventilation.

VI. LENGTH OF TREATMENT

A. Signs of recovery—normal skin color returns, patient may gasp or show other sign of breathing, and the body may move or wiggle.
B. Do not stop heart compressions while patient is being transported to the hospital.
C. When circulation and breathing appear to have returned do not leave patient; watch for need to continue resuscitation in case of relapse.

VII. SEQUELAE

Cardiopulmonary resuscitation must be continued until medical assistance arrives or the patient begins to recover. When the patient is transported to a hospital, resuscitation must continue.

For emergencies that do not require hospitalization, the patient can be moved to a couch for rest, but must be watched carefully. The cause of the emergency must be determined and additional treatment provided when indicated.

The *Record of Emergency* with monitored vital signs should accompany the patient to the medical care facility for reference by the persons assuming responsibility. The carbon copy for the patient's dental files is marked clearly with recommendations for prevention of future emergencies.

AIRWAY OBSTRUCTION[8]

A procedure of subdiaphragmatic abdominal thrusts, the Heimlich maneuver, is recommended for removal of a foreign body obstructing an airway in adults and children.

I. PREVENTION

With thought and planning, care can be exercised to prevent aspiration of objects by a patient during a dental or dental hygiene appointment. A few of the procedures that contribute to safety are as follows:

A. Place the patient in supine position during examination and treatment. The throat is closed (figure 61–4).
B. Use a rubber dam for all appropriate procedures.
C. Use a length of floss to tie to small objects, such as a rubber dam clamp or a bite block. Floss hangs out from angle of lips.
D. Use low-speed handpiece to prevent splashing or spinning masses of agents into the throat.
E. Have assistant use aspirator for various procedures that involve large pieces of calculus, copious blood clots, excess saliva, excess water for ultrasonic scaling, restorative materials, and other potentially inhalable items.
F. Pay attention to mobile permanent or exfoliating primary teeth that could be inadvertently displaced.

II. RECOGNITION OF AIRWAY OBSTRUCTION

Immediate recognition is essential. Differentiation from other emergencies, such as fainting, heart attack, or stroke, in which a sudden respiratory failure may also occur, may be necessary when no object or material was involved that could have been inhaled.

When no doubt exists that an object has been inhaled, medical aid must be obtained. A radiograph may be needed to confirm the location of a radiopaque object.

A. Signs and Symptoms of Partial Obstruction

1. Air exchange
   a. Poor air exchange with gasping and irregular respirations.
   b. Good air exchange with wheezing and forceful coughing.
2. Patient's face is red or cyanotic.
3. Treat poor air exchange as a complete obstruction.

B. Signs of Complete Obstruction

1. No air exchange with attempts at breathing; no sounds from larynx or pharynx.
2. Patient demonstrates the *universal distress signal* (clutches neck with hand).
3. Cyanosis and unconsciousness follow unless emergency care is provided quickly.

III. OUTLINE OF TREATMENT

An airway must be established within 4 to 6 minutes to prevent possible brain damage from oxygen deficiency. With total obstruction, the patient may become unconscious within a few seconds.

Treatment begins with the A-B-C of Basic Life Support, unless inhalation of a specific item was observed. When the inspiration is known, the rescuer can proceed directly to attempt to dislodge the obstructing object.

A. Conscious Adult Patient

1. In good air exchange, let patient cough.
2. Object may become dislodged; follow up with medical examination.
3. If poor air exchange or complete obstruction, apply Heimlich maneuver.
4. Patient may become unconscious; proceed for unconscious patient.

B. Unconscious Adult Patient

1. Initiate A-B-C of Basic Life Support (page 835).
2. When breathing attempt is not successful, readjust airway and attempt again.
3. **Activate EMS.**
4. Proceed with airway obstruction management
   a. Heimlich maneuver—6 to 10 abdominal thrusts.
   b. Examine mouth for object; apply finger sweep.

c. Place resuscitation mask; open airway; give two breaths.

d. Repeat steps a and b until object is expelled.

IV. HEIMLICH MANEUVER: ABDOMINAL THRUST

Manual thrusts are made to the upper abdomen or, in selected cases, the chest. The abdominal thrust should not be used for a woman during pregnancy.

The thrusts are given to provide pressure against the diaphragm that compresses the lungs. In turn, the pressure in the lungs is increased, thereby forcing air through the trachea and perhaps forcing out the obstructing object.

A. Patient Standing or Sitting: Conscious

1. From behind, wrap the arms around the waist of the patient. Make a fist.

2. Hold thumb side of the fist on the patient's upper abdomen above the navel and below the xiphoid. Grab the fist with the other hand.

3. Press the fist into the abdomen with quick upward thrusts until the object is dislodged, or the patient may become unconscious.

B. Patient in Supine Position: Unconscious

1. Open the airway.

2. Stand beside and facing the head of the chair when the patient is in the dental chair. On the floor, a more direct thrust can be applied from astride the patient.

3. Hold the heel of one hand over the upper abdomen, with the other hand on top.

4. Apply 6 to 10 quick upward thrusts followed by a finger sweep and 2 ventilations.

5. Repeat abdominal thrusts, finger sweeps, and ventilations.

V. CHEST THRUST

The chest thrust is not used routinely, but is recommended only when it is not possible to use the abdominal thrust, such as during pregnancy and for very obese individuals.

A. Patient Standing or Sitting with Clinician Behind

1. From behind, wrap arms around the chest of the patient at level of armpits.

2. Make a fist. Position the thumb side of the fist on the sternum. The thrust should definitely not be made on the ribs or on the xiphoid because fracture is possible.

3. Grasp the fist with the other hand and apply quick backward thrusts.

B. Patient in Supine Position

1. Open the airway.

2. Position hands on the lower sternum in the same position as for external cardiac compression (page 837 and figure 61–6).

3. Apply quick downward thrusts.

VI. FINGER SWEEP: UNCONSCIOUS

After each series of 6 to 10 abdominal thrusts, an attempt should be made to remove the offending object by examination of the mouth and throat and by using the fingers, gauze, or suction appropriately. Care must be taken not to force the object deeper.

Finger sweeps are not used for children and infants unless the object is visible.

A. Open the Mouth

Lift the tongue and mandible with the thumb and index finger.

B. Index Finger Sweep

1. Slide the index finger along the buccal mucosa and deep into the throat to the base of the tongue.

2. Anticipate contact with an object, move slowly, with care not to push the object farther into the throat.

3. Hook the end of the finger under and around to remove the object.

C. Repeat

1. Repeat abdominal thrusts, mouth examination, and finger sweep until object is expelled.

2. Place resuscitation mask, open airway, give two ventilations.

VII. INFANT
A. Conscious

1. If good air exchange, encourage coughing.

2. If poor air exchange or complete obstruction, proceed with airway obstruction management.

3. Hold the infant face down over the forearm, with the head supported in the hand. Head is lower than the body.

4. Apply four back blows with the heel of the hand, between the infant's shoulder blades.

5. Turn the infant over by placing the free arm over the back and supporting the infant's head with the hand. Place the infant across the thigh with the infant's head lower than its body.

6. Apply four chest thrusts. The point of pressure is the same as for external cardiac compression in the infant (page 838).

7. Repeat back blows and chest thrusts until object is dislodged or infant becomes unconscious.

B. Unconscious

1. Initiate A-B-C of Basic Life Support (page 835).

2. When breathing attempt is not successful, reposition airway and attempt again.
3. **Activate EMS.**
4. Proceed with airway obstruction management as for conscious infant, with four back blows and four chest thrusts.
5. Examine mouth for object; if visible, use a finger sweep to remove it.
6. Give two ventilations.
7. Repeat steps 3 to 5 until object is expelled.
8. Check airway, breathing, and pulse.

OXYGEN ADMINISTRATION

Oxygen is an important agent, useful in most emergencies when respiratory difficulty is apparent. Oxygen is not indicated for chronic obstructive lung diseases, especially emphysema. Oxygen is also not indicated in the presence of hyperventilation because the patient is receiving increased amounts of air and is in need of carbon dioxide.

The use of oxygen depends on the breathing status of the individual. When breathing is weak, shallow, or labored, *supplemental oxygen* is used. When the patient is not breathing, *positive pressure oxygen* delivery is needed.

I. EQUIPMENT
A. Parts
Oxygen resuscitation equipment consists of an oxygen tank, a reducing valve, a flow meter, tubing, mask, and a positive pressure bag. The *E* cylinder, which can provide oxygen for 30 minutes, is the minimum size recommended. Smaller tanks provide too little oxygen for a real emergency, and larger tanks are less portable.

B. Directions
Clear, readable directions should be permanently attached to the tank. Practice is a definite part of team drills.

II. PATIENT BREATHING: USE SUPPLEMENTAL OXYGEN
A. Apply a full-face clear mask; must fit with a good seal.
B. Supplemental oxygen is started at 4 to 6 L per minute.
C. Monitor breathing; if breathing stops, proceed with positive pressure oxygen.

III. PATIENT NOT BREATHING: USE POSITIVE PRESSURE
For persons not trained in the use of the bag-valve-mask delivery, a mouth-to-mask procedure should be used.

A. Apply full-face clear mask; must fit with a tight seal.
B. Adjust oxygen flow so that positive pressure bag remains filled.
C. Compress the bag manually at 5-second intervals to provide 12 respirations per minute for an adult. For a child, use 4-second intervals.
D. Watch chest rise and fall. When the chest does not rise and fall, recheck airway for obstruction. Proceed with airway obstruction management.
E. Obtain medical assistance.

SPECIFIC EMERGENCIES

Certain systemic disease conditions and physical injuries require specific treatment during an emergency. In table 61–3, the *Emergency Reference Chart,* several conditions are listed with their symptoms and treatment procedures. Some of the same conditions have been described in detail in Section VI of this book.

TECHNICAL HINTS

I. PRECAUTIONS DURING MOUTH-TO-MOUTH VENTILATION
Infection may be transmitted or acquired. Dental personnel may gain proficiency in the use of a face mask with one-way delivery to prevent unnecessary contact with ill, debilitated patients or those known or suspected to be carriers of a disease.

II. CARE OF DRUGS
A. Label each with information about shelf life and due date for replacement. Nitroglycerin, for example, must be changed at 6 months.
B. Check weekly to maintain emergency kit in workable order.
C. Dispose of an outdated narcotic drug in the presence of a witness to prevent question that the drug may have been stolen.

III. EYE SAFETY
In addition to eye protection during working hours, professional people should use protective eyewear for activities outside the practice area, such as for sports, hobbies, and other potentially harmful activities.

IV. MEDIC ALERT IDENTIFICATION
Identification for patients with medical problem. A metal emblem is worn as a bracelet or a pendant to provide specific information pertinent to an emergency that may arise. Information about the emblems is available by writing the Medic Alert Foundation International, Turlock, CA 95380. Note patients who wear the identification and record in the patient history.

TABLE 61–3
EMERGENCY REFERENCE CHART

Emergency	Signs/Symptoms	Procedure

All Cases		1. Determine consciousness (shake and shout); yell for help
		2. Place in supine position (unconscious)
		3. Identify major problem
		   A. Airway
		   B. Breathing
		   C. Circulation
		4. Act in accord with findings
		5. Activate EMS

Respiratory Failure	Labored or weak respirations or cessation of breathing
	Cyanosis or ashen-white with blood loss
	Pupils dilated
	Loss of consciousness
		Position: supine (not breathing)
		        upright (breathing)
		Check for and remove foreign material from mouth
		Establish airway
		Rescue
		  Adult: 1 breath every 5 seconds
		  Child (1–8): 1 breath every 3 seconds
		  Infant (younger than 1 year): 1 breath every 3 seconds)
		Monitor vital signs: blood pressure, pulse, respirations
		Administer oxygen by nonrebreather bag

Airway Obstruction	Good air exchange, coughing, wheezing	Sit patient up Loosen tight collar, belt No treatment; let patient cough
Partial	Poor air exchange, noisy breathing, weak, ineffective cough, difficult respirations, gasping Patient is panicky	Reassure patient Treat for complete obstruction (page 839)

Complete	Gasping with great effort; no noises
	Patient clutches throat
	Unable to speak, breathe, cough
	Cyanosis
	Dilated pupils
		Conscious patient
		  Perform Heimlich maneuver
		  Patient becomes unconscious: proceed for unconscious

		Unconscious patient
		  Initiate A-B-C of Basic Life Support
		  Unsuccessful breathing attempts: proceed with airway obstruction management
		  Perform Heimlich maneuver: 6 to 10 thrusts
		  Examine mouth: apply finger sweep
		  Open airway: give 2 ventilations
		  Repeat manual thrusts and finger sweep until object is expelled
		  Try rescue breathing again
		Obtain medical assistance

Hyperventilation Syndrome	Lightheadedness, giddiness Anxiety, confusion Dizziness Overbreathing (25 to 30 respirations per minute) Feelings of suffocation Deep respirations Palpitations (heart pounds) Tingling or numbness in the extremities	Terminate oral procedure Remove rubber dam and objects from mouth Position upright or best for comfortable breathing Loosen tight collar Reassure patient. Explain overbreathing; request that each breath be held to a count of 10 Ask patient to breathe deeply (7 to 10 per minute) into a paper bag adapted closely over nose and mouth. Never use a bag for a patient with diabetes Carbon dioxide is indicated, NOT oxygen

**TABLE 61–3 (continued)
EMERGENCY REFERENCE CHART**

Emergency	Signs/Symptoms	Procedure

Hemorrhage	Prolonged bleeding
	  a. Spurting blood: artery
	  b. Oozing blood: vein
		Compression over bleeding area
		  a. Apply gauze pack with pressure
		  b. Bandage pack into place firmly where
		     possible
		Severe bleeding: digital pressure on pressure
		  point of supplying vessel
		Watch for shock symptoms

	Bleeding from tooth socket	Pack with folded gauze; do not dab Have patient bite down firmly Do not rinse

	Bleeding of an extremity	Elevate the part: support with pillows or
		  substitute
		Apply tourniquet only when limb is amputated,
		  mangled, or crushed

	Nosebleed	Tell patient to breathe through mouth Apply cold application to nose Press nostril on bleeding side for a few minutes Advise patient not to blow the nose for an hour or more

Syncope (fainting)	Pale gray face, anxiety
	Dilated pupils
	Weakness, giddiness, dizziness, faintness,
	  nausea
	Profuse cold perspiration
	Rapid pulse at first, followed by slow pulse
	Shallow breathing
	Drop in blood pressure
	Loss of consciousness
		Position: Trendelenburg
		Loosen tight collar, belt
		Place cold, damp towel on forehead
		Crush ammonia vaporole under patient's nose
		Keep warm (blanket)
		Monitor vital signs: blood pressure, pulse,
		  respirations
		Keep airway open
		Administer oxygen by nasal cannula
		Keep in supine position 10 minutes after recovery
		  to prevent nausea and dizziness
		Reassure patient, especially during recovery

Shock	Skin: pale, moist, clammy Rapid, shallow breathing Low blood pressure Weakness and/or restlessness Nausea, vomiting Thirst, if shock is from bleeding Eventual unconsciousness if untreated	Position: Trendelenburg Keep quiet and warm Monitor vital signs: blood pressure, respirations, pulse Keep airway open Administer oxygen by nonrebreather bag *Summon medical assistance*

Stroke
(cerebrovascular
accident)
(page 717)
	Premonitory
	  Dizziness, vertigo
	  Transient paresthesia or weakness on one
	    side
	  Transient speech defects
	Serious
	  Headache (with cerebral hemorrhage)
	  Breathing labored, deep, slow
	  Chills
	  Paralysis one side of body
	  Nausea, vomiting
	  Convulsions
	  Loss of consciousness (slow or sudden
	    onset)
		Conscious patient
		  Turn patient on paralyzed side; semiupright
		  Loosen clothing about the throat
		  Reassure patient; keep calm, quiet
		  Monitor vital signs: blood pressure, pulse,
		    respirations
		  Administer oxygen by nasal cannula
		  Clear airway; suction vomitus because the
		    throat muscles may be paralyzed
		  Seek medical assistance promptly
		Unconscious patient
		  Position: supine
		  Basic life support
		  Cardiopulmonary resuscitation if indicated

TABLE 61-3 (continued)
EMERGENCY REFERENCE CHART

Emergency	Signs/Symptoms	Procedure
Cardiovascular Diseases	Symptoms vary depending on cause	*For all patients* Be calm and reassure patient Keep patient warm and quiet; restrict effort Always administer oxygen when there is chest pain. *Call for medical assistance*
Angina Pectoris (page 793)	Sudden crushing, paroxysmal pain in substernal area Pain may radiate to shoulder, neck, arms Pallor, faintness Shallow breathing Anxiety, fear	Position: upright, as patient requests, for comfortable breathing Place nitroglycerin sublingually only when the blood pressure is at or above baseline Administer oxygen by nasal cannula Reassure patient Without prompt relief after a second nitroglycerin, treat as a myocardial infarction
Myocardial Infarction (heart attack) (page 794)	Sudden pain similar to angina pectoris, which also may radiate, but of longer duration Pallor; cold, clammy skin Cyanosis Nausea Breathing difficulty Marked weakness Anxiety, fear Possible loss of consciousness	Position: with head up for comfortable breathing Symptoms are not relieved with nitroglycerin Monitor vital signs: blood pressure, pulse, respirations Administer oxygen by nonrebreather bag Alleviate anxiety; reassure *Call for medical assistance for transfer to hospital*
Heart Failure (page 795)	Difficult or labored breathing Pulmonary congestion with cough May cough up blood Rapid, weak pulse Dilated pupils May have chest pain	*Urgent medical assistance needed* Place patient in upright position Make patient comfortable: cover with blanket Administer oxygen by nonrebreather bag Reassure patient
Cardiac Arrest	Skin: ashen gray, cold, clammy No pulse No heart sounds No respirations Eyes fixed, with dilated pupils; no constriction with light Unconscious	Position: supine Basic life support Check oral cavity for debris or vomitus; leave dentures in place for a seal Begin cardiopulmonary resuscitation: minutes count
Adrenal Crisis (cortisol deficiency)	Anxious, stressed Mental confusion Pain in abdomen, back, legs Muscle weakness Extreme fatigue Nausea, vomiting Lowered blood pressure Elevated pulse Loss of consciousness Coma	*Conscious patient* Terminate oral procedure Call for help and emergency kit Place patient in supine position with legs slightly raised Request telephone call for medical assistance Administer oxygen by nonrebreather bag Monitor blood pressure and pulse *Unconscious patient* Place patient in supine position with legs slightly raised Basic life support Try ammonia vaporole when cause is undecided Administer oxygen *Summon medical assistance* Transport to hospital

TABLE 61–3 (continued)
EMERGENCY REFERENCE CHART

Emergency	Signs/Symptoms	Procedure

Insulin Reaction (hyperinsulinism) (hypoglycemia)	Sudden onset
	Skin: moist, cold, pale
	Confused, nervous, anxious
	Bounding pulse
	Salivation
	Normal to shallow respirations
	Convulsions (late)
		Conscious patient
		  Administer oral sugar (cubes, orange juice, candy or frosting)
		  Observe patient for 1 hour before dismissal
		  Determine time since previous meal, and arrange next appointment following food intake
		Unconscious patient
		  Basic life support
		    Position: supine
		    Maintain airway
		    Administer oxygen by nonrebreather bag
		    Monitor vital signs
		  Summon medical assistance
		  Administer intravenous glucose

Diabetic Coma (ketoacidosis) (hyperglycemia)	Slow onset
	Skin: flushed and dry
	Breath: fruity odor
	Dry mouth, thirst
	Low blood pressure
	Weak, rapid pulse
	Exaggerated respirations
	Coma
		Conscious patient
		  Terminate oral procedure
		  Obtain medical care; hospitalization indicated
		  Keep patient warm
		  Administer oxygen by nasal cannula
		Unconscious patient
		  Basic life support
		  Urgent medical assistance needed

Allergic Reaction
1. Delayed[9]
	Skin
	  Erythema (rash)
	  Urticaria (wheals, itching)
	  Angioedema (localized swelling of mucous membranes, lips, larynx, pharynx)
	Respiration
	  Distress, dyspnea
	  Wheezing
	  Extension of angioedema to larynx: may have obstruction from swelling of vocal apparatus
		Skin
		  Administer antihistamine
		Respiration
		  Position: upright
		  Administer oxygen by nasal cannula
		  Epinephrine
		Airway obstruction
		  Position: supine
		  Airway maintenance
		  Epinephrine
		Summon medical assistance

2. Immediate Anaphylaxis (anaphylactic shock)	Skin
	  Urticaria (wheals, itching)
	  Flushing
	Nausea, abdominal cramps, vomiting, diarrhea
	Angioedema
	  Swelling of lips, membranes, eyelids
	  Laryngeal edema with difficult swallowing
	Respiration distress
	  Cough, wheezing
	  Dyspnea
	  Airway obstruction
	  Cyanosis
	Cardiovascular collapse
	  Profound drop in blood pressure
	  Rapid, weak pulse
	  Palpitations
	Dilation of pupils
	Loss of consciousness (sudden)
	  Cardiac arrest
		Rapid treatment needed (epinephrine)
		Position: supine (except when dyspnea predominates)
		Administer oxygen by nonrebreather bag
		Basic life support
		Monitor vital signs
		Cardiopulmonary resuscitation
		Summon medical assistance; transfer to hospital

TABLE 61–3 (continued)
EMERGENCY REFERENCE CHART

Emergency	Signs/Symptoms	Procedure
Local Anesthesia Reactions 1. Psychogenic	Reaction to injection, not the anesthetic Syncope Hyperventilation syndrome	See earlier in this table Page 843 (syncope) Page 842 (hyperventilation)
2. Allergic (very rare)	Anaphylactic shock Allergic skin and mucous membrane reactions Allergic bronchial asthma attack	See earlier in this table (page 845)

3. Toxic Overdose	Effects of intravascular injection rather than increased quantity of drug are more common
	a. Stimulation phase
	  Anxious, restless, apprehensive, confused
	  Rapid pulse and respirations
	  Elevated blood pressure
	  Tremors
	  Convulsions
	
	b. Depressive phase
	  Follows stimulation phase
	  Drowsiness, lethargy
	  Shock-like symptoms: pallor, sweating
	  Rapid, weak pulse and respirations
	  Drop in blood pressure
	  Respiratory depression or respiratory arrest
	  Unconsciousness
		Mild reaction
		  Stop injection
		  Position: supine
		  Loosen tight clothing
		  Reassure patient
		  Monitor blood pressure, heart rate, respirations
		  Administer oxygen by nasal cannula
		  Summon medical assistance
		Severe reaction
		  Basic life support: maintain airway
		  Administer oxygen by nonrebreather bag
		  Continue to monitor vital signs
		  Cardiopulmonary resuscitation
		  Administration of anticonvulsant

Epileptic Seizure 1. Generalized tonic-clonic (page 743)	Anxiety or depression Pale, may become cyanotic Muscular contractions Loss of consciousness	Position: supine. Do not attempt to move from dental chair Make safe by placing movable equipment out of reach Do not force anything between the teeth; a soft towel or large sponges may be placed while mouth is open Open airway; monitor vital signs Administer oxygen by nasal cannula Allow patient to sleep during postconvulsive stage Do not dismiss the patient if unaccompanied
2. Generalized absence (page 743)	Brief loss of consciousness Fixed posture Rhythmic twitching of eyelids, eyebrows, or head May be pale	Take objects from patient's hands to prevent their being dropped

Burns[10]
1. First degree
2. Second degree (partial thickness)
	Skin reddened
	Swelling
	Pain
	Skin reddened, blisters
	Swelling
	Wet surface
	Pain (more than third degree)
	Heightened sensitivity to touch
		First- and Second-degree Burns
		  Do not give food or liquids; anticipate nausea
		  Be alert for signs of shock
		  Do not apply ointment, grease, or bicarbonate of soda
		  Immerse in cool water to relieve pain; do not apply ice
		  Gently clean with a mild antiseptic
		  Dress lightly with bandage
		  Elevate burned part
		  Obtain medical assistance

TABLE 61–3 (continued)
EMERGENCY REFERENCE CHART

Emergency	Signs/Symptoms	Procedure
Burns, continued 3. Third degree (full thickness)	Leathery look Insensitive to touch	Request medical assistance and transport system Treat for shock Basic life support: maintain airway Check for other injuries Wrap in clean sheet; transport
4. Chemical burn	Reddened, discolored	Immediate, copious irrigation with water for ½ hour Check directions on container from which the chemical came for antidote or other advice Burn caused by an acid may be rinsed with bicarbonate of soda, burn caused by alkali may be rinsed in weak acid such as acetic (vinegar) *Medical assistance needed*

Internal Poisoning[11]	Signs of corrosive burn around or in oral cavity
	Evidence of empty container or information from patient
	Nausea, vomiting, cramps
		Be calm and supportive
		Basic life support: airway maintenance
		Artificial ventilation (inhaled poison)
		Record vital signs
		Call Poison Control Center
		Conscious patient
		    Dilute poison in the stomach with 1 or 2 glasses of water or milk.
		    Induce vomiting by giving 1 tablespoon of syrup of ipecac followed by 1 to 2 glasses of water.
		    Do not induce vomiting if caustic, corrosive, or petroleum products have been ingested
		Avoid nonspecific and questionably effective antidotes, stimulants, sedatives, or other agents, which may do more harm
		Obtain medical assistance

Foreign Body in Eye	Tears Blinking	Wash hands Ask patient to look down Bring upper lid down over lower lid for a moment; move it upward Turn down lower lid and examine: if particle is visible, remove with moistened cotton applicator Use eye cup: wash out eye with plain water When unsuccessful, seek medical attention: prevent patient from rubbing eye by placing gauze pack over eye and stabilizing with adhesive tape
Chemical Solution in Eye	Tears Stinging	Irrigate promptly with copious amounts of water. Turn head so water flows away from inner aspect of the eye. Continue for 15 to 20 minutes
Dislocated Jaw	Mouth is open: patient is unable to close	Stand in front of seated patient Wrap thumbs in towels and place on occlusal surfaces of mandibular posterior teeth Curve fingers and place under body of the mandible Press down and back with thumbs, and at same time pull up and forward with fingers (figure 61–7) As joint slips into place, quickly move thumbs outward Place bandage around head to support jaw

TABLE 61–3 (continued)
EMERGENCY REFERENCE CHART

Emergency	Signs/Symptoms	Procedure
Facial Fracture	Pain, swelling Ecchymoses Deformity, limitation of movement Crepitation on manipulation Zygoma fracture: depression of cheek Mandibular fracture: abnormal occlusion	Place patient on side Basic life support Support with bandage around face, under chin, and tied on the top of the head (Barton) *Seek prompt transport to emergency care facility*
Tooth Forcibly Displaced (avulsed tooth)	Swelling, bruises, or other signs of trauma, depending on the type of accident	Instruct patient or parent to rinse tooth gently in cool water and place in water or wrap in wet cloth Bring to the dental office or clinic *immediately* The longer the time lapse between avulsion and replantation, the poorer the prognosis

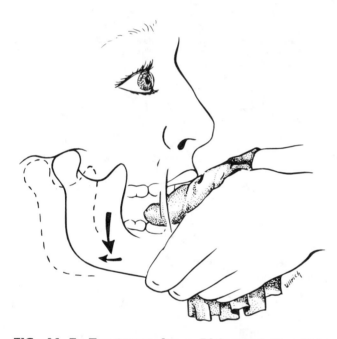

FIG. 61–7. Treatment for a Dislocated Mandible.
With thumbs wrapped in toweling and placed on the buccal cusps of the mandibular teeth, the fingers are curved under the body of the mandible. The jaw is pressed down and back with the thumbs while pulling up and forward with the fingers to permit the condyle to pass over the articular eminence into its normal position in the glenoid fossa. As the jaw slips into place, the thumbs must be moved quickly aside.

REFERENCES

1. **Malamed,** S.F.: *Handbook of Medical Emergencies in the Dental Office,* 4th ed. St. Louis, Mosby, 1993, pp. 44–45.
2. **Cooley,** R.L., Cottingham, A.J., Abrams, H., and Barkmeier, W.W.: Ocular Injuries Sustained in the Dental Office: Methods of Detection, Treatment, and Prevention, *J. Am. Dent. Assoc., 97,* 985, December, 1978.
3. **Roberts-Harry,** T.J., Cass, A.E., and Jagger, J.D.: Ocular Injury and Infection in Dental Practice. A Survey and a Review of the Literature, *Br. Dent. J., 170,* 20, January 5, 1991.
4. **Wesson,** M.D. and Thornton, J.B.: Eye Protection and Ocular Complications in the Dental Office, *Gen. Dent., 37,* 19, January–February, 1989.
5. **Malamed:** op. cit., pp. 50–89.
6. **Biron,** C.R.: Emergency Drugs, *RDH, 13,* 48, July, 1993.
7. **Robbins,** K.S.: Medicolegal Considerations, in Malamed, S.F.: *Handbook of Medical Emergencies in the Dental Office,* 4th ed. St. Louis, Mosby, 1993, pp. 91–101.
8. **American Heart Association:** Guidelines for Cardiopulmonary Resuscitation and Emergency Cardiac Care. Recommendations of the 1992 National Conference, *JAMA, 268,* 2171–2302, October 28, 1992.
9. **Malamed:** op. cit., pp. 347–374.
10. **Clark,** W.R.: Burns, in Rakel, R.E., ed.: *Conn's Current Therapy.* Philadelphia, W.B. Saunders Co., 1993, pp. 1131–1136.
11. **Mofenson,** H.C., Caraccio, T.R., and Greensher, J.: Acute Poisonings, in Rakel, R.E., ed.: *Conn's Current Therapy.* Philadelphia, W.B. Saunders Co., 1993, pp. 1148–1192.

SUGGESTED READINGS

Becker, D.E.: Management of Respiratory Complications in Clinical Dental Practice. Pathophysiological and Technical Considerations, *Anesth. Prog., 37,* 169, July, 1990.

Bhat, M. and Li, S.-H.: Consumer Product-related Tooth Injuries Treated in Hospital Emergency Rooms: United States 1979–87, *Community Dent. Oral Epidemiol., 18,* 133, June, 1990.

Biron, C.R.: Are You Prepared? *RDH, 12,* 10, January, 1992.

Boudoulas, H., Leier, C.V., and Overstreet, J.W.: Syncope in Dental Practice, *Compendium, 10,* 76, February, 1989.

Chandra, N.C.: Mechanisms of Blood Flow During CPR, *Ann. Emerg. Med., 22,* 281, February, 1993.

Deitch, E.A.: The Management of Burns, *N. Engl. J. Med., 323,* 1249, November 1, 1990.

Fagiano, G., Orecchia, C., De Siena, L., and Pandolfi, P.: Prevention and Treatment of Emergencies in Dental Offices, *Anesth. Prog.,* *36,* 221, July–October, 1989.

Hodges, E.D., Durham, T.M., and Stanley, R.T.: Management of Aspiration and Swallowing Incidents: A Review of the Literature and Report of Case, *ASDC J. Dent. Child., 59,* 413, November–December, 1992.

Kawashima, Z. and Pineda, F.R.: Replanting Avulsed Primary Teeth, *J. Am. Dent. Assoc., 123,* 90, October, 1992.

Niemann, J.T.: Cardiopulmonary Resuscitation, *N. Engl. J. Med., 327,* 1075, October 8, 1992.

Pacak-Carroll, D.: Remember, Eye Protection Is Necessary for Patients Too, *RDH, 12,* 14, June, 1992.

Porter, K., Porter, S., Scully, C., and Theyer, Y.: Injuries to Dental Patients and Visitors, *J. Dent., 19,* 127, April, 1991.

Rogers, S.N. and Vale, J.A.: Oral Manifestations of Poisoning, *Br. Dent. J., 174,* 141, February 20, 1993.

Sommers, M.S.: The Shattering Consequences of C.P.R. How to Assess and Prevent Complications, *Nursing 92, 22,* 34, July, 1992.

Swift, J.Q.: How to Handle Office Emergencies. Training Is the Most Important Element, *Dent. Teamwork, 4,* 30, May–June, 1991.

Turcotte, J.A. and Weinberg, A.D.: When Seconds Count, *RDH, 10,* 15, November, 1990.

Willens, J.S.: Strengthen Your Life-support Skills, *Nursing 93, 23,* 54, April, 1993.

Wright, S.: The Pathophysiology of Cardiorespiratory Arrest and Principles of Post-resuscitation Intensive Care, *Br. Dent. J., 173,* 13, July 11, 1992.

proprio- one's own, e.g. *proprio*ceptive
proto- first, e.g. *proto*plasm
pseudo- false, deceptive, e.g. *pseudo*membrane
psycho-, psych- mind, mental processes, e.g. *psycho*somatic
pulmo- lung, e.g. *pulmo*nary
pur- pus, e.g. *pur*ulent
pyo- pus, e.g. *pyo*rrhea
pyro- fever, heat, e.g. *pyro*genic

re- back, again, e.g. *re*gurgitate
-renal kidney, e.g. ad*renal*
retro- back, backward, behind, e.g. *retro*molar
-rhage breaking, bursting forth, profuse flow, e.g. hemor*rhage*
-rhea, (-rhoea) flow, discharge, e.g. pyor*rhea*
rhino-, rhin- nose, e.g. *rhin*itis
rube- red, e.g. *rube*facient

sarco- flesh, muscle, e.g. *sarco*ma
sclero hard, e.g. *sclero*derma
-scopy examination, inspection, e.g. micro*scopy*
semi- half, partly, e.g. *semi*permeable
sero- serum, serous, e.g. *sero*purulent
sial-, sialo- saliva, e.g. *sialo*graphy

somat-, somato-, -some body, e.g. chromo*some*
-squam- scale, e.g. de*squam*ative
stomat- mouth, e.g. *stomat*itis
sub- beneath, under, deficient, e.g. *sub*acute
super- above, upon, excessive, e.g. *super*numerary tooth
syn- with, together, e.g. *syn*drome

tachy- swift, e.g. *tachy*cardia
tact- touch, e.g. *tact*ile
tera-, terato- monster, malformed fetus, e.g. *terato*genic
thermo- heat, e.g. *thermo*phile
thrombo-, thromb- clot, coagulation, e.g. *thromb*in
-thym-, thymo- mind, soul, emotions, e.g. dys*thym*ia
trans- beyond, through, across, e.g. *trans*plantation
tropho-, trophic nutrition, nourishment, e.g., hyper*trophic*
-tropic turning toward, changing, e.g. hydro*tropic*

-ule diminutive, small, e.g. tub*ule*
-uria urine, e.g. glucos*uria*

vaso- blood vessels, e.g. *vaso*dilation
vita- life, e.g. *vita*min

xero- dry, e.g. *xero*stomia

Glossary

INTRODUCTION

Each chapter has included a table of "KEY WORDS" with their definitions. By having the definitions readily available at the lead of a chapter, it is expected that study and learning can be facilitated.

This *Glossary* includes additional words of a general nature. All words that have been defined in this book can be located through the *Index* starting on page 867.

The meaning of words from the basic medical and dental sciences frequently can be determined from the list of word prefixes, suffixes, and combining forms on the previous pages. A medical dictionary is an important adjunct to guide professional reading.

A

Absorption (ab-sorp'shun). taking up of fluids or other substances by the skin or mucous surfaces; passage of substances to the blood, lymph, and cells from the alimentary canal after digestion.

Accessory (ak ses'ō rē). subordinate, attached, or added for convenience.

Acid (as'id). a chemical substance that undergoes dissociation with the formation of hydrogen ions in aqueous solution; pH less than 7.0

Acne vulgaris (ak'nē vul-ga'ris). a chronic inflammatory disease of the sebaceous glands that appears on the face, back, and chest in the form of eruptions.

Acquired characteristics: those obtained after birth, as a result of environment.

Acuity (ă-ku'ĭ tē). sharpness or clearness, especially of the special senses.

Acute (ă kūt'). having rapid onset, short, severe course, and pronounced symptoms; opposite of chronic.

Adenopathy (ad ĕ-nop'ah-thē). swelling or enlargement of lymph nodes.

Adsorption (ad-sorp'shun). the attachment of one substance to the surface or another substance.

Agar (ah'gar). gelatin extracted from seaweed, used as a nutrient solidifying agent in bacteriologic culture media; constituent of a reversible hydrocolloid impression material.

Agglutination (ă-glu'tĭ-nă'shun). state of being united; adhesion of parts; clumping, as of bacteria or other cells.

Alkali (al'kah-lī). a strong water-soluble base; see **Base.**

Allergen (al'er-jen). an antigenic substance that produces hypersensitivity; may be inhaled, ingested, or injected or may produce a reaction upon contact with the skin.

Allergy (al'er jē). a hypersensitive state gained from exposure to a specific substance or allergen, re-exposure to which causes a heightened capacity to react.

Alloplast (al'lo-plast). a graft of an inert metal or plastic material.

Alloy (al'loi). a substance composed of a mixture of two or more metals.

Alopecia (al'ō-pē'shĭ-ah). loss of hair.

Amelia (ah-mēl'ē ah). congenital absence of a limb or limbs.

Ameloblast (ah-mel'-ō-blast). epithelial cell of the enamel organ; functions in the formation of enamel.

Amylase (am'ĭ laze). an enzyme that converts starch into sugar.

Anaphylaxis (an-ah-fĭ lak'sis). an acute, severe, allergic reaction characterized by sudden collapse, shock, or respiratory and circulatory failure following the injection of an allergen; increased susceptibility to an allergen resulting from previous exposure to it.

Anhydrous (an-hī'drus). containing no water.

Anlage (ahn'lah-gheh). earliest primary stage in the development of an organ.

Anodyne (an'ō-dīne). any agent that neutralizes or relieves pain.

Anomaly (ă nom'ă-lē). deviation from the normal.

Anoxia (an-ok'sĭ-ah). oxygen deficiency; a condition in which the cells of the body do not have or cannot utilize sufficient oxygen to perform normal functions.

Antidote (an tĭ-dōte). a medicine or other remedy for counteracting the effects of a poison.

Aphthous ulcer (af'thus ul'ser). aphthous stomatitis; canker sore, vesicle that ruptures after 1 or 2 days and forms a depressed, spherical, painful ulcer with elevated rim.

Aqueous (a'kwē-us). water; prepared with water.

Armamentarium (ar'mah-men-ta'rē-um). the equipment, such as books, materials, and instruments essential to professional practice.

Dental hygiene armamentarium: all the instruments and equipment used during a dental hygiene procedure.

Dental hygiene instrumentarium: set of instruments used for a particular clinical procedure by the dental hygienist.

Arthroplasty (ar'thrō-plas' tē). plastic repair of a joint.
    Total hip arthroplasty: replacement of the femoral head and acetabulum with a prosthesis that is cemented to the bone.
    Acetabulum (as'ĕ-tab' u-lum): the cup-shaped cavity on the lateral surface of the hip bone that receives the head of the femur.

Articulation (ar-tik'ū-la'shun). the place where two or more bones of the skeleton join or unite; bony joint that may or may not be movable.

Artifact (ar'tĭ fact). caused by the technique used, not a natural occurrence; in radiography, a structure, blemish, or an unintended radiographic image that may result from the faulty manufacture, manipulation, exposure, or processing of an x-ray film.

Ascites (ă-sī'tēz). accumulation of fluid in the abdominal cavity.

Aspirator (as pĭ-ra'tor). an apparatus employing suction.

Atom (at'om). the small particle of an element that is composed of protons, neutrons, and electrons.

Attrition (ă trish'un). gradual wearing away of tooth structure, resulting from mastication.

Autograft (aw'tō-graft). a graft in which the tissue is obtained from the same individual.

Autoimmune disease (aw'tō-ĭm-mūn'). disease caused by immunologic action of an individual's own cells or antibodies on components of the body.

Autonomic (aw tō-nom'ik). a division of the nervous system that supplies the sensory innervation for the smooth muscles, heart, and glands. It is divided into the parasympathetic (craniosacral) and the sympathetic (thoracolumbar) systems.

Auxiliary (awk-sil'ē-ar-ē). giving support; helping; aiding; assisting.

B

Bacterial spore. a resistant form of bacteria encapsulated by a thick cell wall that enables the cell to survive in environments unfavorable to immediate growth and division; not a reproductive mechanism.

Bactericide (bak'ter i sīd). capable of destroying bacteria.

Bacteriostatic (bak ter i-o-stat'ik). capable of inhibiting the growth and multiplication of bacteria.

Barodontalgia (aerodontalgia) (bar ō don tal'jĭ ah). the sudden acute pain response in a tooth under reduced atmospheric pressure, notably during high-altitude flying.

Base (bās). a chemical substance that in solution yields hydroxyl ions and reacts with an acid to form a salt and water. A base turns red litmus paper blue and has a pH higher than 7.0.

Bevel (bev'el). the inclination a line or surface makes with another when they are not at right angles.

Bifid (bī'fid). cleft into two parts or branches.

Biocompatible (bi'ō-kom-pat'ĭ b'l). harmonious with life; no toxic or injurious effects on biologic function.

Bruxism (bruk'sizm). a neurogenically related habit of grinding, clenching, or clamping the teeth. Damage to the teeth and attachment apparatus can result.

Buffer (bŭf'er). any substance in a fluid that tends to lessen the change in hydrogen ion concentration (reaction) that otherwise would be produced by adding acids or alkalis.

C

Cachexia (kă kek'sĭ-ah). lack of nutrition; wasting; may occur in the course of chronic disease.

Calcification (kal sĭ-fĭ-ka'shun). the process by which organic tissue becomes hardened by a deposit of calcium and other inorganic salts within its substance.

Cancer (kan'ser). malignant and invasive neoplasm; see **Neoplasm: Precancerous lesion.**

Canker sore: see **Aphthous ulcer.**

Capnophilic (kap-nō-fil'ik). growing best in the presence of carbon dioxide; usually used in reference to bacteria.

Carbohydrate (kar bō-hi'drāte). organic compound of carbon, hydrogen, and oxygen: includes starches, sugars, cellulose; formed by plants and used for growth and source of energy.

Caries: see **Dental caries.**

Carious (kā'rē-us). affected with caries or decay; in dentistry, a carious lesion is a cavity in a tooth that is the result of dental caries.

Cartilage (kar'tĭ lij). firm, elastic, flexible connective tissue that is attached to articular bone surfaces and that forms certain parts of the skeleton.

Caustic (kaws'tik). an agent that burns or corrodes; destroys living tissue; having a burning taste.

Cauterize (kaw'ter īze). to burn, corrode, or destroy living tissue by means of a caustic substance, heated metal, or an electric current.

Cementicle (cē men'ti-k'l). small globular mass of cementum (diameter 0.2 to 0.3 mm); may lie free within the periodontal ligament or be attached to the cementum of the root surface.

Cephalometry (sef ah-lom'ĕ trē). measurement of the bony structure of the head using reproducible lateral and anteroposterior radiographs.

Cheilosis (kē lō'sis). a condition marked by fissuring and dry scaling of the surface of the lips and angles of the mouth; characteristic of riboflavin deficiency.

Chemotaxis (kē mō tak'sis). attraction of living protoplasm to chemical stimuli; for example, movement of neutrophils to an area of inflammation; a host defense mechanism.

Chorea (kō-rē'ah). a nervous disorder characterized by irregular and involuntary action of the muscles of the extremities and the face.

Chronic (kron'ik). characterized by a long, slow course; opposite of acute.

Cicatrix (sik'ah-triks). a scar; fibrous tissue left after the healing of a wound.

Clean (klēn). freedom from or removal of all matter in which microorganisms may find favorable conditions for continued life and growth.

Cleidocranial dysostosis (klī'dō krā'nĭ-al dĭs-os-tō'sis). developmental defect characterized by absence of development of clavicles and abnormal shape of skull.

Coagulation (kō-ag-ū-lā'shun). changing of a soluble into an insoluble protein; process of changing into a clot.

Coaptation (kō-ap-tā'shun). proper adaptation or union of parts to each other, such as the ends of a fractured bone or the edges of a wound without overlap.

Commissure (kom'ĭ-shur). angle or corner of eye or lips.

Communicable (ko-mu'nĭ-kah b'l). capable of being transmitted from one person to another.

Contagious (kon-tā'jus). communicable; transmissible by contact with an infected or sick person.

Contracture (kon-trak'chūr). shortening or distortion; permanent, as from shrinkage of muscles, or temporary, from sudden stimulus.

Corticosteroid (kor'tĭ-kō-ste'roid). hormone produced by the adrenal cortex and synthetic equivalent; various steroids have different physiologic effects.

Glucocorticoid: used in treatment of a variety of conditions, including inflammations, allergies, collagen diseases, and certain neoplasms.

Cryosurgery (krī ō-ser'jerē). surgery performed with the use of extremely low temperature.

Cryotherapy (krī ō-ther'ah pē). therapeutic application of cold.

Cryptogenic (krip tō-jen'ik). of obscure, doubtful, or undeterminable origin.

Current (kur'rent). the number of electrons per second passing a given point on a conductor. Electrons are negatively charged and move toward the positive.

Cuticle, primary (kū'tĭ k'l). a delicate membrane covering the crown of a newly erupted tooth; produced by the ameloblasts after they produce the enamel rods. Also called Nasmyth's membrane.

Cyst (sĭst). a sac, normal or pathologic, containing fluid or other material.

Dentigerous cyst: formed by a dental follicle, containing one or more well-formed teeth.

Radicular cyst: an epithelial-lined sac, formed at the apex of a pulpless tooth, containing cystic fluid.

Cystic fibrosis (sis'tik fī-brō'sis). a generalized hereditary disorder of young children primarily; characterized by signs of chronic pulmonary disease (as a result of excess mucus production in the respiratory tract) and pancreatic deficiency.

D

Defense mechanism. in psychiatry, an unconscious mental process or coping mechanism that lessens the anxiety associated with a situation or internal conflict and protects the person from mental discomfort.

Deglutition (deg'loo tish'un). the act of swallowing.

Dehiscence (dē-his'ens). isolated area in which a root is denuded of bone when the denuded area extends to the margin of the bone. Compare with **Fenestration.**

Dehydration (dē hī dra'shun). removal of water; the condition that results from undue loss of water.

Dental caries (den'tal kar'ēz). a disease of the calcified structures of the teeth, characterized by decalcification of the mineral components and dissolution of the organic matrix.

Dental prosthetic laboratory procedures: the steps in the fabrication of a dental prosthesis that do not require the presence of a patient for their accomplishment.

Dental public health: see under **Public health.**

Denticle (den'tĭ k'l). a pulp stone; relatively large body of calcified substance in the pulp chamber of a tooth.

Denudation (den'ū dā shun). laying bare; surgical or pathologic removal of epithelial covering.

Desensitization (dē-sen'sĭ tĭ zā'shun). process of removing reactivity or sensitivity.

Detritus (dē trī'tus). debris that adheres to tooth, gingival, and mucosal surfaces.

Diagnosis (dī-ag-nō'sis). a scientific evaluation of existing conditions; the process of determining by examination the nature and circumstances of a diseased condition; the decision reached as to the nature of a disease.

Differential diagnosis: the art of distinguishing one disease from another.

Digital (dij'ĭ-tal). of, pertaining to, or performed with a finger.

Dislocation: see **Luxation.**

Distilled water: water that has been subjected to a process of vaporization and subsequent condensation for purification.

DNA (Deoxyribonucleic Acid) (dē ok'sĭ-rī-bō nu-kle'ik as'id). occurs in nuclei (chromosomes) of all animal and vegetable cells; repository of hereditary characteristics.

Donor site (dō'nor sīt). area from which tissue is obtained during surgical procedures such as for a graft.

Dorsum (dor'sum). the back surface or a part similar to the back in position; opposite of ventral surface.

Duct (dukt). a passage with well-defined walls; especially a tube for the passage of excretions or secretions.

Dysarthria (dis-ar'thrĭ-ah). disturbances of articulation as a result of emotional stress or paralysis, incoordination, or spasticity of the muscles used for speaking.

Dyslexia (dis-lek'sē-ah). inability or difficulty in reading, including word blindness and a tendency to reverse letters and words in reading and writing.

Dysmorphism (dis-mor'fizm). abnormality of shape.

Dysplasia (dis-plā'zĭ-ah). abnormal development or growth; an alteration in adult cells characterized by variations in their size, shape, and organization.

Dystrophy (dis'trō-fē). degeneration associated with atrophy and dysfunction.

E

Ecology (ē-kol'ō ji). the science that deals with the study of the environment and the life history of organisms.

Ectopic (ek-top'ik). out of place. An **ectopic pregnancy** is one that occurs elsewhere than in the cavity of the uterus.

Edema (ĕ-dē'mah). collection of abnormally large amounts of fluid in the intercellular spaces, causing swelling.

Pitting edema: pressure on edematous area causes pits, which remain for prolonged period after pressure is released.

Edentulous (e-den'tu-lus). without teeth.

Emaciation (ē-mē sē-ā'shun). condition of excessive leanness or wasted body tissues.

Emesis basin (em'ĕ-sis). a basin, usually kidney shaped, used for receiving material expectorated or vomited.

Emollient (e-mōl'yent). softening or soothing; an agent used to soften the skin or other body surface.

Endemic (en dem'ik). present in a community or among a group of people; the continuing prevalence of a disease as distinguished from an epidemic.

Endodontics (en'dō-don'tiks). that branch of dentistry concerned with the etiology, diagnosis, and treatment of diseases of the dental pulp and their sequelae.

Endometrium (en dō-mē'trĭ-um). the mucous membrane lining the uterus.

Enzyme (en'zīm). an organic compound, frequently protein in nature, that can accelerate or produce by catalytic action some change in a specific substance.

Ephebodontics (e-fē bō don'tiks). dentistry for the individual undergoing the transition from childhood to adulthood; that is, the period of life known as adolescence.

Epidemic (ep'ĭ-dem'ik). the occurrence in a community or region of a group of illnesses of similar nature, clearly in excess of normal expectancy and derived from a common source.

Epithelialization (ep ĭ thē lē al ĭ zā'shun). growth of epithelium over a denuded surface.

Eruption (ē rup'shun). the act of breaking out, appearing, or becoming visible; a visible pathologic lesion of the skin, marked by redness, swelling, or both.

> **Tooth eruption:** the combination of movements of a tooth both before and after the emergence of its crown into the oral cavity, which serves to bring the tooth and maintain it in occlusion with the tooth or teeth of the opposing arch.

Erythrocyte (ē rith'rō sīte). red blood cell; specialized cell for the transportation of oxygen.

Erythroplakia (ē-rith rō pla'kē ah). lesions of the oral mucosa that appear as bright red patches or plaques that cannot be characterized clinically or pathologically as any other disease.

Erythropoiesis (ē-rith rō-poy ē'sis). formation of red blood cells.

Escharotic (es kǎ rot'ik). corrosive; capable of producing sloughing.

Etiology (ē ti ol'o-jē). the science or study of the cause of disease; that which is known about the causes of a disease.

Exfoliate (eks fō'lē āte). to fall off in scales or layers; in dentistry, to shed primary teeth.

Extirpation (eks-tir-pā'shun). complete removal or eradication of a part; in dentistry, the removal of the dental pulp from the pulp chamber and root canal.

F

Febrile (fe'bril). pertaining to fever; feverish.

Fenestration (fen es-trā'shun). isolated area in which a root is denuded of bone when the marginal bone is intact. Compare with **Dehiscence.**

Fermentable (fer men'ta b'l). term applied to a substance that is capable of undergoing chemical change as a result of the influence of an enzyme; usually applied to substances that break down to an acid or an alcohol; applied to carbohydrate breakdown to form acid in bacterial plaque.

Fetus (fē'tus). the unborn offspring in the uterus, after the second month.

Fistula (fis'tū-lah). commonly used term for a narrow passage or duct leading from one cavity to another, as from a periapical abscess to the oral cavity; see **Sinus tract.**

Flora (flō'rah). the entire plant life of a geographic area; used to indicate the microorganisms that live together in a specific location.

> **Oral flora:** the microorganisms that inhabit the oral cavity of an individual, that are usually saprophytic, and that live together in a symbiotic relationship.

Focal infection: infection caused by bacteria or toxins carried in the blood from a distant lesion or focus.

Follicle (dental) (fol'ĭ k'l). the sac that encloses the developing tooth before its eruption.

Forensic dentistry (fo rĕn'sik). the aspect of dental science that relates and applies dental facts to legal problems; encompasses dental identification, malpractice litigation, legislation, peer review, and dental licensure.

Frenectomy (fre-nek'tō-me). complete removal of a frenum.

Frenotomy (fre-not'ō-me). partial removal of a frenum.

Frenum, pl. frena (fre'num) (fre'na). a narrow fold of mucous membrane passing from a more fixed to a movable part, as from the gingiva to the lip, cheek, or undersurface of the tongue, serving in a measure to check undue movement of the part.

Friable (frī'a b'l). easily broken or crumbled.

G

Germicide (jer'mĭ sīd). anything that destroys bacteria; applied especially to chemical agents that kill disease germs but not necessarily bacterial spores; applied to both living tissue and inanimate objects.

Gerodontics (jer ō-don'tiks). that branch of dentistry which treats all problems peculiar to the oral cavity in old age and the aging population. Also called geriatric dentistry.

Gestation (jes-tā'shun). pregnancy.

Gingivectomy (jin'jĭ vek'tō-mē). The surgical removal of diseased gingiva to eliminate periodontal pockets.

Gingivoplasty (jin'jĭ-vō-plas'tē). the surgical contouring of the gingival tissue to produce the physiologic architectural form necessary for the maintenance of tissue health and integrity.

Gnathodynamometer (nath'ō-dī nah-mom'ĕ ter). an instrument for measuring the force exerted in closing the jaws.

Graft (grǎft). tissues transferred from one site to replace damaged structures in another site.

> **Free graft:** tissue for grafting is completely removed from its donor site.

> **Pedicle graft:** the graft remains attached to its donor site. See also **Autograft; Heterograft; Homograft.**

H

Habilitation (hǎ-bilĭ-tā'shun). application of measures that will assist a person in obtaining a state of health, efficiency, and independent action.

Halitosis (hal-ĭ tō'sis). offensive or bad breath, may be related to systemic disease or uncleanliness of the oral cavity.

Health (helth). state of complete physical, mental, and social well-being, not merely the absence of disease.

Hemangioma (hē-man′jĭ-ō mah). a benign tumor composed of newly formed capillaries filled with blood.

Hemorrhage (hem′ŏ rij). bleeding; an escape of blood from the blood vessels.

Hemostat (hē′mo-stăt). an instrument or other agent used to arrest the escape or flow of blood.

Heterograft (het′er-ō-graft). a heterologous graft in which the tissue is obtained from another species.

Homograft (hŏ′mō-graft). a homologous graft in which the tissue is obtained from a different individual of the same species.

Hydrophilic (hī drō-fil′ik). having a strong affinity for water; as opposed to hydrophobic, repelling water.

Hygiene (hī′jēn). the science that deals with the preservation of health.

Hygroscopic (hī grō-sco′pik). capable of readily absorbing and retaining moisture.

Hyperkeratosis (hī′per-kĕr ŭ tō′sis). abnormal increase in the thickness of the keratin layer (stratum corneum) of the epithelium. **Benign hyperkeratosis** is one of the most common white lesions of the oral mucous membrane.

Hyperkinesis (hī per-kĭ nē′sis). excessive motility; excessive muscular activity.

Hyperthermia (hī per ther′mĭa). therapeutically induced hyperpyrexia (high fever).

    Malignant hyperthermia: rapid onset of extremely high fever with muscle rigidity.

Hypertonic (hī per-ton′ik). having excessive tone, tonicity, or activity.

    Hypertonic solution: one that has a higher molecular concentration than another with which it is compared; of greater concentration than isotonic.

Hyperventilation (hī per ven′til ā′shun). increased alveolar ventilation with carbon dioxide pressure below normal.

Hypnotic (hĭp-not′ik). inducing sleep.

Hypocalcification (hī′pō-kal sĭ-fi-kā′shun). deficiency in the mineral content of a calcified tissue, for example in the enamel, results from disturbance in the maturation phase during development; may be caused by systemic, local, or hereditary factors.

Hypodontia (hī pō-don′shĭ-ah). condition of congenitally missing teeth; partial anodontia.

Hypoplasia (hī pō-plā′zĭ-ah). defective or incomplete development; enamel hypoplasia results when the enamel matrix formation is disturbed.

Hypotonic (hī-pō-ton′ik). having diminished tone; tonicity, or activity.

    Hypotonic solution: one that has a lesser molecular concentration than another to which it is compared; of less concentration than isotonic.

I

Iatrogenic (ī-at′rō-jen ik). caused by inadvertent or erroneous diagnosis and/or treatment by a professional.

Idiopathic (id′ē-ō-path′ik). self-originated; of unknown cause.

Idiosyncrasy (ĭd ē-ō-sin′krah-sē). any tendency, characteristic, or the like, peculiar to an individual.

Immunity (ĭ mu′nĭ-tē). an inherited, congenital, or naturally or artificially acquired ability to resist the occurrence and effects of a specific disease.

    Acquired immunity: that possessed as a result of having and recovering from a disease or from building up resistance against vaccines, toxins, or toxoids.

    Natural immunity: that inherited by the child from the mother or from the race.

    Passive immunity: that possessed as a result of injection of antibodies or antitoxins of serum from an immune individual or from an animal.

Implant (im′plant). a material or body part that is grafted or inserted within body tissues.

Implantation (im plan-tā′shun). the placement within body tissues of a foreign substance, for example metal or plastic, for restoration by mechanical means. In dentistry, a foreign material placed into or onto the jawbone to support a crown, partial or complete denture.

Incipient (in-sip′ē-ent). beginning to exist; coming into existence.

Incubation (in kū-bā′shun). the keeping of a microbial or tissue culture in an incubator to facilitate development.

Inert (in-ert′). without intrinsic active properties; no inherent power of action, motion, or resistance.

Infection (in-fek′shun). invasion of the body by pathogenic microorganisms and the body's response to the microorganisms and their toxic products; transfer of disease from one part to another or one person to another.

Infectious (in-fek′shus). capable of being transmitted; producing an infection.

Inflammation (in flah-mā′shun). reaction of living tissue to injury; a defense reaction of the body characterized by heat, redness, swelling, pain, and loss of function.

Inhibitor (in-hib′ĭ-tor). a substance that arrests or restrains physiologic, chemical, or enzymatic action or the growth of microorganisms.

Inoculation (i-nok ū-la′shun). introduction of microorganisms or some substance into living tissues or culture media: introduction of a disease agent into a healthy individual to induce immunity.

Inorganic (in or-gan′ik). not characterized by organization of living bodies or vital processes; also, pertaining to compounds not containing carbon, except cyanides and carbonates.

Insidious (in-sid′e-us). coming on gradually or almost imperceptibly; as in a disease, the onset of which is gradual, with a more serious effect than is apparent.

Intermaxillary (in ter-mak′sĭ-lar ĕ). between the maxilla and the mandible.

In vitro (in vē′tro). outside the living body: in a test tube or other artificial environment.

In vivo (in vē′vo). in the living body of a plant or animal.

Ion (ī′on). an electrically charged atom or group of atoms.

    Anion (an′ī-on). negatively charged ion, which passes to the positive pole in electrolysis.

    Cation (kat′ī-on). positively charged ion, which passes to the negative pole in electrolysis.

I.Q.: Intelligence Quotient; the relationship between intelligence and chronologic age.

Isoniazid (ī′sō-nī′ah-zid). antibacterial compound used in the treatment of tuberculosis.

Isotonic (ī sō-ton'ik). having a uniform tonicity or tension. See also hypertonic, hypotonic.

Isotonic solution: one which has the same molecular concentration as another with which it is compared.

Isotope (ī'sō tōp). any of two or more forms of a chemical element, which have different mass numbers because their nuclei contain different numbers of neutrons. Radioactive isotopes are widely used as tracers in research.

J

Jaundice (jawn'dis). condition in which there are bile pigments in the blood and deposition of bile pigments in the skin and mucous membranes, with resulting yellowish appearance.

Jurisprudence (joor ĭs-proo'dens). the science of law, its interpretation and application.

K

Kaolin (kā'ō-lin). a fine white clay; used in pharmacy in ointments and for coating pills.

Keratin (ker'ah-tin). a protein material formed as a transformation product of the cellular proteins of the flat cells on the surface of the epithelium; form of protective adaptation to function.

Keratinization (ker ah-tin ĭ-zā'shun). process of formation of a horny protective layer on the surface of stratified squamous epithelium of certain body surfaces, including the epidermis and masticatory oral mucosa.

L

Laceration (las er-ā'shun). a wound produced by tearing or irregular cutting.

Latent (lā'tent). concealed, not apparent, potential.

Learning disorders. academic skills disorders; developmental arithmetic disorder (dyscalculia); writing disorder (dysgraphia); and reading disorder (dyslexia).

Lethargy (leth'ar-jē). condition of drowsiness or sleepiness.

Leukoplakia (lu-kō-plā'kē-ah). a white patch or plaque that cannot be characterized clinically or pathologically as any other disease and is not associated with any physical or chemical causative agent except the use of tobacco.

Local (lō'k'l). restricted to one spot or area; not generalized.

Luxation (luk -sā'shun). a dislocation. For example, dislocation of the temporomandibular joint occurs when the head of the condyle moves anteriorly over the articular eminence and cannot be returned voluntarily.

Lymphadenopathy (lim-fad ĕ nop'ah thē). disease process affecting a lymph node or lymph nodes.

M

Maintenance phase: series of appointments after initial therapy for periodic reexamination and additional therapy as needed to keep the teeth and periodontal tissues in health without recurrence of disease.

Malaise (mal āz'). any vague feeling of illness, uneasiness, or discomfort.

Mandrel (man'drel). a spindle, axle, or shaft designed to fit a dental handpiece for the purpose of supporting a revolving instrument.

Manifestation (man'ĭ fĕ-stā'shun). that which is made evident, especially to the sight and understanding.

Oral manifestation: a symptom or sign of a disease in the oral cavity.

Manikin (man'ĭ-kin). model of the human body or a part; used for teaching purposes.

Massage (mah-sahzh'). manipulation of tissues for remedial or hygienic purposes with the hand or other instrument; the systematic application of frictional rubbing and stroking to the gingival tissues for increasing the circulation of blood through the tissues and for increasing the keratinization of the surface epithelium.

Mastication (mas tĭ-ka'shun). a series of highly coordinated functions that involve the teeth, tongue, muscles of mastication, lips, cheeks, and saliva, in the preparation of food for swallowing and digestion.

Matrix (mā'triks). the form or substance within which something originates, takes form, or develops; intercellular substance of a tissue.

Amalgam matrix: a thin metal form, usually stainless steel, adapted to a prepared cavity to supply the missing wall so the amalgam will be confined when condensed into the cavity preparation.

Medication (med ĭ-kā'shun). use of medicine or medicaments for treatment of a disease.

Metabolism (mĕ-tab'ō lizm). the sum total of the chemical changes occurring in the body; chemical process of transforming foods into complex tissue elements and of transforming complex body substances into simple ones, along with the production of heat and energy.

Anabolism (ah-năb'ō-lizm). the building up of tissue; maintenance and repair of the body.

Catabolism (kah-tăb'ō-lizm). the breaking down of tissue into simpler constituents for energy production and excretion.

Micron (mī'kron). unit of linear measurement; one-thousandth of a millimeter.

Milliliter (mil ĭ-lē'ter). one-thousandth part of a liter, usually abbreviated **ml.** It is approximately equal to 1 cubic centimeter.

Miscible (mis'ĭ-b'l). capable of being mixed.

Monitoring (mon'i tŏr ing). the overall surveillance of a patient by methods employing the senses of touch, sight, hearing, or smell or by means of devices that operate chemically, physically, or electronically to measure the adequacy of the various physiologic functions.

Morbidity (mor-bid'ĭ tē). the morbidity rate is the ratio to the total population of individuals who are ill or disabled.

Mortality (mor-tal'ĭ tē). the mortality rate is the death rate; the ratio of the number of deaths to the total population.

Morphology (mor-fol'ō-je). the science that deals with form and structure without reference to function.

Mucin (mu'sin). secretion of the mucous or goblet cell; a polysaccharide protein which, combined with water, forms a lubricating solution called mucous; contained in saliva.

Myotonia (mī'ō-tō'nē-ah). disorder involving the tonic (continuous tension) spasm of a muscle cell.

N

Nasmyth's membrane: see **Cuticle, primary.**

Necrosis (nĕ-kro'sis). cell or tissue death within the living body.

Neoplasm (nē'ō-plazm). a new growth comprised of an abnormal collection of cells, the growth of which exceeds and is uncoordinated with that of the normal tissues; see **Cancer; Precancerous lesion.**

Nidus (nī'dus). the point of origin or focus of a process.

Nosocomial (nōs ō-kō'mĭ-al). denotes a disorder associated with being treated in a hospital, which is unrelated to the primary reason for being in the hospital.

Nostrum (nos'trum). a quack, patent, or secret remedy.

O

Obstetrician (ob'stĕ-trish'un). a physician who specializes in the management of pregnancy, labor, and the period of confinement after delivery.

Obtundent (ob-tun'dent). having the power to dull sensibility or soothe pain; a soothing or partially anesthetic medicine.

Odontalgia (ō-don-tal'je-ah). toothache; pain in a tooth.

Odontoblast (ō-don'tō-blast). connective tissue cell that functions in the formation of dentin.

Odontolysis (ō don tol'ĭ-sis). dissolution or resorption of tooth structure.

Olfactory (ol-fak'tō-re). pertaining to the sense of smell.

Oncology (ong-kol'ō-jē). study or science of neoplastic growth.

Oral and maxillofacial surgery: that part of dental practice which deals with the diagnosis and surgical and adjunctive treatment of the diseases, injuries, and defects of the oral and maxillofacial region.

Orthopnea (or' thop-nē'ah). ability to breathe easily only in the upright position.

Osmosis (oz mo'sis). the passage of a solvent through a semi-permeable membrane into a solution of higher molecular concentration, thus equalizing the concentrations on either side of the membrane.

Osteoblast (os'tē-ō-blast). cell whose activity initiates the formation of new bone.

Osteoclast (os'tē-ō-klast). large multinucleated cell that brings about the resorption of bone; found only during the process of active bone or root resorption.

Osteoectomy, ostectomy (os-tē-ō-ek'tō-mĭ). (os-tek'tō-mĭ). removal of tooth supporting bone for correction of pockets and nonphysiologic bony contours.

Osteomyelitis (os-tē-ō-mĭ-ĕ-lī'tis). acute or chronic inflammation of the bone marrow or of the bone and marrow.

Osteoplasty (os'tē-ō-plas'tē). reshaping of bone; **alveoloplasty,** plastic contouring of the alveolar process to achieve physiologic contours in the bone and gingival tissues.

Otolaryngologist (ō tō-lar-in-gol'ō jist). medical specialist who treats the ears, throat, pharynx, larynx, nasopharynx, and tracheobronchial tree.

P

Pallor (pal'or). paleness.

Palpitation (pal-pĭ-ta'shun). rapid beating of the heart with or without irregularity in rhythm.

Parasympathetic (par ah-sim pah-thet'ik). craniosacral division of the autonomic nervous system.

Pathogenesis (path ō-jen'ĕ sis). the course of development of disease, including the sequence of processes or events from inception to the characteristic lesion or disease.

Pathogenic (path-ō-jen'ik). causing disease: disease-producing.

Pathognomonic (path og-nō-mōn'ik). a sign or symptom significantly unique to a disease to distinguish the disease from other diseases.

Pathosis (path-ō'sis). a disease entity.

Pediatric dentistry (pē dē-at'rik). the practice and teaching of, and research in, comprehensive preventive and therapeutic oral health care of children from birth through adolescence; includes care for special patients beyond the age of adolescence who demonstrate mental, physical, and/or emotional problems.

Pedodontics: see **Pediatric Dentistry.**

Periapical (per ē āp'ĭ-kal). around the apex of a tooth.
> **Periapical tissues:** the tissues surrounding the apex of a tooth, including the periodontal ligament and the alveolar bone.

Pericoronitis (per ĭ kor-ō-ni'tis). inflammation of the soft tissues surrounding the crown of an erupting tooth; frequently seen in association with erupting mandibular third molars and usually accompanied by infection.

Periodontics (per ē ō-don'tiks). the branch of dentistry that deals with the diagnosis and treatment of diseases and conditions of the supporting and surrounding tissues of the teeth or their implanted substitutes.

Periodontology (per ē ō-don tol'ō jē). the scientific study of the periodontium in health and disease.

Periodontopathic (per ē ō-don tō path'ik). refers to an agent able to induce and/or initiate periodontal pathosis.

Periradicular (per ĭ rah-dik'ū-lar). around or surrounding the root of a tooth.

Petri plate (pē trē). a small, shallow dish of thin glass with a loosely fitting, overlapping cover, used for plate cultures in microbiology.

pH: symbol commonly used to express hydrogen ion concentration, the measure of alkalinity and acidity. Normal (neutral) pH is 7.0. Above 7.0 the solution is alkaline; below, acidic.

Phosphorescence (fos-fo-res'ens). emission of radiation by a substance as a result of previous absorption of radiation of shorter wave length; contrasts with fluorescence in that the emission may continue for a time after cessation of the ionizing radiation.

Physiologic saline solution: a 0.9% sodium chloride solution, which exerts an osmotic pressure equal to that exerted by the blood, and thus is compatible with blood.

Pipette (pī pet'). a slender, graduated tube for measuring and transferring liquids from one vessel to another.

Placebo effect (plah-sē'bō). a positive response to a pain-relieving technique that is enhanced through the power of suggestion.

Potentiation (pō-ten′shē-ā′shun). enhancement of one agent by another so that the combined effect is greater than the sum of the effects of each agent alone.

Precancerous lesion: a morphologically altered tissue in which cancer is more likely to occur than in its apparently normal counterpart. A **precancerous condition** is a generalized state associated with a significantly increased risk of cancer.

Precipitate (prē-sip′ĭ tāte). to cause a substance in solution to separate out in solid particles (verb); that which is separated out is called the **precipitate** (noun).

Predisposition (prē-dis-pō-zish′un). a concealed but present susceptibility to disease, which may be activated under certain conditions.

Premaxilla (prē′mak-sil′ah). the intermaxillary bone situated in front of the maxilla proper; carries the incisor teeth.

Premedication (prē med-ĭ-kā′shun). preliminary treatment, usually with a drug, to prevent untoward results that may be effected by the treatment to be performed.

Prescribe (prě skrīb′). to designate or recommend a remedy for administration; to direct in writing the dosage, preparation, and dispensing of a remedy or drug.

Prodrome (prō′drōm). early or premonitory symptom of a disease.

Prognosis (prog-nō′sis). a forecasting of the probable course and termination of a disease and the response to treatment; the prospect of recovery from a disease as indicated by the nature and symptoms of the case.

Proliferation (prō-lif ě-rā′shun). reproduction or multiplication of similar forms.

Prone (prōn). flat, prostrate; **prone position,** lying flat.

Prosthodontics (pros thō-don′tiks). the branch of dentistry pertaining to the restoration and maintenance of oral function, comfort, appearance, and health of the patient by the restoration of natural teeth and/or the replacement of missing teeth and contiguous oral and maxillofacial tissues with artificial substitutes.

Protein (prō′tēn). any one of a group of complex organic nitrogenous compounds widely distributed in plants and animals that form the principal constituents of cell protoplasm. They are essentially combinations of alpha amino acids and their derivatives.

Proteolytic (prō tē-ō-lit′ik). effecting the digestion of proteins.

Protoplasm (prō′tō-plazm). the only known form of matter in which life is apparent; it composes the essential material of all plant and animal cells.

Psychiatry (sī kī′ah-trē). that branch of medicine which deals with the diagnosis and treatment of mental diseases.

Psychosomatic (sī kō-sō-mat′ik). pertaining to the mind-body relationship; having body symptoms of a psychic, emotional, or mental origin.

Ptosis (tō′sis). falling or sinking down; drooping of the upper eyelid.

Ptyalin (tī′ah-lin). an enzyme occurring in the saliva that converts starch into maltose and dextrose.

Public health: the science and art of preventing disease, prolonging life, and promoting physical health and efficiency through organized community efforts.

Dental public health: art of preventing and controlling dental diseases and promoting oral health through organized community efforts.

Pulp stone: see **Denticle.**

Pulpectomy (pul-pek′tō me). removal of the pulp chamber and root canals of a tooth.

Pulpotomy (pul-pŏt′o-me). the removal of a portion of the pulp of a tooth, usually meaning the coronal portion.

Pyorrhea (pī ō-rē′ah). a purulent discharge; discharge of pus. Formerly a name for advanced, severe periodontal disease.

Pyramidal (pĭ-ram′ĭ-dal). shaped like a pyramid.

Pyramidal tracts: collection of motor nerve fibers arising in the brain and passing down through the spinal cord to motor cells in the anterior horns.

Q

Quadrant (kwod′rant). any one of the four parts or quarters of the dentition, with the dividing line of the maxillary or mandibular teeth at the midline between the central incisors.

R

Raphe (rā′fē). a ridge, furrow, or seam-like union between two parts or halves of an organ or structure.

Rarefaction (răr ē fak′shun). being or becoming less dense.

Recurrent (rē kur′ent). returning after intermissions.

Rehabilitation (rē-hă-bil ĭ-tā′shun). restoration to former state of health, efficiency, and independent action; regeneration.

Remission (rē-mish′un). a decrease or arrest of the symptoms of a disease; also the period during which such decrease occurs.

Replantation (rē plăn-tā′shun). replacement into its own alveolar socket of a traumatically or otherwise removed tooth.

Resection (rē-sek′shun). operation in which a part of a tissue or an organ is removed.

Root resection: removal of a root from a multirooted tooth.

Hemisection: removal of half of a tooth.

Resorption (rē-sorp′shun). removal of bone or tooth structure by pressure; gradual destruction of dentin and cementum of the root, as the primary teeth prior to shedding; in orthodontic tooth movement, bone formation on one side compensates for resorption of bone on the other side.

Resuscitation (rē-sus ĭ-ta′shun). restoration of life or consciousness; restoration of heartbeat and respiration.

Rh factor: agglutinogens of red blood cells responsible for isoimmune reactions such as occur in erythroblastosis fetalis and incompatible blood transfusions; erythroblastosis fetalis results when a mother is Rh negative and develops antibodies against the fetus which is Rh positive.

Rheostat (rē′ō-stat). an appliance for regulating the resistance and thus controlling the amount of current entering an electric circuit; the dental unit control usually is located in a device operated by the foot.

Rheumatic (roo-mat′ik). pertaining to or affected with **rheumatism,** which is a general term pertaining to conditions characterized by inflammation or pain in muscles or joints.

RNA (ribonucleic acid) (rī bō-noo-klā′ik as′id). occurs in nuclei and cytoplasm of all cells; stores and transfers genetic information.

Ruga (roo′gah). ridge, wrinkle, fold.

Palatal rugae (roo′gī). the irregular ridges in the mucous membrane covering the anterior part of the hard palate.

S

Scoliosis (skō lē ō′sis). curvature of the spine.

Sedation (sĕ-dā′shun). allaying stress, irritability, or excitement; act of calming, especially by the administration of a sedative drug by inhalation, oral administration, or parenteral injection (intramuscular or intravenous).

Conscious sedation: a minimally depressed level of consciousness that retains the patient′s ability to maintain an airway independently and continuously and to respond to verbal command or physical stimulation; may be produced by pharmacologic or nonpharmacologic methods or a combination of the two.

Deep sedation: a controlled state of depressed consciousness accompanied by partial loss of reflexes, including inability to respond purposefully to verbal command; produced by a pharmacologic or nonpharmacologic method, or combination of the two.

Senescence (se-nes′ens). process or condition of growing old; physiologic aging not necessarily related to chronologic age.

Senility (sĕ-nĭl′ĭ-tē). old age; feebleness of body and mind occurring with old age.

Septum (sep′tum). a dividing wall, partition, or membrane.

Sequestrum (sē-kwes′trum). a piece of necrosed bone that has become separated from the surrounding bone; usually the necrosed bone is being expelled from the body.

Serrated (ser′āt-ed). having a sawlike edge.

Serum (se′rŭm). the clear, liquid part of blood separated from its more solid elements after clotting; the blood plasma from which fibrinogen has been removed in the process of clotting.

Sinus tract (si′nus trakt). a pathologic sinus or passage leading from an abscess cavity or hollow organ to the surface, or from one cavity to another; formerly known as a fistula.

Slough (sluf). a mass of dead tissue in, or cast out of, living tissue.

Spondylitis (spon′dĭ-lī′tis). inflammation of the vertebrae.

Spore: see **Bacterial spore.**

Stabile (sta′bīl). not moving, stationary, resistant; opposite of labile.

Heat stabile (thermostabile): resistant to moderate degrees of heat.

Stomatitis (stō mă-tī′tis). inflammation of the oral mucosa, because of local or systemic factors.

Subclinical (sŭb-klĭn′ĭ k′l). without clinical manifestations; said of early stages of a disease.

Subluxation (sŭb-lŭk-sā′shun). partial or incomplete dislocation; see **Luxation.**

Submerged tooth (sŭb-merjd′). one which is below the line of occlusion and may be ankylosed; intrusion; infraocclusion.

Supernumerary tooth (sū per-nu′mer-ăr ē). extra tooth; one which is in excess of the normal number.

Suppuration (sŭp ŭ-rā′shun). formation of pus.

Sympathetic nervous system: that part of the autonomic (involuntary) nervous system which arises in the thoracic and the first three lumbar segments of the spinal cord.

Syndrome (sin′drom). a group of symptoms and signs which, when considered together, characterize a disease or lesion.

Synergistic (sin er-jis′tik). acting jointly; enhancing the effect of another drug, force, or agent.

Systemic (sis-tem′ik). pertaining to or affecting the whole body.

T

Tactile (tak′til). pertaining to the touch; perceptible to the touch.

Technician, dental laboratory: a technician who performs any type of dental laboratory procedure not requiring the presence of a patient; see also **Dental prosthetic laboratory procedures.**

Teratoma (tĕr ă tō′mah). A neoplasm composed of multiple tissues, including tissues not normally found in the organ in which it arises.

Therapeutic (ther ah-pū′tik). pertaining to the treating or curing of disease; curative.

Therapy (ther′ah-pē). the treatment of disease.

Threshold (thresh′old). that amount of stimulus which just produces a sensation of pain.

Pain threshold: that amount of stimulus which just produces a sensation of pain.

Tic: an involuntary purposeless movement of muscle, which usually occurs under emotional stress; a twitching, especially of facial muscles.

Tincture (tingk′chur). an alcoholic solution of a drug or other chemical substance.

Tone (tōn). the normal degree of vigor and tension; a healthy state of a part.

Tonguetie (tung′tī). abnormal shortness of the frenum of the tongue, resulting in limitation of the motion of that organ.

Topical (tŏp′ĭ-k′l). on the surface; pertaining to a particular spot; local.

Topography (tō-pog′rah-fē). the detailed description and analysis of the features of an anatomic region or of a special part.

Toxic (tok′sik). poisonous.

Toxicity (toks-ĭs′ĭ-tē). the state or quality of being poisonous; degree of virulence of a toxic microbe or of a poison; the capacity of a drug to damage body tissue or seriously impair body functions.

Toxin (tok′sin). any poisonous substance of microbial, vegetable, or animal origin that causes symptoms after a period of incubation; can induce the elaboration of specific antitoxins in suitable animals.

Tracheotomy (trā kē-ot'ō-me). surgical operation to provide an artificial opening into the trachea.

Transdermal medication: drug delivered by patch on skin; a mode for slow release over extended time.

Transmissible (trans mis'sĭ b'l). capable of being carried across from one person to another.

Transplant (trans'plant). tissue removed from one part of the body and placed at a different site.

Transplantation (trans-plan-ta'shun). implanting a tissue or organ that has been taken from another part of the same body or from another person.

    Autotransplant: transfer of a tissue or organ to another place in the same person.

Trauma (traw'mah). an injury; damage; impairment; external violence, producing body injury or degeneration.

Treatment (trēt'ment). the management and care of a patient for the purpose of curing a disease or disorder.

Tremor (trĕm'or). involuntary trembling or quivering.

U

Urticaria (ur tĭ-kā'rē-ah). hives; nettle rash; an eruption of itching wheals usually of systemic origin. It may be caused by a state of hypersensitivity to foods or drugs, foci of infection, physical agents (heat, cold, light, friction), or psychic stimuli.

V

Vehicle (vē'ĭ k'l). a substance possessing little or no medicinal action, used as a medium to confer a suitable consistency or form to a drug.

Ventral (ven'tral). anterior, front surface: opposite of dorsal surface.

Virulent (vir'ū-lent). capable of causing infection or disease.

Viscosity (vis-kos'ĭ-tē). stickiness; ability of a fluid to resist change in shape or arrangement during flow.

Volatile (vol'ah-til). tending to evaporate readily.

Vulcanite (vul'kan-til). a hard rubber prepared by vulcanizing India rubber with sulfur; formerly used for making removable dentures.

W

Wheal (hweel, wēl). an acute circumscribed transitory area of edema of the skin; an urticarial lesion; see **Urticaria.**

Whitlow (hwit'lo). a purulent infection or abscess involving the end of a finger; also called a felon.

X

Xerostomia (zē rŏ-stō mē-ah). dryness of the mouth caused by functional or organic disturbances of the salivary glands.

Appendix

TABLE A-1.
AVERAGE MEASUREMENTS OF THE PRIMARY TEETH (IN MILLIMETERS)

		Overall Length	Length of Crown	Length of Root	Width of Crown (mesial-distal at widest point)
Maxillary	Central Incisor	16.0	6.0	10.0	6.5
	Lateral Incisor	15.8	5.6	11.4	5.1
	Canine	19.0	6.5	13.5	7.0
	First Molar	15.2	5.1	10.0	7.3
	Second Molar	17.5	5.7	11.7	8.2
Mandibular	Central Incisor	14.0	5.0	9.0	4.2
	Lateral Incisor	15.0	5.2	10.0	4.1
	Canine	17.5	6.0	11.5	5.0
	First Molar	15.8	6.0	9.8	7.7
	Second Molar	18.8	5.5	11.3	9.9

(From Black, G.V.: *Descriptive Anatomy of the Human Teeth,* 4th ed. Philadelphia, The S.S. White Dental Manufacturing Company, 1897, according to Ash, M.M.: *Wheeler's Dental Anatomy, Physiology, and Occlusion,* 7th ed. Philadelphia, W.B. Saunders, Co., 1993, p. 58.)

TABLE A–2.
AVERAGE MEASUREMENTS OF THE PERMANENT TEETH (IN MILLIMETERS)

		Overall Length	Length of Crown	Length of Root	Width of Crown (mesial-distal at widest point)
Maxillary	Central Incisor	23.5	10.5	13.0	8.5
	Lateral Incisor	22.0	9.9	13.0	6.5
	Canine	27.0	10.0	17.0	7.5
	First Premolar	22.5	8.5	14.0	7.0
	Second Premolar	22.5	8.5	14.0	7.0
	First Molar	B* L 19.5 20.5	7.5	B L 12 13	10.0
	Second Molar	B L 17.0 19.0	7.0	B L 11 12	9.0
	Third Molar	17.5	6.5	11.0	8.5
Mandibular	Central Incisor	21.5	9.0	12.5	5.0
	Lateral Incisor	23.5	9.5	14.0	5.5
	Canine	27.0	11.0	16.0	7.0
	First Premolar	22.5	8.5	14.0	7.0
	Second Premolar	22.5	8.0	14.5	7.0
	First Molar	21.5	7.5	14.0	11.0
	Second Molar	20.0	7.0	13.0	10.5
	Third Molar	18.0	7.0	11.0	10.0

* B = Buccal measurement; L = Lingual measurement
(From Ash, M.M.: *Wheeler's Dental Anatomy, Physiology, and Occlusion,* 7th ed. Philadelphia, W.B. Saunders Co., 1993, p. 15.)

Index

Note: Page numbers in *italics* indicate illustrations; page numbers followed by "t" indicate tables.

Abbreviations
  emergency care, 835t
  for hepatitis, 20t
  for herpesvirus, 26
  for HIV infection, 29t
Abdominal thrust, 840
Abrasion
  definition of, 334t, 562t
  in elderly patient, 638
  of tooth, 238, *239*
  from toothbrushing, 348–349
Abrasive
  defined, 562t
  in dentifrice, 368, *369*
  for dentures, 386
  fluoride and, 435t
  for stain removal, 565–567
Abscess
  definition of, 537t
  at injection site, 15
  periodontal, 541–543
  staphylococcal, 19t
Absence seizure, 742t, 743, 846t
Absorbable suture, 550
  definition of, 546t
Absorbed radiation dose, 141t
Absorption, 855
  of fluoride, 434
Abstinence, 129, 776t
Abuse
  child, 127–128
  defined, 776t
  substance, 128–130, 129t
Abutment teeth
  definition of, 377t
  plaque removal from, 381–382
Accessibility to wheelchair, *683*
Accessory, 855
  root canal, 232t
Acellular, definition of, 259t
Acid cleaning of dentures, 386
Acidogenic, definition of, 435t
Acidulated phosphate-fluoride, 444–445
Acne vulgaris, 625, 625t, 855
Acquired immunodeficiency syndrome, 29–36. *See also* Human immunodeficiency virus infection
Acquired pellicle, 258–259, 260t
Activation of instrument, 480–481, *481*
Active immunity, 12t

Acyclovir, 27–28
Adaptation of instrument, 479, *479*
  for gingival curettage, 529
  for scaling, 511, *512*, 514
Added filtration, 137
Adenopathy, 855
Adhesive
  debonding and, 594
  denture, 647t
Adolescent patient, 624–628, 625t
  diabetes in, 822
Adrenal crisis, 844t
Adsorption, 259t, 855
Aerobe, 259t
Aerosol
  airbrasive and, 571
  definition of, 12t
  infection and, *16*
  polishing and, 561
  production of, 14–15
  stain removal and, 567
Agglutination, 855
Aging patient, 634–645. *See also* Gerodontic patient
Agoraphobia, 767
Agranulocyte, 806
Agranulocytosis, 810–811
AIDS. *See* Human immunodeficiency virus infection
Aids, self-care, 692–696, *693–696*
Air, in examination, 208–209
Airbrasive, 571
  defined, 562t
Airway
  artificial, 830
  in basic life support, 835
  obstruction of, 839–841, 842t
Akinesia, 712t
Alcohol. *See also* Alcoholism
  consumption of, in history, 97t
  fetal alcohol syndrome and, 751
Alcoholic, 776t
Alcoholics Anonymous, 780
Alcoholism, 775–783
  cancer and, 670
  dental hygiene care in, 780–782
  description of, 775–776
  education about, 782
  systemic effects of, 776–779, *778*
  terminology about, 776t

treatment of, 779–780
  withdrawal syndrome and, 779
Alexidine, 283
Alginate, 169, 172
Alkaline hypochlorite, 386
Alkaline peroxide, 386
Allergen, 855
Allergic reaction
  to anesthetic, 521, 845t
  definition of, 86t
  to drug, 95
  emergency treatment of, 845t
  history of, 97t
Alopecia, 673, 855
Alloy, 394t, 855
Alphabet, American manual, *737*
Alveolar bone
  anatomy of, 183
  attached gingival tissue and, 185
Alveolar crest fibers, 183
Alveolar mucosa, 186, 217
Alveolar process, fracture of, 664
Alveolar ridge, dentures and, 649
Alveologingival fibers, 182
Alzheimer's disease, 635t, 636–637, 637t, 760t
  in Down's syndrome, 754
Amalgam restoration, 580–590
  appointment planning for, 585–587
  discoloration from, 285
  finishing procedures for, 580, 583–585
  fluoride and, 589
  longevity of, 580–581
  marginal irregularities of, *581*, 581–582
  margination and, *587*, 587–588
  mercury and, 583
  overhanging, 582–583
  polishing of, 588–589
Ameloblast, 237, 855
Amelogenesis, 232t
Amelogenesis imperfecta, 236, 281t, 284
Amenorrhea, 625t
  in anorexia nervosa, 769t, 771
American Academy of Periodontology, 290t
American Dental Association
  address of, 53t. *See also* Council on Dental Materials; Council on Dental Therapeutics.
  evaluation programs of, 370
  periodontal screening tool of, 290t

American Dental Hygienists' Association, 6t
American Heart Association
  antibiotic premedication, 102
  address, 800
American manual alphabet, 737
Americans with Disabilities Act, 679
Amniocentesis, 606t
Amniotic sac, 606t
Amorphous, 273t
Amoxicillin, 102t
Ampere, 135
Analgesia, 507t
Anaphylaxis, 845t, 855
Anaplasia, 803t
Anatomic landmarks, radiographic, 158
Anemia, 806–809, *808*
  iron deficiency, 807
  leukemia and, 811
  megaloblastic, 807–808
  sickle cell, *808,* 808–809
Anesthesia
  definition of, 507t
  emergency, reaction to, 846t
  general, preparation of mouth for, 667
  patient history of, 94t
  for scaling and root planing, 519–520
  topical, 519–520
    gagging and, 145
Aneurysm, 785t
Angina pectoris, 98t, 793–794
  definition of, 785t
  emergency treatment of, 844t
Angioneurotic edema, 829t
Angle-bisection technique, 145, *146,* 151–152
  in edentulous patient, 154
Angular cheilitis, 637
  dentures and, 650
Angulation of instrument, 479–480, *480*
  for angle-bisection technique, 152
  of curet, 490
  definition of, 146–147
  for gingival curettage, 529
  for paralleling technique, 150
  procedure for, 145
  for scaling, 491, 511–512, 514
Ankylosis, 224, 249t, 712t
Anode, 135
Anodontia, 647t
Anodyne, 366, 855
Anomaly, 855
  tooth, 240t, 752
  congenital heart, 786
Anorexia nervosa, *769,* 769t, 769–770
Anoxia, 107t, 785t, 855
Antabuse, 780, 776t
Anterior crossbite, 250, *251*
Antibiotic, 16. *See also* Drug therapy
  cardiovascular surgery and, 799–800
  definition of, 86t
  diabetes and, 824
  for elderly patient, 640
  leukemia and, 812
  pacemaker patient and, 798
  premedication, 101–103

for study casts, 165
subgingival irrigation and, 532
Antibody
  definition of, 12t
  hepatitis A, 21
  hepatitis B, 23
  herpes simplex virus, 27–28
  HIV, 32
Anticalculus dentifrice, 278
Anticipatory guidance, 613t
Anticoagulant drug, 785t, 798–799
Antidepressant, 763–764
Antidiabetic agent, 819t, 823
Antigen, 12t
Antihistamine, 97t, 830
Antihypertensive drug, 791
Antimicrobial agent, 367
  definition of, 53t
Antimicrobial soap, 42t
Antimicrobial therapy, 526t
Antiplaque agent, stains and, 283
Antipsychotic medication, 762t
Antiseptic
  definition of, 53t
  surface, 64
Anxiety
  as emergency, 772
  gagging and, 144
Anxiety disorder, 766–768, 767t
Apatite, 273t, 435t
Aperture, of x-ray tube, 135
Aphasia, 712t
Aphtha, 117t
Apical fibers, 183
Aplasia, 803t
Apnea, 107t, 785t
Appliance
  for cleft lip and palate, 621
  debonding of, 591–596, *592,* 592t, *593*
  orthodontic, 376–379, 377t, *378, 379*
  universal precautions and, 65
Appointment
  anxiety disorder and, 768
  bipolar disorder and, 765–766
  bulimia and, 771–772
  for cancer patient, 676–677
  cerebrovascular accident and, 718–719
  charting of, 318–319
  dentures and, 651
  diabetes and, 824–825
  for disabled patient, 682, 684–685
  for elderly patient, 639–640
  emergency prevention and, 828–829
  epilepsy and, 746
  hemophilia and, 815
  major depressive disorder and, 764
  mentally disabled patient and, 762
  presurgery, 657
  sequencing of, 323–325, *326*
    amalgam restorations and, 585–586
    cleft lip and palate and, 621–622
    for infant or toddler, 612–613
    in maintenance phase, 599–600
    pregnancy and, 609, 610t
  sickle cell anemia and, 809
Apron, lead, 143, *144*

for pacemaker patient, 798
  during pregnancy, 609
Arch wire, debonding of, 592
Arkansas sharpening stone, 489t, 503–504
Arm position, with instrument, 477
Arrest, cardiac, 829t
  emergency treatment of, 844t
Arrested caries, 232t
Arrhythmia, 785t, 795, 829t
Arterial blood, 785t
Arteriosclerosis, 785t
Artery, pulse and, 110, *110*
Arthritis, 97t, 726–728
  rheumatic fever and, 787
Artifact, 856
  radiographic, 159t
Asepsis, 53t
Asphyxia, 785t
Aspirin, hemophilia patient and, 816
  medical history and, 97t
Assessment of patient
  for calculus, 272–278
  definition of, 321t
  diagnostic work-up in, 80
  extraoral and intraoral examination in, 116–132. *See also* Examination, extraoral and intraoral
  gingiva and, 180–194. *See also* Gingiva
  history in, 85–105, 86t. *See also* History
  indices for, 287–313. *See also* Indices and scoring methods
  for plaque, 258–271. *See also* Plaque
  procedures for, 80–81
  radiography and, 143
  radiography in, 133–163. *See also* Radiography
  for stains, 280–286
  study casts in, 164–179. *See also* Study cast
  tooth numbering systems for, 81, *82, 83,* 84
  vital signs and, 106–115, 107t, *108, 110, 112,* 112t, *113*
Astigmatism, 732t
Astringent, 366
  definition of, 353t
  disclosing agent and, 408
Ataxia, 712t, 724
Atheroma, 785t
Atherosclerosis, 792, *792*
Athetosis, 723
Atrophy, 712t
Attached gingiva, 185–186
  disease changes in, 189
  probe examination of, 217, *218*
  significance, 201
Attached plaque, 265
Attachment
  of calculus, 260, 276
  definition of, 526t
Attachment apparatus, 181t
Attachment epithelium, 184–185
Attachment level, clinical
  definition of, 181t, 208t
  probe examination of, *215,* 215–216
Attenuation, 134t

Attire, clinical, 42–43
Attrition, *237*, 237–238, 856
   cerebral palsy and, 724
Audiogram, 732t
Audiologist, 732t
Audiometer, 732t
Auditory stimuli, 221–222
Aura, 743
Auscultation, 81
   definition of, 107t
Autism, 754–756, 755t
   definition of, 750t
Autoclave, 58
Autogenous infection, 15–16
Autograph, 856
Autoimmune disease, 856
   myasthenia gravis as, 720–721
Automating film processing, 157–158
Autonomic, 856
   dysreflexia, 714
Autopolymerization, 462
Autotransformer, 135
Auxiliary, 856
Avulsion
   definition of, 232t
   of tooth, 848t
AZT, side effects of, 35

Backscatter radiation, 134t
Bacteremia, 15
   definition of, 86t, 507t
   endocarditis and, 788
   polishing and, 561
   scaling and root planing and, 507
   self-induced, 788
Bacteria. *See also* Infection
   green stains caused by, 281–282
   on hands, 45–46
   morphologic forms of, *259*
   pellicle and, 260, 261
Bacterial plaque. *See* Plaque
Bacterial spore, 856
Bacterial toxin, 196t, 199, 507t, 528
Bacterial zone of necrotizing ulcerative
     gingivitis, 537
Bacteriocide, 856
Bacteriostatic, 856
Balance, of instrument, *474*, 479
Barrier to infection, 41–51
Barrier-free environment, 682–684
Baseplate wax, 172
Basic life support, 829t, 835–837, *836*
Basophil, 806
Bass toothbrushing method, 338–339, *339*
Battery, for power toothbrush, 344
Beading wax of impression, *168*, 168–169
Beam, x-ray, 136
Behavior
   child abuse and, 127–128
   hepatitis B risk and, 22–23
Behavior modification, 412t
Bell's palsy, 725
Benign neoplasm, 671t
Benzocaine, 520
Beta hemolytic *Streptococcus*, 19t

Betel leaf, 283
Bidigital palpation, 118
Bifurcation, 216
Bilateral palpation, 118, *118*
Bimanual palpation, 118, *118*
Binder, in dentifrice, 368
Binge and purge disorder, 770t, 770–772
Bioburden, 53t
Biocidal, 59
Biofilm, 53t
Biohazard, 53t
Biopsy, indications for, 125
Bipolar psychiatric disorder, 764–766
Bismarck brown solution, 409
Bite
   crossbite, 249
   edge-to-edge, 249
   end-to-end, 249
   open, 250
   wax, 166
Bite block (rubber), 702
   film holder, 150
Bitewing survey, 150–151, *151*
   films for, 146
   purpose of, 146
Black, G. V., classification of caries, 232,
     235
Black stain line, 282
Bladder paralysis, 716
   wheelchair transfer and, 685
Blade
   of curet, 488
   offset, 489t
Blanket suture, 550
Bleach. *See* Sodium hypochlorite
Bleeding
   cleft lip and palate and, 622
   gingival
     chemotherapy causing, 674
     in examination, 189t, 192
     follow-up evaluation of, 598
     history of, 97t
     indices of, 299–300
     on Plaque-Free Score, 293, 295
   in hemophilia, 814
   postoperative, 658
Bleeding disorder, 814–816
Blind spot, 732t
Blindness, 731–734
   definition of, 732t
Blister, fever, 28
Blisterform lesion, 122, 123t
Block anesthesia, 507t
Blood
   alcohol levels in, 777
   arterial, 785t
   composition of, 802–806, 804t, 805t
   fluoride and, 434
   venous, 785t
Blood cells, 804–805
   reference values for, 805t
Blood disorder, 97t, 802–817
   alcoholism and, 777–778
   anemia as, 806–809, *808*
   blood composition and, 802–806, 804t,
     805t

   hemophilia as, 814–816
   hemorrhagic, 813–814
   oral findings in, 802
   polycythemia as, 809–810
   terminology about, 803t
   of white blood cells, 810–813
Blood pressure
   definition of, 107t, 111
   equipment for measuring, 112, 830
   hypertension and, 789–791, 790t
   low, 790
   measurement of, 111–114
Blood-borne infection
   hepatitis A as, 21
   hepatitis B as, 22, 23
   hepatitis C as, 25
   hepatitis D as, 25
Body language, 71t
Body mechanics, 71t
   exercises for, 485
Body shield (radiography), 143
Body temperature
   measurement of, 106–109, *108*
   spinal cord injury and, 714
Bone
   aging and, 638
   alveolar
     anatomy of, 183
     attached gingival tissue and, 185
     dentures and, 649
   calculus compared with, 277
   in edentulous mouth, 646
   fluoride and, 440
   initial destruction of, 227
   loss of, *225*
   myelomeningocele and, 716
   normal level of, 225
   osteoporosis and, 635t, 636
   radiation therapy and, 673
Bone marrow
   depression of, 812
   leukemia and, 811
   leukopenia and, 810
   transplant of, 812
Bone marrow failure, 807
Bony ankylosis, 712t
Booster immunization, 42, 42t
   for hepatitis B, 24
Border mold, 546t
Bordetella pertussis, 19t
Bottle caries, 613–614
Bowl, mixing, for impression, 165
Boxing technique for cast, 173
Bracket, debonding of, 591–596, *592*, 592t,
   593
Bradycardia, 107t, 785t
Bradykinesia, 712t
Braille, 732t
Brain damage, alcoholism and, 778
   cerebral palsy and, 722
Breast feeding
   fluoride and, 443
   human immunodeficiency virus
     infection and, 35
Breath odor, 120t, 193, 537t, 858
Breathing, in basic life support, 835–836

Bremsstrahlung radiation, 134t
Brief patient history, 86
Bristle brush, prophylaxis angle with, 569
Bristles of toothbrush, 334t, *335*, 335–336, *336*
Brittle diabetes, 819t
Broad spectrum antibiotic, 53t
Broken instrument, 521–522
Brown stain, 282–283
  fluoride causing, 284
Brush. *See also* Toothbrush
  care of, 55, 349
  for dentures, 387–388
    removable, 384
  for handwashing, 46
  prophylaxis angle with, 569
Brush-on fluoride gel, 453
Bruxism, 238, 856
  definition of, 232t
Buccoversion, 250
Bud, taste, 181t
Budding, of human immunodeficiency
    virus, 30
Buffer, 856
Buffering agent, 366
Bulimia nervosa, 770t, 770–772
Bur, for debonding, 594
  for overhanging margin, 586
Burn, 846t–847t
Burnish, 489t
Burnishing of restoration, 585
Butacaine, 520
Bypass surgery, *793*

Cachexia, 856
Calcite, 566
Calcium
  plaque and, 265
  pregnancy and, 611–612
Calcium carbonate, 566
Calcium fluoride, 437–438
Calculogenesis, 259t
Calculus, 260t, 272–278
  charting of, 317
  classification and distribution of,
      272–273
  clinical characteristics of, 273, 274t, 275
  definition of, 260t, 273t
  dentifrice and, 369
  on dentures, 385
  follow-up evaluation of, 598
  formation of, 275–277
  index of, 306
  prevention of, 278
  radiography and, 227
  removal of, 510–511
  sealant and, 464
  significance of, 277
Calculus plaque, 267
Calculus Score, 306
Calibration, 208t
Cancer, 669–678, 856
  alcoholism and, 778
  characteristics of, 671t
  chemotherapy for, 674

dental hygiene care in, 675–677
description of, 669–670
education about, 677
examination for, 124–125
history of, 98t
HIV and, 33
preparation for treatment of, 670–671
psychological factors of, 674–675
radiation therapy for, *672*, 672–674
surgery for, 671–672
terminology about, 670t
Candida albicans, 19t
  denture related, 650
  HIV and, 34
  leukemia and, 813
Candidiasis, 19t, 31, 34t, 34, 36
  cytologic smear, 125
  denture, 650
  leukemia, 813
Canine, occlusion and, 252
Cannabinoid, street names of, 129t
Cannula, 353t, 526t
Capillary, hemorrhagic disorder and, 813
Capnophilic, 856
Carbohydrate, 856
  diabetes and, 823
  plaque and, 265–266, 268
Cardiac arrest, 829t
  emergency treatment of, 844t
Cardiac valve, endocarditis and, 15
Cardiopulmonary resuscitation, 836–839
Cardiovascular disease
  angina pectoris and, 793–794
  anticoagulant therapy in, 798–799
  classification of, 784
  congenital, 784–787, *786*
  congestive heart failure and, 795–796
  education about, 800
  emergency treatment of, 844t
  history of, 98t
  hypertensive, 789–791, 790t, 791t
  myocardial infarction and, 794–795
  pacemaker for, 796–798, *797*
  prophylactic premedication for, 102,
      102t
  rheumatic, 787
  sudden death and, 796
  surgery for, 799–800
Cardiovascular system, 784–801
  age and, 635
  alcoholism and, 777
Carditis, rheumatic, 787
Caregiver for disabled patient, 696–698
  inservice training, 699–701
Caries
  in adolescent, 626
  autistic patient and, 755
  cerebral palsy and, 724
  charting of, 235t
  cleft lip and palate and, 618
  debonding and, 595
  dentifrice and, 369
  development of, 231–232
  diabetes and, 823–824
  in disabled patient, 689
  education about, 432

elderly patient and, 638, 641
enamel, 232, 234
fluoride and, 439–440. *See also* Fluoride
fracture and, 664
indices of, 308–311
maintenance phase and, 599
mentally retarded patient and, 752
nursing, 234, 236, 613–614
nutrition and, 423–424
overdentures and, 651
overhanging restoration and, 5843
partial dentures and, 384
periodontal abscess and, 543
plaque causing, *267*, 267–268
pregnancy and, 611–612
radiation, 673–674
radiography of, 227
recognition of, 242–243
root surface, 236
sealant and, 463
stain removal and, 564
subperiosteal implant and, 402
xerostomia and, 204–205
Cariogenic plaque, 267
Cariogenic substance, 423, 428–429, *430*
  definition of, 232t, 259t, 435t
  clearance time from mouth, 423t
Cariostatic, 435t
Carious lesion. *See* Caries
Carotid pulse, 110, *836*
Carpal tunnel syndrome, 484t
Carrier of infection
  definition of, 12t
  hepatitis B, 23
Carving of restoration, 584
Cassette, x-ray film, 134t
Cast, study, 164–179. *See also* Study cast
Category, morphologic, 122, 124
Catgut suture, 546t
Catheter, wheelchair transfer and, 685
Cathode, 135
Cavity. *See* Caries
Cavity preparation, particles from, 14
  classification, 232, 235t
Cell
  blood
    reference values for, 805t
    types of, 804–805
  human immunodeficiency virus
      infection of, 30–31
  radiation effects on, 141
Cementicle, 232t, 856
Cementoenamel junction, 200, *200*
  in Periodontal Disease Index, 304–305
  probe examination of, 216
Cementum, 183
  aging and, 638–639
  amalgam restorations and, 586
  fluoride and, 437
  pocket and, 200
  root planing and, 513–516
  ultrasonic scaling and, 518–519
Centers for Disease Control and
    Prevention, 12t
Centigrade thermometer, *107*
Central nervous system depressant, 129t

Central nervous system stimulant, 129t
Centric occlusion, 165t, 249t
Centric relation, 249t
Cephalometer, 249t
Cephalometric analysis, 249t
Cephalostat, 249t
Ceramic, hydroxyapatite, 394t
Cerebral hemorrhage, 717
Cerebral palsy, 722–725, *723*
Cerebrovascular accident, 717–719, *718*
  definition of, 712t
  emergency treatment of, 843t
  history of, 99t
Certainly lethal dose of fluoride, 453–454
Cervical collar, thyroid, 143
Cesarean section, 606t
CEU, 4t
Chair. *See also* Wheelchair
  for disabled patient, 687
  positioning of, 70, 73–76, *73–76*
Characteristic radiation, 134t
Charters toothbrushing method, 341–342, *342*
Charting, 314–319, *316, 318*
  of caries, 235t
  mobility, 224
  periodontal, 217–219, *218*
Cheilitis, angular, 637
  dentures and, 650
Chemical burn, 847t
Chemical dependence, 128–129
Chemical disinfectant, 59–62, 60t, 61t
  items requiring, 63
Chemical indicator for cycle monitoring, *56, 57*
Chemical vapor sterilizer, 58–59
Chemistry of film processing, 157
Chemotaxis, 856
Chemotherapy, 361–370. *See also* Drug therapy
  for cancer, 674
  chlorhexidine for, 367
  definition of, 353t, 526t
  dentifrices and, 367–369
  disabled patient and, 690
  interdental brushing and, 358–359
  leukemia and, 812
  mouthrinses for, 364–367, 365t
  oral irrigation and, 361–364, *362, 363*
  subperiosteal implant and, 402
  for tuberculosis, 17
Chest compression, external, 837–838
Chest pain, 794
Chest thrust, 840
Chickenpox, 26–27
Chief complaint, 321t
Child, 612–614. *See also* Infant; Primary dentition
  calculus in, 273
  chair position for, 75–76
  dentifrice for, *452*
  diabetes in, 822
  external chest compressions on, 837–838
  fluoride and, 434
    toxic doses of, 453, 454

gingiva of, 192–193
hepatitis B immunization of, 23
HIV infection in, 35–36
hypertension in, 791
nursing caries in, 234, 236
radiography in, 153–154
teaching of, 417–418
terminology about, 606t
visually impaired, 733
Child abuse, 127–128
Chin lift, 835, *836*
Chisel scaler, 492, *492*
  angulation of, 511
  sharpening of, 503
Chlorbutanol, 521
Chlorhexidine, 367
  stains and, 283
Chlorhexidine rinse, 64
  necrotizing gingivitis and, 540
Chlorine compounds, 61
Chlorophyll, 281t
Chorea, 856
  rheumatic fever and, 787
Chromogenic organism, 281, 281t
Chronologic age, 281t
Cicatrix, 196t, 856
Circuit, x-ray machine, 135
Circular toothbrushing method, 343, *343*
Circumvallate papilla, 182
Circumferential fiber. *See* Periodontal ligament.
Clasp, of denture, cleaning of, 572
Clasp brush, *384*
Classification
  of anemia, 806–807
  of calculus, 272–273
  of cardiovascular disease, 784
  of caries, 232
  of cleft lip and palate, 617, *619*
  of dental fluorosis, 440t
  of diabetes mellitus, 818, 820t
  of disease, 239
  of fractures, *661*
  of furcations, *201*
  of gingival disease, 198t
  of human immunodeficiency virus infection, 31t, 31–32, 34t
  of inanimate objects for infection control, 63t
  of malocclusion, 250–253, *251–253*
  of periodontal disease, 198t
  of psychiatric disorder, 760t
  of seizures, 742t
Cleaner, interdental, wood, 360–361
Cleaning
  of dentures, 385–389
    by disabled patient, 695–696
    removable, 383–384, 571–572
  of environmental surfaces, 63–64
  fracture and, 666
  of instruments, 55
  interdental, 352–361. *See also* Interdental care
  of prosthesis, 386–389, *388*
  sealant and, 464
  of tongue, 346–347, *347*
  of toothbrush, 349

toothbrushing and, 333–351. *See also* Toothbrushing
Cleaning agent
  in dentifrice, 368
  precleaning, 60, 62–63
  for stain removal, 565–566
Cleanser, denture, 386
Cleft
  floss, 355
  gingival, 190, *191*
Cleft lip and palate, 617–623
  classification of, 617, *619*
  dental hygiene care of, 621–622
  etiology of, 617–618
  general characteristics of, 619–620
  oral characteristics of, 618
  personal factors in, 620
  terminology about, 618t
  treatment of, 620–621
Climacteric, 625t, 630–631
Clindamycin, 102t
Clinical attachment level
  definition of, 181t, 208t
  probe examination of, 215, 215–216
  pocket and, 197
Clinical attire for exposure control, 42–43
Clinical trial, 287
Clinician, position of, 71–73, *72*
Clinician's stool, infection control and, 54
Clock system of toothbrushing, 338
Closed gingival curettage, 526t
Closed instrumentation, 526t
Closed reduction of fracture, 660–661
Clostridium tetani, 14
Clotting defect, 814–816
Coagulation factor, 803t
Coaptation, 546t, 857
Cognitive-behavioral therapy, 768
Coitus, definition of, 625t
Col, 185, *185*
  definition of, 353t
  flossing and, 355
  interdental care and, 352–353
Cold sore, 28
Collagen, 196
Collagenase, 196
Collar, thyroid cervical, 143
Collimation, 137
  protection of clinician and, 142
  protection of patient and, 143
Color
  for disclosing agent, 407
  of gingiva, 187
  stains and, 280–286
Color blindness, 732t
Coloring agent, of dentifrice, 369
Coma
  definition of, 706t
  diabetic, 821t
    emergency treatment of, 845t
Communicability of hepatitis A, 21
Communicable, 857
  period of disease, 12t, 19t
Communication
  with disabled patient, 685
  emergency, 830
  with hearing impaired patient, 736, *737–739, 740*

Community Periodontal Index of Treatment Needs, 307–308
Complete denture, 377t, 384–386, *385*
  definition of, 647t
Complete history, 86
Complete overdenture, 389, *390*
Complete-arch fixed splint, *395*
Compressed air syringe, 209
Compression, external chest, 837–838
Compton scatter radiation, 134t
Computer-assisted maintenance appointments, 600
Conditioning, tissue, 325
Conductive hearing loss, 734
Cone
  for bitewing survey, 151
  sharpening, 499–500, *500*
Cone-cut, 137n
Congenital disorder
  cardiovascular, 784–787, *786*
  cleft lip and palate as, 617–623
  cytomegalovirus infection as, 27
  enamel hypoplasia as, 237
  hepatitis B as, 22
  mental retardation as, 749–758. *See also* Mental retardation
Congestive heart failure, 795–796
Connective tissue, periodontitis and, 197
Conscious patient, airway obstruction in, 839, 840
Consent, informed, 326
  definition of, 321t
  for disabled patient, 681
  endocarditis prophylaxis and, 788–789
  pacemaker patient and, 798
Consultation
  alcoholism and, 781
  disabled patient and, 682
  medical, 101
Contact
  functional, 254
  parafunctional, 254–255
  proximal, 255
Contact lens, 45
Contagious, 857
Contaminated waste, 53t
Contamination, 53t
Continuing education, 4t
Contoured dental chair, 73
Contouring of restoration, 584–585
Contraceptive, oral, 629–630, 100t
Contrast in radiograph, 136–137
Contributing factor, 202
Control, infection, 52–69. *See* Infection control
Controlled release of drug, 361, 526t
Coping denture, 389, *390*
Copper amalgam, discoloration from, 285
Core temperature, 107t
Cowhorn explorer, 221
Coronary bypass surgery, *793*
Coronary heart disease, 791–793, *792*
Corticosteroid, 103, 857
Cortisol deficiency, 844t
Corumdum, 566
Cost of fluoridation, 441

Cotherapist, 4t
Cotton pliers, practice exercise for, 483
Cotton-roll isolation
  amalgam restorations and, 586
  for fluoride application, 446, *446*
  sealant and, 464
Council on Dental Materials, Instruments, and Equipment, 370
  irrigators, 362
  pit and fissure sealants, 462
  power-assisted toothbrushes, 344
  ultrasonic scalers, 516
Council on Dental Therapeutics, 370
  dentifrice approval, 369
  fluorides, 442
  hypersensitivity reduction, 557
  mouthrinses, 364
  periodontal dressings, 545
Counseling
  anticipatory guidance, 613t
  caries control and, 425
  dietary, 423–424, 429–431
  HIV infection and, 36
  ischemic heart disease, 792
  prevention and, 331
Count system of toothbrushing, 338
Craniomaxillary immobilization, 664
Crepitation, 829t
Crestal lamina dura, 226
Crevice, gingival, 184
Cricothyrotomy, 829t
Crisis
  myasthenic, 720–721
  sickle cell, 809
Crossbite, 249
  anterior, 250, *251*
  posterior, *251*
Crown
  anatomy of, 180, *181*
  definition of, 394t
  enamel hypoplasia of, *237*
Crust, 117t
Crutches, 687
Cuff, blood pressure, *112*, 112–114, 830
Cumulative trauma, 71t, 483–486, 484t, *484–486*, 486t
  recommendations for, 486t
  risk factors for, 486t
Cup, rubber, prophylaxis angle with, 568, 569
Curet, 488–490, *489*
  angulation of, 480
  definition of, 489t
  divided into thirds, *512*
  for scaling and root planing, 513–514
  sharpening of, 496, 498
Curettage
  definition of, 526t
  procedure for, 528–530, *529*
Custodial care, hepatitis A and, 21. *See also* Disability
Cuticle, calculus and, 258–259, 276
  primary, 857
Cutting edge of instrument, 489t
Cyanosis, 785t
Cyclosporin, gingival changes from, 203

Cyst, 117t, 857
Cystic fibrosis, 857
Cytology
  exfoliative, 125–127, *126*
  indications for, 125
Cytomegalovirus, 18t, 27
Cytotoxicity of chemotherapy, 674

Day-care center, hepatitis A and, 21
Deaf. *See* Hearing Disorder.
Death
  from cancer, 669
  sudden, 796
Debilitated patient, 27
Debonding, 591–596, *592*, 592t, *593*
Débridement
  definition of, 507t
  necrotizing ulcerative gingivitis and, 540
Debris, food, 260t, 268, 269
  interdental brushing and, 358
  overhanging restoration and, 583
  partial dentures and, 381
  removal of, 330
Decayed, missing, and filled teeth indices, 308–311
Decibel, 732t
Deciduous teeth. *See* Primary dentition
Decontamination, 53t
Decubitus ulcer
  definition of, 712t
  spinal cord injury and, 714
Deep anterior overbite, 250, *251*
Defense against infection, alterations of, 15–16
Defibrillation, 829t
Definition, of x-ray image, 137
Defluoridation, partial, 441
Degenerative joint disease, 727–728
Dehydration, 857
  anorexia nervosa, 769, 770
Delirium, 776t
Delirium tremens, 779
Delta hepatitis, 20t, 25, *25*
Dementia, 636–637, 637t
  in AIDS, 33
Demineralization
  debonding and, 595
  definition of, 435t
Demineralization/remineralization cycle, 437–438
Demyelination, 712t
Density of radiograph, 136
  inadequate, 159t
  milliampere seconds and, 139
Dental ankylosis, 249t
  mobility and, 224
Dental caries. *See* Caries
Dental chair
  infection control and, 54
  positioning of, 73–76, *73–76*
Dental floss, 353–356, *355*, *356*
Dental history, 90, 94t
Dental hygiene
  alcoholic patient, 780–782
  anorexia nervosa and, 770

for anxiety disorder, 768
arthritis and, 727–728
autistic patient and, 755
bipolar disorder and, 765
bulimia and, 771
cancer patient and, 675–677
cerebral palsy and, 725
cerebrovascular accident and, 718–719
cleft lip and palate and, 621–622
definition of, 4t
dentures and, 390
diabetes and, 824–825
for diabetic patient, 824–825
diagnosis of, 4t, 320, 321t
for disabled patient, 679–680, 690
for elderly patient, 639–640
endocarditis and, 789
epileptic patient and, 745–746
fracture and, 664
general surgery and, 666–667
hearing impaired patient and, 736, 740
hemophilia and, 815
for homebound patient, 707
hypersensitive teeth and, 557–558
leukemia and, 812–813
major depressive disorder and, 764
menopause and, 631
menstruation and, 629
mentally retarded patient and, 752
multiple sclerosis and, 722
muscular dystrophy and, 719–720
myasthenia gravis and, 721
myelomeningocele and, 717
necrotizing ulcerative gingivitis and, 540–541
Oral Hygiene Index and, 296–298, 297
oral or maxillofacial surgery and, 657–659
Parkinson's disease and, 726
Patient Hygiene Performance and, 295–296
polycythemia and, 810
pregnancy and, 609–611, 610t
for prosthesis, 390
scleroderma and, 728
Simplified Oral Hygiene Index and, 298–299, 299
spinal cord injury and, 714–715
treatment plan for, 320–327
for visually impaired patient, 733–734
Dental hygiene diagnosis, 4t, 320, 321t
Dental hygienist
  definition of, 4t
  professional, 3–7, 4t
Dental implant, 399, 399–403, 400
Dental lathe, polishing on, 572–573
Dental personnel
  exposure control for, 41–51, 65
  position of, 71–73, 72
Dental Plaque Score, 306–307
Dental plaster, 165t
Dental stone, 165t, 172
Dental tape, stain removal and, 570
Dentifrice, 367–369
  anticalculus, 278, 369
  for dentures, 386

for disabled patient, 692
  fluoride, 452–453
  hypersensitive teeth and, 369, 557
  partial dentures and, 381–382
Dentin
  fluoride and, 437
  structure of, 554–555
Dentinocemental junction, 555
Dentinogenesis imperfecta, 281t, 284
Dentistry, forensic, 86t
Dentition, types of, 232t
Dentofacial orthopedics, 249t
Dentogingival fibers, 182
Dentoperiosteal fibers, 182–183
Denture. See also Prosthesis
  complete, 384–386, 385
  counseling about, 647
  definition of, 377t, 647t
  for disabled patient, 695–696, 696, 700
  education about, 653
  in helpless patient, 708
  identification marks for, 651–653, 652
  partial, fixed, 377t, 381, 381–382
  postinsertion care of, 647–649, 648t
  removable
    cleaning of, 571–572, 695–696, 696
    partial, 377t, 382–384, 383, 384
  as splint, 663
Deodorizing agent, 366–367
Deoxyribonucleic acid, 857. See DNA
Dependence
  alcohol, 775–776
  chemical, 128–129
Deposit
  on dentures, 385
  on tooth, 241, 260t. See also Plaque
    charting of, 317
Depressant, street names of, 129t
Depressed lesion, 123t, 124
Depressive disorder, 763–764, 763t
Depressor, tongue, 702
Depth, probing, 181t, 212
  definition of, 208t
  follow-up evaluation of, 598
  recording of, 218, 218
Desensitization, defined, 857
  of hypersensitive teeth, 556–557
Desensitizing dentifrice, 369
Desmosome, 181t
Desquamation, 196
Detergent, in dentifrice, 368
Detoxification, 779
Developer, film, 157
Developing of film, 156
Developmental disorders, 750t
  cleft lip/palate, 617, 619, 620
  mental disorder, 750t
Dexterity, 481–483
Diabetes mellitus, 818–827
  classification of, 818
  dental hygiene care for, 824–825
  description of, 818–819
  effects of, 820–822
  insulin and, 819–820
  oral effects of, 823–824

patient history of, 100t
  prevention of, 825–826
  terminology about, 819t
  treatment of, 822–823
Diabetic coma, 821t
  emergency treatment of, 845t
Diabetic retinopathy, 732t
Diagnosis, dental hygiene, 4t, 320
  definition of, 321t, 857
Diagnostic cast, 165t
Diagnostic work-up, 80
Diamond particles for polishing, 566
Diaphragm for collimation, 137
Diary, food, 426, 426–427
Diastema, 196
  definition of, 249t
Diastole, 107t
Diastolic blood pressure, 112, 114t
Diet
  adolescent patient and, 625, 627–628
  alcoholism and, 777, 782
  analysis of, 422, 422t, 425–429, 426–428
    definition of, 423
  arthritis and, 728
  blender to prepare, 665, 665
  cancer patient and, 675
  caries and, 423–424, 425
    evaluation of, 431
  counseling about, 429–431, 430
  daily food requirements and, 424, 424–425
  definition of, 423
  dentures and, 649, 651
  diabetes and, 823, 825
  for disabled patient, 698–699
  education about, 431–432
  elderly patient and, 642–643
  fluoride in, 442
  folate deficiency anemia and, 808
  fracture and, 664–666, 665
  for homebound patient, 707
  hypersensitive teeth and, 557–558
  for infant or toddler, 613–614
  iron deficiency anemia and, 808
  liquid diet, 665
  in medical history, 97t
  menopause and, 631
  mucosa and, 423
  myasthenia gravis and, 721
  necrotizing ulcerative gingivitis and, 540, 541
  periodontal tissues and, 422
  phenytoin and, 744
  plaque and, 203, 268, 269
  postoperative, 659
  pregnancy and, 611
  presurgery, 658
  rehabilitated mouth and, 398
  retardation and, 751
  soft solid diet, 666
  staining from, 283
  terminology about, 423t
Differential cell count, 803t
Differential diagnosis, 321t

Diffusion
  definition of, 408t
  disclosing agent and, 408
Digital palpation, 118
Digital subtraction radiography, 134t
Dilantin. *See* Phenytoin
Diplegia, 712t
Diplopia, 732t
Direct infection. *See also* Transmission of
  infection
Direct supervision, dental hygienist, 4t
Disability, 101t, 679–748. *See also* Mental
  retardation; Psychiatric disorder
  care of patient with, 679–704
    appointment scheduling and, 682
    assessment and, 688–689
    barrier-free environment for,
      682–684, *683, 684*
    dental hygiene treatment plan and,
      690
    diet and, 698–699
    disease prevention and, 690–691
    fluoride and, 698
    functioning levels, 691
    group in-service education and,
      699–701
    initial appointment and, 684–685
    instruction for caregiver and, 696–698
    instrumentation and, 701–702
    objectives of, 679–680
    oral manifestations and, 689–690
    plaque control and, 691–692
    positioning and stabilization and,
      687–688
    pretreatment planning for, 680–682
    sealants and, 698
    self-care aids and, 692–696, *693–696*
    terminology about, 680t
    types of conditions and, 680
    wheelchair transfer and, 684–687
  homebound patient and, 705–707
  listing of, impairments, disabilities,
    handicaps, 681t
  physical
    arthritis and, 726–728
    Bell's palsy and, 725
    cerebral palsy and, 722–725
    cerebrovascular accident and,
      717–719, *718*
    maintenance treatment and, 599
    multiple sclerosis and, 721–722
    muscular dystrophy and, 719–720
    myasthenia gravis and, 720–721
    myelomeningocele and, 715–717, *716*
    Parkinson's disease and, 725–726
    power toothbrush for, 344
    scleroderma and, 728
    spinal cord injury and, 711–715
    terminology about, 681t, 712t
  sensory
    hearing impairment as, 734–740, *735,
      737–739*
    terminology about, 732t
    visual, 731–734
Disc, for restoration, 588

Disclosing agent, 267, 407–410, *408*, 408t
  definition of, 408t
  in patient education, 415, 416
Discoloration, 280–286
  of gingiva, 187, 188t
  of pulpless tooth, 284
  of radiograph, 159t
Discrimination, tactile, 208
Disease control. *See also* Infection control
Disease development
  complications of pocket formation and,
    200–201, *201*
  disease classification and, 198t
  factors contributing to, 201–204
  gingival and periodontal infections and,
    195–197, 196t
  gingival and periodontal pockets and,
    197–198
  tooth surface pocket wall and, 198–200,
    199, 200
  xerostomia and, 204–205
Disinfection
  chemical, 59–62, 60t, 61t
    items requiring, 63
  of dentures, 386
  of impression, 171
Dislocated jaw, 847t, *848*
Distance, in radiography, 139, 143
Distocclusion, 252, *253*
Distortion in radiograph, 160
Disulfiram, 780
Diurnal, 107t
DNA, 29t, 30, 857
Dog guide for visually impaired patient,
  734
Dorsal, 117t
Dose, radiation, 141, 141t, 672
Double-pour method of forming cast, 173
Down's syndrome, 752–754
Drainage, of periodontal abscess, 543
Dressing, 545–549, 546t
  anticoagulation therapy and, 799
  chemically-cured, 546
  definition of, 546t
  hemophilia patient and, 816
Drifting of teeth, 255
  space maintenance and, 379–380
Drill, emergency, 832, 834
Droplet, 12t, *16*
Drug abuse, 128–130, 129t
  alcohol, 775–783
Drug interaction, 86t
Drug therapy. *See also* Chemotherapy
  allergy to, 95
  for angina, 794
  anticoagulant, 785t, 798–799
  antihypertensive, 791
  antipsychotic, 762t
  for anxiety disorder, 768
  for arthritis, 727
  for autism, 755
  bipolar disorder and, 765
  cardiovascular surgery and, 799–800
  cerebral palsy and, 724
  cerebrovascular accident and, 718
  defense against infection and, 15

diabetes and, 823, 824
disabled patient and, 699
for elderly patient, 639–640
emergency, 830, 832, 841
emergency prevention and, 829
fetal effects of, 606, 607t, 608, 608t
gingival changes from, 189–190, 203
hemophilia patient and, 815
HIV infection and, 36
for infant or toddler, 614
leukemia and, 812
for major depression, 763–764
over-the-counter medications and, 86t
phenytoin and, 203, 743, 744, 744–745
pregnancy and, 751
prophylactic, antibiotic, 16, 101–103,
  102t, 165
schizophrenia and, 760
scleroderma and, 728
staining from, 283, 285
subgingival irrigation and, 532
sucrose in, 36, 431–432, 614
tuberculosis resistance and, 17
xerostomia from, 204, 762t, 764, 770,
  771
Drug-resistant tuberculosis, 17
Dry heat sterilization, 58
Dry mouth, 204–205. *See also* Xerostomia
Duchenne muscular dystrophy, 719
Dust-borne organism, 14
Dyclonine, 521
Dysmenorrhea, 625t, 629
Dysphagia, 635t, 712t
  myasthenia gravis and, 720
Dyspnea, 785t
Dysreflexia, autonomic, 714
Dystrophy, muscular, 719–720

Ear disorder, 100t
Easlick's disclosing solution, 409
Eating disorder, 768–772, *769*
Ecchymosis, 803t
Echocardiography, 785t
Ectopic, definition of, 273t
Edema
  angioneurotic, 829t
  definition of, 196, 785t, 857
  pulmonary, 796
Edentulous patient, 646–654
  bone and, 646–647
  definition of, 232t, 857
  dentures for, 647–650, 648t
    identification marks for, 651–653, *652*
  fixation in fracture, 663, *663*
  helpless, 708
  mucosa and, 647
  phenytoin overgrowth and, 744
  preventive maintenance for, 650–651
  radiography of, 153, 154
Edge-to-edge bite, 249, *251*
Education
  anticipatory guidance, 613t
  for dental specialty, 5
  factors to teach, 7
  group in-service, on disabled patients,
    699–701

individual planning for, 413–414
learning process and, *412*, 412–413
models for, 419–420
outline for, 413–417
of parents, 418–419, 612–614
patient-centered, 331
planned, 411
of preschool child, 417–418
teaching system for, 419
terminology about, 412t
Educational services of dental hygienist, 3
Elbow position, with instrument, 477
Elderly patient, 634–645. *See also*
Gerodontic patient
Electrical pulp tester, 243–245, *244*
Electrocardiogram, 785t
Electroconvulsive therapy, 764
Electrolyte, 232t
Electromagnetic interference to
pacemaker, 797
Electromagnetic radiation, 134t
Electronic thermometer, 108
Electronic x-ray timer, 136
Element, rare earth, 134t
Elevated lesion, 122, 123t, 124
Embolism
definition of, 785t
pulmonary, 795
stroke and, 717
Embrasure
definition of, 353t, 394t
gingival, *395*
plaque removal from, *396*
Embryo, 606t
Embryology, cleft lip and palate and,
617–618
Emergency care, 828–849
airway obstruction and, 839–841
basic life support and, 835–837, *836*
chemical solution in eye, 847t
epilepsy and, 742, 746–747, *747*, 846t
external chest compression and,
837–839, *838*
of fluoride toxicity, 454
for fracture, 659
for heart failure, 796
oxygen administration in, 841
for pacemaker patient, 798
preparation for, 830, 832, *833*, 834–835,
835
prevention of emergencies and, 828–829
psychiatric, 772
record of, *831*, 832
reference chart for, 842t–848t
rescue breathing and, 837
in sudden death, 796
technical hints about, 841, 848
terminology about, 829t
vital signs in, 829, *831*
Emery, 566
Emphysema, 635t
Emulsion, 140
film processing and, 157
Enamel
debonding and, 595
fluoride and, 437, *438*, 438–439

hypocalcification of, 435t
hypoplasia of, 284
definition of, 232t
pocket and, 200
polishing and, 562
pregnancy and, 608
remineralization of, 435t, 437
Enamel caries, recognition of, 242
Enamel hypoplasia, 236–237, *237*
Enamel-sealant interface, *464*
Encephalopathy, HIV and, 33
Endemic, definition of, 12t, 858
Endemic area of infection, 21
Endocarditis, 788–789
heart valve and, 15
prevention of, 101–103, 787
Endocrine disorder, 100t
alcoholism and, 778
Endodontic therapy
for cancer patient, 671
discoloration from, 285
Endogenous, definition of, 281t
Endogenous stain, 280, 283–285
Endosseous implant, 399, *399*
Endotoxin
definition of, 507t
scaling and root planing, 528
End-rounded filament, 334t, *335*
End-to-end bite, 249, *251*
End-tuft brush, *358*, *359*, 359
Engraving, for identifying dentures, 653
Enlarged gingiva, 191
drugs causing, 189–190
Enolase, 435t
Enteric bacteria, 14
Environmental Protection Agency, 53t
Environmental surface, disinfection of,
63–64, 70
iodophors for, 61
Enzyme
for cleaning of dentures, 386
definition of, 196, 858
Enzyme-linked immunosorbent assay, 12t
Eosin, 408t
Eosinophil, 806
Epidemic, 12t, 858
Epidemiologic survey, 287–288
Epidermis, 117t
Epilepsy, 741–748, *746–747*, *747*
definition of, 742t
emergency treatment of, 846t
patient history of, 100t
Epinephrine, 507t
emergency from 830
Epistaxis, 803t
Epithelium
anatomy of, 184–185
definition of, 181t
interdental care and, 352–353
pocket, 192
formation of, 196
Epithelium-associated plaque, 265
Epstein-Barr virus, 18t, 27
Epulis fissuratum, 650
Equipment, dental, 52
emergency, 830, 832

Ergonomics, 71t
Erosion, 117t, 238
Eruption of tooth, 233t, 858
of first permanent molars, *254*
gingiva and, *185*
sealant and, 463
Erythema, 117t
gingival, HIV infection and, 34–35
Erythema radiation dose, 141t
Erythrocyte, 802, 804–805
Erythromycin, 102t
Erythroplakia, 125, 858
Erythropoiesis, 803t
Erythrosin, 409
definition of, 408t
Ethics
definition of, 4t
principles of, 6, 6t
Ethylene oxide sterilization, 59
Etiologic factor, 202
Eugenol, 545–546, 546t
Euphoria, 776t
Evaluation, 597–599
of blood, 804t
disabled patient and, 692
Examination, extraoral and intraoral,
116–132, 120t–121t
alcoholism and, 781
for cancer, 124–125
child abuse and, 127–128
components of, 116–118, *118*
direct observation, 81, 118
of disabled patient, 688, 700
for elderly patient, 640
gingival, 186–193, 188t–189t, *190–192*
HIV infection and, 34
instruments for, 208t
of lesion, 121–122, *122*, 123t, 124, 124t
objectives of, 116
patient teaching about, 228
procedures for, 80–81
air and, 208–209
clinical attachment level and, *215*,
215–216
explorers and, *219*, 219–222, *220*
fremitus and, 224–225
furcations and, 216
mobility examination and, 223–224
mouth mirror and, 207–208
mucogingival examination and, 217,
217, *218*
periodontal charting in, 217–219, *218*
probe and, 209–210, 211t, *211–214*,
212–215
recording, 223, 314–319
subgingival, 222–223
supragingival, 222
radiographic. *See* Radiography
scaling and root planing and, *509*,
508–510
sequence of, 118–119
special applications for, 127
substance abuse and, 128–130, 129t
technical hints about, 228
of teeth, 239, 240t–241t, 241–242
of tongue, *119*

Excretion, of fluoride, 434–435
Exercise, 485
  dexterity, *482*
  diabetes and, 823
Exfoliation, 232t
  premature, space maintainer for, 379–380
Exfoliative cytology, 125–127, *126*
Exit radiation dose, 141t
Exogenous, 281t
Exogenous stain, 280, 285
Exophytic, 117t
Exostosis, 117t
Explorer
  angulation of, 480
  calculus and, 275
  caries examination and, 242
  definition of, 208t
  dexterity with, 483
  examination with, *219*, 219–223, *220*
  plaque and, 266–267
  sharpening of, 503
Exposure control
  clinical attire for, 42–43
  eyewear for, *44*, 44–45
  face mask for, 43–44
  gloves for, 48–50, *49*
  handwashing in, 45–48, *47*
  immunizations in, 41–42, 43t
  personal protection in, 41
  technical hints in, 50
  terminology about, 42t
External chest compression, 837–838
Extraction, toothbrushing after, 347. *See also* Postoperative Care
Extraoral examination, 116–132. *See also* Examination, extraoral and intraoral
Extrinsic, definition of, 281t
Extrinsic stain, 280
  removal of, 561–575. *See also* Stain removal
Exudate, 192
  definition of, 181t
Eye
  disorder of, 100t
  in Down's syndrome, 753
  emergency, 847t
  examination of, 120t
  foreign body in, 847t
  herpes infection of, 28
  of substance abuser, 129, *130*
  visual impairment and, 731–734
Eyewear, protective, 44–45, *45*, 841
  emergency prevention and, 820
  sealants and, 468

Face
  cleaning of, 67
  deformity of, 619
  of disabled patient, 689
  emergency prevention and, 820
  examination of, 120t
  fracture of. *See* Fracture
Face mask, 43–44
Facet, 232t

Facultative bacteria, 259t
Fahrenheit thermometer, *107*
Familial disorder. *See* Hereditary disorder
Fascioscapulohumeral muscular dystrophy, 719
Fast green as disclosing agent, 409
F.D.I. numbering system, 82, *82*, *83*, 84
Fecal oral transmission, of hepatitis A, 20
Female sexual development, 624
Festoon, 190
Fetal alcohol syndrome, 751, 778–779
Fetor oris, 537. *See also* Halitosis
Fetus
  cytomegalovirus infection in, 27
  defined, 606t, 858
  fluoride and, 440
  HIV infection and, 35
  hydantoin syndrome in, 744
  infections in, 751
  maternal diabetes and, 821
  mental retardation and, 751
  oral development in, 605–606, 617–618
Fever, rheumatic, 787
Fever blister, 28
Fibers
  gingival, groups, 182–183, *182*
  principal groups, 183, *183*
  Sharpey's, 181t, 182
Fibrillation, 829t
Fibroblast, 181t
Fibroplasia, retrolental, 732t
Fibrosis, 181t
Filament, toothbrush, 334t, 335–336, *336*
File, 587
File scaler, 493, *493*
Filiform papilla, 182
Filled teeth, indices of, 309–311
Film
  for angle-bisection technique, 151
  for bitewing survey, 151
  composition of, 139–140
  for periapical survey, 146
  holders, 147, 150
  placement of, 143
  selection of, 145–146
  special, 158
  speed of, 140
Film contrast, 137
Film holder, disposable, *147*, 150
Film packet, 140–141
Film positioning devices, 150, *147*
Filtration
  of face mask, 43
  in radiography, 137
Finger rest, 477–479
  amalgam restorations and, 587
  for disabled patient, 696
  of prophylaxis angle, 569
  for scaling, 5, 514
Finger sweep, 840
Fingerspelling, 736
Finishing
  of amalgam restoration, 580, 583–585
  of study cast, 177
Finishing strip, 570
  restoration and, 587

First degree burn, 846t
First permanent molar, *254*, 255
Fissure
  cavity, 235t, 234
  cleft lip and palate and, 622
  definition of, 117t
Fistula
  definition of, 537, 858
  periodontal abscess and, 541
Fixation, fracture
  external skeletal, *662*, 662–663
  intermaxillary, 661–662, *662*, 664
    in edentulous patient, 663
Fixed appliance, debonding of, 591–596, *592*, 592t, *593*
Fixed partial denture, *381*, 381–382
  definition of, 377t
Fixed prosthesis, 395
Fixed space maintainer, 380, 380–381
Fixing of film, 156, *157*
Flat lesion, 124, 124t
Flat stone
  Arkansas, 503–504
  moving, 496–498, *497*
  stationary, 498–499, *499*
Flavoring, in dentifrice, 368–369
Flexion, 484t
Floor, infection control and, 54
Floor of mouth, examination of, 121t
Flora, 259t, 858
Floss, 353–356, *355*, *356*
  stain removal and, 570
Floss cleft, 190, *191*
Floss holder, 695, *695*
Floss threader, *382*, 383
Flossing
  disabled patient and, 692, 695
  in helpless patient, 708
  partial dentures and, 382
  teaching about, 415
Flowchart, emergency team, 832, *833*, 834, *834*
Fluid, gingival disease and, 184, 192, 196
Fluorapatite, 435t
Fluorescein, 408t, 409
Fluoridation, 438–439
  cost, 441
Fluoride
  action of, 437–438, *438*
  adolescent patient and, 627
  amalgam restoration and, 589
  anticipatory guidance, 613t
  application of, 443–450, 444t, *446–448*
  brush-on gel containing, 452–453
  in calculus, 277
  cancer patient and, 676
  caries and, 236
  debonding and, 593, 595
  in dentifrice, 451–452, *452*
  dentures and, 390
  disabled patient and, 698, 701
  economic benefits of, 441–442
  effects and benefits of, 439–441, 451
  fluoridation and, 438–439, 441
  in food, 442

for homebound patient, 707
hypersensitive teeth and, 557, 558
menopause and, 631
metabolism of, 434–435
in mouthrinse, 450–452
orthodontic appliance and, 379
partial defluoridation and, 441
plaque and, 265
polishing and, 562
pregnancy and, 610–611, 612
rehabilitated mouth and, 397–398
sealant and, 467–468
stain removal and, 563–564, 567
staining from, 283, 285
supplements of, 442–443
systemic, *436*
terminology about, 435t
tooth development and, 436–437
toxicity of, 453–455, 454t, *455*
tray technique, 450, 771
Fluorohydroxyapatite, 435t
Fluorosis, 284, 454–455
    definition of, 435t
    index of, 440t
Fog on radiograph, 159t
Folate deficiency anemia, 808
Foliate papilla, 182
Follow-up evaluation, 81, 597–599
    for disabled patient, 682
    of in-service education, 701
    postoperative, 659
    presurgery, 657–658
Fomite, 12t
Fones toothbrushing method, 343, *343*
Food. *See also* Diet
    cariogenic, 423, 428–429, *430*
    consistency of, 422, 429
    fluoride in, 442
    impaction of, 196
        charting of, 317
        plaque formation and, 202
    staining from, 283
Food and Drug Administration, 53t
Food debris, 260t, 268, 269
    interdental brushing and, 358
    overhanging restoration and, 583
    partial dentures and, 381
    removal of, 330
Food exchange system in diabetes, 823
Food Guide Pyramid, *424*
Food-borne infection, hepatitis A as, 21
Foreign body in eye, 847t
Forensic dentistry, 86t
Form, 86
    for food diary, *426–427*
    for interview, 90, *91–92*
Four-handed dental hygiene, 76–77
    myasthenia gravis and, 721
    for spinal cord injured patient, 714–715
Fracture, 659–666, *660–663*
    emergency treatment of, 848t
    maxillary, 663–664
    of tooth, 238–239, *239*
    skeletal fixation, 662–663
    types of, *660*

Free gingiva, 183–184. *See also* Gingiva;
        Gingival *entries*
    disease changes in, 189
    healthy, 190
Fremitus, 224–225
    definition of, 208t
Frenum, 186, 858
Fulcrum, 361, 477–479, 483
Functional occlusion, 254–255
Functioning level of disabled patient,
        690–691
Fungal infection, HIV and, 34
Fungiform papilla, 182
Furcation, 200, *201*
    anatomic variations of, *508*
    definition of, 507t
    examination of, 216
    pipe cleaner, 360
    probe examination of, 216
    radiography and, 226
Furcation invasion, 394t

Gagging
    prevention of, 144–145
    study cast and, 166
Gamma radiation, 134t
Ganglion, herpesvirus infection on, 26
Gases, blood, 804
Gastrointestinal disorder, 100t
Gastrointestinal system
    age and, 635
    alcoholism and, 777
    fluoride and, 454
Gauze strip, plaque removal, 357, *357*
Gel
    definition of, 435t
    fluoride, 445–446
        cancer patient and, 676
        self-applied, 449–450
Generalized juvenile periodontitis, 626
Generalized seizure, 743
    emergency treatment of, 846t
Genetic disorder. *See* Hereditary disorder
Gentamicin, 102t
Geometric charting form, *316*
Geriatric patient, 634–645. *See also*
        Gerodontic patient
Geriatrics, 635t
German measles, 19t
Germ-free animal, 273t
Gerodontic patient, 634–645
    aging and, 634–636
    dental hygiene for, 639–644, 641t
    diseases in, 636–637
    oral findings in, 637–639
    psychological factors affecting, 639
    terminology about, 635t
Gerontology, 635
Gestation, 605, 606t
Gestational diabetes, 819, 819t, 821
Gingiva, 180–194, *184*
    aging and, 639
    airbrasive and, 571
    alveolar mucosa and, 186
    amalgam restorations and, 586

attached, 185–186
bleeding of. *See* Bleeding
calculus and, 275
of child, 192–193
cleft lip and palate and, 618
dentifrice and, 369
dentures and, 390
of disabled patient, 700
disabled patient and, 689
disease of, 536–544. *See also* Gingivitis
    classification of, 198t
    definition of, 196t
    in disabled patient, 689–690
    factors contributing to, 202–203
    herpetic, 28
    HIV infection and, 34–35
    infection as, 195–197, 196t
    recognition of, 186
education about, 193, 413, 416, 417
embrasures of, *395*
enlarged, 189–190, 191
examination of, 186–193, 188t–189t,
        190–192
fiber groups of, *182*, 183
follow-up evaluation of, 597–598
free, 183–184
interdental, 185
interdental care and, 352–353
junctional epithelium and, 184–185
leukemic infiltrate in, 812
menopause and, 630–631
mucosal anatomy and, 181–182
oral contraceptives and, 630
in Periodontal Disease Index, 304
periodontium and, 182–183, *183*
phenytoin and, 203, 743, *744*, 744–745
    cerebral palsy and, 724
plaque and, 268–269
pockets of, 197–198. *See also* Pocket
polishing and, 563
pregnancy and, 608
probe examination of, 217–219, *218*
scaling and root planing and, 527
tongue and, *182*
tooth anatomy and, 180–181, *181*
tooth eruption and, *185*
toothbrush trauma to, 347–348
Gingival Bleeding Index, 300
Gingival curettage
    definition of, 526t
    procedure for, 528–530, *529*
Gingival index, 302–303, *303*
    disabled patient and, 700
Gingivitis
    classification, 198t
    in adolescent, 626
    definition of, 196
    experimental, 268–269
    fracture and, 664
    irrigation and, 363
    necrotizing ulcerative, 536–541, *537*,
        537t
    toothbrushing and, 347
    orthodontic appliance and, 376
    recognition, 186–192, 188t

Gingivostomatitis, herpetic, 28
Gland, salivary, radiation effects on, 673
Glass ionomer, 435t
Glasses, protective, 44–45, *45*
Glaucoma, 732t
  cause of blindness, 731
Globulin, immune, hepatitis and, 20t
Glossitis, 803t
Gloves, 48–50, *49*
  double gloving, 49
Gluconeogenesis, 819t
Glucose tolerance test, 819t
Glutaraldehyde, 61
Glycerin, defined, 562t
  xerostomia and, 709
Glycolysis, 435t
Goggles, 44–45
Gonorrhea, 19t
Granulocyte, 806
Grasp
  instrument, 475–477, *476*
  of instrument, stroke and, 481
  for mirror, 208
Gray x-ray unit, 140–141
Green stain, 281–282
Group A *Streptococcus*, 19t
Group in-service education, 699–701
Group therapy, for alcoholism, 780
Guard, occlusal, 249t

Habitual occlusion, 165t
Hair, of dental personnel, 43
Halitosis, 120t
  defined, 858, 537t
  NUG sign, 537
  warning sign periodontitis, 193
Hallucination, 761t
Hallucinogen, street names of, 129t
Hand, in Down's syndrome, 753
  in rheumatoid arthritis, 727
Hand care, 45–50, *47, 49*, 481–486
Handle
  diameter, instrument, 475, *475*
  of explorer, 220
  of mouth mirror, 207–208
  of toothbrush, 334, *334*, 335
Handpiece
  maintenance of, 67
  for stain removal, 567–568
Handwashing, 46–48
  gloves and, 49
Hard palate, examination of, 121t
Hawley retainer, 377t, 379
Hazard, radiation, 141
Hazardous waste, 53t
  label for, *67*
Head
  in Down's syndrome, 753
  extraoral examination, 119, 120t
    hydrocephalus, 716, 752
    macrocephalus, 712t
    microcephalus, 712t, 752
  stabilization of, 687
  of toothbrush, 334, *334*, 334t, 335
Head tilt with chin lift, 835, *836*

Headcap, for immobilization, 664
Healing
  definition of, 526t
  diabetes and, 825
  of fracture, 664
  gingival curettage and, 531
  scaling and root planing and, 527
Health, 4t, 6, 859
Health promotion, 4t
Hearing, terminology about, 732t
Hearing aid, *735*, 735–736
Hearing impairment, 100t, 734–740, *735, 737–739*
  cleft lip and palate and, 619
Heart attack, 844t
Heart disease
  anticoagulant therapy in, 798–799
  congenital, 784–787, *786*
  congestive heart failure and, 795–796
  history of, 98t
  hypertensive, 791
  ischemic, 791–793, *792*
  myocardial infarction and, 794–795
  pacemaker for, 796–798, *797*
  prophylactic premedication for, 102, 102t
  rheumatic, 787
  sudden death from, 796
Heart valve, endocarditis and, 15
Heat
  polishing causing, 562
  sterilization with, 57–58
Heimlich maneuver, 840, 842t
Helpless patient, 707t, 707–709, *708*
Hemarthrosis, 803t, 814
Hematocrit, 802, 803t, 804t
Hematoma, in hemophilia, 816
Hematopoiesis, 803t
Hemidesmosome, 181t
Hemiplegia, 712t
Hemoglobin, 803t, 804t, 804
Hemolysis
  anemia caused by, 806
  definition of, 803t
Hemophilia, 814–816
  history of, 97t
  risk for HIV, 32
Hemorrhage, 859
  cerebral, 717
  chemotherapy causing, 674
  emergency treatment of, 843t
Hemorrhagic disorder, 813–814
Hemostasis
  anticoagulant therapy and, 799
  definition of, 635
Hemostat, as film positioning device, 150
Heparin, 785t
Hepatic disorder, 100t
Hepatitis, 17–25, 20t
  abbreviations about, 20t
  in Down's syndrome, 754
  summary of, 18t
Hepatitis A, 20t
  immunity and, 21
  transmission and disease process of, 20–21

Hepatitis B, 20t
  dental personnel exposure to, 66t
  disease process of, 23
  patient history of, 99t
  prevention of, 23–24
  risk of, 22–23
  transmission of, 22
Hepatitis C, 20t, 24–25
Hepatitis D, 20t, 25, *25*
Hepatitis E, 20t, 25
Hereditary disorder
  anemia as, 806–809
  cardiovascular, 785
  enamel hypoplasia as, 236–237
  staining from, 284
Herpes simplex virus, 27–29
Herpesvirus infection, 18t, 25–29, 26t
  clinical management of, 28–29
  cytomegalovirus as, 27
  Epstein-Barr virus as, 27
  herpes simplex virus as, 27–28
  latency of, 26
  patient history of, 99t
  varicella-zoster as, 18t, 26–27
Heterotrophic bacteria, 259t
High functioning level, 691
History
  of adolescent patient, 627
  dental, 90, 94t
  diabetes and, 824
  for disabled patient, 681
  endocarditis and, 788
  form for, *88–89*
  hemorrhagic disorder and, 813
  implants and, 400
  interview in, 87, 90
  items included in, 90, 93, 93t–95t, 95
  of lesion, 121
  medical, 93, 95, 95t–101t
  of pacemaker use, 798
  personal, 90, 93t
  preparation for, 85–87
  purposes of, 85
  questionnaire in, 87
  significance of, 85
Hoe scaler, 491–492, *492*
  angulation of, 511
  sharpening of, 502
Holder
  film, *147*
  floss, 695, *695*
  toothpick, 360, *360*, 360, *360*
    for orthodontic patient, 379
Home infusion program in hemophilia, 814
Homebound patient, 705–707, 707t
Homeostasis, 625t
Hone, 489t
Horizontal angulation
  for angle-bisection technique, 152
  for bitewing technique, 151
  definition of, 146–147
Horizontal toothbrushing method, 343
Hormonal contraceptives, 629–630
Hormonal replacement therapy, 625t

Hormone
    definition of, 625t
    puberty and, 624
Hospice, 706t
Hot flash, 630
Human immunodeficiency virus infection,
        18t, 29–36, *30*
    abbreviations about, 29t
    in child, 35–36
    classification system for, 31t, 31–32, 34t
    clinical course of, 32–33
    dental personnel exposure to, 65, 66t
    establishment of, 30
    fetus and, 606, 608
    life cycle of virus and, 29t
    oral manifestations of, 33–35, 34t
    patient history of, 99t
    prevention of, 36
    replication of, 30
    treatment of, 35–36
Humectant
    definition of, 353t
    in dentifrice, 368
Hydrocephalus, 716, *716*, 752
Hydrodynamic mechanism, 556
Hydrokinetic activity, 353t
Hydrostatic, 353t
Hydrotherapy, 353t
Hydroxyapatite, 435t
Hydroxyapatite ceramic, 394t
Hygiene
    autistic patient and, 756
    dental. *See* Dental hygiene
    dentures and, 649, 651
    peri-implant, 401–402
    personal
        fracture and, 666
        hepatitis A and, 21
        plaque and, 203
    stains and, 280
Hyperactivity, 750t, 769
Hypercholerolemia, 712t
Hyperkeratosis, 181t, 191
Hyperopia, 732t
Hyperplasia
    definition of, 181t
    papillary, dentures causing, 650
Hyperpnea, 819t
Hypersensitive teeth, 554–560
    dental hygiene and, 557–558
    dentin and, 554–555
    desensitization of, 556–557
    education about, 558
    factors contributing to, 554
    pain stimuli and, 555–556
Hypertension, 789–791, 790t, 791t. *See also*
        Blood Pressure
    congestive heart failure and, 795
    essential, 789
Hyperthermia, 107t, 859
Hypertonic solution, 366, 859
    after scaling and root planing, 526
Hypertrophy, 181t
Hyperventilation syndrome, 842t, 859
Hypesthesia, 484t
Hypocalcification, 435t

Hypochloride, 387
Hypoglycemia, 819t
Hypoglycemic agent, 819t, 823
Hypoplasia
    definition of, 281t, 859
    enamel, 236–237
        definition of, 232t
    of enamel, 284
Hypotension, 790
    postural, 71t
Hypothyroidism, 751
Hypoxemia, 829t
Hypoxia, 751, 785t

Iatrogenic, 196t, 859
Ice pack, postoperative, 659
Icteric phase of hepatitis A, 21
Identification
    for dentures, 651–653, *652*
        for disabled patient, 701
    medic alert, 841
Idiopathic lesion, 232t, 859
Immediate denture, 647t
    definition of, 377t
Immersion of dentures, 385, 386, 387
Immersion sterilization, 62
Immobile patient transfer, 686
Immobilization, craniomaxillary, 664
Immune globulin, hepatitis, 20t
    A, 21
    B, 24
Immune system
    alcoholism and, 777
    chemotherapy and, 674
    HIV infection and, 30, 33
    necrotizing ulcerative gingivitis and, 537
Immunity
    definition of, 12t, 859
    hepatitis A and, 21
Immunization, 42t
    for dental personnel, 41–42
    hepatitis B, 23, 24
Immunosuppression
    chemotherapy causing, 674
    cytomegalovirus infection and, 27
Impaction, food, 196
    charting of, 317
    plaque formation and, 202
Impairment, 679. *See also* Disability
Impetigo, 19t
Implant, *399*, 399–403, 399–404, *400, 403,
        404*
    definition of, 394t, 647t, 859
Implant supported partial dentures, 381,
        381
Impression
    beading wax of, *168*, 168–169
    definition of, 165t
    disinfection of, 60, 171
    mandibular, 167–170
    materials for, 169
    maxillary, 167, 168, 170–171
    preparation for, 166–167, *167, 168,*
        171–172
    separation of, from cast, 173

Impulse, radiation, 134t
Incident, exposure, 42t
Incipient lesion, 232, 232t, 234
Incubation period of infection, 19t
    definition of, 12t
    of hepatitis A, 21
    of hepatitis B, 23
    of HIV infection, 35
    for tuberculosis, 17
Indices and scoring methods, 287–314
    on bleeding, 299–300
    Calculus Score, 306
    of caries, 308–311
    clinical trial and, 287
    Community Periodontal Index of
        Treatment Needs, 307–308
    Dental Plaque Score, 306–307
    epidemiological survey and, 287–288
    Gingival Index, 302–303, *303*
    index and, 288
    individual assessment score and, 287
    Oral Hygiene Index, 296–298, *297*
    Papillary-Marginal-Attached Gingiva
        Index, 301–302, *302*
    Patient Hygiene Performance, 295–296
    Periodontal Disease Index, *304,*
        304–307, *305*
    Periodontal Index, 303–304
    Periodontal Screening and Recording,
        289, 289–291, *290*
    Plaque Control Record, *292*, 292–293
    Plaque Index and, 291–292
    Plaque-Free Score, 293, 294t, 295, *295*
    Simplified Oral Hygiene Index, 298–299,
        299
Indirect supervision, dental hygienist, 4t
Induration, 117t
Infant, 612–614. *See also* Child
    airway obstruction, 840–841
    anticipatory guidance, 613t
    cytomegalovirus infection in, 27
    of diabetic mother, 821
    external chest compressions on, 838
    fetal alcohol syndrome and, *778,*
        778–779
    fluoride and, 443
    hepatitis B infection in
        immunization and, 23, 24
        perinatal transmission of, 22
    HIV infection in, 35–36
    terminology about, 606t
Infarction, myocardial, 794–795
    emergency treatment of, 844t
Infection, 11–40. *See also* Infection control
    airborne, 14–15
    alcoholism and, 777
    autogenous, 15–16
    cerebrovascular accident and, 718–719
    chemotherapy causing, 674
    cleft lip and palate and, 619, 622
    diabetes and, 820
    in Down's syndrome, 754
    elderly patient and, 636
    endocarditis as, 788–789
    exposure control and, 41–51
    fetal, 606

Infection (*Continued*)
 hepatitis, 17–25, 20t
 leukemia and, 811, 813
 microorganisms of oral cavity and, 11
 myasthenia gravis and, 721
 patient history of, 99t
 periodontal abscess and, 541–543
 process of, 11, 14
 radiation therapy and, 673
 spinal cord injury and, 714, 715
 summary of, 18t–19t
 transmission of
  chain of, *13*
  definition of, 13t
  hands and, 45
  hepatitis A, 20–21
  hepatitis B, 22–23
  hepatitis C, 25
  herpetic whitlow and, 28
  HIV, 32
  ocular herpes and, 28
 tuberculosis, 16–17
 viral
  cytomegalovirus, 27
  Epstein-Barr, 27
  hepatitis as, 17–25. *See also* Hepatitis
   entries
  herpes simplex, 25–26, 27–29
  human immunodeficiency, 29–36. *See
   also* Human immunodeficiency virus
   infection
  latent, 26
  listing of, 18t
  varicella zoster, 26–27
Infection control, 52–69
 exposure control in, 41–51. *See also*
   Exposure control
 implant and, 401
 inanimate objects, classification of, 63t
 oral, 333–351
  rehabilitated mouth and, 396
  toothbrushing in, 333–351. *See also*
   Toothbrushing
 orthodontic appliance and, 377–378
 in treatment area, 52, 54
  chemical sterilants for, 62
  cleaning and, 55
  disinfectants for, 59–62, 60t, 61t
  instruments and, 54, 64
  needle recapping and, *66*
  objectives of, 52
  packaging and, 55–56
  patient education about, 67–68
  patient preparation and, 64–65
  preparation for appointment and,
   62–64
  presoaking and, 54–55
  radiography and, 144, 154–155
  sterilization and, *55*, 56–59
  for study impression, 171
  technical hints for, 67
  terminology for, 53t
  universal precautions and, 65
  waste disposal and, 67
Infectious mononucleosis, 18t, 27
Infectious waste, 53t, 67

Infiltrate, leukemic, 811
 in gingiva, 812
Infiltration anesthesia, 507t
Inflammation
 dentures and, 650
 early lesion of, 195–196
 gingival, 187–188
  plaque and, 268–269
 leukemia and, 812
 periodontitis and, 197
 toothbrushing and, 347
Influenza virus, 19t
Informed consent. *See* Consent
Infraversion, 250
Infusion, in hemophilia, 814
Inhalant, street names of, 129t
Inhalation, tuberculosis transmission and,
   16–17
Inhalation anesthesia, 667
Inherent filtration, 137
Inherited disorder. *See* Hereditary disorder
Injection, surface antiseptic and, 64
Injection site
 abscess at, 15
 preparation of, 16
Inlay, 394t
Inoculation, 42t, 859
Inorganic elements, 859
 in calculus, 277
 in plaque, 265
Inorganic salts in blood, 804
In-service education, 699–701
Instrument, 473–487
 activation of, 480–481, *481*
 adaptation of, 479, *479*
 for air application, 208–209
 angulation of, 479–480
 broken, 521–522
 cleaning of, 55
 curets, 488–490, *489*
 dexterity with, 481–483, *482*
 disabled patient and, 702
 for examination, 81, 117
 fulcrum of, 477–479
 for gingival curettage, 529
 grasping of, 475–477, *476*
 for home visit, 705–706
 identification of, 473–474
 implant and, 401, 403, *404*
 infection control and, 54, 70
 lateral pressure and, 480
 mouth mirror and, 207–208
 neutral positions for, 477, *477*
 packaging of, 55–56
 parts of, *474*, 474–475
 presoaking of, 54–55
 scalers and, 490–493, *491–493*
 sharpening of, 494–504, *496–504*. *See
   also* Sharpening of instruments
 for stain removal, 567–569
 sterile, 56–59, 64
 terminology about, 489t
 visibility and accessibility of, 481
Instrumentation
 adolescent patient and, 627
 in alcoholic patient, 782

 amalgam restorations and, 586, 587
 arthritis and, 728
 for cancer patient, 676
 cleft lip and palate and, 622
 cumulative trauma from, 483–486,
   484–486, 486t
 for disabled patient, 701–702
 endocarditis and, 788, 789
 fracture and, 664
 hemophilia and, 815–816
 for homebound patient, 707
 pacemaker patient and, 798
 pregnancy and, 610
 presurgery treatment and, 657
 for scaling. *See* Scaling and root planing
Instrumentation zone, 481, 512, 515, 507t
Insulin, 819–820
 definition of, 819t
Insulin reaction, 821t
 emergency treatment of, 845t
Insulin-dependent diabetes mellitus,
   818–819, 820t
Intelligence quotient, 750t
Interdental brush, 358–359, *358, 359*
Interdental care, 352–361
 anatomy of, 352–353
 dental floss and tape for, 353–356, *355,
   356*
 gauze strip for, 357, *357*
 irrigation for, 362
 knitting yarn for, 357, *357*
 orthodontic appliance and, 379, *379*
 partial dentures and, 382
 terminology about, 353t
Interdental gingiva, 185
 healthy, 191
Interdental tip, 359
Interdisciplinary team, 706t
Interface, implant, 401
Intermaxillary fixation, 661–662, *662*, 664
 in edentulous patient, 663
 internal suspension wire, 664
International numbering system, 82, *82,
   83*, 84
Interocclusal record, 166
 definition of, 165t
Interproximal space, 353t
Interstitial implant, 672
Intervention for treatment, 321t
Interview, patient, 87, 90
 form for, 90, *91–92*
Intestine, fluoride and, 434
Intracerebral embolism, 717
Intraoral examination, 116–132, 119,
   120t–121t. *See also* Examation
 HIV infection and, 34
 tuberculosis and, 17
Intrauterine infection, HIV, 35
Intrinsic, 281t
Intrinsic stain, 280, 283–285
Iodine preparation, 408
Iodophor, 61
Ionomer, glass, 435t
Iontophoresis, 558
IQ, 750t
Iron deficiency anemia, 807

Irradiation, 134t
Irrigant, 353t
Irrigation, 361–364, *362, 363*
    definition of, 353t
    gingival curettage and, 530–531
    orthodontic appliance and, 379
    subgingival, *531*, 531–532
Irrigator, 353t
Ischemia, 712t
    definition of, 785t
    stroke and, 717
Ischemic heart disease, 791–793, *792*
Isolation procedure for fluoride
        application, 447
Isotonic solution, 365
    definition of, 353t, 860

Jaw
    dislocated, 847t
    fracture of, 659–666, *660–663*
Jaw thrust, 835
Jeweler's rouge, 566
Joints. *See also* Temporomandibular Joint.
    arthritis of, 726–728
    hemophilia and, 814
    scleroderma of, 728
Joule, 140
Junction
    cementoenamel, 200, *200*
        in Periodontal Disease Index, 304–305
        probe examination of, 216
    mucogingival, 186
Junctional epithelium, 184–185
Juvenile periodontitis, 626
    classification, 198t
    microorganisms of, 264t
Juvenile rheumatoid arthritis, 727

Keratinization, 181t, 860
Ketoacidosis, 819t
Ketone bodies, 819t
Kidney disorder, 100t
Kilovoltage, 138–139
Kilovoltage peak, 135
Knife, amalgam, 587
Knitting yarn for flossing, 357, *357*
    partial dentures and, 382
Korotkoff sounds, 107t
Korsakoff's Syndrome, 778
Kyphosis, 712t

Labioversion, 250
Language, body, 71t
Latency, viral, 26
Latent image, 134t
Latent infection, HIV, 33, 35
Lateral pressure, on instrument, 480
Lathe, polishing on, 572–573
Lavage, 353t
Le Fort classification of fractures, *661*
Lead apron, 143, *144*
    for pacemaker patient, 798
    for pregnant patient, 609
Leakage radiation, 134t, 142
Learning disability, cerebral palsy and, 724

Learning process, *412*, 412–413
Left heart failure, 795
Legal issues, dental hygiene, 6
Lens, contact, 45
Leonard toothbrushing method, 343
Lesion
    agranulocytosis and, 810–811
    cancerous, 124–125
    definition of, 196
    dentures causing, 649–650
    elevated, 122, 123t, 124
    examination of, 121–122, *122*, 123t,
        124, 124t
    idiopathic, 232t
    incipient, 232, 232t, 234
    nutrition and, 423
    oral, HIV, 33, 34t
    subsurface, 435t
Lethal radiation dose, 141t
Leukemia, 811–813
Leukocyte, 802, 805–806
    CD4+ count, HIV, 31
    definition of, 259t
Leukocytes, 805–806
Leukocytosis, 803t, 811
Leukopenia, 803t, 810–811
License, 4t
Lidocaine, 520
Life expectancy, 635
Ligament, periodontal, 182–183
Light cured sealant, 462
Lighting, 76
    for home care, 706
Linguoversion, 250
Lining mucosa, 181–182
Lips
    cleft, 617–623, *619, 620*
    diabetes and, 824
    in Down's syndrome, 753
    in elderly patient, 637
    examination of, 120t
    fetal development of, 605
    seizures and, 743–744
Liver
    alcohol metabolism and, 777
    hepatitis of, 17–25, 20t. *See also* Hepatitis
    leukemia and, 811
Liver disorder, 100t
LLD50/30 radiation dose, 141t
Local anesthesia, 507t
Local factor, 202
Localized juvenile periodontitis, 626
Long axis of tooth, 147
Lozenge, fluoride, 442
Luxation, 857
Lymph node
    examination of, 119, 120t
    leukemia and, 811
Lymphadenopathy, 117t, 811, 860
    in AIDS, 31, 33
Lymphocyte, 806
Lysis, 803t

Macrocephaly, 712t
Macrocyte, 803t

Maintainer, space, 379–381, *380*
    definition of, 377t
Maintenance
    diabetes and, 825
    hemophilia patient and, 816
    implant and, 402–403
    periodontal, 394t
    preventive, 599–601
        cancer patient and, 676–677
        for infant or toddler, 614
        rehabilitated mouth and, 398–399
Maintenance examination, 81, 600
Maintenance phase of treatment plan,
        321–322, 860
Major depressive disorder, 763–764
Malaise, 537, 860
Male sexual development, 624–625
Malignancy, 669–678. *See also* Cancer
    examination for, 124–125
    history of, 98t
Malnutrition, 423
Malocclusion
    cerebral palsy and, 724
    classification of, 250–253, *251–253*
    cleft lip and palate and, 618
    definition of, 248, 249t
    in disabled patient, 689
    fluoride and, 440
    plaque formation and, 202
Mandible, dislocated, 847t, *848*
Mandibular fracture, 660
Mandibular teeth
    cast of, 174–177, *175–177*
    eruption of, 233t
    flossing of, 354
    impression of, 167–168, *169–170*
    loss of, *380*
    numbering of, *83*
    paralleling technique for, *149*
Mandrel, handpiece with, 568
Mandrel mounted stone, 501–502
Manic phase of bipolar disorder, 765
Mantoux test, 42t
Manual, office policy, 67
Manual alphabet, *737*
Manual cleaning
    of denture, 572
    of instruments, 55
Manual toothbrush, *334*, 334–336, *335*
Margin, gingival, 184
Marginal irregularities of restoration, *582*,
        582–583
Margination of restoration, 585, *587*,
        587–588
Marker
    definition of, 181t
    serum, 12t
Marking of dentures, 651–653, *652*
    for disabled patient, 701
Marrow
    depression of, 812
    leukemia and, 811
    leukopenia and, 810
    transplant of, 812
Massage, of mucosa, 389
Mastalgia, 625t

Mastication, 181t
Masticatory mucosa, 181
Materia alba, 260t
    definition of, 259t
Matrix
    calculus and, 273t, 276–277
    plaque and, 262
Maturation
    definition of, 259t, 435t
    fluoride and, 436
    of plaque, 275
Maturity, 625t
Maxillary fracture, 660, 663–664
Maxillary midline projection, 152
Maxillary teeth
    cast of, 174–177, *175–177*
    eruption of, 233t
    flossing of, 354
    geometric charting form for, *316*
    impression of, 167, 168, 170–171
    numbering of, *83*
    paralleling technique for, *148*
    in underjet, 250
Maxillofacial and oral surgery, 655–668
    for cleft lip and palate, 621
    dental hygiene and, 657–659
    for fracture, 659–666
    implant placement, 401
    patient preparation for, 655–656
    terminology about, 656t
Maximum permissible radiation dose, 141t
McCall's festoon, 190
Measles, 19t
Mechanical plaque control, 334t
Mechanical x-ray timer, 136
Mechanics, body, 71t
Median nerve, 483
    definition of, *484*, 484t
Medic alert identification, 841
Medical consultation, 101
Medical history, 93, 95, 95t–101t
Medications. *See also* Drug therapy.
    history of, 96t, 96t–101t
    sucrose in, 36, 431, 614
Megaloblastic anemia, 807–808
Membrane, tympanic, 732t
Menarche, 628
Meningocele, 715–716
Menopause, 630–631
    definition of, 625t
Menstruation, *628*, 628–629
Mental disorder, 101t, 759–774. *See also*
        Psychiatric disorder
    HIV and, 33
Mental health, 6
Mental retardation, 749–758
    autism and, 754–756, 755t
    cerebral palsy and, 724
    characteristics of, 752
    dental instruction and, 752
    Down's syndrome and, 752–754
    etiology of, 751
    maintenance treatment and, 599
    mild, 749
    moderate, 749–750
    profound, 750
    severe, 750
    terminology about, 750t

Merbromin, 409
Mercurochrome preparation, 408
Mercury, in restoration, 583
Mercury hygiene, 584
Mercury manometer, 112
Mercury-column thermometer, 108
Mesioclusion, 253, *253*
Mesognathic profile, 249, *249*
Metabolic disorder, 751
Metabolism
    of alcohol, 776–777
    definition of, 423
Metal plate for fixation of fracture, 661
Metallic stain, 283
Microbial plaque, 260t
Microcephaly, 712t
Microorganism
    in aerosol, 14–15
    black stain line and, 282
    definition of, 259t
    infectious diseases, 18t, 19t
    irrigation and, 363
    plaque formation and, 262–263, *263*,
        265
    scaling and root planing, 527t, 527–528
Migration, pathologic, 249t, 255
Milk, breast, HIV in, 35
Milliamperage control, 135–136
Milliampere seconds, 139
Mineral, pregnancy and, 612
Mineralization
    calculus and, 260t, 273t, 275–276
    fluoride and, 436
    of permanent teeth, 231
Mirror
    dexterity with, 483
    for disabled patient, 684
    mouth, 207–208
Missing teeth, indices of, 309–310
Mixed dentition, 231
    definition of, 232t, *234*
    radiography of, 154
Mixing bowl, for impression, 165
Mobility examination, 223–224
Model, as teaching aid, 419–420
Modified jaw thrust, 835
Modified pen grasp, 476, *476*
Modified Stillman toothbrushing method,
        340, 341
Moist heat sterilization, 57–58
Molar
    bone loss and, *226*
    first permanent, occlusion and, *254*, 255
    occlusion and, 252, *253*
    primary dentition, 254
    probe examination of, 214–215
Molt's mouth gag, 702
Monitoring
    of radiation exposure, 143
    of sterilization, 67
Monocyte, 806
Mononucleosis, infectious, 18t, 27
Mood disorder, 763
Morphologic categories, oral lesions, 122,
        124
Morphology, 117t

Mottled enamel, fluoride and, 438–439
Mounted sharpening stone, 501–502
Mounting of radiograph, 158, 160
Mouth
    clearing of, in CPR, 837
    floor of, examination of, 121t
Mouth mirror, 207–208
Mouth prop, 702
    for disabled patient, 696–697
Mouth-held implements, 715
Mouthrinse, 364–367, 365t
    cosmetic, 365
    fluoride, 442, 450–452. *See also* Rinse
    study cast preparation and, 166
Mouth-to-mouth ventilation, 841
Moving flat stone, 496–498, *497*
Mucogingival examination, 217, *217*, *218*
Mucogingival junction, 186
Mucosa
    abnormalities of, *122*
    alveolar, 186
    anatomy of, 181–182
    dentures and, 649
    diabetes and, 824
    of disabled patient, 700
    disclosing agent and, 407
    of edentulous patient, 647
    in elderly patient, 637
    examination of, 121t
    menopause and, 631
    nonkeratinized, 181t
    nutrition and, 423
    radiation effects on, 673
    underlying denture, 389
Multidrug-resistant tuberculosis, 17
Multiple sclerosis, 721–722
Mumps, 19t
Murmur, heart, 785t
Muscle
    Bell's palsy and, 725
    cerebral palsy and, 724
Muscle coordination, cleft lip and palate
        and, 618
Muscular dystrophy, 719–720
Mutism, 750t
Myasthenia gravis, 720–721
Mycobacterium tuberculosis, 16–17, 19t
Mycoplasma, 259t
Myelocyte, 803t
Myelomeningocele, 715–717, *716*
Myocardial infarction, 794–795
    emergency treatment of, 844t
Myocardium, 785t
Myopathy, 712t
Myopia, 732t

National Council on Radiation, 141
Natural bristle of toothbrush, 336
Necrosis, 537
Necrotic zone of necrotizing ulcerative
        gingivitis, 537
Necrotizing ulcerative gingivitis, 536–541,
        537, 537t
    in adolescent, 626
    clinical recognition of, 536–538

definition of, 537
development of, 538–539
etiology of, 538
HIV infection and, 34–35
microorganisms of, 264t
toothbrushing and, 347
treatment of, 539–541
Needle
    hepatitis B and, 24
    infection prevention and, 16
    marks of, on arm, 129
    recapping, 65, 66
    surface antiseptic and, 64
    for suturing, 550
    universal precautions and, 65, 65
Needlestick, 65
    exposure protocol, 66t
Neglect, 127
Neisseria gonorrhoeae, 19t
Neivert whittler, 500–501, 501
Neonate
    cytomegalovirus infection in, 27
    hepatitis B infection in
        immunization for, 23, 24
        perinatal transmissions of, 22
    HIV in, 35
Neoplasm. *See also* Cancer
    examination for, 124–125
    history of, 98t
    HIV and, 33
Nerves
    Bell's palsy and, 725
    hypersensitivity and, 556, 556
    median, in carpal tunnel, 483, 484, 484t
    shingles and, 27
Neurosurgery, 716, 716–717
Neutroclusion, 252, 253
Neutropenia, 803t
Neutrophil, 806
Neutrophil-rich zone of necrotizing
        ulcerative gingivitis, 537
Newborn. *See also* Infant
    cytomegalovirus infection in, 27
    hepatitis B infection in
        immunization for, 23, 24
        perinatal transmissions of, 22
Nidus
    for bacteria, 260
    definition of, 273t
Nifedipine, 203
Nodule, subcutaneous, 787
Non-A, non-B hepatitis, 24–25
Nonblisterform lesion, 122, 124, 123t
Non–insulin-dependent diabetes mellitus,
        819, 820t
Nonsharp instruments, 474
Nonsurgical periodontal therapy, 196, 507t
Normal occlusion, 248
Normal overbite, 250, 251
Normotensive blood pressure, 107t
NUG. *See* necrotizing ulcerative gingivitis
Numbering system, tooth, 81, 82, 83, 84
Nursing caries, 36, 234, 236, 613–614
Nutrient, 423
Nutrition. *See also* Diet
    definition of, 423
    in medical history, 97t

Nutritional deficiency, 422
    alcoholic patient and, 782
    alcoholism and, 777
    anemia and, 806–807
    anorexia nervosa and, 769
    elderly patient and, 642–643
Nylon toothbrush, 337

Obesity, in disabled patient, 699
Object-film distance, 139
Objective symptom, 81
Objectives for practice, 6–7
Obligate bacteria, 259t
Oblique fiber, 183
Observation, direct, 81, 118
Obsessive-compulsive disorder, 767
Obstruction of airway, 839–841, 842t
Obturator, 377t
    cleft palate for, 621
Occlusal adjustment, 394t
Occlusal brushing, 344–346
Occlusal plane, 146
    definition of, 165t
Occlusal radiographic survey, 152
    in disabled patient, 688
    films for, 146
    purpose of, 146
Occlusal survey, of primary dentition, 154
Occlusion, 248–257
    cardiac, 785t
    centric, 165t
    charting of, 317
    cleft lip and palate and, 618
    in Down's syndrome, 754
    functional, 254–255
    ideal, 248
    malocclusion classifications and,
        250–253, 251–253
    of primary teeth, 253–254, 254
    sealant and, 466, 466
    static, 248–250, 251, 251t
    teaching patient about, 256–257
    terminology about, 249t
    trauma from, 255–256
        definition of, 249t
Occupational Safety and Health
        Administration, 53t
Ocular herpes, 28
Odontoblastic process, 555, 555, 556
Odontoplasty, 394t
Odor, breath, 120t. *See also* Halitosis.
Office policy manual, 67
    emergency procedures, 834
Office Sterilization and Asepsis Procedures
        Research Foundation, 53t
Offset blade, 489t
Oligomenorrhea, 625t
One rescuer in CPR, 838
One-step method of forming cast, 172–173
Onlay, 394t
Open bite, 250, 251
Operating stool. *See* Clinician's stool
Ophthalmologist, 732t
Ophthalmology, 732t
Opioid, street names of, 129t

Opportunistic infection, HIV and, 33,
        34–35
Optician, 732t
Optometrist, 732t
Oral cancer, 669–678. *See also* Cancer
Oral contraceptives, 629–630
Oral epithelium, 181t
Oral flora, 259t
Oral glucose tolerance test, 819t
Oral health, 6
Oral Hygiene Index, 296–298, 297
Oral hypoglycemic agent, 819t
Oral irrigation, 361–364, 362, 363
    definition of, 353t
    fractured jaw and, 666
    professionally applied, 531
Oral manifestations of HIV infection, 33,
        34t
Oral mucosa. *See* Mucosa
Oral prophylaxis, 472
Oral surgery, 655–668. *See also*
        Maxillofacial and oral surgery
    for cleft lip and palate, 622
Oral temperature, 108
    necrotizing gingivitis and, 537
Orange stain, 283
Organic elements
    in calculus, 277
    in plaque, 265–266
Orientation, for disabled patient, 684–685
Orthodontic appliance, 376–379, 377t,
        378, 379
    debonding of, 595
Orthodontic orthopedics, 249t
Orthodontic therapy
    for cleft lip and palate, 621
    maintenance treatment and, 599
    preventive, 377t
Orthopedics
    definition of, 249t
    myelomeningocele and, 717
Orthosis, 712t
Osmotic pain stimulus, 555
Osseous integration, 394t
Osteoarthritis, 727–728
Osteopenia, 635
Osteoporosis, 636
    definition of, 635
    leukemia and, 811
Otitis, 732t
Otologist, 732t
Overbite, 250, 251, 252
Overdenture
    caries and, 651
    complete, 389, 390
    definition of, 647t
Overgrowth of gingiva, phenytoin-
        induced, 203, 690, 724, 743, 744,
        744–745
Overhanging restoration, 582–583
    radiography and, 227
    removal of, 587–589
Overjet, 250, 251
Over-the-counter medication, 86t
Oxygen administration, 841
Oxygen tank, 830

Oxygenating agent, 366
Oxyhemoglobin, 803t

Pacemaker, cardiac, 796–798, *797*
Packaging, infection control and, 55–56
Pain
  angina pectoris, 793
  arthritis, 727
  chest, 794
  myocardial infarction and, 794
  postsurgical, 548t, 659
  sickle cell anemia, 809
Painting
  of disclosing agent, 409
  of fluoride, 445–446
Palate
  cleft, 617–623. *See also* Cleft lip and
    palate
  in Down's syndrome, 753–754
  examination of, 121t
  fetal development of, 605
Palliative treatment, 706t
Palm grasp, 476, *476*
Palmar crease, 753
Palmer system of tooth numbering, *83, 84*
Palpation, 81
  definition of, 117t
  methods, 118
Palsy, Bell's, 725
  cerebral, 722–725
Pandemic, 12t
Panic attack, 766t, 766–767
Panoramic radiography, 152–153
  in disabled patient, 688
Papilla, gingival
  disease changes in, 189
  healthy, 190
  interdental, 185
  of tongue, *182, 182*
Papillary bleeding, on Plaque-Free Score,
    293, 295
Papillary hyperplasia, dentures causing,
    650
Papillary-Marginal-Attached Gingiva
    Index, 301–302, *302*
Papoose board, *688*
Parafunctional condition, 249t
Paralleling technique, 145, *146*
Paralysis
  bladder and bowel, 716
  cerebrovascular accident and, 718
  definition of, 712t
  facial, 689
  spinal cord injury, 713
Paramyxovirus, 19t
Parasite, 259t
Parent
  abusive, 128
  anticipatory guidance, 613t
  of disabled child, 696–698, *697*
  teaching of, 418, 612–614
Parenteral route, 829t
  definition of, 12t, 537
Paresis, 712t
Paresthesia, 484t

Parking, for disabled patient, 683
Parkinson's disease, 725–726
Parotitis, 19t
Partial defluoridation, 441
Partial denture
  fixed, *381,* 381–382
    definition of, 377t
  removable, 377t, 382–384, *383, 384*
Parts per million, 435t
  dentifrice, 452
  fluoridation, *438,* 439
  school fluoridation, 441
  in tooth structure, 437
  water analysis for, 442, 613t
Passive immunity, 12t
  hepatitis A, 21
Paste
  denture, 386, 388
  fluoride, 567
  for coronal polish, 565–567
Patent ductus arteriosus, 785, *786*
Pathogen, definition of, 12t, 259t. *see also*
    Infection
Pathognomonic signs and symptoms, 81
Pathologic migration, 249t, 255
Patient Hygiene Performance, 295–296
Patient preparation, 70
  disabled, 679–689
  infection control and, 64–65
  positioning and, 73–76, *73–76*
  for study casts, 165–166
Pedunculated polyp, 117t
Pellicle
  bacteria attached to, 260, *261*
  brown, 283
  calculus and, 275, *276*
  definition of, 260t
  on dentures, 385
  plaque and, 258–259
  subsurface, 258
Pen grasp, 476, *476*
Penumbra, 134t
Percussion, in examination, 81
Percutaneous, 12t
Periapical survey
  angle-bisection technique for, 151–152
  disabled patient and, 688
  in edentulous patient, 154
  films for, 146
  paralleling technique for, 147, *148, 149,*
    150
  purpose of, 145
Periodontal therapy, charting of, *318*
Peri-implant hygiene, 401–402
Peri-implantitis, 394t
Perimylolysis, 771
Perinatal infection, hepatitis B as, 22
Periodontal charting, 217–219, *218*
Periodontal disease. *See also* Periodontitis;
    Periodontium
  abscess as, 541–543
  case types, 196t
  cerebral palsy and, 724
  in disabled patient, 689–690
  in Down's syndrome, 754

fluoride and, 440–441
fracture and, 664
HIV infection and, 34–35
indices of, 289, 290t, 291
  Community Periodontal Index of
    Treatment Needs, 307–308
  Periodontal Disease Index, *304,*
    304–307, *305*
  Periodontal Index, 303–304
mentally retarded patient and, 752
overhanging restoration and, 583
plaque causing, 267
radiography of, 225–227, *225–227*
rehabilitation and, 394–395
severity and extent of, 212–213
Periodontal ligament
  attachment apparatus, 181t
  gingival fibers, 182, *182*
  mobility and, 223
  pocket formation and, 197, 199
  principal fibers, 183, *183*
  radiography and, 226–227, *227*
Periodontal pocket. See Pocket
Periodontal prosthesis, 393
Periodontal Screening and Recording, *289,*
    289–291, *290*
Periodontal surgery
  gingiva after, 193
  toothbrushing after, 347
Periodontal therapy
  anticoagulation therapy and, 799
  charting of, 315, 317
  definition of, 507t
  elderly patient and, 641
  hemophilia patient and, 815–816, *816*
  maintenance, 394t, 599–600
  mouthrinse after, 364–365
  nonsurgical, 196
    education about, 532
    evaluation for, 525
    gingival curettage as, 528–531, *529*
    gingival irrigation as, *531,* 531–532
    patient instructions about, 526–527
    scaling and root planing as. *See* Scaling
      and root planing
    terminology about, 526t
  overdenture and, 389
  pregnancy and, 609
  treatment plan for, 322
Periodontitis, 197
  adult, 264t
  in child, 192–193
  juvenile, 264t, 626
  classification of, 198t
  definition of, 196
  early-onset, 626
  HIV and, 34t, 34, 35
  necrotizing ulcerative. *See* Necrotizing
    ulcerative gingivitis
  organisms causing, 264t
  plaque and, 268
  rapid progressive, 35, 264t
  refractory, 264t
  types of, 196t

Periodontium. *See also* Periodontal *entries*;
    Periodontitis
    anatomy of, 182–183
    debonding and, 595
    definition of, 181t
    diabetes and, 823
    diet and, 422
    in elderly patient, 638–639
    evaluation of, 597
    infection of, 195–197, 196t
    overdenture and, 389
    probe examination and, 209–210, 211t,
        211–214, 212–215
Periodontometer, 208t
Permanent dentition
    definition of, 232t
    eruption of, 233t
    numbering of, 82, *83*, 84
    occlusion and, *254*, 255
    tooth measurements, 866
Permeability, 196
Permissible radiation dose, 141
Permucosal, 12t
Pernicious anemia, 807–808
Personal history, 90, 93t
Personal hygiene, plaque and, 203
Personal protection against infection, 41
Personal supervision, 4t
Pertussis, 19t
Petechia, 117t, 803t, 813
pH
    definition of, 232t
    demineralization
        dentin, 268
        enamel, 268
    of plaque, 268, 430
Phagocytosis, 803t
Pharmacologic therapy. *See* Drug therapy
Pharyngitis, gonococcal, 19t
Phelan's test, 484t
Phencyclidine, street names of, 129t
Phenolic, 62
Phenylketonuria, 751
Phenytoin
    cerebral palsy and, 724
    gingival changes from, 203, 690, 743,
        744, 744–745
Phobic disorder, 767
Phosphorus, plaque and, 265
Photoelectric effect electrons, defined, 134t
Photopolymerization, 466
Physical health dental hygienist, 6
Physical impairment. *See* Disability
Physician, consultation with, 101
Physicians' Desk Reference, 86t
Physiologic toothbrushing method, 343
Pica, 750t
Piezoelectric scaling, 517
Pigment, stained tooth and, 284–285
Pigmentation, mucosal, 125
Pigtail explorer, 221
Pipe cleaner, 360
Pit and fissure, location of, 462–463
Pit and fissure caries, 234
    recognition of, 242

Pit and fissure sealant. *See* Sealant
Plane
    occlusal, 165t
    sagittal or median, 146
Planing, root. *See* Scaling and root planing
Plaque, 258–271
    acquired pellicle and, 258, 260
    adolescent patient and, 627
    arthritis and, 728
    calculus and, 277
    cancer patient and, 675
    caries and, 231, *267*, 267–268
    cerebrovascular accident and, 718–719
    charting of, 317
    clinical aspects of, 266–267
    composition of, 265–266
    dentifrice and, 369
    on dentures, 385
    diabetes and, 825
    diet and, 269
    disabled patient and, 684, 691–692,
        696–697, 701
    disclosing agent and, 409
    dressing and, 549
    education about, 270, 416
    elderly patient and, 641–642
    fluoride and, 438
    follow-up evaluation of, 598
    food debris and, 269
    formation of, 260, 262, *262*
    gingival and periodontal disease and,
        201
    gingival disease and, 192
    green stains caused by, 281–282
    hemophilia patient and, 815
    hypersensitive teeth and, 557
    implant and, 401–402
    indices of, 291–295, *292*, 294t
        Dental Plaque Score and, 306–307
        disabled patient and, 700
    infant or toddler and, 613
    inflammation and, 195–196
    interdental brushing and, 358
    interdental removal of, 353
    irrigation and, 364
    materia alba and, 269
    maturation of, 275
    mechanical control of, 334t
    microorganisms causing, 262, *263*, 264t
    myasthenia gravis and, 721
    orthodontic appliance and, 377–378
    overhanging restoration and, 583
    partial dentures and, 381–382, 384
    periodontal infections and, 264t,
        268–269
    phenytoin overgrowth and, 745
    postoperative period and, 659
    pregnancy and, 611
    in preschool child, 417
    presurgery treatment and, 657
    rehabilitated mouth and, 396, *396*
    stain removal and, 567
    subgingival, 261t, 262–263, 265
    supragingival, 263t
    technical hints about, 269
    terminology about, 259t, 260t

Plaque Control Record, *292*, 292–293
Plaque Index, 291–292
Plaque-Free Score, 293, 294t, 295, *295*
Plasma, 803–804
Plasma-derived vaccine, hepatitis B, 24
Plaster, dental, 165t
Plastic testing stick, 495
Platelets, 806
    hemorrhagic disorder and, 813–814
Pleomorphism, 259t
Pliers, 483
    debonding, 594
Pneumonia, streptococcal, 19t
Pocket
    calculus and, 277
    complications of, 200–201, *201*
    development of, 197–198
    irrigation and, 363, 531–532
    microorganisms in, 264t
    periodontal abscess and, 542
    probe examination of, 209–210, 211t,
        211–214, 212–215
    radiography and, 227
    scaling and, 513
    subgingival examination and, 222
Pocket epithelium
    formation of, 196
Pocket wall, tooth surface, 198–200, *199*,
    200
Poisoning, 847t
Policy manual, 67, 834
Poliovirus, 19t
Polisher, porte, 576–579, 577t, *578*
Polishing
    of amalgam restoration, 580, 585,
        588–589
    effects of, 561–563
    fluoride and, 456
    of study cast, 165t, 177
Polishing agents
    in dentifrice, 368
    for stain removal, 565–566
Polyarthritis, 726–728
Polycythemia, 809–810
Polydipsia, 819t
Polyp, 117t
Polyphagia, 819t
Polyuria, 819t
Pontic
    definition of, 377t
    shape of, *395*
Porte polisher, 576–579, 577t, *578*
Polyphyromonas gingivalis, 264t
Position
    of clinician, 71–73, *72*
    of film, 150
    of patient, 73–76, *73–76*
        disabled, 687, 697, 697–698
    for study cast, 165
Position-indicating device, 137, *138*
    radiation protection and, 142
Posterior crossbite, *251*
Posteruptive stage of tooth development,
    fluoride and, 436
Postictal phase of seizure, 747

Postoperative care
  anticoagulant therapy and, 799
  cardiovascular surgery and, 799–800
  for cleft lip and palate, 622
  dressing and, 545–547, 549
  instructions for, 548t
  oral surgery and, 658–659
Postpartum mood disturbance, 766
Post-traumatic stress disorder, 767
Postural hypotension, 71t
Powder, denture, 386
Power-assisted toothbrush, 334t
  for disabled patient, 694–695
PPD, 42t
ppm, 435t. *See* Parts per million
Prebook method of maintenance
    appointments, 600
Precautions, universal, 65, *65*
  definition of, 13t
Precleaning of instruments, 54–55
  holding solution for, 60
Predisposing factor, 202
Pre-eruptive stage of tooth development,
    fluoride and, 435–436
Prefixes, 851–853
Pregnancy, 101t, 605–612
  care during, 608–609, 610t
  dental hygiene during, 609–611
  diabetes during, 819, 819t, 821
  drug effects and, 606, 607t, 608, 608t,
    751
  fetal alcohol syndrome and, *778*,
    778–779
  fetal development and, 605–606
  infections in, 751
  oral findings during, 608
  patient instruction during, 611–612
  anticipatory guidance, 613t
  postpartum mood disturbance and, 766
  rubella and, 786
  terminology about, 606t
Preicteric phase of hepatitis A, 21
Prematurity, occlusal, 249t
Premedication. *See also* Drug therapy
  definition of, 86t
  drug abuse and, 130
  for elderly patient, 640
  for endocarditis, 101–103, 102t, 789
  hemophilia patient and, 815
  pacemaker patient and, 798
  prophylactic. *See* Prophylactic antibiotic
  scaling and root planing and, 507
  for study casts, 165
  subgingival irrigation and, 532
Premenstrual syndrome, 625t, 629
Premolar, probe examination of, 214–215
Prenatal fluoride, 440
Prenatal infection, 751
Preparation of patient. *See* Patient
    preparation
Preparatory phase of treatment plan, 321
Preschool child, teaching of, 417–418
Preservative, in dentifrice, 368
Presoaking of instruments, 54–55
Pressure
  in hemostasis, 799

sterilization and, 58
  trauma from occlusion and, 255
Pressure dressing, 546t
Pressure sore, spinal cord injury and, 714
Prevention
  anticipatory guidance, 613t
  of airway obstruction, 839
  of calculus, 278, 369
  cancer patient and, 676–677
  chemotherapy in, 361–370
  counseling about, 331
  of diabetes mellitus, 825–826
  diet and, 422–433. *See also* Diet
  for disabled patient, 685, 690–691
  disclosing agents and, 407–410, *408*,
    408t
  disease control and, 411–421. *See also*
    Infection control
  education about, 331
  elderly patient and, 640–641
  of emergencies, 828–829
  of endocarditis, 787, 788–789
  fluoride and, 434–461. *See also* Fluoride
  of gagging, 144–145
  hemophilia patient and, 815
  implants and, 399–404, *403, 404*
  of infection, 333–351
    cytomegalovirus, 27
    general measures for, 15
    of hepatitis A, 21
    of hepatitis B, 23–24
    of hepatitis C, 25
    of hepatitis D, 25
    human immunodeficiency virus, 36
  interdental care in, 352–361. *See also*
    Interdental care
  maintenance phase of, 599–601
  prosthesis care and, 376–392. *See also*
    Prosthesis
  rehabilitation and, 393–399, 394t, *395,*
    396, 397t
  sealants for, 462–472. *See also* Sealant
  self-cleansing mechanisms and, 330
  steps in, 330–331
  toothbrushing in, 333–351. *See also*
    Toothbrushing
  treatment plan and, 321
Preventive maintenance, dentures and,
    650–651
Preventive orthodontics, 377t
Preventive services, 3
Prevotella intermedia, 264t
Primary dentition
  definition of, 232t
  eruption of, 233t
  formation of, 231
  gingiva and, 192
  numbering of, 82, 84
  occlusion of, 253–254, *254*
  radiography of, 153
  tooth measurements, 865t
Primate space, in primary dentition, 253,
    254
Priority treatment plan, 321
Probe
  angulation of, 480
  calculus and, 275

circumferential probing, 214
  definition of, 208t
  examination with, 209–210, *211–214,*
    212–215
  hemophilia patient and, 815–816
  measuring lesion with, *122*
  periodontal, 289, *289*
  plaque and, 266–267
  scaling and root planing and, 508–509,
    509
  types of, *211,* 211t
Probing depth, 181t, *212*
  definition of, 208t
  follow-up evaluation of, 598
  recording of, 218, *218*
Procedure manual emergencies, 834–835
Processing of x-ray film, 155–158
  panoramic, 153
  patient exposure and, 143
Prodrome, 12t
  of herpes infection, 28
  of schizophrenia, 761t
Profession, 4t
Profile, 249, *249*
  of toothbrush, *335*
Profound retardation, 750
Prognathic profile, 249, *249*
Prognosis, 321t
Progressive systemic sclerosis, 728
Prophylactic antibiotic, 101–103, 102t
  cardiovascular surgery and, 799–800
  pacemaker patient and, 798
  scaling and root planing and, 518
  shunt, 717
  sickle cell anemia, 809
Prophylaxis
  definition of, 472
  for hepatitis B, 24
Prophylaxis angle, for stain removal,
    568–569
Prosthesis
  cleaning of, 386–389, *388*
  for cleft lip and palate, 621
  complete dentures and, 384–386, *385*
  complete overdenture and, 389, *390*
  definition of, 165t, 377t
  disinfection of, 60
  fixed, 395
  fixed partial denture and, *381,* 381–382
  hygiene for, 390
  implant, 647t
  infection and, 16
  mucosa underlying, 389
  orthodontic appliance and, 376–379,
    377t, *378, 379*
  periodontal, 393
  plaque formation and, 202
  removable partial denture and, 382–384,
    383, 384
  space maintainer and, 379–381, *380*
  technical hints for, 390–391
  terminology about, 377t
Prosthodontics, for cleft lip and palate, 621
Protection, radiation, 141–143
Protective gear. *See also* Safety
  for eyes, 44–45, *45*

for pacemaker patient, 798
for stain removal, 567
Proteins, plasma, 803–804
Prothrombin time, 799
Pseudomembrane, 117t
  in NUG, 536, 537t
  pseudomembranous candidiasis, 34t
Psychiatric disorder, 101t
  anxiety disorders as, 766–768, 767t
  bipolar, 764–766
  classification of, 760t
  eating disorder as, 768–772, 769
  emergency and, 772
  major depressive, 763–764
  mood disorder as, 763
  postpartum mood disturbance as, 766
  schizophrenia as, 759–760, 761t, 762
  terminology about, 761t
Psychiatric therapy, for alcoholism, 780
  autism and, 755
Psychological factors
  in aging, 639
  cancer and, 674–675
  cleft lip and palate and, 620
  of diabetes, 822
  for homebound patient, 706
  oral or maxillofacial surgery and, 656
  of spinal cord injury, 714
Psychosis, postpartum, 761t, 766
Psychotherapy
  for anxiety disorder, 768
  for autism, 755
  bipolar disorder and, 765
  for major depression, 763
  for schizophrenia, 760
Puberty, 624–628, 625t
  definition of, 625t
  gingivitis during, 626
Pubescence, 625t
Pulmonary edema, 796
Pulmonary embolism, 795
Pulp
  denticle, 857
  in elderly patient, 638
  vitality testing of, 243–245, 244
Pulpless tooth, discoloration of, 284
Pulse, 109–110, 110
  in emergency care, 836, 836
Pulse pressure, 107t, 112
Pumice, 566
Punctate lesion, 117t
Pupil, examination of, 130
Purging disorder, 770t, 770–772
Purified protein derivative, 42t
Purpura, 803t, 813
Purulent infection, 117t
  definition of, 537
Pus
  definition of, 181t
  gingival disease and, 192
  periodontal abscess and, 541
Putty powder, polishing agent, 566
Pyrexia, 107t
Pyrophosphate, 273t

Quadrant, numbering of, 82, 83
Quadriplegia, 712t

Radial pulse, 110
Radiation
  cumulative effect, 142
  exposure to, 140t, 140–142, 141t
  patient teaching about, 161
  skin dose, 141t
  types of, 134t
Radiation therapy, 101, 672, 672–674
  caries from, 204–205
  disabled patient and, 690
  exposure, 140t, 140–142, 141t
  preparation for, 676
Radiography, 81, 133–163, 463
  analysis of, 158, 159t, 160
  bitewing survey and, 150–151, 151
  caries and, 242–243
  characteristics of radiograph and,
    136–137
  charting of, 317–318
  in child, 153–154
  clinical applications of, 143–145
  definition of, 136, 137
  disabled patient and, 688
  edentulous survey and, 154
  factors influencing, 137–140, 138
  film placement and, 143
  film selection for, 145–146
  fracture and, 239
  hemophilia patient and, 816
  history of, 133
  infection control in, 154–155
  occlusal survey and, 152
  of pacemaker patient, 798
  panoramic, 152–153
  paraclinical procedures and, 154–155
  patient teaching about, 161
  periapical survey and
    angle-bisection technique for,
      151–152
    paralleling technique for, 147, 148,
      149, 150
  periodontal disease and, 225–227,
    225–227
  position-indicating device (PID), 137,
    138, 139
  pregnancy and, 609
  principles of, 146–147
  problems in, 159t
  processing in, 155–158
  protection for, 142, 142–143, 143
  pulp vitality and, 243
  radiation exposure and, 140t, 140–142,
    141t
  scaling and root planing and, 508
  in sickle cell anemia, 809
  technical hints for, 160–161
  trauma from occlusion and, 256
  x-ray production and, 135, 135–136
  x-ray properties and, 133, 135
Radiologic health, 134t
Radiology, 134t
Radiolucency, 136
  in scleroderma, 728
Radiopacity, 136
Rampant caries, 232t
  in elderly patient, 638
  nursing, 234, 236

Rare earth element, 134t
Rash, chickenpox and, 26–27
Ratchet type mouth prop, 702
Reattachment, in periodontal therapy,
  526t
Reception of patient, 70–71
Recession, gingival, 191, 191–192, 192
Recolonization, 526t
Recombinant DNA vaccine, hepatitis B, 24
Recommended Dietary Allowance, 423,
  424, 424–425
  pregnancy and, 611
Records
  calculus and, 275
  charting and, 314–319, 316, 318
    of clinical procedures, 315
    materials for, 315
    periodontal, 315, 317
    purposes of, 314
  on disabled patient, 681
  of emergency care, 831, 832
  examination, 119–121
  forms for patient history, 86
  of immunizations, 42
  indices and scoring methods in,
    287–314. See also Indices and
    scoring methods
  in-service education and, 700, 701
  interocclusal, 165t, 166
  of mobility examination, 224
  patient preparation and, 70
  of plaque, 267
  of pulse reading, 111
  of radiography, 160
  study cast and, 178
  of temperature, 108
  of treatment plan, 322
Rectal temperature, 108
Rectangular collimation, 137
Rectangular position-indicating device, 138
Recurrent caries, 232t
Red blood cells, 804–805
  anemia and, 806–809
  polycythemia and, 809–810
Red lesion, 125
Reference chart for emergency, 842t–848t
Reference values for blood cells, 805t
Referral, for medical consultation, 101
Refractory periodontitis, 196t, 198t, 264t
Regulated waste, 53t
Rehabilitation, oral, 393–399
  of alcoholic patient, 780
  characteristics of, oral, 394–396, 395
  objectives of, 393
  self-care after, 396, 396–399, 397t
  terminology about, 394t
Reimmunization, 42
Remineralization, 234
  definition of, 435t
  demineralization/remineralization cycle
    and, 437–438
  dentifrice and, 369
  perimylolysis and, 771
Remission, of leukemia, 812, 813
Remodeling, of alveolar ridge, 649

Removable dentures, 396
  cleaning of, by disabled patient, 695–696
  in helpless patient, 708
  partial, 377t, 382–384, *383, 384*
Removable orthodontic appliance, 379
Removable space maintainer, 381
Renal disorder, history of, 100t
Replenisher, 156
Replication of virus, 12t
Report. *See also* Record
  of child abuse, 128
  cytology, 126–127
Reproductive system, alcoholism and, 778
Rescue breathing, 829t, 837
Residual ridges in edentulous mouth, 646
Resin, cleaning of, 388
Resorption, 232t
Respiratory disorder, history of, 101t
  contraindication
    for ultrasonic scaling, 517
    for airpolishing, 571
Respiratory failure, 842t
  emergency, 842t–844t
  hyperventiliation, 842t
  cardiovascular disease problem, 794, 795
  sudden death, 796
Respiratory rate, 111
Respiratory system
  age and, 635–636
  spinal cord injury and, 713
Rest
  definition of, 377t
  finger, 477–479
    amalgam restorations and, 587
    of prophylaxis angle, 569
    for scaling, 511, 514
Restoration
  airbrasive and, 571
  amalgam, 580–590. *See also* Amalgam
    restoration
  discoloration from, 285
  fluoride and, 456
  overdenture and, 389
  overhanging, 227, 587–589
  polishing and, 563
  pregnancy and, 609
  rehabilitated mouth and, 393–399, 394t,
    395, 396, 397t
  single tooth, 395
  toothbrushing after, 347
  treatment plan for, 322
Restraint, for disabled patient, 687
Resuscitation, cardiopulmonary, 836–839
Retardation, mental, 749–758. *See also*
    Mental retardation
Reticulation of radiograph, 159t
Retinopathy
  definition of, 732t
  diabetic, 819t
Retraction
  gingival, 191
  mirror for, 208
Retraction system, water, 62
Retrognathic profile, 249, *249*
Retrolental fibroplasia, 732t

Retrovirus, 12t
  human immunodeficiency, 29–36
Rheostat pedal, of prophylaxis angle, 569
Rheumatic heart disease, 98t, 787
  antibiotic premedication for, 102
Rheumatoid arthritis, 726–727
Ribonucleic acid. 863. *See also* RNA
Ridge, alveolar
  dentures and, 649
  in edentulous mouth, 646
Right heart failure, 795–796
Rigidity, in cerebral palsy, 724
Rinse
  after scaling and root planing, 526–527
  cerebrovascular accident and, 719
  chlorhexidine, 367
  dentures and, 383–384, 385
    stain removal and, 573
  disclosing agent as, 409
  in film processing, 156, 157
  fluoride, 442, 450–452
  impression and, 170, 171
  infection control and, 64
  necrotizing ulcerative gingivitis and, 540,
    541
  nonalcoholic, 781
  postoperative, 658–659
  presurgery, 657
  sealant and, 465
  study cast preparation and, 166
  subperiosteal implant and, 402
Risk of infection
  for hepatitis B, 22–23
  for human immunodeficiency virus, 32
    in child, 35–36
RNA, 29t, 30, *30*, 863
Rolling stroke toothbrushing method,
    339–340, *340*
Root
  airbrasive and, 571
  caries of, 236
Root canal, accessory, 232t
Root caries
  in elderly patient, 638
  fluoride and, 440
  radiation therapy and, 673–674
Root planing, 493, 507t, *515, 516*
  effects of, 527–528
  patient instructions, 526
  preparation for, 507–513
  procedures for, 513–516
  prophylactic antibiotic for, 507
  rationale, 506
Rotary stone, 489t
Rouge, jeweler's, 566
Rubber bite block, 702
Rubber cup
  for debonding, 594
  prophylaxis angle with, 568, 569
Rubber dam
  amalgam restorations and, 586
  emergency prevention and, 820
  fluoride application and, 455–456
  hemophilia patient and, 816
  sealant and, 464

Rubella, 19t, 606, 731
  vaccine against, 786
Rubeola, 19t, 606
Ruby sharpening stone, 504
Rumination, 750t

Safely tolerated dose of fluoride, 453–454
Safety, clinician
  dental materials use,
    mercury hygiene, 584
    study cast preparation, 177–178
  eye protection, 44–45, 829
  gloves and, 48
  immunizations, 41
  postexposure protocols HIV, HBV, 66t
  radiation protection, 142–143, 160
Saliva
  examination of, 121t
  functions of, 204t
  xerostomia and, 204–205
Saliva substitute, 205, 676
Salivary gland, radiation effects on, 673
Salts, inorganic, in blood, 804
Sanitation
  definition of, 53t
  hepatitis A and, 21
Saprophyte, 259t
Saturated solution, 273t
Scale. *See also* Indices and scoring methods
Scaler, 493
  angulation of, 480
  curved sickle, 490–491, *490*
  debonding and, 594
  definition of, 489t
  restoration and, 588
  sharpening of, 498–499, 502–503
  types of, 490–493, *490–493*
Scaling and root planing, 506–524
  advantages and limitations of, 519
  in alcoholic patient, 781–782
  anticoagulant therapy and, 799
  clinical procedures with, 518–519
  definition of, 507t, 526t
  diabetes and, 825
  disabled patient and, 702
  education about, 522
  infection control and, 64–65
  leukemia and, 813
  patient instructions about, 526–527
  preparation for, 507–509, *509*
  as presurgery treatment, 657
  procedure for, 509–511, *510*, 510t
  purposes and uses of, 517–518
  rationale of, 506–507
  sonic, 516–517
  stain removal and, 563, 565, 567
  stroke for, 480
  subgingival, 513–516, *515*
  supragingival, 511–513, *512, 513*
  technical hints about, 521–522
  terminology about, 507t
  topical anesthetic for, 519–521
  ultrasonic, 14–15, 516–517
Scar, 117t
Scattered radiation, 134t

Scatterguard, cylindrical, 137
Schizophrenia, 759–760, 761t, 762
School, fluoridation in, 441
Scleroderma, 728
Sclerosis, 117t
    definition of, 785t
    progressive systemic, 728
Scoring methods, 287–314. *see also* Indices
        and scoring methods
Scraper, tongue, 347
Screening, 81
Scrub
    short, 47
    surgical, 48
Scrub brush, 46
Scrub-brush toothbrushing method, 343
Scrubsuit, 42–43
Seal of Acceptance of American Dental
        Association, 370
Sealant, 462–472
    clinical procedures for, 463–466
    definition of, 462
    disabled patient and, 698
    fluoride and, 467–468
    penetration of, 466–467
    retention and replacement of, 467
    selection of teeth for, 462–463
    stain removal and, 563
    terminology about, 463t
Seizure, 741–748, 742t
    alcoholism and, 779
    cerebral palsy and, 724
    emergency treatment of, 846t
    management of, 747
Self-care
    of diabetes, 822
    by disabled patient, 692–696, 693–696
    fluoride and, 449–453
    for rehabilitated mouth, 396–399
Self-cleansing mechanisms, 330
Self-history, 86
Self-induced bacteremia, 788
Senescence. *See* Gerodontic patient
Senility, 636–637, 637t
    definition of, 635
Sensorimotor effects, of spinal cord injury,
        712–713
Sensorineural hearing loss, 734
Sensory disability
    hearing, 734–740, 735, 737–739
    terminology about, 732t
    visual, 731–734
Sensory stimulus, explorer for, 221
Septal defect, ventricular, 784–785, 786
Seroconversion, 12t
Serologic diagnosis, 12t
Serum marker, 12t
Sessile polyp, 117t
Set square tooth numbering system, 83, 84
Sexual development, 624–625
Sexually transmitted disease
    hepatitis B as, 22–23
    patient history of, 99t
Shank, 474–475
    of curet, 488–489
    of explorer, 220
    of toothbrush, 334, 334, 335

Sharp instruments, 474
Sharpening of instruments, 494–504,
        496–504
    of curets and sickles, 496
    dynamics of, 494–495
    of explorer, 503
    facilities for, 494
    of hoe scaler, 502–503, 503
    principles of, 495–496
    of chisel scaler, 503
    stone for, 494, 496–502, 497, 503
        care of, 503–504
        cone for, 499–500
        Mandrel, 501–502
        Neivert whittler for, 500, 500–501, 501
        stationary flat stone and, 498,
            498–499
    testing sharpness, 494–495
Sharpey's fibers, 181t, 182
Shedding, viral, 12t
Shelf life, 53t
Shepherd's hook, 221
Shield, eyewear, 44–45
Shingles, 18t, 26t, 26, 27, 34t
Shock
    anaphylactic, 845t
    emergency treatment of, 843t
    spinal, 712
Short scrub, 47
Shunt, 712t
    antibiotic premedication for, 102, 809
    for hydrocephalus, 716, 716
Sickle, sharpening of, 496, 498–499
Sickle cell anemia, 808, 808–809
    antibiotic premedication for, 103, 809
Sickle scaler, 490, 490–491
    angulation of, 511
Side shield of eyewear, 44–45
Sight, loss of, 731–734. *See also* Eye.
Sign language, 736, 737–739
Signs
    of cancer, 130–131
    of child abuse, 127–128
    of gingival disease, 186–187
    pathognomonic, 81
    Tinel's, 484t
Silex, 566
Silicon dioxide, 566
Silver amalgam, discoloration from, 285
Simian crease, 753
Simplification, work, 71t
Simplified Oral Hygiene Index, 298–299,
        299
Single-tuft brush, 358, 359, 359
Sinus tract
    definition of, 537t
    periodontal abscess and, 541, 542
Sjögren's syndrome, 204
Skeletal fixation, external, 662, 662–663
Skeletal fluorosis, 454
Skeletal system, aging and, 635
Skin, 120t
    acne vulgaris, 625, 855
    age and, 635
    HIV infection and, 34
    scleroderma and, 728

Skin disorder, 625
Sliding board wheelchair transfer, 686
Small intestine, fluoride and, 434
Smear, cytologic, 125
Smith's toothbrushing method, 343
Smokeless tobacco, 203
Smoking, effects of, 203
Snap-A-Ray, 150
Soap
    antimicrobial, 42t
    for handwashing, 46
Sodium bicarbonate solution, 366
Sodium chloride solution, 365–366
Sodium fluoride, 444
    in dentifrice, 452
    hypersensitive teeth and, 558
    topical application, 444–448
Sodium fluoride rinse, 451
Sodium hypochlorite, disinfectant, 61
    for denture cleaning, 386
Soft deposit. *See* Plaque
Soft palate, examination of, 121t
    cleft palate, 618, 619
Soft x rays, 133, 135
Solution
    for denture cleaning, 387
    film processing, 155–156
Sonic scaler, 507t
Sonic scaling, 516–517
Sordes, 706t
Sounds
    Korotkoff, 107t
    respiratory, 111
Source-film distance, 139
Space
    interproximal, 353t
    periodontal ligament, 226–227, 227
Space maintainer, 379–381, 380
    definition of, 377t
Spasticity, 714
    cerebral palsy and, 723
Spatula, for impression, 165
Spaulding classification of inanimate
        objects, 63t
Speech, cleft lip and palate and, 620, 621
Speechreading, 732t, 736, 740
Sphygmomanometer, 112
Spina bifida, 716
Spinal cord injury, 711–715, 713
Spirochetal infiltration zone of necrotizing
        ulcerative gingivitis, 537–538
Spatter, 14–15, 16
    polishing and, 561
Spleen, leukemia and, 811
Splint
    complete-arch fixed, 395
    definition of, 394t
    denture used as, 663
Spoon feeding, 665
Sporicide, 53t
Spot
    blind, 732t
    white
        debonding and, 595
        definition of, 435

Squamous cell carcinoma, 669
Squamous cells, cytologic examination of, 125–126
Squamous epithelium, 181t
Stabilization of disabled patient, 687, 702
Stain, 280–286. *See also* Stain removal
  sealant and, 464
  sharpening stone and, 504
Stain removal, 561–575
  agents for, 565–567
  airbrasives for, 571
  clinical application of, 564–565
  from clothing, 161
  education about, 573
  indications for, 563–564
  instruments used in, 567–568
  polishing and, 561–563
  as presurgery treatment, 657
  procedure for, 567
  prophylaxis angle and, 568–569
  on proximal surfaces, 569–570
  on removal denture, 571–573
Stannous fluoride, 445, 456
  staining from, 283, 285
Staphylococcus aureus, 14, 19t
Stationary flat stone, 498–499, *499*
Stenosis, 785t
Sterile instruments, 64
Sterilization, 56–59
  chemical, 62
  definition of, 53t
  monitoring of, 67
  sharpening of instrument before, 495
  sharpening stone and, 503–504
Stethoscope, 107t, 113
Stiffness of toothbrush, 334t
Stillman toothbrushing method, modified, *340*, 341
Stillman's cleft, 190, *191*
Stimulant, street names of, 129t
Stimulus
  pain, 555–556
  sensory, 221–222
Stippling, 181t
Stone
  Arkansas, 489t
  dental, 165t, 172
  sharpening, 494, 496–499, *497, 498*
    care of, 503–504
    Mandrel mounted, 501–502
    rotary, 489t
Stool, clinician's
  infection control and, 54
  position of, 72, *72*
Storage, of toothbrush, 349
Straight explorer, 221
Straight Mandrel, handpiece with, 568
Straight sickle scaler, 491, *491*
Stray radiation, 134t
Street names of drugs, 129t
Streptococcus mutans, 265
  caries and, 268
  root caries, 236
Streptococcus pneumoniae, 19t
Streptococcus pyogenes, 19t

Stress
  emergency and, 828
  necrotizing ulcerative gingivitis and, 537
Stress reduction, 800
Stretching exercise, 485
Strip
  finishing, 570
  gauze, 357, *357*
Stroke, 712t, 717–719, *718*
  of curet, 490
  emergency treatment of, 843t
  for gingival curettage, 530
  with instrument, 480–481, *481*
  porte polisher and, 578
  probe, 214
  in root planing, 516, *516*
  in scaling, 512, 514–516
  walking, 214, *214*
Study cast, 164–179, 165t, 732t
  criteria for, 174t
  definition of, 165t
  in disabled patient, 688
  disinfection of, 171
  impression material for, 169
  impression trays for, 166–169
  for interocclusal record, 166
  mandibular, 167, 169–170
  maxillary, 167, *167*, 170–171
  paraclinical procedures and, 171–173
  preparation of, 164–166
  purpose of, 164
  as teaching aid, 419
  technical hints for, 177–178
  trimming of, 173–177, 174t, *174–177*
Styrofoam disposable film holder, *147*, 150
Subgingival calculus, 272–273, 275
  mineralization of, 275
Subgingival examination, 508–509, *509*
Subgingival explorer, 220–221
Subgingival irrigation, 362–363, *363*
  definition of, 353t
Subgingival plaque, 261t, 262–263, 265, 266
Subjective symptom, 81
Subperiosteal implant, 399–400, *400*, 402
Substance abuse, 128–130
Substantivity, 353t
Subtraction radiography, 134t
Succedaneous dentition, 232t
Sucrose in medication, 36, 431–432, 614
Suction tip, 830
Sudden death, 796
Suffixes, 851–853
Sugar, in medication, 36, 431–432, 614
Sulcular brushing, 338–339, *339*
  definition of, 334t
Sulcus, 184. *See also* Pocket *entries*
  fluid, gingival, 184, 192, 196
  in disease, 192
  periodontal abscess and, 543
  probe examination of, 209–210
Sulcus Bleeding Index, 300
Sunlight, cancer and, 669–670
Superinfection, hepatitis D and, 25
Supersaturated solution, 273t

Supervision, dental hygienist, 4t
Supine position, 71t
  contraindications for, 74–75
Supplement
  fluoride, 442, 451
  nutritional, 614
Support straps, for disabled patient, 687
Suppuration, 192
  definition of, 181t
Supragingival calculus, 272, 273, 275
Supragingival examination, 508
Supragingival irrigation, *362*, 362–363
  definition of, 353t
Supraversion, 250
Surface
  of calculus, 276
  of denture, 385
  disinfection of, 63–64
  fluoride and, 436–437, *437*
  of mouth mirror, 207
  root, caries of, 236
  sealant and, 463–464
  of sharpening stone, 494
  tooth
    caries in, 234, 242
    irregularities of, 202
    pocket and, 198–200, *199, 200*
    probe examination of, 212, *212*
    scaling and root planing and, 528
Surface absorbed radiation dose, 141t
Surface marker, for identifying dentures, 653
Surface radiation exposure, 140
Surfactant, in dentifrice, 368
Surgery
  for cancer, 671–672
  cardiovascular, *793*, 799–800
  for cleft lip and palate, 620, 622
  coronary bypass, *793*
  dental hygiene prior to, 666–667
  irrigation and, 364
  mouthrinse after, 364
  neurosurgery and, *716*, 716–717
  periodontal, gingiva after, 193
Surgical scrub, 48
Surveillance, 13t
Survey
  dietary, 398
  epidemiologic, 287–288
  radiographic. *See* Radiography
Susceptible host, 13t
Suspension suture, 551
Suture
  anticoagulation therapy and, 799
  definition of, 546t
  removal of, 549, *551*
  types of, 549–550, *551*
Swage, 546t
Swallowing, dysphagia and, 712t
Sweep, finger, 840
Sweetening agent, in dentifrice, 368
  in medications, 36, 431, 614
Symptom, 81

Syncope
  definition of, 829t
  emergency treatment of, 843t
Synergism, 353t
Syphilis, 19t
  congenital, 751
  enamel hypoplasia and, 237
  Treponema pallidum, 19t, 264t
Syringe
  compressed air, 209
  for emergency drug therapy, 830
  hepatitis B and, 24
Systemic factor
  definition of, 202
  in gingival or periodontal disease, 204
Systemic sclerosis, progressive, 728
Systems, in patient history, 86
Systole, 107t
Systolic blood pressure, 112, 114t

Tablet
  disclosing agent as, 409
  fluoride, 442
Tachycardia, 785t
  definition of, 107t
Tactile discrimination, 208, 221
Tactile examination
  calculus and, 275
  for periodontal therapy, 525
Tactile sense, dentures and, 649
Tactile sensitivity, 483
Tank for film processing, 155
Tape, dental, 353–356, *355, 356*
  stain removal and, 570
Tarnish of restoration, 581t, 581
Taste
  dentures and, 649
  radiation and, 674
Taste bud, 181t
Team, interdisciplinary, 706t
Teeth
  abrasion of, 238
  anatomy of, 180–181
  attrition of, *237,* 237–238
  average measurements of, 865–866t
  avulsion of, 848t
  calculus compared with, 277
  caries in, 231–232, 234, 235t, 236. *See
    also* Caries
  cleft lip and palate and, 618
  deposits on, 260t. *See also* Plaque
  of disabled patient, 689
  in Down's syndrome, 754
  education about, 413
  in elderly patient, 638
  enamel hypoplasia of, 236–237
  erosion of, 238
  eruption of, 233t
    gingiva and, *185*
  examination of, 239, 240t–241t,
    241–242
  fetal development of, 605
  fluoride effects on, 435–436
  fracture of, 238–239, *239*
  hypersensitive, 554–560. *See also*
    Hypersensitive teeth

long axis of tooth of, 147
mentally retarded patient and, 752
in periodontal chart, 218
plaque on. *See* Plaque
polishing effects on, 562–563
probe examination of, 214–215
radiation therapy and, 673–674
sealant applied to, 462–463
types of, 231
Telephone medical consultation, 101
Temperature
  amalgam restorations and, 586
  film processing and, 157
  measurement of, 106–109, *108*
  spinal cord injury and, 714
  sterilization, 58, 59
Temporal artery pulse, 110
Temporomandibular joint
  assessment of, 119
  disorder of, 117t
  examination of, 120t
Tension test, 208t, 217
Terminally ill patient, 706t
Tetracaine, 520
Tetracycline
  fetal effects of, 606
  staining from, 284
Tetralogy of Fallot, 785t
Therapeutic dentifrice, 369
Thermal pain stimulus, 555
Thermometer, *107, 108,* 108–109
Thickener, in dentifrice, 368
Third degree burn, 847t
Thompson scattering, 134t
Threader, floss, *382, 383*
Threshold radiation dose, 141t
Threshold radiation exposure, 140
Throat, examination of, 121t
Thrombocyte, 802
Thrombocytopenia, leukemia and, 811
Thrombocytopenic purpura, 803t
Thrombosis, stroke and, 717
Thrombus, 785t
Thrust
  abdominal, 840
  chest, 840
  jaw, 835
  tongue, 249t
Thyroid cervical collar, 143
Tic, 750t, 863
Timer, x-ray, 136
Tin oxide, 566
Tinel's sign, 484t
Tinnitus, 732t
Tip
  interdental, 359
  suction, 830
Tissue conditioning, 325
Titanium, 394t
Tobacco
  cancer and, 670
  NUG and, 537
  plaque and, 203
Tobacco stain, 282–283
Toddler, 612–614. *See also* Child
  terminology about, 606t

Tolerance, drug, 129
Tomography, 152
  definition of, 394t
Tongue
  cleaning of, 346–347, *347*
  in Down's syndrome, 753–754
  in elderly patient, 637
  examination of, *119,* 121t
  in iron deficiency anemia, 807
  papillae of, *182,* 182
  in pernicious anemia, 807
  seizures and, 743–744
Tongue depressor, 702
Tongue thrust, 249t
Tonic-clonic seizure, 743
  emergency treatment of, 846t
  management of, *747*
Tonsil, examination of, 121t
Tooth. *See* Teeth
Tooth numbering system, 81, *82, 83,* 84
Tooth surface pocket wall, 198–200, *199,
  200*
Toothbrush, 333–349
  adaptations for handicap, 692–694
  bristles, 335–336
  brushing plane, 335
  care of brushes, 349
  characteristics effective brush, 334
  claspbrush, 384
  denture, 387, *388*
    adaptations for handicap, 696, *696*
  development of, 333–334
  filaments, end-rounded, 336, *336*
  history of, 333
  interdental brushes, 358–359, *358, 359*
  manual, 334–336, *334*
  orthodontic, 378
  parts of brush, 334–335
  power-assisted, 334t, 344–345
  profiles, trim, 335, *335*
  selelction of brush, 336–337
  single-tuft, end-tuft, 359, *359*
  stiffness, 334t
  suction brush, 708
Toothbrushing, 333–351
  after scaling and root planing, 527
  dentifrices for, 367–369
  of dentures, 387–388
  disabled patient and, 691–693, *694*
  elderly patient and, 642
  evaluation of, 416–417
  guidelines for, 337–338
  in helpless patient, *708,* 708–709
  infection control and, 64
  methods of, 338–343
    Bass, 338–339, *339*
    Charters, 341–342, *342*
    Fones, 343, *343*
    horizontal, 343
    Leonard, 343
    modified Stillman, 341
    rolling stroke, 339–340, *340*
    scrub-brush, 343
    Smith's, 343
  necrotizing ulcerative gingivitis and, 540,
    541

Toothbrushing (*Continued*)
  orthodontic appliance and, 378, *378*
  partial dentures and, 381
  of removable dentures, 384
  for special conditions, 347
  supplemental, 345–347, *347*
  terminology about, 334t
  trauma from, 347–349
Toothless patient. *See* Edentulous patient
Toothpick holder, 360, *360*
  for orthodontic patient, 379
Topical anesthetic
  definition of, 507t
  gagging and, 145
  for scaling and root planing, 519–520
Topical fluoride, 443–444
Torus, 117t
  in edentulous mouth, 646
Total treatment plan, 321t
Tourette's syndrome, 750t
Tourniquet, 830
Toxic waste, 53t
Toxicity
  of fluoride, 453–455, 454t, *455*
  of leukemia therapy, 812
Toxin, 196
Toxoid, 42t
Toxoplasmosis, 751
Trace elements, in calculus, 277
Traditional dental chair, 75
Transcription, viral, 30
Transfer, wheelchair, 684–687
Transformer, step-up, step-down, 135
Transfusion
  hepatitis B and, 23
  HIV and, 35
Transient ischemic attack, 712t
Transillumination, 81
  mirror and, 208
Transmission of infection, 13t. *See also*
    Infection, transmission of
Transosseous wire, 661
Transosteal implant, 400, *400*
Transplant, infection and, 16
Transseptal fiber, 183
Trauma
  child abuse and, 127–128
  cumulative, 71t, 483–486, 484t,
    484–486, 486t
    recommendations for, 486t
    risk factors for, 486t
  disabled patient and, 689
  fracture caused by. *See* Fracture
  from occlusion, 249t
  periodontal abscess and, 542
  postnatal, 751
  seizures and, 743–744
  spinal cord injury and, 711–715
  toothbrushing and, 347–348
Tray, impression, 166–167, *167*, *168*
  preparation of, 169
Tray technique for fluoride, *448*, 448–449,
    449, 450

Treatment plan, 320–327
  appointment sequence and, 323, *324*,
    325
  for cancer patient, 670–671
  consent and, 326
  for disabled patient, 680–682, 691
  planning of, 322
  preparation of, 320–322
  sample of, 325–326
  steps in, 322–323
  technical hints about, 326–327
  terminology about, 321t
Treatment room
  barrier-free, 683–684
  infection control in, 52, 54
Tremor, in cerebral palsy, 724
Trendelenburg position, 71t, 829t
Treponema pallidum, 19t, 264t
Trifurcation, probe examination of, 216
Trimesters of pregnancy, 605–606
Triplegia, 712t
Trismus, 117t
  radiation and, 674
TDD, 732t
Tube, x-ray, 135, *135*
Tube feeding, 665
Tuberculin test, 42t
Tuberculosis, 16–17
  HIV infection and, 32
  isoniazid, 17, 99t, 859
  Mantoux text, 42t
  multidrug resistant, 17
  Mycobacterium tuberculosis, 19t, 32, 42t,
    43
  oral lesion, 17
  patient history, 99t
  rifampin, 17, 99t
  patient history of, 99t
Tubule, of dentin, 554–555
Tuft, toothbrush, 334t
Tufted dental floss, 356
Tumor, 669–678. *See also* Cancer
Tungsten carbide bur for debonding, 594
Tuning fork, 732t
Two rescuers in CPR, 838
Two-step method of forming cast, 173
Tympanic membrane, 732t

Ulcer, 125, 123t
  decubitus, 712t
    spinal cord injury and, 714
Ulceration
  definition of, 537
  dentures causing, 650
Ulcerative gingivitis, necrotizing, 536–541.
    See also Necrotizing ulcerative
    gingivitis
Ultrasonic cleaning
  of denture, 572
  of instruments, 55
Ultrasonic instrument, for restorations, 588
Ultrasonic scaling, 507t, 516–517
  microorganisms and, 14–15
Unattached plaque, 265
Unconscious patient, airway obstruction
  in, 839–840

Underjet, 250, *251*
Unituft brush, *358*, 359, *359*
Universal curet, 489
Universal precautions, 65, *65*
  definition of, 13t
Unwaxed dental floss, 354
Urticaria, 829t
Uvula, examination of, 121t

Vaccine, 19t
  definition of, 42t
  hepatitis B, 24
  rubella, 786
Vallate papilla, 182
Valve, cardiac, 102, 788
  endocarditis and, 788–789
Vancomycin, 102t
Vapor sterilizer, 58–59
Varicella-zoster virus, 18t, 26–27, 26t, 34t
Vasodilator, for angina, 794
Vasomotor reaction, 630
Vector, 13t
Vehicle, infectious, 13t
Veneer, 394t
Venous blood, 785t
Ventilation, mouth-to-mouth, 841
Ventral, 117t
Ventricular fibrillation, 829t
Ventricular septal defect, 784–785, *786*
Ventriculoatrial shunt, 712t
Ventriculoperitoneal shunt, 712t
Verruca, 117t
Vertical angulation
  for angle-bisection technique, 152
  definition of, 147
  for paralleling technique, 150
Vertical toothbrushing method, 343
Vertical transmission of infection, 13t
Vertigo, 732t
Virion, 13t
Virulence, 13t
Virus, 13t. *See also* Infection, viral
Visceral, 712t
Visible light cured sealant, 462
Visible-light cured dressing, 546, *546t*
Visual disability, 731–734
Visual examination, 81
  for periodontal therapy, 525
Visual test, for sharpening, 494–495
Vital signs, 106t, 106–115, 112t
  anorexia nervosa, 769
  body temperature and, 106–109, *108*
  emergency, monitored, 829, *831*, 832
  pulse and, 109–110, *110*
  respiratory rate and, 111
  terminology about, 197t
Vitality testing of pulp, 243–245, *244*
Vitamin
  essential nutrients, 422, 665
  fluoride and, 443
  gerodontic patient and, 643
  pernicious anemia and, 807
Voltage control, 135
Vomiting
  bulimia nervosa and, 770t, 770–772

tooth erosion and, 238
   pregnancy and, 608

Wafer, disclosing agent as, 409
Walking frame, 686
Walkway, barrier-free, 683
Wall, pocket, 198–200, *199, 200*
Washing
   in film processing, 156
   of hands, 46–48, 49
Waste
   film processing and, 155
   infection control and, 54, 67
   infectious, 53t
   label for, *67*
   types of, 53t
Wasting, HIV and, 33
Water
   contamination of, 62
   fluoride in, 438–439, 442–443
   infection control and, 15
Water-borne infection
   hepatitis A as, 21
   hepatitis E as, 25
Wax bite, 166
Wax rim of impression, 168, *168*
Waxed dental floss, 354
Wheelchair
   accessibility to, *683*
   homebound patient and, 707

transfer from, 684–687
   treatment in, 684
White blood cells, 805–806
   disorders of, 810–813
White lesion, cancer and, 124–125
White spot
   debonding and, 595
   definition of, 435
Whiting, 566
Whitlow, herpetic, 18t, 28
Whittler, Neivert, 500–501, *501*
Whooping cough, 19t
Window period, infection, 13t
Wire
   arch, debonding of, 592
   suspension, 664
   transosseous, 661
Withdrawal syndrome, 129
   alcohol, 779
Wood point, porte polisher and, 577
Wood interdental cleaner, 360–361
Work simplification, 71t
World Health Organization classification of
   tooth fractures, 239
Wrist, anatomy of, *484*
Wrist position, with instrument, 477
Written request for medical consultation,
   101

X ray. *See also* Radiography
   angulation of, 145

image, definition, 137
   production of, 135–136
   properties of, 133, 135
X-C-P device, 150
Xeroradiography, 134t
Xerosis, 423
Xerostomia, 204–205
   antidepressant and, 764
   caries and, 236
   definition of, 196t
   dentures and, 649, 651
   diabetes and, 824
   in elderly patient, 637–638
   in helpless patient, 709
   HIV infection and, 35

Yarn for flossing, 357, *357*
Yeast infection, *Candida albicans* and, 19t
   HIV and, 34
Yellow dental stain, 281
   disclosing agent, 409

Zidovudine
   fetus and, 606, 608
   side effects of, 35
Zinc oxide with eugenol dressing,
   545–546, 546t
Zoster, herpes, 18t, 26t, 26–27